AIOS
Ready Reckoner in Ophthalmology

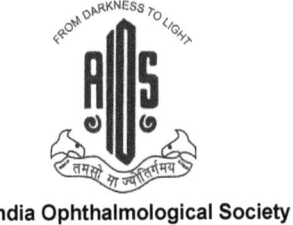

All India Ophthalmological Society

AIOS
Ready Reckoner in Ophthalmology

Third Edition

Editors

Partha Biswas
MS (Ophthalmology)
Medical Director
Trenetralaya
Kolkata, West Bengal, India

Lalit Verma
MBBS MD
Director
Vitreo-Retina Services
Centre for Sight, New Delhi
Formerly Additional Professor
Dr RP Centre
All India Institute of Medical Sciences
New Delhi, India

Harbansh Lal
MS (Ophthalmology)
Director
Delhi Eye Centre, New Delhi
Co-Chairman
Department of Ophthalmology
Sir Ganga Ram Hospital
New Delhi, India

Foreword

Harbansh Lal

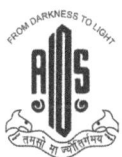

All India Ophthalmological Society

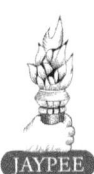

JAYPEE BROTHERS MEDICAL PUBLISHERS
The Health Sciences Publisher
New Delhi | London

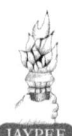 **Jaypee Brothers Medical Publishers (P) Ltd.**

Headquarters
Jaypee Brothers Medical Publishers (P) Ltd
EMCA House, 23/23-B
Ansari Road, Daryaganj
New Delhi 110 002, India
Landline: +91-11-23272143, +91-11-23272703
+91-11-23282021, +91-11-23245672
Email: jaypee@jaypeebrothers.com

Corporate Office
Jaypee Brothers Medical Publishers (P) Ltd
4838/24, Ansari Road, Daryaganj
New Delhi 110 002, India
Phone: +91-11-43574357
Fax: +91-11-43574314
Email: jaypee@jaypeebrothers.com

Overseas Office
JP Medical Ltd.
83, Victoria Street, London
SW1H 0HW (UK)
Phone: +44 20 3170 8910
Fax: +44 (0)20 3008 6180
Email: info@jpmedpub.com

Website: www.jaypeebrothers.com
Website: www.jaypeedigital.com

© 2024, Jaypee Brothers Medical Publishers

The views and opinions expressed in this book are solely those of the original contributor(s)/author(s) and do not necessarily represent those of editor(s) or publisher of the book.

All rights reserved. No part of this publication may be reproduced, stored or transmitted in any form or by any means, electronic, mechanical, photocopying, recording or otherwise, without the prior permission in writing of the publishers.

All brand names and product names used in this book are trade names, service marks, trademarks or registered trademarks of their respective owners. The publisher is not associated with any product or vendor mentioned in this book.

Medical knowledge and practice change constantly. This book is designed to provide accurate, authoritative information about the subject matter in question. However, readers are advised to check the most current information available on procedures included and check information from the manufacturer of each product to be administered, to verify the recommended dose, formula, method and duration of administration, adverse effects and contra indications. It is the responsibility of the practitioner to take all appropriate safety precautions. Neither the publisher nor the author(s)/editor(s) assume any liability for any injury and/or damage to persons or property arising from or related to use of material in this book.

This book is sold on the understanding that the publisher is not engaged in providing professional medical services. If such advice or services are required, the services of a competent medical professional should be sought.

Every effort has been made where necessary to contact holders of copyright to obtain permission to reproduce copyright material. If any have been inadvertently overlooked, the publisher will be pleased to make the necessary arrangements at the first opportunity.

Inquiries for bulk sales may be solicited at: jaypee@jaypeebrothers.com

AIOS Ready Reckoner in Ophthalmology

First Edition: 2010
Second Edition: 2017
Third Edition: **2024**

ISBN: 978-93-5696-189-0

Dedicated to

*Our Teachers,
who inspired hope, ignited imagination, and
instilled the love of learning*

All India Ophthalmological Society

OFFICE BEARERS

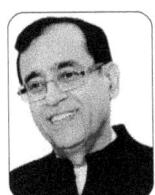
Harbansh Lal
President

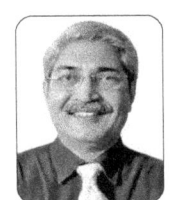
Samar Kumar Basak
President-Elect

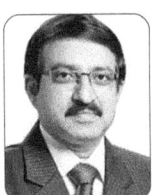
Partha Biswas
Vice President

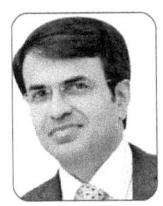
Santosh G Honavar
Honorary General Secretary

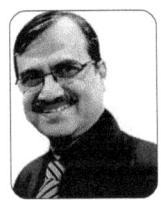
Manoj Chandra Mathur
Honorary Treasurer

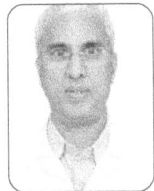
CV Gopala Raju
Joint Secretary

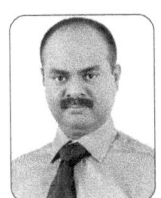
Elankumaran Pasupathi
Joint Treasurer

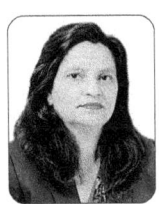
Namrata Sharma
Chairman Scientific Committee

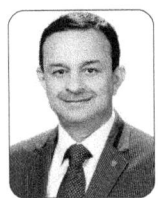
Prashant Keshao Bawankule
Chairman ARC

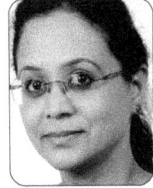
M Vanathi
Editor-Journal

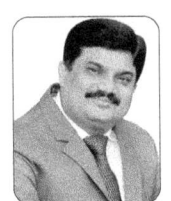
Krishna Prasad Kudlu
Editor-Proceedings

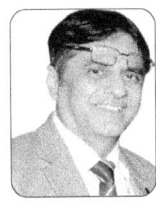
Lalit Verma
Immediate Past President

MEMBERS—SCIENTIFIC COMMITTEE

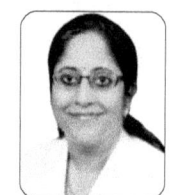
Somasheila I Murthy

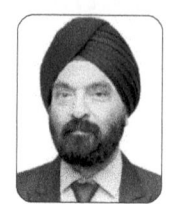
Jatinder Singh Bhalla

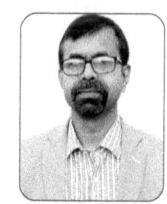
Pradip Kumar Mohanta

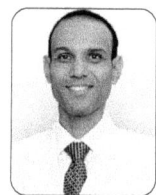
Piyush R Bansal

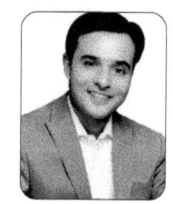
Vardhaman Kankaria

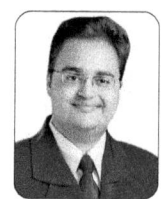
Amit Porwal

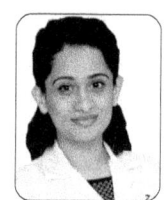
Fairooz Puthiyapurayil Manjandavida

ACADEMIC AND RESEARCH COMMITTEE

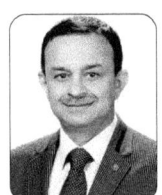

Prashant K Bawankule
Chairman
Academic and Research Committee (ARC), AIOS

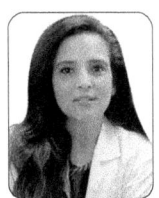

Tinku Bali
Member ARC
(North Zone)

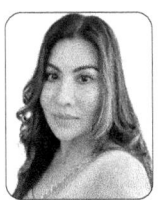

Kasturi Bhattacharjee
Member ARC
(East Zone)

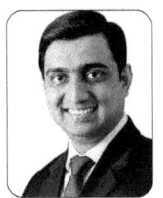

Shrinivas M Joshi
Member ARC
(South Zone)

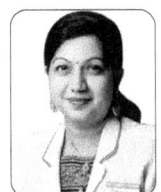

Anagha Heroor
Member ARC
(West Zone)

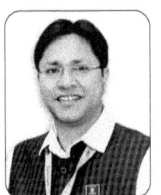

Deepak Mishra
Member ARC
(Central Zone)

Foreword

What you seek is seeking you?
—**Rumi**

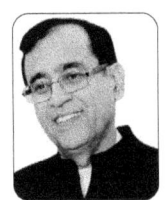

It is a matter of great pride for our fraternity that All India Ophthalmological Society (AIOS) is bringing about yet another informative and an enlightening *AIOS Ready Reckoner in Ophthalmology*, third edition under the aegis of AIOS for all our fellow ophthalmologists.

It is needless to say that with changing times and improvement in our technology and science, a lot of laborious work has gone into this edition by all our editors and authors.

The ready reckoner is well organized and clearly presented and incorporates the use of peer-reviewed evidence.

Numerous world-renowned authors have designed this Ready Reckoner as a quick review of known facts. The chapters have been edited to give as concise a reading as possible on any particular topic.

I hope this Ready Reckoner will help you multiply your knowledge of the science of ophthalmology. Continuous austere practice, along with self-study and devotion in existence are the only tools towards communion in the field of ophthalmology.

I greatly appreciate the efforts of the many talented contributors, who have shared their wisdom and experience.

I take this opportunity to thank Dr Partha Biswas and his entire team, who have worked extremely hard to bring forth the third edition of *AIOS Ready Reckoner in Ophthalmology*.

Harbansh Lal
MS (Ophthalmology)
President, AIOS

Preface to the Third Edition

It is Your Light that Lights the World.
—**Rumi**

The science of ophthalmology is dynamic and evolving throughout the year and there is a constant need to learn and update the newer treatment protocols and management techniques coming up every year to comprehend and treat eye diseases.

Textbooks remain the apex method for a detailed scholarly study of any ocular disease; on the other hand, the Internet can provide swift-search results. However, contents on the Internet are just a quick fix but long-term effects can only be achieved with a Ready Reckoner.

Large portion of clinical medical education takes place, on rounds and in clinics and a Ready Reckoner for a practitioner is always an instant guide in times of need and is the call of the hour and we hope it answers confronted questions while examining patients in the daily practice.

In 2010, the first edition and 2017, the second edition of *Ready Reckoner in Ophthalmology* was published by the All India Ophthalmological Society (AIOS) to address this need.

Doyens in all the subspecialties of ophthalmology came together to bring this Magnum Opus, which could easily be used as in the outpatient department or at the bedside to get an overview of any ocular disease from a clinical viewpoint, along with the latest treatment algorithms. Residents found it useful to answer examination questions both written and in viva voce.

We greatly appreciate the efforts of the many talented contributors who have shared their wisdom and experiences to create this book and update the subsequent editions.

We have received an overwhelming response on the first two editions of the *Ready Reckoner in Ophthalmology*, and we hope that clinicians and practitioners will continue to enjoy this new edition and find it valuable.

Over the last 12 years, ophthalmology has undergone revolutionary changes, and there have been paradigm shifts in the management of various diseases. Thus, we bring forth in the third edition of the *Ready Reckoner in Ophthalmology*, a comprehensive overview of common ocular diseases, updated with the latest advances, along with new chapters.

The book has been divided into 10 sections, with chapters from over 350 authors. Extensive proofreading and plagiarism checks have gone into the preparation of this book. We are very grateful to all our contributors, for having made each chapter as perfect as possible.

We hope our sincere efforts will be able to meet the expectations of our residents in training, practicing ophthalmologists as well as orthoptists and optometrists, and provide them with a companion to serve their patients effectively and efficiently.

Partha Biswas
Lalit Verma
Harbansh Lal

Preface to the First Edition

There is a virtual explosion of knowledge, techniques, and technology in ophthalmology. Concepts, principles of treatments, investigative modalities, and surgical procedures are evolving by the day. Diseases hitherto-considered untreatable are becoming eminently treatable today. While all these developments are most welcome, it really is a challenge to a practicing ophthalmologist to keep up with these developments, involved as they are with day-to-day care of their patients, administrative responsibilities, and keeping their practice or hospital viable and competitive.

While excellent books and journals are storehouses of knowledge, one often feels the need for a quick practical reference when faced with a particular clinical problem. If only there was a "Yellow pages in Ophthalmology" which one could flip through for immediate guidance. The *Ready Reckoner in Ophthalmology* attempts to fill this void and serves as a reference to the multifarious situations faced by us and to handle it, keeping in mind the constraints we often face. This book does not pretend to be an alternative to established textbooks or peer-reviewed journals but a handy table-top guide to practical ophthalmology. It is not expected that every ophthalmologist will be able to treat every condition by referring to this book but at least it will inform them as to what is available and how to guide their patients.

This tome is divided into 9 major sections and more than 300 authors have contributed to this. The topics and questions, based on certain common guidelines were designed by the section editors. Extensive editing, proofreading and in some cases rewriting has gone into the preparation of this book. The author's email ID and a single relevant reference has been given to enable anyone who wants more information on a particular topic to refer or contact the author.

This has been my endeavor to reach from my desk to the desk of every ophthalmologist in our fraternity.

I sincerely hope it is found to be useful and future editions of this book with modifications will emerge to serve as a permanent reference to enhance the practice of ophthalmology.

D Ramamurthy

Acknowledgments

The *AIOS Ready Reckoner in Ophthalmology*, 3rd edition is a result of collaborative efforts of numerous individuals, who have made the publication of this robust handbook possible.

We are overwhelmed in all humbleness and gratitude that this project has finally been completed.

This book would not have been possible without the contribution of our committed authors, who have taken time out of their busy schedules to provide us with pearls of knowledge in every chapter. Our sincere gratitude to all the Section Editors, who are stalwarts in their own spheres. They have collected chapters from their respective authors and edited them meticulously so as to adhere to the required guidelines for this book.

The Governing Council of All India Ophthalmological Society (AIOS) have been a constant source of encouragement, and without their support, this book would not have been possible.

We would like to thank Shri Jitendar P Vij (Group Chairman), Mr Ankit Vij (Managing Director), Mr MS Mani (Group President), Ms Chetna Malhotra (Senior Director—Professional Publishing, Marketing, and Business Development), Ms Pooja Bhandari [Director—Production (Books and Journals)] of M/s Jaypee Brothers Medical Publishers (P) Ltd, New Delhi, India, who printed this book on behalf of AIOS.

Thorough proofreading and strict plagiarism checks have been done to ensure the authenticity of this book.

We would like to acknowledge the support of our own team of comprising of Prajjwal Ghosh, who from the inception has been instrumental in bringing together this project with close assistance from Kingshuk Bhattacharya, Sunny Yadav, Pallabi Dutta, Olivia Rana, Sanjana Singh, Dr Preeyam Biswas, Dr Himani Chatterjee, and Dr Saranya Biswas who have made sure that the project was completed in time.

Finally, we would like to thank every member of AIOS, who have encouraged us with an overwhelming response for previous editions of the Ready Reckoner and we are sure that will meet every expectation in this 3rd edition of *AIOS Ready Reckoner in Ophthalmology*.

Contents

1. **Cornea** 1
   Editor: JK Reddy

2. **Dry Eye and Ocular Surface** 73
   Editor: Somasheila I Murthy

3. **Cataract** 81
   Editors: Jeewan S Titiyal, Sridevi Nair

4. **Glaucoma** 227
   Editor: Krishnadas

5. **Refractive Surgery** 305
   Editors: Chitra Ramamurthy, Shreesha Kumar Kodavoor

6. **Uveitis and Ophthalmic Pathology** 411
   Editor: Jyotirmay Biswas

7. **Retina** 457
   Editor: Mangat R Dogra

8. **Neuro-ophthalmology** 671
   Editor: Rashmin Gandhi

9. **Oculoplasty** 705
   Editor: Kasturi Bhattacharjee

10. **Pediatric Ophthalmology and Strabismus** 891
    Editor: Lav Kochgaway

Index 951

SECTION 1

Cornea

Editor: JK Reddy

1.1 Trichiasis 2
Abhijit Bandyopadhyay
1.2 Chalazion and Stye 3
Jigisha Randeri
1.3 Blepharitis 4
Nikhil Gokhlay
1.4 Lagophthalmos and Exposure Keratopathy 6
Santanu Mitra
1.5 Bacterial Conjunctivitis 7
Praveen Krishna
1.6 Adenoviral Keratoconjunctivitis 9
Prashant Kr Singhal
1.7 Allergic Conjunctivitis 12
Quresh B Maskati
1.8 Keratomalacia 14
Radhika Tandon
1.9 Recurrent Corneal Erosion Syndrome 16
Himanshu Matalia
1.10 Bullous Keratopathy 18
Arun K Jain
1.11 Neurotrophic Keratitis 19
Jayangshu Sengupta
1.12 Toxic Keratopathy 21
MS Sridhar
1.13 Practical Approach in the Management of Bacterial Keratitis 22
Prashant Garg
1.14 Fungal Keratitis 26
Venkatesh Prajna
1.15 Acanthamoeba Keratitis 28
Ajay Dave, R Revathi
1.16 Herpes Simplex Virus Keratopathy 30
Gobinda Mukherjee
1.17 Herpes Zoster Virus Keratitis 33
Ashish Nagpal
1.18 Microsporidial Keratitis 36
Manoranjan Das, Naveen Radhakrishnan, Dhanya Kuppuraj
1.19 Pythium Keratitis 38
Vandhana Sundaram
1.20 Marginal Keratitis 39
Ashok Sharma
1.21 Interstitial Keratitis 41
Ashu Agarwal
1.22 Peripheral Ulcerative Keratitis 43
Ayan Mohanta
1.23 Pellucid Marginal Degeneration 46
Sandeep Arora
1.24 Stromal Dystrophies 47
Jeewan S Titiyal
1.25 Fuchs' Endothelial Dystrophy 49
Samar K Basak
1.26 Keratoconus 51
Rajesh Fogla
1.27 Band-shaped Keratopathy 53
Rishi Swarup
1.28 Keratitis Medicamentosa 54
Falguni Mehta
1.29 Corneal Changes in Contact Lens Users 55
Rajib Mukherjee
1.30 Suture Adjustment and Removal in Penetrating Keratoplasty: Tips and Tricks 58
Jeewan S Titiyal, Ritika Sachdev
1.31 Lamellar Keratoplasty 59
KS Siddarthan
1.32 Corneal Graft Infection 63
Anita Panda
1.33 Graft Rejection 65
Jeewan S Titiyal, Ritika Sachdev
1.34 Episcleritis 69
Saurabh Sanyal
1.35 Scleritis 70
Rupesh V Agrawal

SECTION 1: Cornea

1.1 Trichiasis

Abhijit Bandyopadhyay
Disha Eye Hospitals and Research Centre, Kolkata
disha@cal2.vsnl.net.in

■ RELEVANT CLINICAL FEATURES

Trichiasis is a term used to describe misdirection of eyelashes or ingrown eyelashes, caused by infection, inflammation, autoimmune conditions, or trauma, e.g. burns or eyelid injury. It should be distinguished from distichiasis, which refers to the presence of an accessory row of soft lashes in or along the meibomian orifices. This condition can either be congenital or acquired, due to significant inflammation in the lid structures.

The offending eyelash(es) rub against the sensitive corneal surface and produce irritation, foreign body sensation, reflex watering, superficial corneal erosion, and even corneal ulceration in severe cases. Of the various etiologies, trachoma is one of the most common, especially in endemic areas such as Punjab, Bihar, Haryana, and Rajasthan.

■ IMPORTANT DIFFERENTIAL DIAGNOSES OR ASSOCIATED PROBLEMS

- Lid entropion
- Epiblepharon
- Lid scars
- Cicatricial conjunctivitis.

■ TREATMENT

Treatment of the cause: In trachoma—Surgery for Trichiasis, and Antibiotics to prevent Recurrence (STAR).

Treatment of the underlying causative condition: Like entropion.

Treatment of the aberrant eyelashes:
- Mechanical epilation
- *Electroepilation:* A hair-thin metal probe is passed into each hair follicle and electrical energy is delivered to the follicle, which results in destruction of the follicle by formation of a caustic lye (galvanic method) or overheating (thermolysis method) or by both (blend method).
- *Cryotherapy:* It is performed in segmental trichiasis. A double freeze-thaw technique is performed with a nitrous oxide probe, using a 25-second freeze-thaw-20-second refreeze technique.
- *Argon laser cilioplasty:* Useful if only a few scattered lashes need to be removed.
- *Surgery:*
  - Bilamellar tarsal rotation and transverse tarsotomy with lid margin rotation—these are the recommended surgical procedures for trichiasis from trachomatous scarring in upper lids.
  - Tarsotomy for cicatricial entropion with trichiasis.
  - Eyelid splitting with excision or microhyfrecation (for distichiasis)—eyelid margin is split to expose the distichiasis eyelash follicles. Then each aberrant eyelash follicle is individually excised or microhyfrecated and then removed.
  - Extirpation of hair follicles using radiosurgical technique or a monopolar cautery.
  - Folliculectomy (with or without anterior lamellar resection) for segmental trichiasis and distichiasis.
  - Full thickness pentagonal resection with primary closure of lid, when a segment of a lid is severely affected.

- *Mucous membrane grafting:* Generally, reserved for refractory trichiasis. Eyelid margin is incised and small portion of posterior margin that contains the misaligned eyelash is removed. Then, this defect is replaced with buccal membrane graft in posterior margin to prevent abnormal scarring.

Prevention: In trachoma hyperendemic areas, health education is most important. The WHO recommends SAFE strategy (*S*urgery for trichiasis, *A*ntibiotic treatment, *F*ace washing, and *E*nvironmental improvement) to prevent/control of infection by *Chlamydia trachomatis*.

■ FOLLOW-UP
It depends upon the method used. For mechanical epilation, recurrence is anticipated in every 3–4 weeks.

■ SPECIAL NOTE
Tablet azithromycin, as single dose (1 g), and/or topical tetracycline eye ointment twice daily for 6 weeks after surgery, in trachoma endemic areas.

1.2 Chalazion and Stye

Jigisha Randeri
Rotary Eye Institute, Gujarat
rotaryeye@sify.com

■ CHALAZION
A chalazion is a chronic, nonspecific, and granulomatous inflammation caused by retained sebaceous secretion of meibomian gland or other sebaceous glands into the adjacent stroma.

Clinical Features
Occur at any age; can affect upper and/or lower lid.

Symptoms: Gradually enlarging painless nodule.

Signs: A nontender, round nodule within the tarsal plate. Eversion of the lid may show polypoidal granuloma in case of chalazion ruptured through the tarsal conjunctiva. A "marginal" chalazion is an involvement of a Zeis gland and located at the anterior lid margin.

Differential Diagnosis
Stye (external hordeolum); internal hordeolum.

On Examination
A nontender, round nodule-like swelling of variable size with firm consistency, found anywhere in upper and/or lower lid, away from lid margin. It may be single or multiple. On eversion of the lid, the conjunctiva over the swelling is red. It may be gray at later stage. Large chalazion in upper lid may cause induced astigmatism and distortion of vision.

Management
Treatment may not be required as about one third of all chalazia may resolve spontaneously. Warm compress is also effective in most cases. Persistent lesion may be treated as follows:

Incision and Curettage
Surgery through transconjunctival approach. The eyelid is everted with a chalazion clamp and the cyst is incised vertically parallel to the orientation of meibomian gland and its contents are curetted through the tarsal plate.

Steroid Injection (Intralesional)
0.1–0.2 mL aqueous triamcinolone diacetate diluted with lignocaine with concentration of 5 mg/mL is injected intralesionally transdermally through skin or conjunctiva with a 30-gauge needle. Success rate is about 80%. Second injection can be repeated 2 weeks later. Hard lesions of >6 months durations are less likely to respond.
- In case of recurrence, systemic tetracycline can be given as prophylaxis.
- In case of recurrence of lesion at same site in older individual, a histopathological examination of content is required to rule out malignancy.

■ STYE
It is an acute suppurative inflammation of the eyelash follicle and the Zeis or Moll gland adjacent to it. The most common bacterium is *Staphylococcus aureus*.

Clinical Features
Symptoms: Acute pain and tenderness over the inflamed follicle or gland.

Signs: A localized painful, hard swelling near the lid margin. Signs of acute inflammation are present. An abscess may form which points near the base of the lash. The pain subsides after evacuation of the pus.

Management
Warm compresses helpful in localizing the inflammation in early stage. Evacuation of the pus by pulling the involved lash. Antibiotic eye drops and ointment are applied to control and prevent infection. Systemic antibiotics may be useful in presence of cellulitis. Analgesics and anti-inflammatory drugs to control pain and inflammation are helpful.

Update on Risk Factors
Bortezomib—first-generation proteasome inhibitor for hematological malignancies leads to increase chance of chalazia.

1.3 Blepharitis

Nikhil Gokhlay
Gokhale Eye Hospital and Eye Bank, Mumbai
gokhlay@vsnl.com

■ INTRODUCTION
In clinical use, blepharitis refers to disease of the lid margin which may involve the accessory glands of the eyelid margin, the mucocutaneous junction, and the meibomian glands (MGs).

■ CLINICAL TYPES AND FEATURES
Historically it has been classified by Thygeson into the squamous and ulcerative types. McCulley has classified chronic blepharitis into six major groups to facilitate diagnosis and therapy.
1. *Staphylococcal:* Dry scales and crusts, acute-lid inflammation, short-duration, most common in females.

2. *Seborrheic alone:* Oily or greasy scales and crusts with spotty involvement of glands.
3. *Mixed:* Seborrheic and staphylococcal.
4. *Meibomian seborrhea:* Greasy scales with increased meibomian secretions.
5. *Seborrheic blepharitis with secondary meibomitis:* Greasy scales with patchy meibomitis with solidified secretions and poor expressibility.
6. *Primary meibomitis:* Minimal crusts, associated general dermal involvement in the form of acne rosacea or seborrheic dermatitis. Most severe signs and symptoms. Bron has modified the McCulley classification into anterior blepharitis (types 1, 2, 3, and 5) and posterior blepharitis (types 3, 4, and 6). In clinical practice, patients need not fall into any one category as there is a continuum from one category to the next.

Parasitic infestation may also be associated with lid margin inflammation. *Pthirus pubis* may inhabit the eyelashes and present as blepharitis. *Demodex* (hair follicle mite) may also play a pathogenic role in some cases of rosacea.

Lid margin disease adversely affects the ocular surface due to tear-film disturbance, pathogenic effect of microorganisms involved, inflammatory mediators-released, and the host immune response. The frequency of associated dry eye is as high as 50–80% and is due to unstable tear film and evaporative stress and also to decreased tear secretion. Conjunctival inflammation, phlyctenular inflammation, surface epitheliopathy, limbal infiltrates, marginal keratitis, corneal vascularization, limbal deficiency, and secondary ocular surface failure can be seen in these patients.

TREATMENT

- *Lid scrubs:* Cleaning of the lid margins with dilute solutions of baby shampoos is effective to tackle scales, crusts, and debris that accumulate on the lid margin.
- *Antibiotics:* Staphylococcal control with broad-spectrum antibiotics three to four times a day for 5–7 days is recommended. Application of antibiotic ointments such as erythromycin and tetracycline to the lid margins after lid hygiene also helps these patients.
- *Warm compresses and massage:* Application of local heat to the eyelids helps to thin the waxy meibomian secretions and improves their expressibility. This should be followed by mechanical expression of the secretions by lid massage. This can be done by rolling a finger toward the lid margins so as to press the MGs and express glandular secretions. In the clinic it can be done by squeezing the tarsal plate between two cotton-tipped applicators after topical anesthesia.
- *Tetracyclines (tetracycline, doxycycline, and minocycline):* They reduce lipase production by lid margin staphylococci which reduces production of toxic-free fatty acids, and therefore reduces ocular surface inflammation. They also inhibit collagenases. They have to be used on a long-term basis and are very useful in rosacea.
- *Anti-inflammatory therapy:* Inflammation on the ocular surface can be suppressed by topical cyclosporine and steroids. Cyclosporine is safer to use on a long-term basis and also helps the associated dry eye.
- *Lubricants:* They help to treat the dry eye component and provide symptomatic relief.
- *Nutritional supplements:* Oral supplementation of omega-3 fatty acids has shown to be of benefit in patients with chronic and intractable meibomitis.
- *Hormone therapy:* Androgen support is vital for MG function. In addition androgens are anti-inflammatory on the ocular surface. They are currently under evaluation.
- *Demodex infestation:* 50% tea tree oil eyelid scrubs and daily tea tree oil shampoo scrubs are beneficial if used for minimum 6 weeks. Oral ivermectin has been tried for recalcitrant infections.
- *Meibomian gland dysfunction (MGD):* Single 12-minute treatment with LipiFlow system showed improvement in both signs [tear breakup time (TBUT), corneal fluorescein staining, and MG secretion score] and symptoms [Ocular Surface Disease Index (OSDI) questionnaire] for up to 1 year.

- *Intraductal MG probing:* To reopen MG orifices leading to rapid and long-lasting symptom relief but uncomfortable and inconvenient for patients.
- *Intense pulsed light (IPL):* Treatment with tear substitutes, warm compresses, topical anti-inflammatory agents, and antibiotics often provide acute symptomatic relief; however, they fail to alleviate symptoms in the long term. IPL has been recently introduced in the ophthalmic practice for the management of dry eye disease (DED) due to MGD. The treatment is well tolerated due to its noninvasive nature and adverse reactions are rarely encountered. Moreover, results can be maintained over time with periodic sessions of IPL.

1.4 Lagophthalmos and Exposure Keratopathy

Santanu Mitra
Disha Eye Hospitals, Barrackpore, Kolkata
disha@cal2.vsnl.net.in

RELEVANT CLINICAL FEATURES

Eyelids play a critically important role in the normal tear dispersion over the corneal and conjunctival surfaces. Interruption to the functions of eyelids interferes with this leading to local drying and ocular surface changes collectively known as exposure keratopathy.

Three main eyelid disturbances are seen:
1. Decreased blink-rate associated with several degenerative brain diseases
2. Incomplete blink or lagophthalmos
3. Lid retraction associated with proptosis and thyroid ophthalmopathy. Lagophthalmos, derived from Greek words *lagos* meaning hare and *ophthalmos* meaning eyes, because apparently rabbits sleep with their eyes open.

In the presence of facial paralysis, the levator muscle starts working against a markedly weakened or completely denervated orbicularis muscle, grossly affecting eyelid closure and problems of exposure keratopathy.

Lagophthalmos can occur due to a variety of causes and can be categorized as follows:
- Postsurgical following severe ptosis corrections, eyelid reconstructions, large inferior rectus recession, etc.
- In association with VII nerve palsies—Bell's palsy associated with surgical resection of acoustic neuromas, parotid surgery, etc.
- Thyroid ophthalmopathy with lid retractions
- Lower lid ectropion
- Enophthalmos
- Nocturnal lagophthalmos
- Mechanical factors such as high myopia, proptosis, and buphthalmos
- Systemic inflammatory cicatrization like scleroderma
- Euryblepharon
- Patients under ventilator support
- Patients with exposure keratopathy experience discomfort with grittiness and burning sensation, sometimes increased lacrimation, blurring of vision, and occasional sight threatening problems due to corneal complications.

There is a tear-film instability leading to a decreased tear breakup time (TBUT). The associated epitheliopathy mostly involves the inferior corneal area. Initially it appears as superficial punctuate epithelial erosions. This epithelial disturbance may progress to corneal ulceration leading to visual loss. The more commonly involved inferior ulcer area is horizontally oval in shape. It has basically a smooth and slightly heaped-up edge. In cases of chronic lesions, there is stromal loss with thinning and secondary infective keratitis may supervene.

DIFFERENTIAL DIAGNOSIS

Exposure keratopathy due to lagophthalmos should be differentiated from neurotrophic keratopathies, which are potentially more vision damaging conditions and therefore require closer monitoring. Here corneal hypesthesia is the prime pathophysiology. Dry eye syndrome is another entity which should be carefully ruled out. Also, the different etiological factors of lagophthalmos, as enumerated before, have to be differentiated because often the initial treatment should be directed to cure the root cause.

TREATMENT

Management of exposure keratopathy due to lagophthalmos is directed to prevent the more severe vision damaging corneal complications. Depending on the severity of the root cause of lagophthalmos the management modalities may be of temporary or permanent nature.

Tear Supplements

This forms the baseline of all exposure keratopathy management. Gels and ointments are preferably used particularly during night time.

Temporary Corneal Protection

Therapeutic bandage contact lens (BCL) is not very helpful as lack of corneal sensation and inability to blink properly lead to the loss of the lens. A convenient moist chamber like the use of swimming goggles at night may be helpful. Taping the eyelids shut at night is also greatly beneficial. Use of Frost suture to pull the lower eyelid to forehead is also applicable in postsurgical lagophthalmos correction in the initial period. Recent reports suggest Glad Press'n Seal is a simple method of creating a moisture chamber. Speciality sclera contact lenses like PROSE lens are especially helpful.

Surgical Procedures

- They are employed when correction of a more permanent nature is required.
- Lower lid ectropion may be corrected with an upper lid transposition flap.
- *Upper lid gold weights or Botox injection* for paralysis may induce temporary drooping.
- *Orbital decompression* for thyroid ophthalmopathy has to be undertaken before any lid reconstructive surgery. Two implantable prosthetic devices, a silastic band cerclage of Arion and a stainless-steel wire palpebral spring are used to oppose levator palpebrae superioris (LPS) action.
- *Lateral tarsorrhaphy*, temporary or permanent, is still the most predictable surgical procedure used.

1.5 Bacterial Conjunctivitis

Praveen Krishna
Radhatri Nethralaya, Chennai
ratnagiripk@rediffmail.com

INTRODUCTION

Bacterial conjunctivitis is a microbial infection involving the mucous membrane of the surface of the eye. It is usually self-limiting and benign but at times can be serious signifying an underlying disease.[1]

PREDISPOSING FACTORS FOR CONJUNCTIVITIS

- *Neonate:* Vaginal delivery in infected mother, especially in cases of inadequate prenatal and perinatal care.

- **Infant:** Congenital nasolacrimal duct obstruction is quite often encountered in neonates and infants. Concomitant bacterial otitis media can also cause bacterial conjunctivitis.
- **Child:** Coexisting bacterial otitis media, sinusitis, or pharyngitis and nasopharyngeal bacterial colonization.
- **Adult:** Oculogenital spread, lid malposition, severe tear deficiency, immunosuppression, and trauma. Irrespective of the age, contact with an infected individual is one of the most common causes of bacterial conjunctivitis.

NATURAL HISTORY
Nongonococcal
- **Mild:** Self-limited in adults. In children may progress to corneal infection or preseptal cellulitis.
- **Severe:** Corneal infection may be associated with systemic features such as pharyngitis, otitis media and meningitis.

Gonococcal
- **Neonate:** Manifests within 1–7 days after birth. Rapidly evolves to severe, purulent conjunctivitis. Corneal infection, corneal scarring, and in advanced cases corneal perforation may be seen. Associated septicemia with arthritis, meningitis is usually present **(Fig. 1.5.1)**.
- **Adult:** Quick onset of severe purulent conjunctivitis. Sequelae include corneal infection, corneal scarring, and corneal perforation. Associated systemic features include urethritis, pelvic inflammatory disease, septicemia, and arthritis.

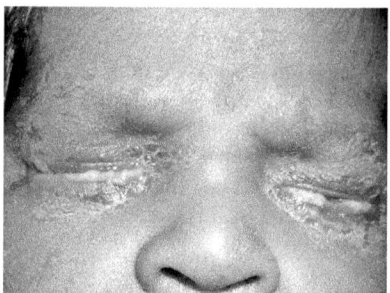

Fig. 1.5.1: Ophthalmia neonatorum (gonococcal).

TYPICAL CLINICAL SIGNS
Nongonococcal
Unilateral or bilateral conjunctival injection with mucopurulent discharge, matting of eyelashes, and lid edema.

Gonococcal
Unilateral or bilateral conjunctival injection with marked eyelid edema, bulbar congestion, marked purulent discharge, and preauricular lymphadenopathy. Corneal infiltrate or ulcer can be seen which often begins superiorly.

DIFFERENTIAL DIAGNOSIS
- Blepharitis, preseptal cellulitis, dacryocystitis, *and* hordeolum
- *Conjunctivitis:* Acute hemorrhagic, allergic, giant papillary, neonatal, and viral
- *Contact lens complications:* Corneal, conjunctival, and tarsal foreign body
- *Keratoconjunctivitis:* Epidemic and pharyngoconjunctival fever (PCF)

DIAGNOSTIC TESTS
History and clinical examination are stand-alone sufficient to diagnose bacterial conjunctivitis. However, in all cases of suspected infectious neonatal conjunctivitis conjunctival cultures may be useful. Bacterial cultures also may be helpful for recurrent or severe purulent conjunctivitis in any age group as well as in nonresponding cases.

TREATMENT

The mainstay of medical treatment of bacterial conjunctivitis is topical antibiotic therapy.

The choice of antibiotic is usually empirical. A 5–7 days course of a broad-spectrum topical antibiotic is usually effective.

Conjunctival cultures and slides for Gram staining should be obtained if gonococcal infection is suspected. The cultures also guide in the choice of antibiotic to be used for treatment.

Only indication for systemic antibiotic therapy is conjunctivitis secondary to *Neisseria gonorrhoeae*. Saline lavage provides comfort and faster resolution of inflammation in gonococcal conjunctivitis. Patients and sexual contacts should be informed about the possibility of concomitant disease and treated appropriately.

Systemic Antibiotic for Gonococcal Conjunctivitis

- *Ophthalmia neonatorum:* Caused by *N. gonorrhoeae*, ceftriaxone 25–50 mg/kg intravenous or intramuscular (IM), single dose, not to exceed 125 mg.
- *Children (<18 years):* Children who weigh <45 kg ceftriaxone 125 mg IM, single dose or spectinomycin 40 mg/kg (maximum dose 2 g) IM, single dose.
- *Adults:* Ceftriaxone 1 g IM, single dose or cefixime 400 mg orally, single dose. For cephalosporin-allergic patients: spectinomycin 2 g IM, single dose.

FOLLOW-UP

Patients with gonococcal conjunctivitis should be seen every day or on alternate days until resolution of signs and symptoms. For other types of bacterial conjunctivitis, patients can be asked to review in 3–7 days.

SPECIAL NOTES

- Patients treated for gonococcal infection should be also treated routinely for *Chlamydia trachomatis* infection.
- A single oral dose of azithromycin 2 g is effective against gonococcal infections, but it is not recommend for widespread use because of concerns about the resistance.
- Sexual abuse must be considered a cause of infection in preadolescent children.
- In gonococcal conjunctivitis parents of neonates and partners of adults should be examined and treated with systemic antibiotics.

REFERENCE

1. Limberg MB. A review of bacterial keratitis and bacterial conjunctivitis. Am J Ophthalmol. 1991;112(4 Suppl):2S-9S.

1.6 Adenoviral Keratoconjunctivitis

Prashant Kr Singhal
Disha Eye Hospitals, Hooghly
p2singhal@sify.com

INTRODUCTION

Adenoviruses are deoxyribonucleic acid (DNA) viruses. There are >50 serotypes affecting the respiratory tract and eye. There is low natural immunity in the general population. Adenoviruses show tissue tropism, i.e., specific subgroups and are associated with distinct clinical syndrome. Epithelial keratitis is due to viral replication and subepithelial infiltrates are immune-mediated.

Transmission: It occurs by contact with ocular or respiratory secretions or fomites. People living in close contact are more susceptible. Transmission by contaminated ophthalmic instruments and eye drops has caused outbreaks.

Incubation period: 2-14 days and *infectivity* lasts 10-14 days after symptoms develop. Virus is also shed 4-10 days even before signs develop.

■ CLINICAL FEATURES

Most adenoviral eye disease present as one of three types:
1. Simple follicular conjunctivitis-most serotypes
2. Pharyngoconjunctival fever (PCF) serotypes 3, 4, or 7
3. Epidemic keratoconjunctivitis (EKC) serotypes 8, 19, and 3 (less frequently 2-5, 7-11, 14, and 16). Simple follicular conjunctivitis is not associated with systemic disease and is self-limiting.

■ HISTORY

Recent exposure or affected family member. Onset is sudden; other eye is affected in almost 50% and is less severe.

■ SYSTEMIC FEATURES

Fever, headache, myalgia, pharyngitis, and characteristic preauricular lymphadenopathy.

■ OCULAR FEATURES

Symptoms
Pain, watering, redness, and photophobia.

Signs
Lid edema and watery discharge.

Conjunctival Sign
- Hyperemia, chemosis with involvement of caruncle; follicular reaction more marked in inferior fornix (earliest and most common sign); papillary hypertrophy; and pseudomembrane and membrane formations (more marked in EKC). These membranes may rarely bleed without conjunctival scarring and dry eye (**Fig. 1.6.1**).
- Conjunctivitis usually resolves by 10-21 days.

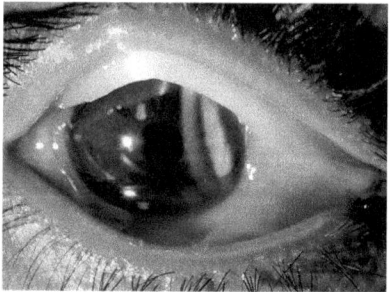

Fig. 1.6.1: Pseudomembrane in adenoviral conjunctivitis.

Cornea
- Cornea involved in 30% cases of PCF and 80% in EKC. Usually bilateral with other eye less severely involved. Keratitis occurs 2-5 days after symptoms develop. Corneal sensation is unchanged. In most cases, keratitis resolves spontaneously in 2-3 weeks.
- In some cases the following stages of keratitis may evolve:
  - *Stage 0:* Mild punctate epithelial erosions develop within the first 2-4 days; stain poorly with rose bengal and fluorescein.
  - *Stage 1:* Fine, diffuse punctate epithelial keratitis (PEK) persists for 2-5 days; may resolve or progress to Stage 2.
  - *Stage 2:* Fine coarse PEK (stains brilliantly with rose bengal) persists for 2-5 days.
  - *Stage 3:* Coarse, granular infiltrates within deep epithelium; appearance of faint subepithelial infiltrates; persists for 2-5 days.
  - *Stage 4:* Classic subepithelial infiltrates: no staining; occurs may persist for weeks to months.
  - *Stage 5:* Punctate epithelial granularity (superficial and deep epithelium) develops late—after weeks to months. May cause permanent scars.

The corneal sensation remains unchanged.

Laboratory workup is not necessary for making the diagnosis. Giemsa stain for intranuclear inclusion is rarely done. Definitive diagnosis can be done on human cell culture.

■ TREATMENT

Primarily supportive. Prevent transmission—highly contagious.

Patient Instructions

- Warn patient about the contagious nature. Need to wash hands frequently, to use towels and soap separate from others, and to avoid direct contact with others. Frequent use of hand sanitizers by the patient's attenders.
- Isolation from work or school for up to 2 weeks or until there is no discharge.
- May get worse before resolving in 2-4 weeks.
- Patient instructions regarding viral shedding for a period up to 12 days from onset.

Ocular Management

- No topical ophthalmic anti-adenoviral drug is approved. Only antiviral drug effective against adenovirus is cidofovir, but is rarely used as it is toxic.
- Cold compresses.
- Artificial tears four to six times daily.
- Remove symptomatic membranes with wet cotton swab or forceps; prescribe antibiotic or steroid ointment.
- Reserve topical steroids for severe conjunctivitis and keratitis. Used in case of severe conjunctival membrane or macroulceration; severe keratitis or prolonged symptoms. Topical steroids reduce the quantity and density of subepithelial infiltrates but exacerbate infiltrates upon discontinuation.
- Cyclosporine 0.05%/0.1% and Tacrolimus 0.03%/0.01% eye ointment are other options for resolution of post adenoviral subepithelial infiltrates. Treatment may be prolonged in severe cases.

Professional Precautions

- Handwashing before and after each examination with use of paper towels and use of hand sanitizers.
- Avoid instrument contact.
- Adequate instrument cleaning and sterilization [immersion in 1-2% solution of sodium hypochlorite (household bleach) or 3% hydrogen peroxide].

■ DIFFERENTIAL DIAGNOSIS

Follicular Conjunctivitis

Trachoma; acute inclusion conjunctivitis; primary herpes simplex conjunctivitis; chicken pox; infectious mononucleosis; neonatal inclusion conjunctivitis; and topical medications.

Subepithelial Corneal Opacities

Herpes simplex virus (HSV) infection; herpes zoster virus (HZV) infection; infectious mononucleosis; Epstein-Barr virus infection; and brucellosis.

■ FOLLOW-UP

Follow-up is only necessary in cases of chronic EKC with conjunctival scarring and keratitis. Rarely surgery may be necessary for symblepharon and entropion.

1.7 Allergic Conjunctivitis

Quresh B Maskati
Maskati Eye Clinic, Mumbai
qureshmaskati@gmail.com

■ INTRODUCTION

Allergic conjunctivitis (AC) is a type I hypersensitivity reaction occurring in response to external allergens, predominantly in males and seen more during the first two decades of life. These may be outdoor allergens such as pollen, or maybe indoor allergens such as house dust, mites, cockroaches, etc. It can be classified into: seasonal allergic conjunctivitis (SAC) and perennial allergic conjunctivitis (PAC); vernal keratoconjunctivitis (VKC), atopic keratoconjunctivitis (AKC), and giant papillary conjunctivitis (GPC). In India, most cases occur year round, unlike the SAC seen in spring and summer in the west.

■ CLINICAL FEATURES

Symptoms

The main symptom in AC is itching. In fact, in the absence of this symptom, the diagnosis may need to be revised. Other symptoms include redness, photophobia, burning, foreign body sensation, pain, discharge, and epiphora. Many patients may also suffer from other allergies such as allergic rhinitis, asthma, atopic dermatitis (strongly-associated with AKC), and eczema, hence a detailed history taking is important. Other members of the family may also suffer from an allergic disorder; hence a family history should be solicited. GPC is usually associated with contact lens wearers. It may rarely be caused by chronic irritation due to silicon tires following retinal detachment surgery.

Signs

Signs of AC include conjunctival congestion, variable amounts of chemosis, and eyelid edema. There is often a ropy discharge seen. The classical feature of AC seen in our country is large or giant papillae, which may either, be at the limbus or in the palpebral conjunctiva, overlying the superior tarsal plate—affection of the lower lid is very rare. The papillae in severe cases resemble cobblestones as they are flat-topped and situated very close to each other. They may be accompanied by evanescent (transient) white dots, comprising of dead epithelial cells and eosinophils. These are known as Horner-Trantas dots. At the limbus, the papillae may coalesce to form a gray-white arc (vernal gerontoxon), resembling an arcus senilis. In long-standing or severe cases, the cornea may develop superficial punctate keratopathy (SPK) and even "shield ulcers", which may arise de novo or due to coalescence of the SPK. These ulcers are more commonly seen in the palpebral variety of AC. Chronic eye rubbing due to itching may result in keratoconus in genetically predisposed individuals.

■ DIFFERENTIAL DIAGNOSIS

Viral and bacterial conjunctivitis may mimic AC. However, the chief symptom in these is watering, discharge, and redness, unlike in AC where itching is the main symptom in over 90% of the patients.

■ TREATMENT

This may be divided into nonspecific and specific treatment. In the former, the child or adolescent should be taught the importance of maintenance of hygiene, frequent hand cleaning, and avoidance of rubbing of eyes as this contributes to worsening of symptoms due to more mast cell degranulation. Cold compresses relieve itching to some extent.

Avoidance of the offending allergen, if known, is an excellent option, though impractical in most cases.

However, the mainstay of treatment is pharmacological. We do have a plethora of drugs to choose from since the last couple of years in India, unlike in the recent past, when the only nonsteroidal drug available was disodium cromoglycate. The following drugs are available:

- *Disodium cromoglycate:* A weak mast cell inhibitor, available as 2% and 4%. Needs to be given in bid dosage as a long-term treatment.
- *Olopatadine:* 1% is available, to be used twice a day. 2% is also available for convenient once a day usage. This drug is a dual-action drug. It acts by stabilizing the mast cells and preventing release of histamine as well as binding with the H_1 receptors preventing the effects of histamine already released.
- *Alcaftadine 0.25%:* This is also a combined histamine blocker + mast cell stabilizer with the advantage of once a day dosing.
- *Epinastine:* Also a dual-action drug, though relatively better antihistaminic than a mast cell stabilizer.
- *Azelastine:* A relatively weak dual-action drug.
- *Ketotifen*: A nonsteroidal anti-inflammatory drug (NSAID). It is a dual-action drug, causing mast cell stabilization as well as nonspecific histamine receptor antagonist.
- *Ketorolac tromethamine:* Also an NSAID. Acts by downregulating the enzyme cyclooxygenase, which is required for prostaglandin synthesis. This causes reduction in the inflammatory response, reducing the symptom of itching.
- *Loteprednol:* This is a smart steroid, available in two strengths, 0.2% and 0.5%. Like with all steroids, it reduces the polymorphonuclear response and the enhanced capillary permeability caused by histamine thus reducing the inflammation. Caution should be exercised as with all steroids. Long-term use can cause cataracts, glaucoma, and dryness and make the eye more susceptible to infections.
- *Topical calcineurin inhibitors:* Cyclosporine eye drops (0.05% and 0.1%) and tacrolimus (0.03% and 0.1%) eye ointments are good alternatives to long-term dual-acting agents for maintenance therapy. Only side effect is stinging sensation on instillation more noticed with tacrolimus than cyclosporine.

FOLLOW-UP

Patients should be encouraged to follow-up at regular intervals. This serves several important purposes:
- Steroid dependence or addiction can be caught early and the patient weaned-off before permanent steroid-induced complications set-in.
- If the drug regime used is not working in a particular patient, he/she can be put on a different regime.
- Reinforcement of instructions on hygiene and avoidance of eye rubbing can be done at each visit, till it becomes a habit.

CONCLUSION

In conclusion, AC is a very common condition in our country and should be tackled in a rational manner to achieve both relief from itching and prevention of complications of the disease and its treatment.

1.8 Keratomalacia

Radhika Tandon
Dr RP Centre for Ophthalmic Sciences, AIIMS, New Delhi
radhika_tan@yahoo.com

■ INTRODUCTION

Keratomalacia (xerophthalmia and xerotic keratitis) is defined as "drying and clouding of the cornea due to vitamin A deficiency and insufficient protein and calories in the diet".

The ocular surface becomes xerotic and the resulting dryness can lead to the development of corneal ulceration and secondary bacterial infections may occur. There occurs an involvement of the tear glands also leading to an inadequate tear film and consequent dry eyes.

Vitamin A is important for dark adaptation and the normal functioning of the rods so night blindness (nyctalopia or poor vision in the dark) may develop because of vitamin A deficiency. The diagnosis is generally made clinically and is essentially based on the presence of a dry or ulcerated cornea in a malnourished person, usually a child, but can also occur in adults at special risk for the same.

Importance of Vitamin A

Essential for normal vision as well as:
- Proper bone growth
- Healthy skin
- Protection of mucous membranes of the digestive, respiratory, and urinary tracts against infection

Causes of Vitamin A Deficiency

- Dietary (i.e., poor intake): Poverty; ignorance; and poor dietary habits
- Metabolic (i.e., absorption)

Vitamin A Deficiency due to Dietary Deficiency

It is seen in developing countries from dietary deficiency:
- Delayed weaning and inadequate nutrition
- Non-breastfed babies with maternal malnutrition so poor liver reserves compounded by unhygienic and inadequate nutritional practices

It is rare in developed countries from dietary deficiency, but can still be seen in some specific situations such as the following:
- Elderly or homeless population with poor diet
- Psychiatric conditions induced dietary restrictions (phobia and anorexia nervosa)
- Alcoholism

Vitamin A deficiency can also occur secondary to conditions associated with impaired absorption, storage, or transport of vitamin A:
- Celiac disease, ulcerative colitis, cystic fibrosis, liver disease, or intestinal bypass surgery and any condition that affects absorption of fat-soluble vitamins
- Uncontrolled phenylketonuria

Severe vitamin A deficiency: Devastating effects in infants and young children.

■ RISK FACTORS

- Protein-caloric malnutrition
- *Precipitated by a systemic illness:*
  - Measles
  - Pneumonia
  - Diarrhea

Keratomalacia is the softening of the corneas:
- May lead to corneal infection
- Rupture (perforation)
- Degenerative tissue changes
- Secondary glaucoma
- Anterior staphyloma
- Resulting in blindness

CLINICAL FEATURES
- Usually bilateral (can be unilateral)
- Centrally located, gray, and indolent corneal ulcers surrounded by dull lack-luster hazy cornea
- Photophobia ±
- The cornea becomes soft and necrotic
- Perforation is common

MANAGEMENT
Vitamin A deficiency treatment regimens along with age, dosage, and dosage schedule are depicted in **Table 1.8.1**.

SPECIAL NOTES
Vitamin A deficiency is basically a public health problem and has to be tackled by proper education, elimination of poverty, malnutrition and ignorance with an improvement in maternal health, encouragement of breastfeeding with proper nutrition of pregnant and nursing mothers, proper weaning practices, and basic amenities of hygiene and sanitation.

The role of ophthalmologists should be to increase awareness in the medical community including general practitioners, obstetricians, pediatricians, health policy makers, and grassroots healthcare workers about the risk factors and preventive measures to prevent blindness from this devastating disease.

TABLE 1.8.1: Vitamin A deficiency treatment regimen.

Age	Dosage	Dosage schedule
0–5 months old	50,000 IU	Day 1, 2, and 14
6–11 months old	100,000 IU	Day 1, 2, and 14
Males >12 months	200,000 IU	Day 1, 2, and 14
Girls: 12 months to 12 years ≥50 years	200,000 IU	Day 1, 2, and 14
Women: • 13–49 years with night blindness ± Bitot's spots • 13–49 years with active corneal lesions	• 10,000 IU (or) 25,000 IU • 200,000 IU	• Everyday (or) Every week for at least 3 months • Day 1, 2, and 14

1.9 Recurrent Corneal Erosion Syndrome

Himanshu Matalia
Narayana Nethralaya, Bengaluru
drhimanshumatalia@yahoo.co.in

■ INTRODUCTION

As the name suggests recurrent corneal erosion syndrome (RCES) is a condition characterized by recurrent and episodic corneal epithelial fallout due to faulty basement membrane complexes.

■ ETIOLOGY

- *Trauma:* Fingernail injury, corneal abrasion, foreign body, contact lens, chemical injury, and lid abnormalities
- *Dystrophies:* Epithelial basement membrane dystrophy (Cogan dystrophy or map-dot-fingerprint dystrophy), lattice dystrophy, and granular and macular dystrophy
- *Systemic causes:* Diabetes mellitus

■ SYMPTOMS AND SIGNS

Symptoms include recurring attacks of pain, foreign-body sensation, photophobia, and tearing, often at the time of awakening or during sleep. Signs are corneal abrasion or localized roughening of the corneal epithelium (negative staining), subepithelial scar, map-like lines, epithelial dots (microcysts), or fingerprint patterns. A healing epithelial defect may look like a pseudodendrite.

■ PATHOPHYSIOLOGY

Recurrent corneal erosion syndrome can occur due to abnormal basement membrane complex with abnormalities of hemidesmosomes, anchoring fibrils, or basement membrane resulting in poor adhesion of epithelial cells. Corneal hydration from lid closure and microsaccades of early morning can "rip-off" this poorly attached epithelium leading to corneal erosion. Gelatinase [matrix metalloproteinase (MMP-2 and MMP-9)] have found to be upregulated in some cases of RCES.

Recurrent corneal erosion (RCE) classification:
- *Hykin et al.:*
  - Small   [0-3 sectors of corneal erosion]
  - Moderate   [4-6 sectors of corneal erosion]
  - Large   [7-9 sectors of corneal erosion]
  - Very large [10-12 sectors of corneal erosion]
- *Chandler:*
  - *Microform erosions:* Milder, short duration, and increased frequency
  - *Macroform erosions:* Persists for days at a time associated with history of trauma

TREATMENT

Management of RCES is usually aimed at allowing the epithelium to heal and thus relieve the symptoms and restore normality in basement membrane complex to avoid recurrence.

Care of an Acute Attack

Lubricants

Mainstay of the treatment of RCES is lubricant drops, gels, or ointments. A higher molecular weight artificial lubricant would help by its "wetting property". Preservative-free lubricants are preferred as the preservative can retard the healing.

Epithelial Debridement
Loosely-attached epithelium should be debrided with dry arrowhead sponge. Debridement helps to remove trapped epithelial cells, which may cause the recurrence. The procedure can be followed by bandage contact lens (BCL) or patching for short period.

Bandage Contact Lens
Bandage contact lens provides the protection to the newly growing epithelial cells against the abrasive action of the lids. It covers the exposed nerve endings thus reduce the symptoms. It also improves the quality of vision by providing a smooth refractive surface and it obviates the need for the eye patching. BCL should be kept in situ for longer duration to allow proper healing of the newly grown epithelium.

Patching
Short duration (<2 days) can be considered if BCL is not available. Benefits are less compared to the risk involved if kept for longer time.

Cycloplegics
In severely symptomatic cases, use of homide or cyclopentolate may be beneficial.

Antibiotics
Prophylactic topical antibiotics can be used but possibility of drug toxicity must be kept in mind.

Prevention of Recurrences
Recurrences are unpredictable. There is currently no treatment, which can claim to prevent recurrence totally. However, there are a few treatment modalities to reduce the chances of recurrence.

Lubricants
Dry eye is hypothesized to be one of the precipitating factors of RCES. Long-term usage of lubricants especially before sleeping and immediately after may help.

Hyperosmotic Agents
Sodium chloride 6% eye ointment has been hypothesized to reduce the swelling of newly forming epithelial cells. However, several studies refute the major advantages of hyperosmotic component of the treatment and suggest that it may just work like a lubricant ointment.

Anterior Stromal Puncture
Anterior stromal puncture (ASP) has a role in the management of recalcitrant and chronic RCES not involving the visual axis. Multiple micropunctures with 25 or 26 G needle through epithelium into anterior stroma in the area of RCES. The epithelial plugs act like anchoring fibrils and reduce the chance of erosion. As it may induce scarring it is best avoided in cases involving visual axis. The same can also be achieved by neodymium-doped yttrium aluminum garnet (Nd:YAG) laser but the scarring induced is more.

Phototherapeutic Keratectomy
Phototherapeutic keratectomy (PTK) has shown to be a promising treatment method to reduce the chances of recurrence. A limited ablation up to anterior Bowman's membrane provides a smoother surface for the newly growing cells. The disadvantage of PTK is chances of hyperopic shift.

Diamond Burr Polishing

Diamond burr polishing involves epithelial debridement with a cellulose sponge and diamond burr polishing of Bowman's membrane. BCL is applied for 10 days along with topical antibiotics. Good treatment option when RCE involves the visual axis.

1.10 | Bullous Keratopathy

Arun K Jain
Advanced Eye Center, PGIMER, Chandigarh
aronkjain@yahoo.com

■ INTRODUCTION

Bullous keratopathy [pseudophakic bullous keratopathy (PBK) or aphakic bullous keratopathy (ABK)] refers to an endothelial cell damage with resulting irreversible corneal edema that occurs commonly after cataract extraction with or without intraocular lens (IOL) implantation.

There are number of other conditions, such as severe viral endotheliitis, uncontrolled glaucoma, and corneal graft rejection, which can lead to endothelial cell loss or failure of corneal endothelial function resulting in bullous keratopathy.

■ ETIOPATHOGENESIS AND CLINICAL FEATURES

The clinical features of bullous keratopathy are chronic corneal edema and leads to scarring and loss of transparency of the cornea. The most common manifestation of PBK is corneal stromal and epithelial edema. Rupture of corneal epithelial bullae often irritates the corneal nerve endings thereby causing severe ocular pain and watering.

Preexisting Low Endothelial Cell Count

Few patients develop corneal edema despite atraumatic surgery, reason being abnormally low endothelial cell counts preoperatively such as seen in Fuchs endothelial dystrophy. Examination of the fellow eye in these cases can give a clue as endothelial dystrophies are bilateral in nature. Presence of central guttae as seen on slit lamp examination and specular microscopy showing evidence of guttae and low cell density can point to a diagnosis of Fuchs endothelial dystrophy.

Surgical Endothelial Trauma

Surgical trauma to the corneal endothelium is often the most common cause of corneal endothelial decompensation. Prolonged use of high ultrasound energy during phacoemulsification or traumatic delivery of the nucleus in extracapsular cataract extraction (ECCE) and small incision cataract surgery (SICS) may cause irreversible endothelial dysfunction in the immediate postoperative period. Use of cohesive and dispersive ophthalmic viscosurgical devices (OVDs) provides excellent endothelial protection during phacoemulsification and IOL implantation.

Toxic Anterior Segment Syndrome

Toxic anterior segment syndrome (TASS) is characterized by limbus to limbus corneal edema 1 day after surgery with a marked inflammatory response and often a hypopyon. An important differential diagnosis is endophthalmitis; hence, it is imperative to differentiate both. Management of TASS includes 1 hourly topical steroids followed by reassessment.

Type of Intraocular Lens Implants

Anterior chamber (AC) angle and iris fixated IOLs are more commonly associated with PBK.

Descemet's Membrane Detachments

Descemet's membrane detachments (DMDs) occur intraoperatively because of improper instrumentation such as use of blunt keratome and improper surgical technique. DMD can be treated with either air injection or perfluoropropane (C_3F_8) or sulfur hexafluoride (SF_6) or in some cases with placement of a full thickness, 10-0 nylon suture to reattach the Descemet's membrane.

■ TREATMENT

Medical Treatments

Therapy for bullous keratopathy is aimed to reduce discomfort and increase visual acuity. Topical hypertonic agents such as sodium chloride (5%) ointment or drops are used to reduce the epithelial edema. Since the edema is more pronounced in the morning while waking up, the hypertonic eye ointment is often prescribed at night to alleviate the symptoms. Bandage contact lens can also be used for symptomatic relief to pain and foreign body sensation. These patients should however be followed up regularly to prevent microbial keratitis.

Surgical Treatments

In eyes without severe stromal scarring, posterior lamellar keratoplasty procedures such as Descemet's stripping endothelial (automated) keratoplasty (DSEK or DSAEK) and Descemet's membrane endothelial keratoplasty (DMEK) have replaced penetrating keratoplasty (PK) as the surgery of choice. However in cases with severe stromal scarring PK is the surgery of choice.[1]

In eyes with poor visual potential other treatment options include bandage contact lenses, anterior stromal puncture, phototherapeutic keratectomy (PTK), amniotic membrane transplantation, and Gundersen conjunctival flap.

■ REFERENCE

1. Narayanan R, Gaster RN, Kenney MC. Pseudophakic corneal edema: A review of mechanisms and treatments. Cornea. 2006;25(9):993-1004.

1.11 | Neurotrophic Keratitis

Jayangshu Sengupta
Priyambada Birla Aravind Eye Hospital, Kolkata
jayanshu@hotmail.com

■ INTRODUCTION

Neurotrophic keratitis is caused by an impairment of trigeminal innervation, leading to a decrease or absence of corneal sensation.[1] The common causes include diabetes, leprosy, vitamin A deficiency, herpes zoster or simplex infections, acoustic neuroma, drug toxicity, and contact lens to mention a few.

Accurate ocular examination must be carried out which include measuring the blink rate and corneal sensitivity apart from routine Schirmer test and vital staining with fluorescein, Rose Bengal, or Lissamine Green dyes. It must be remembered that blink rate is markedly decreased if bilateral neurotrophic keratitis occurs.

According to the Mackie classification, there are three stages of neurotrophic keratitis.

Stage 1 is characterized by punctate keratopathy, epithelial hyperplasia and irregularity, superficial neovascularization, and stromal scarring.

Stage 2 is characterized by a persistent epithelial defect, most frequently localized in the superior half of cornea, surrounded by poorly adherent opaque and edematous epithelium.

This edematous epithelium can spontaneously detach leading to an enlargement of the epithelial defect and inadequate healing of the epithelial edges which eventually become rolled. Descemet's membrane folds and stromal edema is also seen **(Fig. 1.11.1)**.

Stage 3 is characterized by stromal involvement with a corneal ulcer that often leads to stromal melt and corneal perforation.[1]

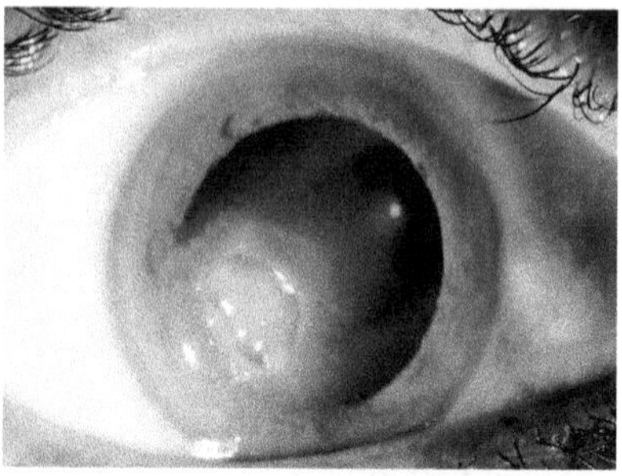

■ CLINICAL FEATURES

Fig. 1.11.1: Neurotrophic keratitis.

Stage 1 of the disease often mimics dry eye, exposure keratitis, topical drug toxicity, contact lens abuse, and corneal limbal deficiency since all of them have punctate corneal erosions and tear film abnormalities. However the hallmark of neurotrophic keratitis is corneal anesthesia.

In vivo confocal microscopy visualizes the affected sub-basal nerve plexus structure and density.

■ DIFFERENTIAL DIAGNOSIS

Neurotrophic keratitis can be infective, toxic, or immune corneal ulcers. They always present with severe symptoms, more signs of inflammation and sometimes with stromal infiltrates. Microbiologic examinations for bacteria, fungi, and viruses are always required.

■ TREATMENT

Medical Treatment

- *Stage 1:*
  - To prevent epithelial breakdown and improve epithelial healing
  - Frequent use of preservative free artificial tear eye drops
  - Punctal occlusion is often helpful
  - In persistent keratopathy, autologous serum tears are considered
  - If no response with mentioned medications, recombinant human nerve growth factor (rhNGF) eye drops [cenegermin (Oxervate and Cacicol)] and a self-retaining cryopreserved amniotic membrane graft (AMG) (Prokera) can be considered.
- *Stage 2:*
  - *Goal:* To hasten the healing of the persistent epithelial defect and prevent the formation of corneal ulcer
  - PF artificial tears/ointments
  - Therapeutic soft contact lenses
  - Topical autologous serum
  - AMG
  - Tarsorrhaphy or botulinum-induced ptosis (chemical tarsorrhaphy)
  - Topical recombinant human nerve growth factor
  - Topical antimicrobial agents to prevent secondary infection
- *Stage 3:*
  - *Goal:* Healing of corneal ulcer and prevention of perforation
  - In addition to above treatment, N-acetyl cysteine, oral tetracycline and medroxy-progesterone also play a role in treating stromal melt.
  - Vitamin C supplementation helps to prevent collagen degradation.

Surgery

- Placement of AMG over the epithelial defect to hasten the healing process. This can be coupled with chemical tarsorrhaphy.

- Tarsorrhaphy and conjunctival advancement flaps are effective surgical procedures in promoting corneal healing.
- Application of cyanoacrylate glue followed by a soft-bandage contact lens is a good treatment option for small perforations.
- Lamellar or penetrating keratoplasty is reserved for larger corneal defects.
- *Corneal neurotization:* This complex procedure involves the transfer of the supraorbital or supratrochlear nerve either directly or indirectly with a nerve graft to the neurotrophic cornea. The nerve graft often used is the sural nerve. This results in good improvement in corneal sensation along with visual acuity with alleviation of symptoms.

REFERENCE

1. Bonini S, Rama P, Olzi D, Lambiase A. Neurotrophic keratitis. Eye. 2003;17(8):989-95.

1.12 Toxic Keratopathy

MS Sridhar
Krishna Institute of Medical Sciences, Hyderabad
srivision@yahoo.co.in

TOXICITY

Damage to structure of ocular tissues or disturbances of function with or without accompanying inflammatory response.

Damage

Direct result of drug, accompanying preservative, and breakdown product of the drug.

Common Medications Causing Surface Toxicity

- *Antivirals:* Idoxuridine, vidarabine, and trifluorothymidine
- *Glaucoma meds:* Pilocarpine, epinephrine, dipivefrin, timolol, and apraclonidine
- Antibiotics and antifungals
- Anesthetics
- *Preservatives:* Benzalkonium chloride, chlorobutanol, and thiomersal

SPECTRUM OF CLINICAL FEATURES

- Conjunctival hyperemia
- Chemosis
- May spare superior conjunctiva
- Follicles
- Mild punctate keratitis and keratinized epithelium
- Coarse and punctate epithelial erosions
- *Pseudodendritic keratitis:* Opaque-degenerated epithelium in dendritic form
- *Severe ulcerative keratopathy:* Oval epithelial defects, primarily in inferonasal quadrant with coarse surrounding lesions, epithelial defect having rolled margins, not heaped
- Whorl-shaped punctate keratopathy
- *Drug-induced cicatricial pemphigoid:* Chronic conjunctivitis, conjunctival shrinkage symblepharon formation, trichiasis, keratopathy, keratitis sicca, and surface keratinization.

MANAGEMENT

- Recognition of toxicity is the key to management
- Consider toxicity if chronic ocular irritation or inflammation does not improve with seemingly appropriate treatment or whose diagnosis is not apparent

- Cessation of offending agent
- If offending drug is required for treatment, use preservative-free medication or consider oral medications
- Nonpreserved lubricating solution or ointment
- Partial or complete tarsorrhaphy
- *Significant thinning:* Tissue adhesive application and conjunctival flap
- *Perforation:* Penetrating keratoplasty and tectonic keratoplasty
- Nutritional and vitamin support
- Punctum occlusion

DIFFERENTIAL DIAGNOSIS

Allergic disease: Chronicity, itching is predominant symptom, lid and periorbital swelling, mucus and stringy discharge, conjunctival redness and chemosis, diffuse distribution, papillary reaction, punctate staining of cornea, and rarely superior ulcers (shield ulcers).

Dry eye disease.

1.13 Practical Approach in the Management of Bacterial Keratitis

Prashant Garg
LV Prasad Eye Institute, Hyderabad
prashant@lvpei.org

INTRODUCTION

Patients with corneal ulcer present both diagnostic and therapeutic challenge. Early diagnosis and appropriate initiation of treatment with antimicrobial agents play a vital role in the management of corneal ulcer.

Causes: In a report published from LV Prasad Eye Institute, Hyderabad, of the culture positive cases 63.9% were bacterial, 33% were fungal, 2.1% were parasitic, and 6.2% were due to mixed infection.

Common Organisms

Staphylococcus aureus; S. epidermidis; Streptococcus: S. pneumoniae; viridans group

Pseudomonas aeruginosa; Enterobacteriaceae; Proteus; Enterobacter: Serratia; Citrobacter

Uncommon Organisms

Actinomycetales: Actinomyces; Nocardia; atypical *Mycobacterium: M. chelonae; M. fortuitum; M. flavescens; Corynebacterium; Peptococcus; Peptostreptococcus; Moraxella; Azotobacter; Bacteroides.*

Common organisms listed above are responsible for 85% or more of bacterial keratitis among reported series throughout the United States and the world.

RISK FACTORS

Traumatic corneal injury, prolonged epithelial ulceration, contact lens, corneal surgery, and herpes simplex keratitis.

CLINICAL EVALUATION

First to know that the suppurative keratitis is due to microbes or sterile, i.e., immune mediated.

Presumed Microbial
Central lesion; >1 mm size; epithelial defect; severe progressive pain; severe progressive suppuration; uveitis.

Presumed Sterile
Peripheral lesions; <1 mm size; intact epithelium; mild nonprogressive pain; mild nonprogressive; no uveitis.

▮ DIFFERENTIAL DIAGNOSIS OF MICROBIAL KERATITIS
Slowly Progressive Localized Infiltrates
- *Gram-positive:* Staphylococcus epidermidis, α-hemolytic streptococci other than S. pneumoniae, Actinomycetales, *Actinomyces, Nocardia,* and *Mycobacterium*
- *Gram-negative:* (1) *Moraxella,* (2) *Serratia*

Rapidly Progressive Diffuse Suppurative Infiltrate
- *Gram-positive:* (1) *S. aureus,* (2) *S. pneumoniae,* (3) + α-hemolytic streptococci
- *Gram-negative:* (1) *Pseudomonas,* (2) *Enterobacteriaceae*
- Mixed infection
- Drug toxicity

Look for Specific Clinical Signs
Gram-positive Cocci
Localized round or oval ulceration with grayish-white stromal infiltrates. The infiltrates often have distinct borders, minimal surrounding stromal haze with associated mild to moderate anterior chamber reaction.
- *S. epidermidis:* Indolent course.
- *S. aureus:* Marked suppuration, deep stromal abscess, endothelial plaque, and large hypopyon.
- *S. pneumoniae:* Focal suppurative stromal infiltrate, serpiginous leading edge (characteristic sign), deep stromal infiltrate, radiating Descemet folds, and retrocorneal fibrin.
- *Other α-hemolytic:* Indolent localized ulceration.
- *Nocardia:* Indolent ulcer, superficial localized infiltrate, calcareous bodies at the edge, hyphate edges, and often described to have a wreath like pattern.
- *Atypical mycobacteria:* Often have a history of trauma with metallic foreign body or surgery. They typically have a slow progression with a waxing and waning course along with lack of response to conventional antibiotics.

Gram-negative Bacteria
The hallmark characteristics are rapid inflammatory destructive course with dense stromal suppuration, ground glass appearance of surrounding cornea, and severe anterior chamber reaction.
- *Pseudomonas:* Rapidly progressive ulcer, severe conjunctival reaction, dense stromal suppuration, copious mucopurulent exudates in addition to the earlier mentioned features.
- *Moraxella:* Indolent ulcer with a superficial focal infiltrate with mild anterior chamber reaction. It is typically seen in a debilitated patient or compromised cornea.
- *Neisseria gonorrhoeae:* Rapidly paced-keratitis in neonate or sexually-active adult; marked conjunctival hyperemia and chemosis, thick copious purulent discharge, and stromal abscess. Preauricular lymphadenopathy is also seen.

LABORATORY DIAGNOSIS

Corneal scraping and microbiological evaluation is necessary in all cases of ulcerative keratitis.

MANAGEMENT

Medical Management

Initial Therapy

The management of suppurative keratitis under the following three headings depending on the availability of laboratory facilities:
1. No laboratory facilities
2. Microscopy available, but no culture
3. Microscopy, culture and sensitivity available

No laboratory facilities: The ulcer is treated with a standard empiric broad-spectrum regimen of one of commercially available fourth-generation fluproquinolones or a combination of fortified antibiotics such as fortified cefazolin and fortified gentamicin. Once empiric therapy has been initiated the patient must be followed-up closely, i.e., within 48 hours.
- *Referral:* The patients with suspicion of nonbacterial keratitis and all severe ulcers must be immediately referred to a specialist who is prepared to undertake more sophisticated evaluation. In addition, any ulcer that either fails to improve within 72 hours or has a suspicious progression must be referred.

Microscopy available: 10% KOH mount to rule out fungal and parasitic infection can be combined with Gram stain if a clinician wants to know about the type of bacteria. If the KOH is negative and there are no characteristic clinical signs of fungal or *Acanthamoeba* infection, the therapy is started with broad-spectrum antibacterial agents irrespective of the results of Gram stain. The patients are followed up closely.
- *Referral:* If a patient does not respond to initial therapy, such cases must be referred to the specialist ophthalmologist having access to detailed microbiology work-up.

Culture and sensitivity available: All cases of suppurative keratitis must have a detailed laboratory work-up. The initial therapy is started based on results of smear examination and the treatment is modified based on the results of culture and sensitivity.

Design for Drug Administration (Table 1.13.1)
- *Drops:* 30-minute intervals for initial 24–48 hours and then reduced to every 2–3 hourly administration. Do not taper antibiotics.
- *Subconjunctival injections:* Once or twice daily for initial 24–48 hours.
- *Intravenous antibiotics:* Only for corneal perforation or scleral suppuration.

Nontuberculous Mycobacterial Keratitis
- Antibiotic options include amikacin-25 mg/mL; ciprofloxacin-*M. fortuitum* sensitive, *M. chelonae* usually not sensitive; clarithromycin or azithromycin—concentrated within cells with C/E ratio of 7–9.
- Prolonged therapy necessary.
- Multiple drug therapy desirable but little information available regarding drug interactions in the therapy of nontuberculous mycobacteria.
- Frequent failure of medical therapy.

Nocardia Keratitis
- *Antibiotic options:* Trimethoprim-sulfamethoxazole (Bactrim® and Septra®—preferable to generic formulations); amikacin (25 mg/mL).
- Prolonged therapy necessary.

TABLE 1.13.1: Modified antibiotic therapy on preliminary identification of selected organisms.

Organisms	Topical	Subconjunctival
Micrococcus, Staphylococcus (penicillin-resistant)	Cefazolin (50 mg/mL)	Cefazolin (100 mg)
Micrococcus, Staphylococcus (methicillin-resistant)	Vancomycin (50 mg/mL)	Vancomycin (25 mg)
Streptococcus	Cefazolin (50 mg/mL) or penicillin G (100,000 units/mL)	Cefazolin (100 mg); penicillin G (500,000 units)
Enterococcus	Vancomycin (50 mg/mL) and gentamicin (14 mg/mL)	Vancomycin (25 mg) and gentamicin (20 mg)
Anaerobic gram-positive coccus	Cefazolin (50 mg/mL) or penicillin G (100,000 units/mL)	Cefazolin (100 mg); penicillin G (500,000 units)
Corynebacterium species	Penicillin G (100,000 units/mL)	Penicillin G (500,000 units)
Mycobacterium fortuitum-chelonae	Amikacin (40–100 mg/mL)*	Amikacin (20 mg)
Nocardia	Amikacin (40–100 mg/mL) or trimethoprim/sulfamethoxazole†,‡ injectable	Amikacin (20 mg)
Neisseria gonorrhoeae/meningitides	Ceftriaxone (50 mg/mL)§	Ceftriaxone (100 mg)
Pseudomonas species	Ciprofloxacin 0.3%; tobramycin or gentamicin 1.4%; or Ceftazidime‖,¶ (50 mg/mL)	Ceftazidime (100 mg)§
Other aerobic, gram-negative bacillus	Ciprofloxacin 0.3%; tobramycin or gentamicin 1.4%; or Ceftazidime‖,¶ (50 mg/mL)	Ceftazidime (100 mg)§

*Consider adding oral azithromycin and surgical debridement.
†Contains trimethoprim (16 mg/mL), sulfamethoxazole (80 mg/mL); use undiluted Septra® intravenous (IV) infusion.
‡Based on severity; consider use of oral trimethoprim or sulfamethoxazole or IV amikacin for severe keratitis and scleritis cases.
§Requires systemic therapy with ceftriaxone intramuscular (IM) 1 g/day for 3 days and oral doxycycline 100 mg twice a day for 14 days.
‖Consider addition of tobramycin or quinolone antibiotic in severe keratitis cases.
¶Consider in severe keratitis.

Surgical Management

The indications for surgical treatment in suppurative keratitis are following:
- Large ulcer with risk of scleral involvement or perforation
- Extreme thinning or perforation
- Worsening in spite of appropriate antimicrobial therapy
- Uncertain etiology with worsening on medical therapy

The options are:
- Tissue adhesive and bandage contact lens
- Lamellar or full thickness patch graft
- Lamellar or full thickness penetrating keratoplasty
- Conjunctival graft

Recent Advances

Photoactivated chromophore for keratitis-corneal crosslinking (PACK-CXL): It has been tried for bacterial and fungal keratitis with different studies showing varying results.

Rose Bengal Photodynamic therapy (RB-PDAT): This procedure is indicated in non-resolving bacterial and fungal keratitis. RB is a photosensitizer that gets excited by green light (500–550 nm) and undergoes a reaction with ambient oxygen to create singlet oxygen (SO) and reactive oxygen species (ROS). SO is the most efficacious element produced by Rose Bengal while riboflavin only produces ROS. SO and ROS react with intracellular components and produce cell inactivation. RB concentration of 0.2% or 0.15% can be used for the procedure. RB-PDAT gives best results only in patients with infiltrates limited to the anterior 300 µm of cornea. This procedure can be repeated and irradiation energy can be adjusted accordingly.

1.14 | Fungal Keratitis

Venkatesh Prajna
Aravind Eye Care System, Madurai
prajna@aravind.org

■ INTRODUCTION

The incidence of fungal keratitis has shown a dramatic increase in the recent years. Filamentous fungi, which includes *Aspergillus* and *Fusarium,* causes the bulk of the fungal corneal infections following corneal abrasion in an agricultural setting in our country.

■ RELEVANT CLINICAL FEATURES

Unlike bacterial infections, there is less pain, conjunctival congestion, discharge and chemosis early in the course of fungal infection and the symptoms are far less than what is expected of the size of the ulcer. Commonly, the patient presents with a central or a paracentral ulcer with feathery stromal margins. With time, the ulcer starts to become larger and elevated above the level of the corneal surface. The surface looks dirty white and dry and has a rough texture. In rare instances, the lesion may be entirely in the posterior aspect of the stroma without an accompanying epithelial defect. In these cases, the posterior stromal lesions also have a feathery-edge like paint sprayed over a wall.

Foci of infiltration can be seen several millimeters away from the main area of involvement. These are called satellite lesions and they may remain isolated from the main lesion or may be connected with the main ulcer by a thin line of stromal infiltration. An endothelial plaque can be an accompanying factor. Like in many other keratitis, a ring infiltrate may surround the primary lesion, most likely representing an antibody response to fungal antigen. Hypopyon is convex and can be present in varying proportions and the amount is not directly proportional to the size of the ulcer.

■ DIFFERENTIAL DIAGNOSIS

Bacterial Keratitis

In the earliest stage and in the very advanced stages, cases of fungal keratitis cannot be clinically distinguished from a bacterial keratitis without the help of microbiological investigations.

Viral Keratitis

In the early forms of fungal keratitis, the feathery margins can be mistaken as dendritic keratitis caused by herpes simplex infections. Fungal pseudodendritic lesions are shorter, stockier, and are associated with surrounding stromal infiltration.

Uveal Prolapse
Ulcers caused by pigmented fungi can mimic a uveal prolapse.

TREATMENT
The initiation of treatment can be performed as soon as the results of the KOH mount and the Gram stain are obtained. If the smears and the culture results are negative, but the clinical features are strongly in favor of fungal keratitis, initiation of topical antifungal therapy is recommended, especially in countries where there is a high prevalence.

Medical Treatment
Natamycin 5% suspension is the gold standard of treatment of filamentous fungal keratitis and should be administered hourly for the initial 24–48 hours and at 2-hour intervals, thereafter. The dosage can then be gradually reduced depending upon the response.

Topical amphotericin B (0.1–0.25%) is found to be efficacious against *Aspergillus* species. Other antifungals include econazole, fluconazole, and 1% voriconazole. The Mycotic Ulcer Treatment Trial 1 (MUTT 1) concluded natamycin to be more efficacious than voriconazole against filamentous fungi. Echinocandins such as caspofungin and anidulafungin are new drugs now available for treatment of nonresolving fungal keratitis.

Lack of progression of the stromal infiltrate is the first sign that the antifungal is effective. This is followed by a rounding of the feathery margins, blunting of the perimeters, and reduction in cellular infiltrate and edema in surrounding stroma. Prolonged conjunctival injection, protracted epithelial ulceration, punctate corneal epithelial erosion, and diffuse stromal haze imply drug toxicity.

While, the appearance of a transient hypopyon in the face of an improving corneal picture has been attributed to hypersensitivity or a toxic reaction, a coexistent bacterial contamination of the antifungal drugs should be considered when a healing ulcer suddenly starts to worsen clinically.

Supplementary therapy includes a cycloplegic-mydriatic agent, such as atropine 1% twice a day. A topical beta-blocker or oral carbonic anhydrase inhibitor should be used to control secondary glaucoma.

For deep stromal keratitis and endothelial plaques, intrastromal injection and intracameral injection of 1% voriconazole and amphotericin B (10 µg) have been tried. Systemic antifungals such as oral ketoconazole (200–600 mg) can be supplemented with topical natamycin, after performing baseline liver function tests in cases with deep stromal keratitis or lesions extending to the limbus and sclera. Prolonged treatments with systemic antifungals are reserved for deep keratitis associated with scleritis and endophthalmitis. Corticosteroids do not have any role in the treatment regimen of fungal keratitis and is not recommended in any stage of the disease.

Surgical Treatment
Regular debridement of the ulcer using a scalpel or a Kimura spatula is an extremely invaluable step to ensure adequate therapeutic levels of the antifungals into the deeper stromal layers. Therapeutic keratoplasty has to be contemplated when the ulcer progresses despite specific antifungal therapy. Indeed, in our experience at least 35% of the patients presenting with a deeper stromal fungal keratitis perforate and require therapeutic keratoplasty to save the globe.

The goals of the therapeutic keratoplasty are to primarily eliminate the infection and restore the integrity of the globe. A recurrence of infection in a graft is more difficult to treat than a rejection. Hence, a large-sized graft, encompassing the infected tissue, should be used without regard for the fear of rejection. Even if one of these transplants is rejected, a second keratoplasty for optical rehabilitation can be performed at a later date. A peripheral iridectomy should be performed in all cases to prevent glaucoma.

FOLLOW-UP

Postoperatively, topical natamycin 5% is continued for a period of 1–2 months. During this time, the usage of topical steroids is not recommended and supplementary topical nonsteroidal anti-inflammatory drugs may be used. Steroids can be used cautiously after the first postoperative month follow-up.

SPECIAL NOTES

Fungal keratitis is fast becoming a silent epidemic, especially in developing countries. The diagnosis should be confirmed with microbiological tests like smears and/or cultures, since it may be difficult to distinguish it from other causes of infectious keratitis in clinical settings, except in the early forms of the disease.

The pharmacological advancements in the field of antifungal therapy have not kept pace with that of newer antibiotics in ophthalmology. In cases, where the disease appears to progress, in spite of adequate and appropriate antifungal therapy, early surgical intervention may be the preferred mode to eliminate the infection.

1.15 Acanthamoeba Keratitis

Ajay Dave
Dave Eye Centre, New Delhi
ajaysdave@gmail.com

R Revathi
Aravind Eye Care System, Coimbatore
revathi@aravind.org

INTRODUCTION

Acanthamoeba keratitis is a rare but potentially devastating infection, accounts for 1% of infectious keratitis. *Acanthamoeba* is a genus of free-living protozoa of the subphyla Sarcodina. They are unicellular and can exist in two forms, (1) active trophozoites and (2) dormant cyst. The cyst form is more resistant to extreme environment, as well as to chlorine and other microbial agents.

Acanthamoeba is ubiquitous, has been found in tap water, bottled water, swimming pool, hot tubs, contact lens solutions as well as soil and air. Though in literature 70–85% of the infections are reported to be associated with contact lens wear, in our country contamination of corneal abrasions by wet soil or water is the common risk factor.

CLINICAL FEATURES

- Young healthy individuals; insidious in onset; often waxing and waning.
- Pain is often severe and out of proportion to the signs of inflammation.
- *Initial epithelial stage:* The superficial infection presents as roughened, irregular epithelium; pseudodendrite, epithelial ridges—raised epithelial lines.
- *Stromal invasion stage:* Linear perineural infiltrates; gray-white infiltrate forming a superficial ring with stromal edema, keratic precipitates, and hypopyon in the later stages. Stromal necrosis occurs in the late stages.
- Radial keratoneuritis occurs in a minority of cases, but seems to be pathognomonic.
- Nodular or diffuse scleritis can be associated with keratitis.

DIFFERENTIAL DIAGNOSIS

- *Viral keratitis:* Both epithelial lesions and perineuritis can mimic viral dendrites. The ring infiltrate is often mistaken for viral stromal keratitis.
- *Fungal keratitis:* Stromal lesions such as perineural infiltrates and ring infiltration with hypopyon can mimic fungal keratitis.

- *In the late-necrotic stage:* This infection cannot be differentiated from any other suppurative keratitis.
- Infection by *microsporidia* may give similar presentation.

DIAGNOSIS

- In the early epithelial stage, the organism can be isolated from vigorous scraping of the epithelial ridges. The hexagonal, double-walled cysts can be seen in 10% KOH wet mount, Gram stain, and Giemsa stain.
- Calcofluor white can facilitate detection in 70% cases. For culture smear specimen should be inoculated on to non-nutrient agar, overlaid with *Escherichia coli*.
- Confocal microscopy gives a presumptive diagnosis. It needs trained mind to discern double-walled structures and round bodies from keratocytes and inflammatory cells.
- A positive corneal biopsy for microscopy and polymerase chain reaction (PCR) for amebic deoxyribonucleic acid (DNA) is diagnostic.

TREATMENT

A prolonged course of antiamebic agents is needed invariably. The early epithelial stage needs a relatively short duration of treatment for 3–4 months, whereas the stromal stage has to be treated for 6–12 months.

Common *antiamebic* agents are *diamidine*—propamidine; *biguanides*—polyhexamethylene biguanide (PHMB) and chlorhexidine; *aminoglycosides*—neomycin; and *imidazole*—itraconazole, ketoconazole, and clotrimazole.

Multiple drug therapy is generally accepted. A combination of 0.02% PHMB or 0.02% chlorhexidine combined with neomycin or 0.1% propamidine is recommended for topical therapy. The drugs should be applied *every hour initially*.

This can be supplemented with oral ketoconazole 200 mg two times or itraconazole 100 mg once a day. Frequency of these medications is tapered over several weeks to months depending on the response.

Long-term prophylactic therapy with PHMB twice a day for a year is recommended. Use of corticosteroids is not recommended generally.

FOLLOW-UP

- Prolonged medical therapy may attain resolution in some cases.
- Cases with no improvement and showing progression with stromal melt would warrant penetrating keratoplasty. The risk of recurrence would be very high.
- It is suggested that the surgical options should be exercised after a full course of maximal medical therapy and a quiescent phase of at least 6 months.

SPECIAL NOTES

- Early diagnosis is very important for the successful management of *Acanthamoeba* keratitis. A delayed diagnosis as well as use of corticosteroids is correlated with poor outcome.
- Disproportionately severe pain due to perineuritis in contrast to hypoesthesia in herpetic keratitis, exposure to contaminated water, soil, or contact lens wear, and failure to respond to earlier antiviral therapy should arouse suspicion about this etiology.
- Practitioners of contact lenses should ensure that the patients do not use nonsterile fluids to rinse, store, or disinfect their lenses. Patients should not swim with their contact lenses.
- Identifying nonresponding cases and performing deep anterior lamellar keratoplasty (DALK) is showing satisfactory results.

1.16 Herpes Simplex Virus Keratopathy

Gobinda Mukherjee
Mukherjee Eye Klinik, New Delhi
mukherjee@eyedoctors.in

■ INTRODUCTION
There are two types of herpes simplex virus (HSV), HSV-1, and HSV-2. In general type 1 causes infections above and type 2 below the waist. HSV-1 is predominantly responsible for ocular HSV disease.

■ SOURCES OF INFECTION
Children with primary disease, adults with recurrent disease, and healthy asymptomatic carriers. Transmission of infection is usually by direct contact, salivary droplets, or direct oral contact.

■ CLINICAL TYPES AND PRESENTATION

Congenital and Neonatal Ocular Herpes Simplex
This is caused by HSV-2 in 80% of cases, due to direct transmission via infected birth canal. Clinical presentation includes conjunctivitis, epithelial keratitis, stromal immune reaction, cataract, necrotizing chorioretinitis, and vesicular skin eruptions.

Primary Herpes Simplex Virus Infection
Presentation: Acute follicular conjunctivitis, keratoconjunctivitis, nonsuppurative preauricular lymphadenopathy, and vesicular periocular skin eruptions.

Primary HSV keratitis, as a rule, has a pure epithelial involvement, with nonspecific diffuse punctate keratitis and multiple scattered microdendrites. Keratitis is seen in 30–50% cases after a few days of follicular conjunctivitis.

Recurrent Herpes Simplex Virus Keratopathy
This is typically a unilateral disease, with bilateral cases forming only 3% of this group. Superficial corneal lesions are associated with presence of live replicating virus, while the deeper lesions appear to be predominantly due to immune response of the host.

Epithelial Keratopathy

Infectious Herpes Simplex Virus Epithelial Keratitis
The earliest epithelial lesions are small "vesicles within epithelium (old name: punctate epithelial keratopathy)". These look like minute-raised clear vesicles, usually found before the patient has recognized his symptoms.

These small vesicles coalesce to form the thin, branching classical *dendritic ulcer,* or the wider branching *dendrogeographic ulcer,* with swollen epithelial borders containing live virus. The linear branches classically end in expansions known as terminal end-bulbs. The presentation may also be a map-shaped epithelial ulceration known as *geographical ulcer* (**Fig. 1.16.1**).

The pathogenesis of this branching dendritic ulcer morphology is believed to be related to the neuronal distribution and lineal viral spread by contiguous cell-to-cell movement.

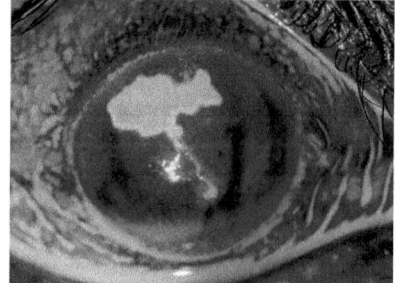

Fig. 1.16.1: Herpes simplex virus (HSV) geographical keratitis.

Differential Diagnosis

The scalloped or geographical borders of HSV geographical ulcer, laden with live virus, are important to recognize and differentiate it from healing *epithelial abrasion* and *neurotrophic keratopathy*, which have smooth borders.

The presenting symptoms include irritation, pain, watering, photophobia and occasional blurring of vision, and thin watery discharge. Corneal sensations are usually temporarily reduced or absent, in the area around the lesion. The raised epithelial borders of the ulcer are not stained by fluorescein, but are well-stained with rose Bengal stain.

One of the most symptomatic, resistant to treatment lesions in the spectrum of HSV epithelial keratitis is the *marginal ulcer* caused due to active viral disease. This lesion is near the limbus with an accompanying blood vessel with significant anterior stromal infiltrates.

Neurotrophic Keratopathy (Metaherpetic Ulcer) (Fig. 1.16.2)

Neurotrophic keratopathy is a serious globe-threatening sequel of recurrent HSV keratitis. It is a chronic, sterile, nonhealing ulcer due to recurrent epithelial breakdown. It is caused by interacting adverse healing factors, such as impaired corneal innervation; abnormal tear film stability; damaged epithelial basement membrane; and chronic insult of topical medications (mostly antivirals).

Stromal ulceration is noticed with gray-white bed and thickened gray heaped-up epithelium at the borders, which is the classical description of neurotrophic keratopathy.

The usual complications of neurotrophic keratopathy are stromal scarring, corneal neovascularization, stromal necrosis, corneal perforation, and secondary bacterial or fungal infection.

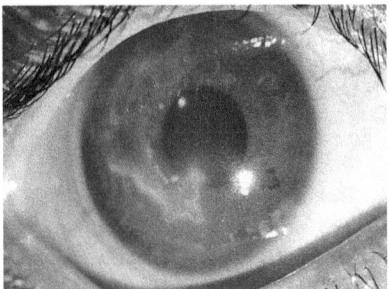

Fig. 1.16.2: Herpes simplex virus (HSV) metaherpetic (neurotrophic) keratitis.

Stromal Keratopathy

It is predominantly immune-mediated. Secondary stromal inflammation can follow epithelial or endothelium involvement.

Viral Necrotizing Keratitis

Generalized or localized ulcerated epithelial defect with necrosis and dense stromal infiltrates in the ulcer bed. It may result in corneal thinning and perforation in a very short period of time.

Stromal Interstitial Keratitis

It accounts for about 20% of all cases of HSV keratitis. It may be focal, multifocal, or diffuse. It may result in anterior chamber inflammation with congestion and the patient often complains of pain. Leashes of blood vessels often move into the cornea in pursuit of these infiltrates.

Immune ring formation in HSV keratitis is a specific immune reaction.

Constant low-grade inflammation with mild fluctuations in severity is the hallmark of this form of HSV keratitis.

Limbal vasculitis presents as a focal limbal edema with hyperemia, without any vascular invasion into the cornea.

Herpes Simplex Virus Endotheliitis

It is an immune-mediated presentation of HSV keratitis, resulting in severe corneal stromal and epithelial edema, caused by local endothelial inflammatory decompensation.

Keratic precipitates (KP) with iritis is always associated with this entity. Three different types are (1) disciform, (2) diffuse, and (3) linear.
1. *Disciform endotheliitis:* The most common type of endotheliitis. The presentation is a round area of stromal edema overlying KPs on the endothelium. The patient experiences photophobia with mild-to-moderate ocular discomfort, and a reduction in visual acuity.
2. *Diffuse endotheliitis:* Diffuse corneal edema with KPs scattered all over the posterior cornea is the feature of diffuse endotheliitis. Mild-to-moderate iritis with dense retrocorneal plaque of inflammatory cells and hypopyon may be seen in severe cases. Patient presents with pain, photophobia, congestion, and decreased visual acuity.
3. *Linear endotheliitis:* Linear endotheliitis presents with a line of KPs which progress centrally from the limbus. There is a sharply demarcated peripheral corneal edema between the line of KPs and the limbus.

Herpes Simplex Virus Trabeculitis
This causes acute, severe rise in intraocular pressure. Iritis is often found in association with trabeculitis.

Herpes Simplex Virus Iridocyclitis
All deeper forms of HSV keratitis can be associated with uveitis. Recurrent nongranulomatous anterior uveitis may be an isolated manifestation of HSV ocular involvement. Clinically, the severity can be varied from mild to severe inflammation, which may result in fibrin formation, hypopyon, hyphema, posterior synechiae, segmental iris necrosis, and inflammatory membrane formation.

■ MANAGEMENT
Antiviral Agents
The topical antiviral agents effective against HSV available are ganciclovir and acyclovir.
Acyclovir is specific to virus-infected cell, with a very low-collateral toxicity. It is a purine analog, is specifically activated by virus-induced thymidine kinase, and initiates phosphorylation.

Indications of Oral Acyclovir
- *Active viral disease (400 mg—5 times a day for 7–10 days):* Primary herpes stromal keratitis (HSK); recurrent epithelial keratitis with atopic disease (eczema); immunocompromised patients; and unable to instill topical antivirals **(Table 1.16.1)**.
- *HSV infection prophylaxis (400 mg—twice a day):* Recurrent infectious disease—twice or more a year; keratoplasty in HSK etiology.

Corticosteroids
Judicious use of steroids is recommended in certain types of HSV corneal manifestations. Oral steroid therapy may be required to control certain severe forms of inflammation. The cases with severe immune-stromal keratitis, linear endotheliitis (all cases), severe disciform, and diffuse endotheliitis do need oral steroids, along with topical steroids, to control the inflammation.

TABLE 1.16.1: Topical antiviral agents.

Drug	Concentration	Dose	Duration
Acyclovir	3% ointment	Five times a day	14–21 days
Ganciclovir	0.15% gel	Four times a day	14–21 days

Specific Treatment

Primary Infection
Acyclovir 3% eye ointment/ganciclovir 0.15% gel must be used four to five times a day for 2–3 weeks.

Recurrent Infectious Epithelial Keratitis
Topical acyclovir 3% eye ointment must be used thereafter, five times in a day, for 14–21 days. Cycloplegics must be used in eyes with photophobia and ciliary spasm. Prophylaxis against secondary infection with a broad-spectrum antibiotic like topical tobramycin eye drops, thrice a day is very important.

Neurotrophic Keratopathy
Discontinuation of all unnecessary topical medication (especially antivirals) should be done immediately. Frequent use of preservative-free artificial-tear substitute drops; gentle debridement of the boggy epithelium; and oral doxycycline (100 mg once a day) may be given to reduce the collagenolytic activity.

Soft-therapeutic bandage contact lens (BCL) is one of the treatment options. Tarsorrhaphy is a very effective option for the treatment of neurotrophic keratopathy. Amniotic membrane grafting may be an option.

Immunologically-mediated Herpes Simplex Virus Manifestations
A topical antiviral, preferably, must be added as a prophylactic measure along with the topical steroid therapy.

Steroids to be used must be of adequate strength (1% prednisolone acetate), and frequency to suppress the stromal inflammation. Oral steroids might be needed in severe stromal reaction.

Iridocyclitis and Trabeculitis
Topical steroids and cycloplegics are indicated. It is advisable to add topical acyclovir. The patients who do not respond to large doses of topical steroids may show resolution with oral acyclovir, 200 mg—five times a day, with topical steroids and cycloplegics. When there is acute severe rise in intraocular pressure, in cases of HSV trabeculitis, topical and systemic antiglaucoma agents must be added to topical steroids.

1.17 Herpes Zoster Virus Keratitis

Ashish Nagpal
Retina Foundation and Eye Research Centre, Ahmedabad
ashish@drnagpal.com

■ RELEVANT CLINICAL FEATURES

Almost a sizable two-thirds of patients with herpes zoster ophthalmicus (HZO) have some corneal involvement **(Fig. 1.17.1)**. Corneal disease may precede, accompany, or follow the acute disease by months to years and may recur in any of its many forms.

The cornea has multiple manifestations of herpes zoster (HZ) keratitis which is probably related to different mechanisms of disease and closely mimics any manifestation of a herpes

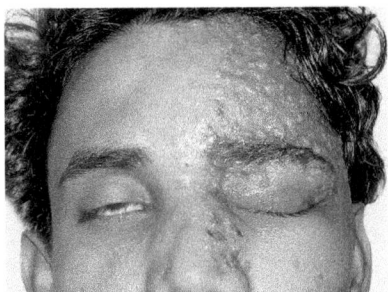

Fig. 1.17.1: Herpes zoster ophthalmicus.

simplex keratitis complex. **Table 1.17.1** lists and describes various clinical manifestations of HZ keratitis.

■ DIFFERENTIAL DIAGNOSIS

It is important to rule out other causes which have similar clinical manifestations; although a past history suggestive of HZO should definitely point us toward it.
- Herpes simplex keratitis
- Interstitial keratitis
- Sclerokeratitis
- Microbial keratitis

TABLE 1.17.1: Spectrum of corneal changes in herpes zoster.

Morphology	Frequency%	Usual onset	Clinical specifications
Punctate keratitis	50	2 days	Coarse punctate epithelial keratitis; usually peripheral, often associated with conjunctivitis
Pseudodendrites	50	4–6 days	Typically in peripheral cornea; multiple dendritic lesions and differ from herpes simplex virus (HSV) that they lack central ulceration and have blunt ends
Anterior stromal infiltrates	40	10 days	Hazy, granular dry infiltrate below Bowman's membrane and leave residual "nummular scars", which are a strong clinical marker of previous herpes zoster (HZ) corneal inflammation
Keratouveitis/ endotheliitis	34	7 days	Sudden-onset Descemet's folds with subsequent stromal edema, and also can have underlying keratic precipitates (KPs). Secondary glaucoma is common association and so is hypopyon or hyphema, if inflammation is very severe
Serpiginous ulceration	7	1 month	Peripheral crescentic corneal thinning with a gray white base may occur and can perforate also
Sclerokeratitis	1	1 month	An extension of keratitis into cornea creates limbal vascular keratitis and eventually may manifest with scleralization, vascularization, and stromal thinning
Corneal mucus plaques	13	2–3 months	• Usually occurs later in a quiet eye with a minimal smoldering keratitis • Elevated, coarse branching lesions which lack terminal branches and stain with rose Bengal but not fluorescein
Disciform keratitis	10	3–4 months	Deep central or peripheral disk-shaped stromal edema may develop with minimal infiltrate and intact epithelium. Immune rings around this edema can be associated finding

Contd...

Contd...

Morphology	Frequency%	Usual onset	Clinical specifications
Neurotrophic keratopathy	25	2 months	Lack of corneal luster, irregular corneal surface, or mild coarse punctuate erosions are indicators of neuropathy. With time if untreated a gray haze develops and horizontal, oval epithelial defects develop in lower aspect of cornea
Exposure keratopathy	11	2–3 months	Cicatricial eyelid changes secondary to herpes zoster ophthalmicus (HZO) causes exposure keratopathy
Interstitial keratitis/lipid keratopathy	15	1–2 years	This occurs secondary to extensive corneal inflammation and is paracentral or peripheral with a vascular leash and lipid deposits
Corneal edema (irreversible)	5	1–2 years	Permanent endothelial decompensation can occur even without scarring and vascularization due to endothelial destruction by varicella virus

■ TREATMENT

Apart from the treatment described for HZO the treatment in HZ keratitis is supportive and requires individual consideration.

Medical
- Topical acyclovir (3%) eye ointment—five times a day for 3–4 weeks—for early punctate epithelial keratitis lesions; for topical antiviral cover when using topical steroids for keratouveitis, endotheliitis, and interstitial keratitis.
- High-dose oral acyclovir 800 mg five times a day for 7 days as early as possible.
- *Topical corticosteroids:* To decrease vasculitis, keratouveitis, endotheliitis, and disciform keratitis.
- *Topical antiglaucoma medications:* To control *intraocular pressure (IOP)* during keratouveitis stage till the trabeculitis is controlled by topical steroids.
- Cycloplegics and preservative-free tear substitute.

Surgical
- *Sometimes needs tissue adhesive with bandage contact lens (BCL):* In case of a corneal perforation.
- *Tarsorrhaphy:* To prevent complications in case of a severe neurotrophic keratopathy or exposure keratitis.
- *Keratoplasty:* Tectonic keratoplasty may be required in large corneal perforations.
- *Penetrating keratoplasty:* For visual rehabilitation necessary to prevent corneal complications.

■ FOLLOW-UP

The patient should be made aware that any redness, pain, and decrease vision in the future he should report to the ophthalmologist immediately.

■ SPECIAL NOTES

The disease morphology might be more severe in immunocompromised individuals and so would be the duration of resolution and in some cases would require a coordinated management with the physician or internist.

1.18 | Microsporidial Keratitis

Manoranjan Das, Naveen Radhakrishnan, Dhanya Kuppuraj

Aravind Eye Hospital, Madurai
mrdas@aravind.org

■ INTRODUCTION

Microsporidia are a diverse group of obligate spore forming intracellular eukaryotes that are closely related to fungi, causing keratoconjunctivitis and stromal keratitis. They are normal flora in the intestine of immunocompetent individuals. Earlier reports documented the occurrence of infections such as gastrointestinal, renal, pulmonary, and ocular infections in immunocompromised individuals, especially human immunodeficiency virus (HIV) infected patients. Increase in the awareness of the disease has led to increased reporting of microsporidial ocular infections in immunocompetent individuals in the last two decades.[1]

Microsporidia belongs to the kingdom—Archezoa/fungi, phylum—*Microspora*, Class—Microsporidiae. Six genera, namely *Enterocytozoon, Encephalitozoon, Pleistophora, Trachipleistophora, Vittaforma,* and *Nosema* have been reported to infect humans. The genus *Encephalitozoon* is usually associated with keratoconjunctivitis and the genera *Nosema* and *Microsporidium* are associated with stromal keratitis. Microsporidia exists as a single, cell spore of size of 1–40 microns. They are transmitted through contaminated water, soil, vegetables, and by zoonotic transmission.

■ MICROSPORIDIAL KERATOCONJUNCTIVITIS

The prevalence of microsporidial keratoconjunctivitis is on the rise worldwide due to the recent increase in the awareness of the disease. Still a majority of the disease goes under diagnosed or misdiagnosed as atypical adenoviral keratoconjunctivitis. Exposure to contaminated water, soil, trauma, swimming in fresh waters, contact lens use, contact sports, etc., are some of the risk factors identified for keratoconjunctivitis. Studies have shown a perennial prevalence with an increase in the incidence during rainy seasons. Patients usually present with a unilateral acute conjunctivitis with symptoms of redness, pain, irritation, discharge, and watering along with a characteristic keratitis with associated defective vision. The corneal lesions present as greyish white coarse, powdery, multifocal, and raised superficial punctate epithelial keratitis, which are larger than the punctate keratitis of viral keratoconjunctivitis **(Fig. 1.18.1)**. They have a characteristic "stuck on" appearance. Unlike the punctate keratitis lesions in adenoviral keratoconjunctivitis, the corneal lesion in microsporidial keratitis can be removed by debridement with a sterile cotton tipped sponge, leaving behind pits in the epithelium. A small subset of patients can also have pearly white and nongranulomatous keratic precipitates on the endothelium. A majority of the cases resolve without scarring and 10–15% of patients may evolve into nummular keratitis with scarring. Limbitis and corneal endotheliitis with diffuse corneal edema have also been reported.

Diagnosis is by smear examination of the corneal scrapings taken with a cotton tipped sponge or Kimura's spatula. Gram stain, Giemsa stain, 1% acid fast (Ziehl-Neelsen stain) and potassium hydroxide with Calcofluor white stain have been used to diagnose microsporidiosis. In Gram stain, they appear as Gram-positive intracellular and extracellular ovoid bodies of 2–3 micron in size with a diagonal or equatorial

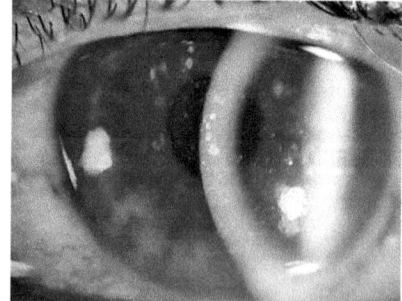

Fig. 1.18.1: Microsporidial keratoconjunctivitis.

band girding the spore. They fluoresce in Calcofluor white stain (**Fig. 1.18.2**). In 1% acid-fast stain, the spores appear as bright red with the characteristic band, against a blue background. In vivo confocal microscopy of microsporidial keratoconjunctivitis shows multiple rosette-like clusters of epithelial cells with spores appearing as hyper-reflective, pinpoint oval intracellular bodies. Polymerase chain reaction (PCR)-based assays are used to detect small-subunit ribosomal ribonucleic acid (rRNA) sequences of microsporidia and have low sensitivity.

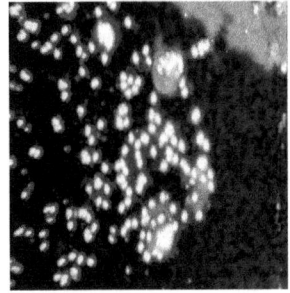

Fig. 1.18.2: Calcofluor white stain.

There is no specific treatment for microsporidial keratoconjunctivitis. Several observational case reports have studied the effects of drugs such as topical voriconazole, itraconazole, polyhexamethylene biguanide (PHMB), fumagillin, moxifloxacin, chloramphenicol, oral albendazole, and procedures like repeated corneal swabbing for the treatment of microsporidial keratoconjunctivitis. Large volume case series have used 0.3% fluconazole eye drops four to six times a day for 1-2 weeks till resolution for smear proven microsporidial keratoconjunctivitis with good clinical outcomes. Low-dose topical steroids might reduce scarring in those cases where the corneal lesions heal with scarring. Randomized control trials have shown that PHMB or corneal debridement did not have any additional benefit over placebo (lubricants) in terms of resolution of the corneal lesions and final visual outcome in clinically diagnosed microsporidial keratoconjunctivitis.[2]

■ MICROSPORIDIAL STROMAL KERATITIS

Stromal keratitis by microsporidiosis follows a long indolent course with recurrences. When compared to keratoconjunctivitis, microsporidial stromal keratitis is relatively uncommon. They usually present with unilateral pain, redness, watering, and defective vision with diffuse multifocal midstromal to deep stromal infiltrates (**Fig. 1.18.3**). They closely resemble viral stromal keratitis, *Acanthamoeba* keratitis, and fungal keratitis. Case reports have documented microsporidial stromal keratitis mimicking acute graft rejection of grafts of penetrating keratoplasty and Descemet's stripping endothelial keratoplasty. The diagnosis of microsporidial stromal keratitis can be challenging due to the midstromal location of the lesion and a high degree of clinical suspicion in nonhealing keratitis is needed. Multiple corneal scrapings may be needed to prove microsporidiosis and in many instances they are diagnosed retrospectively in the histopathology sections of cornea excised during therapeutic keratoplasty. Medical therapy with PHMB, chlorhexidine, fumagillin, fluconazole, voriconazole, oral albendazole, and oral itraconazole has been tried with varying results. They are usually resistant to medical therapy requiring surgical intervention. Recurrence of microsporidial keratitis in the host bed have been reported following deep anterior lamellar keratoplasty and penetrating keratoplasty has been considered as gold standard treatment of microsporidial stromal keratitis.[3]

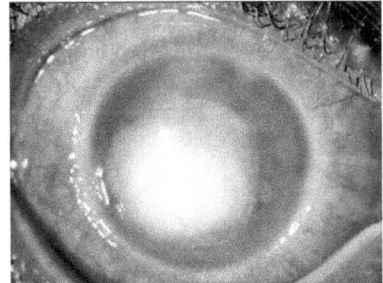

Fig. 1.18.3: Microsporidial stromal keratitis.

■ REFERENCES

1. Agashe R, Radhakrishnan N, Pradhan S, Srinivasan M, Prajna VN, Lalitha P. Clinical and demographic study of microsporidial keratoconjunctivitis in South India: a 3-year study (2013-2015). Br J Ophthalmol. 2017;101(10):1436-9.

2. Sharma S, Das S, Joseph J, Vemuganti GK, Murthy S. Microsporidial keratitis: need for increased awareness. Surv Ophthalmol. 2011;56(1):1-22.
3. Moshirfar M, Somani SN, Shmunes KM, Espandar L, Gokhale NS, Ronquillo YC, et al. A Narrative Review of Microsporidial Infections of the Cornea. Ophthalmol Ther. 2020;9(2):265-78.

1.19 | Pythium Keratitis

Vandhana Sundaram
Sankara Eye Hospital, Coimbatore
Vandhana2011@gmail.com

■ INTRODUCTION

Pythium keratitis caused by fungus-like aquatic oomycete *Pythium insidiosum*. *Pythium* keratitis is a rare form of keratitis and is most frequently misdiagnosed as fungal keratitis. It belongs to the *Phylum* Straminipila, class oomycetes, order Pythiales, and family Pythiaceae. *Pythium* insidiosum is an oomycete commonly seen in the tropical and subtropical regions. It has zygomycetous branching features but unlike fungus its cell wall contains cellulose, β-glucans, and lacks chitin. Absence of ergosterol in the cytoplasmic membrane is also a unique feature which renders most of the antifungal medications ineffective. *Pythium* exists in two forms, such as mycelium and zoospore in freshwater and infection is acquired through motile zoospores pathogenic to humans, horses, and dogs. It can manifest as cutaneous, subcutaneous, ocular, vascular or as disseminated forms of infection.

Importance of *Pythium*:
- Highly virulent
- Late diagnosis due to clinical and diagnostic resemblance with fungal keratitis
- Poor visual prognosis
- Lack of standard treatment
- High recurrence rate
- Severe ocular morbidity

The clinical features consist of stromal infiltrate with feathery margins, subepithelial reticular dot infiltrates, tentacular projections, and peripheral furrowing. Hypopyon with anterior chamber exudates and endothelial plaque are also seen. Though the mentioned features are not seen in all cases their presence helps in early diagnosis **(Figs. 1.19.1 and 1.19.2)**.

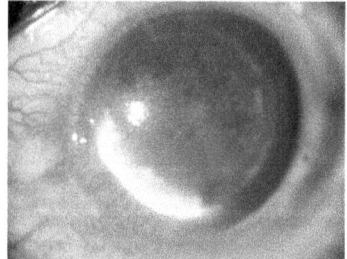

Fig. 1.19.1: Stromal infiltrate with feathery margins and peripheral furrowing.
Courtesy: Dr R Revathy, Aravind Eye Hospital, Coimbatore.

■ LABORATORY DIAGNOSIS

Corneal scraping is done under topical anesthesia with a help of No. 15 blade. The specimen is given for Gram stain, 10% KOH mount, and plated on blood agar, potato dextrose agar, or Sabouraud dextrose agar. Smear examination reveals the presence of long and sparsely septate hyaline hyphae with vesicles and ribbon-like folding pattern of fungal hyphae. Culture plates show growth

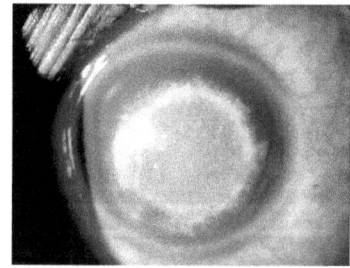

Fig. 1.19.2: Stromal infiltrate with feathery margins, subepithelial reticular dot infiltrates, tentacular projections, and peripheral furrowing.
Courtesy: Dr R Revathy, Aravind Eye Hospital, Coimbatore.

of flat, feathery-edged, partially submerged, colorless, or light-brown small hair-like projections. Confocal microscopy demonstrates the presence of thin and hyper-reflective branching structures with varying angles and plays an important role in early diagnosis in case of recurrence. The potassium iodide-sulfuric acid (IKI-H_2SO_4) stain is another cost-effective and simple test in diagnosing the oomycete of *Pythium* with both good sensitivity and specificity. The *Pythium* hyphae are seen as bluish-black and labeled as positive, and yellow/yellowish brown is considered negative staining. Newer techniques such as deoxyribonucleic acid (DNA) sequencing have also been tried along with polymerase chain reaction (PCR).[1]

■ MEDICAL MANAGEMENT

Owing to close clinical and microbiological resemblance with fungi many patients are usually started on antifungal drugs agents such as natamycin and voriconazole; however, there is poor response due to lack of ergosterol in the *Pythium* cell wall. Once the culture shows evidence of *Pythium* growth or if there is a strong clinical suspicion of *Pythium* then topical and systemic antibacterial must be started. Topical linezolid 0.2% 1 hourly, azithromycin 1% eye drops hourly with oral azithromycin 500 mg BD for 2 weeks is the recommended regimen. A few case reports have also shown good response with topical minocycline along with the mentioned topical agents. A lesser rate of therapeutic penetrating keratoplasty (TPK) was noted in patients taking the mentioned antibacterial agents when compared to antifungal regimen. Patients are reassessed frequently and if favorable response is noted then treatment is continued for a period of at least three months.

■ SURGICAL MANAGEMENT

Patients with early stromal melt, persisting endoexudates, and scleral extension are advocated for early TPK. Other indications include nonresponsive cases, corneal perforation, and limbal extension. Multiple cases of recurrence postkeratoplasty have also been reported hence it is imperative to take at least a 1.5 mm larger size of trephination than the size of the corneal infiltrate. Post TPK the antibacterial regimen is continued at least for a period of 1–2 months. Evisceration and enucleation is advised in advancing keratitis, post multiple recurrences in TPK graft, endophthalmitis, and panophthalmitis. *Pythium* keratitis carries poor prognosis for vision and resolution.[2]

■ REFERENCES

1. Hasika R, Lalitha P, Radhakrishnan N, Rameshkumar G, Prajna NV, Srinivasan M. Pythium keratitis in South India: Incidence, clinical profile, management, and treatment recommendation. Indian J Ophthalmol. 2019;67(1):42-7.
2. Raju RS, Raju CG. A review of the management of Pythium keratitis. J Ophthalmol Clin Res. 2022;2(1):11-7.

1.20 | Marginal Keratitis

Ashok Sharma
Cornea Centre, Chandigarh
asharmapgius@yahoo.com

■ INTRODUCTION

The term marginal keratitis is used to describe noninfectious inflammation of the peripheral cornea and the limbus. The condition occurs as a result of a hypersensitivity reaction to bacterial antigen, especially *Staphylococcus aureus*.

The condition mostly occurs in middle-aged adults but can occur at any age including children. Patients suffering from meibomitis, recurrent chalazia, styes, and rosacea are more prone to development of marginal keratitis. Marginal keratitis has been reported in Behçet's disease.[1]

In a recent report, marginal keratitis has been described as a hypersensitivity reaction to topical dorzolamide. The use of topical pilocarpine has been reported to cause marginal corneal infiltration and limbal ulceration typical of allergic marginal keratitis. Marginal keratitis has been reported after intravitreal injection of ranibizumab.[2] Discontinuation of the offending medication results in complete resolution of the hypersensitivity reaction. Marginal keratitis has also been described in association with dissecting folliculitis of the scalp. Marginal keratitis is postulated to be caused by an enhanced immune response to *Staphylococcus aureus* antigens. It is possible that a similar abnormal response to infection may play role in the pathogenesis of these two conditions.

■ CLINICAL CHARACTERISTICS

The condition presents as irritation, redness, photophobia, and foreign body sensation. Patient usually has marked limbal and conjunctival congestion. The associated peripheral corneal stromal infiltrate can be single or multiple, and present in one or both eyes. The lesion usually has a circumferential orientation, parallel to the limbus and is separated by a clear zone (1–2 mm). As the lesions progress, they maintain the circumferential orientation, in contrast to infective ulcers which progress toward the center of the cornea. If the patient presents in the early stage of the condition, the epithelium overlying the infiltrate is often intact and breaks down during the next 2–3 days, unlike in infections in which the lesion presents with an epithelial defect.

■ DIFFERENTIAL DIAGNOSIS

The condition must be distinguished from the infective peripheral infiltrate due to *Staphylococcus* or any other bacteria. The infective infiltrate is painful, round in shape, and has an overlying epithelial defect. It is invariably associated with anterior chamber reaction. The infiltrate is usually single and nonrecurrent. The material obtained on corneal scraping should be subjected to Gram stain and bacterial culture and sensitivity tests. Patient should be treated with intensive topical broad-spectrum antibiotics.

Peripheral dendritic ulcer and conjunctival ulcer characteristics of herpes simplex keratitis should be excluded.

Marginal keratitis should also be distinguished from keratitis associated with connective tissue disorders, dry eye, Mooren's ulcer, vernal keratoconjunctivitis, and rosacea keratitis.

Fuchs' marginal keratitis is another condition that can result in peripheral infiltrate, stromal thinning, and pseudopterygium formation. Fuchs' superficial marginal keratitis may result in bilateral nasal pseudopterygia encroaching on the visual axis, reducing visual acuity in both eyes.

■ IMMUNOPATHOGENESIS

No active infection by *Staphylococcus* has been demonstrated in marginal keratitis. Marginal infiltrates have been found to demonstrate a sterile neutrophilic response and the immune complex and complement deposition, an indicative of type III hypersensitivity reaction. The peripheral cornea has been demonstrated to have ACE2 receptors, potential source allowing antigen-antibody complex deposition, which is necessary for a type III hypersensitivity. It is the activation of the complement pathway from immune deposits that are thought to result in peripheral corneal opacity seen with marginal keratitis.

Marginal keratitis has been reported after coronavirus disease-2019 (COVID-19) vaccination. Type III hypersensitivity reactions are delayed and may occur between days to weeks following exposure to an antigen. Marginal keratitis has been reported to occur 2.5 weeks after COVID-19 vaccination.

TREATMENT

In mild cases, warm compresses, eyelid hygiene, and topical broad-spectrum antibiotics such as fluoroquinolone four times a day and preservative-free artificial tear drops should improve the condition.

In moderate and severe cases, mild topical steroids should be added in addition to the earlier mentioned treatment. Loteprednol 0.2% or prednisolone 0.25%, four times a day may be prescribed. Once the condition improves, topical steroids should be tapered. During the period when the patient is on topical steroids, intraocular pressure (IOP) should be constantly monitored.

Topical cyclosporine ophthalmic emulsion 0.05% (Restasis) twice daily may be added to control the limbal and eyelid inflammation.

In case of recurrence, oral doxycycline 100 mg twice daily for a month should be prescribed.

REFERENCES

1. Glavici M, Glavici G. Cheratită marginală în boala Behçet [Marginal keratitis in Behçet's disease]. Oftalmologia. 1997;41(3):224-7.
2. Aslan Bayhan S, Bayhan HA, Adam M, Gürdal C. Marginal keratitis after intravitreal injection of ranibizumab. Cornea. 2014;33(11):1238-9.

1.21 | Interstitial Keratitis

Ashu Agarwal
Chaudhury Eye Hospital, New Delhi
ashuagarwal@hotmail.com

INTRODUCTION

Interstitial keratitis (IK) is a broad term used to refer to a nonulcerative and nonsuppurative inflammation of the corneal stroma, characterized by a cellular infiltration **(Fig. 1.21.1)**. It is often associated with vascularization of the stroma, without a primary involvement of the epithelium or endothelium.

Interstitial keratitis is an immune-mediated process believed to be caused by a cellular and humoral response against antigens in the corneal stroma, residual infectious antigens or both.

Although syphilis remains the leading cause of IK, it can be caused due to various bacterial, viral, parasitic, and autoimmune causes. Herpes simplex virus (HSV) has replaced syphilis as the leading cause of IK in some parts of the world (USA).

Interstitial keratitis is often associated with systemic diseases and warrants a comprehensive clinical history, review of systems and physical examination.

CLINICAL PRESENTATION

The inflammatory lesions of IK can present clinically as active or inactive.

Active Interstitial Keratitis

There is an on-going immune-mediated inflammation characterized by stromal infiltration, edema, and sometimes the presence of an immune ring.

Pain, lacrimation, photophobia, and gradual-blurring of vision are the common presentations. In syphilis and occasionally with other causes,

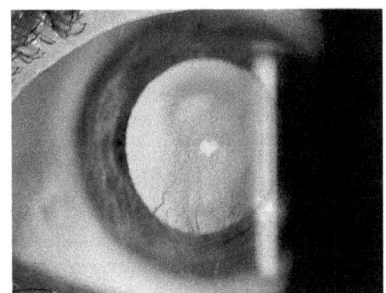

Fig. 1.21.1: Interstitial keratitis.

the entire cornea may develop a ground-glass appearance, obscuring the iris. The vascularization contributes to the orange-red appearance of the cornea called salmon patches. Anterior uveitis and choroiditis may be associated with syphilitic IK. Inflammation and vascularization usually begin to subside after 1-2 months. Some corneal opacity usually remains, causing mild-to-moderate vision impairment.

Inactive Interstitial Keratitis

This refers to a previous episode of the disease, which has remained quiet for a period of at least 1 year. The typical corneal findings include mid-to-posterior stromal scarring, deep vascularization of the cornea (resulting in the formation of ghost vessels), and sometimes reduplication of Descemet's membrane.

DIFFERENTIAL DIAGNOSIS

The differential diagnosis of IK is discussed using the etiological classification: bacterial infections, viral infections, parasitic infections, systemic diseases, and nonsystemic diseases.

Bacterial Infections

- *Congenital syphilis:* Pattern—bilateral, diffuse stromal disease with deep vascularization, 87% of syphilitic IK worldwide is congenital; transmitted from mother with primary, secondary, or early latent *Treponema pallidum* infection; occurs between 5 years and 20 years of ages. Peak: 9-11 years; other ocular findings—iris atrophy, posterior synechiae and salt-and-pepper fundus; systemic manifestations—Hutchinson's triad-comprising of IK, deafness and anomalous teeth; saddle-nose, frontal bossing, and maxillary overgrowth.
- *Acquired syphilis:* Pattern—unilateral, sectoral stromal disease with mild vascularization; occurs about 10 years after infection, usually milder and with less vascularization than the congenital form.
- *Mycobacterial:* Tuberculosis and leprosy.

Viral Diseases

- *HSV:* Pattern—unilateral, diffuse or sectoral involvement, vascularization and associated with iritis; leading cause of IK in the some parts of the world (USA); decreased corneal sensation and iris atrophy; recurrent disease; treatment with topical antiviral agents like acyclovir eye ointment; topical steroids reduce inflammation and edema.
- *Others:* Herpes zoster virus (HZV), Epstein-Barr virus (mononucleosis), mumps; human T-lymphotropic virus type I (HTLV-I).

Parasitic Infections

Leishmaniasis, onchocerciasis (river blindness), and trypanosomiasis.

Systemic Diseases

Cogan's syndrome; other systemic diseases, such as sarcoidosis, lymphoma (Hodgkin's disease), Kaposi's sarcoma, and mycosis fungicides (T cell lymphoma).

TREATMENT

The underlying condition has to be treated for the keratitis to resolve. In addition, treatment with a topical corticosteroid, such as prednisolone acetate 1% eye drops, is often required. These drops are administered at a frequency of six times a day and tapered gradually over the next few weeks to months.

Rarely, the corneal scarring may be dense enough to warrant a keratoplasty subsequently. However, keratoplasty should be performed only when the ocular inflammation has settled down to reduce the chances of postoperative complications such as rejection and graft failure.

The patient should be followed up regularly till the inflammation settles down and scarring has occurred. Thereafter, the patient should be seen periodically (6 months to 1 year).

With appropriate treatment, the visual acuity in IK can generally be preserved or restored.

1.22 Peripheral Ulcerative Keratitis

Ayan Mohanta
Disha Eye Hospitals, Kolkata
ayanmohanta@hotmail.com

■ INTRODUCTION

Peripheral ulcerative keratitis (PUK) is a potentially sight-threatening disorder which usually begins with crescentic destructive inflammation at the corneal periphery and is associated with epithelial defect, presence of stromal inflammatory cells, progressive stromal melting, degradation, and necrosis. It may sometimes lead to perforation.

■ ETIOLOGY

Unlike avascular central cornea the peripheral cornea derives part of its blood supply from the anterior conjunctiva and deep episcleral blood vessels. These blood vessels are a source of immunocompetent cells. Some of the causes of PUK are discussed here.

Noninfectious Conditions

- *Local:* Mooren's ulcer **(Fig. 1.22.1)**, marginal keratitis, blepharitis, acid and alkali injuries to cornea, trauma, and surgery.
- *Systemic:* Rheumatoid arthritis (RA), systemic lupus erythematosus (SLE), relapsing polychondritis (RP), sarcoidosis, progressive systemic sclerosis (PSS), rosacea, Wegener's granulomatosis (WG), polyarteritis nodosa (PAN), giant cell arteritis (GCA), inflammatory bowel disease, and metabolic and neoplastic conditions.

Infectious Conditions (Fig. 1.22.2)

- *Local:* Viral causes include herpes simplex keratitis and varicella-zoster keratitis. Bacterial keratitis, fungal keratitis, and *Acanthamoeba* species have also been reported.
- *Systemic: Shigella* species, tuberculosis syphilis, hepatitis C, human immune deficiency virus (HIV), *Gonococcus, Salmonella* species, and bacillary dysentery.

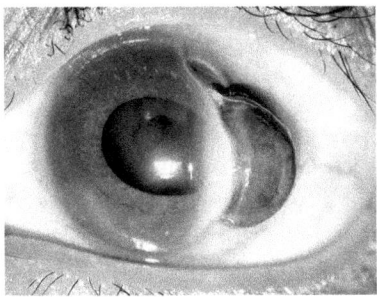

Fig. 1.22.1: Mooren's ulcer with perforation.

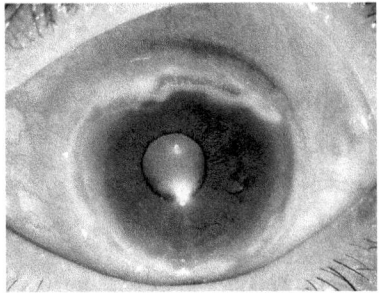

Fig. 1.22.2: Peripheral ulcerative keratitis—infective.

All the earlier mentioned causes lead to inflammatory reaction at the corneal periphery. Inflammation causes immune complex deposition, complement activation, and further increase in vascular permeability. This in turn generates more chemotactic factors (C3a and C5a) for neutrophils. Neutrophils thus recruited at the peripheral cornea liberate proteolytic and collagenolytic enzymes causing destruction of corneal stroma.

CLINICAL FEATURES

Symptoms: Foreign body sensation, severe pain if there is associated scleritis, watering, photophobia, and dimness of vision which is sometimes rapidly progressive. PUK associated with Mooren's ulcer may also cause pain without scleral involvement.

Slit lamp examination: Reveals a crescent-shaped lesion at the juxtalimbal cornea with associated epithelial defect, stromal yellow-white infiltrates, and corneal thinning being a marked feature. Typical "overhanging" edges are seen in Mooren's ulcer. The anterior chamber should be examined for depth and inflammation. Presence of necrotizing scleritis indicates potentially lethal systemic disease.

SYSTEMIC FINDINGS

Systemic signs are sometimes helpful for diagnosis:
- *RA:* Typical swan neck deformity.
- *SLE:* Characteristic butterfly distribution of rashes.
- *PSS:* Shiny and thickened skin effacement of skin margins, tautness of skin leading to sclerodactyly.
- *WG:* Cavitary lung lesions.
- *Sarcoidosis:* Enlarged mediastinal lymph nodes.

Patients with Mooren's ulcer have no diagnosable systemic disorders and suffer from extreme ocular pain without any scleral involvement, marked photophobia, and increased tearing. *It is more a diagnosis of exclusion.*

DIFFERENTIAL DIAGNOSIS

- Marginal keratitis associated with blepharitis
- Dellen
- Furrow degeneration
- Pellucid marginal degeneration

LABORATORY INVESTIGATIONS

- Complete blood count (CBC) and erythrocyte sedimentation rate (ESR)
- *Rheumatoid factor:* Positive in 80% of patients with RA
- *Angiotensin-converting enzyme:* Indicative of sarcoidosis
- *Antinuclear antibodies (ANA):* Positive in SLE and RA
- *Antibody to double-stranded DNA (anti-ds DNA):* Associated with SLE
- *Antibodies to small nuclear ribonucleoprotein-Sm (anti-Sm):* Associated with SLE
- *Antibodies to small nuclear ribonucleoproteins (anti-RNP):* Associated with SLE
- *Antineutrophil cytoplasmic antibodies (ANCA):* C-ANCA: 96% sensitivity for WG
- *Hepatitis B surface antigen (HBsAg):* HBsAg positive 40% patients with PAN
- *Fluorescent treponemal antibody-absorption (FTA-ABS)* for syphilis

Imaging Studies

Chest X-ray and sinus computed tomography (CT) scan to diagnose features of WG, sarcoidosis, and tuberculosis. Radiographic studies of affected joints as a part of systemic evaluation.

Conjunctival Biopsy

Biopsy of adjacent conjunctiva is not a standard diagnostic procedure but can be considered in cases with diagnostic dilemma when conjunctival resection is planned. It may show features of vaso-occlusion or granulomatous inflammation (in WG).

■ TREATMENT

Medical Management

It includes combination of local and systemic therapy. The local therapy helps the epithelium to heal whereas the systemic therapy will quieten down the underlying disease. Certain collagenase inhibitors like topical 20% N-acetylcysteine or collagenase synthesis inhibitor like medroxyprogesterone along with profuse preservative-free lubricating drops help in re-epithelialization of the cornea.

Topical steroids remain the mainstay in the treatment of PUK. Adjunctive treatment includes topical cyclosporine-A 2% and collagenase inhibitors.

Systemic collagenase inhibitors like tetracycline 250 mg qid or doxycycline 100 mg bid may slow progression.

Indications for Immunosuppression

- PUK associated with systemic diseases such as PAN, RA, SLE, PSS, Sjögren's syndrome, RP, and Wegener's granulomatosis.
- PUK associated with necrotizing scleritis.
- Bilateral and/or progressive Mooren's ulcer.
- PUK unresponsive to aggressive conventional medical and surgical therapy. Cyclophosphamide is the drug of choice for PUK associated with connective tissue disorders. Methotrexate, azathioprine, and cyclosporine A are also effective. All these agents are to be used based on the clinical response and adverse effects.

Dosage and Precautions

- *Cyclophosphamide:* 2 mg/kg/day orally; side effect bone marrow depression. Monitor blood counts.
- *Methotrexate:* 7.5–12.5 mg/week oral/IM injection. Monitor CBC, liver function test (LFT), and renal function.
- *Azathioprine:* 1–3 mg/kg/day orally. Monitor absolute platelet count and LFT.

Usually oral prednisolone and an immunomodulatory agent such as cyclophosphamide are initiated at the same time. It takes 4–6 weeks for the effect immunomodulatory agents to set in. Oral prednisolone is used in the interim period to stabilize the patient and control the active inflammatory process until the immunomodulatory agent takes effect. Oral steroids are subsequently tapered and the patient is maintained on the systemic immunomodulatory agent.

Systemic infliximab or rituximab (CD20 antagonists) are useful when patients cannot tolerate cyclophosphamide or methotrexate.

If local or systemic infections are suspected as a cause then appropriate antibiotic medications based on clinical signs of the disease or culture reports are used.

Surgical Management

Conjunctival resection helps to remove the limbal source of collagenases and other factors causing progressive destruction of stroma.

Tissue adhesives (cyanoacrylate glue or fibrin glue) and bandage contact lenses (BCL) application combined with conjunctival resection are helpful in cases of impending perforation.

Conjunctival resection with lamellar keratoplasty and amniotic membrane overlay (Kinoshita et al.) also yields good results in patient's nonresponsive to topical treatment.

Tectonic procedures such as patch grafts full-thickness or lamellar are done to maintain the integrity of the globe in cases of perforations. Elective reconstructive keratoplasty once the disease process is controlled. Amniotic membrane grafting can be done to promote healing in Mooren's ulcer.

■ FOLLOW-UP
Regular and lifelong follow-up is necessary even after complete resolution since relapses may occur. Majority of patients required lifelong immunosuppression to keep the systemic disease under control.

1.23 | Pellucid Marginal Degeneration

Sandeep Arora
Retina Foundation and Eye Research Centre, Ahmedabad
drsandeeparora@gmail.com

■ RELEVANT CLINICAL FEATURES
Pellucid marginal degeneration (PMD) is typically bilateral, nonulcerative, and noninflammatory corneal ectasia with an inferiorly located crescent-shaped thinning of the cornea. The cornea protrudes anteriorly, above the area of thinning, without associated inflammation, vascularization, scarring, or lipid infiltration.

■ ONSET AND PROGRESSION
It occurs in both men and women, presenting between 2nd and 4th decade, with chief complaints of progressive dimness of vision caused by high "against the rule" astigmatism. Episodes of corneal hydrops with resultant pain have been reported.

■ CORNEAL TOPOGRAPHY
The topography usually shows "against the rule" astigmatism, with a sagging bow-tie configuration, oblique inferiorly. The steepest meridian is located 90° to the area of thinning (Butterfly pattern). Bell-shaped appearance of corneal pachymetry map is characteristic of PMD.

■ DIFFERENTIAL DIAGNOSIS
Atypical presentations of PMD have been reported, such as unilateral presentation with the other eye being normal clinically and on topography, in association with keratoconus or keratoglobus, and occurring as isolated superior thinning or a contiguous extension of the zone of peripheral thinning above the horizontal meridian.
- Keratoconus
- Terrien marginal degenerations
- Keratoglobus
- Furrow degenerations
- Peripheral corneal melting disorders (e.g., Mooren's ulcer)

■ TREATMENT
Noninterventional Management
Spectacle correction usually fails early in the course of this disease as the degree of irregular astigmatism increases. In early-to-moderate cases, contact lenses are beneficial in providing visual rehabilitation.

Contact Lenses
Rigid gas permeable contact lenses provide excellent oxygen transmission to the cornea but are harder than the other lenses to fit. Specialized lenses like Rose K or in extreme cases Boston scleral lenses are used.

Corneal Collagen Cross-linking with Riboflavin

A new treatment of applying one-time-only topical dose of riboflavin drops to the cornea and exposing the cornea to a low amount of ultraviolet-A (UVA) light. The activated riboflavin enhances corneal strength and integrity by increasing collagen cross-linking (CXL). Intracorneal ring segments have been tried in mild-to-moderate PMD along with CXL.

Surgical

- Excision of a crescentic wedge of corneal tissue from the inferior cornea, followed by tight suturing, the procedure is usually well-tolerated; however, the effect is typically short-lived
- Crescentic lamellar keratoplasty; crescentic transplant is performed to reinforce the area of thinning
- Intracorneal ring implants with or without CXL
- Penetrating keratoplasty or deep anterior lamellar keratoplasty (DALK) may be done in severe cases
- Intrastromal lamellar keratoplasty where a stromal pocket is created in the thinned out inferior cornea with insertion of donor stromal tissue can be done for disease stabilization

■ FOLLOW-UP

Deterioration of visual function results from the irregular astigmatism induced by asymmetric distortion of the cornea. Until an acute episode of hydrops occurs patient can be routinely followed with twice to thrice consultation a year. Once the disease is stabilized, these patients can be visually rehabilitated with spectacles, scleral contact lenses, or phakic intraocular lenses (IOLs).

■ SPECIAL NOTES

Keratoconus, pellucid marginal corneal degeneration (PMCD), and keratoglobus have all been considered to be associated as part of this spectrum of noninflammatory corneal thinning disorders. PMD is sometimes confused with keratoconus because both involve localized steepening of the inferior peripheral cornea. PMD can usually be distinguished from keratoconus by the extreme peripheral position of the ectasia that has a crescent-shaped morphology.

1.24 | Stromal Dystrophies

Jeewan S Titiyal
Dr RP Centre for Ophthalmic Sciences, AIIMS, New Delhi
titiyal@rediffmail.com

■ INTRODUCTION

Stromal dystrophies largely produce symptoms due to opacification of corneal stroma from deposition of metabolically generated abnormal material **(Table 1.24.1)**.

Other less common stromal dystrophies are Schnyder's crystalline dystrophy, fleck dystrophy, central cloudy corneal dystrophy, congenital hereditary stromal dystrophy, and posterior amorphous dystrophy.

■ TREATMENT

- *For recurrent erosion:* Bandage contact lens (BCL) along with antibiotics or patching with an antibiotic ointment.

TABLE 1.24.1: Tabular outline characteristics of corneal stromal dystrophies.

Names	Other names	Layer	Other layers involved	Heredity	Age at onset	Progression	Laterality	Corneal position	Effect on vision	Other symptoms	Histopathology	H/P stain	Treatment	Recur in graft
Granular dystrophy	Groenouw I	Stroma (pan)	Bowman layer	AD 5q31 TGFβ1	<10 years	Slowly progressive	B/L	Central	Slight at first, moderate after early middle age	Pain or RE uncommon	Rods and filaments of "hyaline"	Masson trichrome red	SK, PTK, LK, PK in early middle age	Yes
Lattice dystrophy	None	Stroma (espant)	epithelium and Bowman's layer	AD 5q31 TGFβ1	<20 years	Slowly progressive	B/L May be U/L	Central	Slight to moderate at first, severe in middle age	Pain or RE	Aligned fibrils of amyloid	Congo red (red and green dichroism), birefringent	MRE; PK in middle age, LK	Yes
Macular dystrophy	Groenouw II	Stroma (pan)	DM and Endothelium	AR16q21 CHST6	<10 years	Progressive	B/L	General	Moderate to severe	None	Excess GAG	Alcian blue Colloidal iron	PK in early middle age, LK	Yes
Central crystalline dystrophy	Schnyder	Stroma (ant)	Bowman layer	AD	<1 year	Slowly progressive	B/L	Central	Slight	None	Cholesterol crystals	Schultz (cholesterol blue green)	Screen for metabolic changes, PTK	Yes

(B/L: bilateral; DM: Descemet's membrane; GAG: glycosaminoglycan; LK: lamellar keratoplasty; MRE: management of recurrent erosion; PK: penetrating keratoplasty; PTK: phototherapeutic keratectomy; RE: recurrent erosion; SK: superficial keratectomy)

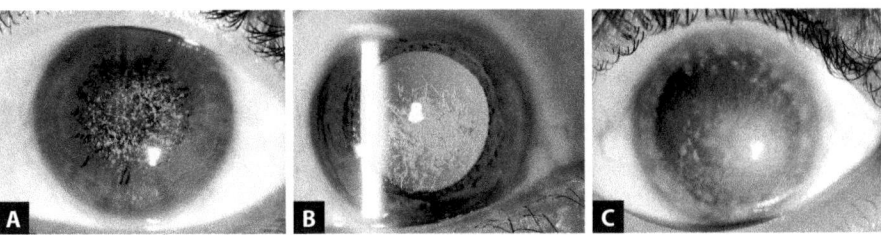

Figs. 1.24.1A to C: (A) Granular dystrophy; (B) Lattice dystrophy; (C) Macular dystrophy.

- Artificial tear lubricating drops (preservative-free), sodium chloride 5% drops during the day and lubricating ointment at bedtime—can be used as preventive treatment for acute state.
- *Excimer laser phototherapeutic keratectomy (PTK):*
  - If recurrent corneal erosions occur despite medical therapy
  - Visual decrease from superficial opacities
- *Lamellar keratoplasty or deep anterior lamellar keratoplasty (DALK):* It can be done in cases with superficial opacity with noninvolved endothelium. Granular and lattice are good candidates for DALK but in macular dystrophy endothelium may be involved and that should be taken into consideration before going for DALK or lamellar keratoplasty in macular dystrophy **(Figs. 1.24.1A to C).**
- *Penetrating keratoplasty:* It is the definitive surgical treatment for dystrophies but carries the risk of open sky surgery as well as the risk of endothelial immune rejection. Dystrophies carry the chance of recurrence after keratoplasty (lattice > granular > macular).

1.25 | Fuchs' Endothelial Dystrophy

Samar K Basak
Disha Eye Hospitals, Kolkata
basak_sk@hotmail.com

■ INTRODUCTION

Fuchs' endothelial dystrophy is most often seen in adult female in fifth to sixth decades of life. It is mostly autosomal dominant. Family history is present in 30% cases. There is an increased apoptosis of corneal endothelium with changes in the collagen composition of the Descemet's membrane.

■ CLINICAL FEATURES

Symptoms
It is a slowly progressive bilateral condition, often without any symptom. Only there is presence of central corneal guttata with "beaten metal" appearance.
- Glare and blurred vision, worse on awakening in the morning.
- Stromal and epithelial edema gradually increases with impairment of vision. Later, severe pain and photophobia due to recurrent erosion from ruptured bullae. In advanced stage—there is gross visual loss but pain is less because of subepithelial scarring.

Signs
Cornea guttata, central stromal edema, epithelial edema with bedewing, bulla-single or multiple, Descemet's wrinkling or folds, hypertrophic epithelium, and lastly subepithelial stromal scarring and vascularization.

Fine pigment dusting on the endothelium may be seen in early stage. It is also associated with nuclear cataract in different grades and higher incidence of *primary open-angle glaucoma (POAG)* among these patients.

■ DIFFERENTIAL DIAGNOSIS

- *Aphakic or pseudophakic bullous keratopathy:* History of cataract surgery.
- *Posterior polymorphous corneal dystrophy (PPCD):* Early in life, endothelium shows—group vesicles, geographic gray lesions, or broad band.
- *Iridocorneal endothelial (ICE) syndrome:* Typically unilateral condition; young to middle age; beaten metal corneal endothelium with corneal edema; raised intraocular pressure (IOP); variable iris atrophy; and thinning and pupillary distortion.
- *Other causes of endothelial dysfunctions:* Blunt trauma, viral endotheliitis, chemical injury, etc.

■ WORK-UP

- IOP measurement
- Pachymetry
- *Specular microscopy:* To measure the endothelial cell count, morphology, and disease state. In case of aphakic bullous keratopathy (ABK) or pseudophakic bullous keratopathy (PBK), the other eye specular is important to get a clue about the preexisting Fuchs' dystrophy.
- Confocal microscopy
- Examination of the family members

■ TREATMENT

Medical

- Sodium chloride (5%) eye drops in daytime and ointment at bedtime.
- Reduction of IOP by antiglaucoma medication if IOP is >20 mm Hg.
- *Bandage contact lens (BCL):* To give temporary relief for painful ruptured corneal bullae.

Surgical

- Descemet's stripping (automated) endothelial keratoplasty (DSEK/DSAEK) is now the treatment of choice. The visual rehabilitation is faster with minimum astigmatism. Cataract surgery [Phaco/manual small-incision cataract surgery (MSICS) with posterior chamber intraocular lens (PCIOL)] is usually combined with DSEK (triple procedure) even in presence of minimal cataract.
- Descemet's membrane endothelial keratoplasty (DMEK) is a more physiological surgery and it is slowly replacing DSEK as the surgery of choice. The visual rehabilitation is even faster than DSEK; there is no hyperopic shift however the initial endothelial cell loss is higher due to more surgical manipulation.
- Penetrating keratoplasty in presence of stromal scarring.
- Newer treatment modalities descemetorhexis without endothelial keratoplasty (DWEK) with injection of cultured human endothelial cells or intracameral injection of Rho-kinase inhibitor.

■ FOLLOW-UP

In early stages: Every 6–12 months to check IOP; to assess the development of corneal edema; and endothelial cell status by specular microscopy. But in presence of epithelial edema, the follow-up may be every 3 months till the surgery is performed.

SPECIAL NOTES

If the patient presents with early Fuchs' dystrophy with significant cataract, every precaution is to be taken to protect the endothelium during phacoemulsification (such as, use of Viscoat or Healon GV, or Healon-5; use of BSS-plus irrigating solution; and higher end phaco machine and less intracameral medicines).

1.26 | Keratoconus

Rajesh Fogla
Apollo Hospital, Hyderabad
dr_fogla@yahoo.com

INTRODUCTION

Keratoconus is a noninflammatory bilateral, asymmetric, and ectasia of the cornea characterized by steepening, distortion, and thinning of the apical cornea and corneal scarring. In most of the patients, keratoconus is diagnosed at an early age, either when spectacles and soft contact lenses are not able to provide sufficient vision or when the patients are evaluated for laser vision correction. Rarely, it may be congenital.

It is most commonly an isolated condition, despite multiple reports of coexistence with other disorders. Commonly recognized associations include vernal keratoconjunctivitis, Down syndrome, Leber's congenital amaurosis, and connective tissue disorders. Keratoconus is a relatively frequent disease with an incidence of 1 in 2,000 in the general population, though 8–10% of reported cases have positive family history or show evidence of familial transmission. Keratoconus is progressive until the third to fourth decades of life, and then it freezes. It may, however, commence at any age in life and may arrest at any age.

These patients seek medical advice because of the high compound myopic astigmatism associated with progressive keratoconus. This is mainly due to the conical protrusion of the cornea. The diagnosis in moderate to advance cases is simply by clinical examination. However, the diagnosis is difficult clinically in very early keratoconus and impossible in subclinical cases. The progressive increase in myopic astigmatism or asymmetric increase in keratometric values inferiorly compared to superiorly might be clinically suggestive of keratoconus.

CLINICAL FEATURES

The clinical signs depend upon the stage of the disease. The signs are Munson's sign and Rizzuti phenomenon. The slit lamp may comprise of stromal thinning; posterior stress lines (Vogt's striae); iron ring (Fleischer ring); scarring—epithelial or subepithelial; and the retroillumination signs are scissoring on retinoscopy and oil droplet sign (Charleaux). The signs on photokeratoscopy are compression of mires inferotemporally (egg-shaped mires) or compression of mires inferiorly or centrally and the videokeratography signs are localized increased surface power, inferior superior dioptric asymmetry, relative skewing of the steepest radial axes above and below the horizontal meridian. The invention of Orbscan IIZ and Scheimpflug imaging provide even the posterior float corneal maps which may help to pick up the subclinical cases also. This is very important as this group of patients should not undergo any form of corneal ablative procedures for the correction of refractive error.

TREATMENT

Keratoconus is a progressive disease in almost all cases at some point of time, though it may get arrested on its own in some patients; however, in 20% of patients, it progresses to a stage that requires full thickness or lamellar keratoplasty.

Corneal Collagen Cross-linking

Recently, a new technique of corneal collagen cross-linking (CXL or C3R) by the photosensitizer riboflavin and ultraviolet A (UVA) has recently been introduced to increase the biomechanical strength of the cornea and arrest the progression of keratoconus. This procedure photopolymerizes the stromal fibers by the combined action of a photosensitizing substance (riboflavin or vitamin B_2) and UVA from a solid-state UVA source. Photopolymerization arrests the progression of the ectasia in keratoconus by increasing the corneal rigidity and might also decrease the severity of the keratoconus. Since all patients do not progress, CXL or C3R should be carried out only in patients in whom progression of keratoconus has been documented.

Contact Lenses

The second aspect of dealing with keratoconus is improving the vision of these patients. The different options of correcting the refractive error are spectacles and soft toric contact lenses in early stages; however, the optimal correction by contact lenses can be provided only by plain rigid gas permeable (RGP) lenses or Rose-K lenses in more advance cases. The later are more specifically designed for keratoconus with two or more relatively flatter peripheral curves incorporated in these lenses. However, advanced cases require scleral contact lens where corneal contact lenses are not stable.

INTACS

Intracorneal segments (INTACS) can be used to decrease the corneal astigmatism or myopia. These segments can be placed or customized according to the cone on topography such as double symmetrical or double asymmetrical or single segment.

Corneal Allogenic Intrastromal Ring Segments

The principle is similar to INTACS but instead of using polymethyl methacrylate (PMMA) segments donor corneal stroma is used. This is advantageous of the fact that there is no extrusion, grade B or C cornea can be used and decreases corneal astigmatism significantly.

Phakic Intraocular Lenses

Phakic intraocular lens (IOL) implant, particularly, implantable collamer lens (ICL) can be used to reduce the refractive error. The toric ICL, though to a limited range can further address to the astigmatism caused by the irregular thinning and protrusion of the cornea. Many Indian companies are customizing high cylinder phakic IOL for keratoconus patients.

Keratoplasty

In some cases, the disease may progress to a stage when corneal grafting becomes inevitable. The ideal form of keratoplasty for keratoconus patients is deep anterior lamellar keratoplasty. The endothelium is healthy in keratoconus unless there is a previous hydrops. If the scarring is involving Descemet's membrane then penetrating keratoplasty is performed.

■ RECENT ADVANCES

Bowman's Membrane Transplant

The donor Bowman's layer transplantation into the mid stroma functions to strengthen and make the anterior corneal surface flatter. This is beneficial in reducing ectasia in advanced keratoconus with minimal intraoperative and postoperative complications.

In short, keratoconus is common eye disease affecting young individuals with varied presentation and the treatment to each patient has to be tailored according to the stage of keratoconus and the need of the individual.

1.27 Band-shaped Keratopathy

Rishi Swarup
Swarup Eye Centre, Hyderabad
rishi@swarupeye.net

■ INTRODUCTION

Band-shaped keratopathy (BSK) refers to a condition in which calcium salts are precipitated on the surface of the cornea, either due to local or systemic causes **(Fig. 1.27.1)**. Systemic causes include hypercalcemic states such as hyperparathyroidism, hypophosphatasia, milk-alkali syndrome, Paget's disease, and sarcoidosis. Local causes include chronic uveitis, phthisis bulbi, end-stage glaucoma, topical use of steroid phosphate preparations, and intraocular silicone oil.

Calcium deposition in local causes may be explained by altered pH, electrolyte imbalance in tears, or endothelial dysfunction. The predominant interpalpebral involvement is explained by increased focal tonicity of tears caused by evaporation in this zone with resultant precipitation of calcium.

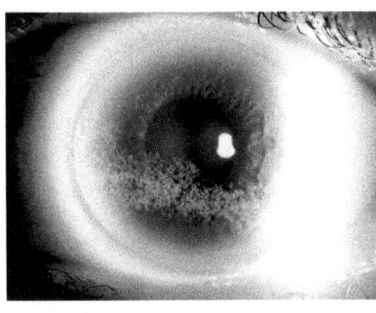

Fig. 1.27.1: Band-shaped keratopathy.

■ CLINICAL FEATURES

The interpalpebral area of the cornea bears a grayish-white plaque in the Bowman's membrane and superficial stroma. Usually there is a peripheral lucid interval which is either due to the lack of Bowman's membrane in the peripheral cornea or due to the buffering effect of limbal blood vessels. Throughout the band are small, clear holes representing areas where corneal nerves traverse the Bowman's membrane, giving it a characteristic *Swiss-cheese* appearance.

■ DIFFERENTIAL DIAGNOSIS

- Spheroidal degeneration
- Primary or secondary calcareous degenerations of the cornea
- Calciphylaxis
- Gout

■ TREATMENT

If no local causes are identified, then serum calcium, phosphate levels, serum angiotensin-converting enzyme (ACE) levels, and parathyroid hormone levels must be checked to rule out systemic causes.

Medical Treatment

It involves treatment of any underlying systemic condition to prevent further calcium deposition.

Mainstay of treatment in BSK is chemical chelation. Initially the epithelium overlying the lesion is mechanically debrided using a spatula or a No. 15 blade. 1% or 2% (0.05 mol) neutral solution of ethylenediaminetetraacetic acid (EDTA) is applied over the lesion either in a water bath or using soaked-cotton-tipped applicator or cellulose sponge for about 5 minutes. After this, scraping with the blade edge will remove the calcium particles. This procedure is repeated till the visual axis is cleared of all calcium and may require 10–30 minutes depending on the density of the plaque.

If the surface is very irregular, phototherapeutic keratectomy (PTK) with an excimer laser can be performed to smooth the surface. It is important that one does not attempt to remove band keratopathy with the excimer laser alone as this will result in significant irregular astigmatism since the cornea, not calcium, will be ablated preferentially.

Amniotic membrane has been used in some situations after surgical removal of BSK to rapidly restore ocular surface stability.

Diamond burr can also be used to debride the calcium deposits without the necessity of chelating agents.

■ FOLLOW-UP

Postoperatively either a bandage contact lens or serial pressure bandages are applied till the epithelium heals. If the underlying condition is not controlled then recurrences are possible, and in such an event, chelation can be repeated.

■ SPECIAL NOTE

Type I Vogt's limbal girdle is thought to represent an early form of BSK.

1.28 | Keratitis Medicamentosa

Falguni Mehta
Rotary Eye Institute, Gujarat
drfalgunimehta@gmail.com

■ INTRODUCTION

It refers to corneal epitheliopathy related to the use of certain topical medications and their preservatives **(Fig. 1.28.1)**.

Topical medications associated with corneal toxicity include antiglaucoma medications (beta-blockers and latanoprost); aminoglycosides; epinephrine compounds; preservatives (benzalkonium chloride and thiomersal); topical steroids; antiviral (idoxuridine, acyclovir, and trifluorothymidine); anesthetics (proparacaine, amethocaine, or tetracaine); miotics (echothiophate and pilocarpine); and topical mitomycin-C.

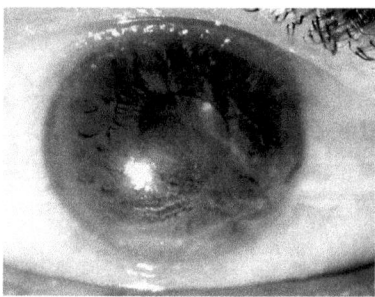

Fig. 1.28.1: Keratitis medicamentosa.

■ PATHOGENESIS

The toxic effects are both direct and indirect.

Directly, damaging epithelial cell organelles, desmosomes, cytoskeletal elements, and/or disruption of cell walls by emulsifying membrane lipids and thus altering cellular metabolism and function.

Indirectly, loss of epithelial microvilli can cause tear film instability, promoting corneal desiccation, and inhibiting re-epithelialization. Secondary neurotrophic changes may then occur.

In severe disease condition, extensive limbal stem cell deficiency evident by effacement of limbal palisades of Vogt can occur. Sometimes immune response can produce subepithelial corneal infiltrates.

■ CLINICAL FEATURES

Symptoms: Persistent redness; ocular irritation; reduced visual acuity, and photophobia.

Signs: Mild form (toxic keratitis): Punctate epithelial erosion of the inferior cornea, persistent epithelial defects, and/or pseudodendrites affecting any area of cornea.

Severe form (vortex/hurricane keratopathy): Diffuse coarse punctate epitheliopathy in a whorl pattern.

Most severe form: Recurrent corneal ulceration, stromal opacification, and neovascularization.

Other manifestations: Peripheral corneal infiltrate in epithelium and anterior stroma with a clear zone between them and limbus; toxic follicular reactions, with or without inflammation, may be associated with pseudodendritic or geographic ulcers and punctal stenosis; pseudopemphigoid/drug-induced cicatricial pemphigoid; toxic ulcerative keratitis (corneal epithelial defects typically oval with gray rolled edges with intense superficial keratitis); and nonprogressive scarring may also occur (pseudotrachoma).

■ DIFFERENTIAL DIAGNOSIS
Ocular cicatricial pemphigoid; herpes zoster ophthalmicus (HZO) keratitis; corneal abrasion; contact lens wear; and *Acanthamoeba* keratitis.

■ DIAGNOSIS
- Careful history critical in establishing a proper diagnosis.
- Proper slit-lamp examination to differentiate especially dendritic pattern from pseudodendrites.
- Staining with both fluorescein and rose Bengal stains.
- Conjunctival biopsy to differentiate, especially between pemphigoid from pseudopemphigoid.

■ TREATMENT
- Early recognition of problem is essential as advanced disease may take 2–3 months to clear and can be sight-threatening.
- Discontinuation of all topical medications.
- Use of nonpreservative artificial tears may relieve symptoms.
- Vitamin supplements and topical lubricants.

■ SPECIAL NOTES
Prevention involves avoiding the use of preservative containing medications or those known to be toxic (i.e., aminoglycosides, some glaucoma medications, and antivirals) in high-risk cases (chronic disease, dry eyes, and previous history of medicamentosa). Polypharmacy must also be monitored.

1.29 | Corneal Changes in Contact Lens Users

Rajib Mukherjee
Mukherjee Eye Klinik, New Delhi
mukherjee@eyedoctors.in

■ INTRODUCTION
First, do no harm, is not only the fundamental principle of medicine, but particularly relevant in contact lens (CL) fitting for nontherapeutic purposes. To understand the problems associated with CL use one must evaluate the changes in corneal physiology associated with it.

Broadly corneal pathophysiology during CL wear is attributed to:
- Hypoxia and hypercapnia
- Allergy and toxicity
- Mechanical effects
- Osmotic effects

■ HYPOXIA AND HYPERCAPNIA

Since the cornea is avascular, oxygen needed by the corneal epithelium is obtained by diffusion from air when the eye is open and from the tarsal conjunctiva when the eye is closed; and the use of a CL markedly reduces this oxygen availability. Oxygen deprivation (hypoxia) on using CL depends on the material of CL and the duration of wear. Along with hypoxia there is carbon dioxide accumulation (hypercapnia) in the cornea. These will suppress the normal aerobic metabolism and furthermore stimulates anaerobic glycolysis, which causes lowered epithelial metabolic rate, decreased epithelial mitotic rate, and increased epithelial lactate production and an acidic shift in stromal pH.

Epithelial thinning and epithelial abrasion—increased susceptibility to injury due to increased fragility of the corneal epithelium.

Epithelial microcysts—small translucent irregularly-shaped dots scattered across cornea, which disappear in 4-12 weeks after discontinuation of CL.

Superficial punctate keratitis—due to compromised junctional integrity.

Microbial keratitis—more common in extended wear as compared to daily wear CL users. Corneal infection associated with rigid gas permeable (RGP) CL occurs less frequently. *Pseudomonas aeruginosa* and *Staphylococcus aureus* are the most common organisms responsible for this catastrophe; while *Streptococcus pneumoniae, Serratia marcescens,* and other bacteria and fungi are occasionally present. Acanthamoeba is an uncommon infection, but at times has been associated with infectious keratitis in CL users.

Stromal edema is because of stromal acidosis consequent to lactate and bicarbonate accumulation.

Stromal striae are observed as fine vertical lines in the posterior stroma.

Posterior stromal folds appear as dark lines in the specular reflection on slit lamp evaluation, or as white lines on direct illumination; seen if stromal edema exceeds 10%.

Endothelial blebs seen in initial CL users as a transient phenomenon appearing about 30 minutes after CL use and subside over several hours. Decreased pH causes patchy endothelial edema which appears as defects on specular reflection.

Endothelial polymegathism—increased variation in cell size is noticed as a long-term change on corneal endothelium. It has a direct relation of material and duration of CL wear.

Corneal warpage—long-term users of *polymethyl methacrylate* (PMMA) CL may develop irregular astigmatism and distortion of central and peripheral cornea. It is attributed to both mechanical molding and hypoxic influences.

Corneal hypoesthesia—alteration in the afferent corneal nervous supply occurs because of hypoxia and hypercapnia.

Superficial vascularization—an apparent increase in limbal vessel penetration is because of reversible dilatation of existing limbal capillaries.

■ ALLERGY AND TOXICITY

Contact lens materials are generally designed to be biologically inert, but several scenarios related to its use may challenge the body's immune system. Provocation of the ocular immune system may be seen if debris accumulates between the CL and the cornea, or if the CL is contaminated with deposits, or due to preservatives of the CL solution.

Immobile lens syndrome, also known as "toxic lens syndrome", which is an inflammatory response believed to be due to debris-trapped behind a CL, seen mostly in extended wear CL users. Patients present with severe pain, photophobia, and lacrimation. There is unilateral limbal hyperemia and peripheral corneal infiltrates with intact epithelium. Keratic precipitates may also be seen in some cases. Discontinuation of CL use with use of lubricants and broad-spectrum topical antibiotic drops usually resolves the condition in 48–72 hours.

Thiomersal hypersensitivity—CL solution preservative. Thiomersal is a low molecular weight chemical which acts as a hapten, by conjugating with carrier protein, in order to act as a complete antigen. It elicits both humoral and cellular immune responses. Patients present with bilateral conjunctival hyperemia and itching. Corneal epithelial punctate staining and superficial infiltrates are features of thiomersal hypersensitivity. Another presentation of thiomersal hypersensitivity is superior limbic keratoconjunctivitis, where one finds congestion of superior bulbar conjunctiva along with superior punctate epithelial staining.

Solution toxicity—the other offending agents in CL solution have been identified as benzalkonium chloride, alkyl triethanol ammonium chloride (ATAC), chlorhexidine gluconate and disodium edetate [ethylenediaminetetraacetic acid (EDTA)]. Principal corneal signs are superficial diffuse punctate-staining associated with stinging and burning sensation. Pseudodendrite formation may be seen in some situations, which are raised branching epithelial plaques that stain very lightly with fluorescein, frequently accompanied with papillofollicular conjunctivitis.

■ MECHANICAL EFFECTS

Cornea is a soft and pliable tissue, very susceptible to injury due to CL, foreign body, fingernails, and eyelashes coming in contact with cornea during lens manipulation.

Lens-edge Imprint

The bearing of a rigid CL on the cornea may leave an imprint following CL removal. Typically the imprint is seen as the outline of the inferior rim of the CL on the epithelium. This manifestation is more often seen in ill-fitting or overnight use of RGP CL.

Epithelial Wrinkling

It is seen in PMMA CL users. It is asymptomatic and recovers rapidly after CL removal.

Air Bubble Dimpling

Entrapment of air bubbles under a PMMA CL is sufficient to cause small indentations on the corneal epithelium. These appear as discrete green dots, because of pooling as seen on fluorescein study.

■ OSMOTIC EFFECTS

Contact lens may alter the tear film osmolarity because of increased tear evaporation, stimulation of reflex tearing, and alteration of the normal blinking rate. Focal depletion of tear film rapidly leads to corneal epithelial desiccation.

3 and 9 O'clock Staining

It is seen in rigid CL users, as staining within the nasal and temporal margin of the cornea adjacent to the area of lens coverage. It is attributed to tear film breakdown adjacent to the CL edge. Refitting with a smaller diameter CL with thinner edge generally solves the problem.

Coarse Punctate Erosions

Mostly occurs in patient using thin high-water content hydrogel CL. Characteristically the erosions are white and coarse punctate appearance, which have been termed as crumb-like and flake-like. Water loss through the CL is thought to be a primary etiologic factor.

1.30 Suture Adjustment and Removal in Penetrating Keratoplasty: Tips and Tricks

Jeewan S Titiyal, Ritika Sachdev
Dr RP Centre for Ophthalmic Sciences, AIIMS, New Delhi
titiyal@rediffmail.com, ritika@centreforsight.net

■ INTRODUCTION

Appropriate and timely management of suture-related complications as well as suture removal and adjustment to reduce astigmatism are key issues in the postoperative care of a case of penetrating keratoplasty and to a large extent determine the final visual outcome of the graft.

Many methods of suturing exist, including single-interrupted, single-continuous running sutures, a combination of the two and double-continuous running sutures.

While interrupted sutures allow earlier removal of individual sutures in case of suture-associated infection or vascularization, continuous sutures allow intra- and postoperative titration to minimize astigmatism.

While each surgeon may have his/her preferred method of suturing, the possibility of removal of individual sutures makes interrupted sutures the preferred technique in pediatric and therapeutic cases as well as in regrafts.

■ SUTURE ADJUSTMENT—CONTINUOUS SUTURES

Timing

It is ideally carried out between 2 and 6 weeks postoperatively. By this time the graft edema usually subsides and an accurate assessment of the corneal topography is possible. Suture adjustment is ineffective if performed before the graft edema has resolved, as with the resolution of the edema and subsequent stromal thinning the suture tension alters.

Suture adjustment carried out after 6–8 weeks, though less likely to jeopardize the wound integrity, will also have less effect on corneal astigmatism.

Indication

Continuous suture titration is usually performed in cases with >3.5 diopters of corneal astigmatism.

Method

The corneal astigmatism is assessed using videokeratography. Under sterile conditions, the continuous suture is gently manipulated with a forceps from the flat meridian, where it is loose, to the tight segments. Slight overcorrection is advisable to account for the regression. On table use of intraoperative keratoscope/keratometer helps in suture adjustment and removal.

■ SUTURE REMOVAL AND REPLACEMENT: INTERRUPTED SUTURES

Indications for Early Selective Removal of Interrupted Sutures

Loose Sutures

All loose sutures should be removed as they do not provide structural support and may be a nidus of infection, and an inciting factor for *vascularization*.

Suture Associated with Infiltrate

Suture-associated infections account for 43% of the cases of graft infection. Loose or exposed sutures along with the mucus strands that accumulate around them are often harbingers of infections that may lead to graft infection and subsequent failure.

Tight Sutures

These may be associated with high *astigmatism*, and may significantly alter the corneal contour causing poor tear film stability and complications like dellen formation.

Timing

- Loose sutures particularly when associated with infection and vascularization should be removed immediately as the entailing complications may risk the very survival of the graft.
- If removal is carried out in the immediate postoperative period (<6–8 weeks) and particularly in cases where adjacent sutures need to be removed, replacement of sutures may be advisable.
- Tight sutures can be removed after 3 months if both adjacent sutures are secure, earlier removal usually warrants replacement.
- Adjacent interrupted sutures should not be removed for 6 months, for fear of causing wound dehiscence.

■ REMOVAL OF ALL SUTURES—CONTINUOUS AND INTERRUPTED

- It is recommend that removal of all sutures by 12 months in vascularized corneas, and 18 months in others to eliminate future suture-related complications. This practice however is not universally adopted.
- As the healing is faster, in pediatric cases it may be as early as 4–6 weeks, and by 6 months all sutures must be removed.
- All sutures must be removed in cases posted for refractive surgery for correction of refractive errors and astigmatism.
- All sutures should be removed prior to contact lens fitting.

■ AFTERCARE

- Increase the frequency of topical steroids temporarily and then taper-off within a month to current level.
- Additional antibiotics may be necessary.
- Extra follow-up is needed in presence of vascularization or infiltration.

■ COMPLICATIONS OF SUTURE REMOVAL

- Wound dehiscence
- Wound infection
- Sudden episode of graft rejection
- Graft ectasia
- Endophthalmitis

1.31 | Lamellar Keratoplasty

KS Siddarthan
Eyemed Eye Hospital, Coimbatore
siddarthanks@gmail.com

■ INTRODUCTION

Replacement of disease-specific cornea rather than the entire cornea has revolutionized corneal transplant surgery.

Lamellar keratoplasty (LK) can be classified into the following:
- Replacement of epithelium and stroma—anterior lamellar keratoplasty (ALK)
- Replacement of Descemet's membrane (DM)—posterior lamellar or endothelial keratoplasty (EK)[1,2]

Anterior lamellar keratoplasty is subdivided into:
- Bowman's membrane transplant
- Superficial ALK (SALK)
- Deep ALK (DALK)[1,2]

Endothelial keratoplasty variants include:
- Descemet's stripping endothelial keratoplasty (DSEK)
- Descemet's stripping automated endothelial keratoplasty (DSAEK)
- Descemet's membrane endothelial keratoplasty (DMEK)
- Pre-Descemet's EK (PDEK)[1,2]

Most of the mentioned procedures can be performed manually or with the assistance of a microkeratome or using the Femto laser to make lamellar cuts at desired planes. LK creates tissue planes that are not just the vertical apposition of the graft edge to the host rim as in PK but also the interface between the graft and host bed in the coronal plane.

Different types of donor-recipient interfaces

S. No.	Surgery	Interface
1.	DMEK	Donor DM to host pre-Descemet's layer (PDL)
2	DSEK/DSAEK	Donor stroma to host PDL
3	PDEK	Donor pre-Descemet's layer to host PDL
4	DALK	Donor PDL to host DM or donor PDL to host PDL or donor DM to host PDL
5	DALK—manual	Donor PDL to host stroma

(DALK: deep anterior lamellar keratoplasty; DM: Descemet's membrane; DMEK: Descemet's membrane endothelial keratoplasty; DSAEK: Descemet's stripping automated endothelial keratoplasty; DSEK: Descemet's stripping endothelial keratoplasty; PDEK: pre-Descemet's endothelial keratoplasty)

■ BOWMAN'S LAYER TRANSPLANTATION

Bowman's layer plays a major role in contributing to the biomechanical strength of the cornea. Thinning and disruption of the Bowman's membrane is postulated in causing corneal ectasia. Thus Bowman's layer transplantation (BLT) will add strength to the anterior cornea thereby inducing flattening, restoring its shape, and hence arresting disease progression.

Technique

The donor cornea is mounted in an artificial anterior chamber (AC) following which the epithelium is removed and air is injected into the donor cornea beneath the Bowman's layer to form the "Bowman's roll". The remnant epithelial cells are removed by immersion of the roll in 70% ethanol. The roll is then stained with trypan blue for better visualization. Recipient preparation can be done either with manual dissection or femtosecond laser where a stromal pocket is created at approximately 60 µm depth. The Bowman's roll is then inserted using a glide and then unrolled as desired.

SECTION 1: Cornea

■ DEEP ANTERIOR LAMELLAR KERATOPLASTY

In pathologies involving the corneal stromal such as granular and lattice dystrophy, stromal scars, corneal ectasias **(Fig. 1.31.1A)**, and vascularized corneas, the DM is often normal and therefore removing only the diseased stroma with sparing of the DM avoids the risk of graft failure due to endothelial rejection.

Technique

Recipient's Preparation

The cornea is marked with a trephine of desired size followed by partial trephination with a guarded knife (350 µm). A type 1 big bubble is created with the help of a 27 gauge DALK cannula, which is used to separate the stroma from the DM (Anwar and Teichmann).[2] Air is injected into the deep stroma in a gentle manner to create a round well-demarcated big bubble which extends to the borders of trephination. Following this the debulking of the anterior two-thirds of the corneal stroma is done with the help of a crescent blade. A partial paracentesis is now done to soften the eye. The big bubble is released with a single slash otherwise called as the "brave slash" using a side port knife. Once the bubble is released, using a fine spatula the plane of cleavage is demarcated and using a blunt scissors the separated stroma is carefully dissected 360° exposing the bare DM.

Donor Preparation

After placing the donor button in the Teflon block, the DM is scored with a Sinskey hook 360° gently stripped. The corneal stromal button is trephined with a Barron's vacuum punch usually 0.25 mm larger than the recipient's button. Trimming of the graft posterior edge is done after punching which enables good approximation. The graft is sutured with 10-0 nylon sutures. The depth of suturing is partial thickness taking care not to perforate the host DM **(Fig. 1.31.1B)**.

■ DESCEMET'S STRIPPING ENDOTHELIAL KERATOPLASTY

Donor Preparation

The donor cornea with its scleral rim is mounted on an artificial AC. Initial 360° limbal corneal incision is made with the help of a 500 µ guarded knife. Using a crescent blade manual lamellar dissection is then proceeded with at two-thirds depth and the dissection is completed with a curved spatula. Once the lamellar dissection is completed throughout the cornea, the donor tissue (endothelial side up) is placed on a Teflon block followed by trephination of desired size.

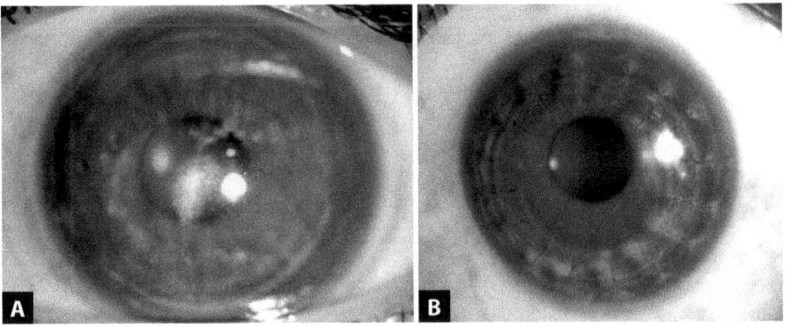

Figs. 1.31.1A and B: (A) Advanced KC; (B) Post DALK.

Recipient Preparation

Conjunctival peritomy is done, a 5 mm sclerocorneal tunnel is made along with two-side ports at 10 and 2 o'clock positions. Cohesive viscoelastics are injected followed by circular scoring of the DM with a reverse Sinskey hook and the DM is removed. A peripheral iridectomy is done. Viscoelastic agent is washed out thoroughly. The donor tissue is then folded into a "taco-shape", (60:40% ratio) and held at the leading edge with an Utrata forceps with 60% side up and inserted through the tunnel into the AC. The AC is filled up by balanced salt solution (BSS) following which the tissue unfolding is noticed. With the help of a 30-gauze cannula from the left side port, air is then injected to unfold the donor lenticule completely. This is followed by interface venting. After a period of 10–15 minutes 40% of the air bubble is then replaced with BSS.

■ DESCEMET'S MEMBRANE ENDOTHELIAL KERATOPLASTY

Donor Preparation

The donor tissue is placed on a Teflon block with the endothelial side up and a 10 mm trephine is used to carefully mark the DM. This is followed by staining of the graft with trypan blue. The marked DM is scored with a Sinskey hook 360° making sure not to create any tags. A Sinskey hook is used to elevate and separate the endothelium-DM all around. The endothelial-DM complex is then stripped under BSS using a single pull technique using a smooth curved forceps. After stripping half of the DM from the donor a "L"-shaped/"S"-shaped, or "F"-shaped mark is made on the stromal side of the complex using a stained stamp. After this, the DM is removed from the rest of the stroma. The DM scrolls on itself with endothelium facing outward. Barron's vacuum punch is used to cut the tissue to a desired size.[3]

Recipient Preparation

Corneal epithelium is removed with a blunt spatula for better visualization **(Fig. 1.31.2A)**. Two paracentesis are made along with a temporal clear corneal incision. The recipient DM is then scored and removed using a reverse Sinskey hook. Peripheral iridectomy is done at 6 o'clock position to prevent pupillary block. The separated DM scroll is then sucked into the DMEK injector using a no-touch technique and the DM scroll is injected into the AC. Following this it is imperative to place a 10-0 nylon suture on the main tunnel incision to secure the DM scroll in the AC. The DM scroll is positioned with injection of saline into the AC. The DM scroll is unfolded over the iris with the L mark seen upright—this confirms the correct graft orientation. Following this air bubble is injected underneath the graft to enable its adherence with the posterior stroma **(Fig. 1.31.2B)**.

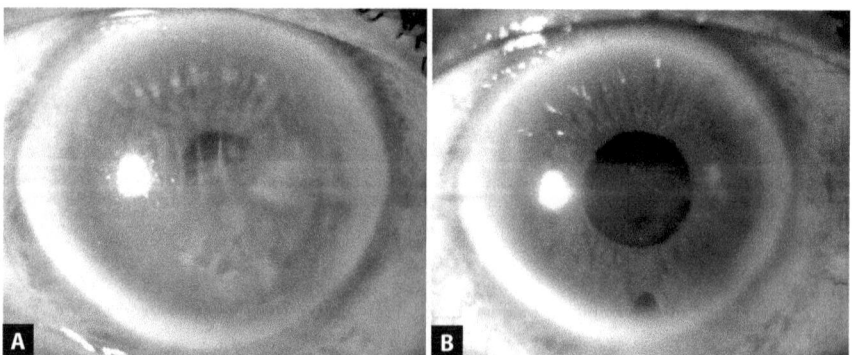

Figs. 1.31.2A and B: (A) Pseudophakic bullous keratopathy; (B) Post DMEK.

PRE-DESCEMET'S ENDOTHELIAL KERATOPLASTY

Donor Graft Preparation
A corneoscleral button with about 2 mm scleral rim is obtained for PDEK. A 5 mL syringe filled with air is attached to a 30 gauge is introduced with the bevel up from the corneoscleral rim into the midperiphery of the corneal stroma. This is followed by gentle injection of air. All the mentioned steps are done with the corneoscleral rim with endothelial side up. A pre-Descemet's bubble or a type 1 bubble is created which spreads characteristically from the center to the periphery. This bubble has a distinct edge thorough out. The cleaved posterior wall of the bubble is the donor tissue which is then trephined to a desired size.

Recipient Preparation
Preparation of the recipient eye is similar to that of DSEK and DMEK. The donor pre-Descemet's is loaded into the Busin glide with forceps or with an injector and inserted into the AC. This donor disk is unrolled with the help of air and fluidics. Similar to DMEK, the PDEK tissue also rolls with the endothelial cells on the outside of the roll. Once unfolded, an air bubble is injected under the graft to enable its adherence to the posterior stroma.[2]

CONCLUSION
Lamellar corneal transplantation offers great advantages and addresses the major risk of endothelial rejection associated with PK. In DALK, the host DM is retained thus eliminating the risk of endothelial rejection. In EK, suture-related astigmatism is eliminated aiding a fast visual recovery to all patients. Also the strength, dosage, and dependence of steroids usage are to the minimum in LK. Another advantage of LK is that it allows disease-specific approach, enabling a single corneal tissue to be used for multiple recipients. LK also needs an experienced corneal hand both during surgery and tissue separation to prevent tissue wastage. With recent modern techniques and eye bank lending support of lamellar tissues to corneal surgeons, LK will be the gold standard for disease specific corneal component surgeries.

REFERENCES
1. Moffatt SL, Cartwright VA, Stumpf TH. Centennial review of corneal transplantation. Clin Exp Ophthalmol. 2005;33:642-57.
2. Singh NP, Said DG, Dua HS. Lamellar keratoplasty techniques. Indian J Ophthalmol. 2018;66(9):1239-50.
3. Siddharthan KS, Agrawal A, Reddy JK. Four in one: Four recipients with a single donor tissue—A novel concept for eye transplantation surgery post-COVID-19. Indian J Ophthalmol. 2020;68(11):2471-4.

1.32 | Corneal Graft Infection

Anita Panda
Dr RP Centre for Ophthalmic Sciences, AIIMS, New Delhi
anitap49@yahoo.com

INTRODUCTION
Though the outcome of penetrating keratoplasty has tremendously improved in the present era, late-graft infection constitutes a significant source of morbidity, more so in developing countries, where patient compliances are very poor due to varied social, economic, and other multiple reasons. The infection in graft also induces the graft rejection besides loss of graft clarity and graft melting.

Rational and intensive medical therapy is required to reduce the graft morbidity and to improve functional status. The reported incidence of nonviral microbial graft infection following penetrating keratoplasty is 1.9–12%; and a serious problem (**Fig. 1.32.1**).

It has been divided into two types—(1) *"early"* and (2) *"late"*. "Early" infection occurs as a host disease recurrence, use of infected donor material or intraoperative contamination and the "late" infection is caused by environmental-acquired pathogens in presence of certain specific risk factors.

■ RISK FACTORS

The most common risk factor is exposed, loose or broken suture, persistent epithelial defect, severe punctate keratopathy, and use of soft contact lens wear including therapeutic lenses.

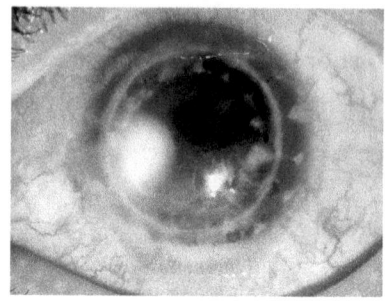

Fig. 1.32.1: Graft infection in penetrating keratoplasty.

It is a significant risk factor for infection if contact lens is used in presence of persistent epithelial defect. Other risk factors are graft hypoesthesia, keratoconjunctivitis sicca, previous herpetic disease, graft failure, and ocular and lid abnormalities. Other factors are due to contaminated donor tissue, poorly preserved donor cornea and intraoperative contamination.

■ ORGANISM INVOLVED

Staphylococcus epidermidis, Staphylococcus aureus, Streptococcus pneumoniae, Haemophilus influenzae, Moraxella, Serratia marcescens, Bacillus subtilis, Corynebacterium, etc.

■ TREATMENT

Concentrated eye drops of cefazolin (50 mg/mL) and tobramycin 14 mg/mL is effective. Treatment can be modified according to culture and sensitivity reports.

To avoid this complication donor tissue must undergo screening and all recipients should be given prophylactic subconjunctival and postoperative antibiotics. All suture removal should be done under aseptic conditions. Any wound dehiscence should be repaired immediately.

■ PREVENTION

To avoid this complication donor tissue must undergo screening and all recipients should be given prophylactic and postoperative antibiotics. Any loose or broken sutures must be taken care of.

Infectious Crystalline Keratopathy

It is a distinctive clinical condition, usually seen in grafted patient. It is an aggregate of gram-positive cocci most notably *Streptococcus viridans* in pattern of crystalline branching opacities. This is associated with long-term steroid use and the presence of epithelial defect. Its laboratory evaluation is done by corneal scraping for smear and culture and sensitivity. But lesions are very deep so it may come negative in scraping. Then corneal biopsy can be done.

Herpes Keratitis

Herpes simplex keratitis remains a frequent cause of recurrence of infection in penetrating keratoplasty. Herpes simplex keratitis can occur as a result of recurrence in patient with herpes keratitis. It occurs as a result of activation of herpes simplex virus (HSV) or by transmission of virus in the donor tissue after penetrating keratoplasty. Systemic acyclovir 400 mg twice-a-day prior to keratoplasty and then for 6 months to 1 year after surgery to prevent recurrence is recommended.

Endophthalmitis

It is a potentially devastating complication after penetrating keratoplasty and can occur in early and late postoperative period.

It is managed by taking vitreous tap for smear examination and culture and sensitivity, after confirming the infiltrates present in the vitreous, intravitreal antibiotics are given after smear and culture and sensitivity. Intensive topical therapy also started immediately.

1.33 | Graft Rejection

Jeewan S Titiyal, Ritika Sachdev
Dr RP Centre for Ophthalmic Sciences, AIIMS, New Delhi
titiyal@rediffmail.com, ritika@centreforsight.net

■ INTRODUCTION

Graft rejection refers to the immunological response of the host to the donor corneal tissue without regard to the effect of the response on graft survival.[1]

It is characterized by a period of graft clarity prior to the appearance of the signs of rejection (differentiating it from primary donor failure). Conventionally, a period of 2 weeks for a primary graft and 1 week for a regraft is taken to define graft rejection. It is possible, however, for rejection to occur prior to this time period if the host has been sensitized to the donor antigens stimulating an immune response.

Factors Responsible for the Immune Privilege of the Corneal Graft

- Corneal avascularity, believed to sequester the graft from the immune response.
- Absence of donor-derived antigen presenting Langerhans cells in the corneal graft.
- Expression of the Fas ligand on the epithelium and endothelium of the corneal allograft.
- Capacity of the allograft to induce immune deviation of the systemic response.[1]

Immune Mechanism Underlying Graft Rejection

A delayed type of hypersensitivity response is postulated in the pathogenesis of graft rejection. Production of donor-specific lymphocytotoxic antibodies is also considered to be important, resulting in antibody-dependent complement-mediated cell lysis.

■ RISK FACTORS FOR GRAFT REJECTION

Age of Donor and Recipient

- Younger patients are more prone to develop rejection due to their more active immune system.
- Donor age >50 years has also been known to increase the risk of graft rejection.

Previous Graft Failure

A regraft is always more prone to failure due to sensitization of the host to alloantigens.

Vascularization

Deep vascularization is more significant than superficial vascularization and is one of the most important risk factors for rejection.

Vascularization in the cornea may be graded as:
- *Grade I:* Only superficial
- *Grade II:* Superficial (2 quadrants) + deep (1 quadrant)
- *Grade III:* Deep 2 quadrants
- *Grade IV:* Extensive and deep.

Graft Size and Eccentricity
Proximity to the limbal vasculature in cases with large or eccentric grafts makes them more prone to develop rejection.

Donor Tissue
Due to higher concentration of human leukocyte antigen (HLA) in the epithelium, it was proposed that the debrided grafts could be better tolerated. This, however, was associated with persistent epithelial defects, which again compromise graft survival. Primary donor graft failure is defined as cornea edema that persists and fails to clear from the immediate postoperative period. This is due to either inherent deficiencies in the donor graft, surgical trauma, or in some cases an improperly stored tissue.

Blood Transfusions
Graft rejections have been reported after massive blood transfusions.

ROLE OF IMMUNE TYPING BEFORE PENETRATING KERATOPLASTY
The Collaborative Corneal Transplantation Study (CCTS) explored the role of immune typing in high-risk cases (defined as corneal vascularization in more than two quadrants or cases with a prior history of graft rejection).

The CCTS demonstrated that for high-risk patients receiving postoperative topical steroid therapy **(Flowchart 1.33.1)**:
- Neither HLA-A, -B or -DR antigen matching substantially reduced the likelihood of corneal graft failure.
- A positive donor recipient cross match did not increase the risk of corneal graft failure.
- ABO blood matching may be effective in reducing the risk of graft failure from rejection.

Graft Rejection pertaining to Endothelial Keratoplasty
Descemet Stripping Endothelial Keratoplasty (DSEK) has a mean endothelial rejection rate of 10% and Descemet membrane endothelial keratoplasty (DMEK) has a low mean rejection rate of 1.9%.

CLINICAL FEATURES OF GRAFT REJECTION

Evaluation
- *Specular microscopy:* Can be used to evaluate the donor endothelium preoperatively. Postoperatively also it helps to assess and follow-up the endothelial cell count.
- *Anterior segment optical coherence tomography:* Helps to evaluate the corneal thickness, level of stromal scarring, thinning and graft attachment in DSEK and DMEK.

Symptoms
Usual symptoms of graft rejection are a period of clear vision after keratoplasty followed by sudden onset of decreased vision, irritation, redness, photophobia, and watering.

Signs
Clinically graft rejection may present as:
- *Epithelial rejection (10–14%):*
  - Characterized by an elevated-epithelial rejection line which stains with fluorescein or rose Bengal.
  - It begins in the periphery and progresses across the graft, representing a zone of destruction of epithelial cells.
  - Corneal thickness is not increased.

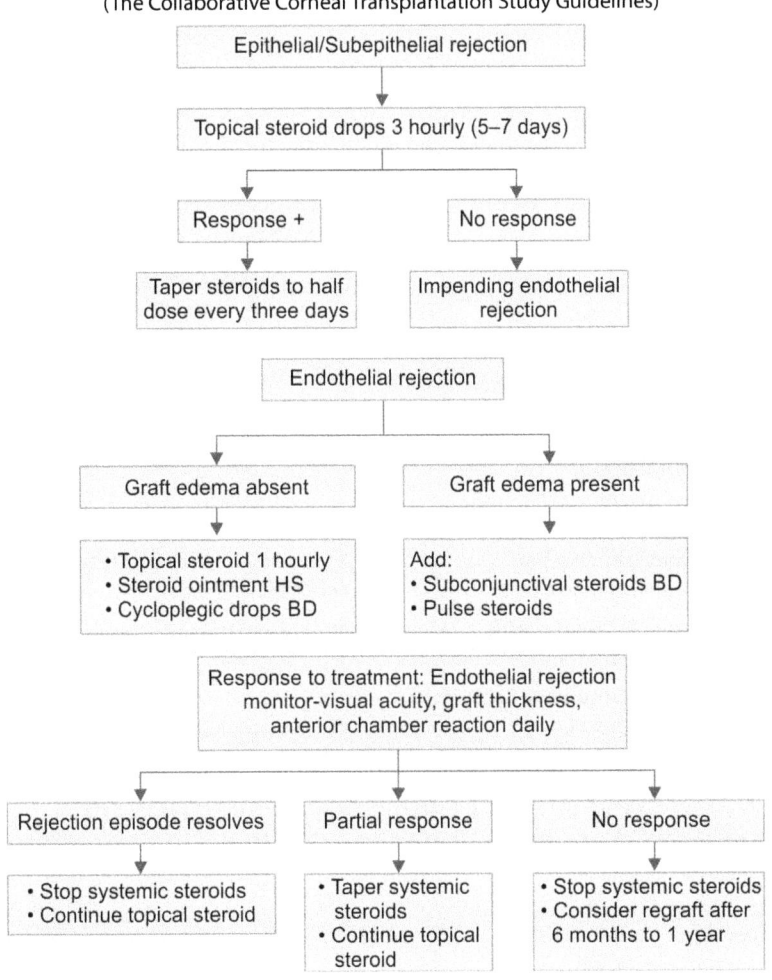

Flowchart 1.33.1: Treatment of graft rejection. (The Collaborative Corneal Transplantation Study Guidelines)

- The eye may be quiet or mildly inflamed.
- The new epithelial cells from the host fill-up the defect produced by the destruction of the epithelial cells.
- *Subepithelial infiltrates (2.4–15%):* Known as Kaye's dots, they are white infiltrates, 0.2–0.5 mm in diameter, seen in the donor tissue beneath the Bowman's membrane, usually close to a loose suture. Patients are often asymptomatic.
- *Stromal rejection:* Presence of full-thickness stromal haze which is sudden in onset in a previously clear graft is characteristic of stromal rejection. Patient may report a sudden decrease in vision. Stromal rejection is rarely seen alone in patients.
- *Endothelial rejection:* It may present as:
  - *Khodadoust line:*
    - Usually originates at a vascularized area of the peripheral donor cornea, or at junction of anterior synechiae with endothelium **(Fig. 1.33.1)**.
    - It advances across the cornea leaving behind damaged endothelium and pigmented keratic precipitates.

- *Diffuse endothelial rejection:*
  - Consists of keratic precipitates throughout the donor endothelium with diffuse stromal edema, Descemet's folds and anterior chamber reaction.
  - The development of an allograft rejection episode is accompanied by an increase in corneal thickness of at least 10%.

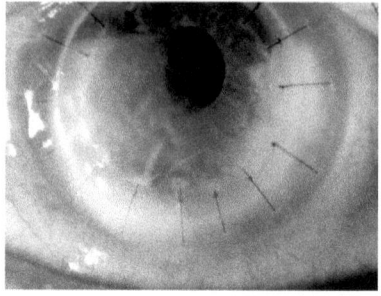

Fig. 1.33.1: Graft rejection (endothelial)—Khodadoust line.

Drugs Recommended by the CCTS

- *Topical steroid drops:* Prednisolone acetate 1%/difluprednate
- *Topical steroid ointment:* Dexamethasone
- *Subconjunctival steroid:* Dexamethasone
- *Pulse steroid:* Intravenous methyl prednisolone 125–500 mg single dose

Role of Cyclosporine

Treatment with specific T-cell immunosuppressant, cyclosporine, may be considered in:
- High-risk grafts
- Repeat episodes of rejection
- One-eyed patients, particularly with large or eccentric grafts

Oral cyclosporine: 8–15 mg/kg/day; monitor liver, kidney functions, and blood counts weekly. Topical 2% cyclosporine in olive oil.

Novel methods of cyclosporine delivery:
- Poly (lactide-co-glycolide polymer placed in anterior chamber
- Subconjunctival cyclosporine in microspheres

NEW AND EXPERIMENTAL DRUGS FOR PREVENTION OR TREATMENT OF CORNEAL GRAFT REJECTION

- Tacrolimus (FK 506)
- Anti-CD 154 monoclonal antibody
- Rapamycin
- Anti-interferon gamma antibody
- Interleukin (IL-2) receptor monoclonal antibody
- CTL A4-immunoglobulin
- Platelet-activating factor antagonists

DIFFERENTIAL DIAGNOSIS OF GRAFT REJECTION

- Sterile or infectious endophthalmitis
- Recurrence of herpetic eye disease in graft
- Late failure due to endothelial cell loss

REFERENCE

1. Panda A, Vanathi M, Kumar A, Dash Y, Priya S. Corneal graft rejection. Surv Ophthalmol. 2007;52(4):375-96.

1.34 | Episcleritis

Saurabh Sanyal
Citizens Eye and Health Care Hospital, Serampore
drsanyal@yahoo.co.in

■ INTRODUCTION
Episcleritis is a mild, self-limiting, and recurrent inflammatory condition of episcleral tissue that lies between conjunctiva and sclera. Most cases are idiopathic, up to one-third have a systemic association. It is more common in females and most common in fourth and sixth decades of life.

Pathophysiology
The inflammatory response is localized to the superficial episcleral vascular network and histopathology shows nongranulomatous inflammation with vascular dilatation and perivascular infiltrates.

Causes
Most cases are idiopathic; however, up to one-third cases are associated with systemic conditions such as rheumatoid arthritis, systemic lupus erythematosus, polyarteritis nodosa, ankylosing spondylosis, inflammatory bowel disease, and gout. Infectious diseases such as tuberculosis, Lyme disease, syphilis, and herpes virus may be associated.

■ CLINICAL FEATURES
Two clinical types are simple and nodular. Simple episcleritis is the most common type presented as intermittent bouts of moderate to severe inflammation. Each episode resolves within 2–3 weeks. Nodular episcleritis have prolonged attacks of inflammation, typically more painful and many are associated with systemic diseases.

Symptoms
Symptoms include acute onset of redness and discomfort. Watery discharge photophobia may be associated. Pain may be present but usually mild.

Signs
The most common signs include localized area of injection of bulbar conjunctiva and freely moveable nodule in nodular episcleritis. Corneal dellen formation as well as peripheral corneal infiltrates may be present. Approximately 10% patients are associated with anterior uveitis.

Complications
Corneal dellen (adjacent to an episcleral nodule) and peripheral corneal infiltrates (adjacent to episcleral inflammation) are the most common complications.

Cataracts and glaucoma could be related to steroid use as part of the management of episcleritis.

■ DIFFERENTIAL DIAGNOSIS
Viral Conjunctivitis
Superior Limbic Keratoconjunctivitis
Scleritis: In scleritis pain is deep, severe, and often radiates toward ipsilateral side of head and face. The sclera may have a bluish hue when observed in natural light; the scleral vessels do not blanch on topical application of 2.5% phenylephrine as seen in episcleritis. Corneal involvement is present as adjacent stromal keratitis is common in scleritis.

LABORATORY INVESTIGATIONS

In most cases with mild self-limiting disease, laboratory studies are not useful. In selected cases, serum uric acid, complete blood count (CBC), erythrocyte sedimentation rate (ESR), antinuclear antibody, rheumatoid factor, venereal disease research laboratory (VDRL), fluorescent treponemal antibody absorption (FTA-ABS), and chest X-ray may be indicated.

MANAGEMENT

- Episcleritis is a self-limiting disease resolves without any permanent damage to the eye. Therefore, most of the cases will not require any treatment.
- Ocular drug therapy may be indicated in cases with prolonged nonresolving situations and in nodular episcleritis.
- Tear substitute and topical corticosteroids and topical are usually used. In milder cases, fluorometholone 0.1% or loteprednol 0.5% may be sufficient. Topical ophthalmic 0.5% prednisolone, 0.1% dexamethasone, or 0.1% betamethasone may be used in more resistant cases.

1.35 | Scleritis

Rupesh V Agrawal
LV Prasad Eye Institute, Hyderabad
rupeshagrawal@lvpei.org

INTRODUCTION

Scleritis is a much more severe ocular inflammation than episcleritis. Scleritis causes pain, may lead to structural alterations of the globe, has a risk of visual morbidity, and is associated with an underlying systemic immunologic disease in the majority of cases. It occurs most often in the second to sixth decades of life and is significantly more common in women. Scleritis is bilateral in more than half of the cases.

CLINICAL FEATURES

The onset of scleritis is usually gradual, extending over several days. Most patients with scleritis develop severe boring (piercing) ocular pain, which may occasionally worsen at night and awaken them from sleep. The pain may be referred to other regions of the head on the involved side. The globe is often tender to touch. Clinical signs aid in diagnosis of scleritis. In scleritis, the sclera assumes a violaceous hue in natural sunlight. It is very essential to examine the patient with suspicion of episcleritis versus scleritis in bright sunlight. Inflamed scleral vessels have a crisscross pattern, are adherent to the sclera, and cannot be moved with a cotton-tipped applicator. Scleral edema often with overlying episcleral edema is noted by slit lamp examination.

DIFFERENT TYPES OF NONINFECTIOUS SCLERITIS

- *Nodular scleritis:* Deep-red to purple immobile scleral nodule.
- *Diffuse anterior scleritis:* Portion of sclera is involved.
- *Necrotizing scleritis:* Patients typically present with severe pain out of proportion to inflammatory signs. Most commonly, a localized patch of inflammation is noted initially, with the edges of the lesion more inflamed than the center. Severe loss of tissue may result if treatment is not intensive and prompt. The sclera may have a blue-gray appearance and show an altered deep episcleral blood vessel pattern after the inflammation subsides.

Scleromalacia perforans, i.e., necrotizing scleritis without signs of inflammation occur predominantly in patients with long-standing rheumatoid arthritis (55% of cases). There are minimal signs of inflammation and generally no pain accompanying this type of scleritis because of destruction of nerves secondary to inflammation.

- *Posterior scleritis:* Patients presents with severe pain, tenderness, proptosis, visual loss, and occasionally restricted motility. Choroidal folds, exudative retinal detachment (RD), papilledema, and angle closure glaucoma secondary to choroidal thickening may develop.

Presence of T-sign on ultrasound B-scan, i.e., fluid in Tenon's sheath around optic nerve is one of the pathognomonic sign of posterior scleritis.

COMPLICATIONS OF SCLERITIS

Corneal changes—segmental anesthesia; acute stromal infiltrates; sclerosing keratitis; limbal guttering; and keratolysis.

Increased scleral transparency and thinning but rarely ever perforate uveitis—anterior, intermediate or posterior—30-35%; cataract—3-4%; glaucoma—especially in limbitis—12-15%; RD—exudative in cases with posterior scleritis; optic nerve head (ONH) swelling and macular edema—both in posterior scleritis; and ectasia with staphyloma.

Infectious Scleritis

This may be bacterial, viral (herpes zoster), fungal, protozoal, or parasitic. Acute infections are mostly by bacteria (staphylococci, *Pseudomonas, and Proteus*). Such processes usually are accompanied by conjunctivitis with purulent exudate. Deep bacterial infiltrates in the presence of scleral necrosis may involve the vitreous. In these cases, gram-negative organisms tend to be present. Staphylococci also can cause chronic infections, with the formation of granulomas or fistulas. Painful nodules may be seen, or conjunctival and scleral ulcers.

The edges of scleritis will give important diagnostic clue. In infectious scleritis, they may be more yellowish-white as against the noninfectious scleritis where they will be more whitish and avascular. Scrapings from this edge can give us clue about the microorganisms present, negative scraping with nonresolving nature of scleritis with high-index of suspicion should prompt one to go for sclera de roofing or scleral biopsy to look for infective microorganism.

SURGICALLY-INDUCED NECROTIZING SCLERITIS

It is a rare complication of ocular surgery. Mostly seen after cataract surgery, but may also be seen after glaucoma, RD, squint, or even pterygium surgery.

It may occur from few days to few decades after surgery. It is consistently seen around the site of the surgical wound on the sclera. The etiology is unknown, but more than half have an underlying autoimmune disorder or metabolic disorders such as diabetes mellitus and dysthyroid status.

Unlike other forms of scleritis, surgically-induced necrotizing scleritis (SINS) is mostly necrotizing in nature and may even be the initial manifestation of serious systemic disease. Thus, all the patients of SINS need to be investigated appropriately. Treatment is very difficult and protracted. Systemic steroids remain the mainstay. They do not respond to nonsteroidal anti-inflammatory drugs (NSAIDs). Pulse intravenous methylprednisolone followed by high-dose corticosteroids along with immunosuppressive agents forms the mainstay of therapy. In severe and rapidly progressive cases, cyclophosphamide is the drug of choice. Even cyclosporine is reported to be effective.

WORK-UP

The work-up of scleritis should include a complete physical examination, with attention to the joints, skin, and cardiovascular and respiratory system. The following laboratory tests are recommended:
- Complete blood count (CBC) with differential and erythrocyte sedimentation rate (ESR)
- Serum antibody screen [antinuclear antibodies, anti-deoxyribonucleic acid (DNA) antibodies, and rheumatoid factors]

- Antineutrophil cytoplasmic antibodies (ANCAs) in cases with bilateral necrotizing scleritis
- Chest X-ray and Mantoux test

Additional laboratory tests may be indicated based on the clinical findings.

■ TREATMENT

Diffuse and Nodular Scleritis

Systemic NSAID—sustained-release indomethacin 75 mg bid. In case of therapeutic failure, high doses of systemic steroids should be given early (oral prednisone 1–1.5 mg/kg/day) tapering slowly every week. When the response is unsatisfactory, methotrexate (7.5–15 mg once weekly) or azathioprine (2 mg/kg/day) should be considered, particularly in patients with systemic lupus erythematosus (SLE). Cyclophosphamide (1–2 mg/kg/day) is mandatory in Wegener's granulomatosis and in polyarteritis nodosa.

Subconjunctival injections of steroids are contraindicated in necrotizing scleritis because of the risk of scleral melting and perforation.

Necrotizing Scleritis

Only its early stages are amenable to medical treatment (i.e., prior to the advent of necrosis, which begins as yellowish avascular nodules). Short-term therapy with methylprednisolone is given as intravenous pulse therapy. Immunosuppressive therapy with cytotoxic drugs is usually required, and the treatment of choice for necrotizing scleritis includes cyclophosphamide (1–2 mg/kg/day), azathioprine (1–2 mg/kg/day), and methotrexate (7.5–15 mg once per week). Wearing of protective goggles is advisable when the sclera is thin. In all cases, consultation with a rheumatologist is advisable. In extreme thinning scleral patch-graft may be done.

Treatment of Infective Scleritis

Intensive antibiotic therapy (topical and systemic) is usually required. *Acanthamoeba* scleritis tends to have a poor prognosis. Any foreign body, either accidentally or surgically introduced, may need to be removed before the infection can be brought under control. *Mycobacterium tuberculosis* is commonly associated with infective scleritis and biopsy of scleral nodule may be necessary to confirm the diagnosis.

Recurrent bilateral scleritis is a serious condition and collaboration with internist/rheumatologist is essential to titrate systemic immunomodulating agents.

SECTION 2

Dry Eye and Ocular Surface

Editor: Somasheila I Murthy

2.1 **Cicatricial Conjunctivitis** 74
    Namrata Sharma, Ritika Sachdev
2.2 **Ocular Surface Squamous Neoplasia** 75
    Anirban Bhaduri
2.3 **Pterygium** 77
    Srinivas K Rao
2.4 **Chemical Injury** 78
    R Revathi

2.1 Cicatricial Conjunctivitis

Namrata Sharma, Ritika Sachdev
Dr RP Centre for Ophthalmic Sciences, AIIMS, New Delhi
namrata.sharma@gmail.com, ritika@centreforsight.net

■ DEFINITION AND ETIOLOGY

Cicatricial conjunctivitis is defined as a chronic progressive ocular affection that produces scarring of the conjunctiva primarily and the cornea sequentially.

Chronic cicatricial conjunctivitis may have varied etiologies according to which it can be grouped into the following broad categories.

Infectious

Chlamydia trachomatis is the most common form of conjunctival scarring worldwide. Some degree of scarring may also occur in cases of *Staphylococcal* blepharitis.

Traumatic

Scarring may follow thermal, chemical, radiation, or surgical trauma. Bilateral cicatricial conjunctivitis has been reported in a patient with psychiatric disturbance (obsessive-compulsive disorder), secondary to self-inflicted trauma.

Immunological

It includes acquired oculocutaneous disorders such as Stevens–Johnson syndrome, cicatricial pemphigoid, erythema multiforme, toxic epidermal necrolysis, dermatitis herpetiformis, linear immunoglobulin A (IgA) disease, chronic atopic keratoconjunctivitis, and porphyria cutanea tarda. Bullous pemphigoid and pemphigus vulgaris are less commonly associated with conjunctival scarring.

- *Ocular cicatricial pemphigoid (OCP):* Usually seen in older women (>60 years), may involve any skin or mucosal surface. The inflammatory response is considered to be initiated by the immunoglobulin or complement components deposited along the basement membrane. Demonstration of the antibasement membrane antibodies by direct immunofluorescence establishes the diagnosis.
- *Stevens–Johnson syndrome, erythema multiforme, and toxic epidermal necrolysis:* These occur in younger patients and are thought to represent the spectrum of a single disease process. These conditions usually have an acute-onset following drug intake or infection.
- *Chronic graft versus host disease:* Ocular graft versus host disease is a common sequela of allogenic hematopoietic transplantation, affecting up to 80% of the chronic graft versus host disease patients.

Drug-induced

Conjunctival cicatrization may occur following systemic (e.g., penicillamine) and topical therapy (described with pilocarpine, adrenaline, timolol, gentamicin, and idoxuridine) use.

Miscellaneous

Inherited conditions like ectodermal dysplasia may present with conjunctival scarring. Cicatricial conjunctivitis may also be a manifestation of a paraneoplastic syndrome.

■ TREATMENT

The treatment entails correction of the etiological agent causing the scarring and correction of the scarring and its sequelae itself.

Infective conjunctivitis is treated with appropriate antibiotics.

Cases with definitely diagnosed active and progressive cicatricial pemphigoid merit treatment with dapsone [exclude sulfa allergy or glucose-6-phosphate dehydrogenase (G6PD) deficiency]. If the response is incomplete, daily azathioprine or weekly methotrexate are added to the regimen.

Patients who fail to respond to this regimen are treated with high-dose systemic prednisone and either daily oral cyclophosphamide or once-monthly intravenous pulse cyclophosphamide. As the inflammation subsides, the therapy is appropriately tapered. Cyclosporine has been found to be ineffective in treatment of OCP.

Continued small trials suggest some role for the expensive intravenous immunoglobulin therapy in OCP where conventional treatment fails. Other agents which have been used for treatment of OCP include oral tacrolimus (FK506), mycophenolate mofetil, and subconjunctival mitomycin. An ongoing trial is evaluating the role of rituximab—a genetically engineered anti-CD20 antibody—in the treatment of OCP.

Topical antibiotic and corticosteroids are commonly used in the acute phase of Stevens-Johnson syndrome. The role of systemic steroids remains controversial.
- *Surgical* correction of lid margin anomalies, trichiasis, and a dry ocular surface should be delayed till the disease is quiescent as surgery may accentuate the conjunctival scarring. Electrolysis, cryoablation, and marginal lid rotation have been used with variable success for treatment of the aberrant lashes. Keratinized posterior lid margin may respond to treatment with topical retinoids.
- *Supportive measures* for treatment of dry eye include tear substitutes (preservative-free), punctal occlusion, and tarsorrhaphy.
- *Ocular surface reconstruction* in severe cases may require surgical measures including amniotic membrane transplant, conjunctival graft, mucous membrane transplant, limbal stem cell transplantation, and penetrating keratoplasty. The outcome of corneal grafts, however, remains dismal. The postoperative course is often complicated with persistent epithelial defects, stromal ulceration, and perforation.
- *Scleral lens therapy* for protection from aberrant lids and lashes and for retention of the precorneal tear film may be useful in chronic cases and for postoperative protection of limbal or corneal transplants.
- *Keratoprosthesis* may be required in severe cases, and may be the only realistic hope for any visual rehabilitation.

2.2 Ocular Surface Squamous Neoplasia

Anirban Bhaduri
Suryadoy Eye Centre, Kolkata
dra_bhaduri@yahoo.co.in

■ INTRODUCTION

Ocular surface squamous neoplasia (OSSN) is an inclusive term that describes the entire spectrum of squamous neoplastic disease from dysplasias to carcinoma in situ and invasive squamous cell carcinoma.

The OSSN is usually associated with old age, ultraviolet (UV-B) exposure, males, and human papillomavirus (HPV) infection. Rule out immune suppression and xeroderma pigmentosum in the young and children.

■ RELEVANT CLINICAL FEATURES

The OSSN usually appear as raised, pearly-gray or pink, and well-demarcated mass with feeder vessels. It usually arises from the limbus, most often within the palpebral fissure. However, lesions may occur elsewhere on the conjunctiva. Patients may be asymptomatic or may have local symptoms or notice a growth **(Fig. 2.2.1)**.

These tumors have a variety of morphological appearances:
- Placoid lesions—gelatinous, papilliform, leukoplakic, and velvety
- Nodular
- Diffuse—which mimics chronic conjunctivitis

CLINICAL FEATURES

The slit-lamp examination findings are:
- Fine keratin nodules
- Intrinsic tumor vessels
- Dilated feeder vessels leading to the mass
- Rose Bengal or Lissamine green staining helps to delineate the extent of the tumor.

Some tumors may be pigmented. Pure corneal OSSN is rare and appears as a nebular opacity with fimbriated edges.

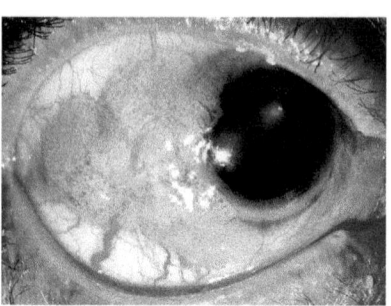

Fig. 2.2.1: Ocular surface squamous neoplasia (OSSN)—large feeder vessels.

DIFFERENTIAL DIAGNOSIS

- *OSSN mimics the following conditions:* Pterygium, pinguecula, hyperkeratotic plaque, Bitot spot, chronic conjunctivitis, episcleritis, and necrotizing scleritis.
- *Other tumors:* Epibulbar choristoma, complex choristoma, pagetoid sebaceous gland carcinoma, amelanotic and melanotic nevi, and melanoma.

TREATMENT

Surgery

Surgical excision with wide margins and edge cryotherapy is the treatment of choice (lowest recurrence rate at 7%). Avoid touching the tumor.
- The conjunctiva is incised 3–4 mm beyond visible tumor. This along with episcleral tissues is dissected en bloc up to the limbus.
- Absolute alcohol is applied to the corneal edge and the epithelium is rolled-off toward limbus. The lesion is then excised by sharp dissection at the limbus.
- The excised tissue is mounted on filter paper after proper orientation for histopathology examination.
- Double quick-freeze-slow-thaw cryotherapy is done to the conjunctival edges.
- Lamellar sclerectomy or keratectomy is performed, along with base cryotherapy if there is scleral or corneal fixity.
- Small wounds are closed with direct repair, but larger wounds need an amniotic membrane graft.

Enucleation with en bloc excision of the conjunctival mass is needed when intraocular invasion is present. Lid-sparing exenteration is done for orbital invasion.

Topical Chemotherapy

- Mitomycin C (MMC) drops are used in corneal OSSN, diffuse OSSN, small recurrences, and an adjuvant in patients with edge-positive for dysplastic disease or carcinoma in situ. MMC (0.04%) eye drops is qid 4 days a week for 4 weeks. Cycles may be repeated after an interval of 2 weeks.
- Topical MMC causes irritation and congestion, but symptoms reduce after cessation of therapy.
- Other topical medications used are 1% 5-FU and interferon $\alpha 2b$.

Radiotherapy

Plaque brachytherapy (ruthenium-106) is useful in treating residual disease where deep sclerocorneal invasion precludes complete excision. A dose of 29–33 Gy is recommended.

FOLLOW-UP

After initial surgery, patients are followed up every 3 months for a year, 6 months for the next 3 years, and then annually. The patients are observed for tumor recurrence, appearance of new tumors, especially at sites of actinic keratosis and lymph node metastasis. Most recurrences occur in the first 2 years.

SPECIAL NOTES

- Patients with pharmacological immunosuppression, human immunodeficiency virus/acquired immunodeficiency syndrome (HIV/AIDS), and xeroderma pigmentosum present at younger age. They often have multifocal, bilateral, and aggressive tumors.
- Aggressive invasive and metastatic behavior is also seen in some rare variants of OSSN—mucoepidermoid carcinoma, spindle cell carcinoma, and adenoid squamous carcinoma.

2.3 Pterygium

Srinivas K Rao
Darshan Eye Hospital, Chennai
srinikrao@gmail.com

INTRODUCTION

A pterygium is traditionally described as a wing-shaped encroachment of the conjunctiva onto the cornea. It is often seen in people who live in tropical climates and hence ultraviolet has been strongly implicated in its causation. However, the reasons for its occurrence in certain individuals and the predilection for the nasal quadrant indicate that other factors are involved in the pathogenesis. The parts of a pterygium include the head on the cornea, the neck at the limbus, and the body, on the bulbar surface of the globe.

PRESENTATION

It can result in irritation and redness, and the patient may suffer from poor vision, either due to induced astigmatism (often with-the-rule) or due to involvement of the visual axis. Cosmetic disfigurement and occasional risk of malignant transformation are other reasons for surgical removal of this lesion. Although the majority of pterygia are idiopathic, they sometimes result from damage to the peripheral cornea, and are termed pseudopterygia, as they are in reality, symblepharon formation.

DIFFERENTIAL DIAGNOSIS

In distinguishing true from pseudopterygia, factors considered important are—location, since pseudopterygia can occur along any meridian of the cornea; shape, pseudopterygia often lack the triangular shape of true pterygia and tend to be more rectangular; finally the classical sign of being able to pass a probe under the body of a pseudopterygium at the limbus is not always seen. Although most pterygia have a single head, sometimes two-headed pterygia can be seen, as also lesions involving 180° of the limbus.

It is important for the clinician to distinguish active, progressing lesions from inactive ones. This will help in the decision to surgically remove these lesions—a process that should not be attempted lightly, since recurrent pterygia tend to be more aggressive and spread faster than the primary lesion. Signs of active pterygia include a fleshy, vascular appearance, poor visualization of the underlying sclera, and the presence of white subepithelial fibrotic lesions at the head of the pterygium-called Fuchs' spots. On the contrary, inactive lesions tend to be thin and atrophic and there is often a pigment line at the head—Stocker's line.

MANAGEMENT

If surgery is decided upon, the procedure to be avoided is bare sclera excision—since complications abound with this procedure including a recurrence rate of 70-90% and a high risk of granuloma formation. The ideal procedures include the use of a free-conjunctival or conjunctival-limbal autograft, the use of intraoperative 0.02% mitomycin C application for 2-3 minutes, or a combination of the two. Varied results have been reported with the use of amniotic membrane transplants, but recurrence rates tend to be higher than with the previous two approaches, and this is best used when extensive conjunctival loss is present. The main problem with the autograft method is the conjunctival disturbance that is created can affect the success of future glaucoma surgery and the time required for the procedure. One can use inferior conjunctiva to preserve the superior bulbar surface for future glaucoma surgery, in case such surgery is required in the future. The time for surgery can be reduced by using fibrin glue to stick the autograft in place. The use of mitomycin is safe if the treated sclera is covered with vascularized tissue. Otherwise, the risks of long-term complications like scleral thinning and melting have been reported.

SPECIAL NOTES

A pterygium is a common problem in India. It is not difficult to diagnose, and the treatment is surgery. While good outcomes are obtained with today's techniques, there have been reports of complications including, infection, granuloma formation, globe perforation during anesthesia, rectus muscle damage and recurrence, and hence the procedure should not be taken lightly.

2.4 Chemical Injury

R Revathi
Aravind Eye Hospital, Coimbatore
revathi@cbe.aravind.org

SOURCES

- *Alkali injuries:* Household cleaners, bleaches, and construction components **(Fig. 2.4.1)**
- *Acids:* Assaults and industrial accidents **(Fig. 2.4.2)**
- *Thermal injuries:* Hot metals or kitchen accidents

SEVERITY

It depends on:
- Penetration—alkalis penetrate deeper
- Concentration of the compound
- Surface area of contact
- Duration of contact.

PATHOPHYSIOLOGY

It depends on depth of penetration:
- OH/H—cell membrane disruption
- Corneal and conjunctival epithelial loss
- Vascular endothelial damage leads on to ischemia
- Lens epithelium—cataract
- Ciliary epithelium—reduced ascorbate secretion in aqueous

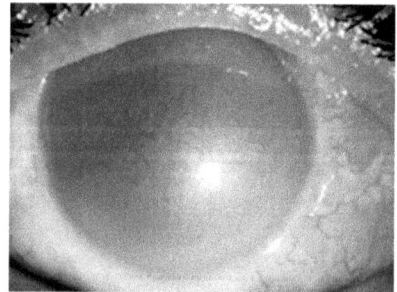

Fig. 2.4.1: Alkali burn with limbal ischemia.

- Cations—damages collagen and glycos-aminoglycan (GAG)
- Episclera—conjunctival scarring
- Corneal basement membrane—affects epithelial healing
- Stroma—scarring
- Trabecular meshwork—glaucoma

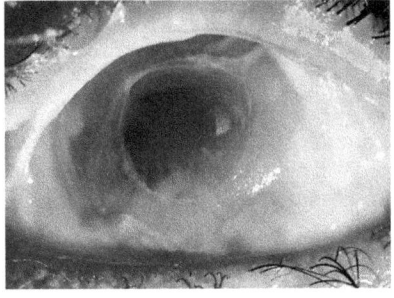

Fig. 2.4.2: Acid burn.

Conjunctival Healing
- Conjunctival healing—epithelium heals from adjacent cells or stem cells from fornices stromal involvement—fibroblastic proliferation—symblepharon
- Episcleral vascular involvement—scleral ischemia and melt

Corneal Epithelial Healing
- Small defect from adjacent cell proliferation
- Large defect from limbal stem cell proliferation and centripetal movement of corneal epithelial cells
- Localized stem cell defect—circumferential movement of stem cells to re-establish barrier
- Large stem cell defect—loss of microenvironment—limbal cell movement slow, conjunctival cells reach limbus and cross over corneal surface—unstable epithelium with goblet cells and vessels. Epithelial regeneration is slowed by:
  - Inflammation
  - Basement membrane damage
  - Stem cell damage

  Epithelial regeneration is enhanced by:
  - Lubrication
  - Controlling inflammation
  - Basement membrane and stem cell restoration

Corneal Stromal Healing
- Stromal edema and keratocyte loss—haze
- Keratocyte repopulation followed by collagen synthesis—ascorbate helps in collagen synthesis
- Type 1 collagenase secreted by keratocytes and polymorphonuclear neutrophils (PMN)—stromal melt
- Epithelial cytokines inhibit type 1 collagenase—early epithelial healing will prevent stromal melt

■ MANAGEMENT
- In acute phase—to promote healing and reduce scarring—mostly medical
- Chronic phase—to restore normal ocular surface and corneal clarity—mostly surgical

Management—Immediate
Prevent Further Damage
- Profuse irrigation—for 20-30 minutes with Ringer Lactate (RL) or any clean water
- Examination under anesthesia and under microscope
- Meticulous removal of all embedded chemical material
- Debride all necrotic tissue

Prevent Infection
Antibiotic prophylaxis four to six times, broad-spectrum, and epithelium friendly.

Control Inflammation
Steroids are the mainstay of therapy as they will not interfere with re-epithelialization and will reduce cellular infiltration and fibrosis. However after second week, may interfere with collagen synthesis—cautious use.

To Promote Epithelial Healing
- Profuse lubrication—preservative free
- Autologous serum—provides growth factors, collagenase inhibitors, retinoic acid, and fibronectin

To Promote Stromal Healing
- Systemic ascorbate—up to 1,000 mg QID
- Doxycycline 100 mg BD—chelate zinc which is necessary for collagenase
- Sodium citrate 10% topical—stabilize PMN and reduce collagenase release
- Citrate and ascorbate—used together to reduce the incidence of stromal ulceration to 4.6% compared to 80% in Grade 3 burns
- Grades 1 and 2—multiple drug therapy can hinder reepithelialization by preservative toxicity.

To Prevent Adhesion
- Coating the raw surface with sodium hyaluronate
- Bandage contact lens (BCL)—risk of infection is there. *Amniotic membrane transplantation* (AMT) will act as biological BCL.

SURGICAL PROCEDURES
- Perilimbal ischemia episcleral mobilization will restore limbal vasculature AMT to cover denuded areas and to promote epithelial healing
- Role of AMT and limbal stem cell grafting
- Immediate stage—biological drape to reduce inflammation, adhesions, infection, and scarring
- Intermediate period—bone marrow (BM) and progenitor cell replacement to achieve normal healing
- Late rehabilitation—to remove scar tissue and get normal ocular surface

SPECIAL NOTES
Surgical interventions like AMT are done in acute phases in Grade 2 or 3 cases. Grade 4 needs episcleral mobilization first. In severe burns repeated-AMT may be needed in addition to punctal occlusion to improve lubrication and tarsorrhaphy to facilitate epithelialization on an anesthetic cornea. Limbal stem cell transplantation can be done as autograft in less severe uniocular cases but in Grade 3 cases, it should be reserved as late rehabilitative procedure. In Grade 4 uniocular injuries and bilateral injuries simple limbal epithelial transplantation (SLET) is preferable.

SECTION 3

Cataract

Editors: Jeewan S Titiyal, Sridevi Nair

3.1 Risk Factors for Age-related Cataract 83
SK Gupta

3.2 How do You Grade Age-related Cataract? 84
Gagandeep Singh Brar

3.3 Preoperative Evaluation of Patients with Age-related Cataract 86
Sudesh Kumar Arya

3.4 Macular Function Tests for Patients Undergoing Cataract Surgery 88
Lingam Gopal

3.5 Informed Consent for Cataract Surgery with or without Implantation of an Intraocular Lens 91
Arun K Jain

3.6 How do You Counsel Amblyopic Adult with Cataract before Surgery? 95
Jaspreet Singh Sukhija

3.7 Sterilization of Operating Room 96
Jagat Ram, Sunil Kumar

3.8 Antibiotic Prophylaxis after Cataract Surgery 99
Sushmita Kaushik, Parul Ichhpujani

3.9 What is the Role of Nonsteroidal Anti-inflammatory Drugs in Patients Undergoing Cataract Surgery? 102
Rupal H Trivedi

3.10 Anesthesia for Cataract Surgery 104
Sunil Kumar, Saurabh Saveria

3.11 Phacodynamics 107
Noshir M Shroff, Haripriya Aravind

3.12 What is Torsional Phacoemulsification and its Advantage? 111
Rohit Om Parkash

3.13 Viscoelastics in Phacoemulsification Surgery 112
Jeewan S Titiyal

3.14 Phaco Incision 116
Ravijit Singh

3.15 How to Proceed if Clear Corneal Incision is Ragged and Incompetent? 118
Arup Chakrabarti

3.16 What are the Various Means of Doing Anterior Capsulotomy? 119
Rupal H Trivedi

3.17 How do You Deal with Hard Cataracts during Phacoemulsification? 122
Rohit Om Parkash

3.18 Zero/Minimal Power Phaco 123
Gaurav Luthra

3.19 What are the Causes of Shallowing of Anterior Chamber during Phaco? How to Prevent it? 126
Cyres K Mehta

3.20 Management of Subluxated Cataract 127
Rajiv Choudhary

3.21 The Capsular Bag is Unexpectedly Mobile during Phaco. How to Manage with a Capsular Tension Ring? 129
Tanuj Dada, Vivek Dave

3.22 How will You Manage a Patient of Visually Significant Cataract with Associated Keratoconus? 131
Sudhank Bharti

3.23 Phaco in High Myopia 133
Sudarshan Khokhar

3.24 Posterior Polar Cataract 134
Divya Agarwal

3.25 Microincisional Cataract Surgery Platform: A Great Leap Forward 140
Mohan Rajan, Sujatha Mohan, Ramya Subramanian

3.26 What should be Done Differently before Cataract and Glaucoma Surgery? 143
Devindra Sood, Aditi Agarwal

3.27 Which Patients with Cataract Need a Combined Glaucoma Procedure? 145
SS Pandav

3.28 90 to 100 Degrees of Iridodialysis during Phaco: What to Do? 146
Mahipal Sachdev, Charu Khurana

3.29 What are the Advantages, Indications, and Limitations of Manual Small Incision Cataract Surgery? 148
Ruchi Goel, KPS Malik

3.30 How to Minimize Corneal Endothelial Cell Damage during Phacosection, a Manual Small Incision Cataract Surgery? 150
MS Ravindra

3.31 Contrast Sensitivity in Pseudophakic Patients 153
Ravi Nabh

3.32 How Important is it to Reduce or Eliminate Spherical Aberration after Phacoemulsification? 155
Amit Gupta

3.33 What should be Done for a Patient Undergoing Phaco and is Suspected to have Globe Perforation during Procedure? 157
Mangat R Dogra, Gaurav Sanghi

3.34 Are Anterior Chamber IOLs Safe for Implantation? Which Anterior Chamber IOLs should be Implanted? 158
Srikant Kumar Padhy, Neelima Aron

3.35 Iris-Claw Lens—Versatility Combines Safety 162
Ravijit Singh

3.36 Scleral-fixated Intraocular Lens 165
Surg Capt (Dr) Srujana D

3.37 How Do You Manage a Patient with Visually Significant Cataract with Associated Uveitis? 173
GS Brar

3.38 What Precautions You Take in Patient of Cataract with Dry Eyes during and after Cataract? 175
KP Chaudhary

3.39 Postoperative Treatment of Uncomplicated Phacoemulsification 177
Tanuj Dada, Vivek Dave

3.40 Following Uneventful Phacoemulsification, the Patient has 4+ Cells and Fibrin on Postoperative Day 1. What should be Done? 178
Reema Bhansal, Amod Gupta, Vishali Gupta

3.41 Postcataract Surgery Cystoid Macular Edema 180
Ramandeep Singh

3.42 Phacoemulsification in Aniridic Eyes 182
Kasturi Bhattacharjee, S Bobby

3.43 Foldable Intraocular Lenses 184
JS Titiyal, Neelima Aron, Bhavya G

3.44 Management of Astigmatism: Toric Intraocular Lenses 189
Abhay Vasavada, Vaishali Vasavada

3.45 Mix and Match Multifocal Intraocular Lenses 191
Gaurav Luthra

3.46 Management of Descemet's Membrane Detachment 193
Jaspreet Sukhija

3.47 When should an Intraocular Lens be Implanted in the Sulcus or Bag or Captured in the Capsular Bag in a Patient Having Posterior Capsular Tear? 195
Suresh Kr Pandey

3.48 Cataract Surgery in Patients with Vitreoretinal Diseases 196
Pranab Das

3.49 Anterior Chamber Deepening during Phacoemulsification 200
GS Dhami

3.50 Phacoemulsification in Pseudoexfoliation with Small Pupil 201
Abhay Vasavada

3.51 What is the Best Way to Prevent and Manage Postoperative Intraocular Pressure Spikes? 203
Sandeep Saxena

3.52 How will You Manage a Case of Visually Significant Cataract with Associated Fuchs' Endothelial Dystrophy? 204
Rajesh Fogla

3.53 How should We Manage Prolonged or Recurrent Uveitis Following Phacoemulsification? 205
Jyotirmoy Biswas

3.54 Management of Posterior Dislocation of Lens Fragment during Phacoemulsification 206
Pranab Das

3.55 Current Surgical Techniques for Pediatric Cataract Surgery 207
Jagat Ram

3.56 Secondary Intraocular Lens Implantation in Children 210
Ashok Sharma

3.57 Femtosecond Laser-assisted Cataract Surgery 212
Deepali Singhal, Sridevi Nair

3.58 What are the Indications for Nd:YAG Laser Capsulotomy in Posterior Capsule Opacification? 215
Suresh Kr Pandey

3.59 An Update on IOL Power Calculation Formulas 216
Ashok Garg

3.1 Risk Factors for Age-related Cataract

SK Gupta
Institute of Clinical Research New Delhi
skgup@hotmail.com, skgupta@icriindia.com

■ INTRODUCTION

Cataract is a condition which is recognized by the opacification of the lens. It may be localized to certain parts or whole of the lens may be affected. It has been found that cataract is a major cause of blindness worldwide, including India **(Fig. 3.1.1)**.

Cataract is a multifactorial disease. The risk factors associated with cataract disease include:
- Socioeconomic status
- Systemic conditions such as dehydration, renal failure, hypertension, low body mass index, and diabetes
- Glaucoma
- *Drugs:* Steroids, cholinesterase inhibitors, spironolactone, nifedipine, analgesics
- Myopia early in life
- Family history of cataract
- Occupational exposure
- Heavy smoking and alcohol consumption
- Use of cheaper cooking fuel
- Working in direct sunlight

■ RISK FACTORS FOR CATARACT (FIG. 3.1.2)

- Several studies conducted in central and eastern India have reported the role of dehydration caused by diarrhea in cataract formulation.
- Steroids have been implicated as an important cause of posterior subcapsular cataract.
- Glaucoma itself as well as medications such as cholinesterase inhibitors used for treating it have been associated with cataract.
- Environmental stress such as cigarette smoking decreases the levels of superoxide dismutase, glutathione, and glutathione peroxidase in lens and leads to oxidative insult as the mechanism of cataract.
- Patients who had quit smoking 25 years or prior have been found to at a 20% lower risk to develop cataract as compared to current smokers. The risk among past smokers was, however, higher than those who have never smoked.

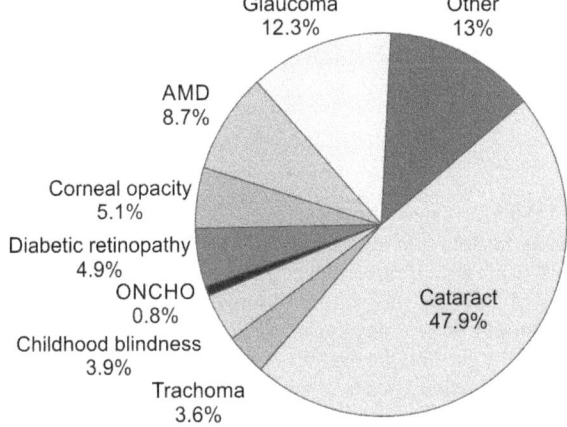

Fig. 3.1.1: Causes of blindness worldwide. (AMD: age-related macular degeneration)

- The role of alcohol in cataract formation is less clear. But in a study, history of alcohol consumption was significant in univariate analysis.
- An association has been found between hypertension and cataract. Patients with high blood pressure (BP) are more prone to cataract.
- The risk of cataract was higher among people belonging to lower socioeconomic status who used cheaper fuel sources such as cow dung, wood, or coal.
- Excessive ultraviolet (UV) light exposure is associated with enhanced risk of cataract possibly due to the oxidative stress associated with the depletion of antioxidants.
- Cortical cataract is generally found in female gender which has been attributed to the hormonal difference.
- Reduced estrogen levels in postmenopausal age group may also be a factor and hormone replacement therapy may play a protective role in reducing the incidence of age-related cataract.

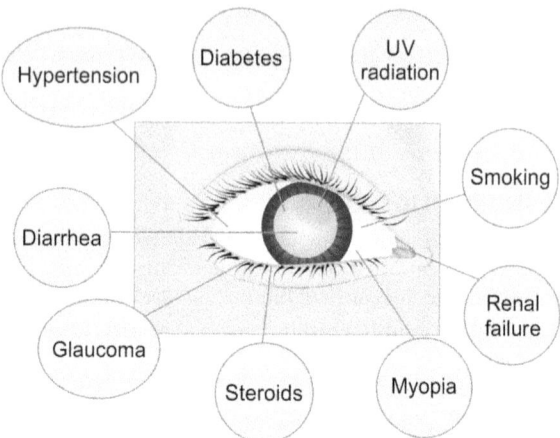

Fig. 3.1.2: Risk factors for cataract.

> **EDITOR'S PEARLS**
> - Age-related cataract is a multifactorial disease. The risk factors for it can be broadly classified into patient-related and environmental factors.
> - Important patient-related factors include increased age, ocular comorbidities, metabolic diseases, and genetic influences.
> - Major environmental factors include ultraviolet light exposure, lower socioeconomic status, drug exposure, and smoking.

SUGGESTED READING

1. Apple DJ, Ram J, Foster A, Peng Q. Elimination of cataract blindness: a global perspective entering the new millennium. Surv Ophthalmol. 2000;45(Suppl 1):S1-196.

3.2 How do You Grade Age-related Cataract?

Gagandeep Singh Brar
Sangam Netralaya Mohali
gsbrarpgi@yahoo.com

INTRODUCTION

Grading of age-related cataract is important for epidemiological and research purposes as well as for planning surgical intervention. In the days of large incision manual cataract extraction, grading of cataract was probably not that important as far as planning of surgery was concerned; but in today's time of phacoemulsification, grading becomes very important especially grading the extent of nuclear sclerosis.

Lens Opacities Classification System III is the standard for grading age-related cataract.[1] This system can be used for assessment both on a slit-lamp biomicroscopy as well as from anterior segment photographs under full dilatation.

METHOD OF GRADING

The pupil is dilated for cataract grading unless contraindicated. After dilatation cataract grading is done with 8X magnification view on slit lamp. The Lens Opacities Classification System III (LOCS) grading transparency is placed behind the patient's shoulder, mounted on X-ray view box and cataract grading is matched with transparency. Patients with nuclear cataract are examined under direct focal illumination for nuclear color and opalescence, whereas cases of cortical and posterior subcapsular are examined under retroillumination and matched with LOCS III transparency. For nuclear cataract, nuclear color (NC) as well as nuclear opalescence (NO) is graded from 1 to 6 whereas patients with cortical and posterior subcapsular cataract (P) are graded from 1 to 5 according to increased density of the cataract **(Fig. 3.2.1)**.

In LOCS III:
- *Severe cataract:* Grades NO ≥4 or NC ≥4 for nuclear cataract, C ≥4 for cortical cataract and P ≥2 for posterior subcapsular cataract.
- *Moderate cataract:* 2 ≥ NO <4 or 2 ≥ NC <4 for nuclear opacity, 2 ≥ C <4 for cortical opacity and 1 ≥ P <2 for posterior subcapsular opacity.
- *Mild cataract:* NO <2 or NC <2, C >2 and P >2.

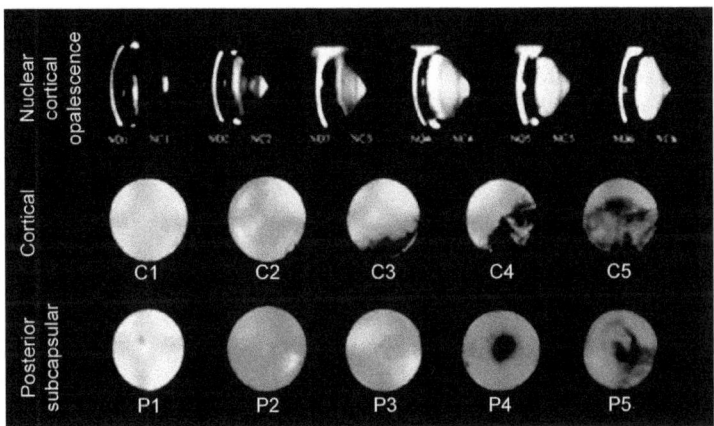

Fig. 3.2.1: Lens opacities classification system III.

NEWER TECHNOLOGIES
- Scheimpflug imaging of the anterior segment of the eye.
- Anterior segment optical coherence tomography (OCT).

The LOCS III criterion as an economic cataract grading system provides data that are in satisfactory concordance with the results obtained using the Pentacam-Scheimpflug system and anterior segment OCT.

EDITOR'S PEARLS
- LOCS III continues to be used as the standard for both research and clinical purposes.
- Objective-automated methods to grade cataract using anterior segment OCT and fundus photography have shown good correlation with LOCS III grading.
- Machine learning and deep learning tools have shown promise in the field of cataract diagnosis and grading.

REFERENCE
1. Chylack LT Jr, Wolfe JK, Singer DM, Leske MC, Bullimore MA, Bailey IL, et al. The Lens Opacities Classification System III. The Longitudinal Study of Cataract Study Group. Arch Ophthalmol. 1993;111(6):831-6.

3.3 Preoperative Evaluation of Patients with Age-related Cataract

Sudesh Kumar Arya
Government Medical College and Hospital, Chandigarh
aryasudesh@yahoo.co.in

■ INDICATIONS OF SURGERY

Presence of glare, diplopia, polyopia or decreased contrast sensitivity may be indications for cataract surgery apart from decreased visual acuity for near or distance. The purpose of cataract surgery is to improve vision and its quality so that quality of life improves. Surgery should be planned on the basis of need, occupation, and lifestyle of the patient. Following examinations should be carried out before cataract surgery.

■ VISUAL ACUITY AND REFRACTION

Distant, near, and intermediate visual acuity (VA) should be recorded with naked eye and with glasses. Power of glasses (POG) should also be checked. If possible refraction should be done in both the eyes to find out the best corrected visual acuity and plan the eye to be operated accordingly.

Dominant eye should be identified before surgery in case the surgeon is planning micromonovision.

External Eye Examination

- Look for deviation of visual axis, eccentric fixation or nystagmus which may be poor prognostic signs even in age-related cataract.
- Pupillary reactions should be carefully checked. Presence of relative afferent pupillary defect may indicate optic nerve disease.
- Enophthalmos, deep set eyes and narrow palpebral aperture may pose problems during surgery. Any eyelid, conjunctival, lacrimal sac, or adnexal infection should be ruled out.
- A thorough examination of fellow eye should be done.

Slit-lamp Examination

Detailed slit-lamp examination is invaluable before any cataract surgery.
- Cornea should be examined for presence of corneal opacity, any irregularity, thinning, ectasia, corneal guttata or any keratic precipitates. Specular reflection should be done to assess the endothelial cell morphology.
- Anterior chamber should be examined for depth and presence of any cells or flare. Gonioscopy is very important in indicated cases to rule out presence of peripheral anterior synechiae or abnormal new vessels in the angle if anterior chamber intraocular lens (IOL) is anticipated.
- Pupillary dilation should be assessed before surgery.
- Presence of posterior synechiae, rubeosis or rigid sphincter may create problem during surgery.
- Lens should be examined for anterior and posterior capsular status, grade of nuclear sclerosis, location of opacity, posterior polar opacity, pseudoexfoliation, phacodonesis, etc. If there is any evidence of zonular weakness, one may plan capsular tension ring or scleral fixated IOLs.
- Vitreous should be examined for presence of any hemorrhage, asteroid hyalosis, opacification or liquefaction.

Posterior Segment Evaluation
- Fundus examination with 90 D lens or indirect ophthalmoscopy should be done to evaluate the macula, optic nerve, retinal vessels, and retinal periphery. Particular attention should be paid to early macular degeneration/maculopathy which may affect visual result after an otherwise uneventful cataract surgery.
- If media is hazy, ultrasonography B-scan should be done to rule out retinal detachment, vitreous hemorrhage, vitreous opacity, posterior staphyloma, and optic nerve head cupping.

Intraocular Pressure
Intraocular pressure (IOP) should be measured to rule out high IOP. If there is suspicion of glaucoma, diurnal variation/visual field's assessment should be done.

Macular Function Tests
Macular function tests by potential acuity meter, laser interferometry, Maddox rod test, photostress recovery time or blue light entoptoscopy should be performed if media is hazy.

Optic Nerve
Optic nerve should be examined for cupping, along with pallor and other abnormality. Visual-evoked potential should be advised for confirming involvement of optic nerve pathway.

Corneal Pachymetry and Specular Microscopy
Corneal pachymetry and specular microscopy is useful for examining the corneal thickness and endothelium respectively thereby assessing indirectly the function of endothelium.

BIOMETRY
- It is preferable to measure axial length and keratometry by optical biometry methods such as the IOL Master and Lenstar due to their higher accuracy.
- Axial length can also be measured by applanation method either by contact or immersion and keratometry can be measured by a calibrated automated keratometer.

Accurate assessment of keratometry is specifically useful for planning location, size of incision, and type of IOLs especially toric IOLs.

INTRAOCULAR LENS POWER CALCULATION
The accurate power of IOL is calculated by keratometry and axial length measurements using various IOL calculation formulas. The Holladay II formula gives accurate results for all eyes. Sanders–Retzlaff-Kraff (SRK)-II is accurate for eyes with axial length 22–24.5 mm. For axial length beyond these limits, a modified SRK-II is used. Short eyes are calculated with Hoffer Q formula and eyes with axial length >26 mm are calculated by SRK-T formula.

For multifocal IOLs and for the patient who has undergone refractive surgery, different formulae are used for IOL power calculation depending upon the choice of the surgeon.

In postrefractive surgery cases Haigis/Haigis-L formula is chosen. Apart from this you should check various online IOL power calculation site, e.g., American Society of Cataract and Refractive Surgery (ASCRS) online calculator, Doctorhill.com.

GENERAL HEALTH OF THE PATIENT
Systemic evaluation should be done for ascertaining fitness for surgery. One must rule out diabetes mellitus, hypertension, ischemic heart disease, chronic obstructive pulmonary

disease, history of allergy to drugs, bleeding disorders, and use of anticoagulants or immunosuppressants. Presence of any musculoskeletal disorder such as kyphosis, scoliosis or excessive obesity, head tremors or nodding may pose difficulty during surgery.

> **EDITOR'S PEARLS**
>
> - Accurate biometry and use of appropriate IOL power calculation formula are keys for achieving optimal refractive outcomes after cataract surgery.
> - Systemic stability must be carefully evaluated in high-risk patients planned for ophthalmic surgery.
> - Clear verbal and written instructions about the operative procedure must be provided to patients in the language of their understanding before surgery.

SUGGESTED READING

1. Bobrow JC, Blecher MH, Glasser DB, Mitchell KB, Rosenberg LF, Isbey EK, III, et al (Eds). Lens and cataract. In: Basic and Clinical Science Course. San Francisco: American Academy of Ophthalmology; 2009. pp. 75-89.

3.4 Macular Function Tests for Patients Undergoing Cataract Surgery

Lingam Gopal
Sankara Nethralaya, Chennai
drlg@snmail.org

INTRODUCTION

Cataract surgery is the most common ophthalmic surgery performed by ophthalmologists. In view of the high expectation, there is need for proper prognostication. Macular diseases are also common in the age group when cataract surgery is needed. In the presence of medial opacity (cataract), the evaluation of the macula by clinical examination may be difficult and can potentially result in less-than-optimal postoperative outcomes. Tests are available to evaluate the macular integrity and function as well as to determine the potential recovery of vision after cataract surgery. It must be emphasized that none of them gives a foolproof prognosis for vision. The errors in estimates can go both ways—under and over estimation.

EYES WITH MILD-TO-MODERATE LENS OPACITIES

Structural Evaluation

1. *Direct macular evaluation:* Slit-lamp biomicroscopic evaluation is the best way of evaluating the anatomical integrity of the macula. Posterior polar opacities may however preclude proper evaluation of the same.
2. *Optical coherence tomography (OCT):* OCT scanning of the macula gives a very good structural evaluation. Features, such as macular hole, epiretinal membrane, foveal thickening, etc. can be detected. With increasing degree of cataract, the quality of the pictures deteriorates and may fail to give proper information. However, considering the infrared wavelength that is used, OCT can surprisingly give clear pictures even in the presence of significant cataracts.

Functional Evaluation

1. *Pinhole acuity:*
    - *Principle:* Pinhole eliminates optical aberrations and improves the vision.
    - *Interpretation:* In the presence of gross opacities, pinhole does not improve the vision. The test is less reliable in eyes with best corrected visual acuity

less than 6/60. Pinhole potential acuity test was found more predictive than potential acuity meter (PAM) for eyes with best corrected vision better than 6/60.[1]

2. *Photo stress test:*
   - *Principle:* The macula is exposed to bright light for 10 seconds (using direct ophthalmoscope light) and the time taken for recovery original minus one line Snellen's vision is measured.
   - Interpretation: Normal recovery time is 20–30 seconds. Prolonged recovery time beyond 50 seconds indicates macular dysfunction.
3. *Blue field entoptoscopy:*
   - *Principle:* When patients are made to look at a bright blue light, they notice flying corpuscles. This effect is produced by the WBC in the perifoveal capillaries and, hence, reflects indirectly the circulation in the macular area.
   - *Interpretation:* A total of 99% of normal subjects visualize at least 15 or more corpuscles seen equally in different quadrants. Abnormal results are indicated by reduced number in one or more quadrants. Reasonable grasp and intelligence is needed to perform the test. Hence, a positive response is of more benefit in interpretation than negative one. This test was found to perform better than two-point discrimination test or Purkinje vascular entopic phenomenon test.[2]
4. *Yellow filter test of Koch:* If a transparent yellow filter is placed over reading material, it is noted to improve vision in eyes with macular degeneration but deteriorate the vision in eyes with only cataract.
5. *Potential acuity meter:*
   - *Principle:* A miniature visual acuity chart is projected on the retina through areas of clarity in the lens and patient asked to read the letters. Focusing of the chart is done to permit patient to see clearly.
   - *Interpretation*: Best results are achieved in cataracts that have not progressed beyond 6/60 level. In general, if more than four-line improvement is predicted, the prognosis after cataract surgery is likely to be good. A predictive capability of 90% and above has been reported.[3] False-positives have been seen with some maculopathies. In general, it is supposed to underestimate rather than overestimate the recovery.
6. *Laser interferometry:*
   - *Principle:* Helium-neon laser provides a collimated beam that is optically split into two. The two beams are projected through clear spaces in the lens to meet behind the lens. This produces interference fringes. The size and orientation of the stripes so produced can be varied.
   - *Interpretation:* The patient is expected to identify correctly the orientation of the stripe as the test is repeated with finer stripes. Unlike the PAM test, focusing is not needed and so the refractive error does not affect the test. However, aphakic eyes are best tested with corrective lens. A conversion table indicates the maximal potential vision. The test tends to overpredict the visual potential in amblyopic eyes.
7. *Lotmar visometer:*
   - *Principle:* This test is similar to laser interferometer but uses white light instead of laser, and hence is less expensive. Moiré fringes are formed using two rotatable equal gratings. The fringes are split into two coherent beams and projected through pupil.
   - *Interpretation:* Interference stripes formed are similar to laser interferometry and interpretation is also similar. The predictions are in general more optimistic especially with macular diseases.
8. *Illuminated near card assessment:*
   - *Principle:* The device is a handheld instrument containing a brightly illuminated vision chart that is transported across a 7 mm by 38 mm viewing window. Visual angle subtended at 16 inches equals that subtended by a letter at 20 feet.

- *Interpretation:* Illuminated near card (INC) was found to be more predictive in eyes with comorbid disease, in contrast to interferometers and PAM.
9. *Vryghem macular function test:*[4]
   - *Principle:* A simplified method of using near vision chart, the Vryghem test uses the Parinaud's near vision chart, a +8.00 diopter lens and the Heine ophthalmoscope. The vision chart is placed 12 cm from the patient. +8.00 diopter lens is placed over the best distance vision correction in a trial frame. The chart is illuminated with the Heine ophthalmoscope light. Those reading the smallest numbers (Parinaud 1) are expected to be having good macular function.
10. *Multifocal electroretinogram (MFERG):* It can potentially indicate the macular function. However, dense cataracts do not permit MFERG.

EYES WITH DENSE CATARACT

In eyes with dense cataract the approach to assess the potential for visual recovery would be different compared to those with mild-to-moderate cataracts. Here one must contend with the possibility of neither being able to see the macula clinically nor being able to image the same. Sometimes even the status of the retina (attached or detached) may not be possible to evaluate clinically and would need ultrasound examination.

Guidance from History

Perusal of old medical records can be of value to decipher previous notifications of macular diseases. History of poor vision since childhood can be due to amblyopia.

Clinical Evaluation

- *Perception of light and accurate projection:* Although accurate projection is encouraging, it excludes only large retinal detachments and absolute field defects and not macular diseases. Similarly, dense cataracts can so scatter light that inaccurate projection can still be compatible with good visual recovery.
- *Two-point discrimination:* Ability to distinguish two lights close together is a good sign but cannot exclude macular disease.
- *Color perception:* Although ability to identify colors is suggestive of potentially good macular function, macular degeneration is known to exist with good color perception.
- *Pupillary assessment:* This is perhaps the best objective evidence for presence or lack of gross posterior segment disease. Both extensive retinal disease and optic nerve disorders will produce afferent pupillary defect. Even total cataracts are known not to produce afferent pupillary defect if posterior segment is normal. However macular disorders are not excluded even if pupils are brisk.
- *Entopic visualization:* Eber and Friedman described a test where in a light is gently rubbed on closed eye lids to-and-fro against the sclera. This can stimulate Purkinje vascular tree images. While some patients can detect the optic disc shadow and macula, others may not appreciate the detail despite having good macular function. It is most useful to compare between the two eyes.
- *Maddox rod test:* If light is shone behind a Maddox rod held in front of the eye, a continuous red streak will be made out. A break in the line indicates possible central scotoma. A high index of suspicion is needed to suspect macular problems when there is mismatch between the vision and the degree of cataract. Information from more than one way of evaluation is needed for proper conclusions.

REFERENCES

1. Melki SA, Safar A, Martin J, Ivanova A, Adi M. Potential acuity pinhole: a simple method to measure potential visual acuity in patients with cataracts, comparison to potential acuity meter. Ophthalmology. 1999;106(7):1262-7.
2. Sinclair SH, Loebl M, Riva CE. Blue field entoptic phenomenon in cataract patients. Arch Ophthalmol. 1979;97(6):1092-5.

3. Ing MR. Potential acuity meter to predict postoperative visual acuity. J Cataract Refract Surg. 1986;12(1):34-5.
4. Vryghem JC, Van Cleynenbreugel H, Van Calster J, Leroux K. Predicting cataract surgery results using a macular function test. J Cataract Refract Surg. 2004;30(11):2349-53.

3.5 Informed Consent for Cataract Surgery with or without Implantation of an Intraocular Lens

Arun K Jain
Advanced Eye Centre, PGIMER, Chandigarh
arooonjain@hotmail.com

■ PATIENT INFORMATION SHEET

A sample consent and patient information brochure is attached:
Name of Patient..
Age/Sex..
Patient ID..
Son/Daughter..of..
....
Address..Tel..

■ WHAT IS A CATARACT?

Cataract is a condition in which the lens in your eye becomes opacified, making it difficult for you to see well enough to carry out your usual daily activities. To correct this, the cataract will need removal with an operation. The natural lens within your eye with a slight cataract, although not perfect, still has some advantages over an artificial lens. In giving permission for cataract extraction with/without implantation of an intraocular lens (IOL) in my eye, I declare that I understand the following information.

■ BENEFITS AND RISKS OF CATARACT SURGERY

Most people find that their eyesight improves considerably after cataract surgery. However, you should be aware that there exists a small risk of complications, either during or after the operation. If you have any questions, you can clarify with your doctor.

The Procedure

- The purpose of the surgery is to replace the opacified lens (cataract) with an artificial lens (implant) inside your eye.
- This artificial lens, usually made of plastic, silicone, or acrylic material, surgically and permanently placed inside the eye, and hence called an IOL. Eyeglasses may be required in addition to the IOL for best vision.
- An experienced eye surgeon will carry out the surgery or may supervise a doctor in training who also performs some operations.
- The surgery is performed under a local anesthetic, you will be awake during the operation. Just before the operation, you will be given eyedrops to enlarge the pupil. After this, you will be given an anesthetic to numb the sensations and decrease the movements of the eye. This may consist simply of eyedrops or injecting local anesthetic solution into the tissue surrounding the eye.
- During the surgery you will be asked to keep your head still and lie as flat as possible. The surgery normally takes 15-20 minutes but may take up to 45 minutes.
- Most cataracts are removed by a technique called phacoemulsification, in which the surgeon makes a very small cut into the eye, softens the lens with sound waves and removes the cataract through a small tube. The back layer of the lens is left behind.

- An artificial lens (implant) is then inserted to replace the cataract. After your natural lens is removed, the IOL is placed inside your eye. In rare cases, it may not be possible to implant the IOL you have chosen or any IOL at all. Sometimes a small stitch is put across cut created in the eye. At the end of the operation, a pad or shield may be put over your eye to protect it.

After the Operation

If you have any discomfort, we suggest that you take a pain reliever such as paracetamol or diclofenac. It is normal to have some watery discharge, feel itching, sticky eyelids, and mild discomfort for a while after cataract surgery. After a few days even mild discomfort should disappear.

In most cases, healing will take about 2-6 weeks, after which new glasses will be prescribed by your optician. You will be given eyedrops to minimize inflammation. The hospital staff will provide necessary instructions regarding the use of various medicines and the precautions to be kept in mind for next few days. Certain symptoms could mean that you need *prompt treatment*, including:
- Excessive pain
- Decrease/loss of vision
- Increasing redness of the eye

Likelihood of Improvement of Vision

After the operation you may read or watch TV almost straight away, but your vision may be blurred. The healing eye needs time to adjust so that it can focus properly with the other eye, especially if the other eye has a cataract. The vast majority of patients have improved eyesight following cataract surgery. Please note that if you have another condition, such as diabetes, glaucoma, or age-related macular degeneration your quality of vision may still be limited even after successful surgery.

Possible Complications during the Surgery

- Tearing of the back part of the lens capsule with disturbance of the gel inside the eye that may sometimes result in reduced vision.
- Loss and drop of all or part of the cataract into the back of the eye requiring another surgery which may require general anesthesia.
- Bleeding inside the eye.

Possible Complications after the Surgery

- Bruising of the eye or eyelids
- High pressure inside the eye
- Clouding of the cornea
- Incorrect strength or dislocation of the implant
- Swelling of the retina—macular edema
- Detachment of retina which can lead to loss of sight
- Infection in the eye, i.e., endophthalmitis, which may lead to loss of sight or even loss of the eye.
- Allergy to the medications used
- Dry eyes symptoms
- New appearance of floaters and/or increase in floaters.
- Risks of cataract surgery include, but are not limited to.

Complications of removing the natural lens may include:
- Hemorrhage (bleeding), rupture of the capsule that supports the IOL and perforation of the eye.
- A cloudy cornea which may or may not settle. This may require further surgery; an acute inflammatory reaction causing pain. This may need further treatment.

- Swelling in the central area of the retina (called cystoid macular edema), which usually improves with time.
- Retained pieces of lens in the eye, which may need to be removed surgically, infection.
- Detachment of the retina, which is definitely an increased risk for highly nearsighted patients, but which can usually be repaired.
- Uncomfortable or painful eye, droopy eyelid, increased astigmatism, glaucoma, and double vision.

These and other complications may occur whether or not an IOL is implanted and may result in poor vision, total loss of vision, or even loss of the eye in rare situations. Additional surgery may be required to treat these complications. Any of these complications may occur, but these complications are now rare.

Complications associated with the IOL may include:
- Increased night glare and/or halo.
- Double or ghost images, and dislocation of the IOL. Multifocal IOLs may increase the likelihood of these problems.
- In some instances, corrective lenses or surgical replacement of the IOL may be necessary for adequate visual function following cataract surgery.

Complications associated with local anesthesia injections around the eye include:
- Perforation of the eye
- Destruction of the optic nerve
- Interference with the circulation of the retina
- Droopy eyelid, respiratory depression, hypotension, and cardiac problems
- In rare situations, brain damage or death

Complications of Surgery in General

As the procedure is generally done under local anesthesia the risk to life is <0.5%.
- If an *IOL is implanted*, it is done by a surgical method. It is intended that the small plastic, silicone, or acrylic IOL will be left in the eye permanently.
- If a monofocal IOL is implanted, either distance or reading glasses or contacts will be needed after cataract surgery for adequate vision.

If complications occur at the time of surgery, the doctor may decide not to implant an IOL in your eye even though you may have given prior permission to do so.

Complications associated with multifocal IOLs. While a multifocal IOL can reduce dependency on glasses, it might result in less sharp vision, which may become worse in dim light or fog. It may also cause some visual side effects such as rings or circles around lights at night. Driving at night may be affected. If complications occur at the time of surgery, a monofocal IOL may need to be implanted instead of a multifocal IOL.

Although you may have opted for phacoemulsification surgery and the same may have been planned by your surgeon after preoperative examination, if during surgery, phacoemulsification is found to be unsafe or not feasible, your surgeon will have the liberty to perform surgery by the conventional technique in the interest of patient safety.

Other factors may affect the visual outcome of cataract surgery, including other eye diseases, such as glaucoma, diabetic retinopathy, age-related macular degeneration, the power of the IOL, your individual healing ability, and if certain IOLs are implanted, the function of the ciliary (focusing) muscles in your eyes.

The selection of the proper IOL, while based upon sophisticated equipment and computer formulas, is not an exact science. After your eye heals, its visual power may be different from what was predicted by preoperative testing. You may need to wear glasses or contact lenses after surgery to obtain your best vision. Additional surgeries, such as IOL exchange, placement of an additional IOL, or refractive laser surgery may be needed if you are not satisfied with your vision after cataract surgery.

The results of surgery cannot be guaranteed. If you chose a multifocal IOL, it is possible that not all the near (and intermediate) focusing ability of your eye will be restored.

Additional treatment and/or surgery may be necessary. Regardless of the IOL chosen, you may need laser surgery to correct clouding of vision. At some future time, the IOL implanted in your eye may have to be repositioned, removed surgically, or exchanged for another IOL.

Since only one eye will undergo surgery at a time, you may experience a period of imbalance between the two eyes (anisometropia). In the absence of complications, surgery on the second eye can usually be accomplished within 2-4 weeks, once the first eye has stabilized.

Condition and Procedure

The doctor has explained that I have the following condition:
(Doctor to document in patient's own words)
The following procedure will be performed to the ....
....eye(s):
(Doctor to document which side)

■ PATIENT CONSENT

- Cataract surgery, by itself, means the removal of the natural lens of the eye by a surgical technique.
- For an IOL to be implanted in my eye, I understand I must have cataract surgery performed either at the time of the IOL implantation or before IOL implantation.
- If my cataract was previously removed, I have been informed that my eye is medically acceptable for IOL implantation.
- I understand that a doctor other than the consultant surgeon may conduct the procedure. I understand this could be a doctor undergoing further training.
- I consent to the administration of anesthesia and to the use of such anesthetics as may be deemed necessary or desirable. I further consent to the administration of such drugs or infusions deemed necessary in the judgment of the medical staff.

The basic procedures of cataract surgery, the reasons for the type of IOL chosen for me, and the advantages and disadvantages, risks, and possible complications of alternative treatments have been explained to me by my ophthalmologist. I understand that if organs or tissues are removed during the surgery, these may be retained for tests for a period of time and then disposed off sensitively by the hospital.

I am fully aware that the surgery is being performed in good faith and that no guarantee or assurance has been given as to the result that may be obtained. I understand that photographs or video footage may be taken during my operation. These may then be used for teaching health professionals. You will not be identified in any photo or video.

Although it is impossible for the doctor to inform me of every possible complication that may occur, the doctor has answered all my questions to my satisfaction.

Based on Above Information

I undersigned (the patient or nearest relative) hereby give my consent for the operation of left eye/right eye with the full knowledge of possible complications and guarded/poor vision prognosis. I certify that I have read this informed consent/it has been read over to me and explained to me in my mother tongue and all blanks or statements requiring insertion or completion were filled in and any inapplicable paragraphs stricken off before I signed. The doctor has answered all my questions to my satisfaction.

Signature/Thumb Impression of Patient/Parent/Guardian: ....
....
Name of Patient/Parent/Guardian................................. Date...
A sample consent and patient information brochure is attached:
Name of Patient...
Age/Sex....................................Patient ID..

Son/Daughter of ....
Address..Tel. ....

■ SUGGESTED READING
1. Informed consent for cataract surgery. San Francisco: American Academy of Ophthalmology; 2008.

3.6 | How do You Counsel Amblyopic Adult with Cataract before Surgery?

Jaspreet Singh Sukhija
Advanced Eye Centre, PGIMER, Chandigarh
jaspreetsukhija@yahoo.com

■ INTRODUCTION

Amblyopia is impaired or diminished vision in one or both eyes due to a maldevelopment of visual pathway arising from strabismus, anisometropia, or form deprivation in infancy or childhood. The visual system is thought to be sensitive to visual inputs only during a limited period of time early in life—the critical period of visual development, when it is immature and plastic.

Hence, therapy for amblyopia does not offer promising results for patients over the age of 9-10 years.

■ INDICATIONS OF CATARACT SURGERY IN AMBLYOPICS

It is of paramount importance to consider these possibilities in a patient with cataract where history is suggestive of amblyopia and as much of the visual input from the amblyopic eye is usually suppressed, so it might be expected that cataract in this eye would not significantly affect the patient's quality of life.

However, patients are frequently symptomatic and request cataract surgery as amblyopic eye is very sensitive at detecting blur (one of the principal effects of cataract) despite reduced visual acuity and contrast sensitivity.

Another indication is a complaint of glare, halos, misty vision, and monocular diplopia.

Diagnosing Amblyopia

1. A history of decreased vision since childhood not fully corrected with refractive aids.
2. Note any misalignment of the eyes which may suggest amblyopia.
3. Also the cataract density will not correlate to the amount of visual loss. This should raise suspicion that the patient is amblyopic after detailed examination reveals no ocular pathology.
4. Presence of a significant refractive error (hyperopia or high myopia) not correlating with the type of cataract would be another indicator of amblyopia.
5. Significant difference in biometry between two eyes.

Correction of amblyopia in cases with senile cataract is a very remote possibility. Thus, counseling such patients regarding the expected visual gain is extremely important. One needs to trace the previous records and compare the best corrected visual acuity. If a significant deterioration in the visual acuity is noted because of the development of cataractous changes, then the vision is expected to improve after surgery.

The benefits of a surgical intervention in patients with sensory amblyopia are further limited. They must be clearly explained the realistic goals of cataract surgery in their case. There is no investigative tool which can quantify the amount of postsurgical visual gain in amblyopic patients.

In young patients, there still exists potential for good visual gain following cataract surgery as there is a possibility that amblyopia therapy may help them. However, those with senile cataract are expected to benefit the least.

Laser interferometry may provide false positive results in amblyopics.

■ SUGGESTED READING

1. Hale JE, Murjaneh S, Frost NA, Harrad RA. How should we manage an amblyopic patient with cataract? Br J Ophthalmol. 2006;90(2):132-3.

3.7 Sterilization of Operating Room

Jagat Ram, Sunil Kumar
Advanced Eye Centre, PGIMER, Chandigarh
drjagatram@yahoo.com

■ INTRODUCTION

Maintenance of asepsis is imperative to ensure safe surgery and to minimize postoperative infection and its disastrous consequences. Postoperative endophthalmitis remains one of the most devastating complications of eye surgery.

Ventilation, cleaning, disinfection, and sterilization are the cornerstones in ensuring operating room (OR) asepsis.

■ VENTILATION IN OPERATING ROOM

The OR should be well-ventilated and the circulating air should be filtered.

- High efficiency particulate air (HEPA) systems remove most microorganisms ranging in size from 0.5 to 5.0 μm. The principle of ventilation in the OR is the delivery of positive pressure filtered air in a vertical unidirectional flow over the operating table. The current United States Public Health Service minimum requirements for optimum OR air is as follows—temperature between 18°C and 24°C, humidity 55–80%, and 25% changes per hour. Laminar airflow curtains or a radial exponential airflow pattern away from the operating field are especially helpful.
- In the surgical OR providing facilities for most forms of surgery, the recommended bacterial count of air should not exceed $1/ft^3$ ($35.5/m^3$). Air entering the OR from filters should not contain $>0.5/m^3$ of bacteria-containing particles. Furthermore, the bacteria-containing particles of air within 30 cm of the operation site should not exceed $10/m^3$ and should not be $>20/m^3$ in the rest of the OR.

■ CLEANING THE OPERATING ROOM

- Cleaning essentially means the removal of foreign matter (e.g., soil and organic matter) from the concerned surface.
- All surfaces should be free from visible dirt. It is normally accomplished with water, mechanical scrubbing, and detergents.
- Cleaning also reduces the bacterial count, though it will not disinfect or sterilize.

■ DISINFECTION AND STERILIZATION OF THE OPERATING ROOM

- Disinfection is a process of freeing the concerned object of all pathogenic microorganisms which may cause infection during its use.
- Sterilization is a process that eliminates all living organisms from the treated object. It is impractical to attempt to sterilize the entire OR and equipment, therefore current practices concentrate on disinfection. The measures commonly used are discussed below.

Chemical Disinfection

Phenolic Compounds
- Good bactericidal and fungicidal action.
- They are sometimes virucidal but are not sporicidal, except at temperatures over 100°C. They are very stable and remain effective after mild heating and prolonged drying.
- However, these agents are not recommended as high-level disinfectants due to their lack of activity against bacterial spores and lack of published efficacy data of available formulations.
- This class of compounds is used for decontamination of the OR and for noncritical medical and surgical items. The floor and 2 m of OR walls should be mopped with phenolic solution. Similarly, wet mopping of all OR tables, mats, instrument trolleys, stools, chairs, and supply shelves with phenol followed by a wipe down with 70% alcohol is an effective daily decontaminating regimen.

Formaldehyde Fumigation
Formaldehyde is an effective agent commonly used to sterilize OR. The efficacy of the process is uncertain at temperatures <20°C and relative humidity <70%.
- For optimum OR disinfection, formaldehyde fumigation is recommended fortnightly as a routine, and at the end of an operating session of a grossly infected case.
- All apertures in the room should be sealed with adhesive tape prior to fumigation.
- The gas is liberated by spraying or heating formalin or solid paraformaldehyde. For each 1,000 ft^3 of space (28.3 m^3), 500 mL of 40% formaldehyde in 1 L of water is put into an electric boiler or a large bowl placed on an electric hot plate with safety cut-out when boiling dry. The OR is sealed after turning on the boiler or hot plate. After fumigation, the room is kept closed for at least 8–10 hours.
- Subsequently, ammonium solution is introduced and left in the room for a few hours to neutralize the formaldehyde (1 L ammonium solution plus 1 L of water for every liter of 40% formaldehyde used).

Other Methods of Formalin Fumigation
- *Permanganate method:* Five ounces of potassium permanganate for every 1,000 ft^3 of space are placed in a jar and on top of this 10–15 ounces of 40% formalin diluted with an equal amount of water is poured. As soon as the reagents are mixed, a violet effervescence takes place and formaldehyde is set free.
- *Paraform method:* On heating formalin, the aldehyde changes into the solid polymeride—paraform. Gas is generated by heating paraform tablets. 25–30 tablets are required for every 1,000 ft^3 of space.
- *Formalin spray/vaporizer:* Aeromax vaporizer can be used to fumigate an OR. 250 cc of 40% formalin dissolved in 5,000 cc tap water makes a dilution of 1:20. 1 L of the solution is used per 1,000 ft^3 of space. This is vaporized for over half an hour. Spraying is not a satisfactory substitute for vaporization of formaldehyde by boiling as the fine aerosol has poor penetration.

Bacillocid Rasant
- It is newer and commercially available compound used for surface and environmental decontamination. It has excellent cleansing properties with bactericidal, virucidal, sporicidal, and fungicidal activity.
- Active ingredients:
  - Glutaraldehyde 100 mg/g
  - Benzyl-C12-18-alkyldimethylammonium chlorides 60 mg/g
  - Didecyldimethylammonium chloride 60 mg/g.

- *Advantages:*
  - Complete asepsis is achieved within 30-60 minutes.
  - Cleaning with detergent or carbolic acid is not required.
  - Formalin fumigation is not required.
  - Shutdown of operation theater (OT) for 24 hours is not required.

Ecoshield
It is stabilized hydrogen peroxide 11% w/v and 0.01% w/v, diluted silver nitrate solution. It can be used for routine mopping of floors and cleaning of OT equipment. It is also used in the form of hydrogen peroxide vapors (fogging) in the disinfection of OT at the end of routine cases, as well as infected cases.

Alkedol
A new method of fumigation:
- *Ingredients:*
  - 6% formaldehyde
  - 6% glutaraldehyde
  - 5% benzalkonium chloride.

Fogging
- Fogging involves nebulization of a disinfectant in a room until all surfaces are wet, followed by wiping off residual fluid from surfaces by masked and gowned personnel. It is not commonly used in recent times.
- Earlier fogging was carried out using formaldehyde. However, due to its carcinogenic effects it is now seldom used. Commercially available disinfectants such as Ecoshield® are now used for fogging.
- The disinfectant is put in a fogger machine and the machine is switched on for 45 minutes in the sealed OT, following which the room is kept sealed for another 45 minutes. Hydrogen peroxide has the advantage of being safer, less irritating, and has shorter cycle times compared with formalin fumigation.

Ultraviolet Radiation
Daily ultraviolet (UV) irradiation for 12-16 hours is recommended and is to be switched off 2 hours before starting OT.

Operation Theater Cleaning Schedule
Before surgery:
- Wet mopping with disinfectants must be done in the morning.
- All equipment, OT tables, walls, and floors must be cleaned and sterilized using appropriate methods.

Between operative procedures:
- Cleaning of operation tables and OT equipment with disinfectant solution is recommended.
- In case of spillage of blood/body fluids decontamination with chlorine solution.
- Wastes should be discarded in recommended color-coded plastic bags.
- Soiled gowns must not be disposed inside the OT.

After surgery:
- Linen and waste material is collected in color-coded bags according to hospital waste disposal protocol.
- Soiled linen is collected separately outside the OT to the dirty utility room, where it is disinfected by soaking in clean water with 0.5% bleaching powder solution for 30 minutes before being dispatched to the laundry facility.

- The OT table is cleaned with water and then carbonized with 0.5 chlorine/70% isopropyl alcohol.

OPERATING ROOM ETIQUETTE

A high standard of discipline is necessary for the safe conduct of any surgery. Minimum number of OT personnel should be allowed to enter the OT complex.
- Anyone with overt infection should be barred.
- All persons entering the OR should change into freshly laundered clothing.
- Hair and beards should be clean and well covered by caps and masks. High-filtration disposable masks are to be worn at all times when within the aseptic zone. All persons must wash their hands thoroughly before entering the OR.

OPERATING ROOM WASTE DISPOSAL

Operating room biohazardous waste including infected linen, disposable syringes, and needles, intravenous (IV) drip sets, IV fluids, and infected and diseased excised pathological tissue poses a significant health hazard to the OR personnel and public. Safe disposal is imperative to prevent the spread of infection and possible recycling of hazardous disposable products.

Thus, proper sterilization of OR with maintenance of high OR etiquette and safe OR waste disposal is mandatory to ensure safe surgery and to minimize postoperative infection and its disastrous consequences.

EDITOR'S PEARLS
- Regular surveillance becomes the most critical measure to keep OR infection free. Taking swabs from walls, microscope handles, floor, AC ducts, OR chairs, and even washing soaps for culture must be the standard practice protocol.
- Adequate disposal of all biomedical wastes should be taught to every healthcare personal with routine drills at regular intervals.
- A dedicated infection control team should ensure that the requisite protocols are enforced and adhered to.

SUGGESTED READING

1. ESCRS Endophthalmitis Study Group, European Society of Cataract and Refractive Surgeons. Prophylaxis of postoperative endophthalmitis following cataract surgery: results of the ESCRS multicenter study and identification of risk factors. J Cataract Refract Surg. 2007;33(6):978-88.

3.8 Antibiotic Prophylaxis after Cataract Surgery

Sushmita Kaushik
Advanced Eye Centre, PGIMER, Chandigarh
sushmita_kaushik@yahoo.com

Parul Ichhpujani
Government Medical College and Hospital, Chandigarh
parul77@rediffmail.com

INTRODUCTION

Cataract surgery is the most common ocular surgery performed in the geriatric population. Although in the current era, endophthalmitis is relatively rare, but the frequency of cataract surgery makes the absolute number of cases significant enough for it to be labelled a public health concern. The incidence rates of acute-onset postoperative endophthalmitis (POE) (presenting within 6 weeks of surgery) range from 0.02 to 0.17%.

Endophthalmitis prevention is difficult to investigate because of the large number of variables associated with even the most routine form of cataract surgery. Common risk factors for POE include old age, blepharitis, ectropion, rural residence, immunosuppressive conditions (diabetes mellitus), clear corneal incisions, use of silicone intraocular lenses (IOLs), and presence of surgical complications, such as posterior capsular rent.

There is no worldwide established approach to prophylaxis of endophthalmitis as cataract surgeons across the globe have their own preferred practice patterns based on extrapolations of the evolving scientific literature.

■ PATHOPHYSIOLOGY OF POSTOPERATIVE ENDOPHTHALMITIS

- Bacteria have been found in normal conjunctival flora without the use of antibiotic agents. Organisms present on the eyelid margin, are transferred to the conjunctiva, because of contamination. Diphtheroids, *Staphylococcus epidermidis, Staphylococcus aureus, Streptococcus* species (*Streptococci viridans*), *Neisseria*, gram-negative bacilli (often *Moraxella* species), *Propionibacterium acnes*, and rarely, fungi may also be present in the conjunctival cul-de-sac.
- Causative pathogens may also arise from tainted intraocular solutions, infected IOLs or surgical instruments, airborne contaminants, and operation theater personnel.
- *Endophthalmitis vitrectomy study (EVS):* EVS reported that gram-positive bacterial infections were more common. Although rare, gram-negative were more virulent and resulted in more dismal outcome.

■ CHARACTERISTICS OF AN "IDEAL" PROPHYLACTIC ANTIBIOTIC

- Potent against common pathogens
- Favorable pharmacokinetic profile
- Least potential for resistance
- Excellent safety profile
- Easy application

Optimal Chemoprophylaxis: Ongoing Debate

The debate amongst ophthalmic surgeons has always focused on the appropriate timing and mode of delivery of prophylaxis—preoperatively, intraoperatively and/or postoperatively, via topical drops or intracameral (IC) route.

Preoperative Prophylaxis in Vogue

Povidone Iodine

- *5% povidone iodine:* This has a broad-spectrum of microbicidal effects against various bacteria, fungi, protozoa, as well as viruses. Therefore, its use prior to surgery is an accepted way to reduce the incidence of POE.
- *Polyvinylpyrrolidone:* It has a high affinity for cell membranes and delivers free iodine (I_2) to the bacterial cell surface. Polyvinylpyrrolidone has rapid bactericidal effects as it acts on the cytoplasmic membrane, even after 1 minute of contact time with skin.

Topical Antibiotics

- *Rationale:* The antibiotic levels exceeding the minimal inhibitory concentration (MIC) of bacteria in the aqueous humor would prevent intraocular infection.
- Currently, moxifloxacin 0.5% and gatifloxacin 0.3% have shown promising results due to wide spectrum of coverage, better tissue penetration, higher potency, and delayed antibiotic resistance.
- Use of topical antibiotics for 3 days prior to surgery has been found to be more effective in eliminating surface bacteria than a 1-hour preoperative instillation, even with concomitant use of 5% povidone-iodine.

Intracameral Antibiotics

The European Society of Cataract and Refractive Surgeons (ESCRS) Study (2007)
- Prospective, randomized, placebo-controlled study that evaluated both topical and IC antibiotics in preventing POE; and showed the benefit of IC antibiotics.
- At the end of cataract surgery, an IC injection of cefuroxime has been shown to lower the risk of endophthalmitis by a factor of five.
- *Salient feature of the study:* Sample size was large enough to yield statistically significant results.
- Patient's potential hypersensitivity to the drug is an important issue as regards an antibiotic's safety.
- Allergic reaction to a topical agent will typically manifest as contact dermatitis or conjunctivitis while hypersensitivity to an IC agent can cause systemic anaphylaxis with associated morbidity and possible mortality.

What is the Indian take on intracameral cefuroxime?
An Indian study did not find strong evidence to support the use of IC cefuroxime to reduce the rate of acute POE (postcataract surgery). Marginal benefit might justify its use by some.

American Society of Cataract and Refractive Surgery (ASCRS) Members Survey (2014)
- This survey showed that only half (47%) of respondents already used IC prophylaxis or planned to use it.
- Half of all the surgeons not using IC prophylaxis expressed concern about the risks of noncommercially prepared antibiotic preparations.
- *Risks with IC antibiotics:* Risk of dilutional error, endothelial toxicity, toxic anterior segment syndrome (TASS), or introduction of contaminated substances into the eye.
- Majority surgeons used topical perioperative antibiotic prophylaxis, either gatifloxacin or moxifloxacin.

All India Ophthalmological Society (AIOS) Members Survey (2017)
- Only 83% respondents prepared the eye with 5% povidone-iodine.
- Most surgeons (90%) used topical antibiotic both pre- and postoperatively, nearly half (46%) used subconjunctival antibiotic at the end of surgery, and 40% used IC antibiotic (46% of them in high-risk patients only).
- Moxifloxacin was the antibiotic of choice (preferred over gatifloxacin) for topical and IC use.

ASCRS Members Survey (2021)
- Numbers of surgeons using IC antibiotic prophylaxis had increased to 66%. Moxifloxacin was the most commonly used antibiotic.
- Irrigation bottle infusion and intravitreal antibiotic injection was each used by only 5% of respondent surgeons.
- Surgeons not using IC antibiotics were either not convinced of its need or were apprehensive of mixing/compounding risk.

Which Antibiotic is Better?
- At dosing levels achieved with IC injections, moxifloxacin has been found to be more effective in killing *Staphylococcus aureus* in culture than cefuroxime.
- Effective antibiotics for IC prophylaxis include vancomycin, cefazolin, and cefuroxime; and the fourth-generation fluoroquinolones viz., gatifloxacin and moxifloxacin.
- Within the cephalosporin class, cefuroxime has a broader spectrum than cefazolin.
- Moxifloxacin is most used. It is easily available in a self-preserved and appropriately concentrated nonpreserved solution.
- Systemic administration of gatifloxacin has been shown to cause dysglycemia.
- If an infection occurs after the use of IC moxifloxacin, it will likely be moxifloxacin-resistant *Staphylococcus*, which is usually very sensitive to the typical POE protocol of vancomycin and ceftazidime.

SECTION 3: Cataract

- Infections that occur with cefuroxime are often destructive, resistant bacteria such as *Enterobacter*. Therefore, it is better to use an agent completely unrelated to the agents used to treat POE.

■ CONCLUSION

There is no global consensus regarding endophthalmitis prophylaxis practices. Intracameral antibiotic therapy along with preoperative 5% povidone iodine is still the most followed regimen for POE prophylaxis among cataract surgeons globally.

■ SUGGESTED READING

1. Althiabi S, Aljbreen AJ, Alshutily A, Althwiny FA. Postoperative endophthalmitis after cataract surgery: an update. Cureus. 2022;14(2):e22003.
2. Chang DF, Braga-Mele R, Henderson BA, Mamalis N, Vasavada A; ASCRS Cataract Clinical Committee. Antibiotic prophylaxis of postoperative endophthalmitis after cataract surgery: Results of the 2014 ASCRS member survey. J Cataract Refract Surg. 2015;41(6):1300-5.
3. Chang DF, Rhee DJ. Antibiotic prophylaxis of postoperative endophthalmitis after cataract surgery: results of the 2021 ASCRS member survey. J Cataract Refract Surg. 2022;48(1):3-7.
4. de Geus SJR, Hopman J, Brüggemann RJ, Klevering BJ, Crama N. Acute endophthalmitis after cataract surgery: clinical characteristics and the role of intracameral antibiotic prophylaxis. Ophthalmol Retina. 2021;5(6):503-10.
5. Endophthalmitis Study Group, European Society of Cataract & Refractive Surgeons. Prophylaxis of postoperative endophthalmitis following cataract surgery: results of the ESCRS multicenter study and identification of risk factors. J Cataract Refract Surg. 2007;33(6):978-88.
6. Kato A, Horita N, Namkoong H, Nomura E, Masuhara N, Kaneko T, et al. Prophylactic antibiotics for postcataract surgery endophthalmitis: a systematic review and network meta-analysis of 6.8 million eyes. Sci Rep. 2022;12(1):17416.
7. Maharana PK, Chhablani JK, Das TP, Kumar A, Sharma N. All India Ophthalmological Society members survey results: cataract surgery antibiotic prophylaxis current practice pattern 2017. Indian J Ophthalmol. 2018;66(6):820-4.
8. Nowak MS, Grzybowski A, Michalska-Małecka K, Szaflik JP, Kozioł M, Niemczyk W, et al. Incidence and characteristics of endophthalmitis after cataract surgery in Poland, during 2010-2015. Int J Environ Res Public Health. 2019;16(12):2188.
9. Reimer K, Wichelhaus TA, Schäfer V, Rudolph P, Kramer A, Wutzler P, et al. Antimicrobial effectiveness of povidone-iodine and consequences for new application areas. Dermatology. 2002;204 (Suppl 1):114-20.
10. Schwartz SG, Grzybowski A, Flynn HW Jr. Antibiotic prophylaxis: different practice patterns within and outside the United States. Clin Ophthalmol. 2016;10:251-6.
11. Sharma S, Sahu SK, Dhillon V, Das S, Rath S. Reevaluating intracameral cefuroxime as a prophylaxis against endophthalmitis after cataract surgery in India. J Cataract Refract Surg. 2015; 41(2):393-9.

3.9 What is the Role of Nonsteroidal Anti-inflammatory Drugs in Patients Undergoing Cataract Surgery?

Rupal H Trivedi
Storm Eye Institute, MUSC, South Carolina, Charleston
trivedi@musc.edu

■ INTRODUCTION

The applications of nonsteroidal anti-inflammatory drugs (NSAIDs) in cataract surgery have grown considerably in the past few years. The current available topical NSAIDs include diclofenac, flurbiprofen, ketorolac, bromfenac, indomethacin, and nepafenac. Most of the topical formulations are US Food and Drug Administration (FDA) approved to prevent inflammation after cataract surgery.

■ PREOPERATIVE

Flurbiprofen is approved by FDA as an inhibitor of intraoperative miosis. One drop every half an hour beginning 2 hours before surgery is recommended for this purpose. Nepafenac 0.1% and bromfenac 0.09% are approved for pain associated with cataract surgery. One drop of nepafenac should be applied beginning 1 day prior to cataract surgery, continued on the day of surgery and through the first 2 weeks of the postoperative period. Starting treatment 1 day before the day of surgery has the potential to inhibit pain more effectively; however, available evidence suggests that it does not affect long-term visual outcomes in routine cataract surgery.

■ INTRAOPERATIVE

Omidria, a 1%/0.3% phenylephrine/ketorolac intraoperative injection (Omeros Corporation, Seattle, Washington, USA) added to irrigating fluid during cataract surgery is FDA-approved for maintaining pupil size by preventing intraoperative miosis and reducing postoperative ocular pain.

■ POSTOPERATIVE

As mentioned above most topical formulations are US-FDA approved to prevent inflammation after cataract surgery. Because cystoid macular edema (CME) is generally associated with postsurgical inflammation, topical anti-inflammatory medications are used to prevent it and to treat established CME. There is evidence that NSAIDs, alone or in combination with topical corticosteroids, decrease the likelihood of postoperative CME, especially in diabetics *(I+, Good, Strong)*. Available literatures suggest a short-term benefit in visual recovery, but no level I evidence of long-term benefit (i.e., 3 months or more). The perioperative prophylactic use of NSAIDs for the prevention of CME has been advocated for high-risk eyes. Administration of NSAIDs before and immediately after surgery may accelerate the postoperative visual recover, however, again, there is no level I evidence that long-term visual outcomes are improved by the routine use of prophylactic NSAIDs at 3 months or more after cataract surgery.

■ POTENTIAL SIDE EFFECTS

Although generally well-tolerated topical NSAIDs may result in significant corneal reactions, including epithelial defects and stromal ulceration and melting, especially with prolonged use.

■ SUMMARY

To summarize, treatment with topical NSAID is dependent on the patient's risk factors and surgeon's preference. Although the use of preoperative and postoperative NSAIDs in preventing clinically significant CME in high-risk patients is advocated, their role in uncomplicated cataract surgery is less clear.

- For uncomplicated surgery and patients who are at low risk for CME, the decision is based on surgeon's preference. For those who prefer to prescribe NSAID for such routine, uncomplicated, low-risk patients, topical NSAID can be started 1 day before surgery and continued until 2-4 weeks postoperatively.
- For patients who are at risk for CME, preoperative treatment can be started 2-7 days before surgery (preexisting ocular inflammation, diabetes mellitus, prior ocular surgery, prior CME in fellow eye, epiretinal membrane, existing macular edema, etc.). Postoperative treatment can also be continued longer for high-risk patients (4-8 weeks).
- In addition to preoperative criteria mentioned above, following intraoperative factors may also be associated with high risk of CME—large incision, prolonged surgical time, iris prolapse, residual cortex, anterior chamber and sulcus intraocular lens, ruptured

capsule, vitreous disturbance, retained lens material, intraoperative bleeding, etc. Postoperative treatment can also be continued longer for high-risk patients (4–8 weeks).

> **EDITOR'S PEARLS**
> - Topical NSAIDs have been found to be more effective than steroids for reducing the incidence of postoperative CME.
> - Topical NSAIDs accelerate visual recovery in the postoperative period.
> - Combination of NSAIDs + Steroids (0.1% dexamethasone) found to be better for lowering incidence of CME as compared to a single drug.
> - No level 1 or level 2 evidence that NSAIDs +/– steroids improve long-term visual acuity outcomes.

Concentration and Dosage of Topical NSAIDs		
Drug	*Concentration*	*Dosage*
Bromfenac	0.07%	Once daily
	0.09%	Once/twice daily
Nepafenac	0.1%	3 times/day
	0.3%	Once daily
Ketorolac tromethamine	0.4%, 0.5%	4 times/day
Flurbiprofen	0.03%	2 hours before surgery
Indomethacin	0.1%	4 times/day
Diclofenac	0.07%	4 times/day

■ SUGGESTED READING
1. Kim SJ, Schoenberger SD, Thorne JE, Ehlers JP, Yeh S, Bakri SJ. Topical nonsteroidal anti-inflammatory drugs and cataract surgery: a report by the American Academy of Ophthalmology. Ophthalmology. 2015;122(11):2159-68.
2. Miller KM, Oetting TA, Tweeten JP, Carter K, Lee BS, Lin S, et al. Cataract in the adult eye preferred practice pattern. Ophthalmology. 2022;129(1):P1-p126.

3.10 | Anesthesia for Cataract Surgery

Sunil Kumar, Saurabh Saveria
Advanced Eye Centre, PGIMER, Chandigarh
eyepgi@sify.com

■ INTRODUCTION
Cataract surgery is the most commonly performed intraocular procedure and has evolved from an inpatient procedure under general anesthesia to essentially a day-care procedure usually done under local or topical anesthesia.

■ TECHNIQUES OF ANESTHESIA FOR CATARACT SURGERY
Following are seven techniques of anesthesia for cataract surgery:
1. Topical anesthesia
2. Peribulbar anesthesia
3. Retrobulbar anesthesia
4. Parabulbar or sub-Tenon's anesthesia
5. Intracameral anesthesia

6. Facial anesthesia
7. General anesthesia

Topical Anesthesia

The first modern use of topical anesthesia was described by Karl Koller in 1884 with cocaine. Currently, the most frequently used agents are tetracaine 0.5%; proparacaine 0.5%; benoxinate 0.4%; amethocaine 0.5-1% both are short acting (20 minutes) and are the least toxic to the corneal epithelium. Lidocaine 4% (lignocaine) and bupivacaine 0.5% and 0.75% have a longer duration of action but an increased associated corneal toxicity. Contraindications to topical anesthesia being a difficult or extended surgery, an uncooperative patient, language barrier, deafness, a hard cataract in a one-eyed patient, allergy to local anesthesia and nystagmus.

Technique
The aim is blocking the superficial corneal and conjunctival sensations. Drops are administered before the placement of the drapes. Preparation of the unblocked eyelid requires the patient to keep the eye closed, but the eye is kept open when the plastic drape is applied in order to secure the lid and lashes. As visual perception is not lost, the patient is asked to focus on the source of the light.

Advantages
No risk, as is associated with needle insertion such as retrobulbar hemorrhage, also the systemic anticoagulation therapy need not be withdrawn.

Disadvantages
- No akinesia of the globe. If intraoperative complications occur the anesthesia may not be adequate.
- Intracameral preservative free xylocard with or without epinephrine can also be used along with topical anesthesia.

Peribulbar Anesthesia

The principle of this technique is to inject the local anesthetic outside the muscle cone in the peribulbar space and avoid proximity to the optic nerve. This utilizes high volumes of anesthetic and the application of a pressure device. Such a block is used for cataract, glaucoma, keratoplasty, vitreoretinal, and strabismus surgeries. The most common mixture used is bupivacaine 0.75% plus lidocaine 2% plus hyaluronidase 150 U. Epinephrine (adrenaline) 5 µg/mL may be added to improve duration of the block. However, it should be avoided in patients who have ischemic heart disease, tachycardia, and hypertension. The lignocaine provides an early onset of action, bupivacaine prolongs the efficacy and hyaluronidase permits diffusion into the orbit more effectively; the required quantity of local anesthetic is, therefore, reduced and the time to onset is decreased.

Technique
A 25- or 26-gauge 2.5-cm long disposable needle is attached to the syringe. The patient is placed in the supine position and asked to look steadily straight ahead. The needle is inserted transcutaneously at the junction of the middle two-thirds and lateral one-third of the lower lid adjacent and parallel to the orbit floor for about 2.5 cm. Gentle aspiration of the syringe is performed to rule out the possible entry of the needle into a blood vessel and then 5-10 mL of the mixture is injected into the lateral adipose tissue of the orbit. Appearance of ptosis of the upper eyelid indicates an effective block. A constant and uniform pressure is then applied to the site for a couple of minutes.

Advantages
The risk of complications is less as compared to retrobulbar block.

Disadvantages
The quality of akinesia and anesthesia may not be as good as with retrobulbar block. It requires more volume. Postinjection orbital pressure rises. Periorbital ecchymoses and conjunctival chemosis may occur.

Retrobulbar Anesthesia
Also called intraconal anesthesia, local anesthetic is injected into the posterior intraconal space. A 22-gauge 3.5-cm long needle is used to enter transcutaneously at the junction of the middle and lateral thirds of the lower orbital margin. The needle is inserted directly backward for about 15 mm and is then angled upward and medially toward the apex of the orbit. As the needle pierces the intermuscular septum between the recti a giveaway feel is felt. After aspiration, 2–4 mL of the anesthetic is injected. This is indicated in all intraocular surgeries as in peribulbar anesthesia but needs an additional facial block.

Advantages
- A retrobulbar block is reliable for producing excellent anesthesia and akinesia. The onset of the block is quicker than with peribulbar; it usually occurs within 5 minutes.
- Low volumes of anesthetic result in less incidence of raised intraocular pressure and less chemosis compared to a peribulbar block.

Disadvantages
The major disadvantage of a retrobulbar block is higher incidence of complications as compared to a peribulbar block. Complications are retrobulbar hemorrhage, ocular perforation, subarachnoid or intradural injection, leading to brainstem anesthesia, respiratory depression or arrest, optic nerve contusion and atrophy.

Parabulbar or Sub-Tenon's Anesthesia
A conjunctival incision 2–3 mm in size is made halfway between the inferior limbus and the fornix to open into the sub-Tenon space. A blunt cannula or needle is used to inject anesthetic into the posterior sub-Tenon space, bathing the nerves, and muscles within the cone. Onset of the anesthesia is rapid. This completely avoids vascular and optic nerve injury, requires lower volumes of the anesthetic, and provides better anesthesia to the iris and anterior segment. This can also be used in all intraocular surgeries.

Complications being conjunctival chemosis and hemorrhage and the potential of damaging one of the vortex veins.

Intracameral Anesthesia
The solution used is 1% isotonic, nonpreserved lidocaine 0.3 mL are administered intracameral, no side effects have been reported, except for possible transient retinal toxicity if lidocaine is injected posteriorly in the absence of a posterior capsule. Adequate anesthesia is obtained in about 10 seconds.

Facial Anesthesia
The most popular are the van Lint and O'Brien techniques.
- *Van Lint technique:* A 22-gauge 3.5-cm long needle is inserted subcutaneously outside the lateral canthus and advanced upward toward the brows, and downward toward the infraorbital foramen, injecting along both the paths.
- *O'Brien techniques:* A needle is placed just posterior to the condyloid process of the mandible and local anesthetic is injected around it to block the facial nerve and its branches.

General Anesthesia

General anesthesia in cataract surgery is generally reserved for pediatric age group but can also be considered in patients who can be uncooperative, such as mentally retarded patients or patients who might have uncontrollable neurological movements, previous complication with local anesthesia, and reported allergy to the local anesthetic agents.

SUGGESTED READING

1. Ram J, Pandey SK. Anesthesia for cataract surgery. In: Dutta LC (Ed). Modern Ophthalmology. New Delhi: Jaypee Brothers Medical Publishers; 2000. pp. 325-30.

3.11 Phacodynamics

Noshir M Shroff
Shroff Eye Centre, New Delhi
shroffey@ndf.vsnl.net.in

Haripriya Aravind
Aravind Eye Hospital, Madurai
haripriya@aravind.org

INTRODUCTION

Refinements in power modulations and advancements in fluidics offer endless programming possibilities for a customized setting. All the parameters should be titrated depending on the hardness of the nucleus and the stage of surgery.

Modulations of phaco power program the way the ultrasonic energy is delivered so as to reduce the risk of thermal injury and increase the efficiency. The basic settings are (**Figs. 3.11.1 to 3.11.3**):
1. Continuous mode
2. Pulse mode
3. Burst mode.

The *continuous* power setting delivers energy continuously with variable power depending on how long the foot pedal is depressed. The maximum power can be preset and one has control of the maximum amount of phaco power delivered.

In *pulse* mode, the power is modulated to turn on and off a certain number of times per second (i.e., pulse per second or PPS). In pulse mode, there is linear power but a fixed interval between pulses. This reduces the phaco power delivery by 50% and maintains a stable anterior chamber. Also allows firmer grasp on the lens material and decreases the chatter at tip because vacuum builds between each pulse.

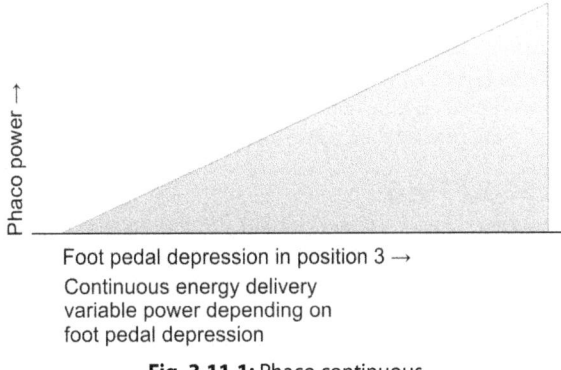

Foot pedal depression in position 3 →
Continuous energy delivery variable power depending on foot pedal depression

Fig. 3.11.1: Phaco continuous.

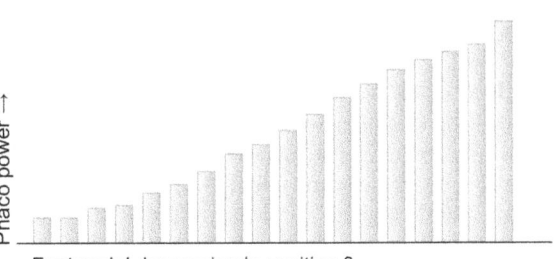

Foot pedal depression in position 3 →
Continuous energy delivery variable power depending on foot pedal depression

Fig. 3.11.2: Phaco pulse.

In *burst* mode, each burst of energy has the same amount of power, but the interval between each burst decreases as the foot pedal is depressed. The longer the pedal is depressed, the shorter the off periods will be between each burst. As the surgeon enters foot position three, the interval between bursts is 2 seconds; with increasing depressions of foot pedal in position three, the interval shortens until there is continuous phacoemulsification at bottom

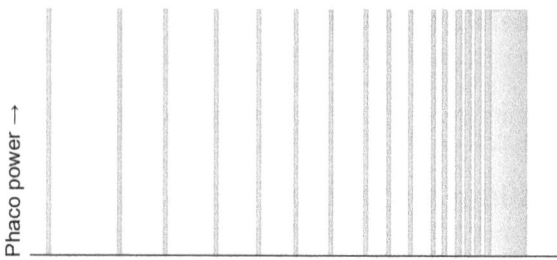

Foot pedal depression in position 3 →
Burst energy delivery
variable burst inter-depending on foot pedal depression
(energy burst will have the same power)

Fig. 3.11.3: Phaco burst.

of foot position three. The total of an on period plus an adjacent off period is the cycle time and a duty cycle is the proportion of the on period relative to the cycle time. In burst mode, the duty cycles are shorter than 50% (i.e., off cycle is longer than the on cycle).

Burst mode is a true phaco-assisted aspiration of lens nucleus. Most of the machines have two settings, viz., single burst and multiple bursts. Single burst delivers just one burst of energy for burying the probe into the nucleus for chopping. In multiple bursts mode, more bursts are delivered with varying intervals on foot pedal depression.

Recently manufacturers of phaco machines have shortened the cycle of on and off time, which smoothens the surgery and has better precision of power delivery. *Hyper settings* in pulse mode can give smoother power delivery. A high pulse rate of 100 PPS results in better cutting ability and yet delivers half of the energy of continuous phaco power. Hyper settings in burst mode allow finer and more precise delivery of bursts of phaco power. Using this we can set a burst mode as small as 4 ms, which is 125 times finer and more precise than using manual control by surgeon.

■ SCULPTING

A low vacuum, low flow rate with a moderate bottle height setting is adequate. The phaco power will depend on the density of the nucleus. The maximum phaco power may be preset at a higher level and titrated with linear pedal control.

Impaling and Chopping

Impaling and chopping requires power and vacuum depending on the density of cataract. As vacuum and flow rate are high, the bottle height should be sufficiently high to maintain anterior chamber depth and stability.

Nuclear Fragment Removal

Initially, the vacuum and aspiration flow rate (AFR) should be moderate to emulsify the fragments. Power can be lowered for emulsification of the nucleus. Higher flow rates are needed to disentangle and attract the nuclear fragments. As the emulsification progresses the parameters should be lowered as the posterior capsule is at a greater risk, with fewer fragments remaining. Vacuum is also lowered to levels sufficient to hold the fragments. Excessive vacuum, AFR, and power may lead to abrupt aspiration, breaking of the vacuum seal, and loss of control.

Epinucleus Removal

Since the capsule is adjacent to the epinucleus, moderate flow rate avoids damage from abrupt, uncontrolled aspiration. A moderate vacuum and minimal power is effective in

SECTION 3: Cataract

maintaining occlusion during epinucleus manipulation without abruptly aspirating and penetrating through the epinuclear bowl.

Tables 3.11.1 to 3.11.3 are settings for the phacoemulsification machines for different steps.

Each surgeon must titrate the settings according to the density of the cataract, the features available in the particular machine used, and more importantly according to his own experience and comfort level.

Active Fluidics System

The introduction of active fluidics system in the Centurion Vision System (Alcon Laboratories) has made a huge impact in improving the efficiency of phacoemulsification.

TABLE 3.11.1: Hard nucleus.

Machine settings	AMO Sovereign		AMO Signature		B & L Millennium	Alcon Infiniti
Sculpting						
Power (%)	70 (linear)		70 (linear continuous)		70	100
Duty cycle/ mode	DB (67%) (linear)		12/4 (75%) (62 PPS) (WhiteStar ICE on)		PPS off (continuous)	Continuous torsional (linear)
Vacuum (mm Hg)	50 (linear)		50 (linear)		45 (fixed)	65 (panel)
AFR (cc/min)	26 (panel)		26 (panel)			34 (panel)
Nucleus removal-I	Unoccluded	Occluded	Unoccluded	Occluded		
Power (%)	35 (linear)	40 (linear)	80 (linear)	95 (linear)	45	80–100
Duty cycle/ mode	CF long pulse (5 PPS)	CD long pulse (5 PPS)	Continuous (Ellipse on)	Continuous (Ellipse on)	35 (87 PPS)	Continuous torsional (linear)
Vacuum (mm Hg)	500*/400** (panel)	500*/400** (panel)	550 (panel)	445 (panel)	90–180 (dual linear)	400 (panel)
AFR (cc/min)	40 (linear)	46 (linear)	40 (linear)	38 (linear)		36 (panel)
Nucleus removal-II	Unoccluded	Occluded	Unoccluded	Occluded		
Power (%)	25 (linear)	30 (linear)	50 (linear)	95 (linear)	45	80–100
Duty cycle/ mode	CF long pulse (5 PPS)	CD long pulse (5 PPS)	Continuous (Ellipse on)	Continuous (Ellipse on)	35 (87 PPS)	Continuous torsional (linear)
Vacuum (mm Hg)	300*/125** (linear)	300*/125** (panel)	350 (panel)	–	90–180 (dual linear)	300 (panel)
AFR (cc/min)	38 (linear)	34 (linear)	38 (linear)	35 (linear)		32 (panel)

*Maximum; **Threshold vacuum
(AFR: aspiration flow rate; CF: constant frequency; CD: current drive; PPS: pulse per second)

TABLE 3.11.2: Soft nucleus.

Machine settings	AMO Sovereign		AMO Signature		B & L Millennium	Alcon Infiniti
Sculpting						
Power (%)	40–50 (linear)		40–50 (linear continuous)		40–50	60–80
Duty cycle/mode	DB (67%) (linear)		12/4 (75%) (62 PPS) (WhiteStar ICE on)		PPS off (continuous)	Continuous torsional (linear)
Vacuum (mm Hg)	50 (linear)		50 (linear)		45 (fixed)	65 (panel)
AFR (cc/min)	26 (panel)		26 (panel)			34 (panel)
Nucleus removal	Unoccluded	Occluded	Unoccluded	Occluded		
Power (%)	25 (linear)	40 (linear)	50 (linear)	95 (linear)	45	60–80
Duty cycle/mode	CF long pulse (5 PPS)	CD long pulse (5 PPS)	Continuous (Ellipse on)	Continuous (Ellipse on)	35 (87 PPS)	Continuous torsional (linear)
Vacuum (mm Hg)	300*/125* (panel)	300*/125** (panel)	350 (panel)	–	90–180 (dual linear)	300 (linear)
AFR (cc/min)	32 (linear)	30 (linear)	38 (linear)	35 (linear)		32 (linear)

*Maximum; **Threshold vacuum
(AFR: aspiration flow rate; CF: constant frequency; PPS: pulse per second)

TABLE 3.11.3: Epinucleus.

Machine settings	AMO Sovereign	AMO Signature	B & L Millennium	Alcon Infiniti
Power (%)	10 (linear)	40 (linear continuous)	20	60
Duty cycle/mode	CL (4 PPS long pulse)	12/4 (75%) (62 PPS) (Ellipse on)	50% 3 PPS	Continuous torsional (linear)
Vacuum (mm Hg)	150 (linear)	200 (linear)	40–100 (dual linear)	150 (linear)
AFR	28 (panel)	32 (panel)	–	20 (linear)

(AFR: aspiration flow rate; CL: clinical level; PPS: pulse per second)

As opposed to gravity-based fluidics systems, active fluidics technology applies pressure directly to the irrigation bag, which is housed inside the machine. The bag is connected to a balanced dual-segment peristaltic pump that allows the Centurion Vision System to constantly adjust to and minimize fluctuations in intraocular pressure (IOP). Furthermore, low-compliance tubing gives a greater pumping efficiency and less occlusion break surge. This helps to maintain a stable anterior chamber with minimum IOP fluctuations throughout the surgery. Moreover, Centurion provides a better control of postocclusion surge enabling the surgeon to operate at higher vacuum settings thereby reducing the effective phaco time.

> **EDITOR'S PEARLS**
> The newer ACTIVE SENTRY Handpiece (Alcon) contains an integrated pressure sensor that measures IOP near the tip, eliminating millisecond delay in adjusting the fluidics. It allows for a more stable chamber with less IOL fluctuations.

SUGGESTED READING
1. Devgan U. Phaco fluidics and phaco ultrasound power modulations. Ophthalmol Clin North Am. 2006;19(4):457-68.

3.12 What is Torsional Phacoemulsification and its Advantage?

Rohit Om Parkash
Dr Om Parkash Eye Institute, Amritsar
drrohit@accuratesight.com

TRADITIONAL VERSUS TORSIONAL PHACOEMULSIFICATION

Traditional phacoemulsification (TrP) uses forward and backward motion at the tip of the phacoemulsification probe. Torsional phacoemulsification (TP) utilizes side-to-side oscillations of an angulated bent tip to change energy profile of the tip and the surgical efficiency. The Kelman tip provides the greatest displacement and shearing action wherein the energy created at the incision is significantly less than at the distal end of the tip.

Advantages
- In TP, the cutting is by shearing action. It rubs and does not push and repel. There is a continuous contact between the tip and the nucleus. The nucleus stays at the tip and disappears. There is no need to reach for nucleus in the periphery. Everything occurs in the middle of the eye. The continuous contact reduces chatter, flow, and turbulence that decrease the number of loose nuclear pieces at the side port incision.
- Torsional phacoemulsification requires footswitch handling dexterity to attain the sweet spot for optimum energy delivery and fluidics. TP uses continuous delivery and the footswitch usage is simple. The nucleus piece starts clinging on to the tip of the needle at foot position two. The nuclear occlusion maximizes at the end of foot position two. The ultrasound activation removes nuclear piece. TP raises the surgical skill.
- Torsional phacoemulsification is an efficient and faster method with no half cycle wastage. One stroke of the tip, one side to another and back, is like two strokes making it effectively 64 KHz. The absence of repulsion with continuous contact decreases the time period.
- There is decreased heat energy produced because of reduced 32 KHz frequency, decreased ultrasound time, decreased energy produced at the incision site and reduced ultrasonic play in position three to embed the nucleus. Wound site thermal injury (WSTI) is no issue with TP in all cataracts.
- Stable anterior chamber (AC) is an advantage because the cold incision site permits the surgeon to work in a tight incision for all cataracts.
- Torsional phacoemulsification utilizes significantly lesser amount of fluid because the continuous contact allows lesser fluid transfer through the eye. Lower fluidic parameters and lesser procedure time decrease fluid consumption.

- Deeper plane emulsification is possible because of less turbulent environment, less fluid flow through the eye and increased efficiency.
- Sculpting is easier, faster, and efficient because with no repulsion the occlusion is maintained continuously.
- Torsional phacoemulsification has clearer corneas because of minimal repulsion, decreased turbulence with better retention of viscoelastic, remarkable chamber stability, improved followability, thermal injury free profile, efficient settings, reduced balanced salt solution (BSS) consumption, and deeper plane of emulsification. Tighter incisions are used in *hard cataracts* because of minimal WSTI. Consequently, there is stable chamber setting. Nonturbulent, repulsion-free environment results in clearer corneas. A 45-degree Kelman tip facilitates emulsification because the quadrants tumble more easily. The foot pedal is pressed fully in position three. If difficulty is encountered, then a combination of TP and TrP is used to avoid occlusion of the handpiece tip by a large sheared-off piece. The short repulsive effect of TrP helps reposition the quadrant and facilitates emulsification.

In *soft cataracts*, it is easier with TP, in the absence of repulsion, to hold thin soft plate of nuclear piece with accurate low fluidics and energy delivery using lower machine parameters.

Posterior polar and subluxated cataracts, small pupil and floppy iris syndrome require low fluid settings with stable chamber. A low aspiration flow prevents vitreous/iris being caught by the phaco tip. A low vacuum setting produces stable chamber setting. These settings cause repulsion, scattering of nuclear pieces and insufficient holding power with TrP. However, with TP, because of absence of repulsive dynamics, the follow ability and holding power is still excellent with very low parameters. The remarkable control enables confident handling of difficult cases.

EDITOR'S PEARLS

- Torsional phacoemulsification has the advantages of reduces cumulative dissipated energy (CDE) and ultrasound time as compared to longitudinal phacoemulsification.
- Results in less endothelial cell loss and less postoperative edema.
- Particularly efficacious in denser cataracts as it produces less chattering of nuclear material.

SUGGESTED READING

1. Berdahl JP, Jun B, DeStafeno JJ, Kim T. Comparison of a torsional handpiece through microincision versus standard clear corneal cataract wounds. J Cataract Refract Surg. 2008;34(12):2091-5.

3.13 Viscoelastics in Phacoemulsification Surgery

Jeewan S Titiyal
Dr RP Centre for Ophthalmic Sciences, AIIMS, New Delhi
titiyal@gmail.com

INTRODUCTION

Ophthalmic viscoelastic devices (OVDs) are used extensively in cataract surgery and play an important role in successful outcome. Different types of OVD with different properties are used at different steps of phacoemulsification.

Ideal OVD should be viscous enough to prevent anterior chamber collapse, yet liquid enough to be easily injected through a small cannula (pseudoplasticity). It should be elastic or shock absorbing and should enhance the coating of surface with minimum surface activity. It should protect the endothelium. It should be noninflammatory, nonpyogenic, nontoxic, and nonantigenic in nature. Till date we do not have a single ideal OVD.

TYPES OF VISCOELASTICS

- *Viscoadaptive viscoelastics:*
  - Healon 5 (sodium hyaluronate 2.3%)
  - 2% hydroxypropyl methylcellulose (HPMC) very commonly used is actually not viscoelastic, it is a viscous material.
- *Viscocohesive viscoelastics:*
  - Healon GV (sodium hyaluronate 1.4%)
  - Healon, Provisc (sodium hyaluronate 1%)
  - Amvisc, Hyal (sodium hyaluronate 1%)
- *Viscodispersive viscoelastics:*
  - Ocucoat (HPMC 2%)
  - Viscoat (sodium chondroitin sulfate 4%—sodium hyaluronate 3%)
  - Visilon (HPMC 2%).

USES OF VISCOELASTIC IN VARIOUS STEPS OF PHACOEMULSIFICATION

Viscoelastic substance is needed to maintain space, helps in pupillary enlargement, capsulorhexis and maintaining anterior chamber, implantation of intraocular lens (IOL), to temponade posterior capsule defect.

Even though all OVDs protect the corneal endothelium during phacoemulsification, some viscoelastics may provide better protection than others. Viscoat (sodium chondroitin sulfate 4%-sodium hyaluronate 3%) is a dispersive OVD with low viscosity at zero shear rate. The dispersive nature causes better adherence of the viscoelastic to the corneal endothelium, possibly resulting in better protection of the corneal endothelium against fluid turbulence and lens fragments during phacoemulsification. Also Viscoat has three negative charges per molecular unit that provide a greater neutralizing effect on positively charged ocular tissue, which better explains the coatability of the corneal endothelium.

Soft shell technique of Arshinoff, first viscodispersive agent is injected in the center of pupillary region then viscocohesive agent is injected below the dispersive viscoelastic which pushes the dispersive agent closer to endothelium. Cohesive viscoelastic in center helps in maintaining anterior chamber as well as pushing the iris lens diaphragm posteriorly. During phacoemulsification even if the cohesive viscoelastic is rapidly aspirated then also dispersive agent pushed to periphery provides the endothelial protection. This technique is especially useful in cases with compromised endothelium such as Fuchs' endothelial dystrophy.

Capsulorhexis

Viscoelastic materials with cohesive property are helpful for performing continuous curvilinear capsulorhexis (CCC). Most viscoelastics including methyl cellulose suffice for this step.

If there is increased convexity of the anterior surface that is associated with positive vitreous pressure or a shallow anterior chamber, prefer using high viscosity OVD such as Healon GV/Healon 5.

Ultra soft shell technique can help in manipulating the flap more comfortably during capsulorhexis under cover of highly viscous cohesive viscoelastic. In this technique, a small layer of balanced salt solution (BSS)/fluid is injected under the layers of viscoelastics.

Nuclear Emulsification

During the emulsification, surgeon requires a viscoelastic that persists in the anterior chamber as well as provides protection to the endothelial cells. Cohesive viscoelastic tends to escape en bloc once the irrigation and aspiration is started. Viscodispersive agents tend to persist in anterior chamber. They, due to low surface tension also, coat the endothelium and provide protection to the endothelium. I personally prefer using Viscoat (soft shell technique) to protect endothelium especially in cases with difficult situations such as poor endothelial status as compared to sodium hyaluronate 1% or 1.4%.

Intraocular Lens Implantation
For IOL implantation cohesive viscoelastic such as sodium hyaluronate 1% or 1.4% are more suitable as they maintain the space better and are easy to remove.

Techniques of Viscoelastic Removal at the End of Procedure
Several techniques have been described for viscoelastic removal after completion of the procedure. It should be remembered that the high cohesive agents are more easily removed whereas complete removal of dispersive agents are difficult. Techniques such as rock and roll, allow aspiration of viscoelastics from behind the IOL. Free movement or rotation of IOL in the bag indicates complete removal.

■ USES IN SPECIAL SITUATIONS
Mixing the lidocaine with viscoelastics prolongs the action of anesthetic agent and has been recently described as *viscoanesthesia*.

Posterior Capsular Rent
After the posterior capsular rent is recognized, one next controls the damage by compartmentalization with a dispersive OVD. After removing the second instrument, viscodispersive viscoelastic (Viscoat) is injected through the paracentesis incision to temponade the tear. Only when anterior chamber is of normal depth can the phaco tip be withdrawn from the eye without anterior chamber collapse. Viscoat does not get mixed with vitreous and allows subsequent manipulations and completion of procedure.

Capsular Bag Dialysis
Viscoelastic substances are helpful for reinflating the dialysed bag and shifting to its position subsequently capsular tension ring (CTR) or capsular tension segment (CTS) can be placed.

Extension of Capsulorhexis
Use of high viscosity viscoelastic such as sodium hyaluronate 1.4% or Healon 5 does help in completion of CCC.

Small Pupil
Apart from other surgical and pharmacological methods to dilate pupil viscoelastic plays an important role. Synechiolysis can be done with the help of high molecular weight cohesive viscoelastics. Also cohesive viscoelastics (Healon 5) are very helpful in enlarging pupil due to mechanical action (viscomydriasis).

Viscoelastic substances, especially dispersive viscoelastic, should always be available in the trolley during phacoemulsification surgery.

■ COMPLICATIONS OF OPHTHALMIC VISCOELASTIC DEVICES
- Raised postoperative intraocular pressure (IOP)
- Capsular bag distension syndrome
- Toxic anterior segment syndrome (TASS)
- Crystallization of OVD over lens surface/IOL calcification.

EDITOR'S PEARLS

Table summarizing the various types of OVDs along with their composition and salient features.

Type of viscoelastics	Example	Composition	Features
Viscocohesives	• Healon • Healon GV • Provisc	• 1% NaHa • 1.4% NaHa • 1% NaHa	• High surface tension and a high degree of pseudoplasticity due to their high molecular weight with long chains. • Create space and flatten the anterior capsule during capsulorhexis
Viscodispersives	• Viscoat • OcuCoat • Healon D	• 4% Sodium Chondroitin Sulfate and 3% NaHa • 2% HPMC • Short chain NaHa	• Low viscosity and high coating ability—better endothelial protective effect • Suitable for lubrication of IOL injector cartridges
Viscoadaptives	Healon 5	2.3% NaHa	Display different behaviors at different flow rates; at low flow rate, it is highly retentive and at high flow rate, its chains fracture and coat the endothelium.
Combination agents	DuoVisc	Combination of a viscodispersive (Viscoat), and a cohesive (ProVisc)	Its dispersive action achieves long-lasting protection of the endothelium while cohesive action facilitates capsulorhexis and IOL implantation
OVD with Lidocaine	VisThesia	Combination of 1% lidocaine hydrochloride and 1 or 1.5% NaHa	Provides the intracameral anesthesia and maintenance of the anatomical space
OVD with trypan blue	Pe-Ha-Blue PLUS	Combination of 1.7% NaHa and 0.020 mg/mL trypan blue	• Allows the surgeon to maintain the chamber, protect the endothelium, and stain the capsule for creation of continuous curvilinear capsulorhexis • Helpful in white cataracts and pseudoexfoliation.

SUGGESTED READING

1. Thirumalai B, Blamires TL, Brooker L, Deeks J. Heavier molecular weight ocular viscoelastic devices and timing of post-operative review following cataract surgery. BMC Ophthalmol. 2007:7:2.

3.14 Phaco Incision

Ravijit Singh
Dr Daljit Singh Eye Hospital, Amritsar
ravijit@yahoo.com

■ INTRODUCTION

Before phaco era, it was so common to hear "small incision big trouble, large incision small trouble". All this changed with the advent of phacoemulsification. Small to smaller to smallest incisions complemented by intraocular lenses that could be passed through these tiny incisions became the order of the day and we still have not stopped dreaming about yet smaller incisions.

As the incisions became smaller the possibility of leaving the incision sutureless also became a reality. From interrupted 8-0 virgin silk sutures to interrupted and continuous 9-0 and 10-0 nylon sutures to no suture at all has been one beautiful journey.

■ EXPECTATIONS FROM A GOOD PHACO INCISION

1. Minimum corneal tissue injury.
2. Should be wide enough to provide a snug fit to the phaco needle.
3. Should not be too tight which could strangulate the infusion of fluid through the coaxial sleeve and cause incision burn.
4. Architecture of the incision should be astigmatically neutral.
5. Should be positioned along the steeper corneal meridian.
6. Should seal well at the end of the surgery.

■ TYPES OF PHACO INCISIONS

Phaco incision types can be divided according to the position, relative to the limbus:

1. *Scleral tunnel incisions*: These were the earliest incisions when we all started doing phaco in the early 90s. The scleral tunnel was supposed to provide a stable incision, much like the suspension bridge. Since there were no foldable lenses at the time, and availability of 5.0 mm optic lenses was also difficult. The usual anesthesia then used to be a retrobulbar block.
2. *Pure clear corneal incision*: This was the next incision in evolution. From scleral to pure clear corneal was a huge leap. Topical anesthesia, no cautery and no patch.
3. *Limbal phaco incision*: Limbal incision is quite like the clear corneal incision but instead of the incision being in the clear corneal tissue, it is made at the limbus. This incision bleeds a little when made though no cautery is needed. This is what is beneficial from the healing point of view.

■ ARCHITECTURE OF THE PHACO INCISION

There are generally three ways that a phaco incision is made:
1. Triplanar incision
2. Biplanar incision
3. Uniplanar incision.

1. *Triplanar incision*: In this, an initial vertical incision is made up to a depth of 300 μm with a guarded knife. A keratome then is used to make the horizontal pocket in the cornea before dipping its tip into the anterior chamber to complete the incision. This triplanar incision is supposed to provide the best seal at the end of surgery (**Fig. 3.14.1**).
2. *Biplanar incision:* The keratome is initially traversed horizontally into some distance within the cornea before proceeding vertically while entering the anterior chamber.

SECTION 3: Cataract

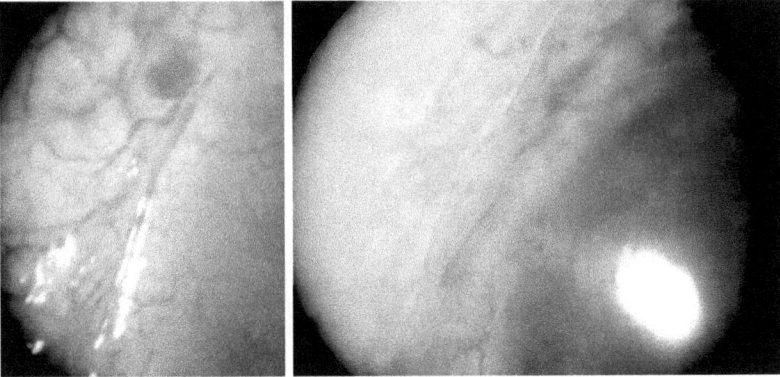

Fig. 3.14.1: Triplanar incision or veiled incision.

3. *Uniplanar incision:* In this, the keratome is positioned at the limbus at an angle and then passed through the cornea obliquely before opening into the anterior chamber.

MAKING THE PARACENTESIS INCISION OR THE SIDE PORT INCISION

The side port incision can be made with a 15-degree blade, microvitreoretinal blade or a diamond knife. The width of the incision is determined by the diameter of the shaft of the chopper being used. A mismatch can cause egress of large volume of fluid and flooding in the surgical field.

INSTRUMENTS FOR MAKING PHACO INCISIONS

- 300 µm preset knife (diamond or steel).
- An appropriately sized keratome to match your phaco needle and sleeve specifications (diamond or steel).
- 15-degree steel blade or a trifacet diamond knife for the side port incision.

HOW TO ENLARGE THE INCISION?

- The initial phaco incision can be enlarged with a 5.0 mm keratome for implantation of a nonfoldable lens. This incision can be extended on either side with gentle cutting movements using the same extender keratome, should a 6.0 mm optic lens need to be implanted.
- If situation demands extending the phaco incision to a full corneal incision, the phaco incision should be left undisturbed and a corneal incision be made (as used to be made for large incision cataract surgery) at the limbus.

SEALING THE PHACO INCISION

A 2-mL syringe fixed to a 27-gauge cannula can be used to inflate the anterior chamber and activate the valvular mechanism of the main phaco incision at the end of the surgery. If need be, hydration of the edges of the main incision as well as the paracentesis incisions may also be done to achieve a good waterproof seal. A cotton-tipped applicator or a Weck-Cel sponge may be used to check the wound.

If at the end of a promised sutureless cataract surgery you find that the phaco incision does not seal properly and the anterior chamber repeated becomes shallow, please do not hesitate to apply a 10-0 nylon suture. The suture may be removed a few days after the surgery.

> **EDITOR'S PEARLS**
>
> Table summarizing the advantages and disadvantages of corneal and scleral incisions.
>
> | | Scleral tunnel incision | Limbal/Clear corneal incision |
> | --- | --- | --- |
> | Site | Scleral incision, beyond limbus | At limbus or clear corneal |
> | Bleeding | Present | Mild or absent |
> | Advantages | • Less rate of endophthalmitis
• Better healing
• Useful in microcornea cases | • Self-sealing
• No need of cautery
• Faster visual recovery |
> | Disadvantages | • Conjunctival incision needed: High chances of bleeding and hyphema
• Slower visual recovery | • Wound leak
• Higher rate of endophthalmitis
• Higher rate of astigmatism
• Risk of Descemet's membrane detachment (DMD) |

■ SUGGESTED READING

1. Baykara M, Ucan G. Modifying the position of cataract incisions in triple procedure. Eur J Ophthalmol. 2008;18(6):891-4.

3.15 How to Proceed if Clear Corneal Incision is Ragged and Incompetent?

Arup Chakrabarti
Chakrabarti Eye Care Centre, Thiruvananthapuram
tvm_meenarup@sancharnet.in

■ INTRODUCTION

Sutureless clear corneal incisions (CCI) were introduced by Howard Fine in 1991. An ideal CCI should have a square or a near square configuration to ensure a watertight closure which can be enhanced by stromal hydration at the conclusion of surgery. CCI created at the temporal limbus usually has a width of 2.8–3.2 mm and a length of 1.75–2.00 mm.

Problems with incision construction are not uncommon. Usually they are minor, requiring the surgeon only to minimally modify the procedure to adjust for the anatomic irregularities created. However dangerous deviation in incision construction may lead to critical alterations in phaco technique and can be the causative factor in multiple subsequent surgical problems eventuating in tears of the posterior capsule and vitreous loss.

■ CAUSES

- *Inaccuracy in wound construction:*
    - External incision unsuitably located anteriorly or posteriorly
    - Internal incision unsuitably located anteriorly or posteriorly
    - Premature entry into the anterior chamber
    - Incision width too broad
- Torn roof or floor
- Wound burns

External incision is too anterior or internal incision is too posterior: It will result in a short corneal tunnel in which watertight closure and wound strength cannot be assured. Though phaco may be uneventful in many cases, postoperative wound leak could lead to hypotony or endophthalmitis. In these situations, one to three 10-0 nylon sutures placed radially and tied adequately to prevent fluid egress should provide satisfactory wound integrity. Stromal hydration should be utilized as an adjunct.

Deep incisions will result in premature entry into the anterior chamber (AC) and a short tunnel. The floor of the tunnel will be thin and may tear. All these will compromise wound integrity so that suture closure will usually be necessary.

If the roof is too thin due to shallow incision, it can tear or buttonhole. A torn roof can be closed with sutures. Usually, it is watertight. However, a buttonhole may lead to a leaking wound which may be impossible to close. In this case, the incision should be abandoned before AC entry, if recognized early. If entry to the AC has occurred, the buttonhole can be closed with an X suture to create downward pressure. The conjunctiva should also be sutured to limit fluid egress. If all else fails, a partial thickness autologous scleral graft or bank scleral patch can be sewn over the buttonhole to create a watertight patch. However, if a thin roof or buttonhole is recognized early enough, one can always return to the original external scleral groove and initiate a fresh tunnel dissection at a deeper plane. The other option would be to relocate to a new site for a fresh CCI or a scleral tunnel incision.

If the incision is too wide, there will be excessive fluid egress around the phaco tip and chamber instability. If AC is difficult to maintain, one or two sutures should be used to partially close it so that the incision is sufficient just for the phaco tip. This will then stabilize the AC and allow an uneventful procedure. Another option would be to close the leaky wound and relocate it to another site (scleral or clear corneal).

Wound burn can result in significant distortion of wound architecture. Multiple tight sutures become mandatory to affect a reasonably watertight closure. Often horizontal mattress sutures are better at approximating the roof and floor of the burned incision to create a watertight incision without the creation of large amounts of astigmatism. Sometimes wound closure becomes impossible, requiring a patch graft.

EDITOR'S PEARLS

- Ragged morphology of a proximal opening of CCI predisposes to incision-site Descemet's membrane detachment (DMD). Once detected care should be taken during intraocular lens (IOL) implantation and stromal hydration to prevent its extension.
- Short phaco tunnels are not self-sealing thus require suture while very long phaco tunnels make maneuvering the instrument within the AC difficult.
- A too posterior wound can lead to ballooning of conjunctiva which results in pooling and distortion of anterior chamber view. Doing a small peritomy in such situations may help in better visualization.

SUGGESTED READING

1. Ernest PH, Fine IH, Fishkind WJ. Complications of wound construction and closure. In: Fishkind WJ (Ed). Complications in phacoemulsification: avoidance, recognition, and management. New York: Thieme Medical Publishers; 2002.

3.16 What are the Various Means of Doing Anterior Capsulotomy?

Rupal H Trivedi
Storm Eye Institute, Medical University of South Carolina, Charleston, USA
trivedi@musc.edu

INTRODUCTION

In order to perform phacoemulsification, an opening in the anterior capsule (anterior capsulotomy) should be created. It aids in hydrodissection and facilitates fixation of the intraocular lens (IOL) implantation.

A number of modalities have been evaluated to open the anterior capsule:
- Manual continuous curvilinear capsulorhexis (CCC) (Utrata forceps, bent 26G needle cystotome)
- Fugo plasma blade
- Vitrectorhexis
- Radiofrequency ablation
- Femtosecond laser-assisted capsulotomy

The ideal anterior capsule opening is of optimum size, centered, round, and continuous. A deep anterior chamber should be maintained by the adequate use of an ophthalmic viscosurgical device (OVD). Use of OVD flattens the anterior lens capsule. Without OVD, anterior chamber becomes shallow and anterior lens capsule becomes dome shaped instead of flattened. Chances of anterior capsule tear are high if capsulotomy is performed in this phase.

Manual anterior CCC is the most commonly performed technique to open an anterior capsule during cataract surgery. It minimizes the risks of inducing radial tears and preserves the integrity of the capsular bag providing a safer environment for phacoemulsification and allows capsular bag IOL implantation. We reported that the manual CCC technique produced the most extensible porcine capsulotomy followed by the Fugo plasma blade, vitrectorhexis, can-opener, and radiofrequency (RF) techniques. Under scanning electron microscope (SEM) examination, manual CCC produced the smoothest edge; vitrectorhexis edge was scalloped rolled over edge; can-opener edge was irregular; RF edge was ragged, rough and irregular; and the plasma blade edge was rough when compared with the manual CCC, but irregularities were less than those of RF edge. The Fugo plasma blade is efficacious when manual tearing is prevented by fibrosis in the capsule such as in delayed surgery for traumatic cataract.

The vitrectorhexis is an alternative anterior capsulotomy method that is used in infants, especially when surgical strategy is to leave an eye aphakic. With the cutting port facing down against the capsule, engage the capsule and enlarge the round capsular opening in a spiral fashion to the desired shape and size. Care should be taken to avoid leaving any right-angle edges, which could predispose to radial tear formation.

The femtosecond laser is used to create anterior capsulotomies of the desired size and reduces the unpredictability associated with manual capsulorhexis. It is now finding wider applications including areas of difficult capsulorhexis such as subluxated lenses. The capsulotomy is created by tiny confluent overlapping zones of photodisruption created by the femtosecond laser. Studies have shown it to produce capsulotomies that are more precise, accurate, reproducible, and stronger than those created with the conventional manual technique.

DYE-ENHANCED CAPSULOTOMY

A report from American Academy of Ophthalmology evaluated currently available data in the published literature to answer the question of whether the use of dye such as indocyanine green (ICG) or trypan blue to stain the lens capsule to improve visualization is safe and effective as an adjunct to cataract surgery. The report concluded that: (1) it is reasonable to use dye when inadequate capsule visualization may compromise the outcome in cataract surgery; (2) more studies are needed to confirm a lack of toxicity of ICG and trypan blue, particularly in the event of posterior segment or longer duration exposure. When injecting under air, the dye should be injected after the paracentesis, but prior to creating the main incision, to help with anterior chamber stability. Staining under air versus under OVD was reported as having similar efficacy and safety. The stained capsule is reported to be less elastic and torn under less stretching force. This change in elastic behavior should facilitate a CCC along with better visualization. Trypan blue can also minimize epithelial cell proliferation. However, the use of dyes is not advised when using hydrophilic IOLs, to avoid permanent discoloration of the IOL.

■ SIZE OF CONTINUOUS CURVILINEAR CAPSULORHEXIS

In addition to its strong edge, the efficacy of capsulorhexis depends on centration, location, and size. It has been suggested that the CCC should be small enough to overlap the edge of the IOL optic for 360°. A CCC that is bigger than IOL optic has been associated with greater posterior capsular opacification (PCO) than smaller capsulorhexis. In contrast, when the CCC is too small, anterior capsular phimosis, decreased visualization of the retina, and decreased effectiveness in the properties of aspheric IOLs can occur.

The ideal capsulorhexis size is around 5–5.5 mm in diameter. Frequent grasping and regrasping of capsular edge help to obtain optimum size of capsulorhexis especially in young children with highly elastic capsule. Forceps with two marks, one 5 mm from the tip and another 2.5 mm from the tip, can be used to create 5 mm capsulorhexis. The mark at 2.5 mm should be placed in the center of the visual axis. The tip of the forceps and the 5-mm mark outline the diameter of an ideal 5 mm capsulorhexis. Corneal markers have been evaluated as a guide for CCC size, but corneal magnification factors decrease their accuracy. Tassignon, et al. proposed a ring-shaped caliper with an internal diameter of 5 mm or 6 mm. They state that it is easy to insert and facilitates capsulorhexis centration.

In eyes where future anterior phimosis is likely to occur, such as eyes with pseudoexfoliation syndrome, retinitis pigmentosa, diabetes, uveitis and eyes with zonular pathology or eyes receiving silicone IOL—slightly larger capsulorhexis (5.5–6.0 mm) may be beneficial. A smaller capsulorhexis may be beneficial when the surgeon wants to ensure that the IOL does not come out of the capsular bag during other concurrent intraocular procedures where shallowing of the anterior chamber or in anticipation of high posterior pressure.

> **EDITOR'S PEARLS**
> - A well centered, adequately sized rhexis is crucial for IOL centration and stability, better estimation of effective lens position and prevention of posterior capsular opacification.
> - It is also important for preventing toric IOL rotation and optimizing outcomes with multifocal IOLs.
> - Femtosecond laser can help in customizing the capsulorhexis and is particularly useful in challenging scenarios such as subluxated and white cataract.
> - Image-guided systems such as Verion (Alcon) and Callisto (Zeiss) are useful intraoperative aids that help ensure proper size and centration of capsulorhexis.

■ SUGGESTED READING

1. Albert DM, Miller JW, Azar DT, Young LH (Eds). Albert and Jakobiec's Principles and Practice of Ophthalmology. Springer, Cham; 2022.
2. Jacobs DS, Cox TA, Wagoner MD, Ariyasu RG, Karp CL; American Academy of Ophthalmology; Ophthalmic Technology Assessment Committee Anterior Segment Panel. Capsule staining as an adjunct to cataract surgery: a report from the American Academy of Ophthalmology. Ophthalmology. 2006;113(4):707-13.
3. Trivedi RH, Wilson ME Jr, Bartholomew LR. Extensibility and scanning electron microscopy evaluation of 5 pediatric anterior capsulotomy techniques in a porcine model. J Cataract Refract Surg. 2006;32(7):1206-13.
4. Wang KM, Jun AS, Ladas JG, Devgan U. Phacoemulsification: Principles and Techniques. In: Albert DM, Miller JW, Azar DT, Young LH (Eds). Albert and Jakobiec's Principles and Practice of Ophthalmology. Springer, Cham; 2022.
5. Wilson ME, Trivedi RH. Pediatric Cataract Surgery. In: Albert and Jakobiec's Principles and Practice of Ophthalmology. Springer, Cham; 2022. pp. 1585-605.

3.17 How do You Deal with Hard Cataracts during Phacoemulsification?

Rohit Om Parkash
Dr Om Parkash Eye Institute, Amritsar
drrohit@accuratesight.com

■ HARD CATARACT PHACOEMULSIFICATION

Hard cataract phacoemulsification is difficult because of different morphology, poor visualization, difficult division and emulsification, excessive wound site thermal injury (WSTI), difficult chamber stability, increased posterior capsule (PC) rupture, and insult to corneal endothelium.

A hard cataract has a thin capsule, scarce cortex and nucleus comprising—a thin epinucleus, a firmer inner nucleus and a hard central core with leathery densely packed fibers.

- The evaluation includes the age, endothelial health, anterior chamber (AC) depth, mydriasis extent, zonular integrity and ruling out deep-set eye.
- Objective recording of endothelial cell count by specular microscopy is indicated.
- Preferably a peribulbar block is administered especially in the hands of beginners.
- The incision width is important as excess energy used causes WSTI. Relatively loose incisions decrease WSTI but unstable AC predispose PC damage. High-end machine takes care of heat and surge.
- A large 6 mm continuous curvilinear capsulorhexis (CCC) helps in decreasing nucleus and anterior capsule contact thereby reducing zonular stress. Trypan blue staining allows anterior capsular edge visualization. This prevents nicking of the CCC edge.
- The hydrodissecting fluid wave is rarely visible. Inject in small amounts. A large single area injection tightens up the eye with a severe focal capsular distention. Cortical decompression predisposes PC rupture. Moving Iris repositor horizontally under the anterior capsular edge in all directions softens the eye and AC deepens as fluid extrudes out.
- It is rarely difficult to rotate a hard nucleus. If nucleus does not rotate in one direction then rotate in the other direction. Avoid two-handed rotation.
- *Endothelial protection:* Soft-shell technique should be used in dealing with hard nucleus cases.
- Bevel down hyperpulsed sculpting is done. Never push the nucleus. A small crater is created. Now chopping is done with burst mode. The nucleus is held firmly by embedding the phaco tip in the deeper part of nucleus. A long pointed chopper is used for chopping in safe zone. If the harder nucleus does not allow full penetration of the chopper, repeat full penetration at a different place before separation force is applied. It is preferable to use the "divide and conquer" technique for dividing the nucleus for emulsification (crater/trench and chop technique).
- The chopper and the embedded tip work in cohesion to totally separate nuclear fibers. If the posterior plate fails to separate, the chopper is moved to a different nuclear plane or to a different place and if still required moved in a different direction to achieve total separation. A complete separation is the key. Chop into small pieces. Do not emulsify and eat up the nuclear piece. Leave them so that they act as a cushion when last piece is being totally separated.
- Occasionally, total separation is not possible. At this stage, continue chopping sequentially through 360°. This gives a central core and partially chopped nuclear pieces. With high vacuum lift the central core and emulsify. Now separate the pieces fully before phacoaspirating.
- Endothelial protection measures include apart from viscoelastic soft shell technique, multiple viscodispersive or visco-adaptive injections at various steps, chopping into

smaller pieces, deeper plane emulsification, stable chamber settings and torsional emulsification/advanced fluidics such as active fluidics.
- High vacuum and flow rate are used to allow the nucleus to remain in contact with the tip thus allowing the ultrasound to be more effective.
- Each machine has its own limitations of parameters, which the surgeon needs to understand. The key lies in the perfect combination of fluidics, energy modulations, and stable AC in managing hard cataracts.
- Torsional emulsification has advantages of minimal WSTI. Hence, routine tight incisions are used. The chamber is stable, turbulence is minimal and emulsification is done in deeper plane. 45° Kelman tip provides deeper sculpting, enhanced cutting, increased cavitations and enhanced aspiration of lenticular material by making the quadrants tumble more easily than with traditional ultrasound.
- The chances of zonular dialysis are very high in such cases. It is always handy to keep a capsular tension ring while operating such cases.
- The cold infusion keeps phaco tip cooler, prevents corneal burns and is said to be endothelial safe.
- The indications for converting back are CCC extension and incomplete separation while chopping or dividing.

EDITOR'S PEARLS

- Meticulous preoperative evaluation and adequate counseling about the condition, prolonged duration of surgery and possible complications are important before operating upon a hard cataract.
- Lack of epinuclear cushion, zonular stress, and fragile capsule make phacoemulsification challenging in these cases.
- Adequate endothelial protection should be ensured. Measures like proper capsule staining and making a marginally large capsulorhexis can help facilitate the nuclear emulsification.
- Use of torsional phacoemulsification, adequate chopping into smaller pieces and their emulsification within the bag or at iris plane is recommended for better outcomes.

SUGGESTED READING

1. Parkash RO. Management of black cataract with phacoemulsification. In: Garg A. Mastering the Techniques of Advanced Phaco Surgery. New Delhi: Jaypee Brothers Medical Publishers; 2007. p. 176.

3.18 | Zero/Minimal Power Phaco

Gaurav Luthra
Drishti Eye Centre and Dehradun Wave Lasik Centre, Dehradun
gaurav.luthra@drishti.org

INTRODUCTION

Phacoemulsification has come a long way from the time Dr Charles D Kelman used a bulky phaco handpiece to perform the first phaco surgery in the early 80s only to be dismissed by the ophthalmic fraternity as a fancy impractical idea. Evolution of surgical skills and recent refinements in phaco machine technology has brought us to a stage where cataracts can now be removed effortlessly utilizing minimal to zero phaco power with excellent results.

Minimizing the amount of phaco energy delivered inside the anterior chamber is crucial to ensuring minimal damage to the corneal endothelium and achieving close to 100% clear corneas postoperative day 1 and beyond. Several strategies can be employed for achieving minimal phaco times including the following.

PEARLS FOR MINIMIZING PHACO TIME

- Gradual transition from trenching to *Chopping* techniques (divide and conquer → stop and chop → direct chop).
- Efficient use of the chopper during segment removal (use chopper to feed pieces to the tip).
- Avoid touching the chopper against phaco tip when delivering phaco power to avoid tip damage.
- Avoid using a *blunt phaco tip*.
- Choose the right phaco tip for your technique:
- 0–15° tips are good for chopping techniques
- 30–45° tips are good for trenching, divide and conquer
- *Old phaco tubings* lose rigidity and decrease vacuum efficiency while also causing surge. Change them regularly.
- Deliver ultrasound (position 3) only when necessary (e.g., when trenching, power should not be delivered on the reverse pass, only on forward passage of tip). Sometimes we are unnecessarily using power when all we need is some more vacuum.
- Use higher vacuum and lower power settings to achieve the same end (see dual linear pedal below).
- *Pulse and hyperpulse* (cold phaco) modes utilize much less energy for the same task (e.g., during segment removal, trenching, etc.).
- Fine tune your chopping technique. With experience embedding and chopping can be combined into a single maneuver. Start chopping even as you are embedding. Saves phaco time.
- *Woodpecker technique in hard cataracts:* When chopping, after embedding the tip and positioning the chopper, a short burst of phaco power while simultaneously chopping helps complete the chop easily.

TECHNOLOGY UPGRADES FOR MINIMIZING PHACO TIMES

- *Kelman* (bent) phaco tips allow better access when direct chopping, Cobra (flared) tips for better grip when chopping especially with microphaco. Mini-flare Kelman tips have been associated with reduced phacoemulsification times.
- The new Intrepid *balanced* tip has two bends in the shaft and is shown to be superior to Kelman tip in terms of increasing the efficacy of phacoemulsification and reducing fluid usage.
- *Dual-linear foot pedal*, available on few machines such as the Millennium (B and L) and OS3 (Oertli) allows linear control in two planes, i.e., pitch (down) and yaw (sideways ↔). This allows setting a basic vacuum in normal pitch movement and additional linear vacuum in yaw ↔ which can be used on demand during crucial steps instead of higher phaco power **(Fig. 3.18.1)**. For example:
    a. When better hold is required during chopping especially in hard cataracts it may be prudent to use more vacuum (yaw) than power (pitch).
    b. When removing a hard fragment one can increase vacuum (yaw ↔) rather than higher phaco power (pitch) to get the same result.
- *Burst mode* available on higher end machines allows embedding when chopping using small bursts of power rather than continuous phaco power.
- *Hyperpulse/cold phaco* involves using power modulation to deliver minimal energy without decreasing cutting efficiency and heat buildup at the tip. This is done by using duty cycles of short millisecond bursts of power, each followed by similar short periods of rest allowing time for the tip to cool. Most new machines are capable of modulated hyperpulse phaco.
- *Torsional ultrasound* (Ellipse-AMO and Ozil-Alcon) is a useful new technology involving sideways movements of the phaco tip rather than conventional linear (backward and forward) movements of the phaco tips. This is thought to improve

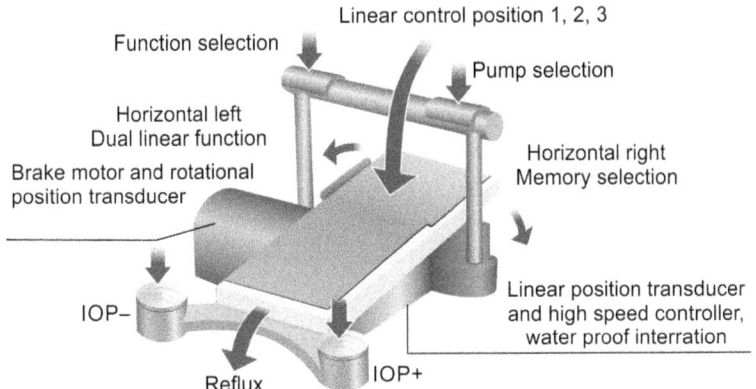

Fig. 3.18.1: Dual-linear foot pedal.

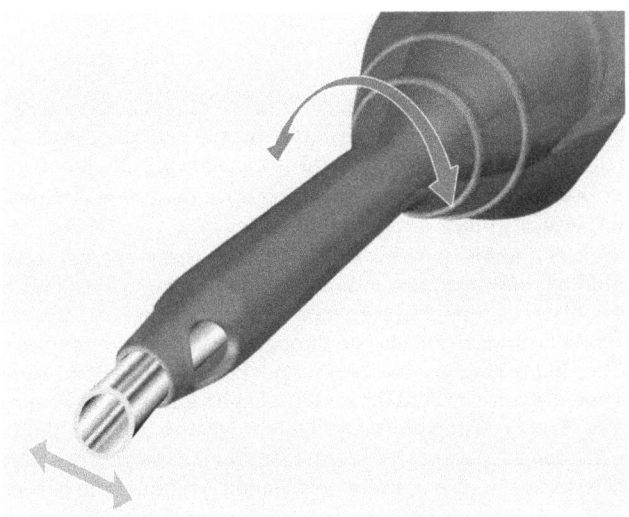

Fig. 3.18.2: Torsional oscillations.

cutting efficiency and at much lower frequencies than traditional ultrasound thereby minimizing use of linear ultrasonic phaco **(Fig. 3.18.2)**.

With experience, innovation, improvisation, and new technology, phaco surgeons can reduce effective phaco times in all but brunescent cataracts to as little as 1–2 seconds. Grade 1–2 cataracts can sometimes be removed without the clock ticking 1 second of effective phaco time, justifying the term—*zero power phaco chop*.

EDITOR'S PEARLS

- Minimal power phacoemulsification can be performed in softer cataracts (mild-moderate nuclear sclerosis) by modifying chopping techniques, increasing vacuum or using larger diameter phaco tips.
- Less phaco energy results in less postoperative corneal edema and faster visual rehabilitation.

SUGGESTED READING

1. Davison JA. Comparison of ultrasonic energy expenditures and corneal endothelial cell density reductions during modulated and non-modulated phacoemulsification. Ophthalmic Surg Lasers Imaging. 2007;38:209-18.

3.19 What are the Causes of Shallowing of Anterior Chamber during Phaco? How to Prevent it?

Cyres K Mehta
Mehta International Eye Institute, Mumbai
cyresmehta@yahoo.com

INTRODUCTION

Shallowing of anterior chamber during phacoemulsification is not uncommon. We need to understand its causes and solution to safely complete phacoemulsification procedure.

The causes of shallowing of anterior chamber during phacoemulsification are as follows:

During Hydrodissection

- If the pupil is small and/or if the rhexis is small, copious hydrodissection without decompression of the nucleus downward with the cannula can make the nucleus pop-up in the bag pushing the iris upward and shallowing the chamber.
  Prevention: Use small aliquots of fluid during hydrodissection and push the nucleus down in the bag every time.
- If the cannula is malpositioned over the anterior rhexis margin (instead of under it as it should be) and hydrodissection carried out the nucleus does not move and there is no fluid wave prompting even more fluid to be injected. Sometimes it can tent the peripheral iris upward and also go through the gaps in the zonules to hydrate the vitreous. Once in the vitreous this fluid cannot come back forward and consequently due to this one way travel of fluid the iris lens diaphragm is pushed forward shallowing the chamber. Several risk factors are likely to give rise to this fluid misdirection syndrome. Anything that causes a disruption in zonular integrity can allow fluid to pass into the posterior segment, e.g., pseudoexfoliation syndrome and old ocular trauma.
  Prevention: Recognize such situations and make sure to hydrodissect in the capsular bag.

During Phacoemulsification of the Nucleus

- On breaking, occlusion during phaco when a piece is aspirated the outflow frequently exceeds inflow into the eye in the phenomenon called surge when the anterior chamber shallows abruptly and the pupil margin will move inward. This was fairly common with older machines which lacked stiff noncompliant tubing and sensors to detect anterior chamber pressure and slow pump speed.
- Microphaco techniques where outflow frequently exceeds inflow and the openings do not seal well, as a metal tube cannot seal an oval opening in the cornea as well as a pliable silicone sleeve, are very prone to surge.
- Mismatch of incision size and phaco accessories such as tip and sleeve.
- Iris hooks if used pull the iris upward shallowing the anterior chamber (AC) and causing more leakage through the four openings they occupy. Use small longer tunnels for the hooks.
- Positive posterior pressure may develop also due to mechanical pressure from a tight speculum which is eased by using a different speculum or a looser one.

- Finally, a suprachoroidal effusion or hemorrhage during phaco can cause shallowing of the AC. Suprachoroidal effusion is caused by the rupture of the short posterior ciliary vessels with a subsequent outpouring of plasma and blood into the suprachoroidal space. This complication commonly occurs upon the withdrawal of the phaco or irrigation and aspiration (I/A) tip in hypertensives. The sudden hypotony thus produced is the driving force for damage to the short, posterior ciliary vessels. Diagnosis is simple, look at the fundus and the glow will be darker, the chamber shallow and a tented up mass will be seen at the posterior pole. Never try to convert to an extracapsular cataract extraction, because an enlarged wound will destabilize the eye and allow a suprachoroidal effusion to become hemorrhagic, leading to an expulsive hemorrhage.

EDITOR'S PEARLS
- In cases of preexisting shallow AC the surgeon should ensure proper maintenance of chamber using a strongly cohesive OVD and minimal distortion of wound during instrumentation.
- Well-constructed incisions help ensure no excessive fluid leakage during surgery.
- In case of sudden intraoperative shallowing of anterior chamber with rise in IOP the surgeon must suspect fluid misdirection syndrome or suprachoroidal hemorrhage.

SUGGESTED READING
1. Cheung CM, Hero M. Stabilization of anterior chamber depth during phacoemulsification cataract surgery in vitrectomized eyes. J Cataract Refract Surg. 2005;31(11):2055-7.

3.20 | Management of Subluxated Cataract

Rajiv Choudhary
Rajas Eye and Retina Research Centre, Indore
choudhary@sancharnet.in
choudharyrajiv14@hotmail.com

INTRODUCTION
Surgical management of cataract associated with zonular dialysis is a real challenge for the ophthalmic surgeon. To aim at better visual outcome, one must do a thorough preoperative evaluation and follow appropriate surgical principle.

One must specifically look for extent of subluxation, vitreous prolapse, and phacodonesis.

SURGICAL PRINCIPLES FOR ANY ZONULAR DIALYSIS
The big and bold surgical paradigm is closed chamber technique.

Incision
I prefer it away from area of zonular weakness so as to decrease stress on existing zonules.

Viscoelastic
Highly retentive viscoelastic material should be used adequately over the area of zonular dialysis so as to help tamponade vitreous and maintain deep noncollapsing anterior chamber (AC).

Capsulorhexis
One should initiate continuous curvilinear capsulorhexis (CCC) in the area remote from dialysis and CCC should be 5.5-6 mm size.

Hydrodissection

It must be done carefully but thoroughly so as to free the nucleus maximally and lessen the stress on zonules during phacoemulsification.

Phacoemulsification

- Capsular hooks/Iris hooks should be placed grasping the anterior margins of the capsular bag to stabilize the lens and minimize the risk of increase in the amount of subluxation.
- Capsular tension segment (CTS)/capsular tension ring (CTR) can be placed after hydrodissection.
- If the amount of subluxation is larger than 5 clock hours, a Cionni ring fixation would be required. In such cases, scleral pockets needs to be pre-prepared before AC entry.
- It is a sort of slow motion phaco. Power should be appropriate for grade of cataract. Vacuum, flow rate, and bottle height should be kept low so as to minimize turbulence. At any stage if vitreous is detected in AC, it should be handled by thorough two-port AC vitrectomy. I prefer chopping in these cases.

Irrigation-Aspiration

I prefer cortical viscodissection so as to decrease stress on the zonules. Bimanual technique is advocated in these cases; however, I personally use coaxial method under cover of high retentive viscoelastic substance. Active fluidics with intraocular pressure (IOP) control will be better if available.

Intraocular Lens Implantation

If capsular bag is retained during phaco, I plan posterior chamber (PC) intraocular lens (IOL) implantation and prefer to orient the haptics of IOL parallel to the dialysis so as to have optimal zonular support and decreased risk of postoperative lens decentration. However, the best would be to use CTR so as to achieve 360° capsular bag expansion and greater stabilization.

■ STEPS TO BE TAKEN ACCORDING TO EXTENT OF SUBLUXATION

Mild (Less than 3 Clock Hours)

In these cases, I do conventional phacoemulsification surgery considering above-mentioned principles.

Moderate (3–5 Clock Hours)

Phacoemulsification in such cases requires the use of CTR. The CTR is inserted after cortical clean up so as to aim at well-centered IOL. The confirmation of CTR in the bag includes dramatic expansion and stabilization of bag. CTR is avoided in cases of break in rhexis or posterior capsular tear (PCT).

Up to 7 Clock Hours

Here, I use modified CTR (MCTR) and fix it to sclera (scleral fixation CTR). 10-0 prolene suture is secured to the eyelet of MCTR; fixation hook is manipulated anterior to the capsulorhexis edge. The double arm suture is passed through the incision between the anterior capsule and under surface of iris and out through the ciliary sulcus and scleral wall and then sutured.

In cases of subluxation >7 clock hours but <9 clock hours, a double Cionni ring can be used to fix the capsular bag to the sclera at two places.

More than 9 Clock Hours
In cases of >9 clock hours of subluxation, after cataract extraction, one can place an anterior chamber IOL, scleral fixated IOL or an iris claw lens (anterior or retrofixation).

Retrofixation of Iris Claw Lens
Main incision is increased to 5.5 mm size, optic held by lens holding forceps in the pupillary area, haptic placed behind the iris and clipping done using dialer through side port, same way the other haptic clipped inserting dialer through the other side port.

> **EDITOR'S PEARLS**
> - During phacoemulsification in subluxated cataract special care should be taken to avoid sudden fluctuation of chamber by the use of appropriate ophthalmic viscoelastic device (OVD).
> - Femtosecond laser-assisted cataract surgery (FLACS) is a useful modality in these cases as the steps of laser capsulotomy and nucleotomy are performed within a closed chamber.
> - The use of CTR/CTS should be avoided in cases with a PC rent or torn rhexis margin.

■ SUGGESTED READING
1. Vasavada V, Vasavada VA, Hoffman RO, Spencer TS, Kumar RV, Crandall AS. Intraoperative performance and postoperative outcomes of endocapsular ring implantation in pediatric eyes. J Cataract Refract Surg. 2008;34(9):1499-508.

3.21 The Capsular Bag is Unexpectedly Mobile during Phaco. How to Manage with a Capsular Tension Ring?

Tanuj Dada
Dr RP Centre for Ophthalmic Sciences, AIIMS, New Delhi
tanujdada@gmail.com

Vivek Dave
LV Prasad Eye Institute, Hyderabad
vivekdave@lvpei.org

■ INTRODUCTION
In cases of zonular dialysis during phacoemulsification, a capsular tension ring (CTR) can provide both intraoperative and postoperative stability of the capsular bag and intraoperative lens (IOL).

■ INDICATIONS FOR USING CAPSULAR TENSION RING
The indication for use of a CTR is in eyes which have a 3-5 clock hour (up to 180°) of subluxation/dialysis. Cases having subluxation of 5-7 clock hours (180-200°) require a Cionni CTR which is sutured to the sclera. Capsular tension segments can be used along with CTR or Cionni ring in greater amounts of subluxation. Double Cionni ring can also be used in subluxations >7-9 clock hours.

■ WHICH DIAMETER TO USE?
The CTR works on the principle of traction-expansion stabilization. The average capsular bag diameter is about 10.5 mm. The diameter of the CTR is more than the bag diameter. The available diameters are given in **Table 3.21.1**. The 14.5 mm is used for high myopes,

TABLE 3.21.1: Types of CTR (Morcher).

Types	Expanded	Compressible	Axial length	Corneal diameter white-to-white
14	12.3 mm	To 10.0 mm	<24 mm	<11 mm
14A	14.5 mm	To 12.0 mm	>28 mm	>12.5 mm
14C	13.0 mm	To 11.0 mm	24–28 mm	11–12.5 mm

13 mm is used for normal eyes and the 12.3 mm is used in pediatric cases and in microspherophakia. As the ring diameter is larger than that of the bag and as the bag is elastic, on injection into the bag, the CTR exerts centrifugal (outward) force on the bag. This supports the deficient zonules and redistributes support to the entire capsule, making the posterior capsule taut and stretched. The diameter can also be selected by the relation of the CTR with the corneal power and the axial length as follows:

$$(3.44 + 0.56 \times P) + (0.71 \times AL) - (0.0135 \times AL \times 2)$$

where P is the corneal power and AL is the axial length.

■ TIME OF INSERTION

The appropriate time of inserting the CTR is variable and depends on the time when capsular bag instability is noted. Generally speaking a CTR can be inserted at any time during nuclear emulsification or after performing the capsulorhexis, though earlier implantation gives better intraoperative safety.

Implanting the CTR *before hydrodissection* allows clear visualization of the anterior capsule and thus proper placement of the ring. The disadvantage is that it precludes adequate cortical clean up as cortex may remain trapped between the capsule and the CTR. If implanted *after hydrodissection* the major advantage is the capsular cortical adhesions are broken and this makes cortex aspiration easier. During phacoemulsification, the CTR keeps the bag stretched and prevents collapse of capsular fornix. It also reduces the possibility of vitreous prolapse and provides better capsular bag stability and IOL centration. If zonular dialysis occurs during automated irrigations aspiration, a CTR should be inserted *prior to IOL implantation*. If a CTR is not available, the nucleus can be prolapsed out of the bag with hydrodissection and a supracapsular phaco performed which causes minimal stress on the zonules, while a dispersive viscoelastic should be used (such as Viscoat) to tamponade the vitreous in the area of zonular dialysis. Nuclear emulsification should be performed gently with low vacuum, low flow, and decreased bottle height.

■ TECHNIQUE FOR INSERTION

The injection of the CTR into the bag is accomplished either manually or using a CTR loaded on an injector (through the main incision). The CTR is introduced into the capsular bag at the area where the zonules are intact to prevent undue capsular instability. It is imperative to ensure that the leading haptic smoothly enters the bag under the anterior capsule. Once this is ensured, the CTR is dialed into the bag with the help of a Sinskey hook or a McPherson forceps. It is important to take care that the eyelet is released only when it is well below the rhexis margin because if it is lost in the sulcus or the anterior chamber angle it becomes very difficult to retrieve the CTR. The final position should be such that the convex part of the ring should about the area of deficient zonules.

In cases with extensive (>200°) zonular dehiscence or with progressive zonular damage, the Cionni modified CTR is used. The Cionni ring has one or two eyelets for fixation of the CTR to the sclera using 9-0 prolene suture. The eyelets are at a higher plane protruding about 0.25 mm forward from the main CTR body and hence, lie over the anterior capsule.

CONTRAINDICATIONS

- Anterior capsular tear
- Posterior capsular rupture
- Incomplete capsulorhexis
- Severely subluxated capsular bag [it is often prudent to enlarge the section and deliver out the cataract intracapsularly, followed by an anterior vitrectomy and an anterior chamber intraocular lens (ACIOL) or a scleral fixated IOL].

EDITOR'S PEARLS
- Capsular tension ring (CTR) is useful in eyes which have a 3–5 clock hour subluxation or intraoperative bag dialysis.
- It is introduced into the capsular bag at the area where the zonules are intact to prevent undue capsular instability.
- It can be inserted at any time, after performing the capsulorhexis, during or after nuclear emulsification, though earlier implantation gives better intraoperative safety.
- CTR should be avoided in cases with posterior capsular rupture or anterior rhexis tear.

SUGGESTED READING
1. Sethi HS, Saxena R, Sinha A. Use of the Unfolder Silver/Sapphire system to inject capsular tension ring during phacoemulsification in cases with subluxated cataract. J Cataract Refract Surg. 2006;32(8):1256-8.

3.22 How will You Manage a Patient of Visually Significant Cataract with Associated Keratoconus?

Sudhank Bharti
Bharti Eye Foundation, New Delhi
drsbharti@bhartieyefoundation.org

CATARACT IN KERATOCONUS PATIENT: MANAGEMENT OPTIONS

Cataract surgery, on a patient of keratoconus, is a challenging job. Cataract surgery can improve the best corrected visual acuity (BCVA) in all severities of keratoconus without significant corneal change.

When to Perform Cataract Surgery?

Phacoemulsification should be performed in these cases when the keratoconus is stable and does not progress further except for cases with white cataracts due to hydrops/C3F8 injection which need to be operated early for visual rehabilitation.

Intraocular lens (IOL) calculation is more predictable in mild keratoconus than in moderate and severe diseases. In mild keratoconus, there is no difference between standard and topography-derived keratometry. However, determining IOL powers with videokeratography-derived K-values might be more accurate than standard keratometry in patients with moderate-severe keratoconus. Another option, if the other eye has no keratoconus, is to use the other eye power to guess estimate the power of IOL. Studies have revealed that the most accurate IOL power was found by using SRKII. Repeated IOL power measurement and using the most frequent of multiple readings is best way to get a good result.

■ MILD-TO-MODERATE KERATOCONUS

Corneal crosslinking, Intacs and Lamellar keratoplasty can be done a few months before cataract removal in a staged procedure and gives good results and also allows better IOL power calculation.

Phacoemulsification with implantation of toric lenses helps to alleviate the excessive astigmatism caused by the keratoconus. Toric IOL technology is slowly gaining popularity, and if used correctly will be a great adjunct to all cataract and intraocular refractive technology. The lens is always oriented along the steep axis of astigmatism, that is, the highest number using the plus cylinder. It is never based on the refraction of the patient as the lens can contribute to that number, skewing the effect of correcting corneal astigmatism only.

■ SEVERE KERATOCONUS

Triple Procedure

When a patient requires both keratoplasty and cataract extraction the two procedures can be performed in combination. The combined or triple procedure (penetrating keratoplasty + cataract removal + IOL implantation) allows faster visual rehabilitation without compromising graft survival when compared with a staged (lamellar keratoplasty followed by phaco + IOL) procedure. However, with recent techniques of lamellar keratoplasty, a single stage lamellar keratoplasty with phacoemulsification can be carried out. Despite the success of the triple procedure, there is still no precise formula available to best predict the IOL power needed to produce postoperative emmetropia though a staged procedure might yield better results.

■ EMERGING CHALLENGES: LOOKING AHEAD

Adaptive Optics in Cataract and Keratoconus

Adaptive optics relies upon a secondary set of mirrors that are in place to adjust for errors within the main optical system. The field of adaptive optics appears to be able to provide many new and interesting discoveries. The measured point spread function in our eyes is far from perfect. In people with keratoconus, these optical errors are even more significant. It is possible, however, to reflect light through a mirror that adapts light to these optical errors and produces a clearer picture on the retina.

Researchers are using adaptive optics to measure the extent of the vision loss in keratoconus that is caused by the cornea and how much is caused by loss of neural information. Keratoconus is one important disease that stands to benefit from the advances in research of adaptive optics. In keratoconus treatment, the progress of the disease can be tracked through the measurements of a patient "wavefront" or point-spread function. In cataract surgery, newer lenses use principles of optics to provide clearer vision through adaptive optics.

> **EDITOR'S PEARLS**
> - Keratometric stability should be looked for before operating.
> - Newer biometers that measure both anterior and posterior corneal curvature should be employed if available.
> - Target slight myopia (1–2D) in moderate-to-advanced cases depending on the severity. Newer formulae such as Haigis, Barrett, and Kane keratoconus have shown promise in producing more accurate refractive outcomes.
> - Implantation of toric lenses can be useful in mild-moderate cases with largely regular astigmatism.

■ SUGGESTED READING

1. Thebpatiphat N, Hammersmith KM, Rapuano CJ, Ayres BD, Cohen EJ. Cataract surgery in keratoconus. Eye Contact Lens. 2007;33(5):244-6.

3.23 Phaco in High Myopia

Sudarshan Khokhar
Dr RP Centre for Ophthalmic Sciences, AIIMS, New Delhi
skhokhar38@yahoo.com

■ INTRODUCTION

These cases present early in life due to enhanced sclerosis. Management depends on phacodonesis, retinal evaluation for coexisting posterior segment problems, and axial length measurement. Aim for postoperative myopia (-1 to -1.50) only. Do not aim for emmetropias, there might be a hyperopic shift (patient has been used to the minified but bigger field of myopic vision).

■ SURGICAL PRECAUTIONS

- High myopes have a thin sclera and hence, the chances of globe perforation are very high while administering peribulbar block. The block should be given carefully by an experienced surgeon. Experts in the field of cataract surgery can perform phacoemulsification under topical anesthesia.
- Since zonules are weak and may be stretched, keep the phaco parameters low. Bottle height—85-90 cm, aspiration flow rate—32 cc, and vacuum—150-200 mm Hg.
- When using infinity, use only Ozil as it is safe. Keep CTR and Iris hooks ready. Myopia causes breathing pupils due to the lack of vitreous support (pupil dilates on starting the flow and constricts on removal of probe from the eye).
- Incision size should be small. I prefer 2.2 mm on infinity and 1.8 mm incision on Stellaris machine. The length of the valve should be <2 mm as it will impede the flow in case you bend the needle posterior. Avoid leaky incisions.
- Use new and hyperflow (Alcon) sleeves. I use the inner silicone sleeve as well for hard cases.
- Rhexis should be large about 6 mm.
- In the bag phaco is possible in moderately hard case. For harder cataracts grade 4 or more on Lens Opacities Classification System (LOCS) the rhexis size is about 7 mm and the lens can be prolapsed into the supracapsular area and emulsified.
- Use Kelman needle as it helps in working more posterior.
- I use stop and chop technique and use Viscodispersive OVD.
- Always put intraoperative lens (IOL) even if the power is zero or negative since that will ensure two separate compartments and reduce the incidence of endophthalmitis and even retinal detachments. Do not hesitate to put suture as the scleral rigidity is low. It can be removed even after first week.

EDITOR'S PEARLS
- Low phaco parameters should be used in high myopes as zonules can be weak and stretched.
- Lens-iris diaphragm retropulsion syndrome (LIDRS) is a common phenomenon seen in high myopes during phaco; it can be simply managed by lifting the iris with a blunt instrument which restores the fluid flow between anterior and posterior chambers.
- While placing a three-piece IOL in sulcus the optic should be preferably captured within the anterior capsulorhexis opening to prevent IOL decentration.

■ SUGGESTED READING
1. Tosi GM, Casprini F, Malandrini A, Balestrazzi A, Quercioli PP, Caporossi A. Phacoemulsification without intraocular lens implantation in patients with high myopia: long-term results. J Cataract Refract Surg. 2003;29(6):1127-31.

3.24 Posterior Polar Cataract

Divya Agarwal
Vikalp Eye and Retina Centre, Bareilly, UP
divyagrm@gmail.com

INTRODUCTION

- Posterior polar cataract (PPC) presents as a round, discoid, opaque mass that consists of malformed and distorted lens fibers located in the central posterior lenticular region.
- Proximity or possibly adherence to posterior capsule is present.
- It is a rare form of congenital cataract.
- It is bilateral in 65–80% cases.[1,2]
- A positive family history has been reported in 40–55% of the cases.
- No gender predilection.
- *Special challenge during surgery:*[1,3]
  - High incidence of posterior capsular dehiscence (7–36%):
    - Tight adherence of plaque to normal posterior capsule
    - Thin posterior capsule underlying the plaque
    - Congenitally absent posterior capsule
  - Increased chances of nucleus drop

PATHOGENESIS

- Posterior polar cataract is associated with hyaloids remnants/tunica vasculosa lentis. It can also arise due to mesoblastic tissue invasion of the lenticular substance.[4-8]
- Hereditary, transmitted as autosomal dominant trait[9-11]
- Various mutations in *PITX3* gene in chromosome 16, *CRY-AB* gene and *CTTP1-5* genes have been postulated.[12,13]
- Sporadic cases have also been reported.
- PPC is thought to be comprised of dysplastic lenticular fibers. These fibers migrate from equator toward the posterior pole of the capsule resulting in central lens opacity.
- PPC has been associated with posterior capsule congenital defects in approximately 20% cases. The posterior capsule is already thin, and when a PPC adheres to it, it results in extreme thinning and a fragile posterior capsule.

CLINICAL PRESENTATION

- The appearance of symptoms might be due to the vacuole such as changes in the vicinity of the central opacity.
  - Intolerance to light
  - Glare
  - Reduced contrast sensitivity
  - Decreased visual acuity
    - Due to forward light scattering (light scattering toward the retina)
- *Causes of delayed presentation:*
  - Increasing density of the opacity
  - Age-related pupillary miosis
  - Increased functional needs or visual expectations

Slit-lamp examination and pupillary retroillumination provide a good evaluation:[5,14]

- Well-circumscribed circular opacity in center of posterior capsule with concentric thickened rings—*Bull's eye appearance/Onion ring appearance*
- Examination of the anterior vitreous may reveal oil-like droplets or particles—preexisting posterior capsular defect—*Fish tail sign*
  - Mean lens thickness in PPC was found to be lower than that of senile cataract.[2,15]

- Other ocular features can be associated like microphthalmia, microcornea, anterior polar cataract.[7,16,17]
- Can be associated with ectodermal dysplasia, psychosomatic disorders, Rothmund disease, scleroderma, incontinentia pigmenti, congenital dyskeratosis, congenital ichthyosis, and congenital atrophy of the skin.[14]
- Detailed clinical examination (including looking for Fish-tail sign) and anterior segment optical coherence tomography imaging can predict the posterior capsular dehiscence preoperatively and prevent dreaded complications such as posterior capsular rupture.
- Anterior segment optical coherence tomography (ASOCT) and intraoperative optical coherence tomography (iOCT) are very valuable imaging modalities to confirm the status of posterior capsule preoperatively or during surgery.[16] Pujari et al. categorized abnormal posterior capsules of PPCs into three morphological types conical, ectatic, and moth-eaten, based on ASOCT appearance.[18]
- Titiyal et al. described the utility of iOCT in seeing real-time integrity of posterior capsule and high-risk morphological features especially during hydrodelineation/hydrodissection maneuvers.[16] They also described one important observation while performing phacoemulsification, the posterior polar cortical disc defect (PPCDD) sign in PPC cases after epinuclear plate removal and plaque aspiration. They proposed that the presence of this sign indicates an intact posterior capsule and the risk of posterior capsular rent (PCR) is comparatively lower in these patients compared to patients without PPCCD signs.

CLASSIFICATION

Duke Elder Classification[14]

- *Stationary form:*
  - More common
  - Well-circumscribed circular opacity in center of posterior capsule with concentric thickened rings—Bull's eye appearance
  - Smaller satellite rosette lesions can also be present.
- *Progressive form:*
  - Opacity appears in the posterior cortex such as radiating rider opacity
  - Feathery and scalloped edges
  - Never involves the nucleus

Singh Classification

- *Type I:* PPC with posterior subcapsular cataract
- *Type II:* Sharply defined round or oval opacity with ringed appearance like an onion with or without grayish spots at the edge
- *Type III:* Sharply defined round or oval white opacity with dense white spots at the edge often associated with thin or absent PC. The dense white spots are a diagnostic sign (Daljit Singh sign) of posterior capsule leakage and extreme fragility.
- *Type IV:* Combination of the above three with nuclear sclerosis.

Schroeder Classification[19]

It is based on pupillary obstruction in the red reflex testing.
- *Grade 1:* A small opacity without any effect on the optical quality of the clear part of the lens.
- *Grade 2:* A two-thirds obstruction without other effect.
- *Grade 3:* The disc-like opacity in the posterior capsule is surrounded by an area of further optical distortion. Only the dilated pupil shows a clear red reflex surrounding this zone.

- *Grade 4:* The opacity is totally occlusive; no sufficient red reflex is obtained by dilation of the pupil. He advocated first step in managing grade 1 should be patching while in grade 2, it should be patching with mydriasis and bifocal glasses.

COUNSELING OF THE PATIENT
- High chances of nucleus dropping intraoperatively due to a posterior capsular rupture
- Relatively long duration of surgery
- Need for any posterior segment intervention
- Delayed visual recovery
- Need for subsequent Nd:YAG capsulotomy in case of residual opacity
- Preexisting amblyopia especially in unilateral PPCs
- Role of genetic counseling and screening of other family members

ANESTHESIA
- Both local and topical anesthesia can be utilized.
- Peribulbar anesthesia with oculodigital pressure is generally preferred—reduces positive vitreous pressure.[1]
- In topical anesthesia,
  - Squeezing the lids with a speculum can distort the globe.
  - Increased eye movement and lack of hypotony would increase the forward movement of the posterior capsule.

SURGICAL TECHNIQUE
- Phacoemulsification is preferred to conventional extracapsular cataract extraction—better control with closed chamber techniques.[21]
- Closed chamber technique minimizes anterior chamber fluctuation and forward bulge of posterior capsule
- Creating a valvular incision
- Injecting viscoelastic prior to retracting any instrument from eye
- Bimanual irrigation/aspiration.

Incision
Temporal clear corneal incision is performed.

Capsulorhexis[2,22]
- Adequate size continuous curvilinear capsulorhexis (CCC) is performed of about 4.5–5.0 mm size.
- If vitreous loss occurs during phacoemulsification, it is easier to manually prolapse the nucleus into the anterior chamber in the presence of a large capsulorhexis without having to further enlarge it.
  - Small size—increases hydrostatic pressure—hampers epinucleus, cortical matter removal
  - Large size—not allow intraocular lens (IOL) implantation in sulcus

Hydrodelineation and Hydrodissection
- Hydrodelineation, which is the separation between the nucleus and the epinucleus, is mandatory to create a mechanical cushion of epinucleus.[2,3,20]
  - Hydrodissection is contraindicated in cases of PPCs, especially in cases where preoperative assessment is suggestive of a defect in the posterior capsule.[2,15]
  - Cortical cleaving hydrodissection is considered a contraindication in eyes with Type 3 and 4 PPCs.[1,2]
  - Vigorous decompression of the capsular bag after the delineation should be avoided.[15]
  - Nucleus rotation should be avoided in all cases.[15]

Inside-Out Delineation[23]
- Described by Vasavada and Raj for PPCs with advanced nuclear sclerosis
- A trench is first sculpted and a right-angled cannula is used to subsequently direct fluid perpendicularly to the lens fibers in the desired plane through one wall of the trench.
  - Avoids subcapsular injection
  - Cannula reaches to adequate depth

Parameters of the Phacoemulsification Machine[1,2]
- Slow motion phacoemulsification with low vacuum, low aspiration, and low inflow parameters, to ensure a more stable anterior chamber.
- Ultrasound energy 40–70%, vacuum 250–270 mm Hg, aspiration flow rate (AFR) 18–20 cc/min, and bottle height of 70–80 cm is recommended.

Nucleotomy Techniques[2,20,24-28]
It depends on grade of nuclear sclerosis:
- *Grade I nuclear sclerosis:* Sculpting followed by sequential *layer-by-layer aspiration* using partial segmentation technique.
- *Grade II and III sclerosis:* Small central trench is made followed by quadrantic division of the nucleus.
- Advanced nuclear sclerosis, a crater and chop technique is used.
- If a posterior capsular plaque is strongly adherent to the capsule that could not be peeled off by viscodissection, the safest option is to leave the plaque untouched for Nd:YAG laser capsulotomy later.
  - Lee and Lee sculpted the nucleus in the shape of the Greek letter lambda "lambda technique", then cracking along both arms and removing the distal central piece.
  - Salahuddin devised "inverse horseshoe" in which after sculpting, he divides the distal end of the nucleus.
  - Lim and Goh developed a technique where they prechop the epinucleus in a piecemeal in situ without getting the chopper to reach all the way down to the depth of the posterior epinucleus.
  - Chee devised a technique for hard PPCs in which she cracks the nucleus in the periphery (partially) avoiding the posterior polar opacity and then chops it into quadrants without rotation.
  - In the absence of hydrodissection, epinucleus delivery poses a challenge in some cases after phaco. Iris spatula-guided epinuclear cleavage can aid in layer-by-layer loosening of epinucleus.

▇ POSTERIOR CAPSULAR DEHISCENCE[1,2,22]
A dispersive viscoelastic, Viscoat, is injected over the area of defect before withdrawing the phaco or irrigation/aspiration probe from the eye.
- If the vitreous face is intact, the cortex is aspirated with bimanual I/A. A posterior capsulorhexis may be performed if the rupture is confined to a small central area.
  - These are distinctly linear defects, not amenable for conversion to a posterior continuous curvilinear capsulorhexis (PCCC) in most cases.
- In case of vitreous disturbance, a two-port limbal anterior vitrectomy with a high cut rate, low vacuum and flow rates, vitrectomy can be safely performed even close to the torn capsule. Typical parameters are cut rate 800–1,200 cuts/min; vacuum 200 mm Hg and AFR 20 cc/min. The vitrector is never placed behind the peripheral posterior capsule. The infusion cannula is directed into the peripheral anterior chamber,
    Once the anterior chamber is free of vitreous, which is confirmed by injecting preservative-free triamcinolone acetonide into the anterior chamber, the remaining cortex is aspirated.

Posterior capsule vacuum polishing is avoided even if the posterior capsule (PC) is intact due to its fragility.
- Sometimes, the posterior cortex displays a classical appearance suggestive of a defect. If the posterior capsule underneath this opaque ring is intact, it is termed as a "pseudohole".

■ INTRAOCULAR LENS IMPLANTATION[1,2,18]

It depends on the nature of posterior capsule rupture and remaining capsular support. It is always better to compress the trailing haptic than capsular bag rotation.
- If there is none or size of the PC tear is small or converted to circular one, single piece IOL can be implanted in the bag.
- If the tear is large, a multipiece IOL in the ciliary sulcus with or without rhexis capture; advantages of rhexis capture—stabilizes IOL, reduces IOL contact with iris.
- Large rupture with doubtful zonular integrity—options include anterior chamber IOL, suturing an IOL to the sclera, or planning an intrascleral haptic fixation of IOL with glue.
  - After intraocular lens implantation, viscoelastic is removed by bimanual methods. Viscoelastic is removed in a piecemeal and gradual manner which reduces the chances of aspiration of vitreous.
  - Main valvular lesion should be sutured in eyes with posterior capsule defect.

■ BIMANUAL MICROPHACOEMULSIFICATION[29]

- Separate infusion and aspiration instruments through watertight incisions of 1.4 mm width:
  - Allowing withdrawal of the phaco-needle first while maintaining the anterior chamber with infusion from the separate irrigating chopper.
  - Easy injection of viscoelastic into the anterior chamber before final withdrawal of the irrigating chopper.

■ POSTERIOR SEGMENT APPROACH[20]

- Indicated for large plaques (>4 mm).
- Primary three ports pars plana vitrectomy is described for PPC.

■ FEMTOSECOND LASER-ASSISTED CATARACT SURGERY[30]

Technique of hybrid pattern of cylinder and chop is safe and effective in managing cases of PPC, specifically for higher grades of nuclear sclerosis grade II–III.
- Titiyal et al. described a hybrid pattern of three cylinders (2, 4, and 6 mm) and three chops (6 mm in length) for nucleotomy.
- Block-by-block emulsification of the prechopped nucleus is done from the center outward.

■ POSTERIOR POLAR CATARACT IN CHILDREN[31]

- Posterior polar cataract occurs as unilateral cataract in a majority of pediatric eyes (93%) as compared to adults.
- *Signs of preexisting posterior capsule rupture:*
  - Well-demarcated defect with thick margins
  - Chalky white spots in a cluster or a rough circle on the posterior capsule
  - White dots in the anterior vitreous that move with the degenerated vitreous like a *fish-tail sign.*
- If there is a need for vitrectomy, the goal is to remove only the central anterior vitreous. No attempt should be made to remove the peripheral or posterior vitreous.

SECTION 3: Cataract

EDITOR'S PEARLS
- Hydrodissection and nucleal rotation to be avoided; performing a good hydrodelineation is important.
- Low flow parameters should be used while minimizing fluctuation of anterior chamber between surgical steps.
- Intraoperative OCT is a useful aid to assess the posterior capsule status and for detecting the subset of cases wherein hydrodissection may be performed safely.
- Intraoperative posterior polar cortical disc defect (PPCDD) sign observed after nuclear emulsification is a sign of safety indicative of intact posterior capsule in PPC.

REFERENCES

1. Osher RH, Yu BC, Koch DD. Posterior polar cataracts: a predisposition to intraoperative posterior capsular rupture. J Cataract Refract Surg. 1990;16:157-62.
2. Vasavada AR, Singh R. Phacoemulsification with posterior polar cataract. J Cataract Refract Surg 1999;25:238-45.
3. Lee MW, Lee YC. Phacoemulsification of posterior polar cataracts—a surgical challenge. Br J Ophthalmol. 2003; 87:1426-7.
4. Luntz MH. Clinical types of cataracts. Duane's Ophthalmology 1996; CD ROM.
5. Gifford SR. Congenital anomalies of the lens as seen with the slit lamp. Am J Ophthalmol 1924;7:678-85.
6. Cordes FC. Types of congenital and juvenile cataracts. In: Haik GM (Ed). Symposium on Diseases and Surgery of the lens. St. Louis: CV Mosby; 1957. pp. 43-50.
7. Greeves RA. Two cases of microphthalmia. Trans Ophthalmol Soc UK. 1914;34:289-300.
8. Szily AV. The Doyne Memorial Lecture: the contribution of pathological examination to elucidation of the problems of cataract. Trans Ophthalmol Soc UK. 1938;58:595-660.
9. Maumenee III. Classification of hereditary cataracts in children by linkage analysis. Ophthalmology. 1979;86:1554-8.
10. Yamada K, Tomita HA, Kanazawa S, Mera A, Amemiya T, Niikawa N. Genetically distinct autosomal dominant posterior polar cataract in a four-generation Japanese family. Am J Ophthalmol. 2000;129(2):159-65.
11. Tulloh CG. Hereditary posterior polar cataract with report of a pedigree. Br J Ophthalmol. 1955;39(6):374-9.
12. Addison PK, Berry V, Ionides AC, Francis PJ, Bhattacharya SS, Moore AT. Posterior polar cataract is the predominant consequence of a recurrent mutation in the PITX3 gene. Br J Ophthalmol. 2005;89(2):138-41.
13. Berry V, Francis P, Reddy MA, Collyer D, Vithana E, MacKay I, et al. Alpha-B crystallin gene (CRYAB) mutation causes dominant congenital posterior polar cataract in humans. Am J Hum Genet. 2001;69(5):1141-5.
14. Duke-Elder S. Congenital deformities. Part 2. Normal and Abnormal Development. System of Ophthalmology; vol. III. St. Louis: CV Mosby; 1964.
15. Kalantan H. Posterior polar cataract: A review. Saudi J Ophthalmol. 2012;26(1):41-9.
16. Titiyal JS, Nair S, Kaur M, Rawat J, Mazumdar SA. Intraoperative posterior polar cortical disc defect: sign of intact posterior capsule. J Cataract Refract Surg. 2021;47(8):1039-43.
17. Harman NB. New pedigrees of cataract-posterior polar, anterior polar and microphthalmia, and lamellar. Trans Ophthalmol Soc UK. 1909;29:296-306.
18. Pujari A, Yadav S, Sharma N, Khokhar S, Sinha R, Agarwal T, et al. Study 1: Evaluation of the signs of deficient posterior capsule in posterior polar cataracts using anterior segment optical coherence tomography. J Cataract Refract Surg. 2020;46(9):1260-5.
19. Schroeder HW. The management of posterior polar cataract: the role of patching and grading. Strabismus. 2005;13(4):153-6.
20. Hayashi K, Hayashi H, Nakao F. Outcomes of surgery for posterior polar cataract. J Cataract Refract Surg. 2003;29:45-9.
21. Das S, Khanna R, Mohiuddin SM, Ramamurthy B. Surgical and visual outcomes for posterior polar cataract. Br J Ophthalmol. 2008;92(11):1476-8.
22. Fine IH, Packer M, Hoffman RS. Management of posterior polar cataract. J Cataract Refract Surg. 2003;29:16-9.

23. Vasavada AR, Raj SM. Inside-out delineation. J Cataract Refract Surg. 2004;30:1167-9.
24. Vajpayee RB, Sinha R, Singhvi A, Sharma N, Titiyal JS, Tandon R. 'Layer by layer' phacoemulsification in posterior polar cataract with pre-existing posterior capsular rent. Eye (Lond). 2008;22(8):1008-10.
25. Salahuddin. Inverse horse-shoe technique for the phacoemulsification of posterior polar cataract. Can J Ophthalmol. 2010;45(2):154-6.
26. Lim Z, Goh J. Modified epinucleus pre-chop for the dense posterior polar cataract. Ophthalmic Surg Lasers Imaging. 2008;39(2):171-3.
27. Chee SP. Management of the hard posterior polar cataract. J Cataract Refract Surg. 2007;33(9):1509-14.
28. Khokhar S, Gupta S, Gogia V. Iris spatula-guided epinuclear cleavage in posterior polar cataracts. Can J Ophthalmol. 2015;50(6):e106-8.
29. Haripriya A, Aravind S, Vadi K, Natchiar G. Bimanual microphaco for posterior polar cataracts. J Cataract Refract Surg. 2006;32(6):914-7.
30. Titiyal JS, Kaur M, Sharma N. Femtosecond laser-assisted cataract surgery technique to enhance safety in posterior polar cataract. J Refract Surg. 2015;31(12):826-8.
31. Mistr SK, Trivedi RH, Wilson ME. Preoperative considerations and outcomes of primary intraocular lens implantation in children with posterior polar and posterior lentiglobus cataract. J AAPOS. 2008;12:58-61.

3.25 Microincisional Cataract Surgery Platform: A Great Leap Forward

Mohan Rajan, Sujatha Mohan, Ramya Subramanian
Rajan Eye Care Hospital, Chennai
www.rajaneyecare.com

■ INTRODUCTION

Modern, cataract surgery has come a long way from the traditional extracapsular cataract surgery to microincision cataract surgery (MICS). With the advent of newer technology it is now possible to remove cataract through a 1.8 mm incision with utmost safety.

Phacoemulsification has become the gold standard for cataract removal for over a decade now.

During phacoemulsification, ultrasonic vibration of the phaco needle which is required to emulsify the cataract gives rise to friction and heat which damages the surrounding wound (in clear corneal incision, damage to the cornea) and the intraocular structures.

In conventional phaco, anterior chamber infusion is provided by a silicone sleeve surrounding the phaco needle. This reduces the transfer of heat energy to the cornea but increases the size of the incision to range between 2.5 and 3.2 mm.

Although the incision size is less compared to the previous surgeries it is still large enough to give rise to intraoperative chamber instability, induced astigmatism, and postoperative wound leak/gape leading to endophthalmitis.

■ BIMANUAL MICROPHACO

In order to reduce the complications related to a temporal clear corneal phaco, the bimanual phacoemulsification was introduced with the size of the wound reduced from standard 2.8 mm to 1.2 mm. However, this led to problems such as wound burns, due to sleeveless needles, increased learning curve, and lastly the need to enlarge the wound to put a foldable intraocular lens (IOL). The IOLs which were recommended for bimanual phaco were plagued by several problems such as increased incidence of PCO, in the bag folding of the lenses due to capsular contraction. These lenses were made extremely thin to be inserted through a small wound and the quality of vision was poorer when compared to standard phaco lenses.

These issues are being addressed by the use of:
- Large bore irrigating choppers
- Low compliance tubing
- Pressurized inflow
- Postocclusion surge reduction (cruise control).

Cruise Control

A 2 cm long flow restrictor with a 0.3 mm internal lumen acts to preferentially limit surge outflow, without affecting the lower flow rates used to attract mobile particles to the phaco tip (<50 cc/min). This clever design features a mesh filter that traps the nuclear emulsate before it can enter and clog the flow-restricting segment (**Fig. 3.25.1**).

The combination of newer instrumentation, longer learning curve, and poor lens technology resulted in the quick death of bimanual phaco.

Microcoaxial Phaco

It was started and propagated by Dr Takayuki Akahoshi. Microcoaxial phaco is performed through one 2.2 mm incision, using standard techniques.

The incision is large enough to accommodate the size of a phaco tip covered with a specially designed sleeve (nanosleeve), which provides sufficient irrigation to maintain anterior chamber stability and offers added thermal protection.

You can inject standard IOLs without enlarging the wound.

Microincisional Cataract Surgery

With the advent of sub-2 mm cataract incisions, the advantages of fantastic chamber stability, safer intraocular structures, greater working space for the surgeon, and minimal learning curve while converting from standard phaco to microincision, it is little wonder that microincision cataract surgery has surely and safely replaced bimanual phaco.

The Bausch and Lomb Stellaris microsurgical system, allows for C MICS through a 1.8 mm wound. Other features which enable working through such a small incision with stable anterior chamber are the *high vacuum flow restrictive tubing (HVFRT), stable flow tip*.

■ THE HIGH VACUUM FLOW RESTRICTIVE TUBING

In phaco during removal of the nucleus pieces there is a postocclusion surge. The lens cortex and capsule fluctuate and move like a trampoline. The HVFRT increases the stability in the anterior chamber and provides stillness of the lens cortex and decreases the fluctuations to next to nil (**Figs. 3.25.2 to 3.25.4**).

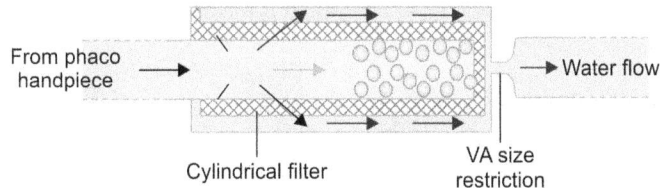

Fig. 3.25.1: Schematic diagram of cruise control.

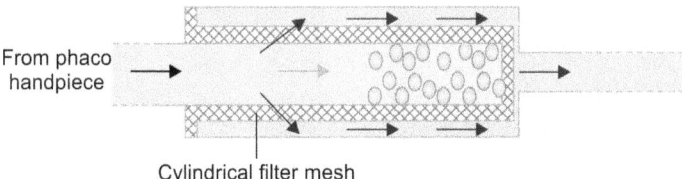

Fig. 3.25.2: Diagram of restricted flow filter.

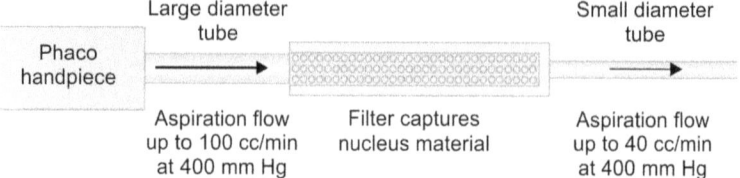

Fig. 3.25.3: Diagram showing working system of a restricted flow filter.

The HVFRT system consists of:
- Tube set with a filter and aspiration tubing with a 1.0 mm/0.040 inch (internal diameter)
- The filter does not allow any particles >0.3 mm (0.012 inch) pass through
- 1.0 mm internal diameter tubing will have <50% of the spikes of a 1.5 mm (0.06 inch) internal diameter tubing
- The smaller internal diameter will allow for things to move faster, while maintaining a very stable anterior chamber.

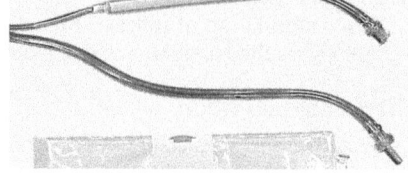

Fig. 3.25.4: High vacuum flow restricted tubing.

How Does it Work?

With a small diameter the flow is restricted thus decreasing the fluctuations/postocclusion surge in the anterior chamber to near zero.
In order to compensate for the reduction in diameter the *vacuum has to be increased*.

■ WOUND STABILITY

It has been well documented that square incisions have good stability and strength and produce very minimal or no astigmatism.

This is also very important to prevent postoperative inflammation and endophthalmitis.

With a 1.8 mm MICS surgery it is possible to make a 1.5 mm long tunnel which in essence gives us a nice and square incision which gives us better anterior chamber stability and extra safety for both the patient and the surgeon **(Figs. 3.25.5 and 3.25.6)**.

■ IMPROVING POSTOPERATIVE OUTCOMES

Vision is 6/6 on day 1 with MICS but takes about a week to get 90% with standard phaco. This is true especially in harder cataracts which is a common scenario in our country

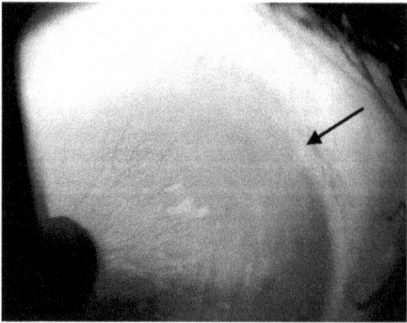

Fig. 3.25.5: Square-shaped wound achieved in microincisional cataract surgery.

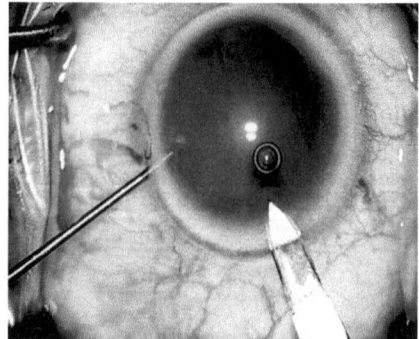

Fig. 3.25.6: Square-shaped entry made by diamond knife.

because of the better fluidics in MICS even in harder cataracts the cornea is clear in day 1. Another important advantage of MICS is that the induced astigmatism is very predictable with an average of 0.2 D with a range of 0 to 0.4 D; whereas in standard phaco the range of induced astigmatism is about 0.5 to 1.25 D. In essence the predictability of astigmatism is much more with S MICS than with standard phaco.

Microincisional cataract surgery is the future in cataract surgery, because of its unique features such as:
- Stability
- Safety
- Super vision

The additional feature of the MI-60 lenses which gives excellent quality of vision, biocompatibility and the ability to be implanted through a small 1.8 mm incision makes MICS the most effective method of cataract removal.

3.26 What should be Done Differently before Cataract and Glaucoma Surgery?

Devindra Sood, Aditi Agarwal
Krishna Netralaya, Gurugram
glaucomacentre@yahoo.com

INTRODUCTION

There are significant numbers of patients where glaucoma is associated with age-related cataract. Once age-related cataract is visually significant, there is need to decide whether to perform phacoemulsification alone, glaucoma surgery first or combined phacoemulsification with glaucoma surgery. A thorough ocular examination is essential for cataract and glaucoma evaluation in each case.

PREOPERATIVE EXAMINATION

Cataract Evaluation
- Type of cataract
- Integrity of zonules
- Presence of pseudoexfoliation
- Presence of posterior synechiae
- Degree of pupillary dilatation
- If possible, potential acuity meter
- Status of macula
- If there is no view of the optic disc, look for relative afferent pupil defect (RAPD) and advise USG B scan to look for optic nerve head (ONH) cupping.

Glaucoma Evaluation
- Type of glaucoma
- Degree of optic nerve damage
- Control of intraocular pressure (IOP)
- Progression of disease
- Number of medication and tolerance
- Compliance

Counseling
- Explain to patients that the visual outcome will depend on the degree of optic nerve damage

- Possible need for glaucoma medications after surgery
- Keep expectations modest
- Explain the possibility of bleb failure

■ PREOPERATIVE CHANGES IN MEDICATION
Ocular Changes
- Discontinue miotics at least 10 days before
- Discontinue adrenergic agonists 1 week before
- Discontinue prostaglandin analogs 1 week before

Systemic Changes
Discontinue blood thinners at least a week before surgery.

Anesthesia
Anesthesia (must for akinesia/absence of sensation/helps to decrease positive vitreous pressure), retrobulbar/peribulbar (avoids adrenaline).

Ensure Good Pupillary Dilatation
- Epinephrine in infusion bottle
- Viscoelastics
- Synechiolysis
- Iris retractors, Malyugin ring, etc.
- Iris sphincterotomies
- Pupil dilators and hooks
- Keyhole iridectomy

Achieve a Soft Eye
Achieve a soft eye to reduce vitreous upthrust/reduce possibility of break in posterior capsule/enable surgical manipulation with precision. Administer intravenous mannitol or oral acetazolamide 20 minutes before surgery to achieve a soft eye.

Intraoperative
- Optimize power used
- Make rhexis through side port before tunnel
- Prevent surge to maintain anterior chamber
  - *Thorough AC wash:* Thoroughly remove the viscoelastic as well as nuclear and cortical material. This will prevent blockage of drainage channels and/or tubes and reduce postoperative inflammation and IOP spikes.
- *Ensure watertight closure:* Do not hesitate to apply sutures if needed. A wound leak will increase the risk of bleb failure and endophthalmitis.

Intraocular Lens Selection
- Multifocal intraocular lenses (IOLs) should be avoided.
- In case of any capsular or zonular compromise, can place a three-piece IOL in the sulcus but avoid AC IOL's as they can directly affect the bleb and produce undue postoperative inflammation.

> **EDITOR'S PEARLS**
> - Preoperatively patients must be counseled regarding guarded visual prognosis, possibility of change in glaucoma medications in postoperative period, risk of snuff-out in advanced cases, and risk of bleb failure.
> - Avoid prostaglandin analogs before surgery and in the early postoperative period due to increased risk of inflammation.

SUGGESTED READING
1. Tham CC, Kwong YY, Leung DY, Lam SW, Li FC, Chiu TY, et al. Phacoemulsification versus combined phacotrabeculectomy in medically controlled chronic angle closure glaucoma with cataract. Ophthalmology. 2008;115(12):2167-73.e2.

3.27 Which Patients with Cataract Need a Combined Glaucoma Procedure?

SS Pandav
Advanced Eye Centre, PGIMER, Chandigarh
sspandav@yahoo.com

INTRODUCTION
- Cataract and glaucoma are both common conditions and are often present in the same patient.
- There is no clear consensus about the appropriate timing of the surgery for either condition, or about the best surgical technique. The indications for combined cataract and glaucoma surgery are generally relative rather than absolute.
- More commonly, a patient with medically well-controlled glaucoma may require cataract surgery and a concurrent trabeculectomy is performed in hopes of reducing the medication burden.
- Alternatively, a patient with a moderate cataract but little or no visual complaints may require trabeculectomy for uncontrolled glaucoma, and concurrent cataract surgery is planned—knowing that filtering surgery often accelerates cataract formation—in order to improve vision and to obviate the need to perform later incisional surgery that might compromise the existing glaucoma filter.
- The effect of a cataract on visual function in a patient with glaucoma may include a reduction in visual field scores as well as in visual acuity. The Advanced Glaucoma Intervention Study (AGIS) demonstrated that, on average, cataract extraction improves visual field defect scores in addition to improving visual acuity.

OPTIONS AVAILABLE FOR COMBINED CATARACT AND GLAUCOMA SURGERY
- Extracapsular cataract extraction with trabeculectomy
- Phacotrabeculectomy
- Phacoemulsification with drainage device
- Combined cataract and nonpenetrating glaucoma surgery

Out of abovementioned options, phacotrabeculectomy is often the procedure of choice.

PREOPERATIVE EVALUATION IN A PATIENT WITH PREEXISTING GLAUCOMA

History
Current and past medication, past lasers [(selective laser trabeculoplasty (SLT), argon laser trabeculoplasty (ALT)], past surgeries (trabeculectomy, drainage devices and peripheral iridotomy).

Examination
Make special note of maximal dilation achieved, anterior chamber depth, gonioscopy (angle architecture and peripheral synechiae), pseudoexfoliation and lens stability.

ADVANTAGE OF COMBINED CATARACT EXTRACTION WITH TRABECULECTOMY

- Only one surgical session is required, reducing hospital visits and the financial burden.
- Less risk of intraocular pressure (IOP) spikes just after surgery. This has implications when we are dealing with advanced glaucoma.
- In addition to visual rehabilitation, combined procedure is effective in terms of control of intraocular pressure and hopefully arrest of progressive glaucomatous damage.

ISSUES DURING SURGERY

- Decision to use antimetabolites
- Location of the surgical incision for the cataract extraction
- Location of the conjunctival incision for the trabeculectomy
- Single-site phacotrabeculectomy, using the same superior scleral incision for both the phacoemulsification and trabeculectomy parts of the operation
- Two-site phacotrabeculectomy, with temporal incision for phacoemulsification, and a superiorly placed trabeculectomy.
- Generally, it is recommended to use antimetabolites during surgery. There are pros and cons to single-site versus two-site trabeculectomy. Overall, no significant difference has been observed in IOP control and need for supplemental antiglaucoma medications between these two approaches.

EDITOR'S PEARLS

- Cataract surgery in patients with glaucoma may be combined with a glaucoma procedure in the same sitting.
- For patients with mild-moderate glaucoma, intolerance, or poor compliance to topical medications or with significant topical medication-related adverse effects, cataract surgery may be combined with minimally invasive glaucoma surgery (MIGS) devices and procedures.
- For patients with significant cataract and advanced glaucoma which is uncontrolled on maximum topical medication—cataract surgery may be combined with trabeculectomy.
- Phacoemulsification has the advantages of smaller wound size, minimal conjunctival manipulation, better anterior chamber depth maintenance and better bleb survival as compared to extracapsular cataract extraction (ECCE) or manual small-incision cataract surgery (MSICS).

SUGGESTED READING

1. Buys YM, Chipman ML, Zack B, Rootman DS, Slomovic AR, Trope GE. Prospective randomized comparison of one-versus two-site Phacotrabeculectomy two-year results. Ophthalmology. 2008;115(7):1130-3.

3.28 | 90 to 100 Degrees of Iridodialysis during Phaco: What to Do?

Mahipal Sachdev, Charu Khurana
Centre for Sight, New Delhi
drmahipal@gmail.com

INTRODUCTION

Damage to the iris occurs most commonly in patients with small pupil or floppy iris when you may inadvertently grab the iris tissue in the phaco-probe. Tearing of the iris may occur during introduction of the phaco tip usually at the beginning of the phaco or when the tip is withdrawn and reinserted when it may catch and drag the iris causing substantial damage and hemorrhage. Patients with a crowded anterior chamber are at greater risk such as those with high hyperopia, phacomorphic cataract, and angle closure glaucoma or if the iris is flaccid after stretching maneuvers. In such patients, it is best to be cautious right from the beginning of the surgery by creating a deep anterior chamber using a dispersive viscoelastic, entering the eye with reflux and if necessary, gently manipulating the incarcerated iris from the phaco tip with a second instrument through the paracentesis to avoid this complication or prevent it from becoming worse.

Once the complication has taken place, stay calm and evaluate the extent of the damage. Use a dispersive or dual-property viscoelastic such as Healon 5 to control any bleeding and reposition the iris tissue. If the bleeding is significant and there is a risk of hyphema, wash out the anterior chamber and quickly refill with balanced salt solution (BSS) or viscoelastic material, raising the pressure high to stop the bleeding. You can use an iris hook to stabilize the iris and complete the surgery making sure that any further disturbance in that region is minimized.

A bimanual irrigation and aspiration decreases anterior chamber (AC) turbulence and may be considered beneficial as there is reduced tendency for iris aspiration into a 0.3 mm irrigation/aspiration (I/A) tip. However, if the surgeon prefers a standard coaxial I/A through the main incision, then a Kuglen hook through the paracentesis can be used to push the iris away from the aspiration tip.

Using a variable vacuum (400 mm Hg) and preset flow (20 cc/min) phaco machine is ideal for aspiration of cortex in the presence of iris. The cortex can be grabbed with low vacuum which is then gradually increased until aspiration occurs and the decreased before aspiration of iris. Phaco machines which control flow and preset the vacuum in I/A, cause a greater postaspiration surge with increased risk of damaging the flaccid iris tissue.

Intraocular lens (IOL) selection is determined by the condition of the capsule and surgical judgment.

The blood aqueous barrier is damaged with increased iris manipulation causing an increase in postoperative inflammation. Hydroacrylic lenses or second-generation material silicone lenses may be preferred in such a situation. Since the pupil may be asymmetric or partially dilated a larger optic IOL (diameter 6 mm) should be chosen to prevent IOL edge exposure and potential glare and other edge effects.

Once the IOL is implanted intracameral pilocarpine may be instilled to help assess iris function and position.

IRIS SUTURES

To repair the iridodialysis, 9-0 or 10-0 prolene sutures can be placed using various techniques, two of which are described below:
- The needle enters the anterior chamber through a convenient paracentesis track, engaging the proximal iris leaflet and then the distal iris leaflet and from there, it passes out through the peripheral cornea. The suture is then tied with sliding knot technique to minimize iris traction. Once the suture has been passed, place a Kuglen hook through the first paracentesis track, engage the suture just beyond the distal iris and draw a loop of the suture out through the first track. Maintaining proper orientation of the sutures, pass the trailing suture through the middle of the loop twice. Draw the trailing strand and the exited strand on the opposite side together pulling the iris leaflets together. This creates the first throw of the knot. Repeat by retrieving the suture loop again for a single locking throw and trim the knot **(Figs. 3.28.1A to E)**.
- A conjunctival limbal peritomy is created over the area of the dialysis. A 10-0 double-armed prolene suture needle is passed through the peripheral cornea 180° away from the middle of the iridodialysis, across the anterior chamber, through the base of the iridodialysis and through the iris root and sclera. A similar second pass is made using the second needle of the double-armed suture and it is brought through the iridodialysis and sclera at the level of the iris root. The free ends of the suture are tied over the sclera and the knot is buried. The conjunctiva is closed in a routine fashion.

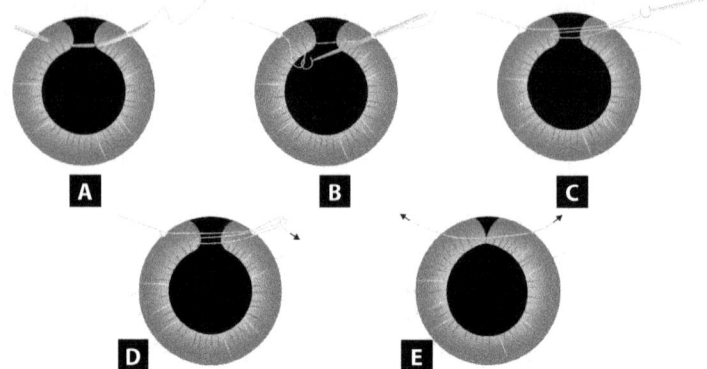

Figs. 3.28.1A to E: Siepser slipknot technique as originally described for repairing an iris defect. Although the free suture end should pass through the loop twice, only the first of the two passes is shown.

■ POSTOPERATIVE CARE

Increased iris manipulation will cause a greater inflammatory reaction; so increased frequency of topical steroids and nonsteroidal anti-inflammatory drugs is indicated. Monitor for any intraocular pressure rise and treat accordingly.

> **EDITOR'S PEARLS**
> - Appropriate management of intraoperative fluidics is extremely important once intraoperative iridodialysis is detected.
> - The decision to repair in the same sitting versus later is determined by the location and extent of the iridodialysis
> - Iris defects may be repaired using a Siepser knot as well as its variations such as Osher–Cionni–Snyder, Condon, Ahmed, and Narang–Agarwal techniques all of which involve externalizing the throws and pulling to tighten over the iris have been described.
> - Sewing machine and Cobbler's technique have also been described for repairing iridodialysis.

■ SUGGESTED READING

1. Chang DF. Siepser slipknot for McCannel iris-suture fixation of subluxated intraocular lenses. J Cataract Refract Surg. 2004;30(6):1170-6.

3.29 What are the Advantages, Indications, and Limitations of Manual Small Incision Cataract Surgery?

Ruchi Goel
Gurunanak Eye Center, Maulana Azad Medical College, New Delhi
gruchi1@rediffmail.com

KPS Malik
Vardhman Mahavir Medical College, Safdarjung Hospital, New Delhi
malikkps@rediffmail.com

■ INTRODUCTION

Manual small incision cataract surgery (MSICS) is now a well-established procedure which offers the safety of closed chamber manipulation and allows an early visual rehabilitation with minimal surgically induced astigmatism. There are various techniques of nuclear delivery in MSICS namely the Blumenthal's, microvectis, phacosandwich, phacosection, and fishhook.

Many of the surgical steps are based on common principles in both MSICS and phacoemulsification such as construction of a triplanar incision, capsulorhexis, hydrodissection, cortical wash, and port hydration. Mastering MSICS aids in learning phacoemulsification in a more controlled manner. It serves as a bail out for phacoemulsification during adverse events such as:
- Improper wound construction with leaking ports and shallow anterior chamber
- Escaped continuous curvilinear capsulorhexis (CCC)
- Phacoemulsification machine failure
- Posterior capsular tear with nuclear pieces still in the anterior chamber
- Prolonged surgery with corneal hydration making visualization of chamber details difficult

By converting to MSICS the surgery can still be completed safely with none or one/two sutures.

MERITS OF MANUAL SMALL INCISION CATARACT SURGERY

The *merits of MSICS* over phacoemulsification are:
- Machine independence
- Low cost of consumables
- Universal applicability to all grades of nuclei
- Lesser chances of vision threatening complications such as nuclear drop
- Shorter learning curve
- Lesser surgical time
- Extremely useful procedure for high volume surgery in remote areas with poor power back up and absence of vitreoretinal surgeon.

FAVORABLE SITUATIONS FOR MANUAL SMALL INCISION CATARACT SURGERY

Preference to adopt any surgical technique depends primarily on its reproducibility and the expertise of the surgeon. For a surgeon well conversant with both the procedures, MSICS is easier to perform in the following situations:
- *Hard brown/black nucleus:* Use of excessive power for trenching/sculpting can cause endothelial cell loss. Also, the bulky unmouldable nucleus causes overcrowding of capsular bag making phacoemulsification difficult. Further, lack of epinuclear plate and use of high vacuum put the posterior capsule at risk. MSICS can accomplish the same task safely and the risk of endothelial damage is obviated by maintaining the anterior chamber deep all the time.
- *Extensive central corneal opacity*: Due to poor visualization of anterior chamber details it is difficult to create a CCC, a must for phacoemulsification. MSICS can be performed with reasonable ease even in a can opener/envelope capsulotomy.
- *Limbal scarring*: Construction of a sclerocorneal tunnel is a better option than making a limbal/clear corneal incision.
- *Morgagnian cataract*: The difficulty in stabilization of nucleus makes phacoemulsification difficult. On the other hand, nuclear prolapse into the anterior chamber is facilitated in MSICS.
- *Traumatic cataract* with torn anterior capsule.

LIMITATIONS

Despite the abovementioned advantages of MSICS it has the following limitations:
- *Scleral disease/thin sclera* where construction of sclerocorneal tunnel is absolutely contraindicated.
- *Preexisting trabeculectomy bleb*: Phacoemulsification may be preferred so as not to disturb the bleb and to preserve the conjunctiva for re-trabeculectomy/glaucoma drainage device implantation.

- An extremely *shallow fornix* can make the nuclear delivery difficult in MSICS, if a superior incision is planned.
- *Anterior chamber depth* <2 mm endangers the endothelium when nucleus is prolapsed into the anterior chamber. In the bag phacoemulsification is a better option in these circumstances.
- An *extensive arcus senilis* obstructs the visualization of nuclear passage through the corneoscleral tunnel. Phacoemulsification is easy as the central cornea is clear.
- Immediate *postoperative redness* at the site of incision is unavoidable in MSICS therefore patients who are particular about cosmesis should be avoided.

Manual small incision cataract surgery is, therefore, a useful procedure by which a sutureless cataract surgery can be performed safely in almost every situation with minimal expenditure.

EDITOR'S PEARLS

Table summarizing the advantages, indications, and limitations of manual SICS

	Advantages	Indications	Limitations
Manual small incision cataract surgery	Machine independent	Hard nucleus	Scleral thinning
	Low cost of consumables	Central corneal opacity	High risk of endothelial cell damage in cases with shallow anterior chamber
	Universal applicability to all grades of nuclei	Limbal scarring	Dense arcus senilis obstructs the visualization of nuclear passage through the corneoscleral tunnel
	Lesser chances of vision threatening complications such as nuclear drop	Morgagnian cataract	Higher wound-related complications
	Shorter learning curve		
	Extremely useful procedure for high volume surgery in remote areas		

■ SUGGESTED READING

1. Goel R, Kamal S, Kumar S, Kishore J, Malik KP, Angmo Bodh S, et al. Feasibility and complications between phacoemulsification and manual small incision surgery in subluxated cataract. J Ophthalmol. 2012;2012:205139.

3.30 | How to Minimize Corneal Endothelial Cell Damage during Phacosection, a Manual Small Incision Cataract Surgery?

MS Ravindra
Karthik Netralaya, Bengaluru
dr.m.s.ravindra@gmail.com, www.karthiknetralaya.com

■ INTRODUCTION

Phacosection is an advanced and safe machineless cataract surgery, performed under topical anesthesia. A single self-sealing sclerocorneal tunnel is created with no sideports.

Gentle fluidics, physiological IOP, minimal posterior bowing of the iris-capsule-zonular diaphragm, no ultrasound, and least intra-bag manipulations are the hallmarks. The overall energy needed is a miniscule. Heat is not generated during the surgery and so the corneal endothelium remains well protected. However, in any manual small incision cataract surgery (MSICS) nucleus delivery needs to be least traumatic and the modern small incision cataract surgery is engineered to minimize direct and indirect endothelial and uveal damage due to mechanical, chemical, thermal, and inflammatory elements.

■ PREOPERATIVE PREPARATIONS

Routine specular microscopy of endothelium is very helpful in all cataract surgeries. If the cell quality and counts are found deficient, MSICS will be the procedure of choice. Whenever any surgical step is modified or a new drug is introduced, a repeat cell count at 1 month becomes useful.

Assess the hardness of the nucleus and document cornea guttata, endothelial diseases, pseudoexfoliation, posterior polar cataract, phacodonesis, subluxation, weak zonules, nondilating pupil, IFIS, etc. during preoperative evaluation. Mild hypotony before surgery is helpful. Dilate the pupil maximally for surgery.

■ INSTRUMENTATION

A surgical microscope with stereo coaxial illumination is essential to perform good surgery. The surgical instruments and tubings need to be the best, without any compromise in their quality. They should not harbor residues of soap, detergents, enzymes, rust, anti-rust agents, blood, cortex, OVD, microbial residues, etc. The scrub nurse needs to flush the cannulas soon after their use while assisting. Soon after the surgery the instruments are transferred into an ultrasound tub containing RO or distilled water, without any additive chemicals. They are then rinsed in RO water and wiped dry immediately. All cannulas and tubings are to be flushed with copious RO water at the earliest. We use a small motor placed inside an RO water container to flush the instruments. All instruments are packed and autoclaved on the same day even if there are no surgeries on the next day. The moisture in tubings and in the crevices of instruments encourages exponential microbial multiplication if they are stored wet overnight. Autoclaving such stored instruments will of course kill the microbes, but the dead microbes can cause toxic anterior segment syndrome (TASS). The B class autoclave should have multiple pre-vacuum and post-dry cycles to ensure complete drying of the load, including the tubings. Avoid all types of chemical disinfection of instruments so as to minimize the TASS. Use powder-free gloves for surgery.

■ DIRECT SCLEROCORNEAL TUNNEL

The sclerocorneal tunnels heal very well, and when well-constructed they will not induce a large surgically induced astigmatism (SIA). Width of the tunnel is not critical like in clear corneal tunnels. The tunnel in Phacosection is created with a 2.8 mm keratome, starting at anterior sclera, about 0.5-1 mm posterior to the limbus. No separate conjunctiva-Tenon's flap is created. The keratome it traverses across the limbus and peripheral cornea and enters AC about 1-1.5 mm anterior to limbus. Visco is infused into AC and a "tunnel floor entry" continuous curvilinear capsulorhexis (CCC) is created. The tunnel is enlarged to 5.2 mm with a keratome. Ensure that the entry and exit of the tunnel are straight, and parallel to each other. For large and hard nuclei, the anterior end of the tunnel is enlarged by about 0.5 mm on either side. This minimizes endothelial damage when the thick and hard hemi-nucleus is extracted from the AC. This technique does not need side pockets.

Any tunnel has to be adequately sized, with a width of 1.5 × diameter of object that go through it. This avoids stretching of the tunnel walls and minimizes damage to the endothelium. Tunnel should not extend too anteriorly into the cornea, as each instrument entering the AC tilts and indents the tunnel, and damages endothelial cells. Ore-locking of the tunnel creates radiating creases in the cornea, and damages the endothelium.

The plane of an instrument in the tunnel needs to be close to the tangent of corneal dome, so that it is tilted, elevated or depressed. This minimizes damage to endothelium. However in certain steps of surgery, one may have to depress the floor minimally.

■ NUCLEUS MANAGEMENT

Endothelial protection is crucial during nucleus management. Hydroxypropyl methylcellulose (HPMC), a dispersive viscoelastic, protects endothelium better than cohesive ophthalmic viscosurgical devices (OVD). Chondroitin sulfate is another OVD that is protective. After the initial keratome entry into the AC, the aqueous in the anterior chamber (AC) is replaced with HPMC, starting away from the main tunnel. Allow the aqueous to escape as you inject. This is to be done before injecting any other drug into the AC. HPMC gets nicely coated to the endothelium and protects it. Replenish HPMC whenever needed, viz., during nucleus management, cortical aspiration, insertion of IOL, etc.

Emulsifying as well as chopping the nucleus inside the bag can be injurious when the zonules are weak and endothelium is compromised. This is even more when it is done at pupil plane or in AC. The removal of the entire nucleus in toto needs a larger rhexis and a tunnel with side pockets. To reduce the width of the tunnel and SIA, the nucleus can be divided inside the eye, either within the capsular bag using a sustainer and a sharp instrument, or in the anterior chamber, under the protection of continuous infusion of HPMC in front of the nucleus. Along with continuous infusion of OVD in front of the nucleus during extraction, move the wire Vectis toward the iris and capsular bag, and depress the posterior lip of the tunnel as the nucleus slides out of AC. This prevents its moving nucleus rubbing against the endothelium.

A good capsule-cortical cleavage hydrodissection is ideal, to ease the cortical aspiration. As against usual belief, this step has nothing to do with nucleus management but greatly assists cortical aspiration. Avoid hydrodelineation and hydrodelamination, as they separate epinucleus and disrupt the nucleus. Epinucleus and most of the cortex are to be removed along with the nucleus. Epinucleus that is left behind is difficult to manage.

Fluidics

Chilled balanced salt solution (BSS) reduces release of cytokines and prostaglandins, stabilizes blood-aqueous barrier, minimizes miosis and constricts uveal blood vessels. Galley pot is not to be used during surgery to minimize environmental contamination, which can lead to TASS and sepsis. Phacosection has gentlest fluidics. Fluid volume, flow, velocity, turbulence, pressure fluctuations and surges are minimal. The total amount of fluid going through the eye during entire surgery can be as low as 20–30 mL. Surges and AC collapses can cause damage to endothelium. The fluid infused and aspirated is very well regulated by using Simcoe bulb and cannula, instead of a continuous infusion. AC is never deepened excessively, and so PC and zonules are not bowed posteriorly and stretched.

Do not direct a jet of fluid toward the endothelium or in between the iris and anterior capsule. The former can be injurious and the latter can cause intraoperative hard eye, which leads to a difficulty surgery, compromising endothelium. Always start infusion before activating aspiration.

Damage to Endothelium

Air if used during surgery, is not to be left behind in the AC. Avoid or dilute and minimize any chemical that is used in the eye. Adrenaline, moxifloxacin and other antibiotics, pilocarpine, lignocaine, trypan blue, etc., infuse them away from endothelium, at pupillary plane. Whenever possible, coat the endothelium with HPMC before infusing a chemical.

Completely remove dispersive viscoelastics at the end of surgery particularly that is stuck to the endothelium, trapped inside the capsular bag, behind the intraocular lens.

Continuous curvilinear capsulorhexis and self-sealing sutureless tunnel are main and salient features of modern cataract surgery. Because of excellent control on various parameters, MSICS is best designed to prevent endothelial cell loss. The cornea should be clear and thin, without any biomicroscopic striate keratopathy on first postoperative day.

EDITOR'S PEARLS

Preventing endothelial damage during manual SICS

Identification of preoperative risk factors	Instruments, solutions, and accessories	Intraoperative considerations
Hard nucleus	Ensure best quality instruments	Adequately sized corneal tunnel to minimize distortion during instrumentation
Corneal guttata and other endothelial disorders	Prefer autoclave, avoid chemical agents as they increase the risk of TASS	Maintained AC depth throughout the procedure
Pseudoexfoliation syndrome	Powder-free gloves	Avoid touching endothelium with lens matter, instruments or even jet of fluid.
Phacodonesis	Chilled BSS solution	Primary chop-preferred technique of nuclear division
Subluxation	Avoid use of chemicals such as adrenaline, lignocaine, trypan blue dye, pilocarpine, antibiotics, etc. wherever possible.	Complete removal of OVD at the end of the surgery
Poorly dilating pupil	Use of dispersive OVDs to coat endothelium during nucleus management	Keep duration of surgery minimal

3.31 Contrast Sensitivity in Pseudophakic Patients

Ravi Nabh
Government Medical College, Chandigarh
ravinabh_pgimer@yahoo.com

INTRODUCTION

- Functional vision describes the effect of sight on quality of life. It is not reflected entirely in the measurement of visual acuity. An individual with 20/20 visual acuity can have deficient functional vision.
- Advances in surgical techniques, intraocular lens (IOL) material, design, and optical quality have made cataract surgery one of the most fascinating and evolving surgery. Major thrust is to provide better functional vision.
- Deficiencies in functional vision are identified with contrast sensitivity testing.

- Many techniques have been used to measure contrast in pseudophakic patients.
- It measures two separate functions:
  - The perceived contrast threshold between object and background.
  - The target size of object subtended on the retina and measured in cycles per degree.
- Contrast sensitivity can be checked by using letter charts and sine wave grating charts.
- Letter optotype charts include that of Terry, Regan and Pelli–Robson.
- Sine wave charts include Vistech and its various versions, second generation Vistech chart (the FACT) and similar charts such as Vector Vision CSV-1000.
- Pelli–Robson chart, FACT CV chart, and Vector Vision CSV-1000 have been used mainly to measure contrast sensitivity in pseudophakic patients.

OUR EXPERIENCE

- Pelli–Robson chart is read at 1 m with spectacle correction under photopic condition.
- It has three decisions per level and step size of 0.15 or 0.10 log units.
- Size of letters is same but there are separate letter chart for both right and left eye.
- Results of the contrast sensitivity are in log contrast units.
- Provides more repeatable measurements of contrast sensitivity or low contrast visual acuity.
- Functional acuity contrast chart uses Gaussian sine wave grating to measure contrast sensitivity at five standard spatial frequencies (1.5, 3, 6, 12, 18 cycles per degree) and contrast levels.
- All measurements are obtained with best corrected spectacle correction under mesopic (3 candelas/m^2) and photopic (85 candelas/m^2) conditions.
- The patient is asked to look at the chart and choose the orientation of sine wave grating pattern in each patch (straight up and down or tilted right or left).
- Last patch on FACT chart that each patient can correctly identify for each spatial frequency is assigned as contrast sensitivity value using a chart by vision sciences research corp. and converted to log scale to obtain log contrast sensitivity value.
- Sine wave grating has been used in visual psychophysics for more than three decades.
- Using computer generated sine wave gratings eliminates the need to control room lights and allow the observer to control the light source and present the target to one eye at a time. These tests have advantage over letter contrast sensitivity charts that they can measure contrast sensitivity at several spatial frequencies. These tests have advantage over letter contrast sensitivity charts that they can measure contrast sensitivity at several spatial frequencies however these test, suffer from poor test—retest repeatability.

EDITOR'S PEARLS
- Reduced contrast sensitivity is one of the manifestations of cataract. Cataract surgery often helps improve this visual function.
- Among the modern-day intraocular lenses, monofocal IOLs fare much better with higher contrast sensitivity scores as compared to multifocal IOLs. Therefore, the former should be preferred in patients with other underlying ocular pathologies such as glaucoma and diabetic retinopathy.
- A postoperative patient with 20/20 vision does not always translate to optimal functional vision. Reduced contrast sensitivity may still be one of the reasons for an unhappy 20/20 patient and must be thoroughly evaluated.

SUGGESTED READING

1. Pelli DG, Robson JG, Wilkins AJ. The design of a new letter chart for measuring contrast sensitivity. Clin Vis Sci. 1988;2:187-99.

3.32 How Important is it to Reduce or Eliminate Spherical Aberration after Phacoemulsification?

Amit Gupta
Advanced Eye Centre, PGIMER, Chandigarh
amitguptaeye@gmail.com

INTRODUCTION

- Wave front analysis is based on the principle that light behaves as a wave rather than a group of single linear waves creating an image. For a perfect image to be formed, all light waves from a single point object must be brought to focus at a single, perfect point of focus.
- However, light travels faster in air than through the relatively dense lens. Also, the surface of the lens (and cornea) is convex, and therefore, not perpendicular to the incoming light waves except in the center. Thus, with the natural (and spheric) lenses, certain portions of the light wave will travel greater distance in air as well as through lesser lens portions compared to the rest of the light waves leading to aberrations.
- Spherical aberration (SA) is a fourth order aberration that varies with the radial distance from the center of the pupil. Quite obviously, it also varies with the pupillary size. Spherical aberrations may be positive or negative. If peripheral portions of a light wave come to a focal point anterior to the paraxial portions, then a positive (or undercorrected) SA is said to exist (the Mexican hat pattern of wavefront aberration) and negative (or overcorrected) if portions of the light wave focus behind the paraxial portions (inverted Mexican hat).
- Young individuals have a lower index of refraction of the central lens compared to the periphery leading to negative SA, thus offsetting the positive SA induced by the cornea and resulting in a more optimal image quality as well as depth of focus. This undergoes a change as we age, the corneal collective positive SA increases with age while the negative SA of the lens becomes less negative or positive. This is an important consideration when implanting a wavefront intraocular lens (IOL) in the young. Several available IOLs incorporate a (usually negative) SA along with an aspheric lens design to correct for the positive corneal SA. The important ones are listed below:
    - *Tecnis Z9000*: Modified *prolate anterior* surface to compensate for the average corneal SA found in the adult eye. It introduces –0.27 µm of SA to the eye measured at 6 mm optical zone.
    - *AcrySof IQ IOL*: The lens has an *aspheric posterior* optic design with a thinner center. It induces –0.20 µm of SA, compared to the –0.27 µm induced by the Tecnis lens leaving a small amount of SA. Koch recently reported that even though optimal ocular and IOL SA varies widely among eyes, most emmetropic eyes achieved the best image quality with a 6.0 mm pupil when total ocular SA is between –0.10 µm and 0.00 µm.
    - *Sofport advanced optics*: This IOL has been specifically designed with zero SA so that it will not contribute to any preexisting higher-order aberrations. As the advanced optics (AO) lens has no relationship to the average or actual SA in the eye, it may be less dependent on centration in comparison to Tecnis or AcrySof IQ IOL.
- One study compared an aspheric monofocal, acrylic noncustomized IOL with aspheric monofocal silicone noncustomized IOL with incorporated negative SA and concluded that even though SA was higher in the first group, three times as many patients perceived more visual disturbances in the latter group. Also, high and low contrast

TABLE 3.32.1: Important strengths and weaknesses of intraocular lens (IOL) types.

IOL type	Depth of field	Contrast sensitivity	Tolerance to defocus	Reduction of HOA
Spheric	+	Neutral	+++	–
Aspheric	+	+	++	+
Custom wavefront	–	++	+	+++

+ = Strength; – = Weakness; ++ = Variable (see bibliography for details)
(HOA: higher order aberration; IOL: intraocular lens)

acuity, photopic and mesopic contrast acuities were also comparable, with the first group reporting better subjective visual quality compared to the "SA compensated" group. The authors suggested that some residual postoperative positive SA may be beneficial by providing better depth of field as well as allowing pseudoaccommodation to occur. It appears, therefore, that visual acuity and contrast sensitivity may not be the most important factors in determining the overall subjective visual performance following cataract surgery.

- A summary of the strengths and weaknesses of several types of IOLs is given in **Table 3.32.1**. A residual positive SA maximizes optical quality in myopic eyes whereas a negative SA optimizes optical quality in hyperopic eyes. Thus, myopic and hyperopic patients may benefit if their SA is not completely corrected.

Microincisional cataract surgery is also an important prerequisite when considering aberrations related to cataract surgery as larger incisions can themselves induce significant aberrations. To conclude, it appears that not all patients would benefit from correction of all presurgical SAs. Further understanding of which higher order aberrations to correct and wavefront analysis may pave the way to provide for the best possible visual outcome after cataract surgery. Further development in wavefront IOL technology will allow the ophthalmologist to provide a more customized approach for many patients undergoing cataract surgery.

HOYA optimized aspheric IOL with aspheric balanced curve (ABC) design: The aspheric balanced curve design of Hoya's negative aspheric IOLs minimizes the aberrations related to decentration and tilt.

EDITOR'S PEARLS

- Spherical aberration in the human eye is a combination of the positive spherical aberration of the cornea and the negative spherical aberration of the crystalline lens.
- As the positive SA of cornea increases with age, most surgeons prefer to implant IOLs with negative SA to minimize the total spherical aberrations of the eye.
- With regard to presbyopia correction strategy some residual spherical aberration may be desirable to increase the depth of focus.

SUGGESTED READING

1. Ruttig NJ, Maria J, Shah SA. Evaluating wavefront analysis application in intraocular lens placement. Curr Opin Ophthalmol. 2008;19(4):309-13.

3.33 What should be Done for a Patient Undergoing Phaco and is Suspected to have Globe Perforation during Procedure?

Mangat R Dogra
Advanced Eye Centre, PGIMER, Chandigarh
Gaurav Sanghi
Sangam Netralaya, Mohali
eyepgi@sify.com

GLOBE PERFORATION
Globe perforation during periocular anesthesia is a devastating complication and can range from *simple perforation* to *globe explosion*.

Risk Factors for Globe Perforation during Periocular Anesthesia
- Large axial length
- Posterior staphyloma
- Shallow orbit
- Previous scleral buckling
- Sharp disposable needle
- Injection by nonophthalmologist

GLOBE EXPLOSION: CLINICAL SIGNS
Suspected Globe Explosion
- Resistance during injection
- Sudden severe pain
- Corneal clouding

Definite Globe Explosion
- Hypotony and "give" in response
- Chemosis
- Subconjunctival hemorrhage and hyphema
- Prolapsed uvea and spontaneous lens extrusion

GLOBE EXPLOSION: WHAT TO DO IMMEDIATELY?
- Do exploration and suture the sclera.
- Do ultrasonography and refer to vitreoretinal surgeon for further management of posterior segment complications.

FURTHER MANAGEMENT AND PROGNOSIS
- Retinal detachment needs to be operated early.
- Vitreous hemorrhage without retinal detachment can be operated after 2–3 weeks.
- Peripheral and equatorial perforations have best prognosis.
- Posterior pole perforations and retinal detachment have poor prognosis.
- Prognosis is worst in cases of globe perforation/explosion with subretinal hemorrhage, retinal detachment, and proliferative vitreoretinopathy **(Flowchart 3.33.1)**.

DO'S AND DON'TS FOR PERIBULBAR ANESTHESIA
Know the risk factors for perforation and be aware if your patient has one!
- Use short and blunt needle with 10 mL syringe.

Flowchart 3.33.1: Immediate management of globe perforation during periocular anesthesia.

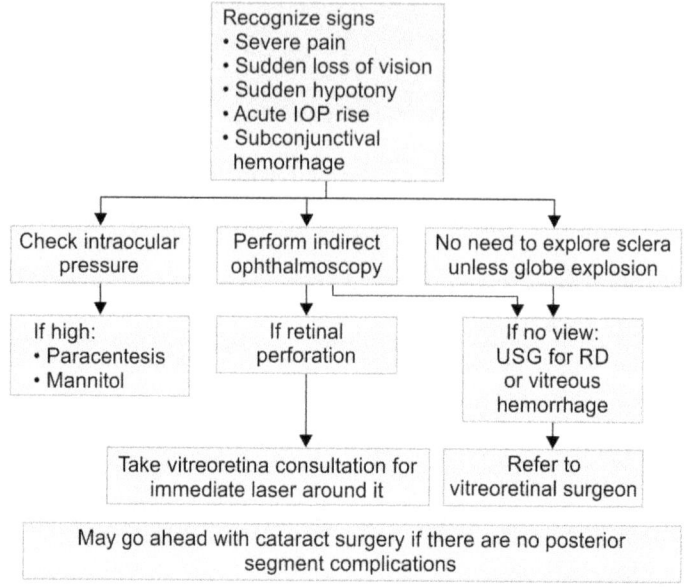

(IOP: intraocular pressure; RD: retinal detachment; USG: ultrasonography)

- Direct needle away from the globe.
- Wiggle the syringe and aspirate the plunger before injection. Discontinue immediately, if resistance to injection, use alternative technique (topical anesthesia).

SUGGESTED READING

1. Brar GS, Ram J, Dogra MR, Pandav SS, Sharma A, Kaushik S, et al. Ocular explosion after peribulbar anesthesia. J Cataract Refract Surg. 2002;28(3):556-61.

3.34 | Are Anterior Chamber IOLs Safe for Implantation? Which Anterior Chamber IOLs should be Implanted?

Srikant Kumar Padhy, Neelima Aron
Dr RP Centre for Ophthalmic Sciences, AIIMS, New Delhi
srikantkumar.padhy19@gmail.com, neelima.aron87@gmail.com

INTRODUCTION

Anterior chamber intraocular lenses (ACIOLs) are lenses which are implanted in the anterior chamber (AC) with the footplates resting in the angle. The intraocular lens (IOL) has undergone several modifications since the time of its development.

FIRST-GENERATION LENSES

The first ACIOL implantation was done in France in 1952 by Baron **(Fig. 3.34.1)**. This IOL was a large convex concave plastic lens resting in the angle. However, this IOL was destined to cause obvious corneal decompensation and failure due to the obvious close contact to the corneal endothelium by the highly vaulted IOL.

SECTION 3: Cataract

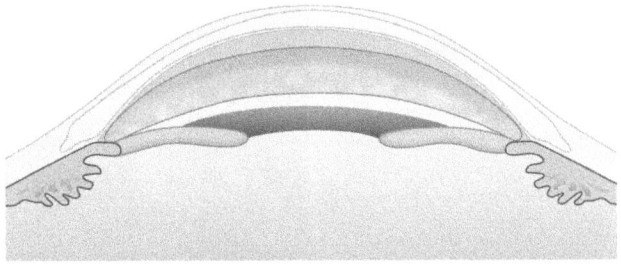

Fig. 3.34.1: Anterior chamber intraocular lens (IOL) (Baron).

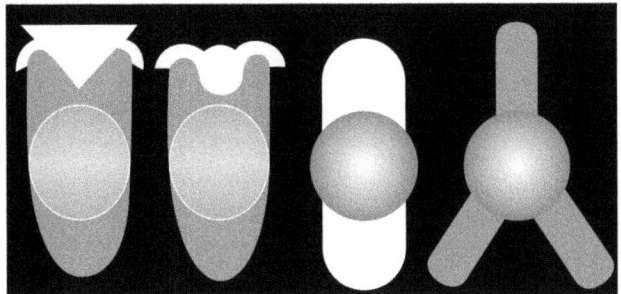

Fig. 3.34.2: Left-to-right—Strampelli tripod anterior chamber intraocular lens (ACIOL) (1953), Choyce Mark I ACIOL (1956), Dannheim ACIOL with closed haptics (1952), Ridley tripod ACIOL (1957–60).

SECOND-GENERATION LENSES
- Rigid AC lenses.
- Derived from early AC lens by further developing them.
- Prototypes are Strampelli tripod ACIOL, Choyce Mark I ACIOL **(Fig. 3.34.2)**.
- Most common complication—corneal decompensation.
- First-and second-generation IOLs come under the category of early ACIOLs. Early ACIOLs can be of following types:
    - Rigid or semirigid ACIOL—BARON lens, Strampelli ACIOL
    - Flexible or semiflexible ACIOL:
        - Open haptic loops
        - Closed haptic loops
        - Peter Choyce lens
    - Barraquer—open loop ACIOL with J-haptics, with nylon loops
- Advantages of early ACIOLs
    - Less decentration
    - Decreased reaction
- Disadvantages of early ACIOLs
    - Corneal decompensation
    - Pseudophakic bullous keratopathy (PBK)
    - Uveitis
    - Secondary glaucoma
    - Uveitis glaucoma hyphema (UGH) syndrome

THIRD-GENERATION INTRAOCULAR LENSES
- Iris supported lenses
- First by Epstein in 1953

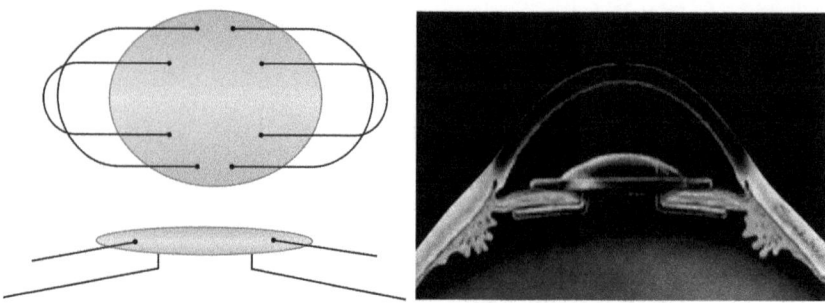

Fig. 3.34.3: Binkhorst lenses—iris clip lenses.

- Prototype lens includes collar stud lens, Maltese cross lens, Copeland lens, iris clip lens, or Binkhorst lens **(Fig. 3.34.3)**, Fyodorov modification lens.
- Advantages
  - Away from angle structure
  - Rate of dislocation was less.
  - Less contact with corneal endothelium
- Disadvantages
  - Iris chaffing
  - Papillary distortion
  - Transillumination defect
  - Cystoid macular edema (CME)
  - Distortion on papillary dilation
  - Intermittent touch leading to corneal decompensation

FOURTH-GENERATION INTRAOCULAR LENSES (1960–1990)
- Had better design and dimension.
- Example: Lusko lens, Cilco Optiflex.
- These IOLs have closed loops which lead to erosion of the chamber angle and to the ciliary body (cheese cutter effect) along with corneal decompensation.

MODERN ANTERIOR CHAMBER INTRAOCULAR LENSES
- Made of flexible loops which are stable in the AC.
- The footplates in the haptics provide minimal but stable areas of contact with the anterior chamber angle.
- The anterior vault prevents the lens from touching the iris and the stability of IOL helps prevent corneal touch.
- Prototype of this type is Kelman multiflex lenses **(Fig. 3.34.4)**.
- Advantages
  - In contrast to a closed loop ACIOL, well-designed open-loop lens has a maintained vault even under high compression preventing IOL touch against the cornea or iris.
  - Sizing is less critical with flexible open-loop designs.
  - Choyce's ACIOL design incorporates broad haptic or footplate fixation elements which makes it tissue friendly as a protective fibrosis around the footplate helps minimize erosion and chafing.
  - As the haptics subtend only small areas of the angle outflow structures point fixation is possible with these.
  - Polished smooth surfaces and rounded edges result in much gentler tissue contact by any part of the IOL (optic or haptic) with lesser possibility of chafing or damage.

SECTION 3: Cataract

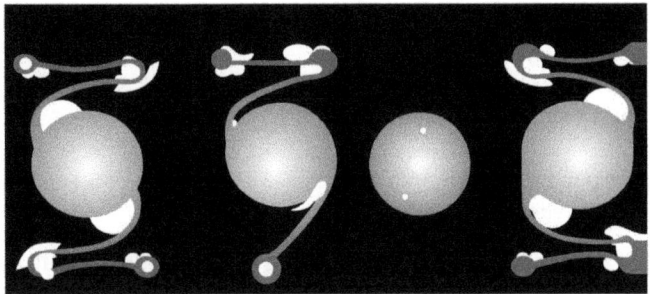

Fig. 3.34.4: From left-to-right: Kelman multiflex ACIOL (1982), Kelman flexible tripod ACIOL (1981), Intermedics Inc Dubroff ACIOL (1981), Modern, one-piece, flexible PMMA ACIOL (Kelman design) with Choyce footplates.

PHAKIC INTRAOCULAR LENSES
- Used to correct high refractive errors in the presence of a normal crystalline.
- May be implanted in the anterior chamber or posterior chamber.
- ACIOLs may either be angle supported, e.g., Baikoff MA20 NuVita phakic lens, Galin lens or iris-fixated lens such as the Artisan myopic lens.

INDICATIONS
- Intra-operative posterior capsular rupture
- Lens or IOL subluxation or dislocation
- Aphakia without any capsular support

CONTRAINDICATIONS
- Uveitis
- Corneal endothelial pathology
- Pediatric eyes
- Shallow anterior chamber
- Presence of peripheral anterior synechiae

PROCEDURE
- Most common indication of implanting anterior chamber IOLs is intra-operative posterior capsular rupture.
- The aim is to implant the IOL in the AC such that it is well-centered. The footplates should rest against the scleral spur and should not capture any iris tissue or interfere with iridectomies.
- IOL power must be determined preoperatively in a planned surgery.
- In case of inadvertent intraoperative posterior capsular rupture, the precludes posterior chamber intraocular lens (PCIOL) implantation the ACIOL power is calculated by subtracting the difference in the A constants of the PC and AC IOLs from the power of originally selected PCIOL.
- The size of ACIOL is calculated by adding 1 mm to the horizontal white-to-white limbal dimension.
- Removal of the cataract must be followed by clearing the vitreous from the anterior chamber.
- The IOL is inserted under a viscoelastic cover or under air.
- A peripheral iridectomy is necessary as it prevents pupillary block.
- There should be no iris tucking.
- The haptics should be positioned away from the iridectomy site.

COMPLICATIONS
- Pseudophakic bullous keratopathy
- Uveitis
- Ocular hypertension and glaucoma
- Hyphema
- Distortion of pupil
- Cystoid macular edema

CURRENT STATUS OF ANTERIOR CHAMBER INTRAOCULAR LENS
- Current ACIOLs are far superior to the older generation ACIOL.
- The flexible loops have decreased the need for exact determination of the IOL size. Oversizing of IOLs has become less of a concern to the surgeon since the haptics accommodate themselves in the smaller AC space.
- The design of haptic loops permits three to four points of contact with the angle which has greatly reduced the risk of developing postoperative glaucoma and synechiae formation.
- The absence of holes in the IOL allows for easy explantation of IOL if required.
- The absence of holes further decreases the iris plugging the holes thereby reducing inflammation, pigment dispersion, synechiae formation, and secondary glaucoma.

CONCLUSION
- Anterior chamber IOLs are a feasible option for IOL implantation in the absence of a posterior capsule.
- It is technically easier and less time-consuming.
- Thus, with the modifications in the design of ACIOLs, the current ACIOLs are found safe for implantation for patients suitable for such lenses.

EDITOR'S PEARLS
- Present day ACIOLs are superior to the older generation and are safe to implant in eyes with lack of capsular support.
- With only three to four points contact with the angle, the risk of developing postoperative glaucoma and synechiae formation is reduced.

SUGGESTED READING
1. Anterior chamber intraocular lenses. Surv Ophthalmol. 2000;45(Suppl 1):S131-49.

3.35 Iris-Claw Lens—Versatility Combines Safety

Ravijit Singh
Dr Daljit Singh Eye Hospital, Amritsar
ravijit@yahoo.com

INTRODUCTION
Perhaps no other design in the history of intraocular lenses (IOLs) has enjoyed a longer innings than the ubiquitous iris-claw lens. Nearly 32 years after the claw fixation principle was conceived by the famous ophthalmologist from the Netherlands, Dr Jan Worst, the basic design continues to remain the same. In India, the iris-claw lens design received unflinching patronage from Dr Daljit Singh and this lens continues to be the design of choice for patients with inadequate or absent capsular support as well as in complicated cases of trauma.

DESIGN OF IRIS-CLAW LENS

- *Worst iris-claw lens:* This was the original design of Dr Jan Worst. A planoconvex optic of 5 mm and a claw mechanism on either side of the optic. The claws were designed diagonally opposite to each other. The optic and the haptics were in a same plane.
- *Singh's modified iris-claw lens:* This lens was basically the same design as above but for the position of the claws. Instead of being diametrically opposite, the claws were at an angle of 45° to optic.

FIXATION PRINCIPLE OF THE CLASSIC IRIS-CLAW DESIGN

- Both the abovementioned designs of the iris-claw lens were fixated to the anterior surface of the iris with the claw mechanism using a lens stabilization forceps and an enclavation needle or a forceps to tuck the iris into the claw. An effort was made to fix the claws to the peripheral iris so that the pupil could function unhindered. In order to fixate the lens to the peripheral iris, the overall length of the lens was nearly 8.5 mm.
- Due to the near absence of viscoelastic materials in the late 70s and all through the 80s, fixation of this lens was carried out under air. The Singh–Worst design needed a relatively smaller incision (than the Worst design) and also a smaller incision would hold an air bubble in the anterior chamber better than a bigger incision, thereby making it a bit easier **(Figs. 3.35.1A to C)**.

"This lens is difficult to implant and even more difficult to explant" was a familiar expression used by many senior surgeons in those days. I admit today that in many ways than one they were quite right.

IMPORTANT FACTS TO BE REMEMBERED ABOUT THE IRIS-CLAW LENS

- The size of the IOL used in the anterior chamber should be much smaller in size as compared to the lenses used in the past, i.e., maximum optic size 4.25 mm with an overall length of 7.25 mm. Yet smaller lenses may be used in children or in other situations. Large-sized lenses run the risk of progressive corneal endothelial damage.
- A sufficient fold of iris must be tucked into the claw for it to hold securely to the iris and to prevent shaking of the lens.

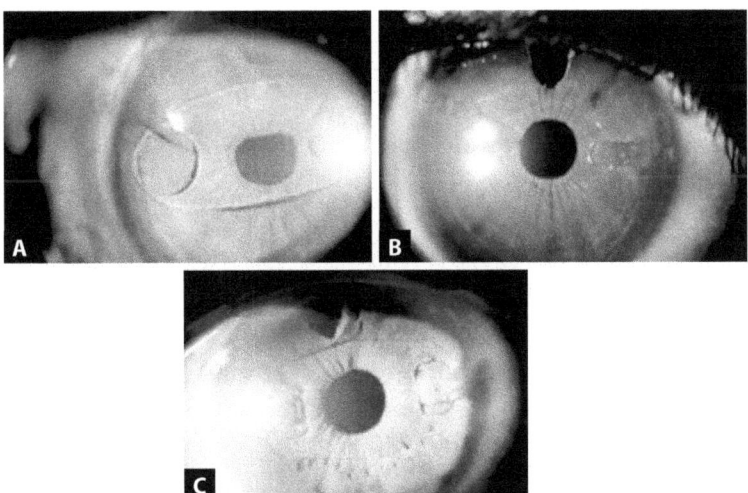

Figs. 3.35.1A to C: (A) Large-sized Singh–Worst design; (B) Small-sized Singh–Worst design; (C) Worst iris-claw lens design.

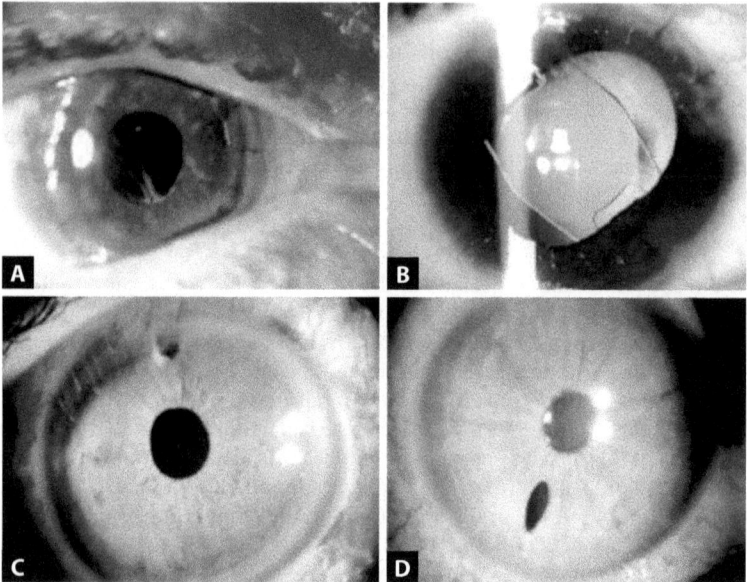

Figs. 3.35.2A to D: (A) Retroiris claw lens in penetrating keratoplasty (PKP); (B) Good pupil dilatation after retrofixation; (C) Retrofixation in megalocornea; (D) Retrofixation after retinal surgery.

- The lens used in aphakic conditions must be plano-convex optic without any haptic vault.
- Lens must be implanted with convexity forwards.
- The A-constant of the iris-claw lens fixed to the anterior surface of the iris is 115.5 mm.
- As far as possible, avoid implantation of the iris-claw lens to the anterior surface of the iris.
- Since this lens design will find application in unusual situations, it is imperative to make sure that vitreous has been handled well and the iris tissue is free, i.e., it should not have adhesions to fibrous or fibrovascular membranes, which may compromise its fixation.

Fixation Sites of Iris-Claw Lens
- Anterior surface of the iris (for which this was designed primarily).
- Retroiris fixation (fixation to the posterior surface of the iris) **(Figs. 3.35.2A to D)**
  - By doing retroiris fixation, we avoid the anterior chamber and the cornea and the related problems.
  - IOL power calculation for the retroiris-fixated lens is done by adding 1 diopter to the IOL power calculation achieved for the anterior-fixated lens.
  - Retrofixation of the iris-claw is our preferred method nowadays.

Instruments Needed for Retroiris-fixated Lens
- Right and left forceps specifically designed for secure gripping of the iris-claw lens for implantation, one for either side of the lens.
- A 27-gauge cannula (three-fourths of an inch long and bent at 45° in the middle), mounted on a 1-mL syringe is used for enclavation of the iris tissue into the claw mechanism.
  The technique is not difficult but needs a bit of perseverance to learn.

CONCLUSION

Progressive loss of endothelial cell count is the only major problem associated with anteriorly fixated iris-claw lens. Other than this, the eyes implanted with the iris-claw lens have shown remarkable tolerance to this lens even after 20 years or more. The technique of retrofixation of the iris-claw lens has helped us to use the iris-claw lens to our advantage by harnessing its versatility and at the same time staying clear of its problems in the anterior chamber.

The greatest boon of the retrofixated iris-claw lens is for the phaco surgeon, who can depend upon this lens as an effective backup in case of compromised capsular support.

Also this lens provides a great option for the cornea surgeons to implant this lens instead messing around with scleral fixation during penetrating keratoplasty (PKP) procedures. I am sure that the iris-claw lens is here to stay and serve for a long time.

SUGGESTED READING

1. Sekundo W. New forceps and spatula for easy retropupillary implantation of iris claw lenses in aphakia: Experience in 4 years of use. Eur J Ophthalmol. 2008;18(3):442-4.

3.36 | Scleral-fixated Intraocular Lens

Surg Capt (Dr) Srujana D
Armed Forces Medical College, Pune
drsrujanabhaskar@gmail.com

INTRODUCTION

Intraocular lenses (IOLs) have undergone lot of changes in the designs, fixation, and indications for their use since their introduction in the late 1940s by Sir Harold Ridley. To implant a routine posterior chamber IOL (PCIOL) intact posterior capsule is mandatory. In the absence of posterior capsule, anterior chamber (AC) IOLs and iris-fixated IOLs have been tried but have been noted to carry high risk of complications (corneal decompensation, iris chafing, and uveitis). To avoid these complications, methods of transscleral fixation of posterior chamber (PC) lenses to the ciliary sulcus have been developed.

Scleral-fixated IOLs (SFIOLs) were first reported by Malbran and coauthors in patients who had previous intracapsular cataract extraction. Later on, various techniques using different kinds of sutures, needles and IOL designs were developed. Maggi and Maggi first reported the technique for sutureless intrascleral fixation of PCIOL. To avoid the suture-related intra- and postoperative problems, Gabor and Pavlidis described a technique for sulcus fixation of the haptics of the IOL. Use of a biological glue to attach the haptic to sclera is a technique described by Agarwal.

INDICATIONS

Indications of SFIOLs include:
- Primary scleral fixation of IOL:
  - Dislocated or subluxated crystalline lenses
  - Capsular rupture during planned extracapsular cataract extraction
- Secondary scleral fixation of IOL:
  - Aphakia with inadequate posterior capsular support
  - Penetrating keratoplasty combined with scleral fixation of IOL
  - Retrieval and scleral fixation of a dislocated or subluxated PCIOL
  - IOL exchange procedures.

PREREQUISITES AND PREOPERATIVE EVALUATION

- Complete eye examination including slit-lamp evaluation to see for health of the corneal endothelial cells, vitreous in AC, evaluation of macula with biomicroscopy

and indirect ophthalmoscopy, especially in eyes for secondary SFIOL wherein there is increased incidence of cystoids macular edema.
- Intraocular pressure (IOP) measurement is important, especially if low, which may indicate the presence of iritis, leaky cataract wound, retinal detachment, or choroidal detachment. On the other hand, a high IOP or a history thereof may necessitate a glaucoma work-up. If the patient has a high cup-to-disc ratio with advanced visual field changes, the surgeon should carefully weigh the benefits versus the risks of secondary lens implantation.
- White-to-white measurement to avoid IOL decentration due to disparity between the globe and IOL.
- Specular microscopy for endothelial cell count and morphology.
- Biometric measurements of axial length and corneal curvature with A-scan ultrasonography and keratometry, respectively, for IOL power calculation in aphakic mode.

MATERIALS FOR SCLERAL-FIXATED INTRAOCULAR LENSES

Flexible materials, such as polypropylene and polymethylmethacrylate with low resistance to deformation, are recommended for the haptics of the IOL which reduces the risk of haptic fracture during surgery.
- Alcon CZ70BD SFIOL (Alcon International, USA), are single-piece polymethylmethacrylate (PMMA) lenses with eyelets with optic and overall diameter of 7.0 mm and 12.5 mm, respectively.
- Aurolab SC6530 (Aurolab, India) single-piece PMMA lens with eyelets with optic and overall diameter of 6.5 mm and 13 mm, respectively.
- Bausch and Lomb Akreos AO60 hydrophilic acrylic lens with four eyelets for four-point fixation. The Bausch and Lomb enVista MX60 IOL hydrophobic acrylic IOL with eyelets at the two haptic-optic junctions.
- Standard three-piece IOL with a haptic design fitting to the diameter of ciliary sulcus can be used for sutureless and glued IOL.

Suture Material
- Polypropylene (Prolene) is a monofilament polymer most commonly used suture material for scleral-fixated IOLs. Rates of suture breakage have been reported from 0 to 27.9% with 10-0 polypropylene. For this reason, 9-0 polypropylene has been increasingly used to reduce the rate of breakage.
- Gore-Tex (WL Gore and Associates, Elkton, Maryland, USA) is a nonabsorbable, polytetrafluoroethylene monofilament suture. It has greater tensile strength and has been reported to have lower suture breakage rates when used in the eye.

TECHNIQUES OF SCLERAL-FIXATED INTRAOCULAR LENSES (FLOWCHART 3.36.1)

Sutured Scleral-fixated Intraocular Lenses

Ab Externo Suture Fixation

Ab externo fixation first introduced by Lewis in 1991 refers to scleral fixation in which sutures are passed from the outside to the inside of the eye **(Fig. 3.36.1)**. The location of the ciliary sulcus is established using external landmarks.

Advantages
- Technically easy as compared to Ab interno technique
- Avoids risk of passing needles out of the eye
- The surgeon's view is not obscured.

SECTION 3: Cataract

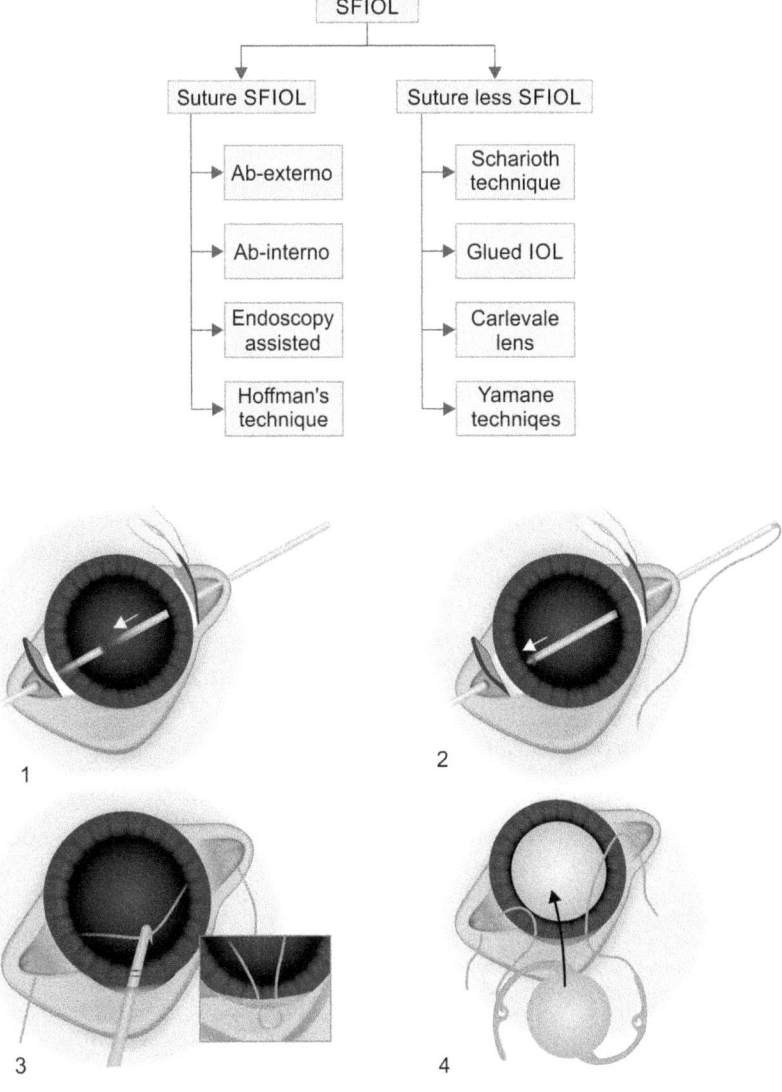

Flowchart 3.36.1: Techniques of scleral-fixated Intraocular lenses (SFIOL).

Fig. 3.36.1: Ab externo suture fixation technique.

Disadvantages
- Requires large incision
- Sutures can erode into subconjunctival space.

Modifications of Ab Externo Technique

Four-point suture fixation: The technique is similar to the external to internal approaches using long straight needle, but here IOL is fixed at four points, two points on each haptic. As in this technique two 10–0 polypropylene sutures are passed, at two places, this will avoid tilt or decentration of IOL.

Small-incision ab externo technique for ciliary sulcus fixation: Regillo and Tidwell published a modified version of the Lewis technique for suturing a PCIOL using a foldable silicone lens to allow for a smaller incision thereby decreasing the risk of intraocular fluid loss and hypotony, improving globe stability during lens insertion and suturing. By obviating the need for limbal-incision suturing, this method requires less time in the operating room and reduces astigmatism.

Knotless ab externo technique for ciliary sulcus fixation: This technique described by Erylidirim in 1995 involves looping the suture around the haptics rather than tying square knots around the haptics. Although Erylidirim's method leaves the surgeon with two lines of suture at each scleral clock hour at the end of the operation, these sutures cannot be used to perform a more stable two-point fixation because the two strands exit through the same port.

Modified technique of Shapirno and Leen: This technique is similar to classic ab externo technique except that it does not require specialized sutures, IOLs, or instruments. Here, same conventional 10-0 polypropylene sutures are required having curved needle which after passing through the sclera is pulled out of the eye with the help of a McPherson forceps **(Fig. 3.36.2)**.

Truly knotless technique for scleral fixation of IOLs: This technique described by Szurman uses ab externo technique for implanting IOL, the needle ends of the 10-0 Prolene suture are then bent and Z-shaped intrascleral passes with at least five indentations are made to secure the IOL **(Fig. 3.36.3)**. The suture is then cut without making any knot and covered by the conjunctiva **(Fig. 3.36.4)**.

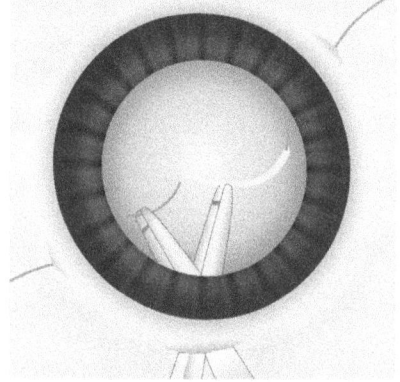

Fig. 3.36.2: Modified technique of Shapirno and Leen.

Ab Interno Technique with Two-point Ciliary Sulcus Fixation

The ab interno technique with two-point ciliary sulcus fixation described by Smiddy and colleagues in 1990, involves passing of suture from the inside to the outside of the eye. Dissect two limbal-based, partial-thickness scleral flaps 180° apart.

Advantages
- Faster than outside-to-inside technique
- Easier with penetrating keratoplasty (PKP)

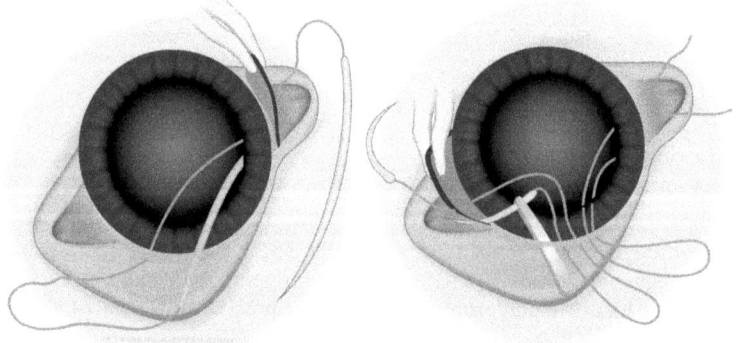

Fig. 3.36.3: Knotless technique for scleral fixation of lenses.

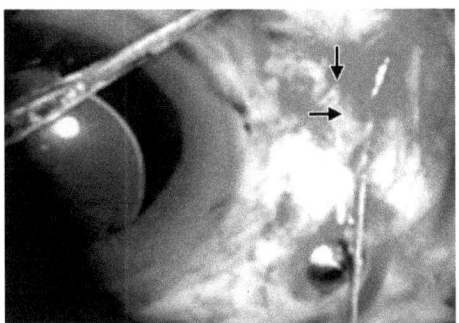

Fig. 3.36.4: No knot at suture ends.

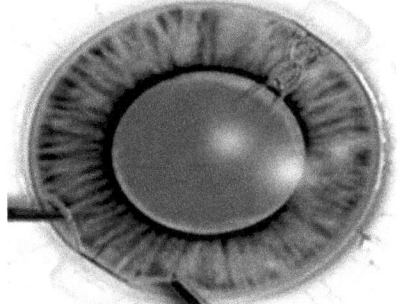

Fig. 3.36.5: Hoffman pockets.

Disadvantages
- Blind procedure of passing needle into ciliary sulcus from behind the iris
- More chance of intraocular bleeding and damage to corneal endothelium

Endoscopy-assisted Scleral-fixated Intraocular Lenses
In this technique, an endoscope inserted through pars plana, or limbus is used for direct visualization of the ciliary sulcus. Further steps of surgery can be done using a bi-manual method or a one-handed technique.

Advantages
- Direct visualization of the ciliary sulcus and needle penetration site
- Exact positioning of the haptics can be done after removal of all vitreous strands.
- Simultaneous posterior segment examination

Hoffman Technique
This technique of suture knot coverage was described in 2006 by Hoffman et al. and avoids the need for conjunctival dissection, scleral cauterization, or scleral wound closure. Although originally described for a subluxated IOL-capsular bag complex it can be used for any IOL or intraocular device that requires transscleral fixation:
- A scleral pocket is created by initiating a scleral tunnel from a clear corneal incision.
- A double-armed suture can then be passed full thickness through the conjunctiva and scleral pocket, and the suture ends can be retrieved subsequently through the external corneal incision (**Fig. 3.36.5**). The knots can then be buried within the pockets.

Sutureless Scleral Fixation

Scharioth Technique
This technique first described by Gabor B Scharioth et al. involves externalization of IOL haptics and their fixation within intrascleral Scharioth tunnels without the use of sutures.
- After peritomy, the eye is stabilized either by pars plana infusion (i.e., 25 g) or by AC maintainer.
- Two straight sclerotomies ab externo are prepared with a sharp 24-G cannula/25-G trocar used for MIVS (microincision vitrectomy surgery) 1.5 mm behind limbus, exactly 180° from each other and directed toward the center of the globe.
- Limbus-parallel intrascleral tunnels are created at about 50% of scleral thickness.
- A standard three-piece IOL with a haptic design fitting to the diameter of ciliary sulcus is implanted with an injector, and the trailing haptic is fixated in the corneal incision.
- The leading haptic is then grasped at its tip with an end-gripping 25-G forceps and pulled through the sclerotomy and left externalized (**Fig. 3.36.6**).
- With the same forceps, the haptic is then introduced into the intrascleral Scharioth tunnel. The same maneuvers are performed with the trailing haptic.

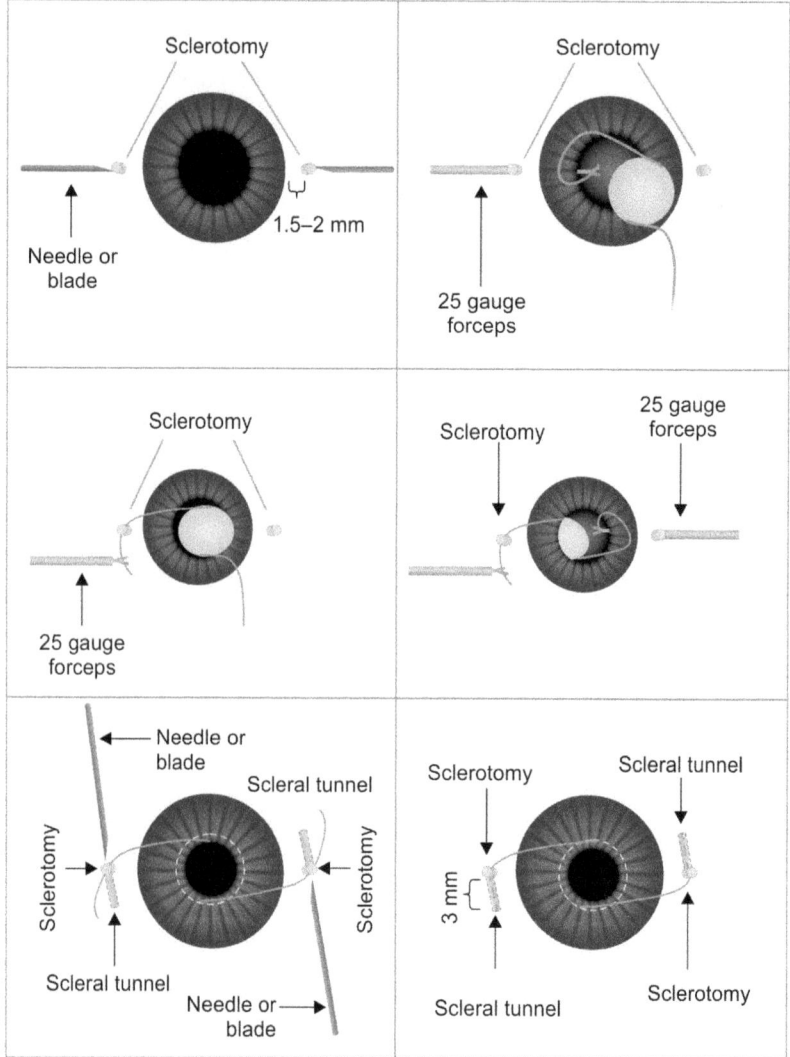

Fig. 3.36.6: Scharioth technique.

- The ends of the haptic are left in the tunnel to prevent foreign body sensation and erosion of the conjunctiva and to reduce the risk of inflammation. The sclerotomies are checked for leakage and, if necessary, sutured.

Glued Intraocular Lens

This technique first described by Agarwal et al. involves the use of fibrin glue for fixation of haptics. The IOLs that can be used are the three-piece foldable IOLs with slightly firm haptics or a three-piece non-foldable IOL.
- Two partial thicknesses scleral flap exactly 180° apart approximately 2.5 mm by 2.5 mm followed by a sclerotomy with a 20-G needle 1 mm from the limbus.
- A 23-G vitrectomy cutter is introduced from the sclerotomy site and thorough vitrectomy is done removing all the vitreous tractions.
- A corneal tunnel is fashioned and then a 23-G glued IOL forceps is passed through the sclerotomy site and the tip of the leading haptic of IOL is grasped, which is then externalized and brought out onto the ocular surface **(Fig. 3.36.7)**.

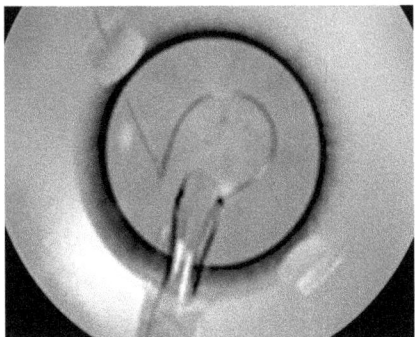

Fig. 3.36.7: Leading haptic externalized through scleral lamella pocket.

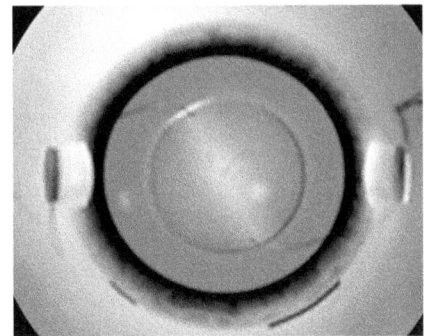

Fig. 3.36.8: Trailing haptic externalized using handshake technique.

- Similarly, the trailing haptic is then externalized using the handshake technique. Scleral pockets are made at the edge of the flap with a 26-G needle just parallel to the sclerotomy site, into which the two haptics are then tucked for additional stability **(Fig. 3.36.8)**.
- The scleral flaps are then glued back (Tisseel, Baxter) into place using biological glue. The glue is then used to seal the conjunctival closure.

Glued Intrascleral Haptic Fixation of an Intraocular Lense in Large Eyes: In eyes with greater WTW (>12 mm), certain adaptations and modifications are adopted for adequate haptic externalization and subsequent tuck. As the vertical diameter of the cornea is lesser than the horizontal diameter, in large eyes with white-to-white (WTW) >12 mm, making vertical flaps gives more haptic to externalize and so gives more tuck.

Performing an anterior sclerostomy at a distance of 0.5 mm from the limbus instead of 1.5 mm has an added advantage of allowing greater haptic externalization. The needle should be inserted vertically to avoid hitting the iris root.

Carlevale Lens

It is a new hydrophilic IOL placed in the ciliary sulcus designed specifically for sutureless scleral fixation **(Fig. 3.36.9)**. It has a system of two haptics with scleral self-anchoring. Two T-shaped "anchors" which are diametrically opposite rest on the sclera in the scleral pocket.

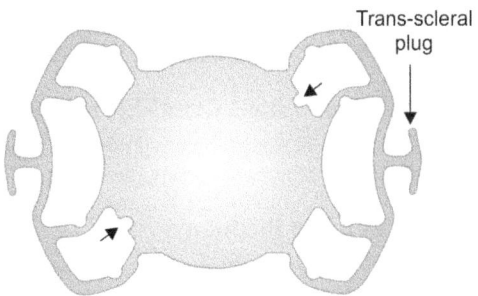

Fig. 3.36.9: Carlevale lens.

Technique:
- Two scleral pockets or flaps are created 180° apart.
- At 2 mm from the limbus two sclerostomies are created under the flap for proper positioning of IOL anchors.
- IOL is implanted into the anterior chamber through a corneal incision <3 mm until first anchor is deployed, which is grasped by a forceps introduced through one of the sclerostomies.
- IOL is now allowed to unfold in the AC while other hand accompanies the exit of anchor under the scleral flap.
- The IOL injection is now completed leaving second anchor in the corneal incision which is grasped using forceps inserted through the second sclerostomy.

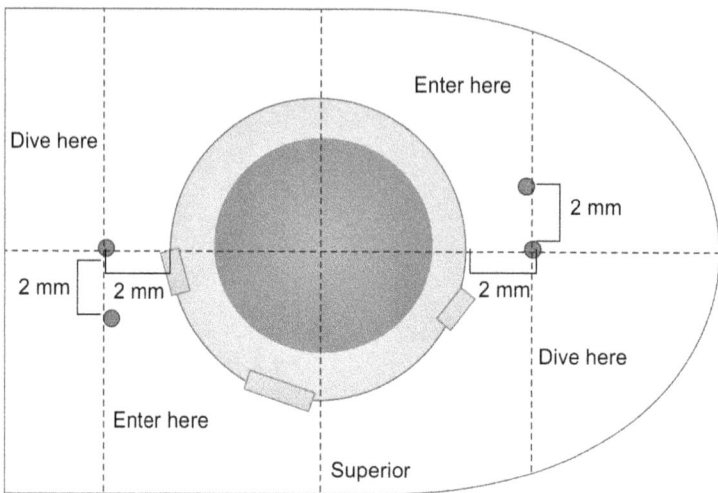

Fig. 3.36.10: Yamane technique.

Yamane Technique

The Yamane technique first described by Shin Yamane et al is a recently developed technique involving sutureless transconjunctival fixation of a three-piece IOL using a 30-G needle.
- A three-piece IOL is inserted into anterior chamber keeping the trailing haptic outside to prevent it from falling into the vitreous cavity.
- At 2 mm from the limbus an angles sclerotomy is made using an ultra-thin walled 30-G needle.
- The leading haptic is threaded into the lumen of the needle using forceps.
- At 180° from the first sclerotomy a second one is made with another 30-G needle (**Fig. 3.36.10**).
- The trailing haptic is inserted into the lumen of the second needle.
- Then, both the haptics are externalized into the conjunctiva.
- The ends of the haptics are cauterized using an ophthalmic cautery device to make a flange of 0.3 mm diameter which is pushed back and fixed into the scleral tunnels.

OUTCOMES AND COMPLICATIONS

Scleral-fixated IOLs have the advantages of remote positioning from corneal endothelium and proximity to the nodal point and rotational axis of the eye.

Suture-related Problems

Erosion of suture knots through the conjunctiva creates communication between the intra- and extraocular environments with attendant risks of toxic or microbial contamination. Once surgeons started to cover the sutures with scleral flaps, the rate of erosion decreased to 15%.

Intraocular Lens Dislocation

Intraocular lens dislocation as a result of suture loosening or rupture has also been reported, and dislocation can occur if there is internal cheese-wiring of the suture, even without disintegration of the polypropylene or disruption of knot integrity. Therefore, removal of the suture if it becomes exposed is not a safe option. Better ways to address this problem include trimming or cautery of the knot and surgical coverage with a corneal or scleral patch graft.

Lens Tilt and Decentration

Without the support of the lens capsule, there is greater potential for a PCIOL to tilt around the points at which it is sutured or to become decentered. Significant lens tilt (>10°) occurs in 11.4–16.7% of patients after two-point scleral fixation of PCIOLs. Techniques that fixate the IOL at two points on one or both haptics may reduce this complication.

Cystoid Macular Edema

This is the most commonly noted complication after scleral fixation of a PCIOL, and most cases are associated with vitreous loss. Light-induced retinal injury may also be a contributory factor.

Hyphema and Vitreous Hemorrhage

The suturing of PCIOLs requires needle passes through vascular uveal tissue. In many cases, associated bleeding is minor and resolves spontaneously. Keeping the suture anterior (1 mm behind the surgical limbus) and avoiding the 3- and 9-O'clock positions are two strategies to eliminate bleeding. In some instances, this complication may lead to ghost cell glaucoma.

Others

Others include pupillary distortion, episcleritis, transscleral haptic erosion through sclera, corneal decompensation, secondary glaucoma, chronic uveitis, endophthalmitis, retinal detachment, and choroidal detachment.

> **EDITOR'S PEARLS**
> - In the absence of adequate capsular support transscleral fixation of posterior chamber IOL in the ciliary sulcus is a viable option.
> - Holds advantage over iris-claw intraocular lens (ACIOLs) and anterior-iris claw IOLs due to lower endothelial cell damage and lower risk of other long-term complications (iris chaffing, iritis, secondary glaucoma)
> - Comparable with retro-fixated iris claw IOLs with respect to final visual outcome and complications such as IOL dislocation, cystoid macular edema (CME), and retinal detachment as per literature.

■ SUGGESTED READING

1. Gabor SG, Pavlidis MM. Sutureless intrascleral posterior chamber intraocular lens fixation. J Cataract Refract Surg. 2007;33(11):1851-4.

3.37 | How Do You Manage a Patient with Visually Significant Cataract with Associated Uveitis?

GS Brar
Sangam Netralaya, Mohali
gsbrarpgi@yahoo.com

■ INTRODUCTION

Cataract is one of the most frequent complications of uveitis, occurring either as a consequence of chronic or repeated episodes of intraocular inflammation or as a complication of the corticosteroids used to treat the inflammation. Despite advances in microsurgery, cataract extraction still poses a formidable challenge in patients with uveitis. Better understanding of the disease process and the risk factors involved has substantially changed the approach toward these patients. With careful patient selection, rigorous pre- and postoperative control of inflammation and meticulous surgery, it now appears possible to obtain a safer and more predictable outcome. Phacoemulsification is now becoming the procedure of choice in these patients as it results in less postoperative inflammation and less complications as compared to conventional cataract extraction. However, posterior synechiae formation, fibrous membranes over the pupil, and poorly dilating pupils make phacoemulsification a challenging task. A small nondilating pupil, along with a cataractous lens, also makes the preoperative evaluation of these patients difficult.

PREOPERATIVE WORK-UP

Preoperative work-up would include establishing specific diagnosis, and control of inflammation (the inflammation should be inactive for at least 3 months prior to surgery). In selected cases, fundus fluorescein angiography and ultrasonography may be required. In assessing the visual prognosis, the potential acuity meter may be overly optimistic while laser interferometer may be overly pessimistic.

Conditions such as Fuchs heterochromic uveitis (FHU) usually do not require any additional therapy. In a subset of patients with recent inflammatory activity, topical steroids started 4-6 times/day 1 week prior to surgery is sufficient. The general response of inflammation to anti-inflammatory therapy in that particular patient is a good guide to the need of preoperative medications.

INTRAOPERATIVE DIFFICULTIES

Intraoperative difficulties during phacoemulsification include:
- Poor visualization due to problems with corneal clarity
- Small pupil due to iris atrophy
- Sphincter sclerosis
- Posterior synechiae
- Hemorrhage from abnormal iris vasculature
- Weak zonular apparatus
- Small pupil may be managed by intraoperative synechiolysis, use of high-viscosity viscoelastic agents, iris hooks, pupillary stretching, sphincterotomy or use of other pupil expansion devices.
- Heparin surface modified intraocular lenses (IOLs) are better tolerated than polymethylmethacrylate (PMMA); lower prevalence of IOL deposits, anterior chamber (AC) cells, and less synechiae. Uveal biocompatibility (AC cells, giant cells on IOL, post-synechiae) is better with hydrophilic acrylic foldables compared to hydrophobic but capsular biocompatibility [lens epithelial cell (LEC) migration, anterior capsule opacification (ACO), posterior capsule opacification (PCO)] is better with hydrophobic acrylic IOLs. Silicone IOLs are best avoided. My choice of IOL material would be a hydrophobic acrylic material. Selective contraindications to IOL implantation would be cases of panuveitis, juvenile rheumatoid arthritis (JRA), pars planitis, and chronic diseases resistant to remission, e.g., sarcoidosis.

POSTOPERATIVE MANAGEMENT

- Patients with uveitic cataract have a higher risk of postoperative inflammation. This can lead to fibrinous reaction in the AC, formation of pupillary membrane, posterior synechiae, and vitreous haze. All these factors can result in poor visual gain postsurgery.
- To circumvent this, it is very crucial to administer topical steroids (prednisolone) in a higher frequency (1-2 hourly) postoperatively along with shorter-acting cycloplegics which will keep the pupil mobile.
- In cases of intermediate or panuveitis, a short course of oral steroids (prednisolone 1.0-1.5 mg/kg) can be given for 7-10 days. Instead, the steroids can also be tapered slowly over every week in severe cases.

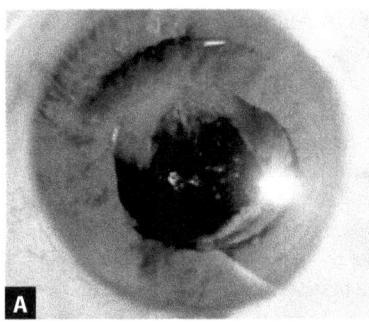
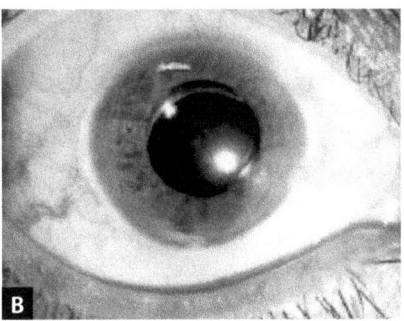

Figs. 3.37.1A and B: On the left side is status 1 year following conventional extracapsular cataract surgery in a patient with bilateral recurrent anterior uveitis and on the right side is status 1 year after phacoemulsification in the other eye of the same patient. Note the significantly better outcome after phacoemulsification and in-the-bag intraocular lens (IOL) implantation.

- Intravenous bolus of dexamethasone can be injected at the conclusion of the surgery which also keeps the inflammation under check.

  Safety of cataract surgery in uveitis is increasing with modern surgical techniques and preoperative management and planning is crucial. Lensectomy with vitrectomy in eyes with significant vitreous involvement/hypotonous eyes may be the procedure of choice whereas extracapsular cataract extraction (ECCE)/phacoemulsification should be performed for well controlled anteriorly localized disease. Main cause of poor visual outcome remains macular edema. One must individualize all decisions for best outcome (**Figs. 3.37.1A and B**).

EDITOR'S PEARLS
A preoperative and postoperative inflammation control with steroids and NSAIDs is the key to achieving optimal outcomes in uveitic cataracts.

SUGGESTED READING
1. Roesel M, Heinz C, Koch JM, Heiligenhaus A. Cataract surgery in uveitis. Ophthalmology. 2008;115(8):1431.

3.38 What Precautions You Take in Patient of Cataract with Dry Eyes during and after Cataract?

KP Chaudhary
Indira Gandhi Medical College, Shimla
kssulbhushanpchaudhary@yahoo.com

INTRODUCTION
In addition to all the relevant investigations as per the protocol in a patient undergoing cataract surgery suffering from dry eye, more precautions are needed to be considered to achieve the best possible surgical outcome.

Slit-lamp examination should include:
- Meniscus height after instillation of fluorescein
- Tear film break-up time (BUT)
- Schirmer's test

A Schirmer value ≤5.0 mm in 5 minutes, and tear-film BUT ≤5 seconds is significant and should be taken into consideration.

Less favorable post-cataract surgery outcomes have been reported in patients with dry eye disease due to the following factors:
- Patients with preexisting dry eye are at risk for developing superficial punctate keratitis, filamentary keratitis, secondary microbial keratitis, persistent epithelial defects, and stromal melt after conventional extracapsular cataract extraction (ECCE).
- In a conventional ECCE or intracapsular cataract extraction (ICCE), a large incision is made at the limbus resulting in denervation of the superior half of the cornea leading to corneal desensitization and subsequent adverse outcomes.
- Additionally, the presence of sutures and prolonged use of topical steroids and postoperative antibiotics, often make the eye susceptible to these complications.
- The use of other ocular medications such as antiglaucoma drugs and oral acetazolamide, can worsen preexisting dry eye or even produce new symptoms. Oral acetazolamide has been found to decrease aqueous tear production.

In patients with dry eye disease, phacoemulsification is more advantageous over conventional ECCE. The significantly smaller incision size in phacoemulsification causes less corneal denervation and desensitization with minimal tear-film surfacing problems and a lower risk of associated complications. Suture-related complications are also avoided due to the self-sealing nature of wounds. The shorter surgical duration and the faster visual rehabilitation with phacoemulsification allows for rapid tapering of topical drops. These patients must be counseled regarding the risk of postoperative complications and the need for intensive dry-eye treatment post-surgery to minimize these complications.

At the time of surgery and postoperatively:
- Rule out blepharitis
- Conjunctival infection
- Culture and sensitivity of conjunctival flora
- Peripheral smear of conjunctiva
- Limbal incision preferred
- Temporary or permanent punctal plug insertion
- Use of specialized goggles or moisture chambers while sleeping
- Omega-3 and omega-6 fatty acid supplement.

EDITOR'S PEARLS
- A thorough preoperative evaluation of dry eye disease, ocular surface optimization and a cautious postoperative management are essential steps for satisfactory outcomes in cases of dry eye disease with cataract.
- Dry eye disease is expected to worsen after cataract surgery and the surgeon must step up treatment for the same in the postoperative period.

SUGGESTED READING
1. Ram J, Gupta A, Brar GS, Kaushik S, Gupta A. Outcomes of phacoemulsification in patients with dry eye. J Cataract Refract Surg. 2002;28(8):1386-9.

3.39 Postoperative Treatment of Uncomplicated Phacoemulsification

Tanuj Dada
Dr RP Centre for Ophthalmic Sciences, AIIMS, New Delhi
tanujdada@gmail.com

Vivek Dave
LV Prasad Eye Institute, Hyderabad
vivekdave@lvpei.org

POSTOPERATIVE MEDICATIONS

The essential postoperative medications to be used after an uneventful phacoemulsification surgery are topical antibiotics and topical steroids which can later be substituted by topical nonsteroidal anti-inflammatory drugs (NSAIDs). Ocular hypotensive medications and cycloplegics may be used as and when required.

Topical antibiotics such as gatifloxacin 0.3% or moxifloxacin 0.5% should be used 4 times/day from the first postoperative day and continued for a minimum period of 7–10 days. It can be continued for a period of 4 weeks. Prednisolone acetate 1% should be given 4 times/day for 1 week, followed by 3 times/day for 1 week and then 2 times/day for the next 2 weeks. The frequency of steroid used may be increased in eyes with significant postoperative uveitis and in pediatric cataract surgery.

The routine prescription for a patient post-cataract surgery is as follows:
- Open pad and bandage after 6 hours of surgery
- Emergency department (e/d) moxifloxacin hydrochloride 0.5% 4 times/day × 1 month
- Eye drop prednisolone phosphate 1% 4–6 times/day × 1 week followed by tapering of dose
- Eye drop tropicamide 1% 3 times/day × 1 week followed by 2 times/day × 1 week.

Patients at a significant risk of cystoid macular edema (CME) (e.g., diabetics, uveitics, vasculopathy, postoperative CME in fellow eye, prostaglandin use and individuals whose surgery was complicated) should use prophylactic NSAIDs such as ketorolac 0.5% (QID), nepafenac 0.1% or bromfenac 0.09% (BD) for a period of 6–8 weeks as the peak incidence of CME is 4–6 weeks following routine uncomplicated surgery.

When phacoemulsification is performed in eyes with glaucomatous optic neuropathy, ocular hypotensive medications (0.5% timolol BD) and oral acetazolamide (1–3 days) should be prescribed in the postoperative period to prevent intraocular pressure (IOP) spikes and further optic nerve damage.

EDITOR'S PEARLS
Topical antibiotics, steroids, and short-acting cycloplegics constitute essential components of post-cataract surgery medications to prevent infection and control postoperative inflammation.

SUGGESTED READING
1. Lorenz K, Dick B, Jehkul A, Auffahrt GU. Inflammatory response after phacoemulsification treated with 0.5% prednisolone acetate or vehicle. Graefes Arch Clin Exp Ophthalmol. 2008;246(11):1617-22.

3.40 Following Uneventful Phacoemulsification, the Patient has 4+ Cells and Fibrin on Postoperative Day 1. What should be Done?

Reema Bhansal, Amod Gupta, Vishali Gupta
Advanced Eye Centre, PGIMER, Chandigarh
eyepgi@sify.com

■ INTRODUCTION

The most dreaded complication of any intraocular surgery is the development of endophthalmitis, especially in India with significantly different rates of endophthalmitis (0.05–0.6%).

- When a patient develops a hypopyon and fibrin on the first postoperative day following an uneventful phacoemulsification, it would be justified clinically to think of infectious endophthalmitis first than anything else.
- Look for any other clinical signs and symptoms of infectious endophthalmitis, such as pain (it may not be present in 25% cases of infectious endophthalmitis), ciliary congestion, lid swelling, conjunctival chemosis or discharge.
- A complete ophthalmic examination is done that includes recording the visual acuity, intraocular pressure (IOP), a careful slit-lamp examination and assessment of media clarity by an indirect ophthalmoscope.
- In case of poor media clarity (grade 4 or 5), an ultrasonography of the posterior segment is mandatory to judge the amount of vitreous involvement because endophthalmitis usually manifests in the entire ocular cavity and is often most severe in the vitreous cavity.
- Although culture of intraocular specimens is the gold standard for both bacterial as well as fungal endophthalmitis, certain percentage of these patients has biopsy samples that are Gram stain and culture negative.
- Once a clinical diagnosis of infectious endophthalmitis is made, it constitutes a true emergency and the patient is admitted in the ophthalmic ward to ensure a close observation after initiation of the treatment, and at least an overnight stay is needed.

■ PROGNOSIS

The prognosis in postoperative endophthalmitis depends not only on the virulence of the microorganisms, but also on early intervention. The patient is started on frequent topical broad-spectrum antibiotics (gatifloxacin 0.3% or moxifloxacin 0.5%), prednisolone 1% and atropine sulfate 1%, while waiting for more definitive treatment. The presenting visual acuity serves as a crucial guide to the most immediate therapeutic intervention. According to the Endophthalmitis Vitrectomy Study (EVS) guidelines, the eyes with visual acuity of hand motions or better are subjected to vitreous tap and intravitreal broad-spectrum antibiotics. The specimens are directly smeared, for Gram stain and potassium hydroxide (KOH), and plated for culture. We use intravitreal vancomycin (1 mg), ceftazidime (2.25 mg), and dexamethasone (400 µg), each in 0.1 mL. Experimental studies have shown that intravitreal dexamethasone has a large safety window and prolongs the half-life of intravitreal vancomycin. Although systemic antibiotics are not recommended by EVS in cases of acute bacterial postoperative endophthalmitis, we usually start broad-spectrum antibiotics (gatifloxacin 400 mg twice daily for 5–7 days) to have an additional beneficial effect because the microbiological spectrum as per the EVS was different from the microbiological spectrum found in our setup where we have higher incidence of fungal and Gram-negative endophthalmitis. Moreover, recent publications justify (or even encourage) use of systemic antibiotics (oral ciprofloxacin or gatifloxacin) in the management of many varieties of infective endophthalmitis. In general, oral prednisolone (1 mg/kg/day) may be given, tapering, and stopping over 4–6 weeks.

The patient is examined during the first several hours, with a complete documentation of the ocular examination as done at the baseline. The intravitreal injection is repeated after 48–72 hours if the clinical picture is more or less the same. If it worsens despite the first intravitreal injection, pars plana vitrectomy with intravitreal antibiotics is done after 48 hours.

If the presenting visual acuity is light perception only, pars plana vitrectomy with intravitreal antibiotics is the initial treatment. Core vitrectomy was the recommended method for endophthalmitis previously. However, a complete but "safe vitrectomy" is recommended now which involves debulking the vitreous cavity of as much exudates as possible. Induction of posterior vitreous detachment is not essential but is not contraindicated. The other indications for pars plana vitrectomy with intravitreal antibiotics are no improvement or deterioration despite intravitreal antibiotics, delayed-onset endophthalmitis or fungal endophthalmitis. The protocol for managing fungal endophthalmitis is pars plana vitrectomy, intravitreal amphotericin B 5 µg and systemic antifungals.

DIFFERENTIAL DIAGNOSIS

Although rare, toxic anterior segment syndrome (TASS) could be thought of as another possibility of such a severe inflammation. It typically occurs within 24 hours; it is almost always limited to the anterior segment; it improves with topical and/or oral steroids and commonly presents with diffuse corneal edema and minimal pain. Iris damage, a nonreactive and irregular pupil and trabecular meshwork damage may be the other associated clinical findings. It may be due to surgical trauma, retained lens material, sterile toxic substances, or other uncommon factors, such as previous uveitis, diabetes, and pseudoexfoliation.

In postoperative endophthalmitis, the patient factors such as patient's own bacterial flora, poor hygiene of the patient, chronic blepharitis, conjunctivitis, canaliculitis, keratoconjunctivitis sicca and compliance with medication play a predominant role. The other important intraoperative risk factors are inadequate eyelid or conjunctival disinfection, prolonged surgery, vitreous loss, inadequate wound closure and the sterility of the operating room complex and its equipment. The surgeon's experience and expertise may also contribute to the level of intraocular inflammation following the surgery.

In our set-up, since there are no definite guidelines for managing a patient with severe postoperative inflammation comprising of hypopyon and fibrin, it is best left at the clinician's discretion to decide the timing and mode of intervention and to change the strategy in high-risk patients. They include one-eyed individuals, immunocompromised patients, and possibly diabetics.

Whatever may be the cause, the diagnosis should be prompt as the most important aspect of management is early recognition and early initiation of therapy. In high-volume cataract surgery such as in camps, epidemic of endophthalmitis is always possible. When such a situation is encountered in a rural or a peripheral setting with inadequate diagnostic and therapeutic facilities, intravitreal antibiotics should be given and the patient(s) should be referred to vitreoretinal services at the earliest for subsequent management.

EDITOR'S PEARLS
Differentiating postoperative endophthalmitis from Toxic Anterior Segment Syndrome is of prime importance as both conditions require immediate yet different lines of management.

SUGGESTED READING

1. Lalitha P, Rajagopalan J, Prakash K, Ramasamy K, Prajna NV, Srinivasan M. Postcataract endophthalmitis in South India: Incidence and outcome. Ophthalmology. 2005;112(11):1884-90.

3.41 Postcataract Surgery Cystoid Macular Edema

Ramandeep Singh
Advanced Eye Centre, PGIMER, Chandigarh
ramandeeppgi@gmail.com

■ INTRODUCTION

Postcataract surgery cystoid macular edema (CME) was first time reported by Irvine in 1953. It represents one of the most common and self-limiting complications following cataract surgery.

■ EPIDEMIOLOGY AND PATHOGENESIS

Cystoid macular edema following cataract surgery is also referred as Irvine–Gass syndrome. The incidence of clinical CME has been reported to be 0–6% and of angiographic CME, 9.15–54.7%. The possible mechanisms by which postcataract surgery CME develops include release of prostaglandin and other inflammatory mediators, vascular compromise, and vitreomacular traction. The leak from the perifoveal vessels is induced by these inflammatory mediators and fluid accumulates in the outer-plexiform layer forming these cystoid spaces, which are characteristic of CME.

The risk factors, which are commonly associated with CME, include rupture of posterior capsule, vitreous loss, iris incarceration, active uveitis, and diabetes. All of these have led to increased release of inflammatory mediators and thus can accentuate CME.

■ OCULAR MANIFESTATIONS

Decreased vision is the major symptom of CME along with others such as metamorphopsia, micropsia, scotoma, photophobia, and conjunctival injection. The typical time of onset of clinical CME is 2–4 weeks postoperatively.

Clinically, CME can be diagnosed on slit-lamp examination using contact or noncontact fundus lens. There is dull foveal reflex because of the edema. The edema causes light scattering which results in the loss of the transparency of the neural retina. Sometimes, intraretinal and intracystic hemorrhages, microaneurysms, and telangiectasias can also be seen. Postcataract surgery CME is also associated with epiretinal membranes in about 10% of the eyes. Chronic CME leads to rupture of the cyst-forming lamellar hole and atrophy of the photoreceptors leading to poor visual outcome.

■ DIAGNOSIS AND ANCILLARY INVESTIGATIONS

Fundus fluorescein angiography (FFA) can detect the CME more efficiently than clinical examination. It reveals a typical petaloid pattern in the central macula as a result of dye leakage from the perifoveal capillaries **(Figs. 3.41.1A to D)**. Optical coherence tomography provides high resolution images which clearly show the individual pockets of the outer-plexiform layer with larger pockets present centrally while progressively smaller cysts peripherally **(Fig. 3.41.2)**. It gives us the quantitative data on retinal thickness which can be used as a tool for serial follow-up to document the response to treatment, thus reducing the need for FFA in the follow-up visits **(Figs. 3.41.3A and B)**.

■ TREATMENT

The treatment of clinical CME is controversial. Spontaneous resolution can occur, so it is difficult to interpret the effectiveness of medications. Hence, there is a lack of randomized clinical trials. In the cases without any predisposing factors, generally conservative approach with close observation is done as CME typically resolves over several weeks in about 90% of the patients. Many studies have studied the use of nonsteroidal anti-inflammatory drugs (NSAIDs) alone or in combination with steroids to treat CME. There

SECTION 3: Cataract

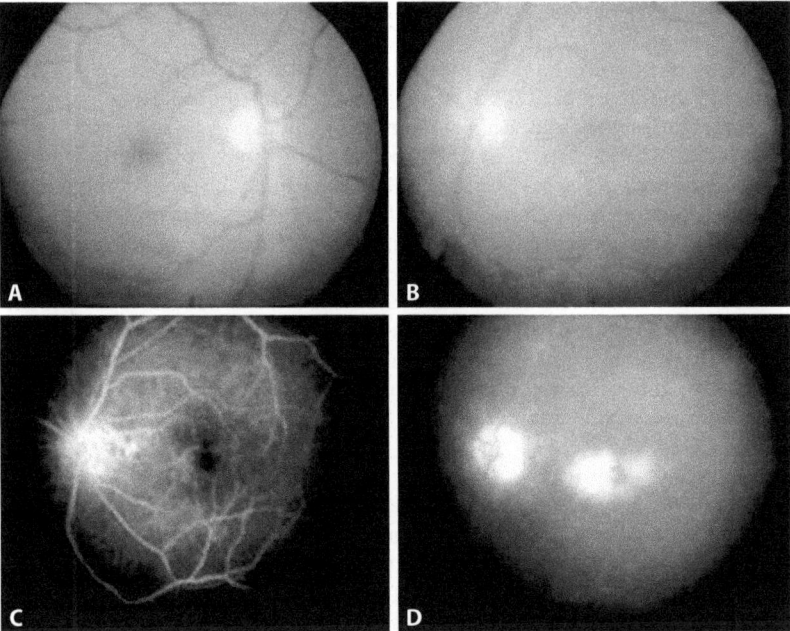

Figs. 3.41.1A to D: (A) Fundus photograph of the right eye showing good foveal reflex; (B) Fundus photograph of the left eye showing loss of foveal reflex; (C and D) Fluorescein angiography is more informative in late phase than early phase showing classic petaloid pattern in the late phase.

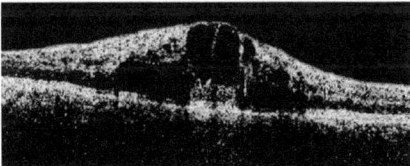

Fig. 3.41.2: Optical coherence tomography line scan showing the individual pockets of the outer-plexiform layer, with larger pockets present centrally and smaller cysts peripherally.

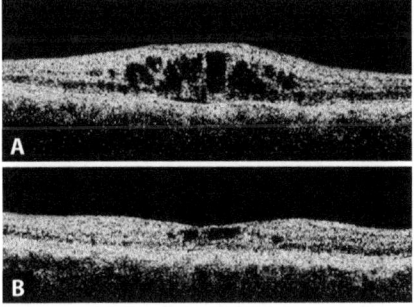

Figs. 3.41.3A and B: (A) Optical coherence tomography line scan showing postcataract surgery cystoid macular edema (CME); (B) Same eye 6 weeks after depot steroid showing near complete resolution of the cystoid spaces.

is theoretical evidence that the two can be used together with beneficial effects, because NSAIDs and steroids inhibit different mediators within the inflammatory cascade, NSAIDs inhibit cyclooxygenase (COX) 1 and 2 and steroids inhibit lipoxygenase and COX 2.

However, the effectiveness of NSAIDs alone or in combination with steroids is variable in various clinical studies.

Management of postcataract surgery of CME involves a stepwise approach. As an initial prophylactic step, topical NSAIDs are given along with the topical steroid drops after cataract surgery to prevent synthesis of inflammatory mediators causing CME.

As a second step for persistent CME, topical steroids are given for long periods to manage postcataract surgery of CME. NSAIDs are usually given in combination with steroids, but sometimes they are given alone for patients who are steroid responders.

As a third step for persistent CME, depot steroids such as triamcinolone (20 mg) can be given in the sub-Tenon's space with good outcome. Intravitreal injection of various steroid preparations may work in refractory cases. Systemic steroids are rarely used to manage postcataract surgery of CME with persistent postoperative inflammation.

Vitrectomy is the last option for the recalcitrant cases with predisposing risk factors such as vitreous adhesions to the iris or a corneoscleral wound and cases with epiretinal membrane vitreomacular traction. Nd:Yag laser treatment to break vitreous may also helpful in selected cases.

EDITOR'S PEARLS

- Any diminution in visual acuity 4–6 weeks after cataract surgery and an unremarkable anterior segment should raise suspicion of Irvine–Gass syndrome.
- Treatment includes topical NSAIDs and steroids (topical/oral/posterior-sub Tenon/intravitreal) based on duration and response to primary management.

SUGGESTED READING

1. Miyake K, Masuda K, Shirato S, Oshika T, Eguchi K, Hoshi H, et al. Comparison of diclofenac and fluorometholone in preventing cystoid macular edema after small incision cataract surgery: a multicentered prospective trial. Jpn J Ophthalmol. 2000;44(1):58-67.

3.42 | Phacoemulsification in Aniridic Eyes

Kasturi Bhattacharjee, S Bobby
Sankaradeva Netralaya, Guwahati
kasturibhattacharjee44@hotmail.com

INTRODUCTION

Aniridia is a bilateral panocular syndrome characterized by extreme form of iris hypoplasia. It can be broadly divided into hereditary and sporadic with an overall incidence of one in 100,000 live births. Besides the defect in iris development, it is associated with multiple ocular abnormalities such as glaucoma, cataract, corneal opacity and pannus, foveal and optic nerve hypoplasia. Cataract may be present from birth as anterior or posterior lens opacities. However, in 50–85% of patients, cortical and subcapsular opacities are found within two decades of life. In most cases, the cataract is progressive and can cause severe visual impairment.

CATARACT SURGERY

Cataract surgery in aniridia eyes is fairly routine with magnificent visualization. Intraoperative fashioning of iris diaphragm is the most important step in cataract surgery as most symptoms of partial or total aniridia ranging from decreased vision and cosmetic concern to incapacitating glare and photophobia is due to absence of the anatomical iris. Thus, the challenge lies in creation of new iris diaphragm during cataract surgery.

The surgical strategy needs to be tailored to each eye since each defect is specific to that patient. Before a prosthetic iris or other device is considered for implantation, the primary repair of an iris defect using methods such as iris sphincterectomy, synechiolysis, iris sutures, and restraining ring or cerclage may be adequate in some cases. These methods are unfortunately not always feasible and might not be sufficient for eyes with substantial iris deficiencies. With suture techniques, iris deficiencies 3 hours (or 90°) can typically be successfully repaired. As the iris tissue in these cases is abnormal, the surgeon should refrain from using overly forceful procedures when treating larger defects. In the region adjacent to the tension pull of the suture, there is a considerable risk of iatrogenic iridodialysis, bleeding, and regional iris atrophy.

■ TECHNIQUES

Though various techniques have been described to overcome the absent or hypoplastic iris by use of colored contact lens, corneal tattooing and iridoplasty, however the use of prosthetic iris implantation during cataract extraction appears a promising alternative. When contemplating use of iris device, the surgeon should first define the clinical situation and then choose the appropriate device based on relevant anatomy.

■ COMMON PROSTHETIC DEVICES

The two common prosthetic devices used during cataract surgery in aniridia are single-piece black diaphragm iridolenticular prosthesis having a clean central optic and opaque periphery and the Morcher endocapsular ring with iris diaphragm.

The single-piece iris diaphragm intraocular lens (IOL) **(Fig. 3.42.1A)** is the implant of choice when the capsular support is inadequate or absent as it can be placed in ciliary sulcus or can be fixated by transscleral sutures. However, it has a significant drawback as it requires a larger incision size which results in increase in postoperative astigmatism and delayed visual rehabilitation.

Morcher iris device prosthesis is preferred by most surgeons as they do not have any optical portion and can be inserted through a relatively smaller incision. Morcher prosthetic iris diaphragm is of two styles. The first style has a single iris fin **(Fig. 3.42.1B)** used for sectoral iris loss. They are often custom-shaped to cover areas of missing iris. The second style has two separate rings with multiple fins **(Fig. 3.42.1C)** that interdigitate on each other and used for creation of a full iris diaphragm, maintaining a pupil size of approximately 6 mm thereby reducing the excess light entering the eye by 75%. This approach offers the advantages of 360° iris diaphragm along with a separate optical system fashioned by placement of an IOL.

Iris diaphragm intraocular lenses are most commonly used modality, however, with disadvantages of a large corneal incision, risk of secondary glaucoma, and chronic iritis. Glare and photophobia are usual symptoms which limit the postoperative visual outcomes. To overcome these limitations, small diameter (3.3 mm) artificial iris implants have been developed which promotes depth of focus, decreases optical aberration, and enhances near vision ultimately resulting in improved photophobia and glare symptoms. Furthermore, the elasticity of the artificial iris implants makes implantation simple and less

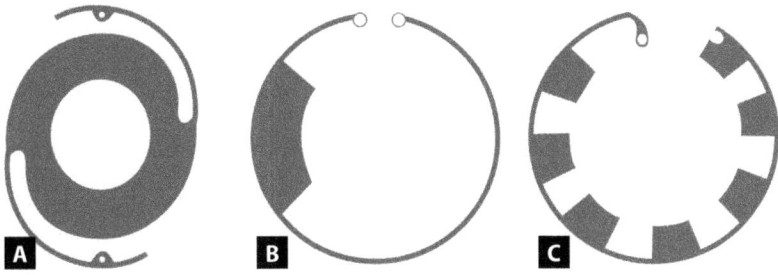

Figs. 3.42.1A to C: (A) Single-piece iris diaphragm; (B) Single iris fin; (C) Multiple iris fin.

traumatic through 2.8–3.0 mm self-sealing tunnel incisions, reducing surgically induced astigmatism that could jeopardize achieving a good final visual acuity.

The capsular tension ring (CTR) with an iris diaphragm [type 50C (Morcher)], which may be built with up to 7 black PMMA multiple fin segments, is an alternative to the diaphragm IOL. These polymethyl methacrylate (PMMA) rings can be rotated above one another and the fins will interlink to form a full diaphragm if two of them are implanted in the bag one after the other. When implanting these exceedingly fragile devices, the surgeon must use the utmost caution because they are extremely prone to cracking.

COMPLICATIONS

The intra- and postoperative surgical complications in aniridic eye are similar to most of the routine cataract surgery except for higher incidence of loss of capsular integrity during capsulorhexis as it has been found that the anterior capsule in eyes with congenital aniridia is often very fragile and there has been reported incidence of postoperative aniridic keratopathy and worsening of preexisting glaucoma. Moreover, intraoperative fracture or breakage of prosthetic iris device is often encountered in early-learning phase. The major advantage of use of prosthetic iris device is the reduction of subjective glare disability resulting in optimum visual acuity in bright light and in extreme contrast setting.

Thus, phacoemulsification along with the use of prosthetic iris device is a safe and effective method of cataract extraction in aniridic eyes. The creation of the iris diaphragm by implantation of artificial iris device offers a safe alternative for those eyes, thereby effectively reducing the glare disability and photophobia.

> **EDITOR'S PEARLS**
> - Aniridic prosthetic devices are a good option for patients with aniridia for rehabilitation from glare, photophobia, and cosmetically.
> - However, regular follow-up is required as it leads to higher incidences of worsening of preexisting glaucoma and aniridic keratopathy.

SUGGESTED READING

1. Burk SE, Osher RH. Surgical management of aniridia. In: Roy FH, Arzabe CW (Eds). Master Technique in Cataract and Refractive Surgery, 1st edition. Thorofare, NJ, USA: Slack Incorporation; 2004.

3.43 | Foldable Intraocular Lenses

JS Titiyal, Neelima Aron, Bhavya G
Dr RP Centre for Ophthalmic Sciences, AIIMS, New Delhi
titiyal@gmail.com, neelima.aron87@gmail.com

INTRODUCTION

During the last two decades there has been dramatic improvement in technology of cataract surgery and intraocular lens (IOL) implantation. The modern surgery consists of small-sized incision (2.2–3.2 mm) for phacoemulsification and insertion of a foldable IOL. In fact, the availability of these foldable IOLs has made microincision phacoemulsification possible.

These foldable implants also enable the surgeon to perform topical cataract surgery eliminating needle injections, patches, and shields.

These small incisions do not induce significant changes in the patient's astigmatism, thus enabling predictable results. Reduction in astigmatism reduces the patient's need for glasses to correct their vision. The available foldable lenses are made of hydrophilic acrylic, hydrophobic acrylic, and silicon. An ideal IOL material is chemically inert, non-carcinogenic, non-allergenic, durable, sterile, and non-inflammatory. It should be light weight, have high-optical quality, high index of refraction, and capsule compatibility and block ultraviolet (UV) radiation.

FOLDABLE INTRAOCULAR LENS MATERIALS IN USE
- Hydrophobic acrylate
- Hydrogel-hydrophilic acrylate
- Silicone

Haptic Materials
Various *haptic materials* such as polymethyl methacrylate (PMMA), polypropylene, polyimide, and polyvinylidene fluoride (PVDF) are available with various IOLs.

Choice of Intraocular Lens Material
Hydrophobic acrylate gives the best results in terms of easy loading, injection, unfolding, capsular compatibility, and less postoperative inflammation. *Silicone IOLs* are not compatible with silicon oil used for VR surgeries. These lenses are slightly difficult to load and inject in the eye. Beginners may require a learning curve.

Designs of Foldable Intraocular Lens
- Multi-piece IOLs
- Single-piece IOLs
- Plate-haptic IOLs

The shape of IOL *lateral surface* can be Square Edge IOL (AcrySof), Round or the OptiEdge technology (Sensar).

Choice of design: Single-piece IOLs are considered the best. Multi-piece IOLs can be used in cases of posterior capsule tear, subluxations, and other related complications. *Surface-modified IOLs* with heparin coating are available which promise lesser inflammation. However, such claims have not been validated in long-term studies.

Aberration Free Intraocular Lenses (Aspheric IOLs)
- *Spherical aberration (SA)* with conventional IOLs.
- *Negative aberration Alcon IQ, Tecnis*: The Tecnis lens with its negative spherical aberration compensates for the average spherical aberration of the cornea and provides improved optical quality of vision. It has a negative spherical aberration of –0.27. AcrySoF® IQ IOL: It is made up of hydrophobic acrylic material with UV and blue light-filtering chromophores. It has a negative spherical aberration of –0.20.

    The *Tecnis Z9000* IOLs (Pfizer, New York, USA) was the first foldable IOL manufactured by integrating wavefront technology into the IOL designs to correct higher order aberrations. In May 2004, the *Tecnis Z9000* aspheric IOL received Food and Drug Administration (FDA) approval for use. The positive spherical aberrations of the cornea get corrected by the anterior surface of IOL with modified prolate shape. It has a modified prolate anterior surface with 6.0 mm biconvex silicone optic and modified square edge design (OptiEdge Design). Tecnis IOL is available with acrylic (single-piece) or PMMA (three-piece) haptics. It reduces spherical aberrations and improves vision in different light conditions. IOLs are available also from Alcon, including the *AcrySof SN60WF* that includes the blue light-blocking feature discussed below and the aspheric version of *AcrySof ReSTOR*.
- *Zero aberration (B and L):* It has zero SA. Conventional IOLs have a spherical design due to its spherical front surface. Aspheric IOLs are designed to compensate the positive spherical aberrations of the cornea by simulating the young human crystalline

---
Authors have no financial interest in this article.

lens to provide improved quality of images. Bausch & Lomb in 2004 launched the first aspheric IOL, *SofPort advance optics* that has a slightly flatter periphery which can provide better contrast sensitivity.
- *HOYA Optimized Aspheric IOL with ABC design*: The aspheric balanced curve design of Hoya's negative aspheric IOLs minimizes the aberrations related to decentration and tilt. The center of the IOL is minimally negative aspheric blended into a standard negative peripheral IOL optic. This makes the IOL more immune to decentration effects.

Choice of these Intraocular Lenses

AcrySof IQ is becoming the preferred choice. It is easy to implant the acrylic IOL and gives superior results.

Advantages: Aspheric IOLs provide good vision quality, better contrast sensitivity and improves night vision.

ACCOMMODATING INTRAOCULAR LENS
- Crystalens Intraocular Lens
- Synchrony Intraocular Lens
- FluidVision Intraocular Lens

AT-45 Silicone Intraocular Lens
It is plate-haptic with 12 mm long made up of third generation nonreflective silicone material (Biosil). It has an A-constant of 119.0 and a hinge at junction.

Crystalens Intraocular Lens

The newer version of *Crystalens* (Bausch & Lomb) gained FDA approval in June 2008. Crystalens is designed to move within the eye, to provide focusing at all distances. When compared to the traditional IOLs, the hinge on either side of Crystalens can be moved by ciliary muscle simulating the natural lens for better focusing of eye at wider ranges of distances.

Synchrony Intraocular Lens

Synchrony (Visiogen Incorporation) is another accommodating IOL with dual optic design that has completed the phase 3 trial but has not received the US-FDA approval. Preexisting astigmatism, improper positioning of IOL while implanting and nighttime symptoms such as halos can result in decreased patient satisfaction.

FluidVision Intraocular Lens

The accommodating IOL has a proprietary hydrophobic acrylic exterior body and is filled with an index-matched silicone oil. As the ciliary body contracts and relaxes, fluid moves in and out of the center of the optic, changing its shape and resulting in seamless vision from near to distance. This provides a 3–4 D (diopter) of accommodation with good visual outcomes across all distances.

TORIC INTRAOCULAR LENSES FOR ASTIGMATISM

Indications

Patients with regular astigmatism above 1–1.25 D are candidates for monofocal toric IOL implantation and regular astigmatism above 0.75 D if you are implanting a multifocal toric IOL. While corneal incisional procedures such as astigmatic keratotomy (AK) or limbal-relaxing incisions have been described, these procedures can correct only a small range of astigmatism with limited precision. Toric IOLs can correct higher degrees of astigmatism with improved precision. US-FDA-approved first toric IOL, *STAAR surgical IOL* in 1998. They have two versions of toric IOLs in full range of distance powers with one correcting till 2.00 D and the other version with astigmatism correction up to 3.50 D of astigmatism. In September 2005 the US-FDA approved AcrySof toric IOL from Alcon. AcrySof® IQ Toric IOLs offer spherical powers in half diopter increments from +6.0 D to +34.0 D and seven-cylinder powers to treat 0.75–4.11 D of preexisting corneal astigmatism. Poor postoperative vision gain can result from lens rotation in the capsular bag, which can be managed by realignment or rarely replacement.

▪ MULTIFOCAL INTRAOCULAR LENSES

Various Types

For clear functional, vision over a range of distance from far to near, multifocal IOLs use the principle of diffraction and refraction.

Refractive Intraocular Lens

Refractive IOLs [ReZoom, Advanced Medical Optics (AMO)] are dependent on pupil size with varying optical zones of IOL powers for near and distance. The center of the lens has an additional +3.5 D to provide an additional power of +2.7 D at spectacle plane.

Diffractive Intraocular Lens

Diffractive IOLs (ReSTOR, Alcon) are pupil independent lenses which has a smooth front surface and multiple concentric rings on the back surface. Other examples are the 3M, and CeeOn 811E IOLs.

ReZoom (AMO)

ReZoom (AMO) is a multifocal refractive design that distributes the incident light through five optical zones to give good distance, intermediate, and near vision.

There are three different distance dominant zones to give excellent sharp vision for distance in low light and bright light conditions. The ReZoom™ IOL can do better distribution of light for intermediate range using 100% of available light. Balanced View Optics™ zones with aspheric transition also add on to the intermediate vision of ReZoom™ IOLs. It has near addition of +3.5 D at the IOL plane to provide a +2.85 D at the spectacle plane. Hydrophobic acrylic material with an OptiEdge™ triple-edge design provides a 360° capsular contact and reduces edge glare. Spectacle independence achieved for distance, intermediate and near vision with ReZoom IOL are 93%, 92%, and 81%, respectively.

ReSTOR

AcrySof® ReSTOR® has been uniquely designed to improve vision at all distances—up close, far away, and everything in-between—giving cataract patients their best chance ever to live free of glasses. The aspheric version of AcrySof ReSTOR got US-FDA approval in 2007. Aspheric designs with flatter periphery can provide better contrast sensitivity and night vision compared to other designs of multifocal IOLs. AcrySof® ReSTOR® IOL was designed to provide quality near to distance vision by combining the strengths of apodized diffractive and refractive technologies.

Apodized Diffractive

Apodization is a modification of IOL design with center to peripheral diffractive steps tapering in a gradual manner to provide a smooth transition of light distribution between the near, intermediate, and far points of foci. Diffraction of light occurs when it passes through the lens material by spreading or bending light into various focal points. The apodized central diffractive optic with multiple steps on AcrySof® ReSTOR® IOL combinedly focusses the light to provide near vision. The light passing through the diffractive portion of AcrySof® ReSTOR® IOL gets bend to give better focusing on the retina. This outer ring of the AcrySof® ReSTOR® The apodized diffractive central region is surrounded by an outer ring which helps to focus light for distance vision. Macular degeneration, diabetic retinopathy, and other eye disorders may prevent a recommendation for this high technology IOL.

Choice of Multifocals
Based on experiences and various studies, it has been shown that ReZoom provides better intermediate vision, especially required in computer users. ReSTOR provides good near and distance vision. Minimal plus add may be required for intermediate vision. A recent study demonstrates that contralateral implantation of +2.5 D and +3 D multifocal IOL provides a good corrected near vision and a noninferior-corrected intermediate and distance vision as compared to bilateral implantation of +2.5 D IOLs.

Problems
Some known side effects of multifocal IOLs are glare, halos, and night vision difficulties, no guarantee of freedom from spectacles. The surgeon cannot predict exact near point distance for best near vision and may choose to place regular monofocal IOL at the time of surgery if he has concern the IOL may not center well in the eye.

Selection of Patients
Professions involving requirements for higher contrast such as drivers and those working in night shift works can have problems with glare. Workers requiring higher contrast, drivers, and night shift workers may have problems due to low contrast sensitivity and glare. Hence these patients should be counseled and may be deferred for implanting a multifocal IOL.

Trifocal Intraocular Lens
The FineVision (Physiol) optic is the first trifocal IOL with diffractive optic. It is a combination of two diffractive parts which can give +1.75 D addition for intermediate vision and +3.5 D addition for near vision. This design will reduce the light energy lost from diffractive designs. The energy gained from dual diffractive design will improve the intermediate vision while maintaining the near and distance vision. The non-apodized PanOptix IOL uses the ENhanced LIGHT ENergy (ENLIGHTEN; Alcon Laboratories, Fort Worth, TX, USA) optical technology that provides high (88%) transmission of light, is less dependent on pupil size, and allows for an excellent near-to-intermediate range of vision.

Extended Range of Vision Intraocular Lens
The Tecnis Symfony IOL gives a continuous extended depth of focus and good visual acuity after cataract removal. The unique pattern of diffraction of these IOLs provides good near vision with incidence of glare and halos similar to a monofocal IOL. These lenses have a wider range of focus compared to multifocal IOLs which work on simultaneous vision where, one image will be in focus when the out of focus image is suppressed.

■ FUTURE

Blue Light-filtering Intraocular Lenses
AcrySof filters out high intensity blue light and UV rays. Blue light in the visible spectrum with 400–500 nm wavelength is found to result in retinal damage and development of age-related macular degeneration.

"Piggyback" Intraocular Lenses
There are situations in which the postoperative refractive outcome may not be optimal after cataract surgery due to errors in IOL power prediction preoperatively. In such situations we can think of placing a new lens with residual power for implantation above the primary lens implanted. This method of a "piggyback lens", can give better refractive outcomes with ease of implantation and improved safety than replacement of an implanted IOL.

Light Adjustable Lens

The Light Adjustable Lens (LAL, Calhoun Vision) corrects the optical aberrations of the eye by using wavefront sensing technology. Myopia, hyperopia, astigmatism, coma, and spherical aberration can be corrected by manipulating the photosensitive materials present in these silicone IOLs.

Customized Implants

Current aspheric implants are available in standard "one-size-fits all" approach. However, custom made implants can be produced to treat several corneal higher- order aberrations (HOAs) for everyone depending on their wavefront pattern. Wavefront aberrations produced after cataract surgery can be due to IOL decentration, IOL tilt and rotation and wound-related factors such as wound size, location, and wound healing process. Customized cornea-based refractive surgical procedures can be done to treat the preexisting higher order aberrations or to treat newly induced aberrations after cataract surgery. This can enhance the outcomes of customized IOLs correcting higher order aberrations.

■ SUGGESTED READING

1. Tognetto D, Sanguinetti G, Sirotti P, Cecchini P, Marcucci L, Ballone E, et al. Analysis of the optical quality of intraocular lenses. Invest Ophthalmol Vis Sci. 2004;45(8):2682-90.

3.44 Management of Astigmatism: Toric Intraocular Lenses

Abhay Vasavada, Vaishali Vasavada
Raghudeep Eye Hospital, Ahmedabad
icirc@abhayvasavada.com

■ INTRODUCTION

As advances in technology and techniques continue to erode the boundaries between refractive and cataract surgery, emmetropia has gone from an exceptional result to an expected outcome.

- Uncorrected corneal astigmatism can result in a poor visual outcome, hence cataract surgeons need to adopt a strategy for the management of astigmatism that is safe, precise and accurate, and yields predictable outcomes.
- Various studies report the incidence of preexisting corneal astigmatism in the cataract population to be anywhere between 30% and 60%.
- Until relatively recently, patients with significant preexisting corneal astigmatism were either left uncorrected or treated with procedures such as incisional corneal surgeries and/or excimer-laser correction. However, incisional technology lacks precision, is unpredictable, has a limited treatment range, and can show regression. On the other hand, astigmatic correction using the excimer laser means an additional procedure to the patient which may not be acceptable by many.
- The use of toric intraocular lenses (IOLs) overcomes these limitations apart from offering a rational, predictable, and stable method of refractive correction. A clear benefit is that it allows surgeons to perform a standard cataract procedure with only a minor variation in the surgical technique.

There are several toric IOLs available in the market. Key points to consider while choosing the toric IOL of choice are rotational stability, predictability, and capsular as

---

Authors have no financial interest in this article

well as uveal biocompatibility. Eligibility criteria for toric IOL implantation include regular corneal astigmatism between 1 D (diopter) and 5 D with no corneal pathology.

- In order to ensure accurate outcomes with toric IOL, following steps are of paramount importance: accurate biometry, precise keratometry, calculating the surgeon's induced astigmatism, marking of the reference axis on the corneal limbus and intraoperative alignment of the IOL axis with the axis marks. Typically, every IOL manufacturer provides an online calculator which is used to calculate the model of the toric IOL as well as the axis of IOL placement. Also, free online calculators are available (Barrett toric calculator), which allows selection of the toric IOL model. I rely on the manual keratometry readings to determine the steep axis of astigmatism.
- Performing corneal topography is invaluable to confirm the regularity of the astigmatism. It is of utmost importance that keratometry is performed by a trained ophthalmologist/technician without instilling any medication in the eye to obtain precise readings. Further, if the patient has an unstable tear film, it should be treated with lubricants prior to deciding the magnitude and axis of astigmatism. More and more emphasis is now being laid on the role of the posterior cornea as a contributing factor in corneal astigmatism. Scheimpflug devices are currently the only means of determining posterior corneal curvature. As a rough guide, posterior cornea contributes to 0.2–0.3 D of astigmatism which is oriented horizontally (i.e., against the rule) in most eyes. Thus, the astigmatism measured on the anterior corneal surface is usually overestimated in with the rule cases, whereas is underestimated by the same degree in against the rule cases.
- On the day of surgery, preoperative reference-axis marking is done with the patient sitting in an upright position, with the head aligned vertically and the patient fixating on a target straight ahead with the other eye. The corneal limbus is marked at the 0° and 180° positions using a specialized corneal marker with an air-bubble. Maintaining the air bubble in the center ensures accurate horizontal positioning of the marker on the limbus.
- However, now, there are several cellphone "apps", such as the toriCAM which allows the surgeon to perform free-hand marking and then verify the position of the 0° and 180° marks. Also, there are image-guided systems such as the Verion (Alcon), Callisto Eye (Zeiss) and intraoperative aberrometry (ORA) that allow precise positioning of the toric IOL based on preoperative and intraoperative imaging which do not require preoperative manual-corneal marking.
- The size and location of the incision can be changed based on the steep meridian of astigmatism. I prefer a 2.2-mm temporal clear corneal incision for all cases irrespective of the orientation of the astigmatism. Intraoperative axis marking is done using a Mendez gauge and a degree marker. For gross alignment, the IOL is rotated clockwise to approximately 20–30° short of the desired position while the IOL is unfolding in the capsular bag. Following viscoelastic removal the IOL is rotated clockwise onto the intended axis of alignment. It is crucial to remove all the viscoelastic from behind the IOL to prevent postoperative rotation of the toric IOL.

In the author's experience, around 60% patients reported 6/9 or better unaided visual acuity (UCVA) on the first postoperative day. At 3 months >90% patients had a UCVA of 6/9 or better. There was a significant reduction in the preexisting astigmatism, with 65% patients having a residual refractive cylinder of 0.25 D or less. For achieving predictable outcomes with toric IOLs, the rotational stability of the IOL is crucial. We have designed a specialized software-based technique that measures rotation precisely in steps of 0.1°.

We found excellent rotational stability with a mean rotation of around 1.6° (time period) with the AcrySof toric IOL, which is currently our preferred toric IOL. The biggest advantage with toric IOLs is that if there is a malpositioning of the IOL due to data entry errors, they can be rotated back to their position, if done within the first 2–6 weeks postoperatively.

Over the years, their applications have extended to several situations, including stable keratoconus, pediatric eyes with significant astigmatism, and also in select cases of pterygium following excision. Thus, in conclusion, toric IOLs significantly reduce preexisting astigmatism with stable long-term results achieving good unaided distance visual acuity.

> **EDITOR'S PEARLS**
> - One should keep a lower threshold to plan for toric IOLs while implanting multifocal IOLs and in cases with against-the-rule astigmatism.
> - Devices that measure the posterior corneal astigmatism as well should be employed if available.
> - Image-guiding tools are a useful aid for optimizing visual outcomes in toric IOL patients

■ SUGGESTED READING
1. Chang DF. Comparative rotational stability of single-piece open-loop acrylic and plate-haptic silicone toric intraocular lenses. J Cataract Refract Surg. 2008;34(11):1842-7.

3.45 | Mix and Match Multifocal Intraocular Lenses

Gaurav Luthra
Drishti Eye Centre and Dehradun Wave Lasik Centre, Dehradun
gaurav.luthra@drishti.org

■ INTRODUCTION

In recent years, with improvements in technology, and increasing demand for good near acuity in pseudophakes, multifocal intraocular lenses (MFIOLs) have become popular with refractive cataract surgeons and patients alike. Most IOL manufacturers caution against using different style multifocal IOLs in the same patient, citing potential problems with neuroadaptation, especially if a diffractive IOL is used in one eye and a refractive in the other.

With bilateral diffractive multifocal IOLs, patients usually have excellent near and distance acuity but compromised intermediate vision, while bilateral refractive multifocal IOLs may result in good distance and intermediate vision but unsatisfactory near vision.

Some surgeons have tried mixing and matching different multifocals and reported encouraging results in patients desiring the whole range of vision from near to intermediate and far.

There are basically three types of MFIOL patient candidates.

The first is "the typical golf player," a patient with predominantly distance vision tasks who occasionally uses a laptop and rarely reads a book. This patient will have the best results with a distance-dominant IOL, such as the ReZoom [Abbott Medical Optics (AMO)] in both eyes and may require glasses for reading **(Fig. 3.45.1)**.

The second type of patient is "the librarian," someone who rarely drives at night and rarely uses a laptop, but who spends several hours reading books each day. A diffractive multifocal IOL like the Tecnis (AMO) in both eyes is the best option. Near vision will be perfect in any lighting condition (and) distance vision is still good, while intermediate vision is somewhat reduced **(Fig. 3.45.2)**.

However, most patients are in between these two extremes and want the best possible vision for a variety of tasks, including reading, driving, playing golf, and using a laptop. For these patients, mixing and matching IOLs is the best option. They should receive a refractive MFIOL like the ReZoom in the dominant eye and a diffractive multifocal like the Tecnis in the nondominant eye.

Most trials have been done with the diffractive Tecnis MFIOL (AMO) in the nondominant eye allowing good near and distance vision and the ReZoom refractive MFIOL (AMO) in

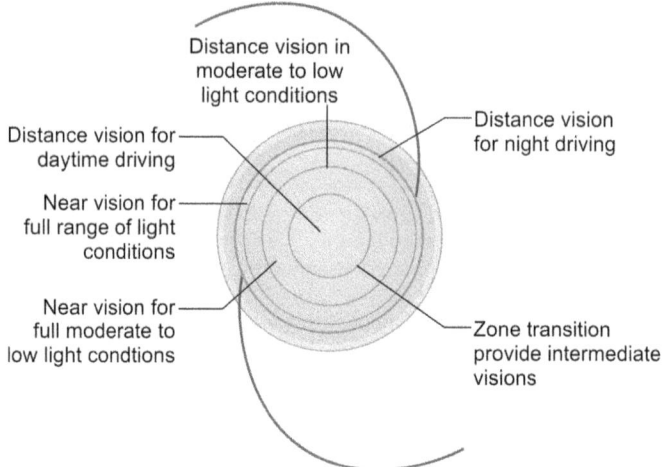

Fig. 3.45.1: ReZoom refractive multifocal intraocular lens (MFIOL).

the dominant eye allowing good distance and intermediate vision, combining to give a full range of vision. Studies quote a spectacles independence rate of 90–100% with this combination as compared to 60–70% with any bilateral MFIOL alone.

Achieving emmetropia with good biometry and considering pupil size are important considerations toward achieving success.

Similar results were reported with a combination of the apodized diffractive ReSTOR MFIOL (Alcon) and the refractive ReZoom IOLs.

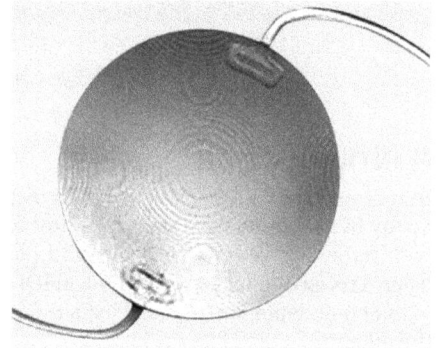

Fig. 3.45.2: Tecnis multifocal intraocular lens (MFIOL).

Some studies have evaluated the mix and match of a diffractive MFIOL with the Crystalens (Bausch & Lomb) accommodating IOL. Results were again satisfactory with patients experiencing less glare and a good range of vision. The Crystalens accommodating IOL gives excellent quality of vision for distance and intermediate while the diffractive MFIOL was good for near and distance.

A recent study used a mix and match of toric monofocal IOL in amblyopic eye of astigmatic amblyopes with diffractive *multifocal* in the fellow eye with encouraging results. The amblyopic eye improved for distance with the toric monofocal while the fellow eye gave good near and distance acuity with the diffractive MFIOL.

■ PEARLS FOR MIXING MULTIFOCAL INTRAOCULAR LENSES

- Patient's satisfaction will depend on realistic and informed expectations.
- Identify the dominant eye.
- Carefully measure the pupil diameter in mesopic conditions to determine whether to use the refractive or diffractive lens in a particular eye (i.e., maximum 5.2 mm for the refractive implant).
- Start by implanting the diffractive IOL in the nondominant eye.
- After the first eye surgery, evaluate patient's satisfaction before deciding which lens to implant in the fellow eye.
- Perform the second surgery within 1 week to push patients to develop bilateral vision rather than search for a "better" eye.

- Provide assistance during the near vision learning curve.
- Perform early yttrium aluminum garnet (YAG) laser capsulotomy.
- Correcting residual refractive errors can significantly reduce or eliminate glare and halo.

The final word has not, however, been said on this issue and further studies will be needed to reach a consensus. Till then one must tread this area with caution.

> **EDITOR'S PEARLS**
> - Patients with realistic expectations are better suited for multifocal IOLs.
> - Patient's needs and requirement should be taken into consideration and adequate chair time provided while planning for multifocal IOLs.

SUGGESTED READING

1. Martínez PA, Gómez FP, España AA, Comas Serrano M, Nahra Saad D, Castilla Céspedes M. Visual function with bilateral implantation of monofocal and multifocal intraocular lenses: a prospective, randomized, controlled clinical trial. J Refract Surg. 2008;24(3):257-64.

3.46 Management of Descemet's Membrane Detachment

Jaspreet Sukhija
Advanced Eye Centre, PGIMER, Chandigarh
jaspreetsukhija@yahoo.com

INTRODUCTION

Localized Descemet's membrane detachment (DMD) is a common occurrence following intraocular surgery but is usually inconsequential as it reattaches spontaneously. On the other hand, extensive separation of the membrane usually persists for a longer period and may require a surgical procedure to reattach the membrane. Several predisposing factors have been implicated for the occurrence of DMD like use of blunt knives, anterior and shelved incisions, anterior chamber entry in a soft eye with a shallow chamber. Another factor, important as far as DMD is concerned, is the technique of corneal lip hydration to aid incision sealing in clear corneal phacoemulsification. Injecting fluid into the deeper stroma may at times strip the membrane.

DIAGNOSIS AND MANAGEMENT

The detection of DMD requires a high index of suspicion on part of the operating surgeon. Prompt recognition of the condition has been suggested in order to decrease the chances of inadvertent removal of the membrane.

Intraoperative

- The diagnosis can be difficult during surgery unless the operating microscope has a slit beam facility, and the surgeon suspects a separation of the membrane.
- Trypan blue dye can assist in identifying the Descemet's membrane (DM) intraoperatively.
- To diagnose a detached DM, the surgeon may instill topical anhydrous glycerin and look for the detached DM adhering to the cornea along a thin, gray, usually oblique line.
- The new microscopes with intraoperative optical coherence tomography (OCT) attachment have enabled the surgeons to visualize the state of the DM in real time which is especially useful in hazy corneas.

Postoperative

Anterior segment OCT helps in visualization of DM postoperatively if the DMD is missed intraoperatively.

Reports are available of the diagnosis being delayed for weeks following surgery. Reattachment of the DM could be spontaneous or may require surgical intervention. The differential diagnosis to consider is a residual piece of anterior capsule that was not removed from the eye during an anterior capsulectomy. If, upon placing an instrument within the eye, the surgeon meets resistance, the instrument should be retracted, and wound size or visualization should be improved before the instrument is again placed into the anterior chamber.

■ TREATMENT

- The best treatment for a large detachment is repositioning it surgically. A patient with this condition usually presents on the first postoperative day with a significant amount of corneal edema that does not resolve. Although reports of spontaneous reattachment of extensive DMD are available, one of the largest series[1] advocates surgical intervention in all cases of subtotal or total DMD.
- Injection of long-standing gases, such as intracameral sulfur hexafluoride (SF6) and perfluoropropane (C3F8), has been suggested as a modality for reattachment of DM. Sodium hyaluronate carries the risk of elevated intraocular pressure (IOP) but can be used when other measures fail to reattach the membrane.
- Patients who required a surgical intervention are those with >50% involvement, marked separation of the membrane from the stroma along with folding of the membrane which had to be unrolled surgically with the use of air/or sodium hyaluronate.
- If it encompasses one-third to one-half of the corneal surface area, the DM can be reattached to the cornea using 10-0 monofilament sutures passed through the cornea. The surgeon makes a paracentesis site at the limbus, inferior and temporal to the previous wound; injects air or a viscoelastic substance to force the detached DM into its proper position; places the sutures in a reverse fashion, starting at a point posterior to the limbus, passing anteriorly into the anterior chamber, through DM and into the cornea stroma; and ties the suture in a way that does not distort the DM. Sutures may not be needed to correct a detached DM if it is recognized intraoperatively.
- The surgeon should be careful when using a clear corneal incision, especially when attempting to hydrate the lips of the incision at the end of surgery.
- Follow a conservative approach when there is limited separation of the DM from the stroma without any folding/scrolling of the membrane. All cases where there is infolding or curling of the membrane should be managed early with surgical intervention. Corneal clarity can be maintained in majority of cases of DMD provided the condition is recognized early and managed adequately.

EDITOR'S PEARLS

- Early intervention should be considered in significant DMDs to achieve better visual outcomes.
- Intracameral air injection may be sufficient in superior non-planar DMDs.

■ REFERENCE

1. Banitt MR, Malta JB, Shtein RM, Soong HK. Delayed-onset isolated central Descemet membrane blister detachment following phacoemulsification. J Cataract Refract Surg. 2008;34(9):1601-3.

3.47 When should an Intraocular Lens be Implanted in the Sulcus or Bag or Captured in the Capsular Bag in a Patient Having Posterior Capsular Tear?

Suresh Kr Pandey
SuVi Eye Hospital and Research Centre, Kota
suvieye@gmail.com

INTRODUCTION

The primary objective of cataract surgery is to ensure the placement of the intraocular lens (IOL) within the capsular bag, ideally in cases where there is an intact capsulorhexis continuous curvilinear capsulorhexis (CCC) and an intact posterior capsule. Understanding how to address complications arising from less-than-ideal surgical conditions is crucial for achieving the best possible results for our patients. When faced with the challenge of implanting an IOL in the presence of a torn posterior capsule, several options are available for consideration.

INTRAOCULAR LENS IMPLANTATION IN THE CAPSULAR BAG

Many surgeons restrict in-the-bag implantation in eyes where posterior capsular tear is converted to a true posterior capsulorhexis. Optic capture can also be achieved in pediatric cases to delay posterior capsule opacification.

HAPTICS IN SULCUS WITH RHEXIS-OPTIC CAPTURE

In cases of an unconverted posterior capsular tear with an intact anterior capsulorhexis, it is appropriate to consider the implantation of a three-piece IOL into the ciliary sulcus with a technique known as rhexis-optic capture, as initially described by Neuhann. The CCC must have a diameter that is at least 1 mm smaller than the optic's diameter and should be centered correctly.

When faced with a torn posterior capsule while the CCC remains intact, the surgeon can proceed by initially implanting the lens into the ciliary sulcus. Gentle posterior pressure is then applied to the surface of the optic, positioned 90° away from the optic-haptic junctions. A sweep or lens manipulator is employed, focusing first near the distal edge and then the proximal edge, to guide the optic beneath the edge of the CCC. This maneuver leads to the optic settling within the capsular bag, causing the CCC to become slightly oval-shaped. This method effectively secures the optic-haptic junctions at the apex of the oval, offering an optimal level of stability.

One key advantage of this technique is that it does not rely on the relationship between the haptic diameter and sulcus length for centration, making it compatible with any three-piece foldable lens. Additionally, if the CCC is appropriately centered, the optic will remain in a centered position over time. Notably, as the optic is drawn backward toward the plane of the anterior capsule, it results in minimal changes to the effective lens positioning (ELP). Therefore, there is generally no need to modify the lens power for lower IOL powers. However, for IOLs with powers exceeding 23.00 diopters, the altered lens position may necessitate a 0.50 diopter decrease in the power of the implanted lens.

Furthermore, complications such as pigment dispersion, often observed in cases of pure sulcus implantation, are less likely to occur with optic capture, as the optic is drawn back and its edges are shielded by the anterior capsule. Optic capture also serves as a preventive measure against the undesired fusion of the leaves of the anterior and posterior capsules, which can lead to early capsular opacity and the need for a capsulotomy.

CILIARY SULCUS FIXATION

In cases where it is not feasible to employ either in-the-bag implantation or optic-capture techniques, the surgeon must carefully plan the placement of both the haptic and the optic in the sulcus. It is essential to note that the sulcus diameter typically approximates the white-to-white measurement plus an additional 2 mm. To rely solely on the sulcus for lens fixation, there must be capsular support at two opposing points on the sulcus circumference, along with adequate zonular stability. This approach raises two primary concerns—centration and compatibility with the uveal tissue.

Single-piece AcrySof® lenses are not suitable for sulcus placement due to their short length, thickness, lack of angulation, and tackiness. Similarly, many three-piece IOLs measure 13 mm or less in width between their haptics, making them unsuitable for certain eye anatomies. An ideal lens for sulcus fixation should have angulated haptics with excellent memory, a haptic diameter ranging from 13.5 to 14.0 mm, a third-generation silicone composition, a 6.5 mm optic for optimal compatibility with uveal tissue, and a margin of safety in case of minor decentration. Additionally, the lens should feature rounded edges to minimize irritation of the iris pigment epithelium. It is important to note that pupillary capture may be more common following the primary implantation of IOLs in pediatric cases.

Finally, it is crucial to remember that sulcus fixation results in a more anterior effective lens position (ELP) compared to bag fixation, which is assumed by our current power calculation formulas. When the calculated lens power falls within the range of 15.00 D–23.00 D, it is advisable to reduce the power of the sulcus lens by 1.00 D. For lenses with powers below 15.00 D, the surgeon should consider reducing by 0.50 D, and for IOLs with powers exceeding 23.00 D, a reduction of 1.50 D should be considered to approximate the refractive target more accurately.

EDITOR'S PEARLS

- Adequate capsular rime support is a prerequisite for implantation of IOL in ciliary sulcus.
- A three-piece IOL is preferred choice for implantation in ciliary sulcus.
- Posterior optic capture of IOL ensures better stability by avoiding its capture in pupillary plane.

SUGGESTED READING

1. Gimbel HV, DeBroff BM. Intraocular lens optic capture. J Cataract Refract Surg. 2004;30(1):200-6.

3.48 Cataract Surgery in Patients with Vitreoretinal Diseases

Pranab Das
Calcutta Medical Research Institute, Kolkata
drdaspranab@yahoo.co.in

INTRODUCTION

Cataract and retinal diseases frequently are associated with one another. Progression of cataract can occur following surgical procedures for vitreoretinal diseases. Conversely cataract surgery may aggravate retinal diseases such as diabetic retinopathy and uveitis. Thus, cataract surgery is frequently necessary in patients with underlying retinal diseases.

OPTIONS AVAILABLE TO TACKLE CATARACT ASSOCIATED WITH VITREORETINAL DISORDERS

- *Simultaneous cataract and vitreoretinal surgery:* In certain cases, it is advisable to perform a combined surgical procedure to address both cataract and vitreoretinal disorders in a single operation.
- *Cataract surgery preceding vitreoretinal assessment and treatment:* When dealing with cases where the cataract is dense enough to hinder the proper evaluation of vitreoretinal pathology and its impact on visual function, a staged approach is warranted. This involves initiating cataract surgery followed by a thorough assessment of the posterior segment and subsequent treatment of any underlying vitreoretinal conditions.
- *Treatment of vitreoretinal disease prior to cataract surgery:* In specific situations, it may be more appropriate to address vitreoretinal diseases before proceeding with cataract surgery.

Numerous studies have demonstrated the safety and efficacy of employing techniques such as phacoemulsification or manual extracapsular cataract extraction in combination with pars plana vitrectomy.

The combined surgery approach offers several advantages, including a shorter postoperative recovery period, enhanced visualization of the posterior pole during vitrectomy, and the convenience of a single surgical intervention. By removing the cataract at the time of vitrectomy, patients are spared the need for an additional cataract surgery, which can be more technically challenging due to the absence of vitreous support following vitrectomy.

However, it is important to acknowledge potential challenges associated with simultaneous surgery, including difficulties in visualizing the capsulorhexis due to a reduced or absent red reflex, instability of the cataract wound during globe manipulation, intraoperative miosis following cataract extraction, bleeding from anterior structures, loss of corneal transparency due to corneal edema and Descemet's folds, and optical effects and undesirable light reflections during vitreoretinal surgery caused by the implantation of the intraocular lens (IOL) prior to posterior segment procedures. Moreover, postoperative complications such as fibrinous reactions, synechiae formation, IOL decentration, pupillary capture, and posterior capsular opacification tend to be more common with combined procedures.

Patients with proliferative diabetic retinopathy and limited visibility of the posterior capsule are at an increased risk of posterior capsule rupture, which, in turn, raises the likelihood of postoperative neovascular glaucoma. Careful consideration of these factors is crucial when determining the most suitable approach for each patient's unique circumstances.

COMBINED PROCEDURE

A combined procedure can be performed under either general anesthesia or local infiltration, but it is essential to consider that it may require a longer duration, which could make general anesthesia more preferable. The sequence of the procedure typically involves the following steps:

- *Phacoemulsification:* The surgery begins with phacoemulsification, carried out through a limbal or clear corneal incision. Surgeons can opt for either the divide and conquer or phaco chop technique to emulsify the cataract nucleus.
- *Viscoelastic and wound closure:* Following successful phacoemulsification, the anterior chamber is filled with viscoelastic. Depending on the extent of globe manipulation anticipated during the surgery, it may be necessary to suture the corneal or limbal incision with 10-0 nylon to ensure its integrity.

- **Pars plana vitrectomy:** Subsequently, a three-port pars plana vitrectomy is performed. During this step, the vitreous humor in the posterior segment of the eye is carefully removed, facilitating the treatment of vitreoretinal disorders.
- **Intraocular lens (IOL) implantation:** After the vitrectomy, the IOL is implanted into the capsular bag while viscoelastic is used to maintain space and stability. The decision on whether to perform internal tamponade, if required, is typically made after the IOL implantation.

It is important to note that there may be variations in the sequence, and some surgeons may prefer to implant the IOL before the vitrectomy, depending on the specific circumstances of the case and their preferred surgical technique.

Retinal Detachment

Successful retinal detachment surgery requires the removal of vitreoretinal tractions and the implementation of a comprehensive internal tamponade. In phakic eyes (those with a natural lens), eliminating peripheral cortical vitreous can be challenging due to difficulties in manipulation and limitations in visibility. Therefore, lens removal is necessary for a significant portion of patients undergoing pars plana vitrectomy for retinal detachment.

The surgical procedure should follow a specific sequence to ensure optimal outcomes:
- **Lens removal:** The surgery begins with the removal of the natural lens. This step is essential in phakic eyes to facilitate the removal of peripheral cortical vitreous.
- **Vitrectomy and membrane peeling:** Following lens removal, the surgeon proceeds with vitrectomy and membrane peeling. These actions address the vitreoretinal tractions and any membranes that may be contributing to the retinal detachment.
- **Buckle placement:** After vitrectomy and membrane peeling, a retinal buckle is carefully placed to provide support and stabilization to the retina.
- **Intraocular lens implantation:** The IOL is implanted into the eye, typically following the completion of vitrectomy and buckle placement. This step helps restore proper vision and is a critical aspect of the surgery.
- **Intraocular tamponade:** Finally, an intraocular tamponade is introduced as needed to maintain retinal reattachment. The choice of tamponade depends on the specifics of the case and the surgeon's judgment.

To ensure the stability and integrity of the procedure, it is advisable to secure the main incision, created during the lens emulsification, with a 10-0 nylon suture. This precaution is particularly important due to the anticipated globe manipulation during vitreous surgery for retinal detachment.

Retinitis Pigmentosa

Apart from the typical risks associated with cataract surgery, it is important to recognize that individuals with retinitis pigmentosa (RP) may face specific factors that can lead to suboptimal visual outcomes following the surgery. These factors include:
- **Outer retinal atrophy at the macula:** RP patients may exhibit outer retinal atrophy at the macular region, which can impact visual function.
- **Macular edema:** Macular edema, a condition characterized by the accumulation of fluid in the macular area, can be a concern in RP cases.
- **Posterior capsular opacification:** The development of posterior capsular opacification, a clouding of the posterior capsule, can affect visual clarity.
- **Aggressive anterior capsule contraction in RP:** RP patients may experience more aggressive anterior capsule contraction, which can pose challenges.

To optimize outcomes for RP patients undergoing cataract surgery, the following considerations are essential:
- **Large anterior capsulorhexis:** Surgeons should aim for a relatively large anterior capsulorhexis to address the specific challenges associated with RP. This approach can improve surgical outcomes.

- *Avoidance of silicone IOLs:* It is advisable to refrain from using silicone IOLs in RP cases due to the increased risk of anterior capsular contraction and the potential for posterior dislocation if an early capsulotomy becomes necessary.

These tailored measures take into account the unique characteristics of RP and aim to enhance the visual results and overall success of cataract surgery for individuals with this condition.

Macular Hole

The conventional surgical approach for managing a macular hole involves a pars plana vitrectomy, which includes the removal of the posterior hyaloid, peeling of the internal limiting membrane (ILM), and the use of gas tamponade, followed by a strict postoperative face-down position for 7-14 days. To achieve successful ILM peeling, it is imperative to have an unobstructed view of the posterior pole. However, the presence of cataract or the accumulation of blood on the lens surface from the scleral port can compromise visibility, making ILM peeling a challenging task.

To address this issue, an increasing number of ophthalmic surgeons are advocating for a combined procedure instead of the traditional sequential surgery. In a combined procedure, a more comprehensive vitrectomy is performed, ensuring a more effective gas fill. This increased gas fill duration may result in a longer tamponade effect, enhancing the closure rate of macular holes.

During a combined procedure, there are varying approaches regarding the timing of cataract surgery and IOL implantation in relation to the posterior segment surgery. Some surgeons prefer to complete the emulsification of the lens and the implantation of the IOL before commencing the posterior segment surgery. In contrast, others opt to delay IOL implantation until the conclusion of the posterior segment surgery. This approach minimizes the creation of disruptive light reflexes and prismatic effects caused by the IOL's edge, which can otherwise hinder the visualization of the retinal periphery. These modifications to the surgical process aim to optimize outcomes and enhance the overall success of macular hole treatment.

Postvitrectomy Eye

Cataract surgery in eyes that have undergone a vitrectomy presents unique challenges due to the absence of vitreous support, weakened zonules, and fluctuations in both anterior chamber depth and the presence of posterior capsule plaques. These factors can increase the risk of various complications during the surgical procedure.

To mitigate these challenges, it is crucial to take several measures:
- *Precise incision construction:* Accurate sizing and construction of incisions are vital. This includes creating a clear corneal incision for the phaco tip and a side port for nucleus manipulators. Properly sized incisions help prevent leakage of irrigation fluid and minimize fluctuations in the anterior chamber.
- *Infusion bottle placement:* It is advisable to keep the infusion bottle at a lower height in these cases. This placement helps maintain stability and control of the anterior chamber during surgery.
- *Optimal phaco machine settings:* Keeping the settings on the phaco machine at lower levels is prudent, as it reduces the risk of complications in vitrectomized eyes.
- *Management of posterior capsule fibrosis:* Many vitrectomized patients develop primary posterior capsule fibrosis, often taking on an annular or plaque-like shape. This fibrosis can be addressed by carefully peeling it off with forceps or through meticulous polishing and vacuuming of the posterior capsule. If these methods prove ineffective, performing a posterior continuous curvilinear capsulorhexis (CCC) is a recommended alternative.

These precautions and techniques are essential to navigate the challenges associated with cataract surgery in vitrectomized eyes and ensure a successful surgical outcome.

> **EDITOR'S PEARLS**
>
> In cases with vitreoretinal disease and cataract, a first-staged phacoemulsification with IOL implantation in the bag is a good option. It may aid in better planning of the second stage procedure.

■ SUGGESTED READING

1. Lahey JM, Francis RR, Fong DS, Kearney JJ, Tanaka S. Combining phacoemulsification with vitrectomy for treatment of macular holes. Br J Ophthalmol. 2002;86(8):876-8.

3.49 Anterior Chamber Deepening during Phacoemulsification

GS Dhami
Dhami Eye Care Hospital, Ludhiana
gsdhami@gmail.com

■ INTRODUCTION

Anterior chamber (AC) deepens during phaco surgery in rupture of the posterior capsule (PC) with hyaloid, rupture without luxation of nucleus into the vitreous, rupture of PC and the hyaloid face with total or partial luxation of the nucleus into the vitreous.

Other conditions are:
- Postvitrectomized eyes
- High myopia
- Optical phenomenon in cases of keratoconus
- Traumatic cataracts
- Posterior polar cataract without preexisting PC defect.

■ MANAGEMENT

- Assess the depth of AC
- Evaluate the PC integrity
- Assess the hardness nucleus
- If the nucleus is very hard, it is advised to convert into extracapsular cataract extraction (ECCE)
- If the nucleus is soft, medium hardness (Grade I-III), inject viscoelastic such as Viscoat under the nuclear to block the capsular tear
- Move the nucleus away from the place of tear, or into the iris plane in AC
- Fill the remaining bag with more Viscoat but do not inject too much as to extend the capsular tear. Perform vitrectomy through the side port incisions.

If the AC collapses, inject more viscoelastic agents, continue till the nucleus is free from the vitreous bands. The nucleus now can be carefully emulsified with phaco tip and settings of phaco machines are changed to reduced vacuum, low-flow rate, and low power. The vitreous in AC tends to block the aspiration up of the phaco but a performing good vitrectomy is helpful. The cortical matter then can be removed with irrigation aspiration or with vitrector in aspiration mode. Then the PC support is assessed and intraocular lens (IOL) is implanted in the capsular bag or in case of inadequate PC support IOL is implanted over the capsulorhexis in the sulcus. If there is no AC or PC support then transscleral fixation of IOL is planned for next sitting.

When there is complete or partial luxation of the nucleus in the vitreous, this can occur:
- During hydrodissection
- During rotation of the nucleus
- During cracking of the nucleus

- During chopping of the nucleus
- A preexisting capsular defect as in posterior polar cataracts.

At this stage, our aim is to save the nucleus from dropping into the vitreous. This is very brief moment that occurs with deepening of AC accompanied by shifting of the nucleus to one side. This requires a support of the nucleus with Viscoat acting as mechanical raft to elevate the nucleus. Any delay in the nucleus drop may require the vitreoretinal surgeon to help the anterior segment surgeon to come out of the crisis.

Before closing the case, a nice cleaning of the AC of cortical matter, viscoelastic, and vitreous is done to prevent secondary glaucoma and uveitis till further intervention is done by the vitreoretinal (V-R) surgeon.

EDITOR'S PEARLS

- Fluctuating anterior chamber depth and reverse pupillary block are the most common problems encountered during phacoemulsification following pars plana vitrectomy in cases of cataracts.
- The sudden deepening of the anterior chamber makes the surgical procedure more cumbersome and increases the risk of intraoperative complications.

SUGGESTED READING

1. Cheung CM, Hero M. Stabilization of anterior chamber depth during phacoemulsification cataract surgery in vitrectomized eyes. J Cataract Refract Surg. 2005;31(11):2055-7.

3.50 Phacoemulsification in Pseudoexfoliation with Small Pupil

Abhay Vasavada
Raghudeep Eye Hospital, Ahmedabad
icirc@abhayvasavada.com

INTRODUCTION

Phacoemulsification is always a challenge in patients with dense cataract with pseudoexfoliation. However for cataract surgeons the syndrome poses intraoperative challenges due to coexisting poor pupillary dilatation and zonular weakness. The operating surgeon has to cope with challenging task of minimizing iris trauma and at the same time safety removing the cataract by avoiding endothelial trauma. Serious complications caused mainly by zonulopathy manifest as zonular dehiscence, capsule tear or rupture, vitreous loss and dropped nucleus or fragment. In addition, a higher incidence of postoperative inflammation and increased anterior capsule opacification (ACO) and posterior capsule opacification (PCO) are found in these eyes.

- The surgery is initiated by performing two paracentesis incisions using an angled dual bevel 1 mm knife.
- First Viscoat is injected into the anterior chamber to coat the corneal endothelium. This is followed by injection of Provisc or Healon GV using the soft shell technique. This ensures that the Viscoat is pushed toward the cornea.
- A 2.2 mm uniplanar temporal clear corneal incision is fashioned. An anterior capsulorhexis is initiated by making a nick with a 26-G (gauge) cystotome and thereafter completed using Utrata forceps.
- By adhering to principles of closed chamber and slow motion techniques, author prefers to perform phacoemulsification using Ozil technology. Phacoemulsification is initiated by keeping low bottle height and low aspiration flow rate and phaco power according to the density of the cataract. The parameters which routinely use for different stages of phacoemulsification are as follow: Ozil amplitude (linear) varying

from 80 to 100%, present vacuum from 500 to 350 mm Hg, aspiration flow rate varying from 25 to 18 cc/min and bottle height varying from 60 to −90 cmH$_2$O.
- After starting phacoemulsification by creating a trench, subsequently step-by-step chop in situ and lateral separation techniques are used to create multiple small fragments which are removed by using the step-down technique. This allows for safe posterior plane emulsification away from the endothelium.
- Before initiating the fragmental removal, inject Viscoat to avoid endothelial injury from the hard nuclear fragments during fragment removal. The use of viscoelastic such as Provisc or Healon GV and Viscoat also offers several advantages to the surgeon while performing phacoemulsification.
- Constant anterior chamber depth is maintained using viscoelastic agent before removing any instrument from the eye. Ozil technology enhances the effectiveness of phacoemulsification multifold. Ozil incorporates the use of a torsional ultrasound with a 0.9 mm mini-flare Kelman tip. The oscillatory movement of the Kelman tip creates a shearing motion bringing it in constant contact with the nucleus.
- The use of Ozil lends the following advantages to the surgeon—by increasing follow ability, reducing turbulence and chatter, and increasing the efficiency of energy delivery.
- Subsequently, bimanual irrigation and aspiration (I/A) was performed through two paracentesis incisions for cortex removal.
- Author prefer to use AcrySof (model: SN60AT, Alcon Laboratories, Forth Worth, Texas, USA) IOL for implantation in the capsular bag.
- Later, residual viscoelastic substance is removed by bimanual irrigation and aspiration by tapping on the IOL surface for removal of the viscoelastic substance which has been trapped under the IOL.
- Author prefers to perform stromal hydration including the two paracentesis incisions and the main incision including edges of the clear corneal incision and also the internal entry to help seal it.
- It is safe to carry out phacoemulsification with fewer complications by using Ozil technology or other phacoemulsification machines and appropriate ophthalmic viscosurgical devices.

EDITOR'S PEARLS
- Small pupil and zonular weakness need to be addressed in cases of pseudoexfoliation during phacoemulsification.
- Adjunctive use of capsular tension ring may provide better IOL centration and long-term stability of IOL bag complex.

SUGGESTED READING
1. Susic N, Kalauz-Surac I, Brajkovic J. Phacoemulsification in pseudoexfoliation (PEX) syndrome. Acta Clin Croat. 2008;47(2):87-9.

3.51 What is the Best Way to Prevent and Manage Postoperative Intraocular Pressure Spikes?

Sandeep Saxena
King George's Medical University, Lucknow
sandeepsaxena2020@yahoo.com

■ INTRODUCTION

Cataract surgery is known to result in a reduction in intraocular pressure over the course of several months to years after the procedure. However, one common side effect during the early postoperative period, particularly within 24 hours of surgery, is an increase in intraocular pressure. The reasons behind this rise in intraocular pressure can be attributed to factors such as the presence of retained lens material, postoperative inflammation, and the retention of viscoelastic substances in the anterior chamber.

For patients with glaucoma who are contemplating cataract extraction, the potential risks associated with sudden pressure spikes are a cause for concern. In contrast, patients without a history of glaucoma or exfoliation syndrome who undergo cataract surgery are unlikely to experience a clinically significant elevation in intraocular pressure in the postoperative period.

However, individuals with glaucoma and exfoliation syndrome may encounter elevated intraocular pressure, which can be managed with topical pressure-lowering medications after surgery. The extent to which spikes in intraocular pressure contribute to progressive damage to the optic nerve head in comparison to sustained elevated pressure levels is not entirely clear. Nevertheless, most experts recommend preventing or treating such pressure spikes as a precaution.

Moreover, it is believed that patients with more advanced glaucoma and severe visual field loss are at a higher risk of experiencing progression, including the potential for central and paracentral visual loss following a postoperative increase in intraocular pressure.

It is worth noting that the use of Viscoat (sodium chondroitin sulfate 4% – sodium hyaluronate 3%) has been associated with a significantly greater increase in intraocular pressure and more frequent intraocular pressure spikes in the early postoperative period after small incision cataract surgery compared to OcuCoat (hydroxypropyl methylcellulose 2%).

To prevent an elevation in intraocular pressure due to retained ophthalmic viscosurgical devices (OVD), the most straightforward approach is to ensure complete removal of the OVD from the eye at the end of the surgery. This can be achieved by using an irrigation/aspiration probe with a high flow rate of 50 cc per minute or higher, combined with a high vacuum level of at least 500 mm Hg. This approach facilitates the easier removal of viscoelastic substances. However, in some instances, traces of viscoelastic material may still remain in the angle of the eye. To address this, the angle sweep technique can be employed, using balanced salt solution, a 27-gauge blunt cannula, and a 3-cc syringe. This technique involves forcefully irrigating the angle of the eye opposite the paracentesis and employing a sweeping motion to wash out any remaining OVD.

In terms of prophylactic treatment to manage intraocular pressure after phacoemulsification surgery, it has been found that the dorzolamide-timolol fixed combination is more effective than brimonidine in reducing intraocular pressure at both the 6-hour and 24-hour postoperative marks.

■ SUGGESTED READING

1. Zamvar U, Dhillon B. Postoperative IOP prophylaxis practice following uncomplicated cataract surgery: a UK-wide consultant survey. BMC Ophthalmol. 2005;5:24.

3.52 How will You Manage a Case of Visually Significant Cataract with Associated Fuchs' Endothelial Dystrophy?

Rajesh Fogla
Apollo Hospitals, Hyderabad
dr_fogla@yahoo.com

INTRODUCTION

Current management of bullous keratopathy associated with Fuchs' endothelial dystrophy would be endothelial keratoplasty (EK) procedure such as Descemet's stripping endothelial keratoplasty (DSEK) or Descemet's stripping automated endothelial keratoplasty (DSAEK). Both of these procedures allow selective replacement of dysfunctional endothelium through a 5.5-mm scleral incision. When compared to conventional full thickness penetrating keratoplasty, EK procedures have several advantages. As the corneal topography is relatively undisturbed, visual recovery is faster following EK. Tectonically the wound is more secure following EK. With eye banks starting to provide precut donor tissues, corneal surgeons will be able to perform EK procedures without having to make a huge investment in newer instruments.

As the corneal topography is relatively unaffected by EK procedure, cataract removal with intraocular lens implantation has significantly better visual outcome when simultaneously performed at the same time. EK has been noted to induce a hyperopic shift of +0.75 to +1.25 D postoperatively, which is secondary to change in the posterior curvature of the cornea. This has to be taken into consideration during intraocular lens power selection to avoid postoperative hyperopia.

Cataract Surgery in Patients with Fuchs' Endothelial Corneal Dystrophy: When to Consider a Triple Procedure?
Of all preoperative and intraoperative parameters, only central corneal thickness (CCT) and corneal backscatter at the basal epithelial cell layer (EV) were identified as significant factors, predictive of the need for EK.

As optimal cut-off points, the following cut-off points were chosen:
- 1,894 scatter units for EV and
- 630 mm for CCT
- Both cut-off points correspond with a specificity of 94% and represent sensitivity of 63% for EV and 40% for CCT.

SURGICAL PROCEDURE

- Cataract surgery can be performed through a 2.75-mm scleral tunnel, 1 mm behind limbus.
- Corneal epithelium can be debrided to improve visualization.
- Under cohesive viscoelastic cover both capsulorhexis and Descemet's stripping can be performed easily although some surgeons recommend use of anterior chamber maintainer for this procedure.
- After hydrodissection, ensure adequate rotation of the nucleus. Phacoemulsification can be performed as per surgeon's preferred technique. Nuclear fragments can be brought into the anterior chamber and then emulsified, as there is no risk of endothelial damage.
- Foldable intraocular lens is placed in the bag, followed by complete removal of viscoelastic from the eye.
- The wound is enlarged to 5.5 mm. Donor tissue can be inserted either folded using a pair of forceps, or without folding using a pair of intravitreal forceps introduced into

the eye from the opposite quadrant. Busin glide is preferable to forceps. Donor tissue is positioned and supported using a large air bubble. Scleral wound is secured with interrupted sutures. Venting incisions can be placed in the midperipheral cornea to drain interface fluid, if present.

Visual recovery is noticed from the 3rd or 4th day, and by 1 month most patients have an average visual acuity of 6/12 in the operated eye. EK has become the procedure of choice for patients undergoing combined cornea and cataract surgery. The other option in this clinical scenario would be femtosecond laser-guided penetrating keratoplasty. A top hat configuration of the donor and recipient wound edge helps improve wound apposition, reduced astigmatism, and early removal of sutures. However, the postoperative refractive outcome is less predictable when compared to EK. Recently attempts are being made to transplant donor Descemet's membrane for endothelial dysfunction, Descemet's membrane endothelial keratoplasty (DMEK). Once perfected this may become the procedure of choice for management of endothelial disorders in future.

EDITOR'S PEARLS

- While performing phacoemulsification in Fuchs' endothelial corneal dystrophy (FECD) phaco chop with a torsional phaco tip and use of soft shell technique is recommended.
- Intraocular lens (IOL) selection and power calculation are important—a hydrophobic acrylic IOL with slight myopic target is preferable.
- Patient should be counseled about the need for EK in future.

SUGGESTED READING

1. Fogla R, Padmanabhan P. Initial results of small incision deep lamellar endothelial keratoplasty (DLEK). Am J Ophthalmol. 2006;141(2):346-51.

3.53 How should We Manage Prolonged or Recurrent Uveitis Following Phacoemulsification?

Jyotirmoy Biswas
Sankara Nethralaya, Chennai
drjb@snmail.org

INTRODUCTION

The causes of prolonged recurrent uveitis following phacoemulsification most commonly occur due to organisms with low virulence, which are often sequestered in the capsular bag. However, other causes include the lens implant itself, malposition of the intraocular lens (IOL) haptic and retained lens material, especially cortical remnants. Newer lenses with their improved design very rarely produce inflammation. Patients with preoperative uveitis are at increased risk of chronic postoperative inflammation. Diabetes also tends to produce chronic inflammation. Occasionally, haptics may erode uveal tissue causing inflammation; capture of lens optic by the pupil can also cause iritis.

MANAGEMENT

A careful slit-lamp examination should be done to find out the position of posterior chamber IOL, any residual cortex and plaques of organisms. An ultrasound biomicroscopy can be done to find out chronic irritation due to malpositioning of the IOL. Low-grade inflammation due to IOL displacement can be controlled with a low dose of topical corticosteroids such as prednisolone and does not require surgical intervention, unless there is uncontrolled inflammation, glaucoma, hyphema, etc., where lens reposition or exchange, removal of residual cortex from the anterior chamber or release of iris from the wound is needed.

Presence of a plaque or abscess requires injection of antibiotics such as vancomycin, ceftazidime within the capsular bag or in the vitreous cavity. Any case of postoperative uveitis not responding to topical steroids should be suspected to have low-grade infection. An anterior chamber tap is advised in these situations and subjected to polymerase chain reaction for eubacteria, *Propionibacterium acnes (P. acnes)* and other organisms. In refractory cases, IOL explant with vitrectomy may be required for *P. acnes* infection.

■ SUGGESTED READING
1. Roesel M, Heinz C, Koch JM, Heiligenhaus A. Cataract surgery in uveitis. Ophthalmology. 2008;115(8):1431.

3.54 | Management of Posterior Dislocation of Lens Fragment during Phacoemulsification

Pranab Das
Calcutta Medical Research Institute, Kolkata
drdaspranab@yahoo.co.in

■ INTRODUCTION

Dislocation of lens fragments into the vitreous cavity during phacoemulsification is a relatively uncommon but potentially sight-threatening complication as it may lead to elevated intraocular pressure (IOP), corneal edema, intraocular inflammation, retinal detachment (RD), and other complications. Various ocular and systemic factors predispose posterior capsular rupture and lens fragment dislocation during phacoemulsification. Among these posterior polar cataract, pseudoexfoliation syndrome, hard nucleus, non-dilating pupil, deep seated eye, very old age, traumatic cataract, postuveitic cataract, post-vitrectomized eye are common predisposing conditions. So, identifying these factors preoperatively with meticulous examination and taking appropriate measures during surgery may lower the incidence of this devastating complication.

The primary management of retained lens fragments in the vitreous cavity by the cataract surgeon is controversial. Primary surgeon should minimize attempts at retrieving intravitreal lens fragments to reduce the risk of secondary complications such as vitreous hemorrhage, corneal edema/decompensation, retinal tears, and detachments. Cortex and small nuclear remnants may be carefully observed without surgery. No attempts should be made to impale or aspirate a partially descended nucleus with the phaco tip because it can be extremely hazardous. The downwardly directed infusion can repel the nucleus further, and aspiration of vitreous with the large diameter of the phaco tip can lead to giant retinal tear and detachment.

It is very important to identify posterior capsular rupture at the earliest to prevent posterior dislocation of lens fragments. Once the posterior capsule rupture is noted intraoperatively, surgeon's first priority should be safe removal of nucleus, epinucleus, and cortex. The next priority is the appropriate excision of anteriorly prolapsed vitreous using an automated vitreous cutter. At this stage surgeon should try to preserve enough anterior or posterior capsule for posterior chamber intraocular lens (IOL) implantation. Some anterior segment surgeons advocate the technique called posterior-assisted levitation for lifting a descending nucleus, with a cyclodialysis spatula inserted through a pars plana sclerotomy with variable result. Instead of spatula one can use Viscoat for the same purpose. These techniques can be applied only when nucleus is at posterior chamber or in anterior vitreous.

If the nucleus dislocates into the posterior vitreous or onto the retina, the anterior segment surgeon should not try to retrieve it. If enough capsular support is there posterior chamber IOL can be implanted in the sulcus after clearing the anterior chamber of any lens matter and prolapsed vitreous. Then case is to be referred to vitreoretinal surgeon for pars plana vitrectomy and lens fragment removal. If vitreoretinal set up is available, pars plana vitrectomy can be done in the same sitting if corneal clarity permits to do so. It will allow to avoid second surgery and early recovery of vision.

The timing of the vitrectomy-lensectomy has been debated. Some authors advocate early vitrectomy to reduce the rate of glaucoma and intraocular inflammation. Various studies had shown equally good results even if the surgery is delayed for 1–2 weeks.

SUGGESTED READING
1. Lai TY, Kwok AK, Yeung YS, Kwan KY, Woo DC, Yuen KS, et al. Immediate pars plana vitrectomy for dislocated intravitreal lens fragments during cataract surgery. Eye. 2005;19(11):1157-62.

3.55 Current Surgical Techniques for Pediatric Cataract Surgery

Jagat Ram
Advanced Eye Centre, PGIMER, Chandigarh
drjagatram@yahoo.com

INTRODUCTION
Pediatric cataract is an important cause of childhood blindness. The prevalence of childhood cataract has been reported as 1–15 cases in 10,000 children. It is estimated that globally, there are 200,000 children blind from bilateral cataract.

CURRENT SURGICAL TECHNIQUES
The aim of the surgical technique is to provide a long-term clear visual axis by preventing posterior capsule opacification (PCO) or secondary membrane. Most of the pediatric cataract can be aspirated using two-way irrigation-aspiration (IA) cannula or automated IA; however membranous or calcified cataract may need phacoemulsification. The best current technique for pediatric cataract is *"Phacoaspiration with primary posterior capsulotomy with or without anterior vitrectomy and capsular bag implantation/optic capture of intraocular lens."*

PREOPERATIVE EVALUATION
A thorough history from the parents is useful to understand whether the cataract is congenital, developmental, or traumatic in origin. One must ascertain if there is any history of maternal drug use, infection, or exposure during pregnancy. Each child should be examined by a pediatrician for thorough systemic workup to rule out systemic associations, anomalies, or congenital rubella.

INTRAOCULAR LENS POWER CALCULATION
Intraocular lens (IOL) power calculation for the growing pediatric eye poses several problems. Most reports have recommended undercorrection of the IOL power for pediatric cataract, anticipating the myopic shift following IOL implantation. The axial length and keratometry readings should be measured for IOL power calculation in children. Dahan et al. have suggested to aim for undercorrection in children aged between 2 and 8 years, and to perform biometry and undercorrect them by 10%. For children younger than 2 years, perform biometry and undercorrect them by 20% or use the axial length only.

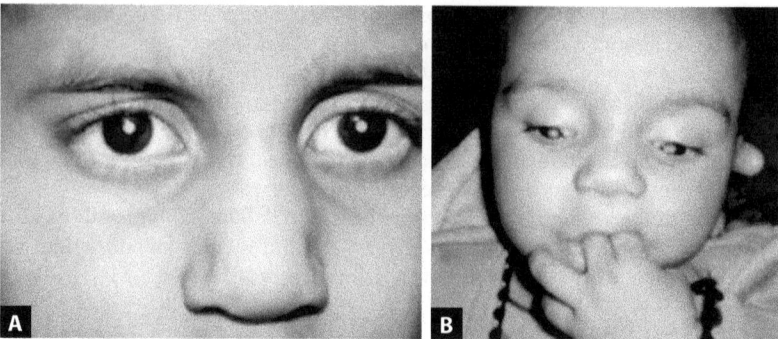

Figs. 3.55.1A and B: Bilateral visually significant cataract in children.

IOL power suggested for 21 mm is (22.00 D), 20 mm (24.00 D), 19 mm (26.00 D), 18 mm (27.00 D), and for 17 mm axial length 28.00 D.

INDICATIONS FOR CATARACT SURGERY FOR PEDIATRIC CATARACT

- *Child with visually significant cataract:* Cataracts, which occupy visual axis and occupy 3 mm or more of the pupil is an indication for cataract surgery.
- *Unilateral partial or complete cataract:* It needs early surgery to prevent amblyopia.
- *Poor retinoscopic reflex:* If during retinoscopy through dilated pupil reflex is poor due to cataract, it is an indication for surgery.
- *Congenital or developmental cataract with strabismus, nystagmus/unsteady fixation.*
- *Children with bilateral cataract where one eye has been operated:* Second eye with cataract should be operated preferably within 1–2 weeks to prevent amblyopia **(Figs. 3.55.1A and B)**.

WHEN TO OPERATE PEDIATRIC CATARACT?

The timings of cataract surgery depend on the indications and factors influencing visual outcome. Once indicated, the child may be operated as early as 2 weeks of age considering the safety of general anesthesia. Unilateral cataract needs early surgery and in bilateral cataract, after operating first eye, second eye may be operated within a week or two to prevent amblyopia.

PREOPERATIVE COUNSELING

Preoperative counseling is most important. Parents must understand that surgery is only the first step of management. The child needs follow-up for a long period for repeated correction of residual and changing refractive error and occlusion therapy. The possibility of postoperative complications and need of secondary intervention must be emphasized.

SURGICAL STEPS

Surgery is performed under general anesthesia.

Incision Construction

The main limbal incision is fashioned superiorly with a 1.0–1.5 mm entry into the cornea to create a valve. With the availability of soft-foldable lenses which require incisions of 3.0 mm or less, some surgeons are shifting to clear corneal incision with good results. Two paracentesis incisions are made in the clear cornea.

Anterior Capsulotomy

A continuous curvilinear capsulorhexis (CCC) is the gold standard for pediatric cataract surgery. A small initial opening is made in the center of anterior capsule with the help of needle cystotome. The capsulorhexis is performed with the help of Utrata's forceps which greatly facilitates the control of capsulorhexis. We aim at a rhexis as small as possible because the elasticity of a pediatric capsule creates an opening that is larger than expected. In total cataracts or where the red reflex is very poor, trypan blue staining of the anterior capsule is extremely helpful.

Another alternative to manual CCC is to perform a vitrector-mediated anterior capsulotomy. Other alternatives for fashioning CCC are use of radiofrequency (RF) diathermy and plasma blade may also be used to achieve CCC. The desirable size of CCC is 5.0–5.5 mm in diameter.

Hydrodissection

Hydrodissection is essential to ensure maximum removal of lens cortex and lens epithelial cells (LECs) from the equatorial region.

Lens Substance Removal

The cortical material is aspirated using two-port IA. Two-port IA helps to remove the cortex completely and it also maintains the anterior chamber during the procedure.

Posterior Continuous Curvilinear Capsulorhexis

Posterior capsule opacification (PCO) is the most common complication after a successful cataract surgery in children. In younger children PCO is almost inevitable if posterior capsule management is not performed at the time of primary surgery. The general consensus is to perform a posterior capsulotomy, especially in younger children. We perform posterior CCC (PCCC) of 3 mm in children undergoing cataract surgery at age <6 years.

Anterior Vitrectomy

Most surgeons prefer to perform anterior vitrectomy along with primary PCCC to decrease the incidence of PCO. Anterior vitreous acts as a scaffold and helps in LEC migration and proliferation. The vitrectomy may be performed using limbal or pars plana route. The aim is to remove only the central anterior vitreous and not for a complete peripheral vitrectomy.

Intraocular Lens Implantation

Capsular bag implantation of IOL is the best choice to reduce the contact of IOL with uveal tissue and to achieve IOL centration.

Although polymethylmethacrylate (PMMA) IOL has the longest safety record, hydrophobic acrylic, foldable IOL are preferred nowadays. We prefer single-piece AcrySof IOL over others.

Incision Closure

Because of lower scleral rigidity in children with a consequently greater risk of fish mouthing of the incision with resultant anterior chamber collapse, all incisions should be closed with a suture, especially the main incision.

■ POSTOPERATIVE MANAGEMENT

Postoperatively, a child's eye tends to show more tissue reactions. The inflammatory response can be managed with the use of intensive topical steroid (as frequently as 6–12 times a day). The steroids are tapered over a period of 6–8 weeks. Topical antibiotics are instilled four times a day for 10-14 days. Cyclopentolate eye drops 0.5% or atropine eye ointment should be used for about 4 weeks to prevent posterior synechiae formation.

Postoperative amblyopia therapy should be instituted meticulously. Occlusion therapy for unilateral cataract after surgery should be instituted early as these children are at higher risk of developing amblyopia.

VISUAL OUTCOME FOLLOWING PEDIATRIC CATARACT SURGERY

Pediatric cataract, if not treated early, may be associated with dismal results. However, early surgery combined with appropriate refractive correction and aggressive amblyopia therapy usually provides encouraging results (Fig. 3.55.2).

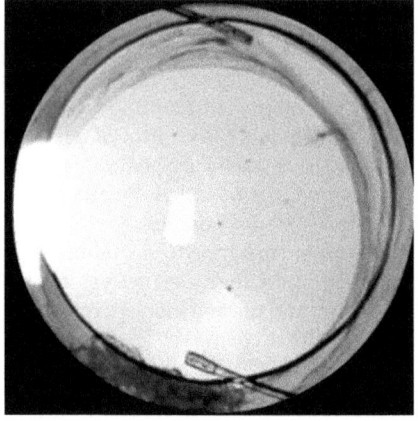

Fig. 3.55.2: Clear visual axis after 8 years of phacoaspiration with primary posterior capsulotomy with AcrySof (MA60AC) implantation in an infant's eye.

EDITOR'S PEARLS
- Timing of surgery can influence the development and severity of amblyopia in pediatric cataract patients.
- Decision to implant an IOL depends on the age, ocular biometry, anatomical considerations, and fellow eye status.
- Amblyopia therapy and optical rehabilitation are the keys to achieving optimal visual outcomes in children after cataract surgery.

SUGGESTED READING
1. Ram J, Brar GS. Textbook of Pediatric Cataract Surgery. New Delhi, India: Jaypee Brothers Medical Publishers (P) Ltd.; 2006.

3.56 Secondary Intraocular Lens Implantation in Children

Ashok Sharma
Cornea Centre, Chandigarh
asharmapgius@yahoo.com

INTRODUCTION

Intraocular lens (IOL) implantation is considered as most widely used option for visual rehabilitation of pediatric cataract patients. At times, the primary surgery option of implanting IOL in the pediatric eye may not be executed because of the extensive posterior capsule rupture, in complicated cataracts [uveitis/juvenile rheumatoid arthritis (JRA)] or in traumatic cataracts. Patients undergoing pars plana vitreous surgery and/or lensectomy for major retinal problem are also left aphakic at the time of primary surgery. Secondary IOL implantation is considered as a better option in both unilateral and bilateral pediatric aphakes.
- Patients having adequate posterior capsule support should be considered for sulcus-supported posterior chamber IOL implantation. Rarely one may be able to separate anterior capsular from postcapsule and lens may be placed in the bag.
- For patients having inadequate posterior capsule support several options including angle-supported anterior chamber IOL (ACIOL), iris-fixated ACIOL, and suture-fixated

iris IOLs and scleral-fixated posterior chamber IOL (PCIOLs) exist. Iris-supported ACIOLs being closer to endothelium have been associated with corneal endothelium decomposition. Angle-supported ACIOLs have been reported to cause similar problems. In addition angle-supported ACIOLs may be contraindicated in patients with angle recession, iridodialysis, inadequate iris support, and glaucoma. The sutured PCIOL procedure specifically, the transsclerally sutured PCIOL procedure is may be considered in patients with inadequate posterior capsule support. Recent surgical and technological advances, including the technique of burying the suture knot in sclera and use of an ab externo approach have significantly improved the results.

A patient undergoing secondary IOL implantation needs comprehensive ophthalmological work-up including detailed retina evaluation. Several variations in the technique of passing sutures in transscleral fixated posterior chamber IOL (TSFPCIOL) have been advocated. Care is taken to avoid exact 3 o'clock and 9 o'clock positions and previous sclerostomy sites. We prefer to make partial thickness scleral flaps. Some authors make scleral groove and bury the suture directly. We performed TSFPCIOLs in 21 eyes of 21 children who had undergone pars plana vitrectomy and lensectomy and were aphakic. Sixteen (76.2%) eyes achieved best-corrected visual acuity (BCVA) of 20/40 or better, and five (23.8%) eyes between 20/200 and 20/60.

We observed that decrease in visual acuity in one eye was due to cystoid macular edema and in another patient due to cellophane maculopathy. Complications including transient intraocular hemorrhage in 13 eyes (52%), transient choroidal effusion in two eyes (8%), late endophthalmitis in one eye (4%), and retinal detachment in one eye (4%) have been reported. The key in the long-term success of TSFPCIOLs is to make thicker partial thickness scleral flap (**Fig.3.56.1**). This precaution also avoids the extrusion of the end of 10-0 propylene sutures. In addition meticulous vitrectomy at the base of vitreous should be performed.

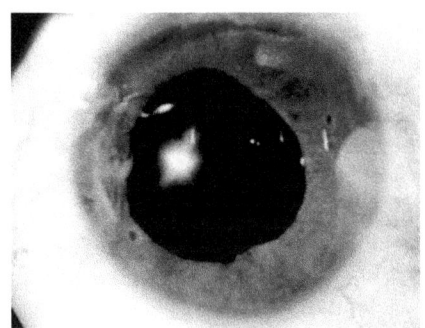

Fig. 3.56.1: Long-term (12 years) successful visual rehabilitation with TSFPCIOL.

This takes care of the traction at vitreous base and eliminates the possibility of cystoid macular edema. Late IOL dislocation due to breakage of polypropylene sutures in six eyes (24%) after 7-10 years of TSFPCIOLs has been reported. The late IOL dislocation has been attributed to the degradation of polypropylene suture material. The use of larger diameter (9-0 instead of 10-0) polypropylene suture material and placement of the haptic and a suture in the ciliary sulcus to promote formation of scar tissue has been advocated. This may enhance the long-term stability of scleral-fixated PCIOLs. Nowadays, the intrascleral fixation of haptics with fibrin glue has led to avoidance of all suture-related complications.

Several authors have reported excellent visual outcome following secondary sulcus PCIOL. Some of the investigations have found that visual results are comparative to primary PCIOL implantation. In our experience also the results of secondary sulcus PCIOLs were encouraging.

A secondary PCIOL implant is safe and effective for management of unilateral or bilateral pediatric aphakic. Treatment of amblyopia is made easier and possible. Secondary PCIOLs in sulcus may provide as good vision as in primary PCIOLs. Scleral-fixated IOL is a viable option for patients with inadequate posterior capsular support. In our experience scleral-fixated IOLs have also been found effective in patients with severe ocular trauma who had undergone pars plana vitrectomy and lensectomy. The option should be used in selective patients. However, these patients should be monitored for long-term complications.

SUGGESTED READING

1. Gimbel HV, Venkataraman A. Secondary in-the-bag intraocular lens implantation following removal of Soemmering ring contents. J Cataract Refract Surg. 2008;34(8):1246-9.

3.57 | Femtosecond Laser-assisted Cataract Surgery

Deepali Singhal, Sridevi Nair
Dr RP Centre for Ophthalmic Sciences, AIIMS, New Delhi
deepali.singhal88@gmail.com, srideviaiims@gmail.com

INTRODUCTION

Cataract surgery is the most commonly performed surgical procedure worldwide.[1] The advent of femtosecond laser (FSL) technology revolutionized the field of ophthalmic surgery. Major advantage being decreased energy requirements and reduced unintended destruction of collateral tissue which is due to its ultrafast pulses in the range of 10^{-15} seconds, it has been recently approved for cataract surgery in 2010.

The use of lasers was introduced for a variety of different applications within the field of cataract surgery during the 1970s. Neodymium-doped yttrium-aluminum-garnet (Nd:YAG) laser for posterior capsulotomy for treating posterior capsular opacification was first described in 1980. Lasers have also been used for phacopuncture, anterior capsulotomy before cataract extraction and photolysis of the cataractous lens. However, these applications are not in practical usage.

MECHANISM

Femtosecond laser is an infra-red laser using neodymium—glass 1,053 wavelength light, that allows the light to be focused at a 3 μm spot size, accurate within 5 μm in the anterior segment. Unlike the slower excimer and neodymium:YAG lasers the ultrashort pulses (10^{-15} seconds) prevent collateral damage to surrounding tissues due to minimal heat generation.

Photodisruption

As with the Nd:YAG laser, FSL cuts tissue through a process of photodisruption (the process of converting laser energy into mechanical energy). Absorption of laser by the tissue results in plasma formation, which is made of free electrons and ionized molecules, that rapidly expands, to create cavitation bubbles. The force of the cavitation bubble formation separates the tissue.

PROCEDURE

Currently, five FSL technology platforms are commercially available for cataract surgery: (1) Catalys (OptiMedica), (2) LenSx (Alcon Laboratories, Incorporation), (3) Lensar (Lensar, Incorporation), (4) VICTUS (Technolas), and (5) Femto LDV Z8 (Ziemer Ophthalmic Systems).

Preoperative Planning

A complete ocular examination is performed including parameters such as pupil diameter, anterior chamber depth, and thickness of the lens and cornea. The size of the capsulotomy and intraocular lens (IOL) to be implanted is selected. Lens fragmentation pattern is selected and parameters for the location, structure, and depth of the clear corneal incisions (CCIs) are entered. The depth, length, and axis of arcuate keratotomies when required are determined by traditional nomograms.

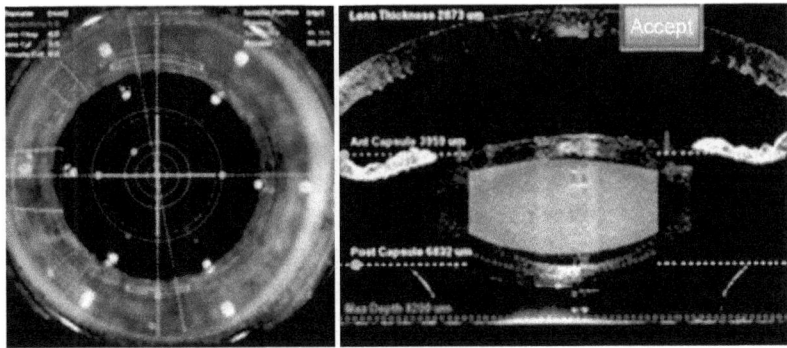

Fig. 3.57.1: Optical coherence tomography (OCT) image-guided femtosecond laser-assisted cataract surgery (FLACS).

Docking
The patient's eye is docked into the laser platform which is known to cause a significant rise in intraocular pressure (IOP 80 mm Hg), which can increase the risk of ischemic retinal and optic nerve injury, particularly in elderly patients. LenSx circumvents this by using a curved contact lens to applanate the cornea that produces a much lower rise of IOP of about 40 mm Hg. OptiMedica's Liquid Optics interface produces an IOP increase of about 15 mm Hg.

Intraoperative Anterior Segment Imaging
Detailed assessment of the cornea, iris, iridocorneal angle, and lens (including anterior and posterior capsule) is done using high-resolution, three-dimensional, wide-field imaging **(Fig. 3.57.1)**. Two systems utilized for this purpose include Fourier-domain optical coherence tomography (OCT) incorporated in LenSx, Catalys (OptiMedica), Femto LDV Z8 and VICTUS (Technolas Perfect Vision) and Scheimpflug imaging in LensAR.

Treatment Stage
After visualization, the treatment is initiated. Construction of laser incision is performed in the posteroanterior planes, which limits the energy transmission to retina. Since the bubbles are maintained posterior to the laser target, the focus of the laser beam is preserved and avoids scatter before the target tissue.

At present, FSL can be utilized for following applications in cataract surgery: (1) Creation of corneal arcuate incisions, (2) Corneal wound construction, (3) Anterior capsulotomy, and (4) Lens fragmentation.

Limbal-relaxing Incisions
Femtosecond laser allows for the creation of highly accurate, reliable, and more predictable LRIs which help to correct low astigmatism.

Corneal Wound Construction
Femtosecond laser allows creating more precise and reproducible three-dimensional corneal cuts resulting in multiplanar self-sealing incisions **(Figs. 3.57.2 and 3.57.3)**. The wounds are self-sealing, which reduces the incidence of leakage. Manual incisions are known to commonly require stromal hydration and are unstable at low IOP. An increased incidence of postoperative infections is associated

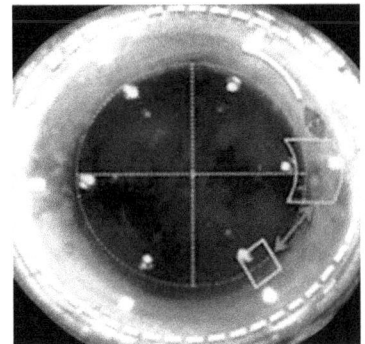

Fig. 3.57.2: Corneal incision placement.

with CCIs. Thus, the corneal incision can be customized in terms of geometry, angle, depth, and width with precise wound architecture. They have been found to result in fewer corneal higher order aberrations and lower incidence of posterior wound gap, wound-site DM detachment, and ragged DM morphology.[2]

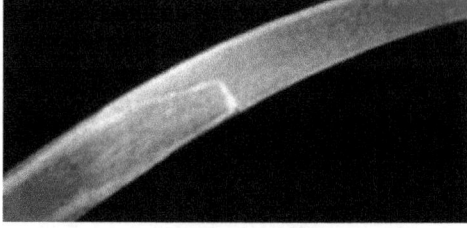

Fig. 3.57.3: Optical coherence tomography (OCT) image of biplanar corneal incision.

Capsulorhexis

Femtosecond laser creates capsulotomies which are more precise, accurate, reproducible, and more robust than those created with the conventional technique. Thus, the capsulotomy is more regular with a more constant and reproducible effective lens position (ELP). It also helps to maintain good IOL centration, which is important for premium IOL implantation. It also facilitates a more consistent overlap between the edge of the capsulotomy and the edge of the IOL reducing the incidence of PCO. Since the FSL cuts inside out in a circular manner, it can provide a precise control over CCC during capsulotomy in complicated scenarios such as white cataract and subluxated cataracts.

Lens Fragmentation

Femtosecond laser machine uses two patterns for lens fragmentation (**Fig. 3.57.4**):

- *Liquefy pattern:* Spherical-based fragments are produced and no phaco power required, mainly works for soft nucleus.
- *Chop pattern:* Pie-shaped fragments are produced, mainly work for hard nucleus, allow for less duration of surgery and reduced phaco power being used. Recently, a hybrid pattern including three cylinders (2 mm, 4 mm, and 6 mm) and three chops (6 mm in length) has been described with no risk of posterior capsule tear.

So, a major advantage of FSL is less phaco power leading to minimal corneal endothelial damage and no risk of posterior capsule damage.

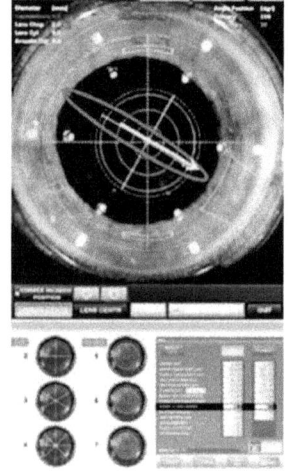

Pretreatment of nucleus with FS laser helps significantly reduce the amount of phacoemulsification energy delivered intraocularly which may translate into reduced endothelial cell loss that may be particularly advantageous in patients with hard cataracts.

Fig. 3.57.4: Lens fragmentation patterns and placement.

■ SURGICAL TECHNIQUE

Following laser application, the eye is undocked, and patient is shifted (ideally should not be moved) to main operation theater (OT). The incisions are opened with the spatula so-called as blade-free cataract surgery. The anterior capsule is separated along the precut groove and nuclear emulsification is completed with minimal phaco power. IOL implanted in bag and anterior chamber (AC) formed with balanced salt solution (BSS). No hydration of the incisions is required.

■ CONTRAINDICATIONS

Corneal pathologies, that hamper the applanation of the cornea or transmission of laser including descemetocele with impending corneal perforation, hypotony and glaucoma are relative contraindications.

Patients with poorly dilating pupil that is smaller than intended diameter for the capsulotomy, shallow AC depth resulting in inadequate clearance between the intended plane of capsulotomy and endothelium are important contraindications for capsulotomy using the FSL.

Any residual, recurrent, active ocular, or eyelid disease including recurrent corneal erosions is contraindication for the use of procedure.

This device is not intended for use in pediatric surgery.

COMPLICATIONS

Suction loss if occurs during capsulorhexis creation, the surgeon should revert to traditional phacoemulsification since the bubbles formed could obstruct further imaging.

An incomplete capsulotomy may be created, incidence being <1%. Also, radial tears can be difficult to identify. So, it is recommended that the surgeon should ensure that the capsule is free before proceeding with phacoemulsification.

Intraoperative miosis may be observed with FLACS owing to prostaglandin release during laser application. The use of non-steroidal anti-inflammatory drugs preoperatively has been recommended its occurrence.

CONCLUSION

Femtosecond cataract surgery is an advanced technology that can increase surgical precision and safety, though further studies are required to establish its cost effectiveness in routine cases. It is advantageous in cases with premium IOL implantation and in complex scenarios.

EDITOR'S PEARLS
- Advantages of FLACS include standardized corneal incisions, perfectly centered and round capsulorhexis, lens nucleus fragmentation even in eyes with hard cataracts.
- FLACS has particularly useful role in complicated scenarios such as subluxated cataract, white cataract, and posterior polar cataracts.

REFERENCES

1. Trikha S, Turnbull AM, Morris RJ, Anderson DF, Hossain P. The journey to femtosecond laser-assisted cataract surgery: new beginnings or false dawn? Eye. 2013;27(4):461-73.
2. Titiyal JS, Kaur M, Ramesh P, Shah P, Falera R, Bageshwar LMS, et al. Impact of clear corneal incision morphology on incision-site descemet membrane detachment in conventional and femtosecond laser-assisted phacoemulsification. Curr Eye Res. 2018;43(3):293-9.

3.58 What are the Indications for Nd:YAG Laser Capsulotomy in Posterior Capsule Opacification?

Suresh Kr Pandey
SuVi Eye Hospital and Research Centre, Kota
suvieye@gmail.com

INTRODUCTION

Posterior capsule opacification (PCO) (secondary cataract) remains the second most common cause of visual loss worldwide. Neodymium-doped yttrium-aluminum-garnet (Nd:YAG) laser capsulotomy is the simplest intraocular surgical procedure we perform as ophthalmologists. PCO remains the most common complication after cataract surgery. Advances in surgical techniques, intraocular lens (IOL) designs/biomaterials have been instrumental in bringing about a gradual and unnoticed decrease in the incidence of PCO. In pediatric cases, it can become very dense and cause as much or more vision loss as the original cataract.

Clinically PCO can be of two major types: Elschnig's pearls are a proliferation of cells on the outside of the capsule. This type of PCO can be several layers thick and develops months to years after cataract surgery. Elschnig's pearls can also appear along the margins of a previously performed Nd:YAG laser capsulotomy. A secondary cataract will also form from wrinkling of the lens capsule, either secondary to contraction of the myofibroblasts on the capsule or because of stretching of the capsule by IOL haptics.

Neodymium-doped yttrium-aluminum-garnet laser capsulotomy is usually performed in an ophthalmologist's office as an outpatient procedure. It is important to perform a careful complete ocular examination before proceeding Nd:YAG laser posterior capsulotomy to rule out other causes of decreased vision. Before beginning the capsulotomy, the patient is given an *informed consent* for the procedure. *The decision to perform Nd:YAG laser posterior capsulotomy procedure is based on the same criteria as the decision to have the original cataract surgery:*

- Clinically significant PCO causing vision problems and are affecting patient's work or lifestyle.
- Significant glare caused PCO by bright lights while driving.
- Inability to pass a vision test required for a driver's license or other employment.
- The difference in vision between two eyes is significant.
- Patients have another vision-threatening retinal disease, and it is important to have clear media to view retina.

Beside clinically significant PCO, Nd:YAG laser posterior capsulotomy is also indicated into create an opening in the posterior capsule, in some cases of capsule blockage syndrome. It is also indicated to create "relaxing" anterior capsulotomy in capsule phimosis. In cases of pigments deposition on the surface of IOL, Nd:YAG laser is also used to "sweep" pigments from IOL surface. The procedure is not necessary unless vision loss caused by clouding of the lens capsule is seriously affecting the person's vision and lifestyle.

EDITOR'S PEARLS

- Nd:YAG laser capsulotomy is minimally invasive and considered safer than conventional surgical procedure; however, one should perform a thorough evaluation before performing the laser.
- Complications such as IOL decentration and shift, IOL pitting, uveitis, IOP spike, macular edema, and retinal detachment have been associated with the procedure.

SUGGESTED READING

1. Apple DJ, Ram J, Foster A, Peng Q. Elimination of cataract blindness: a global perspective entering new millennium. Surv Ophthalmol. 2000;45(Suppl 1):S1-196.

3.59 An Update on IOL Power Calculation Formulas

Ashok Garg
Garg Eye Institute and Research Centre, Hisar
drashok_garg@yahoo.com

INTRODUCTION

Both classical and modern formulas have been used for the power calculation of regular intraocular lens (IOL) or accommodative IOL in aphakic, pseudophakic, and phakic eyes. The modern formulas include that of Haigis, Hoffer Q, Holladay, Olson, SRK/T, SRKI and II, and the more recent formulas by Odenthal et al. (the historical method), Aramberri et al.

(the double-K method), Rosa et al. (the R-factor method), and Jin et al. (the adjusted-K method). Most of these efforts were to improve the prediction of IOL-power by a better prediction of the postoperative anterior chamber depth (ACDpost) or the effective lens position (ELP) defined by ACDpre, corneal height and curvature, lens thickness, and axial length (AL). All the existing IOL-power calculations (except Lin's new formulas) are based on the classical vergence formulas (CVFs) of Fyodorov (1975), and Van der Heijde (1976) or their revision, the Hoffer Q formula (1981).

The CVFs assume a thin-lens (for both corneal and IOL) and are all based on a 2-optics system (the cornea and the IOL) which, strictly speaking, can only apply to aphakic eyes. For pseudophakic or phakic eyes, the 3-optics systems are much more complex and the oversimplified 2-optics CVF suffers the following possible drawbacks. It excludes the effects of IOL thickness and shape (configuration) and the role of natural lens or primary IOL. Major error may result from the use of the keratometric power (Kpre or Kpost) rather than the true postoperative corneal power which requires accurate measurement of both the anterior (r_1) and posterior radius (r_2). In addition, the CVF assumes paraxial ray and spherical surface for the cornea and IOL. Therefore it also excludes the effects due to corneal surface asphericity change after refractive surgery.

One of the major pitfalls of the existing IOL power calculations is the ignoring of individual true corneal power and using a mean-zero error for the postoperative refraction. Except the Haigis formula and the Lin Z^2-formula, all other optimization formulas are based on one-constant such as the surgeon factor, the A-constant, the ACDpost or the ELP. The mean-zero error might be the result of the balanced errors of short and long eyes. Therefore, the validity range of AL for various existing formulas under a linear empirical-fit could not justify their accuracy when they are applied to individual eyes. A true personalized IOL power prediction, in our opinion, should at least individualize the following parameters—the postoperative ELP, AL, corneal anterior and posterior surface, and the IOL types (or configurations).

In this chapter, I shall update the IOL formulas and address the critical issues covering four subjects:
1. IOL-power formulas
2. Corneal power after refractive surgery
3. Piggyback IOL power, and
4. Accommodating IOL (AIOL).

INTRAOCULAR LENS POWER FORMULAS

1. *Theoretical formulas:* All the theoretical formulas (except Lin's formulas) for IOL power are based on a two-lens systems, i.e., the cornea and the pseudophakic lens focusing images on the retina, where thin lens is also assumed. **Table 3.59.1** summarizes these formulas.
   a. Basic theoretical formulas: These include Colenbrander's, Fyodorov's, Van der Heijde's formula, and the Hoffer 1974-formula which yield approximately the same IOL powers. Binkhorst's formula yields 0.50 D stronger lens power.
   b. Modified theoretical formulas: These include Hoffer's 1983-formula, Shamma's fudged formula, and Binkhorst's adjusted formula. These formulas are modification of Colenbrander's formula.
   c. The modern formulas: These include formulas of Holladay I and II, Hoffer Q, SRK/T formula. The more recent formula of Haigis using 3-constant optimization for all ranges of eye length and IOL types. In Lin's new formulas presented in this chapter, the effective anterior chamber depth (ACD), corneal power, and IOL types are personalized.
2. *Regression formulas:* These formulas are derived empirically from retrospective computer analysis of data of patients who have undergone surgery before. The factors on which IOL power calculation depends are:

TABLE 3.59.1: For emmetropic intraocular lens (IOL) power calculations.

For calculation of IOL power in emmetropia:

Colenbrander's formula
$$P = \frac{1336}{L-C-0.05} - \frac{1336}{\frac{1336}{K} - C - 0.05}$$

Fyodorov's formula
$$P = \frac{1336 - LK}{(L-C)\frac{(1-CK)}{1336}}$$

Van der Heijde's formula
$$P = \frac{1336}{L-C} - \frac{1}{\frac{1}{K} - \frac{C}{1336}}$$

Binkhorst's formula
$$P = \frac{1336(4R\,L)}{(L-C)(4R-C)}$$

Lin's S-formula (I)
$$Z'P = \frac{1336}{(L-S)} - \frac{1336}{\frac{1336}{DC} - S}$$

Modified formulas for ametropia:

Shamma's fudged formula
$$P = \frac{1336}{L - 0.1(L-23) - C - 0.05} - \frac{1}{\frac{10125}{K} - \frac{C+0.05}{1336}}$$

Binkhorst's adjusted formula
$$P = \frac{1336(4R - L)}{(L-C)(4R-C)}$$

Hoffer's formula
$$P = \frac{1336}{L-C-0.05} - \frac{1336}{1336 - C - 0.05}$$
$$K + E$$

Lin's S-formula (II)
$$Z'P = \frac{1336}{(L-S)} - \frac{1336\ qE\ Pn}{\frac{1336}{DC} S}$$

$q = (1 + kP)/Z^2$

$Z = 1 - S\,(Dc/1336),\ Z' = 1 - p'(Pn/1336)$

a. *Axial length measurement:* This is the most important step in calculation of lens power. The IOL Master is a recent method using partial coherence interferometer (PCI) which gives high accuracy in measurement of AL. An error of 1 mm affects the postoperative refraction by 1.2–2.5 D approximately. It is measured in millimeters (mm).
b. *Corneal power:* It is measured either in diopters or in mm (radius of curvature). Keratometer measures the radius of curvature of the central part of anterior corneal surface (r_1) and given by $K = 337.5/r_1$. All the conventional formulas for corneal power (K_c) is given by **(Table 3.59.2):**

$$K_c = 1.114\,K - C$$

With C given by a mean value of 5.1 D, 5.5 D or 6.5 D to count for the mean posterior surface power. The Lin's formula using the personalized p–C = $41/r_1$ to count for the role of individual posterior corneal surface (r_2) which may deviate significantly from the commonly used mean value of 6.5 mm. As pointed out by Lin, each 1.0 D of corneal power would result in an error of about 1.3–1.6 D of IOL-power calculation.

c. *Postoperative ACD:* It is the least important factor in calculation of lens power. An error of 1 mm affects the postoperative refraction or IOL-power by approximately 0.6–2.5 D depending on the ocular conditions based on Lin's M-formula.

■ THE ESTIMATED INTRAOCULAR LENS POSITION (ELP)

The main part of highly accurate IOL power calculation is able to correctly predict the estimated IOL position (defined as ELP = d) for any given patient and IOL. Various formulas have been presented as follows:

SRK/T,
    d = A constant
Hoffer Q,
    d = pACD
Holladay I,
    d = Surgeon factor
Holladay II,
    d = ACD
Haigis,
    d = $a_0 + (a_1 \times ACD) + (a_2 \times AL)$
Lin,
    S = d + gT + Gp **(Table 3.59.3)**.

In actual practice, the two eyes with same AL and keratometric reading may have different lens power. This may be due to:

TABLE 3.59.2: Corneal power (Dc) calculation after refractive surgery.

1.	Clinical-history method	Dc = Kpre–RC, RC = Refractive correction of LASIK
2.	Contact lens method	Dc = B + P + Rw – Rno B = base curve; P = power of CL; Rw = Refractive error; Rno = bare refraction
3.	Shamma's method	Dc = 1.114 Kpost – 6.8
4.	Maloney topography method	Dc = 1.114 Ktopo – 5.5
5.	Koch method	Dc = 1.114 Ktopo – 6.1
6.	Shamma's refraction method	Dc = (1.114 Kpost – 6.8) – 0.23 (RC)
7.	Hoffer mean-value method	Dc = 337.5 $(1/r_1 + 1/r_2)/2$
8.	Lin Gaussian-optics i. ii.	Dc = 1.117 Kpost – $41/r_2$ Dc = $(377/r_1)[1 – 0.109 (r_1/r_2)]$
	where	r_1 = Cornea front surface radius (postoperative) r_2 = Cornea back surface radius (postoperative) Kpost = Postoperative keratometry Kpre = Preoperative keratometry

TABLE 3.59.3: Lin's formula for intraocular lens (IOL)-power in aphakia and phakia.

A.	2-optics aphakia/IOL:	
	Effective ACD:	$S = d + gT$
	Thin-IOL:	$d = ELP$ (for $T = 0$)
	Thick-IOL:	$g = 1/(1+Z''P1/P2)$
		$Z'' = 1 - T(P2/1336)$
B.	3-optics phakia/IOL	$S' = (d + gT) + Gp'$
		$p' = p + 2.4$ mm
		$G = 1/(1+Z'P/Pn)$
		$Z' = 1 - p'(Pn/1336)$
C.	Piggyback-IOL	$S' = (d + gT) + g'p'$
D.	IOL-power (the most generalized format for 3-optics system):	
		$Z'P = 1336 [1/X - 1/Y]-Pn - q'E$
		$X = L - S - 0.05$ mm
		$Y = 1336/Dc - S'$
		$q' = (1 + kP)/Z^2$
		$Z = 1 - S'(Dc/1336)$

Where:

d = Separation of cornea and IOL (or ELP, ACD)

p = Separation of piggyback and primary IOL, or IOL and natural lens

T = Thickness of piggyback-IOL

P = IOL power (thin lens), or P1/P2 for front/back power (thick-lens)

Pn = Power of natural lens (or primary-IOL)

Dc = Corneal power

E = Refractive error to be corrected (on corneal plane)

(g, G) = Geometry factor for (thick-IOL, subsystem)

- Effective (or optical) lens position (S) which may be different from the ELP (or d)
- Individual geometry of lens types
- Presence of the natural lens or the primary-IOL.

Hoffer Q formula is best for short eyes. Holladay for long eyes and SRK/T is best for very long eyes. Overall SRK/T is probably the most accurate in majority of cases. It, however, ignores the role of IOL thickness and types and only good for 2-optics aphakic-IOL like others. The Lin's formula is good for all AL and IOL types.

ACCURACY OF INTRAOCULAR LENS POWER CALCULATION

In spite of recent advances in technology, there is no single method to accurately determine the net central power of the postrefractive surgery of eyes. The current method available is limited by lack of clinical experience on large scale and by the theoretic nature of all the calculation methods.

The factors, which significantly affect the accuracy of IOL power calculations, are:
1. The error in preoperative biometry with regard to the difference between post- and preoperative AL measurements

2. The position of the implantation of IOL
3. The style of IOL
4. The preoperative corneal astigmatism
5. Surgically-induced corneal astigmatism
6. The postoperative astigmatism
7. The true corneal power [post-LASIK (laser in situ keratomileusis)]
8. The formulas used to find IOL-power
9. Assumption of thin lens or 2-optics system.

■ THE NEW GENERATION FORMULAS

Formulas to be detailed in the following include: SRK (I, II), SRK/T, Hoffer Q, Holladay (I, II), Olson and the more recently formulas of Haigis d-formula, and Lin's S-formula.

1. *SRK formula:*
   a. *SRK I formula:* It is basic regression formula. It is given by:
   $P = A - 0.9 K - 2.5 L$
   where P = IOL power for emmetropia
   K = Keratometric power reading
   A = A constant
   L = Axial length (in mm).
   b. *SRK II formula:* In this formula, the A constant is adjusted to different AL ranges. It is given by:
   $P = A1 - 0.9 K - 2.5 L$
   A1 = Adjusted constant
   A1 = A + 3, if axial length (L) <20 mm
   A1 = A + 2, if L = 20–21 mm
   A1 = A + 1, if L = 21–22 mm
   A1 = A, if L = 22–24.5 mm
   A1 = A – 0.5, if L >24.5 mm.
   c. *SRK/T formula:* Regression formula for ACD (or ELP) is used to calculate IOL-power based on Fyodorov formula. This formula is more accurate than SRK I and II.
   $$ACDpost = ACD - 3.336 + \text{Corneal height (H)}$$
   where ACD is related to the manufacturer's A-constant by:
   $ACD = 0.62467 A - 68.747$.
2. *Hoffer Q formula:* The Hoffer Q formula was published in 1993 (Hoffer, 1993) and gives the IOL-power:
   $P = f(A, K, R_x, pACD)$
   which is a function of:
   A: Axial length
   K: Average corneal refractive power (K-reading)
   R_x: Refraction
   pACD: Personalized ACD (ACD – constant)

   Likewise, the Hoffer Q refractive error R_x:
   $R_x = f(A, K, P, pACD)$, which depends on A, K, P, and pACD.
   For the calculations, K = 337.5 divided by the average radius of curvature the cornea.
   The personalized ACD (pACD) is set equal to the manufacturer's ACD-constant, if the calculation was selected to be based on the ACD-constant. In case the A-constant was chosen, pACD is derived from the A-constant (Hoffer, 1998) according to (Holladay et al. 1988):
   pACD = ACD–const = 0.58357 × A-const – 63.896.
3. *Holladay formulas:* The components of the three-part Holladay system are:
   a. Holladay (I) formula:
      i. Data screening criteria to identify improbable AL and keratometric measurement.

ii. The modified theoretical formula, which predicts the effective position of the IOL based on the AL and the average corneal curvature.
iii. Personalized surgeon factor (PSF) that adjusts for any consistent bias on surgeon from any source. It is advance method, which requires patient refractions.
   The initial formula uses the "Basic Surgeon Factor". It can be calculated from the A-constant provided by lens manufacturer.
   b. Holladay (II) formula: The IOL-power is calculated based on the Binkhorst formula as in the Holladay I.
4. *Olson formula:* Olson proposed his 2003 regression formula for the predicted ACDpost as follows:
$$ACDpost = ACDmean + 0.12H + 0.33 ACDpre + 0.3T' + 0.1L - 5.18$$
Where H is the corneal height, T' is the natural lens thickness. This formula, however, can only apply to phakic eyes. For aphakic or pseudophakic eyes, the coefficients will change.
5. *Haigis formula:* It uses three constants to set both the position and shape of a power prediction curve. The IOL calculation according to Haigis is based on the elementary IOL formula for thin lenses.
$$d = d = a_0 + (a_1 \times ACD) + (a_2 \times AL)$$
Where
d = Effective (or optical) lens position
ACD = Measured ACD of the eye
AL = Axial length of the eye.
a_0 constant = Same as lens constants for the different formulas given before
a_1 constant = Tied to ACD
a_2 constant = Measured AL.
Thus the value ford is determined by a function rather than a single number.
   The a_0, a_1, and a_2 constants are derived by multivariable regression analysis. The Haigis formula IOL constants will appear different than normal as they interact with the ACD and the AL.
   The conventional optimization based on one-constant (A-constant, surgeon's factor, ACD) which could only "parallel shift" the calculated curve to fit the measured data for a predicted mean zero error. Therefore, the validation range of the AL is limited, where improvement for long eye results more errors for short eye, and vice versa. For example, SRK/T is accurate for long eye (L >26 mm), but not for very short eye (L <22 mm) which requires the Hoffer formula. Haigis 3-constant optimization allows the curve-fit by both parallel shift and rotation of the curve such that it covers wider range of AL. However, the above Haigis formula also assumed thin-IOL and excludes the role of IOL configurations for different IOL types.
6. *Lin's S-formula:* Based on a generalized effective ACD ("S") derived from Gaussian optics in thick-lens for 2-optics and 3-optics system valid for all ranges of AL and IOL types. It also includes the effects due to natural lens and primary-IOL which are totally neglected in all the other formulas presented in above A to E. An effective (or optical) ACD is introduced as S given by, for the case of thick IOL in aphakic eye:

$S = ELP + gT$,	(1.a)
$g = 1/[1 + Z'' (P1/P2)]$	(1.b)
$Z'' = 1 - T (P2/1336)$	(1.c)

Where T is the IOL thickness, and the geometry factor (g) is determined by the ratio of the IOL front and back surface power P1/P2. Note that g could be positive (for P1/P2 >0) or negative (P1/P2 <0). Therefore "S" could be myopic or hyperopic shifted. Other formulas for "S" are summarized in **Table 3.59.3** for both phakic and piggyback IOL.

■ INTRAOCULAR LENS POWER IN APHAKIC EYE

This is a simple 2-optics system consisting of the cornea and IOL (with natural lens removed). The IOL-power calculation based on S and the true corneal power (Dc) is also developed by Lin as follows:

$$P = 1336/X - 1336/Y - qE, \quad (2.a)$$
$$X = L - S + 0.05 \quad (2.b)$$
$$Y = 1336/Dc - S \quad (2.c)$$

where $q = (1 + kP)/Z^2$ is a nonlinear term, with k about 0.003 and $Z = 1-S(Dc/1336)$. E is the remaining refractive error after IOL implant. The above Lin's new formula contributes two improvements—the S function, defined by Eq. (1) to include the IOL configuration and the true corneal power calculated by:

$$Dc = 1.117K - 41/r_2, \quad (3)$$

In which the true corneal power after refractive surgery is personalized by its measured front and back surface radius (r_1 and r_2). The K-reading is further defined as $K = 337.5/r_1$. Because that both S and Dc are personalized, accurate IOL power may be calculated for individual cases without the use of "fudge factors" to fit for mean zero error.

The individual effective ACD (the "S") may be calculated from Eq. (1) for a given function of f (P, L, Dc, E) by solving a quadratic equation of S, similar to the d-function of Haigis. The 3-constant optimization such as Haigis, but using S rather than d, allows us to obtain the minimal mean error not only for all ranges of axial length (L), but also for all IOL types via the g-factor in Eq. (1).

INTRAOCULAR LENS POWER IN PHAKIA AND PIGGYBACK INTRAOCULAR LENS

For phakic IOL or piggyback IOL, the IOL power calculations involve with a 3-optics system which has been recently formulated by Lin by generalizing the Eq. (2) of 2-optics (aphakic-IOL) as follows:

$$Z'P = 1336/X - 1336/Y - q'E - Pn \quad (4)$$

Which has the following revisions to count for the effects from the presence of the natural lens or the primary IOL (having a power Pn) and the separation between the cornea and IOL (ACD or ELP); and IOL and natural lens or primary-IOL (p).

1. A reduction factor $Z' = 1-p'$ (Pn/1336), with $p' = p + 2.4$ mm, is introduced and has a value of $Z' = 0.95$, for $p' = 6.0$ mm for a typical phakic-IOL implanted in front of a natural lens power of 21 D and separated by $p = 1.0$ mm or $p' = 1.0 + 2.4 = 3.4$ mm. In comparison, Z' is about 0.99 for the case of piggyback IOL (with $p' = p = 1.0$ mm). Therefore a reduction of about 5% and 1% is expected in the IOL-power term (Z'P).
2. A new $S' = S + Gp'$ is introduced, with a system geometry factor given by:

$$G = 1/[1 + Z'(P/Pn)] \quad (5)$$

Where P and Pn are the IOL-power and the natural lens (or primary-IOL) power, respectively. The above system geometry factor (G) may be compared to the IOL geometry factor given by $g = 1/[1 + Z''(P1/P2)]$, with $Z'' = 1-T(P2/1336)$ and for thick-IOL case $S = ACD + gT$. Therefore $S' = ACD + gT + Gp'$, for the general case of thick-IOL implanted in phakic (or primary-IOL) eye.
3. A new nonlinear term q' is introduced and given by:

$$q' = (1 + kP)/Za^2 \quad (6.a)$$
$$Za = 1-S' (Dc/1336) \quad (6.b)$$

Which reduces to the 2-optics (aphakia) $q' = q$, when $p' = 0$, $S' = S$, and $Z' = Z$ as expected. The new 3-optics Za may be further related to the Z in 2-optics aphakic-IOL by:

$$Za = Z - Gp' (Dc/1336) \quad (7)$$

Where the second term is due to the shifted distance of the second principal plane of the IOL-natural lens or piggyback-IOL and primary-IOL subsystem.

4. Conversion function (CF), one may define Zeff derived from $Zeff^2 = Z'Za$ to obtain:

$$Zeff = 1 - Seff (Dc/1336) \quad (8.a)$$
$$Seff = S + 0.5p' (Pn/Dc) \quad (8.b)$$

Where Seff is defined as the shifted S by an amount proportional to p' and the power ratio (Pn/Dc) of the natural lens or primary-IOL(Pn) and the cornea (Dc). For typical values of p' = 3.0 mm, Pn = 20 D, Dc = 43 D, one obtains Seff = S + 0.7 mm. This 0.7 mm shift may result in IOL-power difference about $(0.7/S)^2$ or about 3–5%, for S = 3–4 mm. Above Eq. (8) allows us to calculate a conversion function (CF), defined by:

$$CF = -(dE/dP)$$

Which may be derived from the derivative of Eq. (4) and using Eq. (8) as follows:

$$CF = (1 - 2k'E)Zeff^2 \quad (9)$$

Therefore, the CF in 3-optics is lower due to the natural lens (or primary IOL) about 5–10% less than 2-optics formula. In other words, the conventional 2-optics formulas overestimate the IOL-power when it is implanted in phakia or pseudophakia, but simplified as aphakia.

▪ PIGGYBACK INTRAOCULAR LENS POWER

Given the CF, the piggyback IOL power to correct a residual ametropia power (E), on the corneal plane (not spectacle plane), may be calculated by:

$$P = E/CF \quad (10)$$

Where CF is given by Eq. (9) in general. Comparison of various formulas is shown in **Table 3.59.4**. Several critical issues on the previous formulas may be addressed as follows:
- All the formulas, except Lin's, are based on the spectacle power (E) converted to IOL-power (P). The Es of Lin is defined as E on the corneal plane.
- Formulas of Sanders–Kraff and Feiz–Mannis are comparable. However, both are based on a mean value of CF = 0.7 which may be valid only for average clinical data. Individual CF value could be 10–20% deviate from this mean value and would require Lin's formula.
- Gills formula is only good for hyperopia and it is also based on average case.
- Shamma's formula might be good for low IOL power, say 5.0 D or less. It includes the dependence of ACD (or the A-constant). However, it does not include the effects due to corneal power or individual IOL types. It also assumes thin IOL and a 2-optics system or aphakic IOL.
- Holladay II based on Binkhorst uses AL, K, ACD, LT, CD, preoperative R_x, and age to calculate the ELP and needs numerical method versus the analytic formula of Lin which also revises ELP by S.
- Lin's new formula based on Gaussian optics might be the only one which includes most of the effects due to individual ocular parameter and IOL types, where the effective ACD (S, or Seff) has been rigorously defined for various systems of aphakic, aphakic or pseudophakic and for both thin and thick IOL. The roles of natural lens or primary-IOL are also included in the new formula **(Table 3.59.4)**.

▪ ACCOMMODATING INTRAOCULAR LENS

The accommodating rate function (M) defined as the accommodation amplitude increase per 1.0 mm forward movement of a plus AIOL may be expressed by the Lin's M-formula:

$$M = (Z/1336)P[2Dc + ZZ'P] \quad (11)$$

Above formula is a general form for both phakia and aphakia and also for dual-optics AIOL. For the thick-IOL single-optics case, the M value is higher for convex-concave IOL configuration (having front and back surface power of P1 and P2) which has higher P1 for a given P1 + P2, when P2 <0 (concave). Depending on ocular conditions, M ranges from 0.5 D/mm to 2.5 D/mm for AIOL-power of 10–20 D.

TABLE 3.59.4: Piggyback intraocular lens (IOL)-power (P) formulas for residual ametropia error.

1.	Sanders and Kraff (1980) based on empirical data of over 2,500 IOL lens	$P = E/0.67 = 1.49E$
2.	Feiz and Mannis (2001)	$P = E/0.7 = 1.43E$
3.	Holladay II (1993) based on Hoffer (1981),	$P = (IOL)1 - (IOL)2$
		$(IOL)j = 1336/[1336/Kj - ELP]$
	Colenbrander (1973)	Kj ($j = 1,2$), for pre- and postoperative corneal power
	For plus IOL,	$P(+) = 1.5E,$
	For minus IOL,	$P(-) = 1.0E;$
		E is the postoperative refractive error at spectacle plane
4.	Shammas (2001)	$P = (E/a)/(138.3 - A) - 0.5$
	where	
	$a = 0.03$ for plus IOL,	
	$a = 0.04$ for minus IOL.	
	A = A-constant = $(ACD + 63.896)/0.5836$	
5.	Gills (1996) only for hyperopic correction	$P(+) = 1.4E + 1.0$
6.	Lin (2005)	$P = Ec/(CF) = (1.25 - 1.7) Ec$
	The Z^2-formula*	$CF = (1 - 2kE)(Ec/Z^2)$
	For both plus and minus IOL.	$Z = 1 - S(Dc/1336)$
		Typical value: $CF = (0.6$ to $-0.8)$

Where:

Dc is the corneal power and k is a nonlinear term.

S is the effective (optical) lens position, $S = ELP + gT + Gp'$

E(Ec) is the refractive error on the spectacle (corneal) plane and may be related by another conversion factor $Ec = E/Zs^2$, with $Zs = 1 - 0.012E$.

*For simplified 2-optics system, see Eq. (9) in the text and **Table 3.59.3** for 3-optics system.

■ CONCLUSION

The existing IOL-power (except Lin's) based on 2-optics system could only apply to aphakia. For phakia or piggyback IOL, a 3-optics system based on Gaussian optics is required.

The Lin's new formulas provide more accurate calculations for both phakia and aphakia presented by:
- The S-formula (to include IOL thickness and types)
- The Seff-formula (to include the role of natural lens and primary-IOL)
- The personalized r_2-formula (including corneal posterior surface power post-LASIK)
- The M-formula (for AIOL efficiency)
- The Z^2-formula (for conversion of IOL-power in 3-optics system of phakia or piggyback IOL).

■ SUGGESTED READING

1. Atchison DA, Smith G. Optics of the Human Eye. Woburn, MA: Butterworth-Heinemann; 2000; pp. 14-16, 143-7, 160-2.

> *"Education is not the learning of facts, but the training of the mind to think"*
>
> —**Albert Einstein**

SECTION 4

Glaucoma

Editor: Krishnadas

- 4.1 Acute Angle-closure Glaucoma 228
  Devindra Sood, Aanchal Rathore
- 4.2 Aqueous Misdirection Syndrome 231
  Kavita Prasad, George V Puthuran
- 4.3 Bleb Fibrosis 234
  L Vijaya
- 4.4 Bleb Leaks 236
  Tanuj Dada, Shibal Bhartiya, Neha Midha
- 4.5 Blebitis 238
  SS Pandav
- 4.6 Traumatic Glaucoma 240
  Rengaraj Venkatesh
- 4.7 Glaucoma Following Vitreoretinal Surgical Procedures 243
  Ganesh Raman, Parthasarathy Sathyan
- 4.8 Glaucoma Following Cataract Surgery 246
  R Ramakrishnan
- 4.9 Postoperative Ocular Hypotony 252
  JC Das
- 4.10 Neovascular Glaucoma 256
  Sushmita Kaushik, Parul Ichhpujani
- 4.11 Overfunctioning Blebs 259
  Murali Ariga, Sangeetha R, Nishanth M
- 4.12 Chronic Primary Angle-closure Glaucoma 262
  Vinay Nangia
- 4.13 Primary Congenital Glaucoma 264
  Sapna Sinha, R Krishnadas
- 4.14 Pseudoexfoliation Syndrome/ Exfoliative Glaucoma 267
  Prashanth R, Krishnadas SR
- 4.15 Steroid-induced Glaucoma 270
  Prashanth R, Krishnadas SR
- 4.16 Visual Field Defects in Glaucoma 273
  Murali Ariga, Malarchelvi Palani, Nivean Madhivanan
- 4.17 Trabeculectomy 279
  Swati Upadhyaya
- 4.18 Glaucoma Drainage Implants 289
  Swati Upadhyaya
- 4.19 Minimally Invasive Glaucoma Surgery 297
  Swati Upadhyaya

4.1 Acute Angle-closure Glaucoma

Synonym: Acute Angle-closure Crisis

Devindra Sood
Glaucoma Service, Krishna Netralaya, Gurugram
glaucomacentre@yahoo.com

Aanchal Rathore
Glaucoma Service, Alakh Nayan Mandir Eye Institute, Udaipur
aanchalrathore@gmail.com

■ DEFINITION

It is a rapid increase in intraocular pressure (IOP) from abrupt blockage of trabecular meshwork by peripheral iris because of a pupillary block. Since most episodes of acute angle-closure glaucoma present acutely with no evidence of characteristic glaucomatous optic nerve damage, episodes of acute rise in eye pressure is often referred to as acute angle-closure crisis rather than glaucoma.

■ CHARACTERISTIC SIGNS AND SYMPTOMS

Symptoms

Sudden onset of pain or aching on side of affected eye accompanied by blurred vision, colored halos, redness and occasionally by nausea, vomiting, and sweating. Pain is usually in trigeminal distribution and referred to the eye, orbit or teeth.

Signs

Diminished vision, ciliary congestion, corneal edema, shallow anterior chamber, anterior chamber flare and cells, moderately dilated and sluggishly reactive pupil, markedly elevated IOP, closed angles on gonioscopy and hyperemic optic disks. Features suggestive of previous episodes of acute angle closure include posterior synechiae, peripheral anterior synechiae, glaucomflecken, sector or generalized iris atrophy, pupillary sphincter atrophy, optic nerve cupping or pallor, and visual field defects. Moderate amount of flare and anterior chamber cells and inflammation, and posterior synechiae are not uncommon. Keratic precipitates (KP) are conspicuous by their absence. Presence of KP suggests anterior uveitis rather than acute angle-closure glaucoma. In addition, a dilated pupil is a typical sign of acute angle closure, in contrast to a small, miotic pupil which characterizes uveitis.

If corneal edema precludes examination, topical glycerin or 5% NaCl may be used for clarity.

■ FELLOW EYE: EXAMINATION MANDATORY AND OFTEN CONFIRMS DIAGNOSIS

- Shallow anterior chamber.
- *Gonioscopy:* Critically narrow, occludable anterior chamber angles with iridocorneal contact and appositional angle closure.
- *Ultrasound biomicroscope (UBM):* It can help in identifying underlying mechanism, but not mandatory.
- *Visual field examination:* In view of emergency situation, it is practically not feasible to perform perimetric examination.

■ DIAGNOSIS

It is based on symptoms and signs (on slit lamp examination) with raised IOP (preferably by applanation tonometry) and iridocorneal contact on gonioscopy. Examination of unaffected fellow eye for shallow anterior chamber and gonioscopy for confirmation of status of angle outflow status is mandatory.

■ DIFFERENTIAL DIAGNOSIS
- *Uveitic glaucoma:* Characterized by anterior chamber flare, cells and KP, deep anterior chamber with open angles on gonioscopy (focal PAS in inferior angle may be present) and small irregular pupil with posterior synechiae.
- *Posner–Schlossman syndrome:* Minimal reaction, occasional small KP around inferior cornea, deep anterior chamber with open angles on gonioscopy.
- *Neovascular glaucoma:* Acute rise in IOP from closure of angle from contracting fibrovascular membrane, evident rubeosis on iris/angle. It is often useful to identify cause for ischemia and examine the other eye.
- *Malignant glaucoma:* Associated with misdirection of aqueous into anterior chamber with the lens iris diaphragm pushed forward. Both central and peripheral anterior chambers are extremely shallow, in the presence of a patent iridectomy.
- *Dislocation of natural crystalline lens:* It can be associated from trauma or systemic associations: Marfan syndrome, homocystinuria, Weill–Marchesani syndrome, and acquired syphilis. Identifying dislocated/subluxated lens is the key factor.
- *Steroid-induced glaucoma:* Acute rise in IOP seen typically in high responders. Likely to be bilateral and anterior chamber is usually deep with history of steroid usage.
- *Lens-induced glaucoma:* Phacomorphic glaucoma in particular presents with features identical to acute angle-closure glaucoma with pain and ocular congestion, corneal epithelial edema, shallow anterior chamber and dilated, fixed pupils. A hypermature, swollen cataract lens is characteristic. Rarely, an immature but intumescent lens presents as acute angle-closure glaucoma either spontaneously or following penetrating trauma. A hypermature leaking Morgagnian cataract can also present with acute onset of glaucoma mimicking acute angle closure. The anterior chamber, however, is very deep in these eyes.

■ TREATMENT
Immediate medical therapy is indicated to reverse acute angle closure and minimize damage to optic nerve and trabecular meshwork.
- Protection of the fellow eye with miotic therapy.
- Definitive treatment is laser iridotomy in both eyes.
- Management of long-term sequelae of acute angle closure.

■ MEDICAL MANAGEMENT
A combination of beta blockers, alpha agonists, topical or oral acetazolamide and hyperosmotics is initially recommended to effect reduction of intraocular pressures although the primary aim of therapy is to produce miosis and pull the peripheral iris away from apposition to the trabecular meshwork. This is achieved by use of miotics such as pilocarpine, but when the intraocular pressures are very high, the iris sphincter may be unresponsive to the miotics. Initial treatment with aqueous suppressants and hyperosmotics reduce the IOP to a level which permit pupillary constriction by miotics. Primary treatment with miotics may be ineffective in reversing acute angle closure, especially when IOP is very high, and exceed the diastolic pressures in the iris vasculature. Very high IOP causes iris ischemia and papillary sphincter is unresponsive to the action of miotics **(Table 4.1.1)**.

■ FOLLOW-UP
Reassess half hourly.
Additional measures to break the attack include:
- Patient can lie supine to facilitate lens iris diaphragm moving back.

TABLE 4.1.1: Drugs and their doses.

Drug	Dose and administration	Comments
Beta blockers (timolol or levobunolol)	0.5%, twice a day	Use in absence of systemic contraindication
Pilocarpine	1% or 2% three/four times a day	Constricts pupil, pulls peripheral iris away from trabecular meshwork. Helps break attack. Excess use can aggravate pupillary block and cause systemic toxicity
Brimonidine	0.15–2%, twice a day	
Systemic acetazolamide	250 mg three to four times a day	Rule out relevant contraindication
Syrup glycerol	1–1.5 g/kg. One stat and then three times a day	Rule out relevant contraindication in diabetics, 45% isosorbide may be substituted
I/V mannitol	1.5–2 g/kg 60–90 drops/minute	Rule out relevant contraindication. Dehydrate vitreous and allow lens iris diaphragm to shift posteriorly. Most effective means to control acute angle closure
Steroid drops	3–4 times/day	Reduce inflammation
Analgesics and antiemetics as required.		

- *Mechanical compression:* Digital massage/depressing anesthetized central corneal with moistened cotton applicator.
- Laser peripheral iridoplasty (rarely required).
- Paracentesis may be considered to relieve pain in acute angle closure unresolved by conservative treatment.

Lasers

When IOP is normalized/peripheral chamber, deep Nd:YAG laser iridotomy can be done which is the definitive treatment to address relative pupillary block. It may take more than one sitting as the iris is usually boggy from inflammation.

Surgery is considered only if medication and laser iridotomy have had no effect or laser is unable to penetrate, surgical iridectomy is preferred. If peripheral anterior synechiae are formed from prolonged acute angle closure, trabeculectomy may be considered.

Note: It is mandatory to treat the unaffected eye with a laser iridotomy.

■ SUGGESTED READING

1. Sood D. Advances in the Management of Primary Adult Glaucoma, CME Series No: 10. New Delhi: All India Ophthalmological Society, 2004. pp. 41-68.

4.2 Aqueous Misdirection Syndrome

Synonyms: *Malignant Glaucoma, Ciliary Block Glaucoma, Direct Lens Block Angle Closure, Ciliolenticular Block Glaucoma, Cilio-Vitreo-Lenticular Block Glaucoma, Posterior Aqueous Diversion Syndrome*

Kavita Prasad, George V Puthuran
Aravind Eye Hospital, Madurai
george@arvind.org

■ DEFINITION

Aqueous misdirection syndrome (AMS) is a secondary angle-closure glaucoma characterized by shallowing or flattening of the central and peripheral anterior chambers, elevation of the intraocular pressure (IOP) and aggravation by miotics but frequent relief with cycloplegic-mydriatic therapy, with a patent iridotomy and the absence of suprachoroidal fluid or blood.

■ MECHANISM

The commonly accepted theory of aqueous misdirection states that the aqueous is secreted and sequestered in the vitreous cavity, pushing the lens, hyaloid face and the iris forward collapsing the anterior chamber, and blocking the trabecular outflow. Following surgery in anatomically predisposed eyes, the ciliary processes rotate forward sealing the posterior zonules and the lens (cilio-vitreo-lenticular block) allowing aqueous to be secreted into the vitreous in pockets and behind the detached vitreous body. The hyaloid moves forward in contact with ciliary processes, iris or lens and it becomes impermeable to aqueous. Pressure in the vitreous increases and compacts the vitreous which further increases resistance to fluid flow.

Factors contributing to aqueous misdirection include:
- Swelling of ciliary processes
- Angle closure
- Hyperopic eyes
- Vitreous inflammation
- Miotic use
- Slack zonules seen in exfoliation syndrome
- Wound leak following intraocular surgery

■ CLINICAL FEATURES

The usual presentation is that of a postoperative patient following glaucoma filtration surgery, combined glaucoma surgery or cataract surgery presenting with *axial shallowing* of the anterior chamber, *elevated IOP* and the presence of a *patent iridectomy/iridotomy*. It may also occur following suturelysis, bleb needling, and discontinuation of postoperative cycloplegics.

Though elevation of IOP >21 mm Hg is classically seen in aqueous misdirection syndrome, IOP may be normal or even low, especially if associated with overfiltration, which may mask the increased IOP effect which otherwise should have occurred due to secondary angle closure. In fact, a good rule is that a flat or shallow anterior chamber associated with IOP in the teens after filtration surgery is malignant glaucoma (MG) until proven otherwise. There is an absence of other causes of chamber shallowing such as suprachoroidal hemorrhage or choroidal effusion or less common causes including gross retinal detachment or other causes acting as a mass and pushing the lens–iris diaphragm.

■ DIFFERENTIAL DIAGNOSIS

- *Pupillary block glaucoma:* This is the chief differential diagnosis. These cases generally tend to have a relatively deeper central anterior chamber depth with peripheral shallowing and an elevated IOP. Characteristic iris bombe is usually apparent. Pupillary block is relieved by a patent iridectomy/laser iridotomy.
- *Suprachoroidal hemorrhage:* It leads to axial shallowing with accompanying severe, acute pain; choroidal elevation on fundus examination or ultrasound; high IOP acutely which usually subsides within 12-24 hours.
- *Choroidal effusion:* Eye is usually hypotonous with peripheral anterior chamber shallowing. Axial shallowing is usually less prominent but may progress as the effusion enlarges. Pain is unusual and the choroidal effusion is generally visible by fundus examination or ultrasound.

Secondary postoperative angle closure following vitreoretinal surgery may occur in which the axial depth may be reduced (especially after scleral buckling procedures). However, this reduction in depth is only moderate and not progressive in nature. They may have choroidal effusion in addition.

■ WORK-UP

Aqueous misdirection syndrome is a diagnosis of exclusion. It can occur at any time in the postoperative period from days to weeks to months.

Evaluate and assess the filtering bleb and any incisional wound for evidence of leak.

Assess patency and function of peripheral iridectomy/iridotomy and exclude role of any pupillary block component.

Look for axial depth of anterior chamber and contour of iris on slit lamp.

Gonioscopy should be performed to confirm closure of the angle, assess the contour of the iris as well as to look for retroiridal abnormalities.

Indirect ophthalmoscopy should be performed to rule out any posterior segment pathology.

Ultrasound [A scan, B scan as well as ultrasound biomicroscope (UBM)] aids in the confirmation of the diagnosis.

■ MANAGEMENT

The approach to the management in these cases must be methodical.
- Rule out choroidal hemorrhage or effusion → fundus examination and/or ultrasound.
- Rule out overfiltration or wound leak → Seidel test; oversized contact lens, pressure patch or Simmons shell in hypotonous eyes.
- Rule out pupillary block → Nd:YAG laser iridotomy if functional iridotomy not present.

Medical Therapy

It is usually successful in around 50% of cases.
- *Mydriatic:* Cycloplegic—atropine 1% qid, phenylephrine 2.5-10% qid. They tighten the zonules, pull the lens-iris diaphragm, and move the ciliary body ring outward, away from the hyaloid.
- *Aqueous suppressants:* Timolol 0.5% bid/or brimonidine 0.15% tid/or acetazolamide 250 mg PO qid. These agents decrease aqueous production and thus decrease the amount of aqueous that is misdirected into the vitreous cavity.
- *Osmotics:* Glycerine 50% or isosorbide 45% (1-1.5 g/kg) PO q12h or intravenous mannitol 20% (1-1.5 g/kg) q12h. These agents dehydrate the vitreous volume and pressure.
- *Steroids:* Prednisolone acetate 1% qid. Prevents peripheral anterior synechiae (PAS) formation and permanent adhesions of hyaloid to the ciliary body.

Medical therapy should be continued until the anterior chamber forms and IOP normalizes. Medications are gradually withdrawn over several days, as there is a significant risk of recurrence following discontinuation of cycloplegics.

In cases where laser or surgical therapy has been ineffective, continued treatment with atropine 1% daily is recommended.

Surgical Management

Laser Therapy

- Hyaloidotomy with Nd:YAG laser in aphakic or pseudophakic patients should be performed concomitantly with medical therapy in patients who have had cataract surgery. Disruption of the anterior hyaloid face allows flow of misdirected aqueous from posterior to anterior segment. Care must be taken to perform the hyaloidotomy peripheral to the lens optic.
- Direct argon laser photocoagulation of ciliary processes can be tried. It presumably works by causing laser shrinkage of ciliary processes thus relieving ciliohyaloidal block of anterior flow of aqueous humor.
- Cyclodestructive procedures (cyclocryotherapy and cyclophotocoagulation) have been reported as treatment for aqueous misdirection.

Surgical vitrectomy is essential to disrupt the hyaloid face and confirm that the normal anterior chamber depth has been restored at the end of the surgery. In phakic eyes, anterior vitreous is difficult to remove without damaging the lens; therefore, treatment is less likely to succeed. Vitrectomy is often combined with lens extraction to deepen anterior chamber and reverse aqueous misdirection.

FOLLOW-UP

Periodical evaluation and assessment to ensure reversal of aqueous misdirection.

PREVENTION

- Trabeculectomy surgery modification, including releasable sutures, the use of viscoelastics during surgery, and postoperative use of atropine has been proposed to prevent malignant glaucoma. Tight wound closure to prevent wound leak, shallow chambers, and hypotony is crucial to prevent aqueous misdirection in eyes at risk.
- Releasable suture removal or laser suture lysis following glaucoma filtering surgery need to be performed cautiously to prevent overfiltration or wound leak which predisposes to aqueous misdirection. Not more than one suture is to be released or lysed at any given time. Any wound leak or shallow chamber following suture release needs to be treated aggressively, if necessary with additional sutures in the operating room.
- The fellow eye is at increased risk of developing malignant glaucoma postoperatively. Hyperopic eyes and eyes with short axial length also are at increased risk. Prophylactic laser iridotomy is recommended in cases with evidence of chronic angle closure or an occludable angle, preferably with avoidance of the use of miotics.

If surgery in the fellow eye is required, preoperative cycloplegics and osmotic agents must be used, with close observation postoperatively for the development of aqueous misdirection. Prophylactic vitrectomy with zonulo-hyaloido-iridectomy or vitrectomy with posterior tube shunt placement can be done.

PROGNOSIS

Prognosis depends on the length and the severity of the attack. In patients with relatively healthy optic nerves, the prognosis can be good if the attack is abated and IOP is controlled.

SUGGESTED READING

1. Ian C, Joel S, David E. The malignant glaucoma syndromes. In: Malik K, Schuman MD, Joel S (Eds). Chandler and Grant's Glaucoma, 5th edition. Thorofare, NJ, USA: Slack Incorporated; 2013, pp. 289-304.

4.3 Bleb Fibrosis

L Vijaya
Sankara Nethralaya, Chennai
drlv@snmail.org

■ DEFINITION
Bleb fibrosis is associated with inadequate intraocular pressure (IOP) control with obstruction to aqueous outflow. Subconjunctival and episcleral scarring account for the majority of late failure of bleb function that characterize bleb fibrosis. Gonioscopy will reveal patent sclerostomy. Healing response of the individual may be responsible for bleb fibrosis. Several factors have been identified as predisposing factors for bleb fibrosis. These include younger age, history of multiple ocular surgeries, uveitis, trauma, and neovascular glaucoma. Histologically early bleb fibrosis is characterized by hypercellular response with active fibroblasts; whereas late bleb fibrosis shows features of "microkeloid" appearance with collagen and few cells. The overlying conjunctiva will be normal. Failed or fibrosed filtering blebs have dense and thick collagenous tissue with abundant collagen, few fibroblasts, and blood vessels.

■ DIFFERENTIAL DIAGNOSIS
Early bleb fibrosis should be differentiated from other causes of bleb failure such as trabeculectomy ostium obstruction and tight wound closure. Trabeculectomy ostium obstruction can be diagnosed with gonioscopy. Obstruction is usually due to blood or fibrin clot, vitreous, iris, incompletely excised Descemet's membrane or scleral tissue.

■ WORK-UP
Following trabeculectomy postoperative evaluation is crucial. In each visit IOP should be measured. One of the causes for raised postoperative IOP is bleb fibrosis. Careful slit-lamp examination is essential to identify bleb fibrosis and rule out tight wound closure. Gonioscopy helps in differentiating bleb failure due to internal ostium obstruction from bleb fibrosis.

■ TREATMENT
Topical Corticosteroids
Following trabeculectomy topical corticosteroids are used routinely in a tapering dose for 6-8 weeks. Use of topical corticosteroids reduces wound healing response by reducing cellular tissue infiltration, fibrinous exudation from capillaries and minimizes fibroblastic activity. Beneficial effects of subconjunctival and systemic steroids are not known. They may be useful in eyes with severe inflammation. Nonsteroidal anti-inflammatory drugs are not effective in reducing the healing response; on the contrary they have been associated with an adverse outcome.

Antimetabolites
To reduce postoperative bleb fibrosis adjunctive antimetabolites are used. Use of these drugs is very important in eyes with high-risk of failure. Commonly used antimetabolites are mitomycin C (MMC) and 5-fluorouracil (5-FU) and they inhibit fibroblast proliferation and subsequent scar tissue formation. MMC acts on both proliferating and nonproliferating cells and inhibits cell synthesis. MMC is hundred times more potent than 5-FU and is mainly used intraoperatively. 5-FU is cell specific and interferes with only replicating cells. It can be used intraoperatively as a soak at the scleral flap or as a subconjunctival injection at conclusion of surgery. It also can be used in the postoperative period as

subconjunctival injections. In case of early bleb fibrosis subconjunctival administration of 5-FU during the first 2-3 weeks are recommended.

Step for 5-Fluorouracil Injections

1. Before injection of 5-FU the eye should be examined to rule out any corneal epithelial toxicity and bleb leaks.
2. Good topical anesthesia.
3. The dose is 5 mg (0.1 mL of 50 mg/mL solution).
4. Injected mainly 180° away from trabeculectomy site, occasionally close to bleb. Avoid injections into bleb.
5. Injected using 1 mL tuberculin syringe with a 30-gauge needle.
6. One drop of povidone iodine to be instilled at conclusion.

Maximum dose should be 50 mg in 10 injections during the first 2-3 weeks; complications associated with 5-FU include corneal and conjunctival epithelial toxicity, conjunctival wound leaks, subconjunctival hemorrhage and corneal ulcers.

Adjunctive Measures with Antifibrotic Therapy

- Digital ocular compression and focal compression can be used to elevate the bleb and to reduce the IOP in the early postoperative period. Digital ocular compression is done through the inferior eyelid while patient is looking up. Moderate pressure is applied for 5-10 seconds and then the bleb is examined. The procedure can be repeated until elevation of bleb occurs with reduction in IOP. Focal compression is done with a moistened cotton tip applicator at the edge of scleral flap after anesthetizing the conjunctival cul-de-sac. If necessary patient can be trained to do digital ocular compression. Potential complications of digital ocular compression include hypotony, flat anterior chamber, hyphema, iris incarceration into trabeculectomy stoma, choroidal effusion, and aqueous misdirection.
- Wound modulation with suture lysis (laser) and release of releasable sutures. If there are tight sutures coexisting with bleb fibrosis sutures can be either released or cut with laser to facilitate more filtration flow. Since this is done along the antimetabolite use only one suture at a time should be tackled to avoid hypotony and its related problems.

Needling of Bleb

In late bleb fibrosis that occurs beyond 1 month following trabeculectomy external revision of bleb by needling is recommended.

Steps of Needling of Bleb

1. Can be done as an outpatient procedure at the slit-lamp or preferably in Operation Theater under asepsis.
2. Topical anesthesia, cotton tip applicator soaked in local anesthetic is applied over the bleb for 1 minute to enhance anesthesia effect.
3. Local instillation of povidone iodine.
4. Lid speculum is used.
5. 5-10 mm from bleb site conjunctiva is penetrated using 27-gauge or 30-gauge needle on a tuberculin syringe.
6. The needle is advanced into the bleb sweeping motion is done with the needle till all the resistance disappears.
7. Same procedure is done under the scleral flap.
8. The end point is elevation of bleb with reduction in IOP.
9. Subconjunctival administration of 5-FU (5 mg) away from bleb site.
10. Postoperative topical steroids and 5-FU subconjunctival injection in the postoperative period.

FOLLOW-UP

Trabeculectomy with evidence of failing blebs requires very meticulous postoperative follow-up to 8–10 weeks. Any evidence of early bleb fibrosis should be identified and treated in initial 2–3 weeks to prevent long-term failure. Periodical evaluation and assessment of bleb function is indicated to identify bleb fibrosis and planning appropriate intervention. In case conservative methods to salvage filtering function fail to control IOP adequately, additional medical therapy to reduce IOP or additional surgical procedures such as a repeat trabeculectomy or glaucoma drainage devices is considered.

SUGGESTED READING

1. Lanco AA, Katz LJ. Dysfunctional filtering blebs. Surv Ophthalmol. 1998;43(2):93-126.

4.4 Bleb Leaks

Tanuj Dada, Shibal Bhartiya, Neha Midha
Dr RP Centre for Ophthalmic Sciences, AIIMS, New Delhi
tanujdada@hotmail.com

DEFINITION

A breach in the structural integrity of the conjunctiva/filtering bleb leading to an egress of aqueous from the defect is termed as bleb leak.

CLASSIFICATION

Leaking blebs can be divided into two groups:
1. *Early onset:* Occurring within 3 months after surgery and related to improper wound closure or healing.
2. *Late onset:* Any time after 3 months and are related to thin-walled, cystic, and avascular blebs in which adjunctive antifibrotic agents, such as mitomycin C (MMC) and 5-fluorouracil (5-FU) have been used.

RISK FACTORS

Intraoperative and perioperative use of antimetabolites including MMC and 5-FU; full-thickness filtration, exposed bleb, argon laser suture lysis, exposed scleral flap sutures, limbus-based conjunctival flaps, conjunctival retraction following filtering surgery, inadequate wound closure, buttonholing of the conjunctiva, and trauma to the bleb are significant risk factors for bleb leaks.

SIGNS/SYMPTOMS

The bleb leak may be asymptomatic while some patients may report increased tearing, fluctuating vision or blurred vision.

A positive Seidel testing is diagnostic and must be performed in all suspect cases. In this test, 2% fluorescein solution or a sterile fluorescein strip is placed on the bleb, and dilution of the fluorescein caused by the aqueous flow is observed under cobalt blue slit-lamp illumination. In addition, hypotony may be observed in patients with bleb leakage. Decreased vision due to hypotony, hypotony maculopathy, corneal folds, and irregular astigmatism from lid pressure may be characteristic (**Fig. 4.4.1**).

COMPLICATIONS ASSOCIATED WITH BLEB LEAKAGE

A bleb leak if not managed on time can lead to serious sight-threatening complications such as hypotony maculopathy, blebitis, endophthalmitis, bleb failure, flat anterior chamber, cataract formation, corneal decompensation, synechiae formation, choroidal effusions, macular edema, and loss of vision. The Collaborative Bleb-related Infection Incidence and Treatment Study (CBIITS) had observed an incidence of infections to be about 7.9% in eyes with bleb leaks as compared to 1.7% in those without.

DIFFERENTIAL DIAGNOSIS

Other causes of hypotony such as over-filtration, choroidal effusion, cyclodialysis cleft, and aqueous suppressant therapy are to be excluded.

TREATMENT

Early-onset Bleb Leaks

Conservative management with topical antibiotics (fourth generation fluoroquinolones), aqueous suppressants, and rapid tapering of corticosteroids may help to heal the fistula and stop the leakage. A shield should be worn to protect the bleb from injury especially at night. Tissue adhesives, fibrin glue, cyanoacrylate glue, large diameter contact lenses, collagen shields to cover the leak can be used. Bleb leaks which have not resolved with conservative treatment could be closed by using 9/10-0 Vicryl sutures on a tapered needle.

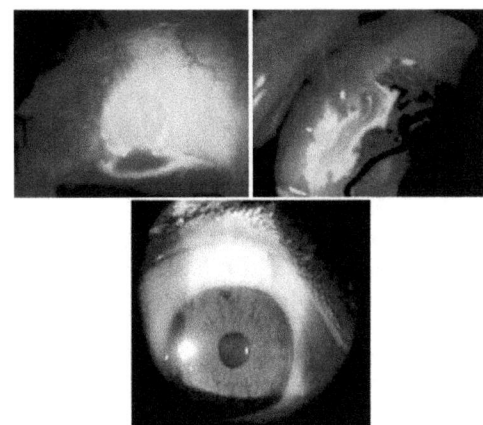

Fig. 4.4.1: Thin cystic bleb with leak showing a positive Seidel's sign.

Small postoperative leak with elevated bleb and formed anterior chamber can be observed and conservative measures can be used. However, a brisk leak with flat bleb and shallow anterior chamber warrants early surgical intervention. Prolonged periods of observation and tapering of steroids to promote healing may lead to scarring of the conjunctiva and bleb failure. Resuturing of the bleb should be performed using a 9/10-0 Vicryl suture on a tapered needle.

Late-onset Bleb Leaks

Although a number of methods such as autologous blood injection; trichloroacetic acid, laser therapy (argon, holmium or Nd:YAG), cyanoacrylate glue, compression sutures, etc. have been tried for managing late leaks, incisional repair of these blebs with conjunctival mobilization is the preferred approach. (A) Advancement of the conjunctiva with a conjunctival relaxing incision in the fornix, (B) Rotating or sliding conjunctival pedicle flap or (C) A free conjunctival autograft from the same or the fellow eye if there is a large defect (>4 mm from limbus). Amniotic membrane transplantation can be used if conjunctival tissue is not available. If the sclera is necrotic or there is a full thickness defect, a scleral reinforcement with a scleral patch graft must be performed with conjunctival mobilization. Donor corneal patch graft, fascia lata, preserved pericardium, and Tenon fascia may also be employed to reinforce devitalized sclera/conjunctiva.

FOLLOW-UP

The main problem associated with bleb revision procedures is that they all increase the risk of bleb failure and can lead to loss of intraocular pressure (IOP) control with subsequent progression of glaucomatous optic neuropathy. A careful monitoring of IOP is required in the postoperative period and recommencement of medical therapy if required to achieve desired target IOP. Rarely, repeat filtering procedures are indicated if intraocular pressures are persistently about target despite medical therapy.

SUGGESTED READING

1. Lanco AA, Katz LJ. Dysfunctional filtering blebs. Surv Ophthalmol. 1998;43(2):93-126.

4.5 Blebitis

SS Pandav
Advanced Eye Centre, PGIMER, Chandigarh
sspandav@yahoo.com

INTRODUCTION
- The spectrum of bleb-associated infection severity ranges from infection limited to the filtering bleb to intraocular extension leading to endophthalmitis.
- Brown et al. introduced the term blebitis in 1994 to describe a presumed infection in or around the filtering bleb without vitreous involvement. It may be associated with mild to moderate anterior chamber inflammation.
- The presence of inflammatory cells within the vitreous is a key for differentiating endophthalmitis from blebitis.
- Blebitis is a severe, potentially vision threatening infection that should be treated aggressively.

INCIDENCE
- The incidence of blebitis and endophthalmitis after glaucoma filtration surgery is higher than most other intraocular procedures.
- The overall incidence of acute-onset postoperative endophthalmitis after any type of intraocular surgery has been reported around 0.093%, while 0.124% after glaucoma filtering surgery.
- Rate of blebitis increases by a factor of four if the patient wears contact lenses. Therefore, contact lenses, especially soft lenses are not recommended after a trabeculectomy.

RISK FACTORS
- *Inferior bleb:* Inferiorly located blebs are thought to be less protected by the upper lid, more susceptible to mechanical irritation from the lower lid, and are immersed in the lacrimal lake and its endogenous bacterial flora potential of causing bleb infections.
- Thin bleb.
- Bleb leak.
- *Antifibrotic agents:* Migration of bacteria across the filtering bleb is recognized to be the initial step in the development of blebitis[1] and ordinarily such spread is prevented by the physical properties of the bleb together with the eye's innate immune response. The thinner and relatively avascular blebs that result with use of antifibrotic agents frequently have areas of absent conjunctival epithelium.
- *Type of surgery:* Bleb-related infections were reported to be lower with combined phacoemulsification and trabeculectomy than trabeculectomy alone.
- *Postoperative complications:* Major complications in the early postoperative period such as flat anterior chamber, early wound leak, and suprachoroidal hemorrhage have been associated with the development of late-onset bleb-related infection.
- *Blepharitis and conjunctivitis*
- *Chronic use of antibiotics:* Use of prophylactic topical antibiotics beyond the immediate postoperative period has been reported to be associated with an increased risk of bleb-related infections with intermittent use (risk ratio 2.1) and even more with continuous use (risk ratio 5.94).
- *Juvenile glaucoma.*
- Nasolacrimal duct obstruction and the use of punctual plugs
- Fully functioning blebs or eyes with low intraocular pressure (IOP) on no medications are at the greatest risk.
- If a bleb leak leads to blebitis and continues to leak, it should be repaired to prevent recurrence of blebitis and bleb-related infections.

ORGANISMS
- Most studies reported *Staphylococcus (S.) epidermidis* (more common) or *Staphylococcus (S.) aureus* as common organisms to cause blebitis.
- These organisms are known to be a part of normal flora of eyelids and conjunctiva. *Staphylococci* are less virulent organisms and unlike *Streptococcal* species, they do not produce exotoxins and do not have the ability to penetrate intact conjunctiva.

SYMPTOMS
- Suddenly develops in an eye, which has been quiet for months or years after filtration surgery.
- Initially, most patients report sudden onset of red eye without warning. Later eye pain, photophobia, discharge, and decreased vision can develop.
- The prodrome (brow ache, headache or external eye infection) in blebitis is often several days or longer.

SIGNS
- In early stage, conjunctival injection localized to the region of filtering bleb may be noted. Later bleb appears milky, with loss of translucency.
- Turbid fluid inside bleb may be visible, possibly with frank purulent material in or leaking from the bleb depending on the severity of infection.
- Inflammatory cells may spill over into the anterior chamber. Hypopyon in the presence of signs of external bleb infection indicates endophthalmitis until proven otherwise.

WORK-UP
- *Slit-lamp biomicroscopy:* Bleb area, presence of inflammatory cells in anterior chamber and vitreous.
- Seidel test should be performed to detect any bleb leak.
- *Gonioscopy:* Look for the microhypopyon.
- Ultrasound B-scan of vitreous should be performed if fundus examination is obscured due to inflammation.
- *Microbiologic procedure:* A swab of conjunctiva over the bleb and an anterior chamber tap should be performed for Gram stain and culture sensitivity before starting antibiotic therapy.
- Forster demonstrated >25 years ago that the yield of organisms from the anterior chamber tap is frequently less than the yield obtained from vitreous taps.

TREATMENT
- Early diagnosis and prompt intensive treatment of blebitis are critical in view of rapid deterioration and potential risk of progression to endophthalmitis, which has relatively devastating outcome.
- Intensive topical treatment alone may be appropriate for patients with blebitis, without evidence of vitreous involvement or hypopyon.
- *Either of following two regimens of topical drops:*
  - *Regimen 1:* Combination of fortified vancomycin (25-50 mg/mL) and tobramycin (14 mg/mL) or cefazolin (50 mg/mL) and tobramycin (14 mg/mL); alternating every half an hour for 24-48 hours after a loading dose.*
  - *Regimen 2:*
    - Fourth generation fluoroquinolones (gatifloxacin 0.3% or moxifloxacin 0.5%) every 1 hour after a loading dose.*

---
*Loading dose: One drop every 5 minutes, to be given four times.

- Start topical steroids 24 hours after antibiotics use and clinical improvement.
- Taper fortified antibiotics to regular strength after about 48 hours on clinical evidence of improvement of infection.
- Device removal is not necessary in the treatment of blebitis after EX-PRESS glaucoma filtration device implantation under a scleral flap, and this condition may be treated in the same way as blebitis after trabeculectomy.
- No difference has been found in relative incidence of blebitis when trabeculectomy is performed with adjuvant mitomycin or ologen implant.
- Studies have found that once a patient has had an episode of blebitis, the risk of having a second episode is much higher. Therefore, a late-onset bleb leak must be closed, preferably by conjunctival advancement.

Presence of white blood cells in the vitreous in the setting of blebitis is considered endophthalmitis and immediate intravitreal antibiotic administration is indicated. Bleb-associated infections are usually caused by very virulent organisms and thus pars plana vitrectomy is warranted once the vitreous is involved.

PREVENTION
- Routine checkup for leaks in functioning filtering blebs to identify eyes at high risk for acquiring an infection.
- Educate the patient to be on the lookout for any new or unusual redness, pain or worsening of vision.

REFERENCE
1. Aaberg TM Jr, Flynn HW Jr, Schiffman J, Newton J. Nosocomial acute-onset postoperative endophthalmitis survey. A 10-year review of incidence and outcomes. Ophthalmology. 1998;105(6):1004-10.

4.6 Traumatic Glaucoma

Rengaraj Venkatesh
Aravind Eye Care System, Puducherry
venkatesh@pondy.aravind.org

DEFINITION
Traumatic glaucoma refers to a heterogeneous group of post-traumatic ocular disorders with different underlying mechanisms that lead to the common pathway of abnormal elevation of intraocular pressure (IOP) and increased risk of optic neuropathy.

TYPES OF OCULAR TRAUMA
1. *Mechanical injury:*
   a. Direct
   b. Nonpenetrating (blunt) trauma
   c. Penetrating trauma
   d. *Surgical trauma:* Following cataract surgery, penetrating keratoplasty, sclera buckling, pars plana vitrectomy, Nd:YAG laser procedures
   e. Indirect
   f. Head injury
2. *Chemical injury:*
   a. Alkali burns
   b. Acid burns
3. Radiation, electrical, and thermal injury.

MECHANISM OF TRAUMATIC GLAUCOMA

Traumatic glaucoma can be either open angle or closed angle. In the open angle type, the obstruction to aqueous outflow can be pre-trabecular (e.g., epithelial down growth), trabecular (hyphema and ghost cell glaucoma) or post-trabecular (elevated episcleral venous pressure following carotid cavernous fistula). Angle closure happens following adherence of peripheral iris to the trabecular meshwork or peripheral cornea. In the anterior (pull) mechanism, an abnormal tissue in the angle contracts and pulls the iris into the angle (e.g., fibrovascular membrane associated with neovascular glaucoma). Posterior (push) mechanisms include pupillary block (e.g., by a swollen cataractous lens) and forward movement of lens iris diaphragm (secondary to ciliochoroidal effusion or ciliary block).

CLINICAL FEATURES

Nonpenetrating (Blunt) Trauma

Glaucoma following blunt trauma can occur immediately after injury or be delayed by months and years as in angle recession. Immediate cause for glaucoma can be either due to hyphema, inflammation or changes in the position of the lens.

- *Hyphema:* Blunt trauma causes distortion of anterior chamber angle, which can result in vessel rupture in iris and ciliary body and bleeding into the anterior chamber. The blood can mechanically block outflow channels or the erythrocytes and blood products can block the trabecular meshwork. As the IOP rises, bleeding is arrested and a clot forms. Clot lysis and retraction occur 2–5 days after the trauma, and the maximal risk of rebleeding from the site occurs at this time. Rebleeding is reported in 0.4–35% of patients, and can result in subtotal or total hyphema (eight-ball hyphema). Rarely subtotal hyphema can result in pupillary block glaucoma. Total hyphema is associated with sudden loss of vision, high IOP, extreme pain and nausea. Long-standing total hyphema poses the risk of both optic nerve damage due to raised IOP, and blood staining of cornea. Very rarely, ghost cell (hemolytic) glaucoma can occur after vitreous hemorrhage associated with perforating or nonperforating ocular trauma. About 2–3 weeks after the injury, normal blood cells in the vitreous transform into rigid, khaki-colored ghost cells and migrate into anterior chamber. These cells block the trabecular meshwork and raise the IOP.
- *Inflammation:* In case of inflammation, inflammatory cells or trabeculitis can lead to open angle glaucoma. If inflammation is uncontrolled it can result in 360° posterior synechiae, iris bombe, and secondary angle-closure glaucoma.
- *Angle-recession glaucoma:* Past history of trauma can be elicited in many cases. These patients have characteristic gonioscopic findings—an uneven iris insertion, an area of torn iris processes, and a posteriorly recessed iris, revealing a widened ciliary band. In addition to widened ciliary body band, sclerosis and fibrosis of the trabecular meshwork are observed. Raise in IOP can occur anywhere between 1 year and 10 years or even later after the trauma. So good counseling about the risk of glaucoma and close follow-up of these patients is very important.
- *Position of lens:* Subluxation or dislocation of lens can cause either an open angle or closed angle glaucoma. Subluxation or dislocation can result in pupillary block by the lens or vitreous or if there are ruptured lens materials in the anterior chamber it can clog the trabecular meshwork and result in glaucoma. Lenses dislocated into the vitreous could leak proteins due to phacolysis resulting in phacolytic glaucoma several years after injury and lens dislocation.

Glaucoma Following Penetrating and Perforating Trauma

All mechanisms that can elevate IOP after blunt trauma can also lead to increased IOP in eyes that have had penetrating or perforating injuries. In addition, eyes that have been ruptured may have fibrous in growth, epithelial down growth or retained foreign bodies that may cause elevated IOP by different mechanisms. Injury to lens from penetrating trauma could cause rapid progression of cataracts, intumescence and secondary angle-closure glaucoma from a swollen crystalline lens and papillary block. Leakage of lens proteins and cortex due to injury to the lens capsule could also result in phacoantigenic uveitis associated with glaucoma. All penetrating injuries with corneal tears/perforations and loss of chamber depth need to be repaired immediately. Long-standing collapse of anterior chambers and iridocorneal adhesions could result in peripheral anterior synechiae with secondary angle-closure glaucoma if penetrating corneal tears are not repaired in time.

CHEMICAL INJURY

Glaucoma is more common after alkali burns but also seen after severe acid burns. IOP elevations in the early phase are caused by scleral shrinkage and in the intermediate phase by inflammation. The eyes can be treated with aqueous suppressants, cycloplegics, and topical steroids. Late elevations of IOP are usually caused by trabecular damage and formation of peripheral anterior synechiae (PAS) or other intraocular scarring.

WORK-UP

- Detailed present/past history about injury
- Detailed slit-lamp examination and look for all the complications of blunt trauma
- Cyclodialysis
- Iridodialysis
- Iridoschisis
- Anterior synechiae
- Iris sphincter tears
- Mydriasis
- Iris atrophy
- Transillumination defects
- Iritis
- Zonular breaks
- Careful gonioscopy to rule out angle recession and look for other signs of angle damage following a trauma. Comparison with the angles in the injured and uninjured eyes is important, particularly in cases with subtle findings. Documented asymmetry supports the diagnosis.
- *Look for signs of lens trauma such as:*
  - Phacodonesis
  - Subluxated lens
  - Cataract
  - Detailed examination of the posterior segment to look for abnormalities, which may signify prior episodes of trauma, includes the following:
    - Vitreous opacities
    - Chorioretinal scars
    - Macular hole
    - Retinal breaks
    - Retinal detachment
    - Optic atrophy
    - IOP measurement
- Snellen visual acuity and visual field testing is of critical importance in diagnosing and monitoring the disorder.

TREATMENT

- *Hyphema:* The goals of treatment of hyphema are to prevent rebleed and to control IOP. Minimal hyphema can be managed by complete rest, aqueous suppressants, and steroids. Subtotal or total hyphema has to be evacuated by surgery/anterior chamber wash to prevent secondary complications including corneal staining and amblyopia in young children. One proposed guideline is that an IOP threatening the optic nerve such as 60 mm Hg for 2 days, 50 mm Hg for 5 days or 35 mm Hg for 7 days is a definite indication for surgical evacuation of blood clot. Always keep in mind the risk of rebleed in traumatic hyphema and the rebleed can sometimes be worse than the original bleed resulting from ocular injury.

- *Inflammation:* Usually managed with aqueous suppressants, cycloplegics and anti-inflammatory agents like steroids. Keep in mind the risk of steroid response in these cases. If there is posterior synechiae or iris bombe, a laser iridotomy will be very important to break the angle closure stage.
- *Angle recession glaucoma:* Management is with antiglaucoma medications, other than aqueous suppressants, drugs which enhance the uveoscleral outflow can be tried. Argon laser trabeculoplasty can be done with caution, but the results are not satisfactory, and in uncontrolled glaucoma filtering procedures are indicated.
- *Position of lens:* Management will be to control the IOP and remove the lens in most cases of gross subluxation or dislocation. Placement of IOL can be difficult in these cases, and most of them would require a scleral-fixated IOL as a primary or secondary procedure. In minor subluxation with pupillary block even a peripheral iridotomy can help to tackle glaucoma.

FOLLOW-UP

An injury severe enough to cause hyphema also causes an angle recession in >60% of eyes. Glaucoma may develop in 6% of eyes that have angle recession (>240°). Patients with angle recession and normal IOP should be examined annually for the rest of the life. Penetrating injury and chemical injury also need lifelong follow-up for screening of glaucoma.

SUGGESTED READING

1. Campbell DG. Traumatic glaucoma. In: Singleton BJ, Hersh PS, Kenyon KR (Eds). Eye Trauma. St. Louis: CV Mosby; 1991. pp. 117-25.

4.7 Glaucoma Following Vitreoretinal Surgical Procedures

Ganesh Raman, Parthasarathy Sathyan
Aravind Eye Hospital, Coimbatore
dr.sathyan.p@gmail.com

DEFINITION

Increase in intraocular pressure (IOP) with or without glaucomatous optic disk damage and visual field loss following vitreoretinal surgery or retinal laser procedure. Incidence of IOP elevation following vitreoretinal surgical procedures varies depending on the procedure performed and several risk factors. The overall incidence is approximately 35%.

RISK FACTORS

Risk factors for IOP elevation following vitreoretinal procedures include preexisting glaucoma, scleral buckle, use of silicon oil or expansile gas injection, lensectomy, proliferative vitreoretinopathy, use of endolaser, intravitreal triamcinolone, excessive tissue manipulation, prolonged or complicated surgery, intraoperative complications, postoperative inflammation, and steroid response.

MECHANISM

The mechanism of glaucoma depends upon the preoperative, intraoperative, and postoperative status of the eye. Causes of open-angle glaucoma associated with vitreoretinal procedures include—inflammation, steroid induced (intravitreal triamcinolone), angiogenesis, mechanical obstruction of the trabecular meshwork by silicon oil, blood or triamcinolone crystals, gas expansion or silicon oil without angle closure and idiopathic mechanisms associated with trabecular dysfunction and outflow obstruction. Angle closure mechanisms contributing to elevated IOP include pupillary block associated with an intraocular gas, especially in aphakic eyes, silicon oil, also in aphakic eyes without a patent inferior iridotomy, fibrin, IOL and without a pupillary block in cases of uveal congestion, ciliary body edema and iridocorneal apposition, mechanical shifting of the iris lens diaphragm anteriorly, angle neovascularization, peripheral shallowing with normal central anterior chamber as in tight buckle syndrome.

CLINICAL FEATURES

Symptoms

Severe pain, redness, blurred vision, tearing along with nausea, and vomiting may be present although the surgical procedure itself may be the cause of many of the symptoms. Irrespective of the mechanism of glaucoma after vitreoretinal surgery the severity of symptoms is almost always directly related to the raised IOP levels.

Signs

- Corneal edema
- *Anterior chamber:* May be shallow or deep depending upon the causes mentioned.
- *Pupil:* May be semi-dilated, dilated if good mydriasis is achieved or irregular with posterior synechiae. Frank Iris Bombé can be a presenting feature in the absence of a patent iridotomy and papillary block.
- The lens iris diaphragm can be pushed forward, shallowing the chamber.
- Intraocular lens position: Has to be verified as it may cause pupillary block glaucoma if placed in the sulcus.
- *Fundus examination* is important to assess the status of the retina and to exclude vitreous hemorrhage, choroidal effusion, and choroidal hemorrhage. The presence of intravitreal gas complicates the examination and one may have to resort to the use of B-scan ultrasonography in rare cases.
- Intraocular pressure can be measured with Goldman applanation tonometer (tonopen, pneumotonometer can also be used, noncontact tonometer is not recommended in the presence of corneal edema) keeping in mind that corneal edema underestimates IOP.

DIFFERENTIAL DIAGNOSIS

- *Suprachoroidal hemorrhage:* Painful eye, reduced visual acuity, congested conjunctiva, edematous cornea, shallow anterior chamber. Brown, dome-shaped choroidals seen on slit-lamp biomicroscopy. B-scan ultrasonography reveals hemorrhagic choroidal detachments.
- *Vitreous hemorrhage:* Diminution of vision or decrease in vision, quiet eye, normal anterior chamber, pupil and lens and faint red glow. Fundus view will be very hazy and B-scan ultrasonography will reveal the vitreous hemorrhage.
- *Malignant glaucoma:* Severe pain, nausea and vomiting, corneal edema, uniform shallow anterior chamber, forward movement of IOL/lens iris diaphragm. B-scan ultrasonography may show aqueous pockets in the vitreous cavity. No response to iridotomy, but temporarily responds to atropinization.

4. *Endophthalmitis:* Reduction of visual acuity, lid edema, discharge, chemosis, anterior chamber and vitreous cavity inflammation, vitreous abscesses and exudates in the anterior chamber.

■ MANAGEMENT

The initial steps of management include the medical treatment aimed at reduction of the IOP and surgical correction of any cause of the same. In the majority of cases the medical treatment is sufficient because of the transient nature of glaucoma. Medical therapy usually begins with topical beta-blockers (timolol maleate 0.5%), topical alpha-2 agonists (brimonidine 0.15-0.2%, twice daily) or topical carbonic anhydrase (dorzolamide 2%, twice daily) depending on the magnitude of IOP rise. Medical treatment with topical aqueous suppressants is supplemented with oral carbonic anhydrase inhibitors (acetazolamide 250 mg thrice a day) for a short duration of time and intravenous (mannitol 20%) or oral (oral glycerol) hyperosmotic agents are often employed to achieve immediate but transient reduction in IOP if the patient is very symptomatic. Prostaglandin analogs (latanoprost 0.005%, travoprost 0.04%, bimatoprost 0.03%, applied once a day) can be used in the absence of intraocular inflammation. Steroid-antibiotic combination eye drops are applied routinely but in case of severe inflammation of the eye, frequent steroid eye drops (1-2 hours during the day and eye ointment at night) are used. Cycloplegics (atropine 1% eye ointment thrice daily) to break the papillary synechiae and also pull the lens iris diaphragm backward are useful in angle-closure glaucoma with nonpapillary block mechanisms.

Glaucoma not responding to the above treatment may require additional intervention:
- Paracentesis to reduce IOP in idiopathic secondary glaucoma.
- Laser iridotomy or surgical peripheral iridectomy in patients with pupillary block.
- Partial removal of intraocular gas.
- Partial removal of silicon oil.
- Release of tight buckle in tight buckle syndrome.
- Anterior chamber wash for blood or emulsified silicon oil.
- Adequate panretinal photocoagulation for neovascularization.
- Pars plana vitrectomy for removal of triamcinolone crystals.
- Glaucoma filtering surgery/shunt procedures may be required if the IOP is not controlled for more than 4-8 weeks or if progressive glaucomatous disk damage is documented.
- Destructive procedures such as cyclocryotherapy or cyclophotocoagulation may be required in intractable glaucoma following vitreoretinal surgery, especially if conventional surgical procedures are not feasible. These procedures may also be indicated for symptomatic relief when visual potential is poor.

■ CONCLUSION

Glaucoma following vitreoretinal procedures is usually transient and generally responds to medical therapy. Aggressive treatment of glaucoma and appropriate follow-up is required to achieve good functional outcome and maintain good quality of life for the patient.

■ SUGGESTED READING

1. Costarides AP, Alabata P, Bergstrom C. Elevated intraocular pressure following vitreoretinal surgery. Ophthalmol Clin North Am. 2004;17(4):507-12.

4.8 Glaucoma Following Cataract Surgery

R Ramakrishnan
Aravind Eye Care System, Tirunelveli
drrk@tvl.aravind.org

INTRODUCTION

The advent of newer biocompatible intraocular lenses has led to the optimism of acquiring a normal postoperative vision without being exposed to the minimal, but possible hazards of an artificial lens in the eye. Along with the numerous advantages, the intraocular lenses do result in some unwanted postoperative incidences, glaucoma being one of them. However, the term pseudophakic glaucoma should not be used, because it is not a single mechanism that leads to glaucoma; it is preferable if the cause of the rise in intraocular pressure (IOP) or glaucoma is included in the definition to designate the proper scenario.

INCIDENCE

The incidence of postoperative glaucoma following cataract surgeries is dependent on the methodology; type of intraocular lens (IOL) used and associated premorbid factors. Different studies show that there is a lowering of IOP by as much as 1.1–2.5 mm Hg for at least 6 months. However, any kind of IOL surgery complications relating to elevated IOP occur in the early as well as late postoperative period and have been found to be around 29% in some studies. Chronic glaucoma was found to occur in 4% of eyes in one series and 2.1% of eyes in another. However, comparing incidences from different studies is irrational as each study has its own definition of glaucoma and different instruments to measure the IOP.

MECHANISM OF INTRAOCULAR PRESSURE ELEVATION AND DIFFERENTIAL DIAGNOSIS OF THE CAUSE

With any cataract procedure, early and late postoperative IOP elevations can occur by a wide variety of mechanisms **(Fig. 4.8.1)**.

Early (First Postoperative Week)

Transient Intraocular Pressure Elevation

In the immediate postoperative period there may be a transient increase in the IOP even in an uncomplicated cataract surgery.

Distortion of the Anterior Chamber Angle

A white ridge resembling "inverted snow bank" lines the inner margin of the corneoscleral section. Cause of this has been thought to be tight corneoscleral sutures or edema of the deeper corneal stroma. Whatever be the cause, the ridge is known to cause peripheral anterior synechiae, vitreous adhesions and hyphema along with a transient rise in IOP **(Fig. 4.8.1)**.

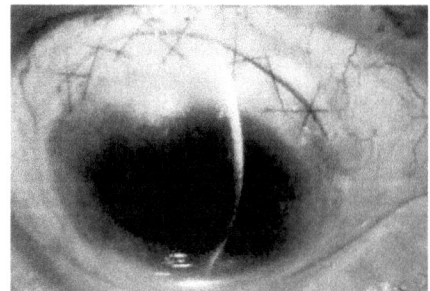

Fig. 4.8.1: Tight sutures cause transient intraocular pressure elevation. Wound gape and leak predispose to aqueous misdirection glaucoma.

Influence of Viscoelastic Substances

Of all the modern viscoelastics in use, high molecular weight viscoelastics are thought to be associated with a transient increase in

IOP even after meticulous anterior chamber (AC) wash. Healon, Healon GV, Healon-5, chondroitin sulfate, polyacrylamide (discontinued), etc. are known to cause a rise in IOP. However, methyl cellulose [1-2% HPMC (hydroxypropylmethylcellulose)] is found to be the safest among these with a good function of protecting the corneal endothelium. These substances are also notorious in causing increased inflammation and associated IOP rise. Mechanical obstruction of trabecular meshwork with reduced outflow facility is most likely primary mechanism for all types of viscoelastics.

Inflammation and Hemorrhage

Any form of cataract surgery may lead to inflammation. When the inflammation is excessive, the IOP rises because of inflammatory debris clogging the trabecular meshwork and also due to increased protein concentration of the aqueous following breakdown of blood aqueous barrier. One such condition is the uveitis-glaucoma-hyphema (UGH) syndrome where severe uveitis occurs with accompanying bleeding. The source of the bleeding may be the lens or the haptic rubbing against the ciliary body or the iris, or from the new vessels in the corneoscleral section. This condition was more common with anterior chamber and iris fixated lens though it has been reported after posterior chamber lens implantation when the haptic is placed in the sulcus and results in chronic irritation of the ciliary body. Most of the postoperative hemorrhages associated with cataract extraction are self-limited. The source of hemorrhage is from the corneoscleral wound or the iridectomy. Mechanism of IOP elevation is due to clogging of meshwork with red blood cells **(Fig. 4.8.2)**. Recurrent bleeding from cataract wound neovascularization (*Swan's syndrome*) rarely may present with secondary open angle glaucoma.

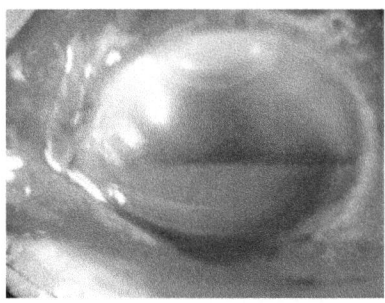

Fig. 4.8.2: Hyphema.

Inflammation and lens particle glaucoma: Cortical lens fragments may be retained sometimes in the anterior chamber if thorough intraoperative cortical wash was not attempted or missed due to small pupil. This can obstruct the trabecular meshwork in the form of free lens particles or macrophages swollen with lens material. However, glaucoma does not occur in all eyes which contain cortical remnants and the inflammatory response may be more pronounced and prolonged in eyes which contain a higher amount of lens material. When inflammation is severe enough, keratic precipitates and sometimes a hypopyon may be present. Differentiation between this sterile inflammatory endophthalmitis and infectious endophthalmitis can be difficult and may depend on the initial response to therapy **(Figs. 4.8.3 and 4.8.4)**.

Enzyme glaucoma: It is also known as zonulolytic glaucoma. Usually occurs 2-5 days postoperatively. This entity has been reported in around 27% of cases following use of alpha-chymotrypsin enzyme used to lyse the zonules following ICCE (intracapsular cataract extraction). IOP elevation is more common in patients with preexisting open angle glaucoma. IOP elevation is thought to occur due to blockage of trabecular meshwork with lens zonule fragments.

Acute infection: Early IOP elevation can occur in patients with endophthalmitis particularly of bacterial origin as early as 1st postoperative week. Main treatment for IOP control should be aimed at controlling the underlying infection. The mechanism of IOP elevation is most likely secondary to outflow obstruction from inflammatory cells and debris, and appropriate antimicrobial treatment should aid in clearing this particulate load.

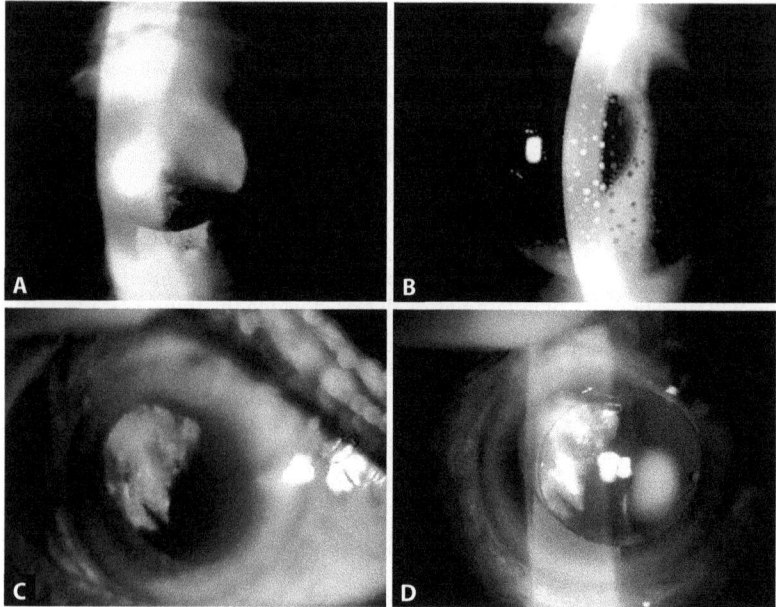

Figs. 4.8.3A to D: (A and B) Residual cortex in anterior chamber and inflammatory keratic precipitates; (C and D) Fluffy cortex behind intraocular lens.

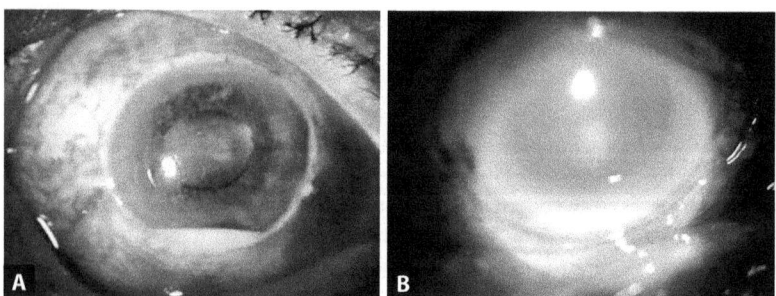

Figs. 4.8.4A and B: Uveitis with hypopyon.

Intermediate (After First Operative Week)

Pigment Dispersion (Pseudophakic Pigmentary Glaucoma)

Pigment dispersion with pseudophakia occurs because of the same mechanism that leads to phakic pigment dispersion syndrome though a typical Krukenberg's spindle is rare. It mainly occurs when the haptic of the IOL is in the sulcus and rubs against the pigment epithelium; previously used to be common with iris fixated and anterior chamber lenses. The diagnostic clue of a pigment dispersion mechanism is a transillumination defect in the iris.

Vitreous Filling the Anterior Chamber

Vitreous may peak into the anterior chamber in aphakic eyes (commonly) and in eyes where the IOL is placed over a capsular rent. This may lead to pupillary block or mechanical distortion of the anterior chamber leading to a rise in IOP. It is reversed by mydriasis, iridotomy or vitrectomy **(Figs. 4.8.5A and B)**.

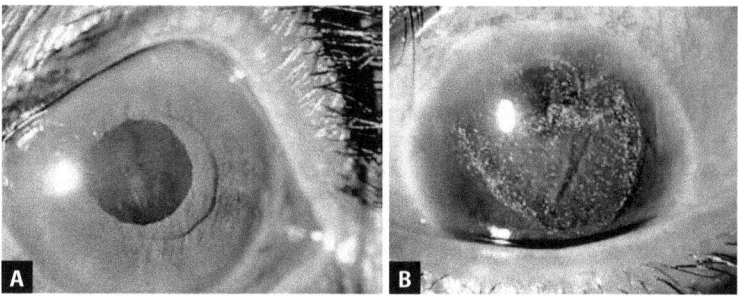

Figs. 4.8.5A and B: Vitreous in anterior chamber.

Pupillary Block

Pupillary block glaucoma may occur after IOL implantation. Previously, in AC lenses, the posterior rough surface got adhered to the iris. In posterior chamber IOL (PCIOL), the iris may form synechiae with the anterior lens surface or the anterior lens capsular rim usually due to excessive inflammation which leads to formation of posterior synechiae. The AC is also shallow, but, unlike aqueous misdirection syndrome, the central AC depth is deeper than the periphery (**Fig. 4.8.6**). Pupillary block can also be caused due to vitreous blocking the pupil, though this was common during the ICCE era. Often in such cases there is a slow development of synechial closure and permanent secondary angle-closure glaucoma.

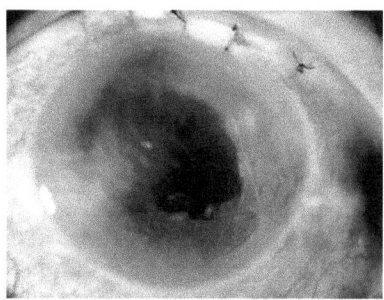

Fig. 4.8.6: Pupillary block glaucoma in pseudophakia.

Malignant glaucoma: It may occur rarely after cataract extraction in cases with preoperative shallow anterior chamber more commonly if the patient is left aphakic but may occur in pseudophakic patient as well. It may occur hours to days or even months after surgery.

Peripheral Anterior Synechiae and/or Trabecular Damage

Peripheral anterior synechiae (PAS), generally results after a flat AC postoperatively, which might be due to overfiltration or wound leak. This leads to chronic contact of the peripheral iris forming anterior synechiae. PAS can also form over the haptics of an anterior chamber IOL. Trabecular damage may occur directly due to surgery or due to increased inflammation postoperatively or due to a preexisting mechanism which crossed the critical threshold postsurgery.

Steroid-induced Glaucoma

This is one of the commonly overlooked causes of increase in IOP. It is suspected after all other causes have been excluded. It is managed by gradual tapering of steroid under the cover of antiglaucoma medications.

Late Postoperative Phase (After 2 Months)

Nd:YAG Laser Posterior Capsulotomy

Glaucoma may occur after YAG laser capsulotomy mainly in eyes with preexisting glaucoma or a preoperative pressure above 20 mm Hg, larger capsulotomies, and in sulcus rather than capsular fixed PCIOL. The pressure rise may be detected within the first few hours and usually returns to baseline within a week, although some may last for several weeks with some studies showing late and persistent rise in 0.8–6%.

Epithelial and Fibroblast Downgrowth

These factors may also lead to blockage of the trabecular meshwork resulting in rise of the IOP. Mainly occurs through the wound site and due to improper apposition of the surgical wound **(Fig. 4.8.7)**. The argon laser produces characteristic white burns on the epithelial membrane over the iris surface (known as popcorn sign) which aids in confirming the diagnosis of epithelial downgrowth and also to determine the extent of involvement.

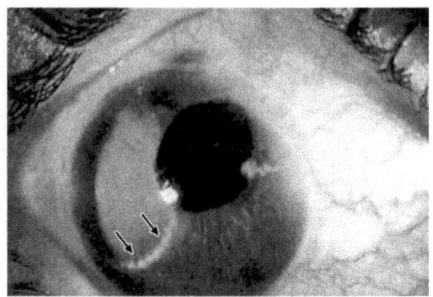

Fig. 4.8.7: Epithelial downgrowth.

Preexisting Open-angle Glaucoma

A preexisting open-angle glaucoma (POAG) may be discovered postoperatively and considered as pseudophakic glaucoma. Generally, a comparison with the contralateral eye and a proper history excludes or confirms the condition.

Irreversible Trabecular Meshwork Damage

After cataract surgery, the IOP usually returns to normal within 1 week. However, if the patient has a history of preexistent glaucoma, the resolution may be prolonged. In any patient, as a result of myriad insults of cataract surgery on the trabecular meshwork, the IOP elevation can become sustained or permanent. Such type of chronic glaucoma in aphakia or pseudophakia should be initially evaluated for other causes of sustained IOP elevation such as because of steroid use, recurrent hemorrhages, persistent inflammation, or angle closure.

■ CLINICAL FEATURES

Symptoms

These patients may present with the complaint of the accompanying cause of rise in IOP. This may range from mild discomfort, watering, photophobia to severe pain, blepharospasm to loss of vision.

Signs

- *IOP:* Increased
- *Cornea:* Edema, presence of keratic precipitates
- *AC depth:* Shallow or flat if the cause is pupillary block or aqueous misdirection, respectively
- *AC reaction:* Cells and flare, presence of hyphema
- *Gonioscopy:* Iris bombe, flat peripheral AC, PAS, new vessels, and haptic eroding the angle
- *Wound dehiscence:* Aqueous misdirection, iris prolapse
- Epithelial ingrowth
- Fibrous downgrowth
- *Fundus:* May show glaucomatous cupping
- Iridectomy
- Posterior synechiae

■ WORK-UP

The work-up consists of a routine ophthalmological examination starting from history, diffuse light examination, slit-lamp examination, IOP, gonioscopy (should never be withheld if an angle closure is remotely suspected) and fundus evaluation. However, in acute cases such as pupillary block, initial management should be started as soon as the diagnosis is made without waiting for a detailed examination. Special investigations including fundus photograph, ultrasound including ultrasound biomicroscopy, detailed fundus examination or retinal nerve fiber analysis can be carried out. The main aim behind the work-up is to delineate the specific mechanism in each case so that the appropriate therapy can be instilled sooner than later.

PREVENTIVE MEASURES
Preoperative Considerations
- Avoid epinephrine during local anesthesia
- A good massage to the eye to make the eye soft, reduce vitreous volume and IOP.

Intraoperative Considerations
- Minimal intraocular manipulation
- Sclerocorneal tunnel incision
- Judicious use of viscoelastics and thorough viscoelastic aspiration
- Thorough cortical clean up
- Prefer PCIOL rather than ACIOL (anterior chamber IOL) and prefer in the bag placement than sulcus placement.

MANAGEMENT
Early and Intermediate Postoperative Period
- No intervention in modest pressure rise if AC is deep and the eye is nonglaucomatous.
- If there is pain or a threat to the optic nerve head, cornea, or cataract incision, temporary medical measures should be employed. For example, with topical carbonic anhydrase inhibitors, β-blockers or α-2 agonist for glaucoma; steroids to control inflammation and NSAIDs (nonsteroidal anti-inflammatory drugs) to block prostaglandin synthesis.
- UGH syndrome is managed with mydriatics or miotics in mild cases and steroids with antiglaucoma medications in severe cases.
- Pigment dispersion can be managed medically.
- Pupillary block glaucoma has to be reversed immediately by performing Nd:YAG (neodymium-doped yttrium aluminum garnet) laser iridotomy.
- Malignant glaucoma is treated with aqueous suppressants, strong cycloplegics such as atropine and Nd:YAG laser hyaloidotomy may be attempted to relieve the ciliary block. 50% of cases will reverse with medical management within 5 days. However, some may need surgical intervention.

Late Postoperative Period
- Most of the chronic patients can be managed medically.
- In patients requiring YAG capsulotomy, treatment with α-2 agonist, both preprocedure and postprocedure, helps in preventing the IOP spike.

SURGICAL MANAGEMENT
Surgical management becomes necessary once the medical option is exhausted. **Table 4.8.1** provides the indications for surgery in glaucoma following cataract surgery. The choice of the procedure depends on the presenting condition and expected visual potential. In cases of intractable glaucoma with useful visual potential glaucoma drainage devices are usually preferred such as Ahmed, Baerveldt or AADI (Aravind aqueous drainage implant). AADI which resembles Baerveldt in its working principle is available at economical price which would be more suitable choice in our Indian scenario. In cases with poor or no visual potential diode laser cyclophotocoagulation may be done to relieve the pain.

TABLE 4.8.1: Indications for surgical techniques for glaucoma following cataract surgery.

Trabeculectomy with antimetabolites	Seton	Laser cyclophotocoagulation
Mobile conjunctiva	Scarred conjunctiva	Scarred conjunctiva
Good visual potential (20/100 or better) or only eye	Visual potential fair to good (20/200 or better)	Fair to poor visual potential (20/200 or worse)
Little or no ocular inflammation or active neovascularization	Active ocular inflammation or neovascularization	Not a candidate for more invasive procedure

Source: Chandler PA, Grant WM, Epstein DL. Chandler and Grant's Glaucoma. 4th edition. USA: Lippincott Williams and Wilkins; 1996. p 354.

■ FOLLOW-UP AND PROGNOSIS

These depend on the antecedent cause and the mechanism of glaucoma. In a noneventful surgery, the follow-up is done as per routine cataract surgeries. If preoperative evaluation and surgical maneuvers' indicate a possible rise in IOP, immediate and frequent follow-up is needed. Once diagnosed, the follow-up depends on the nature of glaucoma and the seriousness of the condition and also the effect of the initial intervention.

■ SUGGESTED READING

1. Allingham RR, Damji KF, Freedman S, Moroi SE, Shafranov G (Eds). Shield's Textbook of Glaucoma: Glaucoma after Ocular Surgery. USA: Lippincott Williams and Wilkins; 2004. pp 415-21.

4.9 Postoperative Ocular Hypotony

JC Das
Shroff Eye Centre, New Delhi
drjcdas@yahoo.com

■ DEFINITION

It is defined as having an intraocular pressure (IOP) <6 mm Hg, below which deleterious effects on the eye are common. However, it represents a range of IOP in single digits that is usually deleterious to the function of the eye. Some patients develop severe hypotony maculopathy with an IOP of 6 mm or more, whereas others may have good vision despite the IOP of 3 mm Hg. Hypotony (transient or prolonged) associated with shallow or flat anterior chamber (AC) (intraoperative or postoperative) is one of the serious complications following glaucoma filtering surgery. Hypotony even if transient induces a cascade of events with profound effects on visual outcome.

■ INCIDENCE

- 17–41% in full thickness filtering surgery
- 3–33% in trabeculectomy without antifibrotic agent
- 15–30% after trabeculectomy with mitomycin C (MMC) and 5-fluorouracil (5-FU)
- 2–32% after aqueous shunts
- 7–24% after cyclodestructive procedures

Hypotony maculopathy occurs in 1.3–7% (average: 4%) of cases of trabeculectomy with adjunctive MMC/5-FU. However, hypotonous maculopathy is very rare in Black Africans despite the use of high doses of MMC.

Eyes Predisposed to Ocular Hypotony

- Surgery on eyes with inadequately controlled chronic angle-closure glaucoma.
- Aphakia/pseudophakia.

- High myopia and posterior vitreous detachment.
- Nanophthalmos.
- Vitrectomized eye.
- Marked inflammation.
- Shunt surgery in an eye which has undergone multiple procedures.
- Increased episcleral venous pressure (e.g., Sturge–Weber syndrome).
- Advanced age, hypertension, and diabetes.
- Fellow eye has developed shallow AC hypotony in the past.
- Use of antimetabolites in high concentration and for longer duration.
- Sudden decompression during surgery.

CLINICAL FEATURES

Anterior chamber is usually shallowest on postoperative day 2 or 3 and gradually deepens over 2 weeks. It may present in two forms:
1. Hypotony with shallow or flat AC.
2. Hypotony with normal or deep AC.

HYPOTONY WITH SHALLOW OR FLAT ANTERIOR CHAMBER

It is important to distinguish between shallow AC with iridocorneal touch and flat AC with lenticular-corneal touch because the management and prognosis differ significantly. Spaeth has graded the shallowness of the AC into three grades: Grade 1—Peripheral Iris Corneal Touch, Grade 2—Central Iridocorneal Touch, and Grade 3—Lenticulocorneal Touch.

In shallow AC with iridocorneal touch, the cornea is typically clear and iris stroma has not been flattened by gentle touch with the cornea, whereas in flat AC with lenticulocorneal touch, cornea is edematous and iris stroma is flattened and in contact with cornea.

In grades 1 and 2 of shallow AC, chamber deepens spontaneously in 2 weeks' time and no special management is necessary. A prolonged shallow AC >2 weeks may be associated with corneal damage and peripheral anterior synechiae. It also interferes with bleb formation resulting in bleb failure. This necessitates surgical intervention to reform the AC. Flat AC with lenticulocorneal touch (grade 3) results in corneal decompensation, cataract formation and posterior segment changes and therefore needs immediate surgical intervention to reform the AC.

EFFECTS OF HYPOTONY

The process of hypotony starts right at the operation table, when the AC is entered. Preventing hypotony after the beginning of surgery and maintaining it throughout by deepening the AC either with viscoelastic or AC maintainer results in deep AC postoperatively. Just deepening the AC at the end of surgery does not prevent postoperative shallow AC and its complications. Even transient hypotony may lead to serious complications in vulnerable eyes and may include suprachoroidal effusion, ciliochoroidal detachment, suprachoroidal hemorrhage, ciliary body rotation, and aqueous misdirection.

DIFFERENTIAL DIAGNOSIS

When hypotony is associated with shallow or flat AC, one should consider following situations and associated features since it is essential to address these for management of hypotony:
- Wound leak
- Overfiltration
- Choroidal effusion (ciliochoroidal detachment)
- Pupillary block with existing hyposecretion but nonpatent peripheral iridotomy (PI)
- Ciliary body shutdown due to antimetabolite toxicity and severe inflammation
- Cyclodialysis (inadvertent).

WORK-UP

- *Assessment of anterior chamber depth and inflammation:* According to Spaeth grading of 1, 2, and 3. Chamber depth assessment facilitates better management and prevents long-standing complications such as bleb failure, cataract progression, and corneal decompensation. A severe degree of inflammation leads to further lowering of IOP because of increased uveoscleral outflow. It also worsens the choroidal effusion contributing to further hypotony. Post-trabeculectomy hypotony with normal or deep AC is not considered a complication. If hypotony persists for a longer time it can cause the serious complication of maculopathy with characteristic features of macular striae, choroidal folds, tortuous retinal veins but with no evidence of vascular leak on fluorescein angiography (hypotony maculopathy).
- *Assessment of wound leak:* Siedel's test with fluorescein dye is the simplest way to demonstrate a leaking bleb. Anesthetize the conjunctiva with a fresh solution of paracaine—touch the area of suspected wound leak with sterile fluorescein strip soaked with a drop of paracaine. With the patient seated on slit-lamp examine the area with blue filter—a stream of clear aqueous lined on both sides with fluorescein line is a positive sign of aqueous leak. In an extremely hypotonic eye with flat AC the leak may be temporarily closed and the Siedel's test may be negative on casual examination. A mild pressure over the eye may open up the leaking area and Siedel's test may be demonstrated positive.
- *Assessment of overfiltering bleb:* An overfiltering bleb is large in size, diffuse, unusually raised with flat/shallow AC and extreme hypotony (sometimes unrecordably low).
- *Assessment of IOP:* If the postoperative IOP is in high single digit with shallow or flat AC (where it is expected to be much below the 6 mm Hg) always reconsider diagnosis and exclude aqueous misdirection glaucoma or pupillary block (with hyposecretion) or late onset suprachoroidal hemorrhage in its early phase. It has to be kept in mind that in presence of flat AC IOP reading with applanation tonometer tends to be higher as it applanates the crystalline lens (or pseudophakos) with the cornea.
- *Choroidal effusion:* Some amount of choroidal effusion in the periphery is common after filtering surgery which resolves on its own. However, if it is massive it is easily visible with ophthalmoscope. Choroidals are dark, raised, smooth swellings unlike serous retinal detachment which is much paler. Ultrasonography distinguishes ciliochoroidal effusion from suprachoroidal hemorrhage on B-Scan.
  Effusions are dome-shaped with highly reflective anterior border and little internal reflectivity on A-Scan. The suprachoroidal hemorrhage has high internal reflectivity on A-Scan. UBM (ultrasound biomicroscopy) can yield more information including the presence of cyclodialysis cleft which has been inadvertently created during surgery.
- *Degree of inflammation:* Severe uveitis results in breakdown of blood aqueous barrier, decreased aqueous production, and increased uveoscleral outflow leading to further hypotony.

TREATMENT

Preventing incidence of postoperative hypotony is crucial because it is difficult to treat. Anticipation and recognition of predisposing factors is important. And meticulous technique in each step of trabeculectomy is crucial to minimize chances of hypotony in the postoperative phase l. Utmost care during surgery to avoid intraoperative hypotony by maintaining deep AC from the beginning to the end of surgery, as for instance, by use of AC maintainers or viscoelastics. Preoperative IOP control with intravenous (IV) mannitol, hyperosmotic drugs, and digital compression is also mandatory. Meticulous wound closure to avoid wound dehiscence and leak and judicious use of antimetabolites and titrating the concentration and time exposure of antimetabolites, especially mitomycin prevents ocular hypotony and associated complications.

Address the Specific Cause
The treatment of postoperative hypotony is directed at the underlying cause:

Overfiltration Leading to Immediate Postoperative Shallow Anterior Chamber
If the bleb is well-formed and the eye is quiet, a patient with grade 1 or 2 of iridocorneal touch may be observed for 5-7 days or even longer if improvement occurs. It is only the grade 3 or flat AC with lenticulocorneal touch which needs immediate intervention starting with conservative management for 48-72 hours.
- Limit the use of corticosteroids—use cycloplegics, aqueous suppressants, and hyperosmotic agents to promote the wound healing by reducing aqueous flow.
- Pressure patch
- Large size bandage contact lens (CL) (17.5-24 mm).
- Simmonds shell and pressure patching with ointment or collagen shield under the shell.
- If this fails in 48-72 hours AC formation with BSS (balanced salt solution) or sodium hyaluronate/large-sized sterile air bubble or gas (15% perfluorocarbon or 50% sulfur hexafluoride) with scleral flap resuturing.
- Injection of autologous serum or haem/autologous fibrinogen concentrate inside the bleb is advocated for persistent hypotony without leak.

Conjunctival Defect or Wound Leak
Small wound leak especially from fornix-based edges respond favorably to conservative treatment:
- *Pressure patch:* A fusiform-shaped cotton ball is placed over the closed lid in area of the fistula and held in place with gauze pads to act as tamponade. Patient is instructed not to go to sleep as with Bell's phenomenon eyeball rotates upward and the pressure is applied over the cornea, worsening the condition. Application of pressure patch for few hours during the daytime in the office hours for few days is sufficient to close the small leaks.
- Large diameter (17.5-24 mm) bandage CL or hollow bandage CL or Simmonds scleral shell tamponade may be used.
- Cyanoacrylate tissue adhesive covered with collagen shield has been tried in some cases. However, it is less effective in conjunctival leaks than on corneal leaks because no stroma is available to adhere to.
- Autologous fibrin glue over the wound.
- Blue green argon laser application after pretreatment with Rose Bengal has been advocated.
- If the leak is large, conjunctival suturing with 10-0 monofilament nylon or even free conjunctival flap may be needed.

However, a late wound leak/bleb leak occurring months or even years after filtering surgery (especially after use of antimetabolites) is more problematic to deal with. No conservative treatment is likely to work with, though injection with blood/autologous serum around/into the bleb has been tried, compression sutures from the cornea to the Tenon capsule behind the bleb works better. If the bleb is big enough not to respond surgical bleb revision is the only option.

Serous Choroidal Effusion/Ciliochoroidal Detachment
Causing hypotony and shallow AC:
- If the effusion is small conservative management to take care of inflammation and hypotony is sufficient.
- Surgical drainage is warranted only when the effusion is massive coming to the central area as there is "kissing choroidals" or suprachoroidal hemorrhage or associated retinal detachment. Drainage of the suprachoroidal fluid with vitrectomy, injection of gas tamponade with formation of AC is undertaken.

Cyclodialysis Cleft Detected by Gonioscopy or Ultrasound Biomicroscopy
- Closed by argon laser application spot size 100 μm, duration of 0.1–0.2 seconds, and power of 400–1,000 MW.
- Penetrating diathermy, cryotherapy, and placing buckling elements at the limbus are other modalities.

Hypotonic Maculopathy
One of the dreaded complications is hypotony persisting for >6 weeks. Permanent visual loss is more likely if maculopathy persists >6 weeks. Hypotony persisting for nearly 6 weeks should be dealt with conservatively such as pressure patch, bandage CL, and Simmonds shells and no steroid drops.
- If not responding, more aggressive treatment in the form of injection of autologous serum/blood/autogenous fibrinogen concentrates in and around the bleb.
- If fails, the scleral flap may be resutured with tighter sutures.
- If the sclera is friable preserved sclera/pericardium may be used.

SUGGESTED READING
1. Weinreb RN. Glaucoma in 21st Century. Philadelphia: Harcourt Health Communications; 2000.

4.10 | Neovascular Glaucoma

Sushmita Kaushik, Parul Ichhpujani
Advanced Eye Centre, PGIMER, Chandigarh
sushmita_kaushik@yahoo.com, parul77@rediffmail.com

DEFINITION
Neovascular glaucoma (NVG) is a secondary angle-closure glaucoma caused by neovascularization of the angle and a fibrovascular membrane contracting to result in peripheral anterior synechiae. Vascular endothelial growth factors (VEGF) stimulated by retinal ischemia from several disorders [retinal vein occlusions and diabetic retinopathy (DR)] are the primary cause of the fibrovascular membrane and ocular neovascularization. NVG has been also known as rubeotic glaucoma, congestive glaucoma, thrombotic glaucoma, hemorrhagic glaucoma, and hemorrhagic glaucoma.

SIGNS AND SYMPTOMS
- *Presentation:* Longstanding angry looking red eye with painful vision loss. Rarely, asymptomatic.
- *Intraocular pressure (IOP):* Markedly elevated IOP (>40 mm Hg) with or without corneal edema.
- *Course of neovascularization:*
  - Early NVI is seen as small tufts of blood vessels at the pupillary ruff, but can be easily missed.
  - NVI can also begin at the edges of a peripheral iridotomy.
  - Neovascularization then follows over the iris surface toward the anterior chamber angle in an irregular radial meandering fashion **(Fig. 4.10.1)**.
  - At the angle, fine new vessels cross the scleral spur and ramify over the trabecular meshwork. Fibrosis of these vessels leads to development of ectropion uveae.
  - NVA may develop without NVI, on rare occasions.

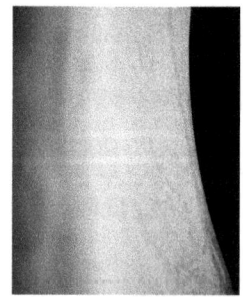

Fig. 4.10.1: Neovascularization of iris.

SECTION 4: Glaucoma

- *Gonioscopy:* Total or near-total angle closure with zippering, with or without NVA.
- *Posterior segment:* Evidence of retinal vessel occlusion (either artery or vein), ocular ischemic syndrome (OIS) or DR. If the fundal view is poor, a B-scan ultrasound may be carried out to rule out vitreous hemorrhage, retinal detachment, or tumor.
- *Ocular association:* As highlighted earlier, prior history of a retinal vascular occlusion, DR or chronic uveitis.
- *Systemic association:* Associated with systemic vascular diseases such as diabetes mellitus (DM), hypertension (HTN), carotid artery disease, or giant cell arteritis (GCA).

PATHOPHYSIOLOGY

- *Ischemia:* The most common causes of NVG include ischemic central retinal vein occlusion (CRVO), DR, and carotid artery disease and OIS. NVG may also be seen in patients with hemi- and branch retinal vein occlusion, retinal artery occlusion, and GCA. NVG typically develops within 3 months of CRVO while in retinal artery occlusions develop within 4 weeks of the occlusion.
  Perfusion pressure and ocular blood flow (perfusion pressure/vascular resistance) are key players in the cascade of events. Therefore, it is imperative not to markedly lower the systemic arterial blood pressure while lowering the IOP in such patients.
- *Role of VEGF:* In ischemic retinal disease, hypoxia induces VEGF, which acts upon the healthy endothelial cells of viable capillaries to stimulate the vasoproliferation in form of a fragile new vascular plexus. Multitude of other substances are involved in the angiogenesis such as the insulin-like growth factors I and II, insulin-like growth factor binding proteins 2 and 3, interleukin-6 (IL-6), placental growth factor (PGF), basic fibroblast growth factor (BFGF), and platelet-derived growth factor (PDGF).
- *Role of erythropoietin (EPO):* EPO is important for the initiation and control of the ocular neovascularization. Hypoxia induces retinal EPO expression and eventually this results in high EPO concentration in anterior chamber in NVG eyes. In NVG, the elevated EPO might result from retinal ischemia as well as due to an elevated IOP-induced self-regulated neuroprotective mechanism of the eye.
- *Neovascularization of iris:* The angiogenic factors diffuse into the aqueous and interact with the vascular structures in areas where the greatest aqueous-tissue contact occurs. The capillaries of the posterior iris sprout to form neovessels, which then grow along the posterior iris surface and ascend through the pupil, running on the anterior surface of the iris (NVI), and then over the angle, resulting in NVA.
- *Peripheral anterior synechiae (PAS):* It may cause a radial traction along the surface of the iris and pull the pigment layer around the iris pupillary margin anteriorly (ectropion uveae).
- *Secondary angle-closure glaucoma:* NVA along with the fibrovascular membrane, physically bridges and occludes the angle. It also physically pulls the iris and cornea into apposition, thus blocking the trabecular meshwork.

MANAGEMENT

- *Work up:* Gonioscopy, fundus fluorescein angiography and/or B-scan ultrasound. Recently, the OCT-Angiography (OCTA) has been used to delineate the extent and depth of NV and may be used as a follow-up tool to document regression of NV. In young patients with NVG, ultrasound biomicroscopy must be done to rule out ciliary body tumors.
- *Definitive management:* Eradication of the new vessels
  - Stage 1 (preglaucoma with abnormal blood vessels in the pupillary margin): Neovascularization must be addressed before the elevation of IOP. Panretinal photocoagulation (PRP) helps to attain this goal by destroying ischemic retina and thereby minimizing the oxygen demand as well as reducing the amount of VEGF being released. PRP tends to be effective in causing regression and involution of anterior segment neovascularization.

- Stage 2 (open angle but the IOP is elevated because of NVA): PRP needs to be done along with an intravitreal anti-VEGF. Elevated IOP is addressed with standard topical and/or oral glaucoma medication. Glaucoma surgery is resorted to medical therapy fails.
- Stage 3 (angle is closed with elevated IOP): PRP with an intravitreal anti-VEGF injection, reduction of inflammation and treatment with anti-glaucoma drugs and/or surgery is the mainstay. Intraocular inflammation may be treated with topical corticosteroids and cycloplegics such as atropine.

- *Medical treatment:* Aqueous suppressants, topical steroids and cycloplegics are the mainstay of treatment. Topical medications to lower IOP include carbonic anhydrase inhibitors, beta-blockers, and alpha-2 agonists, which lower aqueous production. Prostaglandin analogs (PGAs) are not effective because access to the uveoscleral route is generally compromised from angle closure. Additionally, PGAs and pilocarpine are proinflammatory, hence avoided.
- *Laser treatment:* Prompt PRP and other relevant treatment of the underlying disease are crucial to effective management and control of NVG and preservation of vision. PRP is ideally performed 2–3 weeks prior to glaucoma surgery to allow for regression of neovascularization and inflammation so that results are optimal. In patients with poor view of the fundus, adequate PRP cannot be done, therefore, laser can be applied surgically. PRP may reverse IOP elevation in the open-angle stage and in some cases of early angle-closure stage of NVG. Caution needs to be exercised with PRP as it can lead to ciliochoroidal effusions and increased IOP.
  Pars plana vitrectomy (PPV) and lensectomy (if necessary) with endolaser application may be considered.
      In patients with OIS, carotid endarterectomy for the carotid artery stenosis may cause a dramatic increase in postoperative IOP because of reperfusion of the ciliary body. Therefore, PRP and topical medications must be started prior to carotid endarterectomy.
- *Anti-VEGF therapy:* Intravitreal bevacizumab or ranibizumab or aflibercept injection appears to be beneficial as an adjuvant treatment in NVG and rubeosis due to its antiangiogenic properties; reduces both VEGF-A and placental growth factor. Anti-VEGF has a role as a bridge to PRP and surgery.
  Despite regression of neovascularization from effective PRP or anti-VEGF therapy, additional medical treatment or surgery is needed to control residual glaucoma from angle closure.
- *Trabeculectomy:* Poor outcome of glaucoma filtration surgery is more likely in patients with younger age, extensive PAS, pseudophakia, prior PPV, and postoperative hyphema.
- *Glaucoma drainage device (GDD) surgery:* It is a preferable option in inflamed eyes as augmented trabeculectomy has a high chance of failure. These implants can be inserted either in the anterior chamber or in pars plana if combined with pars plana vitrectomy. Variable success rates have been described with drainage implants and it decreases over time. No significant differences have been noted among the various types of implants. In quiet eyes with regressed new vessels, trabeculectomy with adjunctive, high-dose mitomycin may also be effective in controlling IOP.
- *Palliative measures:* For painful blind eyes with refractory IOP control: Cyclodestruction/transscleral cyclophotocoagulation are done. Endocyclophotocoagulation (ECP) may also have a role as an adjunct therapy.

PROGNOSIS
- Prognosis is highly guarded and dependent on the prevention as well as the treatment of the underlying disease process resulting in NVG early in its course.
- Intensity and frequency of follow-up care depends on the systemic conditions predisposing the patient to the development of NVG.

SUGGESTED READING
1. Brown GC, Magargal LE, Schachat A, Shah H. Neovascular glaucoma. Etiologic considerations. Ophthalmology. 1984;91(4):315-20.
2. Senthil S, Dada T, Das T, Kaushik S, Puthuran GV, Philip R, et al. Neovascular glaucoma: a review. Indian J Ophthalmol. 2021;69(3):525-34.
3. Sun C, Zhang H, Jiang J, Li Y, Nie C, Gu J, et al. Angiogenic and inflammatory biomarker levels in aqueous humor and vitreous of neovascular glaucoma and proliferative diabetic retinopathy. Int Ophthalmol. 2020 Feb;40(2):467-75.

4.11 | Overfunctioning Blebs

Murali Ariga, Sangeetha R, Nishanth M
MN Eye Hospital, Chennai
muraliariga@gmail.com

ETIOLOGY AND DEFINITION
For a successful surgical outcome after formation of a well-functioning bleb is essential. After conventional trabeculectomy, when trabeculectomy, there is excessive leakage through the surgical fistula and/or lack of resistance in the boundary layers of the evolving bleb, it leads to an overfunctioning bleb.

SIGNS AND SYMPTOMS
Overfunctioning blebs usually result in ocular hypotony and a large diffuse bleb. Anterior chamber (AC) is usually shallow and there may be peripheral iridocorneal apposition. Intraocular pressure (IOP) may be low (single digit) with associated anterior or annular choroidal effusion. Longstanding hypotony may cause sight-threatening complications. Chorioretinal folds in the macula, choroidal hemorrhage, and cataract result in visual loss. In severe cases there may be lens-cornea touch with "kissing choroidals".

Symptomatic patients present with decreased vision, foreign body sensation, and epiphora. Visual loss may be due to intermittent astigmatism induced by the upper lid in case of hypotony, induced astigmatism caused by the pressure of the upper lid on a large cystic bleb extending over the limbus or induced astigmatism caused by a scleral flap that is too loose. Ocular surface disturbances may also be noted due to dellen formation when the bleb is steep walled.

CLINICAL EVALUATION
Visual acuity should be checked at every visit. Slit-lamp evaluation is to look for the bleb height, extent and vascularity. Seidel's test should be performed to check for bleb leakage in thin-walled blebs. IOP by applanation tonometry is recorded and monitored periodically. Dilated fundus examination is necessary to look for choroidal effusion and macular changes.

Brightness scan (B-scan) ultrasound is useful to exclude the presence of hemorrhage in choroidal effusion. Occasionally diffuse choroidal effusion without bullous elevation that is not seen on clinical examination may be obvious on B-scan and could explain the forward displacement of the lens-iris diaphragm. Ultrasound biomicroscopy (UBM) is another useful diagnostic modality to document changes in the AC depth, angle, and ciliary body. However, because it involves contact with the eye it may not be suitable in the immediate postoperative period. Anterior segment optical coherence tomography (OCT) can be used to classify bleb characteristics (diffuse, cystic or encapsulated, etc.) and are useful in immediate postoperative period.

MANAGEMENT

Early Postoperative Period
- To promote inflammation and development of increased resistance in the developing bleb, the topical corticosteroids can be decreased or temporarily withdrawn.
- Topical cycloplegic agents will move the lens-iris diaphragm back and help the ciliary body restart the production of aqueous.
- *Torpedo patch:* Pressure patching by placing a small fusiform-shaped cotton ball over the lid in the area of trabeculectomy flap. This cotton ball is held in place with cotton pads to act as a tamponade.
- Placement of a large bandage soft contact lens or a symblepharon ring may help to reduce outflow through the bleb and also deepen the AC.
- Anterior chamber shallowing due to overfiltration may be reversed by injection of air or viscoelastic such as sodium hyaluronate into the AC.
- Persistent shallow AC with choroidals necessitates drainage along with AC reformation.

INTERMEDIATE TO LATE POSTOPERATIVE PERIOD

The following can be attempted:
- Compression mattress sutures over the bleb
- Autologous blood injection into the bleb
- Continuous wave Nd:YAG (neodymium-doped yttrium aluminum garnet) laser application over conjunctiva
- Cryotherapy to shrink the bleb.

Compression Sutures
Under topical anesthesia a 9-0 nylon suture is passed 1-2 mm of clear cornea close to the limbus. This suture goes over the bleb and is passed through conjunctiva-Tenon capsule posterior to the bleb and parallel to limbus. This suture is then draped over the bleb and tied tightly to the free end in the cornea (knot is buried).

Autologous Blood Injection
Under topical anesthesia viscoelastic is injected into the AC (this will prevent backflow of blood from the bleb into the AC in eyes with low IOP). 1 mL of freshly drawn autologous blood is taken in a sterile 1-mL syringe with a 30G needle. Under strict aseptic precautions this needle is introduced subconjunctivally a few millimeters away from the bleb and the needle tip advanced into the bleb. 0.2-0.5 mL of blood is then slowly injected. One should wait till the blood clots before the needle is withdrawn. IOP increase may be observed after 2 weeks. A small amount of this injected blood may trickle into the AC and this may not need any further intervention.

The Nd:YAG laser (continuous wave) has been used with power of 4 J and an offset of 3-4 (0.9-1.0 mm) so as to deliver energy at the level of the episclera. Approximately, 30-40 spots in a grid pattern starting in the periphery are applied till the end point of blanching and wrinkling of the conjunctiva is reached.

Although autologous blood injection and laser bleb revision have demonstrated modest success in the management of overfiltering or dysfunctional blebs **(Figs. 4.11.1A and B)**, the exact mechanism by which these methods work has not been well understood (presumed to cause cellular proliferation).

Surgical revision and repair is the most reliable and definitive treatment when all else fails. Resuturing the scleral flap and/or placing a donor graft (sclera, amniotic membrane, pericardium or dura) over the fistula are the options available. Conjunctival grafting either free or sliding may be necessary to replace thin avascular conjunctiva that may overly the flap in cases when mitomycin was used.

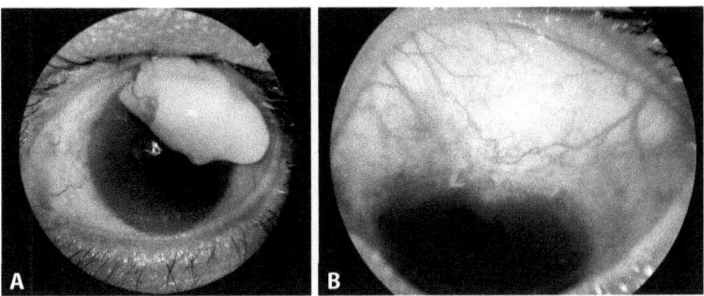

Figs. 4.11.1A and B: Overfiltering blebs.

Circumferential Blebs

Blebs, which are functioning well, can extend inferiorly even to 360°. Once the bleb starts to extend downward from the superior quadrants, its downward expansion is favored by the relative thinness of the Tenon layer laterally. When bulging, these blebs can cause symptoms as they interfere with blinking and tear flow. Management can include lubricants and tear supplements, as well as staged removal of the sectors of the conjunctiva, away from the functioning upper quadrant.

Corneal Dissecting Blebs

The anterior edge of the bleb extends over the cornea within the epithelium, forming a white, nonvascularized, multiloculated, and spongy tissue, which can protrude for several millimeters. The Bowman layer and the stroma remain intact. This condition can cause symptoms when it interferes with blinking or tear flow, causes bubble formation or irritates corneal nerves. Management can include topical lubricants and tear substitutes. If not effective, the part of the bleb lying over the peripheral cornea can be excised under topical anesthesia. Simple excision without suturing or grafting is usually sufficient.

Dellen

Corneal dellen develop in front of steep-walled blebs usually when placed either nasally or temporally. The bulk of the bleb impedes the contact of the inner surface of the upper lid with the peripheral cornea. Lubricants and tear substitutes are indicated for management, and they need to be used intensively. Ointments and patching are the next levels of intervention. Conservative measures such as these are effective in most cases. When symptoms persist, compression mattress sutures may be tried. Surgical revision is to be considered when all these measures fail.

■ FOLLOW-UP

Treatment of overfiltering blebs may incite cellular proliferation and subconjunctival fibrosis causing filtration failure and elevation in IOP. Periodical monitoring of IOP helps early identification of bleb fibrosis and prompt institution of ocular hypertensive therapy.

■ SUGGESTED READING

1. Doyle JW, Smith FM. Complications of glaucoma filtering surgery. In: Yannof M, Duker JS (Eds). Ophthalmology. St Louis: Mosby; 2004. pp. 1610-15.

4.12 Chronic Primary Angle-closure Glaucoma

Vinay Nangia
Suraj Eye Institute, Nagpur
nagpursuraj@gmail.com

■ DEFINITION

A chronic asymptomatic form of primary angle-closure glaucoma (CPACG) with features indicating trabecular obstruction by peripheral iris, such as peripheral anterior synechiae, elevated intraocular pressure (IOP), iris whirling, glaukomflecken, lens opacities, pigment deposition in angle or on the trabecular surface, with glaucomatous optic disk damage or optic disk damage in association with visual field loss.

■ CLINICAL FEATURES

Symptoms

A patient with CPACG may be asymptomatic and may present like primary open angle glaucoma (POAG). When symptomatic he may complain of blurring or loss of vision, haloes when the IOP is elevated with corneal edema, and pain and redness when the IOP is very high for a longer period of time or in a situation which resembles an acute on chronic episode.

Signs

The IOP is elevated and sometimes may even be normal when examined. The cornea may be clear or edematous depending on the IOP and duration of chronic angle closure. The anterior chamber will be shallow with a narrow peripheral anterior chamber depth on Van Herick's test. The pupils may be irregular and mid-dilated, with iris atrophy, whirling and sometimes glaukomflecken if the patient has had intermittent attacks of elevated IOP. Gonioscopy will show anterior synechiae, which may be intermittent, scattered throughout the angle or involving certain quadrants or involving the entire 360°. The areas without peripheral anterior synechiae will show increased pigmentation and varying degrees of the angle structures may be visible. Visual field loss and optic disk damage may be present in varying degrees of severity.

■ EVOLUTION

The development of CPACG may occur following creeping angle closure when the angle may close circumferentially and without causing any symptoms. It may follow several attacks of intermittent angle closure or may develop following an unresolved episode of acute angle closure.

■ WORK-UP

All patients should undergo a routine ophthalmic evaluation, including visual acuity, refraction, and slit-lamp biomicroscopy, with special emphasis on assessing the anterior chamber depth, the pupil, the iris, and the lens surface. Van Herick's test should be a routine part of the evaluation. Applanation tonometry should be performed. Gonioscopy should be performed with a single mirror, three-mirror or the magnaview gonioscopy lens. Indentation gonioscopy is a must and may be done with the Zeiss indentation gonioscope, posner gonioprism or Sussman four-mirror indentation gonioscope. Anterior segment optical coherence tomography will give further details of the angle. Automated perimetry should be done. Optic disk evaluation should be done using a 90 D or 78 D lens for stereoscopic evaluation. Pupillary dilatation may be considered for better optic disk and retinal evaluation with due precautions or may be done following laser peripheral iridotomy (PI). Optic disk photography and use of spectral domain optical coherence tomography for assessing the optic nerve and retinal nerve fiber layer damage may be helpful.

DIFFERENTIAL DIAGNOSIS

A subluxed lens giving rise to shallow anterior chamber and closed angles and elevated IOP, plateau iris syndrome which goes unrecognized and develops longstanding elevated IOP, an eye with pseudoexfoliation and shallow anterior chamber with varying degrees of angle closure, the presence of a ciliary mass, or a retinal volume increase pushing the iris-lens diaphragm forward and leading to a rise in IOP are conditions to be considered in the differential diagnosis.

TREATMENT

Medical Treatment

The medical treatment of a patient with CPACG would be generally similar to POAG. One would use the same principles of treatment. One may opt to start with a beta-blocker or an alpha agonist or a prostaglandin. The degree of pressure reducing efficacy of prostaglandins in presence of closed angles may be considered. Pilocarpine may also be used. For long-term use it would be indicated in certain selected situations, since it has a tendency to move the iris-lens diaphragm forward. Systemic carbonic anhydrase inhibitors may also be used depending on the indications.

Laser Treatment

Laser iridotomy may be done with the Nd:YAG (neodymium-doped yttrium aluminum garnet) laser alone or in combination with argon laser. It will help to deepen the anterior chamber and relieve the pupillary block. Laser iridotomy may or may not reduce the IOP in all cases of CPACG but may influence the further progressive closure of the angle and/or shallowing of the anterior chamber. Laser trabeculoplasty does not have a clear indication in CPACG. The use of peripheral iridoplasty in CPACG in India is not well-documented. In patients where surgery is not considered initially the use of laser PI with medical management would be the indicated therapy.

Surgical Treatment

Trabeculectomy is the surgical procedure of choice in patients of CPACG. One may give consideration to surgical management especially when the disk is significantly damaged. In early or moderate disk damage a combination of laser PI and medical management may be utilized. With severe disk damage, surgery may be considered even as the initial line of management. Patients undergoing trabeculectomy should be asked to discontinue pilocarpine at least 1–2 weeks, prior to surgery, to prevent a higher possibility of shallow anterior chamber post-surgery. Caution should be exercised when considering the use of mitomycin-C in patients of CPACG undergoing trabeculectomy. Combined glaucoma and cataract surgery may provide additional benefit by significantly deepening the anterior chamber and improving the visual acuity and may be used when indicated. Combined surgery or cataract surgery alone has been shown to be effective in the management of uncontrolled PACG and even in patients controlled with medical therapy. The possibility of developing malignant glaucoma may be higher when only trabeculectomy is done versus when combined surgery or only cataract surgery is done. Cataract surgery requires significant skills and phacoemulsification is the only technique that should be used in such a situation. It is most preferable that a 2.2-mm incision should be used for surgery. A shallow anterior chamber is a major challenge in cataract surgery and the surgeon needs to be extremely cautious.

FOLLOW-UP

A patient with CPACG needs lifelong follow up. The duration between follow-up visits will vary with the clinical decision of the individual physician, the stage of management, and the method of treatment. A patient on follow-up may undergo the complete eye examination including applanation tonometry, gonioscopy, and disk evaluation.

SUGGESTED READING

1. Ritch R, Lowe R. Angle closure glaucoma: Clinical types. In: The Glaucomas—Clinical Science, 2nd edition. St. Louis, MO: Mosby; 1996. pp. 821-40.

4.13 Primary Congenital Glaucoma

Sapna Sinha, R Krishnadas
Aravind Eye Care System, Madurai
dr.sapnasinha@outlook.com, krishnadas@aravind.org

DEFINITION

Primary congenital glaucoma (PCG) refers to a specific form of developmental glaucoma characterized by isolated maldevelopment of the trabecular outflow apparatus (trabeculodysgenesis) of the anterior chamber angle unassociated with other developmental ocular anomalies or ocular diseases that can elevate the intraocular pressure (IOP). PCG with onset at birth to <1 month old is referred as the neonatal/newborn onset PCG while late onset PCG is defined as PCG with its onset after 2 years of age. Children suffering from infantile onset PCG would have an onset between neonatal/newborn and late onset glaucoma (i.e., between 1 month and 24 months old).

EPIDEMIOLOGY

Primary congenital glaucoma occurs in about 1 out of 10,000 births and results in blindness in approximately 10% of the affected children and reduced vision (worse than 20/50) in about half of all those affected. Most are sporadic, but there is an autosomal recessive inheritance pattern reported in 10% of children with variable penetrance and expressivity.

The prevalence is higher in cultures with consanguinity, particularly those with a high carrier rate of *CYP1B1* gene (GLC3A locus on chromosome 2p21). The only known risk factors are genetic, consanguinity, and affected siblings. The risk of congenital glaucoma in the second child is approximately 5%, and the risk increases to 25% with two affected siblings.

PATHOPHYSIOLOGY

Isolated trabeculodysgenesis is the hallmark of PCG attributed to arrest in development of the anterior segment structures derived from neural crest cells late in gestation. In eyes with PCG, the iris and the ciliary body have the appearance of the anterior chamber in the 7th or 8th month of gestation, rather than that of full term development at birth. The iris and ciliary body fail to recede posteriorly, with the insertion of the peripheral iris and the ciliary body overlapping the posterior aspect of a poorly developed trabecular meshwork. Such poorly developed aqueous outflow pathway renders them functionally incompetent, causing obstruction to the flow of aqueous humor and elevation of IOP.

CLINICAL FEATURES

The classic triad of symptoms includes epiphora, photophobia, and blepharospasm as a consequence of corneal irritation secondary to corneal epithelial edema caused by elevated IOP. The condition may present as red eye mimicking conjunctivitis. High IOP causes corneal clouding, rapid enlargement of the globe, and limbal stretching. A corneal diameter >11 mm in a newborn and 12 mm in an infant <1 year is very suggestive of raised IOP and congenital glaucoma. A measurement of >13 mm in a child of any age is abnormal, as is marked asymmetry in corneal diameters. The cornea can enlarge up to 16–17 mm Hg in most severe of congenital glaucoma. There is corneal haze due to edema, which is intermittent to begin with and precedes breaks in Descemet's membrane (Haab's striae). Persistent elevation in IOP causes stromal scarring, chronic stromal corneal edema, and irregular corneal astigmatism. Increased distensibility of the sclera causes scleral thinning and blue sclera. Ocular enlargement and buphthalmos often are irreversible even with normalization of IOP. Myopia and astigmatism are caused by increased length of the globe. Anisometropia and amblyopia are common in unilateral or asymmetric PCG.

Examination under anesthesia or sedation is useful to detect the characteristic features of congenital glaucoma:
- Longer axial length on A-scan
- Large corneal diameter >12 mm in full term infants
- Evaluation by hand held slit lamp reveals cloudy cornea or Haab's striae.
- Cycloplegic streak retinoscopy reveals progressive myopia or loss of hyperopia.
- IOP estimation before induction of deep planes of anesthesia with Tonopen or Perkins tonometer reveals normal infant IOP to be 10–15 mm Hg. IOP under anesthesia in congenital glaucoma appears to be typically between 25 and 35 mm Hg.
- Gonioscopy is characteristic for an abnormal, high insertion of iris and indistinct, poorly developed trabecular meshwork.
- Ophthalmoscopy reveals concentric optic nerve cupping with pink neural rim tissue to begin with, which later becomes sloped and excavated as in adult glaucoma.

■ DIFFERENTIAL DIAGNOSIS

Tearing and redness are also caused by nasolacrimal duct obstruction, conjunctivitis, corneal epithelial defects and abrasions, ocular inflammation (keratitis and iridocyclitis), and corneal dystrophies (Meesman, Reis Bucklers, etc.). Axial myopia and isolated megalocornea also cause corneal enlargement.

Corneal haze and edema simulating congenital glaucoma may also be caused by obstetric trauma, corneal ulcers from neonatal rubella, herpes virus or syphilis, metabolic diseases such as mucopolysaccharidoses, congenital hereditary stromal and endothelial dystrophy, sclerocornea, and corneal dermoids. Secondary glaucomas and elevated IOP associated with anterior segment dysgenesis and phacomatosis are also included in differential diagnosis.

■ WORK-UP

In young infants, anterior segment evaluation and fundus assessment with a direct ophthalmoscope set at +10 diopters may be performed under sedation with choral hydrate (25–50 mg/kg). If children are unable to cooperate additional evaluation under anesthesia may be scheduled.

Corneal diameter is measured and cornea examined under magnification to document corneal edema, Haab's striae and corneal enlargement. A corneal diameter >12 mm in the 1st year of life is diagnostic of congenital glaucoma. Assessment of refractive error establishes a baseline to judge progression, as increasing myopia indicates ocular enlargement from uncontrolled glaucoma. IOP is measured by Tonopen or Perkins tonometer. Ophthalmoscopy documents optic nerve head changes.

All anesthetic agents alter IOP of infants with infantile glaucoma. Rapid lowering of IOP is observed with halothane and sevoflurane, while cyclopropane, succinylcholine, and ketamine rapidly elevate IOP. Most accurate IOP measurements are achieved by intramuscular ketamine and in case of inhalational anesthesia, immediately prior to intubation before deep levels of anesthesia are achieved. The normal IOP in children under inhalational anesthesia such as halothane is observed to be approximately 9–10 mm Hg and a pressure of 20 mm Hg or higher should arouse suspicion of abnormal elevation of IOP. The most reliable IOP estimation in children is, however, obtained while they are awake and cooperative. Perkins tonometer provides a suitable mode of measurement of IOP in children under anesthesia, while noncontact tonometry or a Tonopen could be used to estimate IOP in children who are awake and cooperative. Mean IOP in unanesthetized infants is known to be approximately 11.4 ± 2.4 mm Hg.

A-scan and B-scan mode ultrasonography is used to measure the axial length of the globe (normal 18–20 mm in infants) and increasing axial length indicates progression from uncontrolled glaucoma.

■ TREATMENT

Medical Therapy

Medications are used as a temporizing measure to lower IOP, and reduce corneal edema prior to surgical management, which is the mainstay of therapy since glaucoma is due to a structural developmental abnormality. Long-term medical therapy is also difficult in children due to difficulties in compliance as well as possible adverse effects of the drugs used in reduction of IOP. Medications may also be used adjunctively following surgical treatment.

- Topical carbonic anhydrase inhibitors (dorzolamide and brinzolamide) can be safely administered in children.
- Topical beta-blockers (timolol, levobunolol, or betaxolol) can also be used in children provided there are no known contraindications to their use. Lowest effective doses when available are recommended and it is preferable to use these medications once daily with nasolacrimal duct obstruction following their administration to prevent their systemic absorption and adverse effects.
- Fixed combinations of dorzolamide and timolol may be used when monotherapy is inadequate to control IOP when beta-blockers are not contraindicated.
- Prostaglandin analogs although systemically safe in children, their efficacy in congenital and development glaucoma is largely unproven.
- Alpha agonists such as brimonidine are not recommended for use in children. These drugs are contraindicated in infants/small children weighing <40 lb as it may cause bradycardia, hypotension, hypothermia, hypotonia, and apnea due to CNS depression. Brimonidine may also prolong anesthetic recovery or precipitate respiratory failure in young and premature infants. Although may be used with caution in older children, alpha agonists are generally not recommended for use in children and young adults since it causes drowsiness and lethargy.
- Oral acetazolamide in the dosage of 5–10 mg/kg every 6–12 hours may be used in children requiring IOP lowering therapy as short-term measure. Long-term therapy with oral acetazolamide predisposes to systemic adverse effects, including metabolic acidosis and is not recommended.

Definitive treatment of congenital glaucoma is surgical, while medical therapy is frequently useful as a temporizing IOP, lowering treatment prior to surgery, or as adjuvant therapy after partially successful surgical procedures in refractory childhood glaucoma. Decision on the right choice of surgery initially is of paramount importance as the first operation has the greatest chance of success.

Angle surgery (trabeculotomy and goniotomy) is usually the preferred first-line treatment with the best success rates and low complication rates. When cornea is relatively clear, goniotomy with visualization of the angle by a direct gonioscope results in clinical success in about 80% of children with congenital glaucoma. If visualization of the angle is precluded by corneal edema and scarring, ab externo trabeculotomy may be performed.

Combined trabeculotomy-trabeculectomy is more successful than either procedure performed alone and is primary procedure of choice in patients with greater risk of failure. It is generally accepted that in eyes with corneal diameter <14 mm, angle surgery is generally successful in controlling the IOP better over long term. In children presenting late with severe glaucoma and corneal diameter >14 mm, angle surgery alone is seldom sufficient for long-term success. In such instances, combined trabeculotomy—trabeculectomy is the procedure of choice. Trabeculectomy is associated with a high risk of failure due to excessive scarring. Use of adjunctive mitomycin has little benefit in prevention of conjunctival scarring. Occasionally, thin blebs associated with use of antimetabolites increase risk of hypotony and bleb-related endophthalmitis. Recent studies have also investigated the role of 360° trabeculotomy with 6-0 Vicryl or canaloplasty with illuminated catheters as initial surgery in PCG and have been reported to result in enhanced success.

Glaucoma drainage device is important part of the therapeutic repertoire in childhood glaucoma, especially refractory glaucoma. It is preferable to trabeculectomy when conjunctival scarring is evident, or in buphthalmic eyes with very thin sclera and when initial angle surgery has failed to control IOP.

Cyclodestruction procedures are reserved until both angle procedures and other surgical modality have failed resulting in refractory glaucoma.

Concurrent with controlling IOP, ametropia correction, and amblyopia management are essential to optimize long-term visual outcome.

■ FOLLOW-UP

Long-term prognosis in children with congenital glaucoma has generally improved with superior microsurgical techniques, especially in children diagnosed early and generally asymptomatic at diagnosis or if corneal enlargement, edema or scarring is not severe. Prognosis for vision and surgical success is generally poor with corneal diameter >14 mm and if associated with corneal scarring and stromal edema. Children whose IOP is controlled by surgery may experience vision impairment due to amblyopia, corneal scarring, strabismus, anisometropia, cataracts, filtration failure, and recurrent glaucoma. Such children require an integrated approach to treatment with visual rehabilitation and education. Children with congenital glaucoma require lifelong follow-up and therapy.

■ SUGGESTED READING

1. Mandal AK, Netland P. The Pediatric Glaucomas. St. Louis: Elsevier; 2006.

4.14 Pseudoexfoliation Syndrome/Exfoliative Glaucoma

Prashanth R, Krishnadas SR
Aravind Eye Hospital, Madurai
loweriop@yahoo.com

■ DEFINITION

Pseudoexfoliation syndrome (XFS) is characterized by the production and progressive accumulation of a fibrillar extracellular material in ocular and systemic tissues. It is the most common identifiable cause of glaucoma worldwide.

Glaucoma occurs more commonly in eyes with XFS than in those without it. Elevated intraocular pressure (IOP) with or without glaucomatous damage occurs in approximately 25% of persons with XFS, or about 6-10 times the rate in eyes without XFS. Pseudoexfoliative glaucoma has a more progressive clinical course and worse prognosis than primary open-angle glaucoma (POAG). There is a significantly higher frequency and severity of optic nerve damage at the time of diagnosis, worse visual field damage, poorer response to medications, more severe clinical course, and more frequent necessity for surgical intervention. Persons with elevated IOP and XFS are much more likely to develop glaucomatous damage on long-term follow-up than those without XFS.

■ SIGNS AND SYMPTOMS

Patients with XFS remain asymptomatic until advanced glaucoma develops. The condition is most common in the sixth to eighth decade of life. There is no racial, sexual, or geographic predilection. Exfoliation syndrome often occurs unilaterally, but within 5 years, 14-41% of those afflicted may develop the bilateral form.

The patient presents with a fine, flaky material on the anterior lens capsule, pupillary margin of the iris, and throughout the inner surface of the anterior chamber (**Figs. 4.14.1 and 4.14.2**). Over time, this coalesces into a characteristic "bulls-eye" pattern seen in pseudoexfoliation. There is often increased transillumination of the iris at the pupillary margin and there may be pigment granules on the endothelium and iris surface. Within the angle, there may be observable pigment or clear flaky material. Initially, IOP is unaffected; however, elevated IOP develops in up to 80% of patients. In these cases, glaucomatous cupping and visual field loss may ensue.

Other signs of XFS are insufficient mydriasis, posterior synechiae, pigment deposition on the iris surface, deposition of pigment and pseudoexfoliation material on the corneal endothelium, pigment liberation after pupillary dilation and pseudoexfoliation material covering the ciliary processes and the zonules. Phacodonesis, lens subluxation, and corneal endothelial decompensation can be present. An associated nuclear cataract is a common finding.

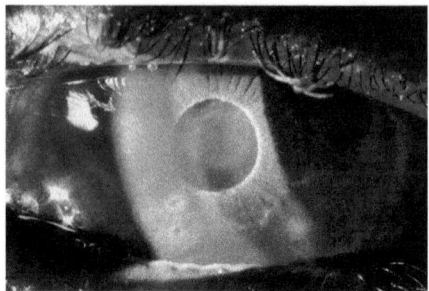

Fig. 4.14.1: Exfoliation in pupillary area.

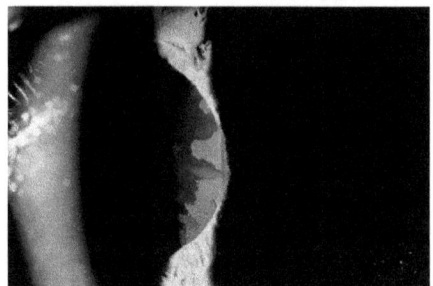

Fig. 4.14.2: Exfoliation on the anterior lens capsule.

■ PATHOPHYSIOLOGY

Pseudoexfoliation syndrome is a common ocular manifestation of a systemic disease, known to cause disease primarily in the eye. Exact etiology of this condition remains unknown. Defects in elastin metabolism have been postulated to result in synthesis of pseudoexfoliative material. It has been shown that specific mutations of the lysyl oxidase-like protein 1 (*LOXL1*) gene which is important in elastin metabolism are strongly associated with the development of PXF and secondary glaucoma. Two single nucleotide polymorphisms have been identified. Pseudoexfoliative material can be identified preclinically with transmission electron microscopy which shows fibrillar elastotic material. Histochemically, pseudoexfoliative material is a glycoconjugate surrounding a protein core. These aggregates are synthesized intracellularly in multiple different cell types in the anterior segment including nonpigmented ciliary epithelial cells, trabecular endothelial cells and pre-equatorial lens epithelial cells. This is thought to be a result of oxidative stress. The material is then released into the extracellular space and deposited around the cells that produced the material, and also other structures such as the zonules, pupillary margin, and anterior lens surface.

Open-angle Glaucoma

Potential causes of elevated IOP in eyes with XFS include trabecular cell dysfunction, blockage of the meshwork by exogenous and endogenous exfoliation materials, blockage of the meshwork by liberated iris pigment, trabecular cell dysfunction, and coexisting POAG.

Angle-closure Glaucoma

Characteristics of eyes with XFS which predispose to angle-closure glaucoma include the predisposition to posterior synechia formation, zonular weakness and associated forward lens movement, iris stiffness and rigidity, pupillary block, and a smaller pupil.

WORK-UP

- *History:* Patients may be asymptomatic, or they may complain of decreased visual acuity secondary to cataract or glaucomatous visual field changes.
- Complete ophthalmic examination, including gonioscopy of the anterior chamber angle and IOP determination. Peripupillary iris transillumination defects can be characteristically observed in some eyes.
  Gonioscopy shows a discontinuous pigmentation of the trabecular meshwork. Also, pigment is characteristically deposited on the Schwalbe line or anterior to the Schwalbe line (the Sampaolesi line).
      The most commonly recognized feature is the three-ring sign on the anterior lens capsule, formed by a central disk, a peripheral ring and a clear zone, which separates the two. The clear zone varies in diameter and may exhibit curled edges.
- *Imaging Studies:* Optical coherence tomography (OCT) and Heidelberg retinal tomography (HRT) have shown a high correlation between the retinal nerve fiber layer thickness and the visual field mean defect during achromatic perimetry. GDx nerve fiber analyzer has been reported to be a valuable tool in helping the clinician to discriminate between healthy eyes and glaucomatous eyes.

DIFFERENTIAL DIAGNOSIS

- *Uveitis:* Corneal endothelial deposits can be present in both exfoliative and uveitic glaucomas. The ragged volcano-like peripheral anterior synechiae of some inflammatory glaucomas are not seen in exfoliation syndrome, but angle closure due to narrow angles is not rare in exfoliation syndrome. Photophobia is common with uveitis.
- *Pigmentary glaucoma:* Krukenberg spindle and mid-peripheral iris transillumination defects are characteristic clinical signs, and this form of open-angle glaucoma is common in young males with myopia.
- *Capsular delamination (true exfoliation):* Trauma, exposure to intense heat (e.g., glass blower), or severe uveitis can cause a thin membrane to peel off the anterior lens capsule. Glaucoma is uncommon in this condition.
- Primary amyloidosis.
- Primary open-angle glaucoma.
- Fuchs heterochromic uveitis.

MANAGEMENT

Glaucoma associated with XFS tends to respond less to medical therapy than does POAG. XFS without a pressure rise requires only periodic monitoring of IOPs, disks, and visual fields. The treatment of pseudoexfoliation glaucoma is the same as that of POAG; however, topical medications tend to be less effective. Adjunctive therapy with other medications or laser treatment is often necessary. In exfoliative glaucoma prostaglandin analogs effectively reduce the 24-hour IOP from baseline. It is preferable to use medications that increase aqueous outflow, such as prostaglandin analogs and mitotic, if tolerated. Aqueous suppressants, when used to control IOP in exfoliation glaucoma tend to cause sledging of aqueous due to suppression of aqueous humor inflow and sluggish flow of aqueous. This results in increased deposition of exfoliation in the trabecular outflow pathway and progression of glaucoma due to increase in aqueous outflow resistance. Moreover, prostaglandin analogs, owing to their inhibitory effect on matrix metalloproteinases also reduce formation of exfoliation fibrils, which has a favorable outcome on IOP and glaucoma progression.

    Laser trabeculoplasty has been reported to be particularly effective in PXF glaucoma, due to relatively pigmented angles. However, the duration of IOP lowering is limited with more than half of patients failing after 5 years.

If medical therapy and laser therapy (trabeculoplasty) are unsuccessful to control the glaucoma, trabeculectomy can be performed with similar success rates to that of POAG.

Cataracts occur more commonly in patients with XFS. Weakness of the zonular fibers, spontaneous lens subluxation, and phacodonesis also can be present. Therefore, in these patients, cataract surgery alone or combined cataract surgery and glaucoma filtering surgery is associated with a higher incidence of intraoperative complications, most notably zonular dialysis, posterior capsular breaks, vitreous loss (5-10 times more common), lens dislocation, loss of residual lens material in vitreous, and intraocular lens (IOL) decentration. The increased intraoperative posterior capsule complication rate appears to correlate with the level of cataract maturity.

Postoperatively, complications can occur after uneventful cataract extractions due to continued destabilization of the zonules and capsular contraction with consequent IOL decentration and dislocation.

Note:
- An initially normal IOP measurement does not preclude prior IOP elevation with subsequent field loss and disk damage. Remember that pseudoexfoliative glaucoma undergoes periods of exacerbation and remission. Serial photographs and automated visual fields are more appropriate for managing this condition than IOP measurements, since the patient may experience progression yet manifest normal IOP if measured during remission.
- Argon laser trabeculoplasty/selective laser trabeculoplasty and filtration surgery are more effective in controlling IOP in cases of pseudoexfoliative syndrome than in POAG.

FOLLOW-UP

Patients with XFS should have annual eye examinations for early detection of glaucoma. Exfoliative glaucoma patients are followed up at more frequent intervals than POAG, since progression can occur far more rapidly. It has been observed that eyes with exfoliation have elastotic degeneration of the lamina cribrosa which predisposes these optic nerve heads to damage at lesser IOP than eyes without exfoliation. Moreover, eyes with exfoliation are also subject to higher intraocular pressures.

SUGGESTED READING

1. Ritch R, Schlötzer-Schrehardt U. Exfoliation syndrome. Surv Ophthalmol. 2001;45(4): 265-315.

4.15 | Steroid-induced Glaucoma

Prashanth R, Krishnadas SR
Aravind Eye Hospital, Madurai
loweriop@yahoo.com

DEFINITION

Corticosteroid-induced glaucoma is an iatrogenic, secondary form of open-angle glaucoma resulting from prolonged use of topical, periocular, intravitreal, inhalational or systemic corticosteroids. It resembles primary open-angle glaucoma (POAG) in its presentation and clinical course, with increased resistance to trabecular outflow of aqueous humor. Though one-thirds of patients administered corticosteroids demonstrate some responsiveness to steroid use, only a small percentage have significant intraocular pressure (IOP) elevation with resultant glaucomatous optic nerve damage and visual field loss.

A high percentage of patients with POAG demonstrate steroid responsiveness. The type and potency of the corticosteroid drug, frequency of its administration, and susceptibility of the patients affect magnitude of IOP rise and its duration.

SIGNS AND SYMPTOMS

Signs and symptoms of steroid-induced glaucoma resemble POAG. Infants treated with corticosteroids may develop buphthalmos resembling that of congenital glaucoma. Acute rise in IOP to high levels following steroid administration may cause symptoms of colored haloes, blurred vision, and corneal edema. Prolonged rise in IOP causes typical optic nerve damage characteristic of glaucoma and corresponding retinal nerve fiber bundle type of glaucomatous visual field loss. The cause of elevation of IOP is not always related to use of corticosteroids and may be due to underlying disease such as uveitis. Whereas IOP rise reverses after discontinuing steroids, it may remain persistently elevated depending on trabecular damage or dysfunction necessitating continued medical therapy or surgical intervention.

An increase in IOP in response to the local or systemic use of corticosteroids but the response varies among individuals. Usually it takes 2–4 weeks after initiation of topical steroids, though rarely there can be an acute rise of IOP within hours in association with systemic use of steroid or adrenocorticotrophic hormone (ACTH). If the ocular hypertension is of a significant magnitude, not recognized, and not treated, subsequent glaucomatous optic neuropathy can develop (i.e., steroid-induced glaucoma).

In vernal keratoconjunctivitis (VKC), steroid-induced glaucoma is a common complication as patients require long-term therapy and steroids are often used to provide early relief of symptoms. Patients may also develop raised IOP after periocular injection of steroids. Although many respond to glaucoma medical therapy, some may require excision of depot of corticosteroid or filtering surgery. Intravitreal corticosteroid injections are associated with IOP rise in close to 50% of patients requiring medical therapy to prevent glaucomatous disk damage. Glaucoma progression may be severe enough in 1–2% of such individuals necessitating filtering surgery.

The popular use of intravitreal triamcinolone acetonide (IVTA) for subretinal fluid, macular edema, and adjunctive therapy in the treatment of choroidal neovascularization has led to an increased incidence of corticosteroid-induced ocular hypertension and glaucoma. Intravitreal implants that release corticosteroids are more frequently associated with rise in IOP often requiring excision of the implants with filtering surgery.

PREDISPOSING RISK FACTORS

Preexisting POAG, glaucoma suspect, or a first-degree relative with POAG are important risk factors for corticosteroid-induced ocular hypertension and glaucoma. Age may be a risk factor; increased risk appears to occur in a bimodal distribution peaking first at 6 years of age. As one progresses through adulthood, age may not be a factor until late adulthood when the risk again rises. Finally, those with connective-tissue disease, type-1 diabetes mellitus, and high myopia should all be considered high risk, and prudent follow-up should be pursued during periods of corticosteroid use in these individuals.

TYPES OF STEROIDS

1. *Topical ocular preparations:* IOP rise may occur with corticosteroid drops or ointment applied to the eye or with steroid preparations applied to the skin of the eyelids. The risk of IOP rise increases with duration of use and may be directly correlated to its anti-inflammatory effect.
2. *Periocular:* This route of steroid delivery includes subconjunctival, sub-Tenon, or retrobulbar injections. The elevation in IOP noted cannot always be predicted by the patient's response to topical steroid treatment. Sometimes, it is necessary to excise the depot of steroids in order to control the intraocular pressures.
3. *Intravitreal:* IOP elevation develops in about half the patients that receive intravitreal triamcinolone, usually developing between 2 and 4 weeks after the injection. In eyes that are pseudophakic or have undergone vitrectomy, the rise can happen

more rapidly. Steroid implantation in the vitreous can also cause IOP elevation and necessitate treatment for glaucoma.
4. *Dermatologic:* Steroid-induced glaucoma may develop after application of steroid preparations applied to the skin of the eyelids. This elevation occurs most frequently with chronic use, such as in patients with atopic dermatitis.
5. *Systemic steroids* can elevate the IOP as well. The elevation appears to be correlated to the patient's IOP response to topical steroids. Though not common, elevation of IOP has also been noted with the use of inhalational and nasal corticosteroids.

■ PATHOPHYSIOLOGY

Evidence supports three independent potential mechanisms of increased resistance to the outflow of aqueous humor that can act synergistically to produce corticosteroid-induced ocular hypertension:
- Accumulation of polymerized glycosaminoglycans in the trabecular meshwork from reduced availability of lysosomal enzymes in response to corticosteroid-induced stabilization of lysosomal membranes.
- Suppression of phagocytosis by trabecular endothelial cells with resultant accumulation of trabecular debris and increased outflow resistance.
- Genetic influences, with possible upregulation of myocilin, optineurin, and other factors with resultant increase in aqueous outflow resistance.

■ DIAGNOSIS

Diagnosis of steroid-induced glaucoma requires a high index of suspicion and the questioning of patients specifically about their use of steroid eye drops, ointments, skin preparation and pills. History should also include duration of steroid use, and family history of glaucoma. Complete ocular examination should be done including measurement of IOP, gonioscopy, and optic disk evaluation. Fundus photographs and optic disk imaging are desirable for documenting progression, though not mandatory.

■ TREATMENT

In individuals with an IOP >20% above their baseline measurement or in those for whom there is clinical or functional evidence of damage to their optic nerve during or after treatment with corticosteroids, any or all of the following may be necessary to reduce IOP.
- Determine if steroid use (in any form) is truly needed, stop or taper steroids.
- Reduce the concentration or dosage of the steroid.
- Change to a steroid with a lesser propensity for IOP elevation (e.g., fluorometholone and loteprednol).
- Switch to a topical nonsteroidal anti-inflammatory drug (e.g., ketorolac 0.4% and bromfenac 0.09%).
- Start antiglaucoma therapy. All drugs, including aqueous suppressants, prostaglandin analogues, and miotics may be used as appropriate. Treatment of elevated IOP and indications for surgery usually follow general treatment guidelines as applied in management of POAG.
- Obtain baseline visual fields and/or optic nerve photography or peripapillary retinal nerve fiber layer measurements.

If the IOP is very high (>50 mm Hg, even in the case of an optic nerve that appears healthy), surgical intervention with either a tube or a filter may be appropriate. These surgeries are required in fewer than 2% of patients receiving an intravitreal injection. Surgeons should consider a vitrectomy or the explantation of the steroid implant for patients who have received intravitreal injections or intraocular implants of a corticosteroid.

■ FOLLOW-UP

Close and regular monitoring of the IOP of patients treated with corticosteroids is required (especially those with a personal or family history of POAG or steroid-induced glaucoma).

The frequency of IOP monitoring should match the patient's risk factors for steroid-induced spikes in pressure as well as the medication's potency, dosage, route of administration and half-life, and the duration of treatment.

High-risk patients who receive intravitreal injections require examinations 1 day and 1 week after treatment and at least monthly follow-up examinations after the medication's cessation.

■ SUGGESTED READING
1. Jones R, Rhee DJ. Corticosteroid-induced ocular hypertension and glaucoma: a brief review and update of the literature. Curr Opin Ophthalmol. 2006;17(2):163-7.

4.16 | Visual Field Defects in Glaucoma

Murali Ariga, Malarchelvi Palani, Nivean Madhivanan
MN Eye Hospital, Chennai
muraliariga@gmail.com, malarchelvipalani@gmail.com, nivean69@gmail.com

■ DEFINITIONS

Visual field is defined as that part of the environment that is visible to the steadily fixing eye. It has been described by Traquair as "an island of vision surrounded by a sea of darkness". It is portrayed as "a hill of vision" with the peak at the fovea due to the high density of photoreceptors and tapers off toward the periphery in a steep fashion nasally than temporally. The normal visual field extends 60° superiorly, 60° nasally, 80° inferiorly, and 90° temporally. The blind spot, anatomically the location of the optic nerve head is located 10°–20° temporal to fixation.

Perimeters have evolved from Bjerrum screen to the present state of the art, fast, and accurate automated static perimeters (SAP) such as Humphrey field analyzer (HFA-Carl Zeiss), Octopus (Haag Streit), Dicon, Oculus, Opto, and many others.

Scotoma is an area of visual field loss or depression surrounded by an area of normal or less depressed vision. This can further be absolute or relative scotoma. An absolute scotoma is defined as an area of total loss of vision in which even the brightest and largest target cannot be perceived and a relative scotoma is an area of partial visual loss where brighter lights or larger targets are seen but smaller or dimmer ones are not.

■ EXAMINATION STRATEGIES

Choosing Test Patterns

In glaucoma it is usually sufficient to test the central 30° or 24° (called 30-2, 24-2 in HFA or G program in Octopus machines). In the 30-2 test 76 test points with a uniform 6° paraxial grid within central 30° are examined while in the 24-2 tests 54 points are examined. The 10-2 program tests 68 points 2° apart in the central 10° and the macula program examines 16 points which are 2° apart in the central five degrees. In advanced glaucoma it is useful to do the 10-2 or macula program to check for split fixation. G program of the Octopus tests 59 locations in the central field which are concentrated in the central, arcuate and nasal midperiphery. The M program tests 45 locations in the central 4° which are 0.7° apart.

Threshold Estimation

In static perimetry which is now employed in all automated perimeters a fixed size stimulus is varied in brightness in different locations in the visual field and the threshold is determined for each tested point by a bracketing strategy. The obtained threshold value (expressed in decibels or dB) may vary within 1–2 dB when tested twice during a field test (fluctuation).

Newer Strategies

Full threshold determination at each point of the visual field is time consuming and may fatigue the patient. Newer techniques such as Swedish interactive threshold algorithm (SITA) in the HFA are based on the fact that a response at one location has implications not only for that tested location but also for neighboring points. SITA program can be SITA-standard and SITA-fast of which SITA-standard is the recommended program for glaucoma. Tendency-oriented perimetry (TOP) in Octopus machines is similar to SITA wherein it analyses the location where the stimulus is presented and assesses the threshold of the four neighboring locations by interpolation.

STEPWISE INTERPRETATION OF SINGLE VISUAL FIELD DATA: THE TEN STEPS

Step 1: Patient Data

The name, age, ID number, and refraction data must be entered correctly as the patient's raw data will be compared with age-matched normative database. The visual acuity will correlate with the foveal threshold (foveal threshold is estimated in HFA machines). Proper correction of patient's near vision and placement of trial lenses is important. The ideal pupil size should be between 3 and 4 mm.

Step 2: Test Data

The test data gives information about the strategy (full threshold/SITA in HFA and normal/TOP in Octopus) and extent of field tested.

Step 3: Reliability

The reliability of the test result can be estimated by analyzing three parameters—false positive, false negative and fixation loses, and the gaze tracking plot available in modern HFA models. The percentage of fixation losses (>20%), false positive, and false negative responses (exceeding 1/3) indicates unreliability. High false-positive areas will show as white scotomas and high false-negative will show clover-leaf pattern. An unreliable field test should be repeated. Also a test done for the first time should not be considered as baseline test because most patients have a learning curve and do better on repetitive testing.

Step 4: Numerical or Raw Data (Called as Values in Octopus Printouts)

The raw data is the exact retinal sensitivity in dB units of selected points calculated by the field analyzer. A sensitivity of 0 indicates absolute scotoma—no response to the brightest light stimulus.

Step 5: Gray Scale

The gray scale in the printout gives us a general impression of the tested visual field. It can be used to describe the damage to the patient or relatives. To develop a gray scale printout, interpolated threshold values are assigned to locations between test points and threshold sensitivities are combined into groups of 5 dB in width so that the range from 1–40 dB is assigned to 8 levels of gray.

Step 6: Total Deviation and Pattern Deviation Maps and Probability Plots (Termed Comparisons and Corrected Comparisons in Octopus Printouts)

The total deviation is the difference between patient's measured thresholds (raw data) and the age-matched normal value at each tested location. The statistically significance of the deviation at each location is plotted on the underlying total deviation probability map and represented by darker symbols with greater deviation and greater significance. A key to the probability plot is shown here. For example, a test location with the symbol <1% means that <1% of reliable normal fields in the age-related database have a low sensitivity. The pattern deviation adjusts for generalized depression due to cataracts or refractive errors and helps to expose a localized scotoma. There is a probability plot below the pattern deviation.

Step 7: Global Indices or Statistical Indices

These five main indices give information on the amount of damage the visual field has:
1. *Mean deviation (mean defect in Octopus):* It signifies the average severity of field loss. It is the average of all the numbers shown in the total deviation numerical plot except the points in the area of the blind spot. The mean deviation is expressed in terms of dB units with P value. A positive value indicates that the patient's overall sensitivity is better than the average normal individual whereas a negative value indicates it is worse than the normal person.
2. *Pattern standard deviation (loss variance in Octopus):* It is calculated to estimate the amount of localized loss a given visual field has. It is an index of the degree to which the numbers in the total deviation plot differ from each other. "P" values are assigned to if pattern standard deviation (PSD) exceeds that found in 90% of normals.
3. *Short-term fluctuation (SF):* It is the standard deviation of multiple measurements of threshold within a test session at 10 standard locations and weighted according to the variance of the normal population. SF is usually 1–2 dB in normal reliable fields. SF is not derived in SITA in order to shorten the test time.
4. *Corrected pattern standard deviation (corrected loss variance in Octopus):* This index is obtained from PSD by correcting for SF, i.e., corrected pattern standard deviation (CPSD) = PSD - SF. The CPSD or corrected loss variance (CLV) is useful in identifying a local scotoma.
5. *Visual field index (VFI):* It is an index developed to reflect the amount of remaining functioning ganglion cells. It is centrally weighted; the depressed central points are given more importance than the depressed peripheral points. It is less affected by cataracts and other media opacities. Normal visual fields have values close to 100%. It is used to measure the rate of progression of glaucoma.

Step 8: Glaucoma Hemifield Test, Defect or Bebie Curve (Octopus)

The glaucoma hemifield test (GHT) compares five zones in the upper hemifield with mirror image locations in the lower hemifield. These zones are in the areas where glaucomatous defects are most likely to be seen. A score is assigned to each zone based on percentile deviations in the pattern deviation plot of points. The difference in scores between the upper and lower zones is compared with age-related normal. Five possible inferences appear—outside normal limits, borderline, generalized reduction, abnormally high sensitivity, and within normal limits.

Defect Curve or Bebie Curve

The defect curve is derived by ranking all tested points (59 points in the G1 test) and plotting them in a curve with the least deviated points to the left and most deviated points to the right of the curve. The normal range is shown with the confidence limits.

Step 9: Is the Test Report Abnormal?

The minimal criteria for glaucomatous damage in HFA—Anderson's criteria are:
- The localized defect should be a cluster of at least three or more nonedge points in an expected location such as the arcuate or paracentral area, which have sensitivities occurring in <5% of the population and one of which has a sensitivity occurring in <1% of the population.

- The CPSD or PSD has a value that occurs in <5% of the population.
- The glaucoma hemifield test is abnormal.

In the Octopus printouts of a reliable field an MD (mean deviation) value >2 or LV (loss variance) value >6 can be considered as criteria for abnormality.

Step 10: Is it Glaucoma?
Interpretation of visual field defects must be correlated and supported by optic disc changes/nerve fiber layer defects and other clinical findings.

TYPICAL FIELD DEFECTS IN GLAUCOMA
- Follow an arcuate pattern corresponding to the pattern of nerve fiber bundle loss.
- Asymmetrical field defects respecting the horizontal midline.
- Located in midperiphery in early-to-moderate cases.
- 5–25° from fixation.
- Should be reproducible.
- Not attributable to other pathology.
- Usually clustered or localized in neighboring test points.
- Defect should correlate with the appearance of the optic nerve head.
- Do not affect visual acuity except in advanced glaucomatous optic atrophy or due to cataract.

Figures 4.16.1 to 4.16.3 depict the single visual field printouts of HFA and **Figures 4.16.4A and B** show the Octopus perimetry printout, both giving importance to the structural and functional correlation and clinical significance.

How Often Fields should be Performed?
It is generally advisable to obtain at least two reliable visual fields to establish a baseline before commencing definitive therapy. The field defect must be reproducible. Glaucoma suspects and relatives of glaucoma patients may be tested once every year. In compliant patients with good IOP control and stable glaucoma the visual field may be tested every 6 months. Glaucoma patients with unstable high IOP or other risk factors for progression may be subjected to testing every 3–4 months.

Assessing Visual Field Progression
One method would be to obtain an "overview" print in which up to 16 previously tested visual fields can be shown in single printout without any statistical interpretation. For statistical analysis one may use the recently available progression analysis software such as GPA II in HFA machines or Eyesuite in Octopus perimeters.

PEARLS AND PITFALLS
There is a learning curve in a patient undergoing visual field testing especially with the first few tests. Miotic pupils (pupil size should be at least 3 mm) and cataracts can cause generalized depression. Cataracts and high refractive errors (>6 diopters) can cause diffuse field loss which is usually determined by the total deviation plot. In patients with high refractive errors visual field test should be performed with contact lenses to avoid the artifacts associated with trial lenses. Trial lenses used for perimetry must be full aperture lenses and must be properly centered. The patient should also be properly positioned on the chin rest with forehead touching the forehead band. Unexplained or atypical visual field defects must raise the suspicion of a nonglaucomatous cause for the defect. Always consider the complete clinical picture including the role of coexisting conditions. Never interpret the visual field in isolation. A visual field is a subjective test. It is important for the technician to encourage and monitor the patient throughout the test.

SECTION 4: Glaucoma

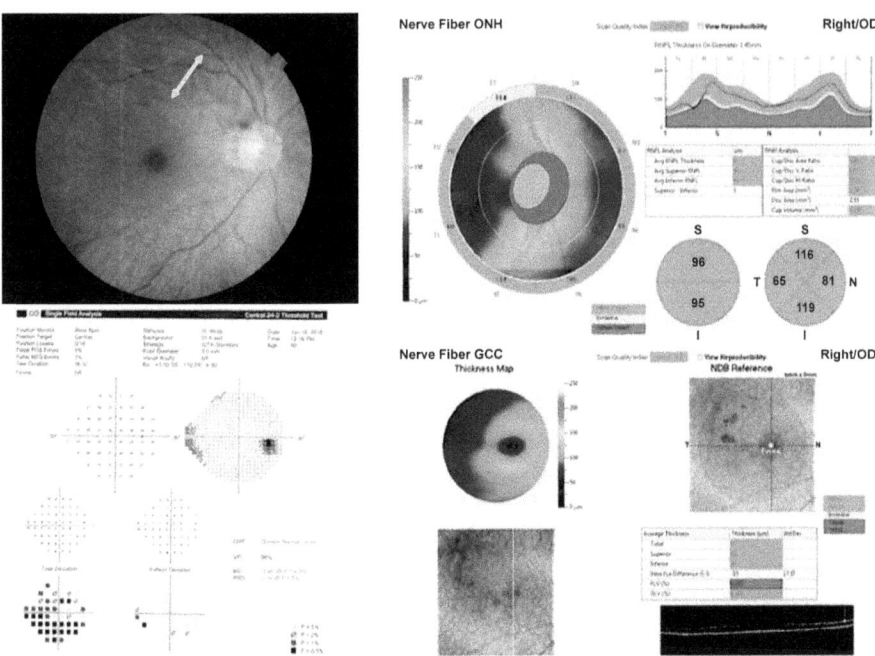

Fig. 4.16.1: Fundus photograph shows disk hemorrhage with superior wedge-shaped retinal nerve fiber layer (RNFL) defect and focal thinning of superotemporal neuroretinal rim. Visual field shows early field defect—nasal step. Optical coherence tomography optic nerve head (OCT ONH) analysis shows borderline changes in the superotemporal quadrant with corresponding depression in the TSNIT graph (denoting the thickness profile of temporal, superior, nasal, inferior, and temporal areas) and ganglion cell complex (GCC) thickness.

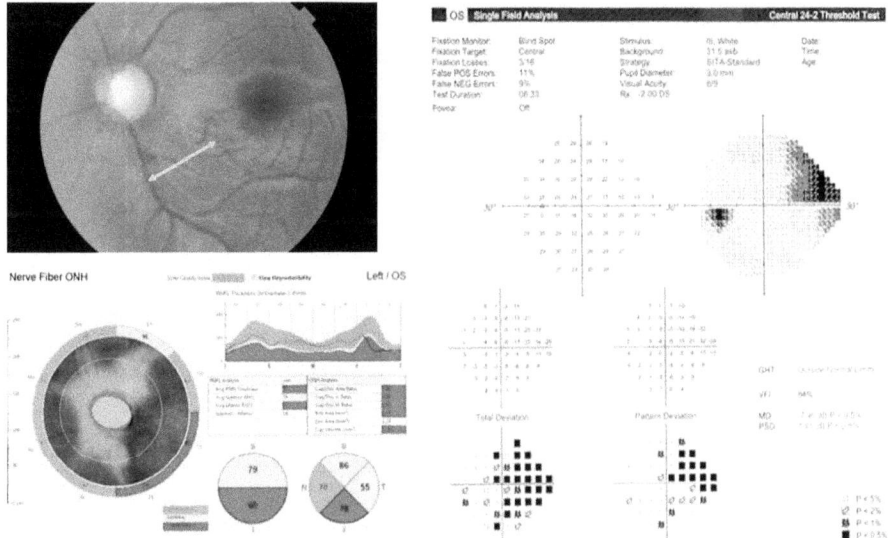

Fig. 4.16.2: Fundus photograph shows vibrational circular dichroism (VCD) ratio 0.7 with wedge-shaped inferior retinal nerve fiber layer (RNFL) defect. Visual field shows superior arcuate scotoma with few areas of depressed sensitivity along the inferior quadrant. Optical coherence tomography optic nerve head (OCT ONH) analysis shows reduction in RNFL thickness in the inferior quadrant.

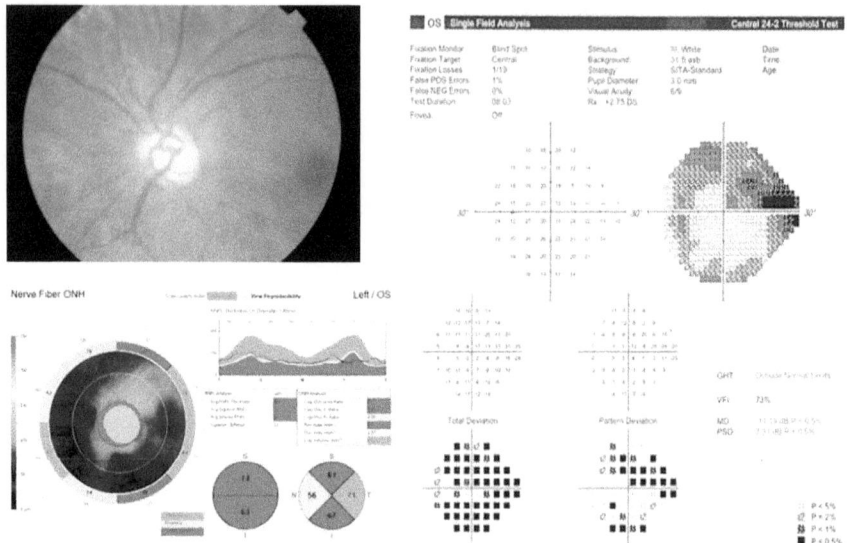

Fig. 4.16.3: Fundus photograph shows vibrational circular dichroism (VCD) ratio with thinning of superior and inferior neuroretinal rim. Visual field shows a corresponding superior arcuate scotoma with areas of depressed sensitivity along the inferior arcuate area. Optical coherence tomography optic nerve head (OCT ONH) analysis shows reduction in superior and inferior retinal nerve fiber layer (RNFL) thickness.

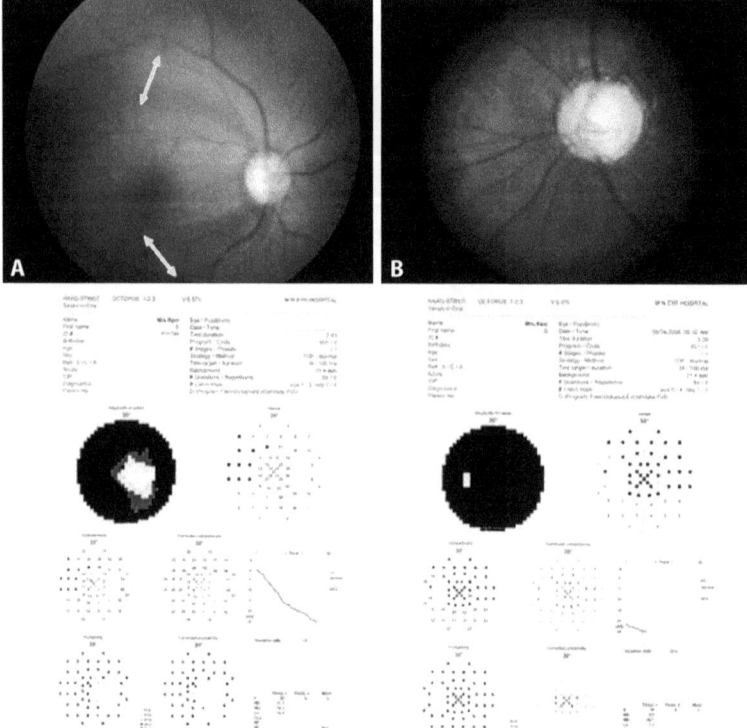

Figs. 4.16.4A and B: (A) Fundus photograph shows glaucomatous disk with superior and inferior retinal nerve fiber layer (RNFL) defects with biarcuate scotoma and abnormal Bebie curve in Octopus printout; (B) It depicts a near total glaucomatous optic neuropathy with severely depressed visual fields.

SUGGESTED READING
1. Bhartiya S, Ariga M, Puthuran GV, George R. Practical Perimetry. 1st edition, New Delhi; Jaypee Brothers Medical Publishers; 2016.

4.17 | Trabeculectomy

Swati Upadhyaya
Aravind Eye Hospital and PG Institute of Ophthalmology, Puducherry
swati.dr@aravind.org

INTRODUCTION
Trabeculectomy is a partial thickness fistulizing procedure which creates a pathway between the anterior chamber and the subconjunctival space, bypassing the normal aqueous outflow pathway. It is the most commonly performed filtering surgery, which was introduced by cairns in 1960s. It replaced the full thickness filtering surgeries which were associated with several complications such as persistent flat anterior chamber, cataract formation, corneal decompensation, synechiae formation, and endophthalmitis due to thin, over filtering blebs.

INDICATIONS
- Uncontrolled glaucoma with maximal medical therapy and laser treatments
- Progression of glaucoma despite adequate intraocular pressure (IOP) control
- Rapid deterioration in advanced glaucoma with threat to fixation
- Poor compliance to medical therapy
- Intolerance to antiglaucoma medications
- Socioeconomic reasons

CONTRAINDICATIONS
- Blind eye
- Extensive conjunctival scarring and scleral thinning
- Active anterior uveitis
- Active anterior segment neovascularization

RISK FACTORS FOR FILTRATION FAILURE
- Young patients
- African, Asian, and Hispanic ancestry
- Diabetes
- Aphakic and pseudophakic patients with prior conjunctival incision surgery
- Secondary glaucomas such as uveitic and neovascular glaucoma
- Previous failed trabeculectomy
- Recent intraocular surgery— <3 months

The abovementioned risk factors are associated with excessive conjunctival scarring which can decrease the success rate of trabeculectomy. Antimetabolites such as 5-fluorouracil (5-FU) and mitomycin-C (MMC) are used as adjuncts to prevent the conjunctival scarring and to improve the surgical outcome.

STEPS OF TRABECULECTOMY
Anesthesia
Local anesthesia such as retrobulbar, peribulbar, and sub-Tenon can be used. General anesthesia is preferred in certain situations such as pediatric patients, uncooperative patients, and patients with altered mental status. Ocular massage should be avoided in cases with advanced glaucomatous damage.

Traction Sutures

Corneal or superior rectus traction suture **(Fig. 4.17.1)** can be used for adequate exposure of the surgical field. Clear corneal traction suture is preferred as the latter is associated with increased trabeculectomy failure. A 7-0 or 8-0 vicryl or silk suture is passed through the superior cornea 1 mm from limbus at a depth of three-fourth thickness with width of 2–2.5 mm which helps in rotating the eyeball inferiorly.

Conjunctival Flap

Superior or superonasal quadrant leaving the adjacent area for future surgery is usually preferred. Inferior placement is usually avoided due to increased risk of endophthalmitis.

Limbal or fornix-based conjunctival flap can be made. Blunt instruments should be used to avoid conjunctival injury. In fornix-based flap **(Fig. 4.17.2A)**, two clock hours (6–8 mm) limbal peritomy is made in the desired quadrant and dissected posteriorly. Fornix-based flaps are easier to make and are associated with more diffuse blebs. Limbal-based flaps are made by making an incision 8–10 mm away from the limbus and dissected anteriorly to expose the corneoscleral junction. It is associated with decreased early wound leak compared to fornix-based flaps.

Adequate and minimal cautery should be done to achieve hemostasis.

Adequate and minimal cautery **(Fig. 4.17.2B)** should be done to achieve hemostasis.

Application of Antimetabolites

Antimetabolites are used to reduce subconjunctival fibrosis especially in cases at high risk for failure. MMC (0.2–0.5 mg/mL) or 5 FU (50 mg/mL) is applied for 1–5 minutes using cellulose or polyvinyl alcohol sponges. Sponges are kept below conjunctival-Tenon flap carefully not touching the margins **(Fig. 4.17.3)**. Application time is usually individualized in each case. Sponges are removed and irrigated thoroughly with balanced salt solution (BSS). It can also be done after creation of scleral flap but before opening into anterior chamber.

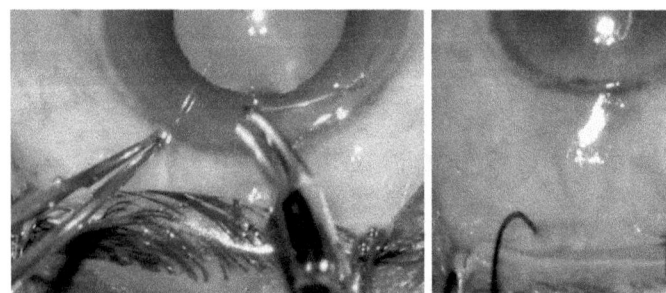

Fig. 4.17.1: Clear corneal and superior rectus traction suture.

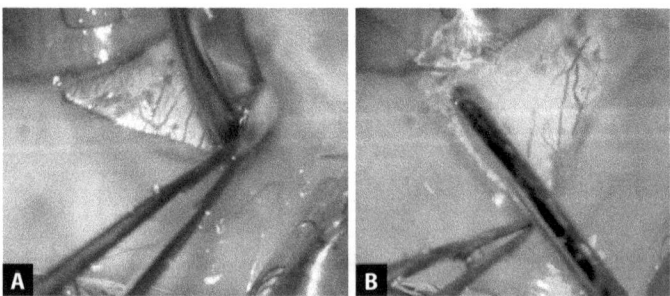

Figs. 4.17.2A and B: (A) Creation of fornix-based conjunctival flap; (B) Cautery.

Scleral Flap Creation

A partial thickness scleral flap is created in the desired quadrant preferably at 12 O'clock. It should be half to two-thirds thickness of sclera. Thin flaps may tear or avulse during closure. Shape can be triangular, rectangular, or trapezoidal.

A triangular flap of 4 × 4 × 4 mm with base at limbus is usually preferred by many surgeons **(Figs. 4.17.4A to E)**. Flap is outlined by number 11 Bard-Parker blade and undermined using number 15 Bard-Parker blade. Apex of the flap is held gently with blunt forceps and lamellar dissection is carried out till the blue-gray zone. A crescent blade is used to continue dissection into the clear cornea to create the entry site for sclerostomy anterior to scleral spur and ciliary body. A paracentesis is made before sclerostomy and anterior chamber is filled with BSS or viscoelastic. This helps in reforming the anterior chamber.

Sclerostomy

A block of tissue at the sclerocorneal junction is excised either manually or by using a punch. Two radial incisions are made 2 mm apart using a sharp blade or knife at the anterior margin of the corneal dissection and

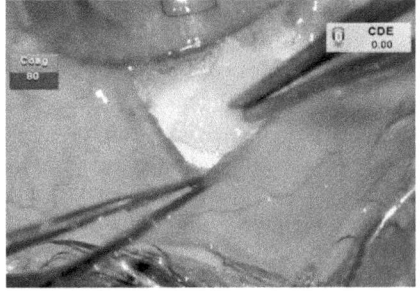

Fig. 4.17.3: Application of antimetabolite.

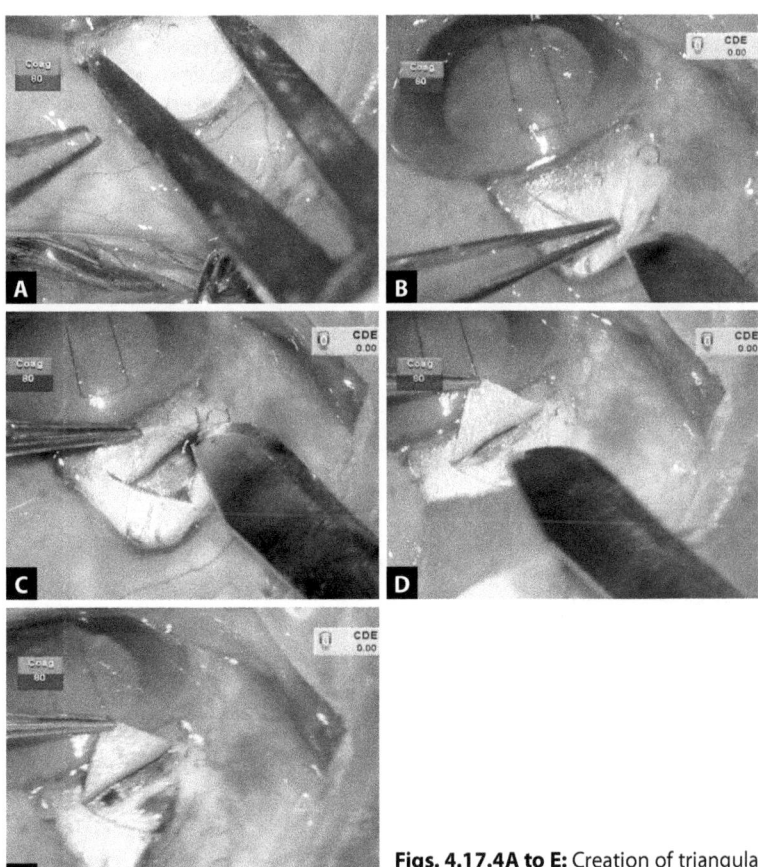

Figs. 4.17.4A to E: Creation of triangular scleral flap.

extended posteriorly to 1–1.5 mm. Vannas scissors or sharp blade is used to connect the incisions resulting in removal of rectangular piece of tissue. Alternatively, anterior chamber is entered using a 1 mm V-shaped lancet blade and Kelly's punch (**Fig. 4.17.5**) is used to excise the tissue.

Peripheral Iridectomy

A peripheral iridectomy (**Fig. 4.17.6**) helps in preventing the occlusion of sclerostomy by iris tissue. Iris is grasped near its root and brought out through the sclerostomy. It is then cut by Vannas or Dewecker scissors keeping it parallel to limbus. Base of the iridectomy should be larger than the sclerostomy to prevent the incarceration of iris. Bleeding can result from cutting the iris root or ciliary body.

Closure of Scleral Flap

Scleral flap is closed with 9-0 or 10-0 nylon suture in an interrupted fashion. The edges of the rectangular flap or apex of triangular flap are sutured first (**Fig. 4.17.7**). The additional sutures can be placed to regulate the flow. Slip knots can be used to titrate the flow. Balanced salt solution is injected through the paracentesis. If the flow is excessive, slip knots need to be tightened or additional sutures are placed. If aqueous flow is low or does not flow, slip knots can be loosened or replaced with looser ones. Sutures are buried to the scleral side. These sutures can be lysed by laser postoperatively whenever required. Alternatively releasable sutures are placed which can be easily removed at the slit lamp.

Conjunctival Closure

Usually, conjunctiva is closed with absorbable suture such as 8-0 vicryl. In case of limbus-based flap, a running suture is used to achieve a watertight closure (**Fig. 4.17.8**). Fornix-based flaps can be closed using a purse-string suture at both ends. Mild to moderate bleb raise and any leakage is looked for after injecting BSS through paracentesis.

One drop of atropine and antibiotic-steroid eye drops or inferior subconjunctival antibiotic-steroid injection are administered at the end of the surgery.

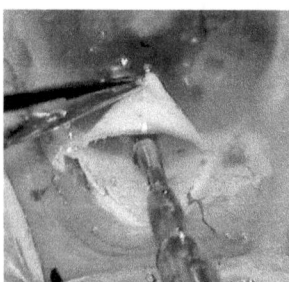

Fig. 4.17.5: Sclerostomy using Kelly's punch.

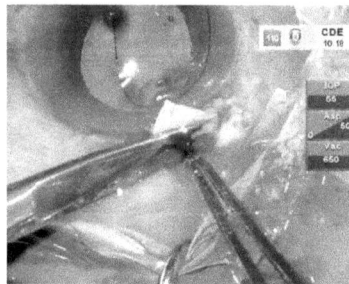

Fig. 4.17.6: Peripheral iridectomy.

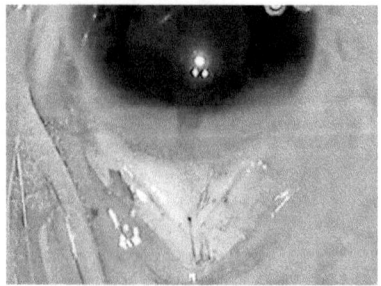

Fig. 4.17.7: Scleral flap closure.

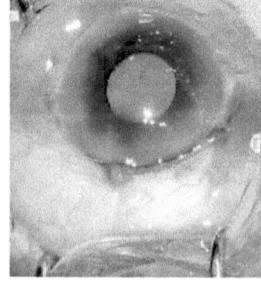

Fig. 4.17.8: Conjunctival closure.

■ MOORFIELDS SAFER SURGERY SYSTEM (FIG. 4.17.9)

It is designed by Peng T Khaw and Sumit Dhingra to improve the surgical outcome of trabeculectomy by minimizing complications and maintaining adequate control of IOP.

Site of Surgery

Superior half of the globe is preferred as it is fully covered and protected by upper lid. Upper lid also covers the peripheral iridectomy and also provides mechanical protection. It is associated with fewer incidences of endophthalmitis, inflammation, and recurrent subconjunctival hemorrhages. If superior site is not available, glaucoma drainage devices should be considered.

Traction Suture

Corneal traction suture is preferred instead of superior rectus traction suture. This is to avoid superior rectus hematoma, subconjunctival hemorrhage which can trigger excess wound healing response resulting in bleb failure. The vector force of corneal traction suture is superior to superior rectus suture. 7-0 black silk suture on a 3/8 curve needle is used. Corneal suture should be placed at appropriate depth to prevent cheese wiring and anterior chamber penetration.

Conjunctival Incision

Limbal-based flaps were made in the past to prevent wound leakage. But limbal based resulted in cystic blebs with ring of steel. Fornix-based flaps are preferred as they are associated with diffuse posterior bleb. It is technically easier to perform than limbal-based flaps.

Scleral Flap

Rectangular partial thickness scleral flap measuring 3.4 × 4.5 mm is preferred. Horizontal incision is made parallel to the limbus and partial thickness scleral pockets are made. Two side incisions are then made. The incision is not made all the way to the limbus which helps in posterior aqueous flow resulting in more diffuse blebs. Scleral flap should not be too thin to avoid cheese wiring, button holing, flap dehiscence and it should be thick enough to provide resistance. Any area with potential aqueous vein should be avoided.

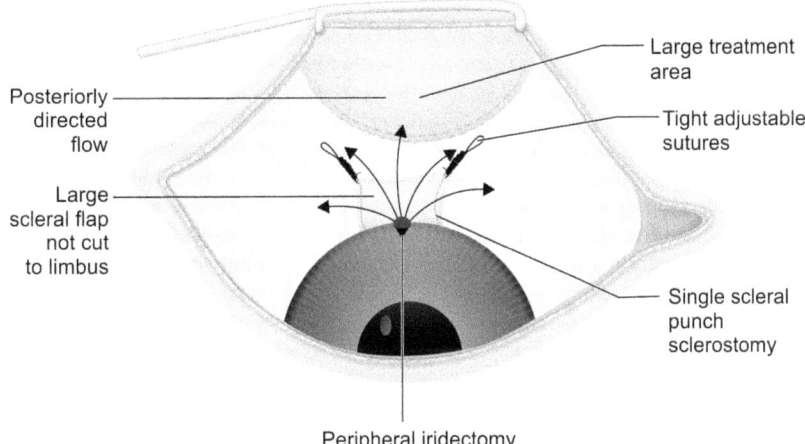

Fig. 4.17.9: Moorfields safer surgery system.

Conjunctival Pocket

Wide conjunctival pockets are made for applying antimetabolite sponges using Westcott scissors. Care should be taken while dissecting over superior rectus.

Antimetabolite Treatment and Duration

Wide area of application of antimetabolite is encouraged to reduce the development of ring of scar tissue. MMC is applied at a concentration of 0.3–0.5 mL for 3 minutes or alternatively 5-fluorouracil 50 mg/mL can be used. The antimetabolite should be washed thoroughly at least with 20 mL BSS.

Three circular medical grade alcohol sponges are used as they do not frame. Alternatively custom-made conjunctiva clamps are used to insert and remove sponges. Care should be taken not to touch the conjunctival margins to prevent postoperative wound leakage.

Paracentesis and Infusion

Paracentesis is used to maintain the anterior chamber. It is placed obliquely and parallel to limbus to prevent the lens damage. It can be placed inferiorly which can be used postoperatively to form the anterior chamber. An anterior chamber maintainer can be used to continuously maintain the chamber.

Sclerostomy

Manual block removal can be done. Alternatively, specially designed punch (Khaw small Descemet membrane punch) can be used. It results in the formation of functionally adequate small sclerostomy with less astigmatism.

Peripheral Iridectomy

It prevents the incarceration of iris. Small and broad-based peripheral iridectomy is preferred to avoid glare and diplopia. Using an infusion, iris is made to come out through the sclerostomy by depressing the wound. This avoids manipulation which reduces iris trauma and need for an assistant.

Scleral Flap Sutures

Sutures are placed to secure the flap and to form adequate tension which creates a resistance for aqueous flow. These are particularly useful in cases where antifibrotic agents are used and in cases of angle closure. Two sutures are placed at the corners of rectangular flap. The further flap sutures are placed after assessing the amount of aqueous flow by inflating the eye through the paracentesis. Preplacing sutures while the globe is firm is easier and can be easily tied during closure which shortens the duration of intraoperative hypotony.

Postoperative adjustment of sutures is required to increase the flow. Laser suture lysis can be done though there is risk of suddenly lowering the pressure. Releasable or adjustable sutures can be used. A subsequent adjustable suture technique which allows transconjunctival adjustment of scleral flap using a specially designed forceps with smooth edges (Khaw transconjunctival adjustable suture control forceps No. 2-502).

Conjunctival Closure

Traditionally, conjunctiva is closed with interrupted suture at the ends of conjunctival incision. Purse-string sutures, interrupted horizontal mattress sutures, sutures with corneal groove are the newer techniques. Conjunctival retraction, wound leaks, suture discomfort are almost eliminated by these techniques. Round bodied needle is preferred over spatulated needle.

Postoperative Care

Topical medications: Steroids such as prednisolone acetate 1% are given in tapering doses over 8–12 weeks. Antibiotics are given for 1–2 weeks. Cycloplegics such as atropine or homatropine are used for 2–3 weeks especially in cases of shallow anterior chamber and intense inflammation.

Digital ocular compression can be done in the early postoperative period to reduce the IOP. It is applied to inferior sclera or cornea through the inferior lid. Alternatively, it can be near the posterior edge of the flap to elevate the bleb.

Laser suturolysis using argon or Nd:YAG laser can be done in cases of raised IOP, flat bleb, and deep anterior chamber. It should be done within a few weeks of surgery. Pulling of releasable sutures under slit lamp can also be done.

Subconjunctival 5-FU can be injected in cases of early failure with thickened, vascularized bleb.

COMPLICATIONS

Intraoperative

Conjunctival Button Holes

Tears or holes in conjunctiva and Tenon capsule can result in filtration failure if not recognized and treated intraoperatively. It can result from improper handling of conjunctival tissue and usage of toothed or serrated forceps. Limbal-based flaps are difficult to create and can result in tears. Previous conjunctival scarring can lead to multiple conjunctival tears. Conjunctival holes and tears should be sutured with 10-0 nylon interrupted horizontal mattress or purse-string sutures using an atraumatic needle. Tenon capsule should be included in the suture for additional support. Large buttonhole in the middle of the flap is difficult to treat and another site should be chosen. Small button holes near flap edge can be excised. At the end of the surgery, leaks should be checked and treated appropriately. Button holes or tear can result in shallow anterior chamber, hypotony, and bleb failure.

Scleral Flap-related Complications

Thin or thick flap can both result in complications. Thin flaps can predispose to flap tear, buttonhole, avulsion, and over filtration. Thick flaps can lead to premature entry and under filtration. If button hole or tear occurs before sclerostomy, another site should be chosen. If it occurs after sclerostomy, tear can be sutured with 10-0 nylon or sealed with Tenon, donor sclera or dura mater graft. Premature entry resulting from thick scleral flap is treated by superficial scleral dissection and advancing it into the clear cornea. Flap shrinkage can occur due to excessive cautery and additional sutures should be placed to prevent excess leakage. Flap amputation can occur during flap dissection, peripheral iridectomy, vitrectomy, and flap suturing. It should be treated with scleral patch graft.

Intraoperative Bleeding

Hyphema: Bleeding can occur during conjunctival dissection, sclerostomy, and iridectomy. Patients on anticoagulant and antiplatelet drugs are at high risk of bleeding, hence to be stopped with physicians' advice. Iridectomy is the most common cause of hyphema intraoperatively and can result when it involves iris root and ciliary body. Bleeding occurs from the cut end of radial iris vessels and greater arterial circle. It can be stopped with gentle compression or irrigation. Persistent bleeding can also be stopped with air tamponade or viscoelastic. Bleeding from the scleral flap should not be cauterized as it can lead to flap shrinkage and can be stopped by direct pressure with cotton-tipped applicator. Scleral flap should not be sutured until the active bleeding stops, otherwise blood clot can block the ostium.

Suprachoroidal hemorrhage: It is a rare complication of filtration surgery, which occurs intraoperatively or within 48 hours of surgery. Risk factors are high preoperative IOP, generalized atherosclerosis and prolonged hypotony. It is recognized by sudden shallowing of anterior chamber, loss of red reflex, and expansion of dark choroidal mass. Immediate closure of the wound is recommended which is followed by intravenous mannitol. Rarely, sclerostomy is needed for drainage of hemorrhage. Visual potential is usually good if the wound is closed without loss of uveal or retinal tissue. It can be prevented by preplacing sutures, good preoperative IOP control, slow decompression of anterior chamber and using punch instead of block dissection.

Others

Iridectomy complications include bleeding, large iridectomy, iridodialysis, and inadvertent cyclodialysis cleft. Vitreous loss and lens injury can occur during peripheral iridectomy and sclerostomy. Vitreous loss occurs due to the damage to the zonules and is managed by anterior vitrectomy. Descemet membrane detachment can occur from the limbal wound or from the paracentesis. It is managed by air tamponade.

■ POSTOPERATIVE COMPLICATIONS

Early Postoperative Complications (Flowchart 4.17.1)

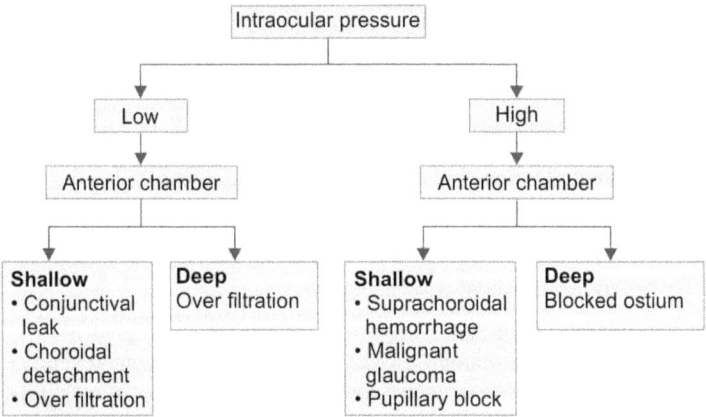

Flowchart 4.17.1: Early postoperative complications.

Shallow Anterior Chamber

Shallow anterior chamber (AC) is one of the most common complications seen in the immediate postoperative period. It is more commonly seen in patients with hyperopic eyes and angle-closure glaucomas. Cause of shallow AC should be identified and treated appropriately.

Shallow Anterior Chamber with Low Intraocular Pressure

Common causes include conjunctival leaks and serous choroidal detachments.

Conjunctival leaks: It is the most common cause of shallow AC in the immediate postoperative period. Seidel's test is used to identify the leaks. Small leak near suture site with deep chamber can be observed. Leaks can lead to shallow AC, hypotony, and choroidal detachment, hence should be treated appropriately. Topical antibiotics with or without the use of topical aqueous suppressants can be administered in cases of small leak. If the leak persists, bandage contact lens is kept in place for 2 weeks. Simmons shell, symblepharon ring, autologous tissue glue can also be tried. If the leaks persist despite these measures and in cases of large leaks, bleb revision with conjunctival advancement, rotation flap or conjunctival autograft is needed.

Choroidal detachment (CD): If the AC is shallow with normal to low IOP and negative Seidel's test, choroidal detachment should be suspected. Hypotony is the most common cause of CDs. Shallow CDs are usually asymptomatic. Large CDs can push the lens-iris anteriorly resulting in shallow AC. Fundus examination can reveal large multiple mounds of CDs. It is usually treated conservatively with topical steroids and cycloplegics. Rarely surgical drainage of CDs is required in cases of lens-corneal touch and kissing choroids.

Shallow Anterior Chamber with Raised Intraocular Pressure

Causes include suprachoroidal hemorrhage, malignant glaucoma, and pupillary block.

Suprachoroidal hemorrhage: It usually occurs within the first postoperative week. Prolonged hypotony is the most common cause of postoperative suprachoroidal hemorrhage. There is sudden onset of severe pain with shallow anterior chamber, high IOP, loss of red reflex with choroidal elevation. Conservative management is done initially with topical aqueous suppressants, steroids, and cycloplegics. Choroidal drainage can be done after 2 weeks which allows liquefaction of blood clot and proper evacuation.

Pupillary block: It occurs if the peripheral iridectomy is not patent or lamellar, and in cases with posterior synechiae. Blockade can due to blood clot, fibrin or vitreous. Flat bleb with normal or elevated IOP is the usual presentation. It is treated with aqueous suppressants, mydriatics to break posterior synechiae, and peripheral laser iridotomy.

Malignant glaucoma: It is usually diagnosed after excluding all other causes of postoperative shallow AC with raised IOP. Cases of angle-closure glaucomas and nanophthalmos are at risk of developing malignant glaucoma. There is posterior misdirection of aqueous leading to collection of aqueous in vitreous cavity which results in anterior movement of iris-lens diaphragm. It presents with uniformly shallow AC, high IOP, and patent peripheral iridotomy. Conservative management with topical cycloplegics, aqueous suppressants, systemic hyperosmotic agents and carbonic anhydrase inhibitors is usually effective. Laser hyaloidotomy and surgical management such as pars plana vitrectomy with or without lensectomy is done in cases where medical therapy fails.

Over filtration: It can present with normal or shallow AC with hypotony and a large, diffuse bleb. It usually results from loose scleral flap suture. It may resolve spontaneously. Persistent hypotony and development of choroidal effusions needs intervention. Conservative management includes topical cycloplegics with or without aqueous suppressants and pressure patching. Symblepharon ring or Simmons shell can also be tried. Anterior chamber reformation with balanced salt solution, viscoelastic, air or expandable gases can be done in cases which are not responding to medical treatment. Other options include compression sutures, injecting autologous blood into bleb, cryo or laser therapy to decrease the bleb size. Bleb revision may be needed in some cases.

Normal anterior chamber with high IOP: It occurs due to blockade of sclerostomy ostium by blood, fibrin, iris, steroid-induced IOP raise, tight scleral flap sutures, and early bleb failure. It is usually associated with low or flat bleb. Management includes laser disruption of blood, fibrin and iris blocking the ostium, suture release or lysis of tight scleral flap suture. Failing bleb can be treated by increasing the frequency of topical steroids, ocular massage, antimetabolite therapy, and bleb needling.

Snuff out: Severe, unexplained vision loss is a very rare complication in post-trabeculectomy patients. It occurs in patients with advanced glaucomas with fixation split. Snuff out can be minimized by giving sub-Tenon anesthesia, avoiding epinephrine in anesthetic mixture. Postoperative IOP spikes should be managed promptly.

Late Postoperative Complications

Bleb failure: Filtration failure is the most common late postoperative complication. It could be due to blockage of external and internal ostium. Blockade of external ostium at Conjunctival-Tenon-episcleral interface is the most common cause of bleb failure. Tight scleral flap resists the aqueous flow in the early postoperative period which allows contact between conjunctiva and episcleral resulting in vascularization, leucocyte infiltration, and connective tissue proliferation. This process can result in subconjunctival scarring which is the main pathology behind the late bleb failure. Functional bleb appears diffuse, avascular with microcysts. Early signs of bleb failure include vascularized, inflamed bleb along with increasing IOP. Late signs include flat fibrosed bleb or thick walled, elevated dome shaped Tenon cyst. Gonioscopy should be done to rule out blockade at internal ostium such as blood, fibrin, iris and should be treated appropriately by Nd:YAG laser. In cases with patent ostium, ocular massage along with increased frequency of topical steroids can help in early stages of bleb failure. Suture lysis or release should be done in cases where ocular massage does not elevate IOP. Bleb needling is advised if other measures fail in treating failing bleb. Bleb revision is the last resort in cases of bleb failure.

Bleb-related infections: Blebitis and bleb-related endophthalmitis are two clinical entities of bled-related infections. These are potentially devastating complications of trabeculectomy. It can occur from months to years after surgery. Risk factors include leaky, thin-walled cystic blebs, usage of MMC, conjunctivitis, blepharitis, and chronic antibiotic usage. Patient usually presents with sudden onset pain and redness in blebitis and associated decreased vision in cases of endophthalmitis. Bleb appears whitish in color along with surrounding congestion with mild to moderate anterior reaction in cases of blebitis. Hypopyon can be seen in some cases. Vitreous is not involved in blebitis. If the vitreous is involved, it is termed as bleb-related endophthalmitis. Seidel's test is done to rule out bleb leakage. B-scan (brightness scan) is done to assess the vitreous involvement. Conjunctival swab, anterior chamber, and vitreous taps are done to find out the causative organisms. *Staphylococcus* and *Streptococcus* are the most common causative organisms. Treatment includes topical fortified antibiotics and intravitreal antibiotics. Topical steroids are started after the antibiotic has been used for 12–24 hours. Vitrectomy can be done to debulk the organism.

Leaking blebs: Thin, cystic blebs with the usage of antimetabolites are at risk of bleb leakage. These blebs are at high risk of bleb-related infections. Seidel's test helps in identifying the leak. Small leaking blebs can be treated with aqueous suppressants alone. Other options include bandage contact lenses with antibiotic cover, application of cyanoacrylate glue or autologous fibrin glue, cryo or cautery to bleb and injection of autologous blood into bleb. Finally, bleb revision with resection of thin-walled bleb with conjunctival transposition or conjunctival autograft, scleral graft can be done.

Overhanging blebs: Large, diffuse blebs covering the cornea are commonly associated with the usage of antimetabolites and superonasal blebs. These blebs can cause irritation, foreign body sensation, dellen formation, astigmatism, and cosmetic unacceptance. Treatment includes lubricant eye drops, compression sutures, autologous blood injection, and bleb revision with resection and conjunctival grafting is required.

Chronic hypotony: When the IOP is <6 mm Hg for >3 months, it is called chronic hypotony. Risk factors include young patients, myopic, usage of antimetabolites, over filtration, and leaking blebs. Visual acuity is usually maintained well in hypotony. Hypotonic maculopathy is a condition where there is a sudden drop in visual acuity along with choroidal folds and retinal striae in macula. Conservative management is usually tried first. Surgical management such as bleb revision and scleral patch is usually needed.

Cataract formation: It is very common after trabeculectomy. The causes include direct lens trauma, shallow anterior chamber with lens-corneal touch, hypotony, inflammation, usage of steroids, and intraoperative MMC.

4.18 Glaucoma Drainage Implants

Swati Upadhyaya
Aravind Eye Hospital and PG Institute of Ophthalmology, Puducherry
swati.dr@aravind.org

■ DEFINITION

Glaucoma drainage devices (GDD) are being increasingly used in the surgical management of patients with refractory glaucoma.

They are employed more commonly as second-line of management after failed glaucoma filtration surgery.

In recent times they are increasingly being used as a primary procedure in refractory glaucomas secondary to pars plana vitrectomy (PPV), penetrating keratoplasty, uveitis, and neovascular glaucoma.

■ HISTORY

- *Baerveldt:* In 1992, introduced nonvalved single plate Baerveldt implant.
- *Ahmed:* In 1993, introduced the first valved single plate AGV (Ahmed glaucoma valve) implant.

■ CLASSIFICATION

Nonvalved/Nonrestrictive Implants

Tubular structure which allows the passive movement of aqueous:

Nonvalved

- Molteno
- Baerveldt
- AADI (Aurolab aqueous drainage implant)
- Ahmed clear path

Valved Implants

Tubular structure with valve which allows unidirectional flow:

Valved

- Ahmed glaucoma valve
- Krupin valve

Molteno Implant

Prototype implant

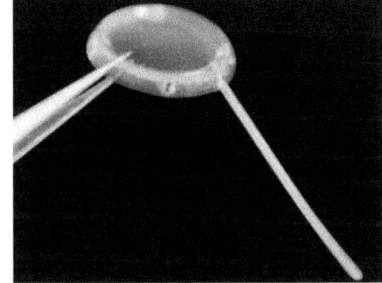

Fig. 4.18.1: Molteno implant.

Single Plate (Fig. 4.18.1)

- Acrylic plate with diameter 13 mm with surface area 137 mm²
- Silicone tube with inner diameter of 0.3 mm and outer diameter of 0.6 mm

Double Plate (Fig. 4.18.2)

- Two plates, one of which is attached to the silicone tube in the anterior chamber (AC).
- A second tube connects the two plates

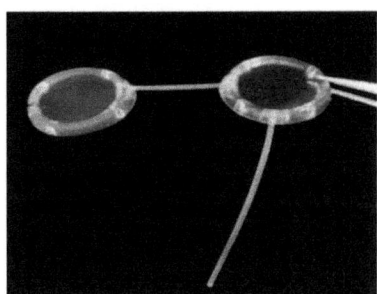

Fig. 4.18.2: Molteno double plate implant.

- Increased surface area of 270 mm²
- Better pressure control than single plate with risk of hypotony

Baerveldt Implant
- A silicone tube is attached to a soft barium-impregnated silicone plate with a surface area of 250 mm² or 350 mm² (**Fig. 4.18.3**).
- Large surface area
- Designed for easy insertion in a single quadrant
- Has fenestrations that allow growth of fibrous tissue
- Reduces the height of the bleb, which reduces the risk for diplopia.
- Helps secure the implant.
- *Hoffman elbowed Baerveldt implant:* For patients undergoing vitrectomy/in corneal grafts (**Fig. 4.18.4**)

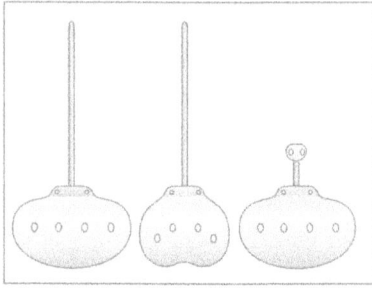

Fig. 4.18.3: Baerveldt implant.

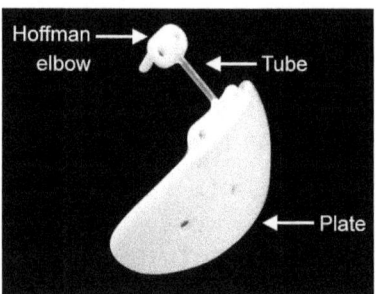

Fig. 4.18.4: Hoffman elbowed Baerveldt implant.

Aurolab Aqueous Drainage Implant
- Nonvalved Baerveldt 350 mm² type implant (**Fig. 4.18.5**)
- Manufactured by Aurolab since June 2013
- Low cost (being 5 times cheaper than AGV and 15 times cheaper than Baerveldt)
- More flexible than Baerveldt

Ahmed Glaucoma Valve
- Developed by Mateen Ahmed and was approved by the Food and Drug Administration (FDA) in 1993 (**Fig. 4.18.6**)
- Consists of three parts
- Silicone, polypropylene plate
- Surface area of 184 mm² and is 1.9 mm thick
- A second plate can be connected to the reservoir plate to increase the surface area by 180 mm²
- Drainage tube in silicone
- Thin silicon elastomer membranes which act as a valve.

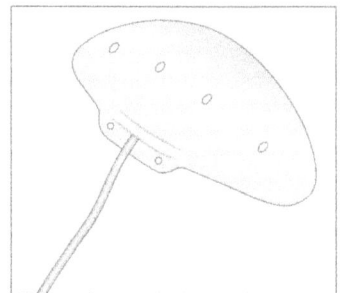

Fig. 4.18.5: Aurolab aqueous drainage implant (AADI).

Valve
- Consists of two thin silicone elastomer membranes, 8 mm long and 7 mm wide
- Allows unidirectional flow and maintains intraocular pressure (IOP) between 8 and 10 mm Hg.
- Closes below 8 mm Hg.
- Hypotony is least in Ahmed.

MECHANISM
Acts like a Venturi chamber:
- After implantation, aqueous flows slowly and continuously into the trapezoidal chamber of the valve.

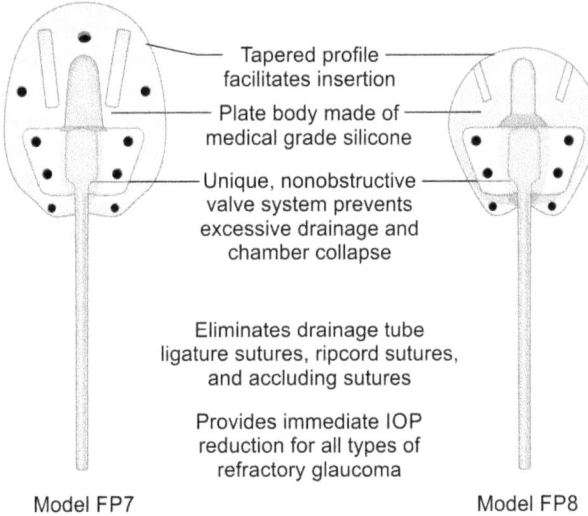

Fig. 4.18.6: AGV FP 7 (Adult) and FP 8 (Paediatric).

- The inlet cross section of the chamber is wider than the outlet.
- Enable the valve to remain open even when only a small difference in pressure exists.
- The velocity of aqueous increases significantly as it exits the smaller outlet port of the tapered chamber.
- The increased exit velocity helps in evacuating the aqueous from the valve, in effect reducing the valve.

INDICATIONS
- Failed trabeculectomy
- Uveitic glaucoma
- Neovascular glaucoma
- Traumatic glaucoma
- Sturge–Weber syndrome
- Penetrating keratoplasty with glaucoma
- Retinal detachment surgery with glaucoma
- Iridocorneal endothelial syndrome
- Refractory infantile glaucoma
- Aphakia/pseudophakia glaucoma

CONTRAINDICATIONS
Absolute
Ciliary block glaucoma

Relative
- Corneal decompensation
- Vitreous in AC
- Scleral thinning
- Extensive conjunctival scarring

PATHOPHYSIOLOGY—FUNCTIONING OF GDD (FLOWCHART 4.18.1)
- Implantation of GDD
- Fibrous capsule forms around the end plate over several weeks

Flowchart 4.18.1: Pathophysiology—functioning of glaucoma drainage devices.

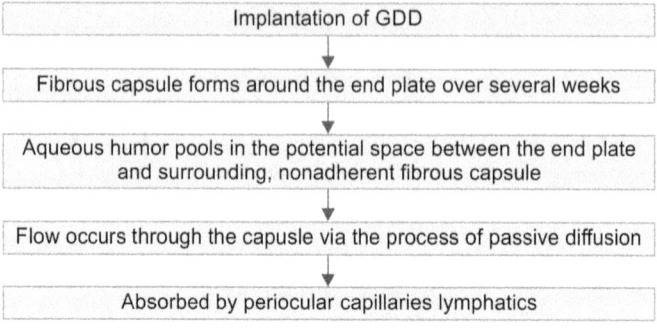

(GDD: glaucoma drainage devices)

- Aqueous humor pools in the potential space between the end plate and surrounding, nonadherent fibrous capsule
- Flow occurs through the capsule via the process of passive diffusion
- Absorbed by periocular capillaries lymphatics

■ PREOPERATIVE ASSESSMENT

Selection of Glaucoma Drainage Devices

Ahmed glaucoma valve/valved implants is favored in:
- Patients with higher risk of hypotony [uveitic glaucoma, prior cyclophotocoagulation (CPC)]
- Higher risk of suprachoroidal hemorrhage
- Immediate IOP reduction needed (IOP >40 mm Hg)
- Poor compliance to medications

Baerveldt glaucoma implant/nonvalved implants such as AADI favored when low IOP is targeted.

Preoperative Considerations

- *Lens status:* Aphakia/pseudophakia/cataract
- Pars plana vitrectomy in cases where pars plana approach is planned.
- Antiplatelet and anticoagulant drugs should be stopped 1 week prior to surgery.
- Antiglaucoma medications (AGM) should be continued till the morning of the surgery.

Preoperative Assessment

- Conjunctival mobility, scarring
- Scleral thinning
- Corneal endothelial status
- Corneal graft
- AC depth
- Vitreous in AC
- Gonioscopy to look for peripheral anterior synechiae (PAS), neovascularization of angles (NVA)
- *Iris:* Neovascularization of iris (NVI)
- *NVI/NVA:* Preoperative anti-VEGF (vascular endothelial growth factor) injection should be given.

■ SURGICAL TECHNIQUE

- *Anesthesia:*
  - Retrobulbar/peribulbar/sub-Tenon are preferred.
  - General anesthesia is rarely required.

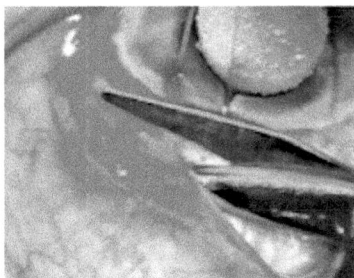

Fig. 4.18.7: Conjunctival peritomy.

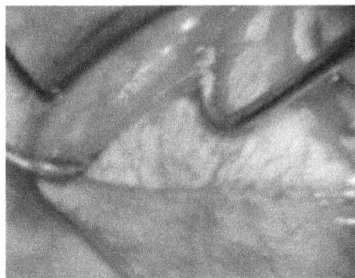

Fig. 4.18.8: Identification and isolation of recti.

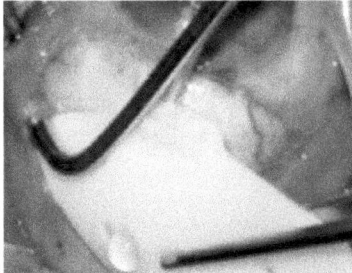

Fig. 4.18.9: Wings of GDD placed under the recti.

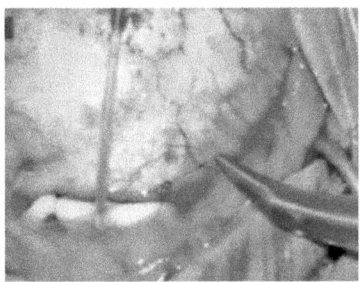

Fig. 4.18.10: Securing the plate on the sclera.

- *Quadrant selection:*
    - Superotemporal quadrant—preferred for its better surgical exposure and less postoperative strabismus
    - Inferonasal quadrant in case of an existing superotemporal GDD or extensive conjunctival scarring from prior surgery, trauma, or inflammation.
    - Superonasal quadrant usually avoided due to postoperative strabismus and acquired brown syndrome.
    - Inferotemporal quadrant avoided due to presence of inferior oblique muscle.
        - Inferior GDD placement is generally preferred in eyes with silicone oil or that are likely to require retinal detachment repair with silicone oil in the future.
        - Silicone oil can enter into tube and can cause subconjunctival inflammation.
- *Surgical steps:*
    - Traction suture-corneal/scleral
    - Creating a conjunctival-Tenon flap-fornix based **(Fig. 4.18.7)**
    - *End plate attachment:*
        - Identification and isolation of recti **(Fig. 4.18.8)**
        - Placed 8–10 mm from the limbus
        - Wings of Baerveldt implant are tucked under the bellies of both recti **(Fig. 4.18.9)**.
        - Ahmed, single plate Molteno are narrow and can be placed between the recti.
        - Double plate Molteno occupies two quadrants and connecting silicone tube is placed under or over the superior rectus.
    - Securing the plate using interrupted nonabsorbable sutures (typically, 9-0 nylon on a spatulated needle) **(Fig. 4.18.10)**
        - Passed through each of two eyelets on the anterior edge of the plate
        - The suture knots are buried within the eyelets to prevent future erosion through overlying conjunctiva.
    - Implant preparation

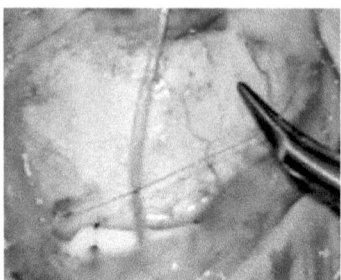

Fig. 4.18.11: Tube ligation.

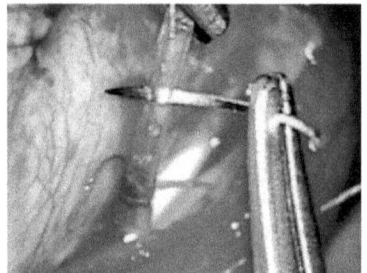

Fig. 4.18.12: Venting slits.

AHMED VALVE
- Priming of the valve to break the surface tension of the valve leaflets
- Done before the attachment of plates
- Using balanced salt solution through 30-gauge cannula
- Patency is confirmed when flow is observed within the device's trapezoidal chamber
- The endplate should be handled delicately to avoid damaging the valve mechanism: No-touch technique

NONVALVED IMPLANTS
- To prevent postoperative hypotony and temporary restriction to flow while capsular fibrosis occurs around the endplate tube ligation is done using absorbable (6-0 polyglactin/Vicryl) or nonabsorbable (polypropylene) suture **(Fig. 4.18.11)**.
- Ligating sutures are placed 5 mm anterior to the tube plate junction to facilitate visualization at the slit lamp for laser suturolysis
- Intraluminal stent 4-0 or 5-0 polypropylene or nylon suture
- Venting slits or fenestrations—in patients with higher preoperative IOP **(Fig. 4.18.12)**

TWO-STAGE IMPLANTATION
- The external plate is placed in the subconjunctival space without inserting the tube into the AC.
- The tube is inserted 6–8 weeks later, after the fibrous capsule has formed around the external plate.
- *Tube insertion:*
  - A paracentesis made inferotemporally and ophthalmic viscosurgical device (OVD) is injection for the maintenance of AC depth.
  - The tube is then cut to permit its extension of 2–3 mm into the AC.
  - Tubes are trimmed with an anterior bevel for AC and pars plana entry and with a posterior bevel for sulcus entry.
  - Scleral fistula and scleral tunnel **(Fig. 4.18.13)**
  - Advancement of the tube using nontoothed forceps/tube inserter
  - Placing it above and parallel to the iris plane
  - Securing the tube with interrupted or figure of eight sutures **(Fig. 4.18.13)**
- *Pars plana insertion:*
  - Indicated in cases of conjunctival scarring, corneal endothelial decompensation, severe PAS
  - Done in aphakia/pseudophakic eyes
  - Prior pars plana vitrectomy or a combined procedure should be done.
  - Devices: AGV with pars plana clip, Baerveldt implant with Hoffman elbow
- *Scleral patch (Fig. 4.18.14):*
  - To minimize the risk of conjunctival erosion and subsequent tube exposure
  - Materials—cornea, sclera, pericardium, dura, and fascia lata
  - A longer scleral tunnel may obviate the need for a patch graft.

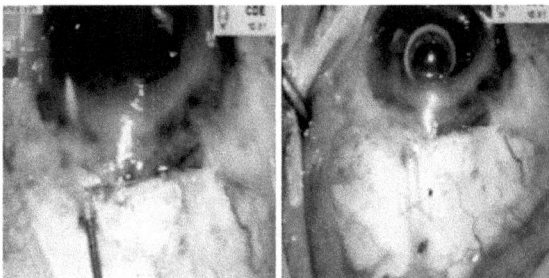

Fig. 4.18.13: Scleral tunnel, tube insertion in AC and securing the tube on sclera.

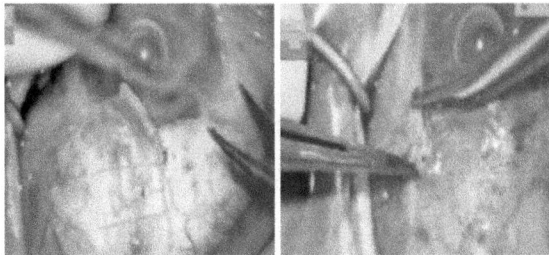

Fig. 4.18.14: Corneal patch graft and conjunctival closure.

- *Conjunctival closure (Fig. 4.18.14):*
  - Closed using 7-0 or 8-0 Vicryl-running or interrupted fashion
  - Additional mattress sutures at the limbus help prevent conjunctival retraction.

POSTOPERATIVE MANAGEMENT
- Topical antibiotics and corticosteroids are initiated.
- Antibiotics in the first postoperative week
- Corticosteroids are continued for 2–3 months postoperatively.
- AGM is resumed on the first postoperative day after insertion of a nonvalved GDD unless fenestrations or slits were placed.
- Tube opening after nonvalved GDD surgery with an absorbable ligature occurs spontaneously between postoperative weeks 4 and 6.
- May lead to fibrinous AC reaction and hypotony
- *Late postoperative period:*
  - Nonabsorbable sutures can be removed around 4 weeks using laser.
  - Argon laser suturolysis a spot size of 50 μm, duration of 0.02–0.05 seconds, and power of 250–800 MW
  - A Hoskins lens aids in visualization of the ligature.

COMPLICATIONS
Intraoperative
- Cheese wiring of the cornea
- Conjunctival buttonholing
- Rectus muscle disinsertion/damage
- Scleral tear/perforation
- Hyphema
- Flat AC and hypotony
- Short tube/tube truncation
- Suprachoroidal hemorrhage

Postoperative

- *Hypotony:*
  - More common in nonvalved implants
  - Due to incomplete occlusion of the tube, leakage from the sclerostomy site, larger fenestrations, spontaneous tube ligature lysis results in hypotony, flat AC, corneal tube touch, and corneal lens tube.
  - Can result in dreaded complications such as choroidal effusion, choroidal hemorrhage, and hypotony maculopathy.
  - Corneal endothelial decompensation, cataract formation can occur.
- *Management:*
  - *Medical in the early postoperative period:*
    - Cycloplegics
    - Oral steroids
  - *Surgical when hypotony does not resolve in 72 hours:*
    - *Tube relegation:*
      - Ab interno stenting using supramid suture
      - Tube religation and choroidal effusion drainage
- *Suprachoroidal hemorrhage:*
  - Seen with hypotony and patient with high preoperative IOP
  - Also seen in elderly hypertensives
  - Should be drained surgically
- *Hypertensive phase:*
  - IOP >21 mm Hg during the first 3 months in the absence of tube obstruction
  - Secondary to bleb encapsulation
  - Elevated cystic bleb
  - To rule out:
    - Blockage of the tube by fibrin, blood, iris tissue, and vitreous
    - *Fibrin and blood:* Increase the topical steroids
    - Intracameral injection of tissue plasminogen activator
    - *Iris tissue:* Topical pilocarpine/argon laser/surgical management
    - *Vitreous:* Seen in cases of pars plana approach where incomplete vitrectomy has been done.
    - Or vitreous in AC
    - Removed by neodymium-doped yttrium aluminum garnet (Nd:YAG) vitreolysis
  - Valve malfunction
  - Aqueous misdirection
- Migration of the plate can occur
- *Migration of the tube:*
  - Posterior migration of the tube when the tube is not secured properly to sclera
  - Anterior migration due to displacement of the implant
- *Retraction of the tube:*
  - Seen commonly in pediatric patients as the eyeball grows with age
  - Treated by repositioning or by tube extension
- *Erosion:*
  - Erosion of the conjunctiva overlying a tube
  - Results from eyelid rubbing, repetitive eye movements, poor ocular surface lubrication, and immunological factors
  - Major risk factor for endophthalmitis
  - Scleral patch can be placed over the erosion
  - Tube repositioning through a new scleral fistula
  - GDD removal in case of large erosion/erosion over the plate
- *Overhanging bleb:*
  - When the patch graft is too thick or the plate is too anterior
  - Prevented by appropriate plate and patch graft placement during surgery

- *Strabismus and diplopia:*
  - Pseudo-Brown syndrome
  - Result of scarring, mass effect of the endplate, a large resulting bleb, and fat fibrosis
  - Resection of large bleb, prism, strabismus surgery, and rarely implant removal
- *Endophthalmitis:*
  - Rare
  - Risk factors are tube erosion, needling of the bleb
- *Corneal decompensation:*
  - Poor tube placement with lens-cornea touch or persistent flat chamber from hypotony
  - In eyes that have undergone penetrating keratoplasty, the risk of graft failure in eyes is high.
  - Repositioning of the tube is done.

SUGGESTED READING

1. American Academy of Ophthalmology. (2023). Glaucoma Drainage Devices. [online] Available from https://eyewiki.aao.org/Glaucoma_Drainage_Devices [Last accessed July, 2023].
2. Hong CH, Arosemena A, Zurakowski D, Ayyala RS. Glaucoma drainage devices: a systematic literature review and current controversies. Surv Ophthalmol. 2005;50(1):48-60.

4.19 | Minimally Invasive Glaucoma Surgery

Swati Upadhyaya
Aravind Eye Hospital and PG Institute of Ophthalmology, Puducherry
swati.dr@aravind.org

DEFINITION

Term coined by Dr Ike Ahmed in early 2000s.

Cardinal Features
- Ab interno microincisional approach.
- Minimal trauma to normal anatomy and physiology.
- Demonstrable/reliable intraocular pressure (IOP) lowering and reducing medication use.
- High safety profile.
- Rapid recovery with minimal need for follow-up.

CLASSIFICATION

Based on different mechanisms by which minimally invasive glaucoma surgery (MIGS) work they are classified into:
- *Increasing trabecular outflow:*
  - iStent and iStent inject trabecular micro-bypass
  - Gonioscopy-assisted transluminal trabeculotomy (GATT)
  - Trabectome
  - Kahook dual blade (KDB) glide
  - Ab interno canaloplasty (ABiC)
  - Hydrus microstent
- *Increasing suprachoroidal drainage:*
  - iStent Supra
- *Increasing subconjunctival outflow:*
  - XEN gel implant
  - InnFocus MicroShunt

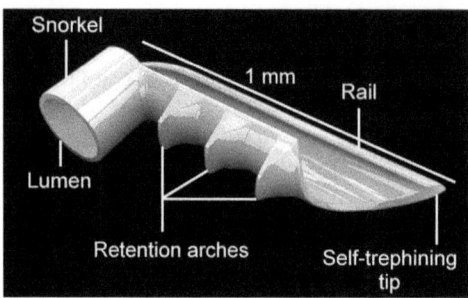

Fig. 4.19.1: iStent.

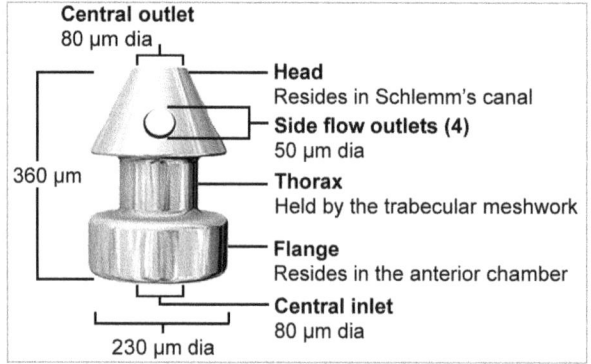

Fig. 4.19.2: iStent inject.

- *Decreasing aqueous production:*
  - Endocyclophotocoagulation
  - Micropulse laser

iSTENT TRABECULAR MICRO-BYPASS (GLAUKOS) (FIG. 4.19.1)

iStent trabecular micro-bypass (TMB) is the first generation device from Glaukos which was Food and Drug Administration (FDA) approved in 2012. It is snorkel shaped, heparin-coated titanium device which measure 1 mm in length and 0.3 mm in height. It has three retention arches for preventing device migration and to ensure stability. It enhances trabecular outflow. It is implanted into the canal by gently incising the trabecular meshwork and then stenting the canal.

iStent Inject **(Fig. 4.19.2)** is the second generation implant and the tiniest implant in the world, measuring 0.3 mm. It comes in a pair with two implanted loaded in one single injector.

GONIOSCOPY-ASSISTED TRANSLUMINAL TRABECULOTOMY (FIG. 4.19.3)

It was first described by Dr Davinder Grover and Dr Ronald Fellman of Glaucoma Associates of Texas, Dallas, in 2014. Originally done with an illuminated microcatheter (iTrack, Ellex), the alternative option for the developing world is by using 5-0 or 6-0 Prolene suture with a blunted tip, which is called as Suture GATT. The blunted tip of the Prolene suture is introduced into the Schlemm's canal after making an initial 1–2 clock hour goniotomy in the nasal angle. With gentle stokes using a microsurgical forceps, the suture is advanced into the canal till it appears at the initial goniotomy site after traversing 360°. Finally the suture is pulled away from outside using McPherson forceps, thus creating a 360° trabeculotomy. Postoperative hyphema is the most common complication after GATT.

SECTION 4: Glaucoma

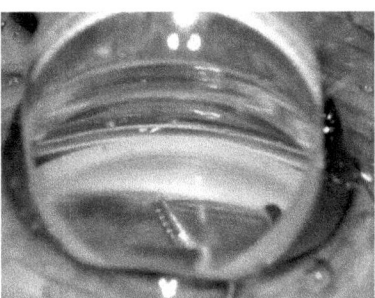

Fig. 4.19.3: Suture GATT.

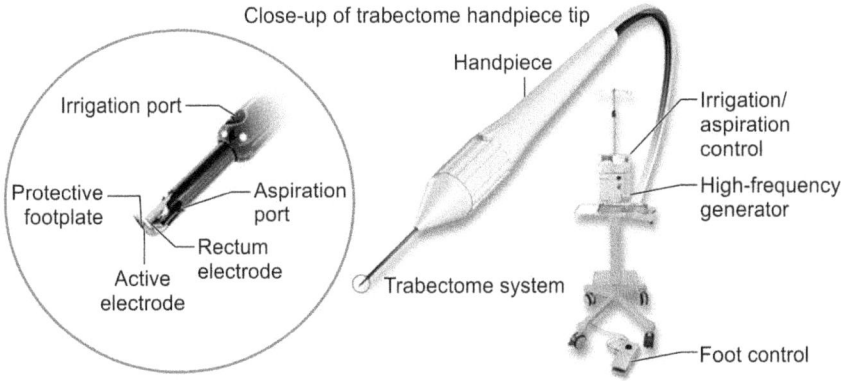

Fig. 4.19.4: Trabectome machine and handpiece.

■ TRABECTOME (NEOMEDIX INC.) (FIG. 4.19.4)

Got FDA approved in 2004. It is a single use, disposable 19.5-guage hand piece that has an electrocautery, irrigation, and aspiration.

Wire delivers a radiofrequency current at 550 kHz that ablates the intervening TM for up to 180° between the wire and the tip-plate (which is bent at 90° to protect the outer wall of Schlemm's canal. It thus removes a strip of trabecular meshwork and the inner wall of Schlemm's canal.

■ KAHOOK DUAL BLADE GLIDE (NEW WORLD MEDICAL) (FIG. 4.19.5)

It is an elegant, single-use, stainless steel blade which makes parallel incisions in the trabecular meshwork (TBM) and inner wall of the Schlemm's canal. The sharp tip pierces TM under gonioscopic visualization; the ramp lifts and stretches the tissue as the device is advanced. The two blades precision manufactured through laser cutting technology produce simultaneous incisions in treated tissues. Up to 180° of TM can be removed using KDB. Unlike in trabectome, there is no need for additional machinery for electrocautery.

■ BENT AB INTERNO NEEDLE GONIECTOMY (FIG. 4.19.6)

Originally described by Dr Arsham Sheybani, bent ab interno needle goniectomy (BANG) involves the excision of 3–4 clock hours of TM using a 25-guage hypodermic needle, bent at 90° at the tip (bent toward the needle hub, not in opposite direction as for cystitome). It is the low cost alternative to KDB with similar mechanism of action.

■ AB INTERNO CANALOPLASTY (FIG. 4.19.7)

It involves the use of ophthalmic viscosurgical device (OVD) to viscodilate the Schlemm's canal and proximal collector channels. An illuminated microcatheter is required for this procedure. Initial steps are just like GATT, but instead of pulling out the catheter, the catheter is slowly withdrawn in the opposite direction ab-internally with simultaneous injection of a high viscosity OVD. This dilates the canal and collector channels, thus enhancing the natural pathway of aqueous drainage. Ab interno canaloplasty (ABiC) can be a better option for patients on anticoagulants, as it involves minimal disruption of TM with lower rates of hyphema.

■ HYDRUS MICROSTENT (IVANTIS, INC.) (FIG. 4.19.8)

Food and Drug Administration approved in 2018, this is an 8-mm long curved device, made of Nitinol, a nickel-titanium alloy that possesses super elastic properties. This device comprises alternating spines for structural support and windows for aqueous outflow. It is implanted ab- internally into the Schlemm's canal. It dilates the canal to 4–5 times its natural width countering the collapse caused by high intraocular pressure.

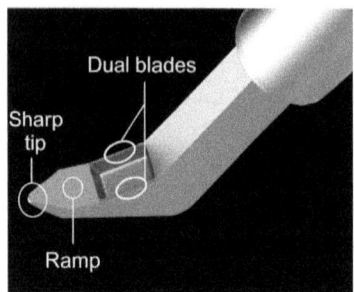

Fig. 4.19.5: Kahook dual blade glide.

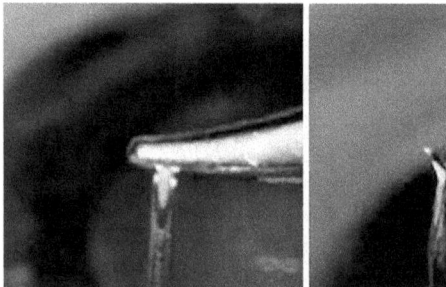

Fig. 4.19.6: Bent 25-gauge needle.

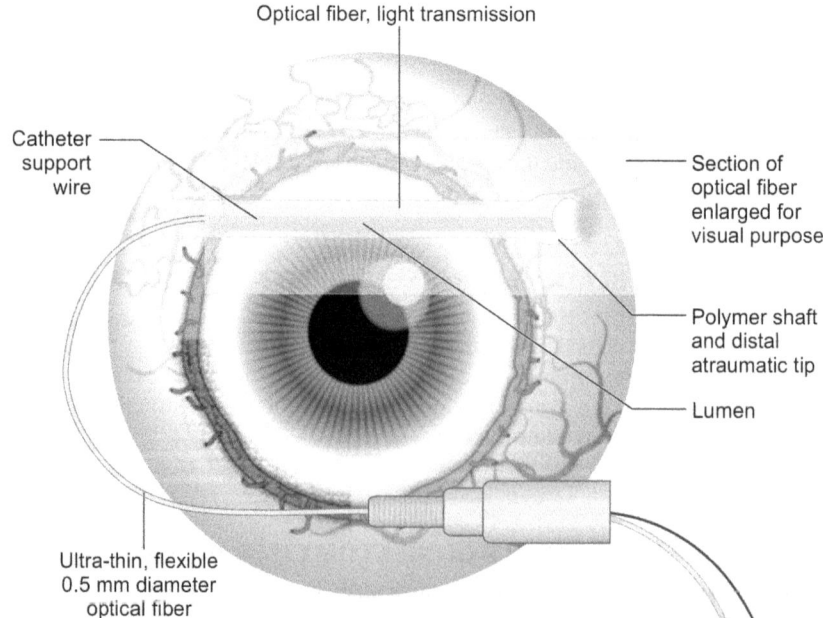

Fig. 4.19.7: Ab interno canaloplasty.

iSTENT SUPRA (GLAUKOS) (FIGS. 4.19.9A AND B)

The iStent Supra is a third generation stent from Glaukos. It is designed to reduce IOP by accessing the suprachoroidal space in the eye. Approximately 4.0 mm in length and curved to follow the eye's anatomy, this device is made of polyethersulfone (PES) and has a titanium sleeve and retention ridges to provide stability to the implant. It is implanted through an ab interno approach.

XEN GEL STENT (ALLERGAN) (FIGS. 4.19.10A AND B)

Food and Drug Administration approved in 2016, this is a 6-mm long soft flexible implant composed of gelatin derived from porcine dermis, formed into a tube and then cross-linked with glutaraldehyde. It enhances aqueous outflow into the subconjunctival space. It can be implanted both by ab interno as well as ab externo approach, with or without antimetabolites. Its outer diameter is 150 μm and the internal diameter is 45–60 μm.

INNFOCUS MICROSHUNT (SANTEN) (FIG. 4.19.11)

The PreserFlo MicroShunt (previously known as InnFocus Microshunt) is an 8.5-mm device, made from poly-styrene-block-isobutylene-block-styrene (SIBS), which is a biocompatible and bioinert material. It is implanted ab-externally and helps in reducing IOP by increasing sub-conjunctival/sub-Tenon drainage of aqueous humor.

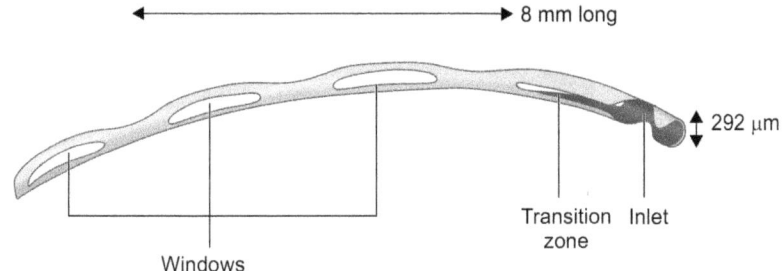

Fig. 4.19.8: Hydrus Microstent.

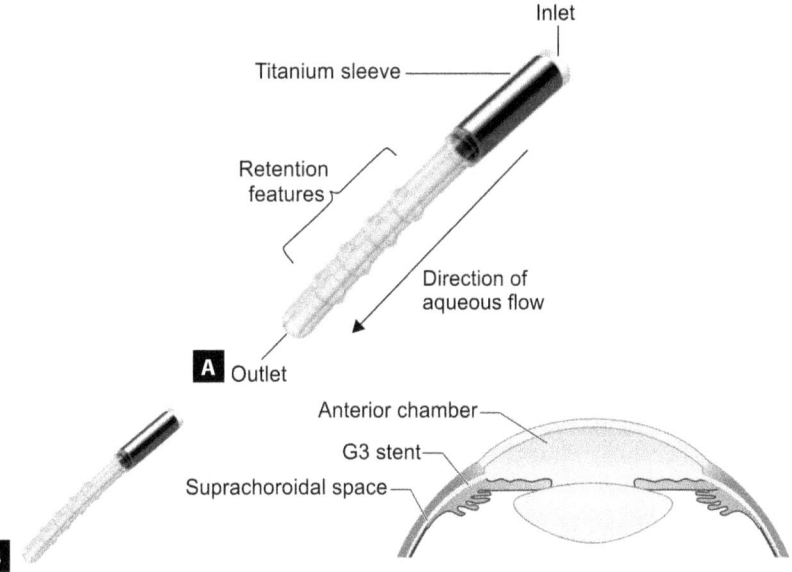

Figs. 4.19.9A and B: (A) iStent Supra; (B) iStent Supra in the eye.

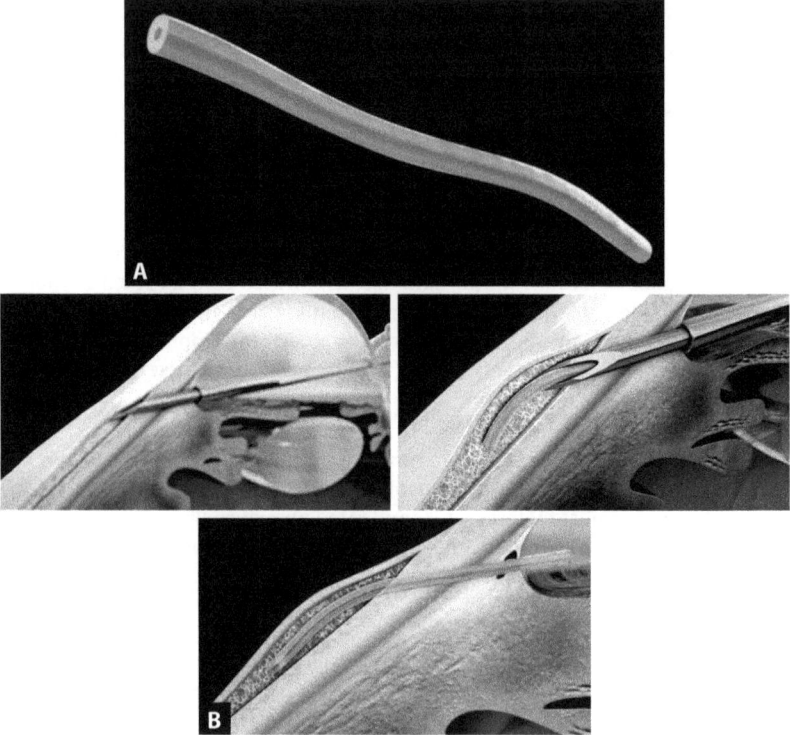

Figs. 4.19.10A and B: (A) Xen Gel Stent; (B) Xen Gel Stent in the eye.

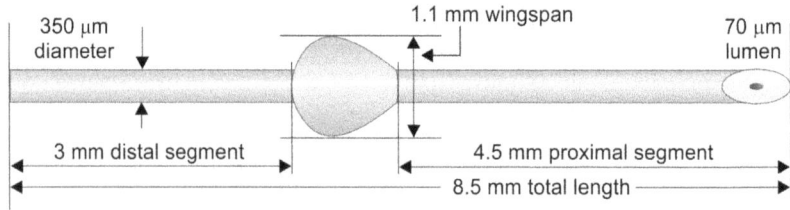

Fig. 4.19.11: PreserFlo MicroShunt.

ENDOCYCLOPHOTOCOAGULATION (FIG. 4.19.12)

The principle of endoscopic cyclophotocoagulation (ECP) is to reduce aqueous production by destroying the ciliary processes (cyclodestruction).

The 20 gauge ECP probe consists of a light pipe, a video endoscope, and an endolaser. It can be introduced in the anterior chamber through a clear corneal/scleral incision, after injecting OVD in the anterior chamber and behind the iris. Under the videoendoscopic view, the 810 nm laser is delivered to the ciliary processes, which can be seen shrinking and becoming white after laser delivery.

Endoscopic cyclophotocoagulation is very useful in eyes with narrow angles, in eyes with glaucoma in aphakia/pseudophakia.

Conventionally, a power of 100 MW for 0.1–0.2 seconds is used.

Pop sounds signify eruption of ciliary processes, so we should reduce the energy settings.

■ MICROPULSE LASER (FIGS. 4.19.13A AND B)

Micropulse transscleral cyclophotocoagulation (MP-TSCPC) has recently emerged as a viable alternative for traditional continuous wave diode TSCPC procedure in the treatment of refractory glaucoma. MP-TSCPC uses a series of repetitive short pulses of energy (On cycle) interspersed with rest periods in between the pulses (off cycle) to allow for thermal dissipation within the ciliary body. This prevents reaching of coagulation temperatures, as in continuous mode diode laser, reducing collateral damage to ciliary body. Such non-selective and diffuse ablation of ciliary processes can cause prolonged hypotony or even phthisis bulbi. More selective ablation of ciliary processes results in reduction of aqueous humor. Apart from cilioablation resulting in aqueous humor and IOP reduction, an increase in uveoscleral outflow pathway has also been described that can significantly reduce intraocular pressures. Additionally, micropulse effect on the longitudinal fibers of the ciliary muscles, with displacement of the scleral spur, and expansion of trabecular spaces, also causes an increase in trabecular outflow, similar to that caused by cholinergic drugs like pilocarpine. MP-TSCPC has been performed with significant IOP reduction in several types of refractory glaucoma. Evidence available from published literature seems to suggest that MPTSCPC can cause considerable reduction in IOP as well as in need of glaucoma medications as compared to preoperative period. Despite intermittent delivery of laser to the ciliary body, MP TSCPC can cause significant adverse effects, including pain, anterior chamber inflammation, transient rise in IOP and corneal edema. Rarely, the procedure can cause persistent hypotony, choroidal detachment, permanent visual loss and pthisis bulbi.

■ INDICATIONS

- Mild to moderate glaucoma cases
- Uncontrolled IOP on maximum medical and laser therapy
- Primary open angle glaucoma (POAG), pigmentary glaucoma, and pseudoexfoliation glaucoma (PXFG)

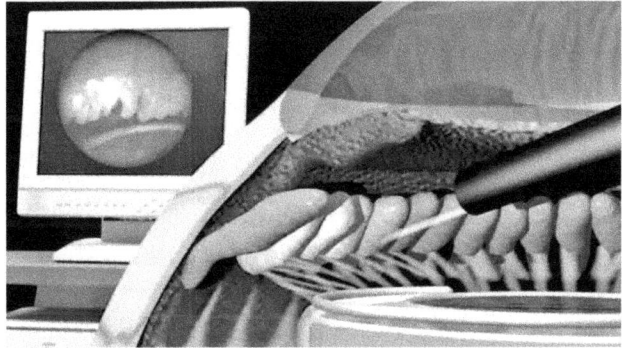

Fig. 4.19.12: Endocyclophotocoagulation.

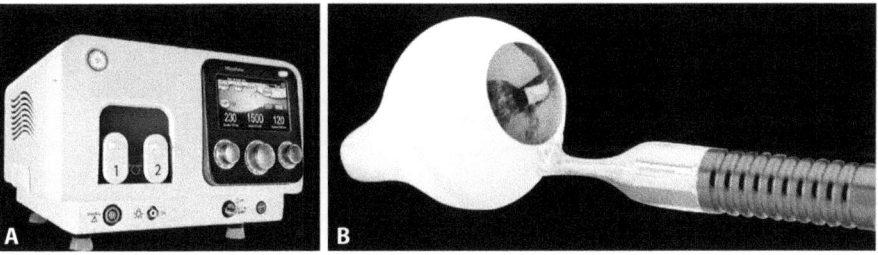

Figs. 4.19.13A and B: (A) Micropulse Laser machine; (B) Micropulse Laser machine.

- Noncompliance to treatment
- Adverse drug reaction

CONTRAINDICATIONS
- Neovascular glaucoma (NVG)
- Primary and secondary angle-closure glaucoma (not for Micropulse laser and ECP)
- Abnormal angle anatomy
- Coexisting corneal pathology
- High episcleral venous pressure conditions such as Sturge–Weber Syndrome

COMPLICATION OF MINIMALLY INVASIVE GLAUCOMA SURGERY
- For stenting procedures such as iStent, Hydrus—stent displacement, stent malposition, stent obstruction, stent migration, and stent fragmentation.
- For GATT, BANG, KDB, ABiC, Trabectome—hyphema (most common), hypotony, PAS, choroidal/retinal detachment (with GATT in the event of false passage)
- Common to all MIGS—postoperative inflammation, transient IOP elevation, and posterior capsular opacification.

CONCLUSION
Minimally invasive glaucoma surgery is proving to be a bridge between lasers on one side and more invasive filtering surgeries on the other side. It requires sound knowledge of angle structures, mastery over intraoperative gonioscopy, diligent maneuvers, and a little practice to effectively use these devices. As no size fits all, the choice of MIGS should be based upon patient's factors, target IOP and affordability. Trabeculectomy still remains the gold standard treatment for glaucoma, but MIGS can be useful for mild to moderate glaucoma.

SUGGESTED READING
1. Dhingra D, Bhartiya S. Evaluating glaucoma surgeries in the MIGS context. Rom J Ophthalmol. 2020;64(2):85-95.
2. Francis BA, Singh K, Lin SC, Hodapp E, Jampel HD, Samples JR, et al. Novel glaucoma procedures: a report by the American Academy of Ophthalmology. Ophthalmology. 2011;118(7):1466-80.
3. Grover DS, Godfrey DG, Smith O, Feuer WJ, De Oca IM, Fellman RL. Gonioscopy-assisted transluminal trabeculotomy, ab interno trabeculotomy: technique report and preliminary results. Ophthalmology. 2014;121(4):855-61.
4. Gurnani B, Tripathy K. Minimally Invasive Glaucoma Surgery. In: StatPearls [Internet]. 2022. StatPearls Publishing.
5. Saheb H, Ahmed II. Micro-invasive glaucoma surgery: current perspectives and future directions. Curr Opin Ophthalmol. 2012;23(2):96-104.
6. Vera V, Sheybani A, Wustenberg W, Romoda L, Camejo L, Liu X, et al. Compatibility and durability of the gel stent material. Expert Rev Med Devices. 2022;19(5):385-91.
7. Yook E, Vinod K, Panarelli JF. Complications of micro-invasive glaucoma surgery. Curr Opin Ophthalmol. 2018;29(2):147-54.

"With our THOUGHTS, we make the WORLD."

—Buddha

SECTION 5

Refractive Surgery

Editors: Chitra Ramamurthy, Shreesha Kumar Kodavoor

5.1 Preoperative Work-up for Refractive Surgery 306
Soundarya B

5.2 Applications of Scheimpflug Principle in Ophthalmology 309
Pranessh, Shreesha Kumar Kodavoor

5.3 Corvis ST: Utility and Interpretation 313
Gitansha Shreyas Sachdev

5.4 Microkeratomes in Today's Practice 317
Divya Giridhar, RR Sudhir

5.5 Femtosecond Laser: Applications in Modern Refractive Surgery 321
Kumar Doctor, Shivani P Pattnaik

5.6 Femtosecond Lasers for Flap Making 324
Mahipal Sachdev, Charu Khurana, Raghav Malik

5.7 Intraocular Lens Power Calculation Postrefractive Surgery 332
Anagha Heroor, Vikram Vaidee

5.8 Phakic Intraocular Lens: Indications and Preoperative Evaluation 337
Shreesha Kumar Kodavoor, Ashalyne James

5.9 Phakic Intraocular Lens: An Overview 342
Partha Biswas, (Lt Col) Billal Hossain, Sneha Batra

5.10 Wavefront-guided and Optimized Ablations: What We Need to Know? 348
Ananth D

5.11 Contoura Vision 352
Shreesha Kumar Kodavoor, Neha K Rathi, Gopal R

5.12 Topography-guided Ablations in Normal and Abnormal Corneas 355
Jagadesh C Reddy

5.13 Complications of Small Incision Lenticule Extraction 357
Neha K Rathi, Shreesha Kumar Kodavoor, Ramamurthy Dandapani

5.14 Small Incision Lenticule Extraction 362
Krishana Prasad Kudlu, Aparna Nayak N

5.15 Refractive Lens Exchange: Current Perspective 368
Ritika Sachdev, Kanika Bhardwaj

5.16 Retreatment Options Following Refractive Surgery 372
Chitra Ramamurthy, Soundarya B

5.17 Corneal Procedures for Correction of Presbyopia 376
Sri Ganesh, Sheetal Brar

5.18 Surface Ablation 381
Komal B Patekar, Shreesha Kumar Kodavoor

5.19 Corneal Collagen Cross-linking in Refractive Surgery 383
Pooja Khamar, Sailie Shirodkar, Ritica Mukherji

5.20 Complications of Collagen Cross-linking 386
Ashalyne James, Shreesha Kumar Kodavoor

5.21 Newer Procedures in Refractive Surgery 391
Rupal Shah

5.22 Phototherapeutic Keratectomy 393
JK Reddy

5.23 Refractive Surprise after Cataract Surgery 394
Rishi Swarup, Samita Moolani

5.24 Complications in Laser-assisted In Situ Keratomileusis 399
Madhuvanthi Mohan, Sujatha Mohan

5.25 Posterior Segment Complications after Refractive Surgeries 407
Shrinivas Joshi, Giriraj Vibhute, Rajashree Salvi

5.1 Preoperative Work-up for Refractive Surgery

Soundarya B
The Eye Foundation, Coimbatore
soundslikeme@gmail.com

■ INTRODUCTION

Any form of surgery or ocular procedure carries its own set of risks and complications, and refractive surgery is no exception to this. Preoperative assessment plays an important role in choosing the type of procedure that is ideal for each individual patient in order to avoid these complications. It also becomes important for the surgeon to understand the patient's needs and expectations and counsel them appropriately regarding the risks, benefits, and limitations of each procedure.

■ BASIC EVALUATION

History

Evaluation begins with proper elicitation of history, to rule out any systemic or ocular contraindications such as collagen vascular disorders, glaucoma, past ocular herpes, dry eye, family history of keratoconus, etc. History regarding past ocular procedures and contact lens use also provide useful information for planning. In case of contact lens wear, topography must be repeated after stopping the use of contact lens for at least a week in case of soft contact lenses. Age is an important factor and age <18 years is a contraindication for refractive procedures.

General Ocular Examination

A comprehensive ocular examination should include a thorough slit lamp examination to rule out any ocular pathologies involving the eyelids/cornea/lens, intraocular pressure measurement, and fundus examination which includes peripheral retinal examination especially in cases of high myopes. It is important to look for corneal scars which could indicate past viral infections and also helps in deciding the type of procedure that would be suited for these eyes. A complete squint evaluation should also be done when indicated.

Cycloplegic Refraction

A thorough cycloplegic refraction is very important to assess and rule out latent hyperopia. A stable refraction for at least 1 year is mandatory to proceed with refractive surgery. It has to be kept in mind that refractive errors—usually a myopia of up to -12 D, astigmatism up to -5 D and a hyperopia of up to $+6$D can be corrected by keratorefractive procedures.

It may also be sensible to do an orthoptic evaluation preoperatively in these patients to rule out disorders of accommodation which may manifest postoperatively.

Dry Eye Evaluation

This plays a major role in preoperative assessment as it helps in detecting patients who might require perioperative management with lubrication and other modalities and also helps in avoiding postoperative patient discomfort and the higher chances of regression associated with dry eye.

Evaluation includes dry eye questionnaires, Schirmer's test, tear film break up time, ocular staining scores, and meibomian gland analysis/imaging. Any patient with dry eye needs to be treated adequately prior to taking up for surgery with preservative free lubrication and anti-inflammatory agents such as steroids/cyclosporine. Meibomian gland dysfunction should also be addressed with lid hygiene, antibiotics or in-office methods such as LipiFlow.

CORNEAL TOPOGRAPHY

Corneal topography has evolved significantly over the years. The *first generation* topographers were placido-based devices which project a system of concentric light circles onto the corneal surface. The major drawback was the lack of data from the posterior corneal surface. The term "tomography" then developed, which refers to sectioning of the cornea, thus allowing assessment of the posterior corneal surface as well. This includes the *second generation* corneal tomographers like Orbscan® (Bausch and Lomb, USA), which combines placido disc and slit scanning technologies.

The technology of the *third generation* tomographers uses the Scheimpflug principle with a rotating camera which allows analysis of both anterior and posterior surfaces of the cornea by direct imaging. Examples include Pentacam (Oculus, Germany), TMS-5 (Tomey Corporation, Japan), Sirius (CSO, Italy), and Galilei (Ziemer, Switzerland). Currently, the two most commonly used tomography devices for refractive surgery screening are the Orbscan and Pentacam.

The main indices to look for in the refractive display maps are significant inferior-superior (I-S) asymmetry and skewing of axis in the sagittal/curvature map, mean K-value to rule out too flat or too steep corneas, values on the elevation maps, central corneal thickness and thinnest pachymetry values to determine the expected residual stromal bed thickness postprocedure. **Figure 5.1.1** shows a normal Pentacam map.

Anterior and posterior elevation maps, constructed in relation to a reference shape such as a best fit sphere or ellipsoid are used to indicate the presence of ectasia. Values of the highest elevation point in the central zone of approximately more than +12 in the anterior float and +15 to +18 in the posterior float maps are considered abnormal.

Indices in the Belin–Ambrósio enhanced ectasia display page of the Pentacam that are most useful for screening include the Belin–Ambrósio enhanced ectasia display-total deviation value (BAD D), Ambrósio relational thickness (ART) values and the pachymetric progression index (PPI).

CORNEAL BIOMECHANICAL ASSESSMENT

The ocular response analyzer (ORA, New York) and Corvis ST (Oculus, Germany) are two devices used to assess the corneal biomechanics. In combination with the Pentacam, corneal biomechanics has shown potential to modify refractive screening.

The tomographic and biomechanical index (TBI) which is a combination of Scheimpflug-based corneal tomography and biomechanical strength is used as one of the red flag indicators and has 90.4% sensitivity and 96.0% specificity for detecting subclinical ectasia.

Aberrometry

Wavefront analysis and aberrometry help in identifying preexisting corneal higher order aberrations. In eyes with very high preexisting aberrations, a wavefront-guided or a topography-guided approach may be a better option to reduce these aberrations.

Mesopic pupil size measurement preoperatively also becomes important as it gives an idea of the postoperative visual quality in terms of increased glare and halos in patients with larger pupil sizes.

ECTASIA RISK SCORING

Although rare, ectasia remains one of the most vision-threatening complications following refractive surgery, whose incidence ranges from 0.033 to 0.60%, and can present months or years after the procedure. So it is of paramount importance to rule out the presence of forme fruste keratoconus before proceeding with refractive surgery.

The definition of *forme fruste keratoconus* (FFKC) is not consistently established, although it widely includes any tomographically normal eye which has frank keratoconus in the fellow eye or any eye with subtle tomographic changes not amounting to frank keratoconus.

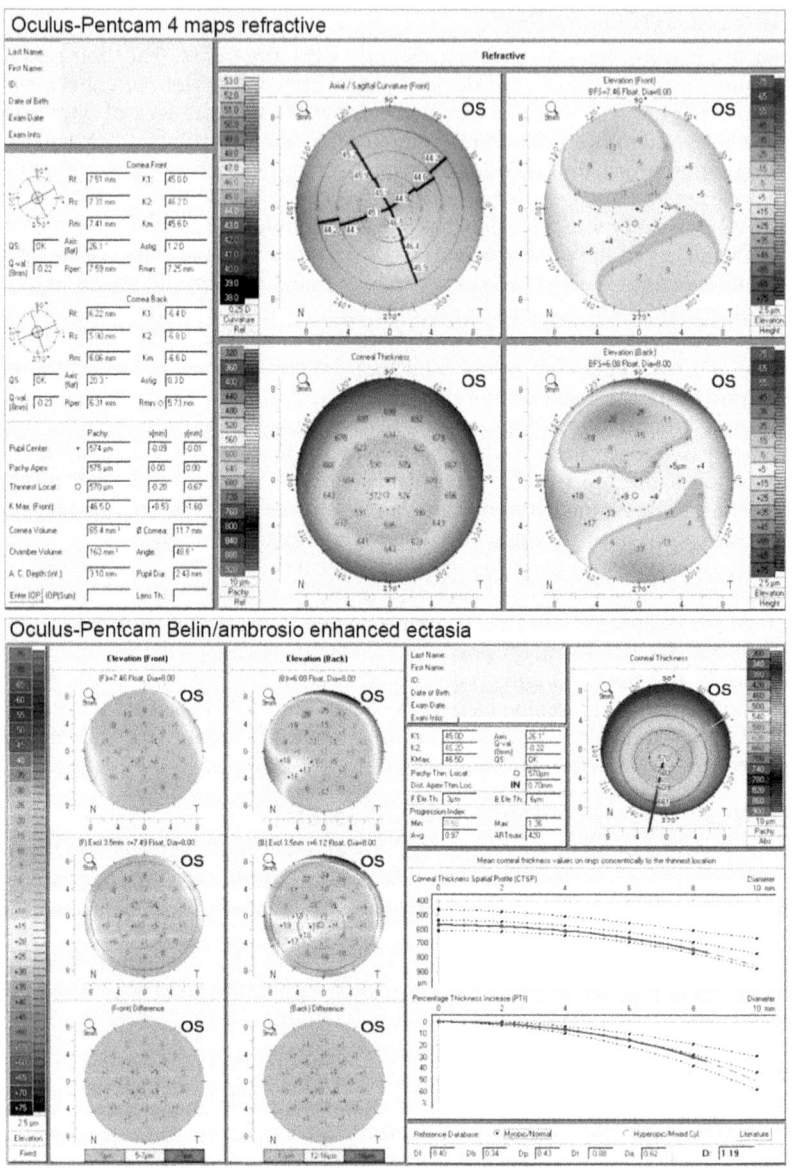

Fig. 5.1.1: Normal pentacam map.

Percentage of tissue altered (PTA) is an important factor to look at before proceeding with refractive surgery. It is derived as PTA = (FT + AD)/CCT (FT = flap thickness, AD = ablation depth, and CCT = preoperative central corneal thickness). A value of >40% is usually considered a risk factor for developing ectasia.

Multiple risk scoring systems have been developed. The Ectasia Risk Score System (ERSS) includes multiple factors such as patient age, gender, spherical equivalent of manifest refraction, pachymetry, and topographic patterns. It also takes into consideration the operative factors such as the type of procedure, flap thickness, ablation depth, and residual stromal bed thickness.

Newer indices like the Pentacam Random Forest Index (PRFI) use artificial intelligence and utilize machine learning to improve detection of ectasia susceptibility and subclinical keratoconus, however more research is needed in the future for these indices to be incorporated into everyday clinical practice.

■ CONCLUSION

Multiple factors have to be put together and analyzed before considering a patient for refractive surgery, the major factors being age, stable refractive error, absence of other ocular and systemic contraindications and a normal tomographic and biomechanical assessment. Any single abnormal index in tomography should not always be considered a red flag without correlating with other factors such as perioperative parameters. Finally, it is very important to understand the patient's specific needs and expectations and cater the treatment according to it and counsel them appropriately before taking up for the procedure.

■ SUGGESTED READING

1. Ambrósio R Jr, Lopes BT, Faria-Correia F, et al. Integration of Scheimpflug-based corneal tomography and biomechanical assessments for enhancing ectasia detection. J Refract Surg. 2017;33:434-43.
2. Ambrósio R Jr. Post-LASIK ectasia: twenty years of a conundrum. Semin Ophthalmol. 2019;34:66-8.
3. Bohac M, Koncarevic M, Pasalic A, et al. Incidence and clinical characteristics of post-LASIK ectasia: a review of over 30,000 LASIK cases. Semin Ophthalmol. 2018;33:869-77.

5.2 Applications of Scheimpflug Principle in Ophthalmology

Pranessh, Shreesha Kumar Kodavoor
The Eye Foundation, Coimbatore
eskay_03@rediffmail.com

■ INTRODUCTION

Scheimpflug principle, as described by Theodor Scheimpflug states that three planes (the film, subject, and lens planes) must converge along a single line. The images taken during the study are digitized in the main unit and all image data is transferred to the computer interface bus. Scheimpflug's principle **(Fig. 5.2.1)** has been particularly useful in ophthalmic imaging over the past decades. Several devices were used to obtain cross-sectional images of the anterior segment using a Scheimpflug camera perpendicular to the slit beam. The most commonly used Scheimpflug device in ophthalmology is currently the Pentacam (Oculus Wetzlar, Germany).

■ APPLICATIONS OF THE SCHEIMPFLUG PRINCIPLE

In Corneal and Refractive Surgery

Scheimpflug-based topographers play a vital role as an anterior segment diagnostic and interventional modality. Currently, the topographers using Scheimpflug-based imaging are Pentacam, Galilei, and Sirius.

Advantages of using Scheimpflug-based imaging systems
- Precise measurement of the central cornea
- Ability to correct for small eye movements
- Easy fixation for patient
- Short examination time

The Scheimpflug device does not appear to be as limited as the slit scanning in terms of postrefractive measurement.

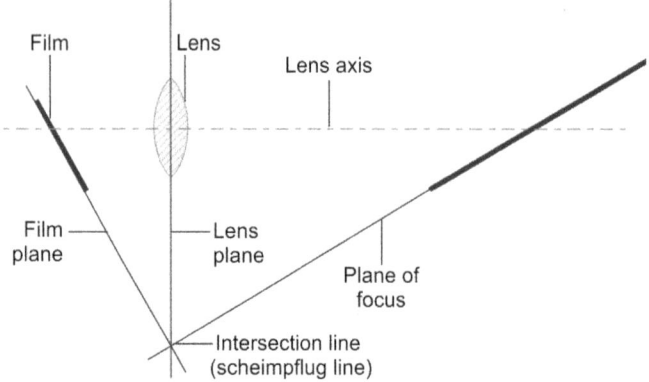

Fig. 5.2.1: This figure illustrated the intersection of the film, subject and the lens plane to obtain Scheimpflug image.

Variations in Scheimpflug-based Systems

Single Scheimpflug imaging: Pentacam™ (Oculus GmbH) utilizes a single Scheimpflug imaging camera. It rotates around the central axis and captures 50 meridian images, each passing through the same point in the center of the cornea. Pentacam software extracts 500 high-quality points from each image, achieving 25,000 data points, the true surface area of each corneal surface. A visit takes less than 2 seconds, and the system can adjust the center of each image before reconstructing the corneal image, reducing any movement. Pentacam's software adds a ray-tracing algorithm to build and calculate a three-dimensional mathematical image of the entire anterior segment. Image analysis is performed by linear densitometry and correlates density with a layer of the cornea and lens.

Corvis® ST (Oculus) uses a high-speed Scheimpflug camera to take over 4,300 images/second in order to capture the cornea's deformation in response to a defined air pulse. The acquired Scheimpflug pictures enable accurate determination of intraocular pressure (IOP) and corneal thickness. The cornea's biomechanical properties can be investigated in greater detail and have important implications for the treatment of corneal pathologies and keratorefractive surgery.

Dual Scheimpflug imaging: Two Scheimpflug cameras (used in Galilei Dual Scheimpflug Analyzer, Ziemer Ophthalmology) oriented at 90° are used, which rotate around a shared central axis housing the slit beam light source. Upgradation to dual imaging systems enables the comparison and averaging of related corneal data from each channel to account for inadvertent misalignment and eye movement. It is unaffected by angular surfaces, enabling correct pachymetry to be determined even when the degree of decentration from the corneal apex is unknown. In contrast to single Scheimpflug systems, which must estimate the changing surface inclination before calculating the correct thicknesses or posterior heights, it is possible to place each averaged thickness and posterior height value in the cornea to its suitable location using dual cameras. Due to the reciprocal dual-camera views, any inaccuracy resulting from the misalignment can be fixed by averaging these corresponding data. This technique makes it easier to map the cornea and anterior section with more accuracy because of how naturally human eyes move in real life. The latter can obtain an accurate and reliable pachymetric analysis compared to the single imaging system.

Incorporation of placido topography: Scheimpflug devices would give erroneous data while processing the anterior and posterior curvature of the cornea on moving toward the periphery, as the curvature is only a small part of the anterior segment imaging. This can be avoided by combining dual Scheimpflug imaging with infrared Placido topography.

Several devices combine the two approaches to improve precision in readings [CSO Sirius Topographer® (CSO, Firenze, Italy)].

Comparison of Three Scheimpflug Topographers

Topographer	Pentacam	Galilei	Sirius
Principle	Single Scheimpflug	Dual Scheimpflug with placido	Single Scheimpflug with placido
Acquisition speed	25 scan images in 2 sec	25–50 scan images in 2 sec	25 scan images in 2 sec
Points mapped	25,000 points	122,000 points	21632 anterior and 16000 poterior points
Principle	Single Scheimpflug	Dual Scheimpflug with placido	Single Scheimpflug with placido

Topographic Indices in Various Scheimpflug Topographers

Topographer	Notable Indices

Pentacam (Oculus, Wetzlar, Germany)	• Belin-Ambrósio enhanced ectasia display total deviation value (BAD-D)
	  – The Belin/Ambrósio Enhanced Ectasia Display I—enhanced visualization of the cone by enhancing the reference surface
	  – Also gives the corneal thickness spatial profile (CTSP) and percentage thickness index (PTI)—plot points outside the outlier are suggestive of keratoconus
	  – Belin/Ambrósio Enhanced Ectasia Display II—calculated final D using 5 parameters [Df (front), Db (back), Dp (pachymetry progression), Dt (thinnest value), and Da (thinnest displacement)]
	  – BAD III—added additional 4 parameters to the latter
	• Pachymetric progression index (PPI):
	  – Ambrósio relational thickness (ART)—412 µm is the cut-off value for ART max
	  – Keratoconus index (KI)—reliable screening parameter

Sirius (Costruzione Strumenti Oftalmici, Florence, Italy)	• Root mean square (RMS) lower the RMS, the more regular the surface. Belin/Ambrosio enhanced ectasia total derivation (BAD-D) similar to the 4.5 mm root mean square per unit area. • Symmetry index of curvature—measures vertical asymmetry • Baiocchi-Calossi-Versad front and back index (BCVf) (highly specific for keratoconus) and (BCVb)—analyzes the coma and trefoil components of elevations in the zones
Galilei (Ziemer, Biel, Switzerland)	Asphericity asymmetry index (AAI), or Kranemann-Arce index

In Fuchs Endothelial Corneal Dystrophy: The FECD (Fuchs endothelial corneal dystrophy) tomographic patterns that are indicative of the presence of edema can be found using Scheimpflug imaging. These recurring patterns, which may be detected in the posterior elevation and pachymetry maps, can be utilized to forecast how FECD will progress. An objective, quantitative index for evaluating the optical health of the cornea in FECD can be provided by corneal backscatter (two spiking humps in densitogram) detected by the Pentacam.

In phakic intraocular surgery: During the preoperative evaluation, the 3D chamber analyzer is useful for surgeons implanting phakic intraocular (IOLs). Pentacam uses a rapid, reproducible, noncontact approach to show where implanted contact lenses (ICLs) should be placed in reference to the cornea and crystalline lens. This enables the ophthalmologist to monitor these patients' cataract risk by following up with them using ICL.

In Corneal Pathologies

Scheimpflug imaging is helpful for managing post-PKP (penetrating keratoplasty) patients (on suture removal), as well as for planning and screening Intacs for patients with keratoconus. It aids in keeping track of any corneal haze that surface photorefractive keratectomy (PRK) and opacities that postadenoviral-conjunctivitis patients may experience. High-resolution Pentacam can aid in delineating the flap—bed interface, allowing for the visualization of diseases present at the interface, such as Interface Fluid Syndrome, which may develop in post-LASIK steroid responders.

In Cataract Surgery

It has been demonstrated that Scheimpflug's calculation of lens density correlates with the Lens Opacities Classification System (LOCS) III grading, enabling it to identify the progression of cataractogenesis more subtly. A recently introduced software (using densitometry) called Pentacam Nucleus Staging (PNS) offers an accurate and exact evaluation of lens density based on features providing a nuclear cataract score in five stages (0-5). Even in posterior capsular opacification, since Pentacam tomograms are free of flash reflections, they make objective PCO quantification simpler than with slit-lamp retroillumination images.

In Glaucoma

The anterior chamber volume is an effective screening method for identifying eyes with narrow angles, which is highly sensitive and specific. Based on the central corneal thickness, various IOP correction formulas are built within the Pentacam software. In contrast to the anterior segment optical coherence tomography (OCT), it is inefficient in assessing the anterior chamber angle. This is because the scleral surface's reflectivity makes it difficult to see the sclera spur.

Limitations/Disadvantages of Scheimpflug Imaging Device

- Confusion in data interpretation in color-coded maps when comparing Scheimpflug versus Placido-based imaging system as in the earlier red depicts the higher location, whereas in Placido system, the steepest is marked red.
- It is impossible to compare the precision of the many Scheimpflug devices. As, each machine extrapolates and calculates data based on a separate set of algorithms and systems. Galilei (Ziemer, Biel, Switzerland) reduced the corneal power's value by around 3% compared to earlier versions by moving the optical reference plane to the anterior corneal surface. With respect to the posterior corneal surface, Pentacam determines the total corneal refractive power.
- Care must be taken when cross-comparing the variable between each system as they are not mutual.
- Epithelial abnormalities and defects in corneal clarity may influence Scheimpflug imaging, leading to false-positive alterations in the posterior corneal surface and pachymetry.

Using additional Placido-based systems may be able to negate some of the earlier mentioned issues.

■ SUGGESTED READING

1. Chu HY, Hsiao CH, Chen PYF, Ma DHK, Chang CJ, Tan HY. Corneal Backscatters as an Objective Index for Assessing Fuchs' Endothelial Corneal Dystrophy: A Pilot Study. J Ophthalmol. 2017;2017:8747013.

2. Doctor K, Vunnava KP, Shroff R, Kaweri L, Lalgudi VG, Gupta K, et al. Simplifying and understanding various topographic indices for keratoconus using Scheimpflug based topographers. Indian Journal of Ophthalmology. 2020;68(12):2732.
3. Mirzaie M, Bahremani E, Taheri N, Khamnian Z, Kharrazi Ghadim B. Cataract Grading in Pure Senile Cataracts: Pentacam versus LOCS III. J Ophthalmic Vis Res. 2022;17(3):337-43.
4. Roberts CJ. Importance of accurately assessing biomechanics of the cornea. Curr Opin Ophthalmol. 2016;27(4):285-91.

5.3 | Corvis ST: Utility and Interpretation

Gitansha Shreyas Sachdev
The Eye Foundation, Coimbatore
gitansha@theeyefoundation.com, sachdevgitansha@gmail.com

■ INTRODUCTION

Hysteresis, a term coined in 1980 by Sir James Ewing denotes the property of a physical system wherein it reacts slowly to an applied force. Corneal hysteresis measurement is a relatively new tool introduced in the armamentarium of keratorefractive preoperative work-up. The Ocular Response Analyzer (ORA, Reichert Inc, NY, USA) and Corvis ST (Oculus, Optikgeräte, GmbH) are the two available devices for corneal hysteresis measurement.

Ocular Response Analyzer (ORA, Reichert Inc, NY, USA) utilizes a rapid air impulse and an advanced electro-optical system to measure two applanation pressure measurements, the first while the cornea is flattened inward and the second as the cornea resumes its original form.[1] The Corvis ST (Oculus, Optikgeräte, GmbH) includes a dynamic applanation tonometry to deform the cornea and a Scheimpflug camera to image the various stages of deformation.[2]

■ INTERPRETATION OF CORVIS ST PARAMETERS

The device calculates and provides the following measurements:
- The tonometry and pachymetry evaluation
- Dynamic corneal response
- Vinciguerra screening report
- Biomechanical or tomographical assessment

Tonometry and Pachymetry Evaluation

The device allows a dynamic measurement of the corneal deformation following an air puff application. The pressure of the air puff required to flatten the cornea provides the tonometric data. The device takes six measurements and provides the mean value.

Additionally, the corrected intraocular pressure (IOP) is displayed using various nomograms such as biomechanical corrected IOP values, Dresden, Ehlers. The IOP correction is based on the age, corneal thickness and the biomechanical response. Moreover, the IOP measurements are not influenced by the tear film properties.

Corneal pachymetry evaluation is done prior to corneal deformation. Measurements can be taken with the help of calipers along the central 8 mm of the corneal diameter. The pachymetry progression map provides the corneal thickness along the horizontal meridian, along with two standard deviation values (**Fig. 5.3.1**).

Dynamic Corneal Response

The corneal deformation secondary to the air puff is measured using a high speed camera to provide the dynamic corneal response. The device captures around 140 images within 31 ms. The first or "initial stage" is the original corneal shape prior to deformation (**Fig. 5.3.2A**). Applanation 1 is the next stage of transition from convex to concave,

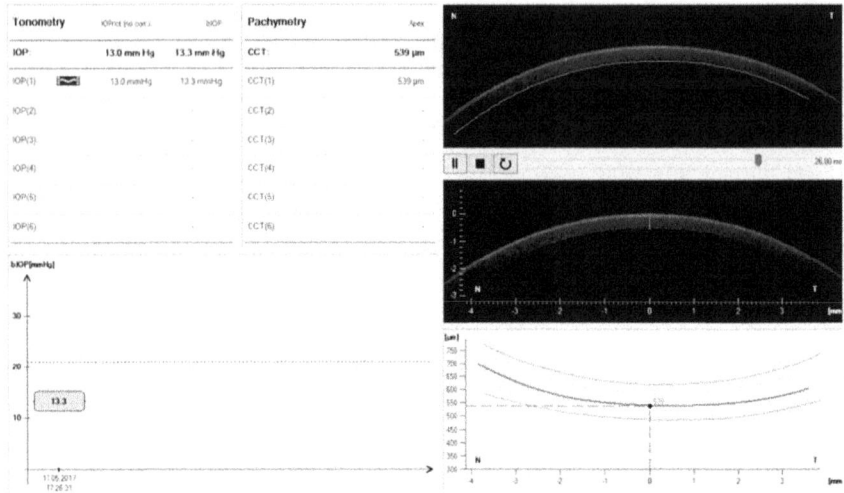

Fig. 5.3.1: Tonometry and pachymetry assessment.

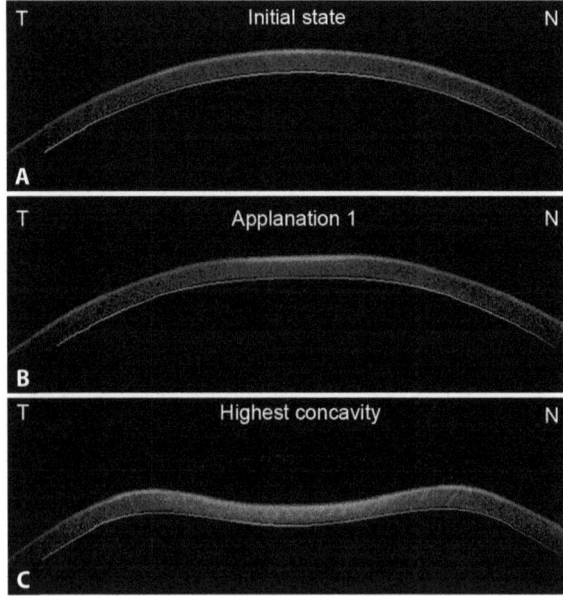

Figs. 5.3.2A to C: Stages of corneal deformation. (A) Initial stage; (B) Applanation stage; (C) Stage of highest concavity.

when the central corneal surface is flat **(Fig. 5.3.2B)**. The length of the "flat" corneal surface is called the applanation length. The force of the air puff at this step measures the IOP. The next step is that of highest concavity wherein the corneal apex is farthest from the original position **(Fig. 5.3.2C)**. The distance of the corneal apex from the original point to the point of maximum concavity is called the deflection amplitude and the length of the curve the bend radius.

Weaker corneas have a shorter applanation length, increase deflection amplitude and smaller bend of radius **(Fig. 5.3.3)**.

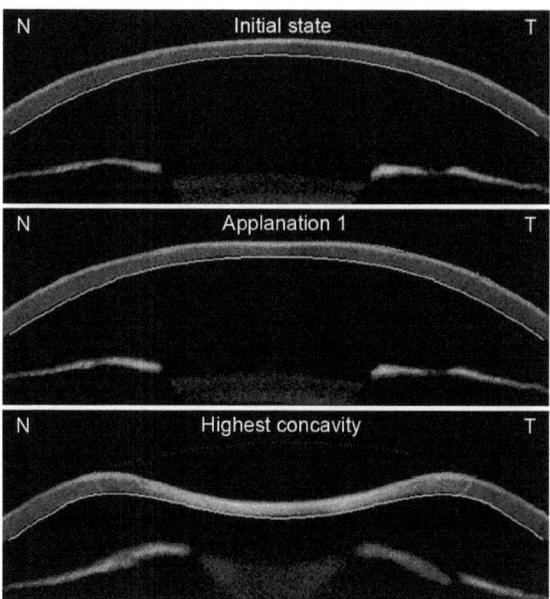

Fig. 5.3.3: Shorter applanation length, increased deflection amplitude and smaller bend of radius in weaker corneas.

Deformation amplitude is the deflection amplitude at center and periphery. DA ratio provides the ratio of deformation at the apex to the 2 mm zone. Inverse concave radius (ICR) is the inverse of the bend radius. Softer corneas bend or deform more in the middle with relatively lower movement in the paracentral regions, thereby displaying a higher DA ratio vis-à-vis stronger corneas. Similarly, as the bend radius is lower, the ICR is higher in softer corneas.

Vinciguerra Screening Report

The Vinciguerra Screening Report includes the dynamic corneal response pattern and compares it to the IOP-adjusted standard deviations. Higher standard deviations denote a softer cornea **(Fig. 5.3.4)**.

Additional parameters provided include SPA1 stiffness parameter which describes the corneal rigidity and ARTh or the Ambrósio relational thickness horizontal. The device combines these values to provide the corneal biomechanical index (CBI). CBI value ranges from 0 to 1, wherein a lower value (i.e., 0) denotes a stronger cornea.

Biomechanical or Tomographical Assessment

The device uses artificial intelligence provides the tomographic biomechanical index (TBI) combining the CBI (Vinciguerra Screening Report) and BAD-D (corneal tomography, Pentacam) values **(Fig. 5.3.5)**. Similar to CBI, TBI values range from 0 to 1, wherein a lower value denotes a stronger cornea.

■ CLINICAL SIGNIFICANCE AND UTILITY

Preoperative corneal biomechanics measurement combined with corneal tomography, affords an improved sensitivity and specificity in detection of eyes with significant risk of ectasia development postkeratorefractive procedures or early cases of subclinical ectasia.

Additionally, the device allows an early screening for normal tension glaucoma (NTG) using the biomechanical glaucoma factor (BGF). Studies have demonstrated

SECTION 5: Refractive Surgery

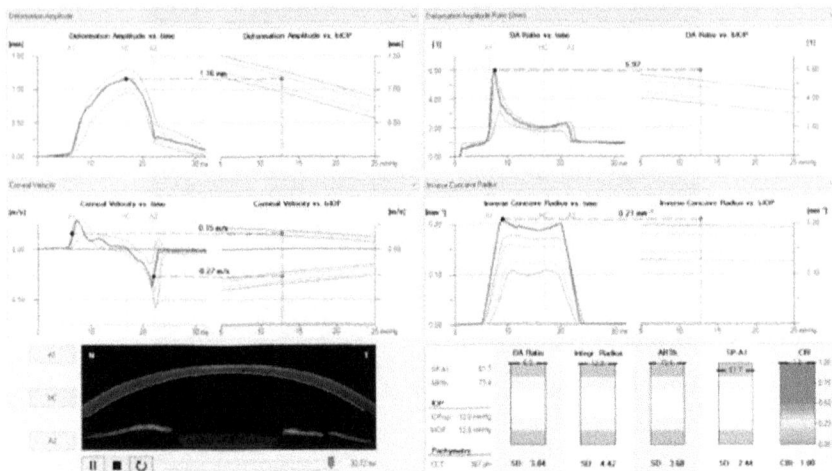

Fig. 5.3.4: Vinciguerra screening report showing higher standard deviation values in a softer cornea.

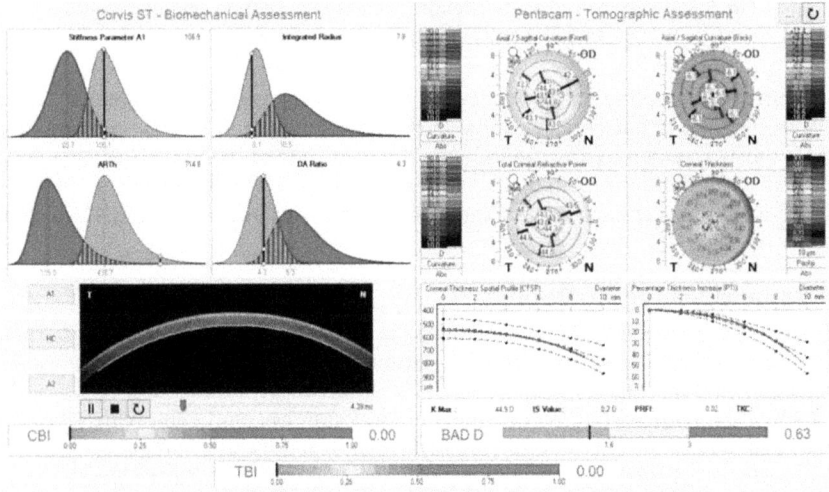

Fig. 5.3.5: Biomechanical and tomographic assessment.

that corneal biomechanical properties may serve as an independent risk factor for NTG development.

In conclusion, the Corvis ST is a promising screening tool for refractive and glaucoma surgeons. Further studies and software developments will allow a more extensive and sensitive application in varying clinical scenarios.

■ REFERENCES

1. Kirwan C, O'Malley D, O'Keefe M. Corneal hysteresis and corneal resistance factor in keratoectasia: findings using the Reichert ocular response analyzer. Ophthalmologica 2008;222(5):334-7.
2. Ambrosio et al: integration of Scheimpflug-Based corneal Tomography and Biomechanical Assessment for Enhancing ectasia detection. J Refract Surg. 2017;33(7):434-43.

5.4 Microkeratomes in Today's Practice

Divya Giridhar, RR Sudhir
Sankara Nethralaya, Nungambakkam, Chennai
divg1212@gmail.com, drrrs@snmail.org

■ HISTORY

Jose Ignacio Barraquer created the first microkeratome in 1958, with keratophakia and frozen keratomileusis in mind. He discovered that the cornea may be applanated, allowing for treatment with a tool similar to a Carpenter's plane. Barraquer created the first manual microkeratome based on this principle.[1]

Castroviejo electrokeratome was the prototype of a motorized microkeratome, which began operations in 1991.[1] The Carrazio-Barraquer pivoted rotating microkeratome (CB) was launched in 1996, which had the benefit of permitting the hinge to be placed where desired. The Hanastome automated microkeratome, which produces a corneal flap with a superior hinge, was introduced by Chiron in 1997. In 2001, Carriazo unveiled the first generation of pendular microkeratomes (Carriazo-Pendular, SCHWIND).[1]

The cornea is made firm by increasing the intraocular pressure, which is accomplished by all contemporary designs having a suction ring that attaches to the eye. The oscillating blade is advanced through the tissue with an offset of 130, 160, 180, or 200 μm after the applanation blade flattens the cornea. The oscillating blade creates a smooth incision, whereas the advancing microkeratome creates the corneal section. By stopping the oscillating blade at a predetermined location, a successful hinge of flap is produced.[1]

■ CLASSIFICATION[1]

Microkeratomes can be either manual or mechanical.
- First generation microkeratomes had linear cutting action, 0 degree plane and fixed thickness
- Second generation had pivoted rotational cutting action.
- Third generation has a pendulum-like cutting action.
- Fourth generation include blade less microkeratomes, e.g., Hydrokeratome, Visijet keratome

1. *Head propulsion:* There are two options: Automated or manual [the Carriazo-Pendular microkeratome (SCHWIND) provides both]. The advantage of automated propulsion is that it provides a consistent pace of cut.
2. Head translation
   a. *In linear translation:* The cutting head can only generate a nasal hinge because it is supported by two parallel rails in the horizontal plane. For instance, Moria-LSK One-Use Plus
   b. *Arciform translation:* The cutting head is moved in an arc like fashion along an eccentric axis. For instance, Moria M2.
   c. *Pendular movement:* The Carriazo-pendular microkeratome cuts in a pendulum-like motion along a horizontal axis located above the corneal apex.
3. Single-use and reusable microkeratomes.

■ MECHANICAL MICROKERATOMES

Summit-Krumeich-Barraquer-Microkeratome (SKBM)

The handpiece of the Barraquer microkeratome (**Fig. 5.4.1**) has two motors that separately control the pace of blade translation and oscillation and a drive band regulates the blades traverse across the cornea. The preview window is an applanation plate that is calibrated and transparent, enabling surgeons complete visibility of the cornea and the diameter of the flap. By simply changing the ring position, the hinge can be placed superiorly or nasally with the new automated Carriazo-Barraquer microkeratome has a dual motor technology.[1]

Amadeus

The Amadeus design **(Fig. 5.4.2)** offers complete flap visualization during the cutting process and software that does ongoing checks of several operation parameters, thus providing additional safety. By adjusting the ring and plate diameters, it is possible to alter the hinge width and translation speed. There are two rings—8.5 and 9.5 mm. Plates are available in 140, 160, and 180 μm depths, 220 and 300 μm plates will be added to the lineup.[1]

MK-2000

The MK-2000 (Nidek) is an automated microkeratome that is FDA approved **(Fig. 5.4.3)**. The device is safe and created flaps of predictable thickness and is suitable for eyes with prominent brows and tight apertures. The head of the device has a polished leading edge that is gentle on the epithelium. The device has no external gears/tracks and thus less chance of mechanical obstruction during the pass.[1]

Hansatome Microkeratome (Bausch & Lomb)

The Hansatome microkeratome **(Fig. 5.4.4)** has a simple three-step assembly with a rolling gear for smooth transition. The elevated gear track features a nasal location, away from the lid and speculum.[1]

This device creates somewhat larger flaps, thus can be utilized for expanded zone treatment, for example, in hyperopes and in those with large pupils.

Carriazo Pendular

This Carriazo Pendular microkeratome **(Fig. 5.4.5)** has a unique pendular movement.

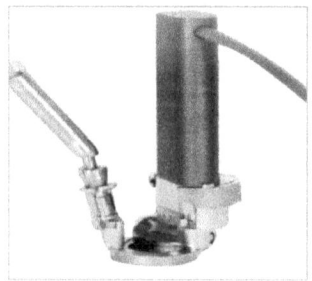

Fig. 5.4.1: Summit-Krumeich-Barraquer-Microkeratome.

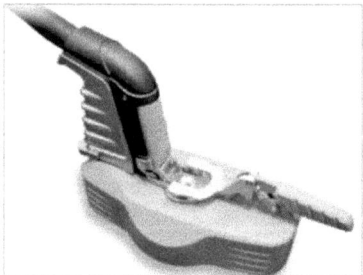

Fig. 5.4.2: Amadeus microkeratome.

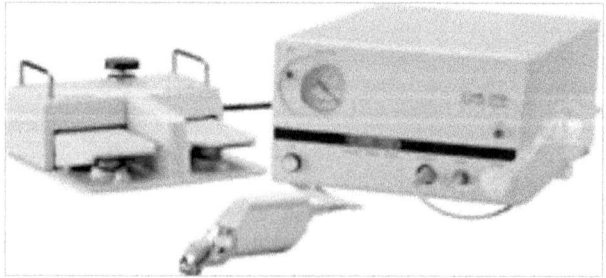

Fig. 5.4.3: MK-2000 (Nidek) microkeratome.

SECTION 5: Refractive Surgery

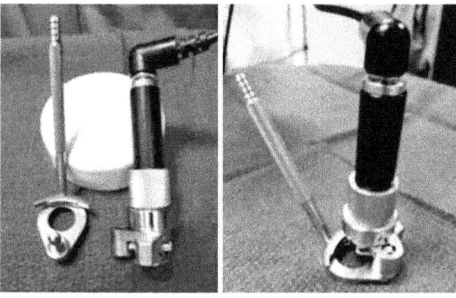

Fig. 5.4.4: Hansatome microkeratome.

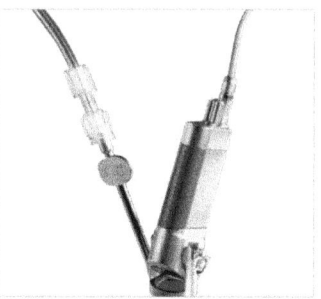

Fig. 5.4.5: Carriazo pendular microkeratome.

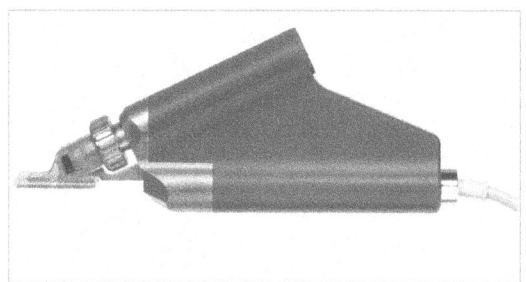

Fig. 5.4.6: Moria One-Use Plus microkeratome.

This device has a convex-shaped head that creates greater central applanation as the device is passed over the cornea, thus ensuring even applanation. The device also has multiple built in safety measures.[1]

Moria One-Use Plus

The One-Use Plus (**Fig. 5.4.6**) is a linear propulsion automated microkeratome device.

The One-Use Plus has the advantage of being easy to use. Rotating blades are not present. It makes only one pass at the cornea to create a flap.[1]

▪ ADVANTAGES
- Microkeratome is >20 years old and thus a familiar procedure for many surgeons compared to Femto LASIK which is a recent technology.
- Microkeratome-assisted LASIK is more economical than Femtolaser LASIK.
- The time duration for LASIK flap creation using a microkeratome is less compared to Femto LASIK.
- Ability to create flap in eyes with anterior stromal opacity or scar—since the microkeratome is a mechanical device, it has the ability to cut through opacities in most cases without much difficulty in contrast to Femtolaser, which is susceptible to vertical gas breakthrough in such eyes with scars. Also the use of microkeratome depends on the size, depth, and location of the scar.[2]
- Less inflammation—flap creation in Femto LASIK causes inflammation in the lamellar interface which is absent in a microkeratome-assisted flap.[2] Also the duration of visual recovery is faster with use of a microkeratome.

▪ DISADVANTAGES
Microkeratome devices can result in buttonhole flaps/free flaps in eyes having a steep or flat cornea respectively. Also mechanical obstruction of the device can cause incomplete or partial flaps.

Also the chance of epithelial ingrowth is more in microkeratome LASIK, since the angle between the side cut and interface shallower and flatter compared to laser.[3]

■ FLAPS CHARACTERISTICS

The flaps created in the femtosecond laser are more precise, with a predefined thickness and predictable length of hinge. For better flap stability and position, these flaps have steep border cuts.

The microkeratome creates meniscus-shaped flaps, which are thin in the center and have a thicker periphery.[2,3]

Nowadays, microkeratomes like the Moria SBK One-Use Plus creates more uniform flaps similar to femtosecond lasers.

■ NEW CUT TECHNOLOGIES

Waterjet System (Hydrokeratome; Visijet)

The waterjet system (which substitutes conventional blade) creates a flap by the application of continuous flow of water under high pressure onto the cornea. This technology involves the use of 33 μm diameter circular beam of saline water moving at a very high speed which cuts between the corneal lamellae. Also, this action helps remove any debris from the cut.[4]

Unfortunately, this technology has not been widely accepted among refractive surgeons.

Disposable Microkeratomes

The use of disposable microkeratomes reduces the possibility of error during cleaning and reassembling.

To be able to use a presterilized new head for each patient and reduced problems with care, safety and maintenance are added advantages.[4]

■ CONCLUSION

The first generation microkeratomes experienced issues with suction loss, the production of flaps with uneven margins and a broad range of flap thickness.

With uniform edges and a preset thickness and shape, the last generation of microkeratomes allows for accurate flap creation.

Today's microkeratomes have advanced safety features such as voice confirmation, battery power backup, automatic vacuum loss shutoff, software-driven flap centering, and real time monitors to detect motor resistance.

In the forecast period of 2022–2028 the global microkeratome market is expected to grow at a steady rate.

Both microkeratome and femtosecond laser are safe to correct refractive error, but the use of microkeratome has the following added advantages:
- Economical
- Less inflammation
- Faster visual recovery compared to Femto LASIK (since there is less inflammation)
- Used in eyes with anterior stromal scar
- Less suction

■ REFERENCES

1. Azar DT. Refractive Surgery, 2nd edition. Mosby, Elsevier: Philadelphia, PA, USA; 2007.
2. Xia LK, Yu J, Chai GR, Wang D, Li Y. Comparison of the femtosecond laser and mechanical microkeratome for flap cutting in LASIK. Int J Ophthalmol. 2015;8(4):784-90.
3. Kahuam-López N, Navas A, Castillo-Salgado C, Graue-Hernandez EO, Jimenez-Corona A, Ibarra A. Laser-assisted in-situ keratomileusis (LASIK) with a mechanical microkeratome

compared to LASIK with a femtosecond laser for LASIK in adults with myopia or myopic astigmatism. Cochrane Database Syst Rev. 2020;4(4):CD012946.
4. Maldonado MJ, Fernández JCN, Pinero DP. Advances in technologies for laser-assisted in situ keratomileusis (LASIK) surgery. Expert Rev Med Dev. 2008;5(2):209-29.

5.5 Femtosecond Laser: Applications in Modern Refractive Surgery

Kumar Doctor, Shivani P Pattnaik
Doctor Eye Institute, Mumbai
drkumardr@gmail.com

■ INTRODUCTION

The femtosecond laser has become an indispensable and vastly utilized technology for refractive surgeons. Advanced models of machinery and improvised laser software have given it a sharper clinical edge and good safety outcomes. This review aims to outline the current surgical applications of the femtosecond laser in corneal refractive surgery.

■ THE BEGINNING

In the early 1980s, Mourou and Strickland introduced the concept of chirped pulse amplification (CPA), a method that amplified short laser pulses to ultrahigh peak powers. This seminal development paved the way for the birth of femtolaser technology.[1] The ability to predetermine laser delivery patterns allows treatment in a specified pattern and delivery of laser at a required intrastromal depth. As the energy can be focused at a desired depth, even though mild opacities, creation of numerous adjacent cavitation bubbles in a specified pattern provides a precise and powerful tool for tissue dissection.

■ MECHANICS

The pulse duration of the femtosecond laser is in the 10^{-15} second range. With a wavelength of approximately 1,053 nanometers, femtolaser technology produces ultrafast laser pulses that are capable of operating at the femtosecond scale or one quadrillionth of a second and is not absorbed by optically transparent tissues. The area of focus can be preset within the cornea and the energy can be dialed to a threshold to generate plasma. This further generates a shock wave of rapidly expanding cloud of free electrons and ionized molecules and further results in disruption of the target tissue. This process involves generation of free electrons and ions in plasma state which in turn displace the surrounding tissue matter by high velocity expansion. This high velocity displacement spreads through the target tissue as a well-defined shockwave (Fig. 5.5.1).

The vaporized tissue now formed a cavitation bubble in the focal volume of the laser beam and the rapidly expanding plasma drops in temperature. The cavitation bubble is composed of water (H_2O), nitrogen (N_2), and carbon dioxide (CO_2) which diffuses out of the tissue. This non-thermal ablation occurs because the interaction time is less. An infrared scanning pulse of 1,053 nm wavelength with 1 μm precision cutting capacity now creates flaps, incisions, and patterns of fragmentation.

■ ADVENT IN REFRACTIVE SURGERY

In the year 2000, the Food and Drug Administration (FDA) approved an ultrafast laser, thereafter the femtosecond laser has meteorically transformed the creation of flaps for laser-assisted in situ keratomileusis (LASIK).[2]

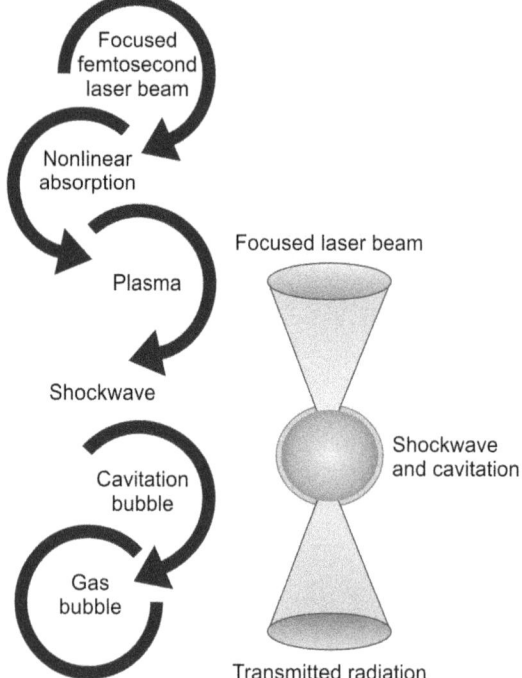

Fig. 5.5.1: Femtosecond laser photo disruption.

CLINICAL APPLICATIONS

Femtosecond technology, along with its approval for LASIK, was swiftly picked up for various other corneal and refractive procedures such as:
- Customized creation of a channel for implantation of intrastromal corneal ring segments (ICRS), for both allogenic and inert synthetic implants. With the help of the advanced Femto technology, donor cornea can also be customized to any width, length, and size.
- Limbal relaxing incisions (LRI)
- Small-incision lenticule extraction (SMILE)/corneal lenticule extraction for advanced refractive correction (CLEAR)
- Intrastromal presbyopia correction (INTRACOR)
- Anterior and posterior lamellar keratoplasty and cutting of donor buttons

CURRENTLY AVAILABLE FEMTOSECOND LASERS

There are a number of US FDA-approved femtosecond laser platforms for use in corneal refractive surgery. Namely the Victus (Bausch and Lomb Surgical), ELITA (Johnson and Johnson), ATOS (Schwind), IntraLase FS laser (Abbott Medical Optics Inc., Santa Ana, California, USA) the WaveLight FS laser (Alcon Laboratories Inc., Fort Worth, Texas, USA) the VisuMax (Carl Zeiss, Meditec AG, Jena, Germany), and Femto LDV Z8 (Ziemer Ophthalmic Systems, Port, Switzerland). Detailed comparison of the laser systems is shown in **Table 5.5.1**.

LIMITATIONS OF FEMTO APPLICATION IN LENTICULAR EXTRACTION

- Corneal wavefront-guided or ocular wavefront-guided laser surgery is not possible.
- Hyperopia and hyperopic astigmatism is yet not possible.

TABLE 5.5.1: Comparison of femtosecond machines.

Parameter	IntraLase FS	Technolas/Femtec	Femto LDV	WaveLight	VisuMax
Pattern	Raster	Spiral	Segmental	Raster	Spiral
Applanation	Planar	Curved	Planar	Planar	Curved
Mobility	No	No	Yes	No	No
Wavelength	1,053 nm	1,053 nm	1,045 nm	1,045 nm	1,043 nm
Type of laser	Amplifier	Amplifier	Oscillator	Oscillator-amplifier	Fiber-optic amplifier

- Cyclotorsion compensation is possible in new generation femtolasers but multiple adjustments can be made and techniques are innovated to make the same possible.

ADVANTAGES IN FEMTOSECOND LASER-ASSISTED CORNEAL FLAP CREATION

In femtosecond LASIK, the femtolaser is used to create a flap in the cornea with unparalleled precision. By leveraging the accuracy of femtolaser technology, ophthalmologists are able to correct refractive errors such as myopia, hyperopia, and astigmatism more effectively and safely than with a microkeratome.

Following is a compilation of various advantages of femtosecond laser LASIK surgery over traditional blade/microkeratome-assisted LASIK surgery:
- Less cases of dryness reported by the patient and diagnosed on follow-up.
- Minimize buttonhole flap or free cap formation.
- The flap diameter to hinge ratio is consistently the same, which is why when the flap is reposited, it falls back uniformly.
- The size of the hinge is consistent, unlike variable hinge size in microkeratomes.
- The side cut can be made from 70 to 150°, therefore the apposition of the side cut is far superior than the microkeratome.
- More uniform flap thickness resulting in uniform flap weight resulting in perfect placement of the flap.
- Superior consistency in flap diameter, thickness accuracy, and reproducibility.
- Thinnest flaps of 90 μm and creation of thinner planar flap are possible with femtosecond laser whereas microkeratomes fashion meniscus corneal flaps which have a thin configuration centrally and thick peripherally.
- Reduce clinically significant epithelial ingrowth due to better apposition of angulated flaps.
- The capacity to revisit an inadvertent incomplete lamellar corneal flap after suction loss or unpredictable technical error, and even while creating a secondary flap on a different plane below a primary flap of inadequate quality with insignificant repercussions as the new machines have a built in Optical Coherence Tomography (OCT), so the original flap thickness can be analyzed and recut.
- Biomechanical tissue stability, i.e., the ability to cut ultrathin flaps with no effects on stromal architecture.
- The cavitation bubbles produced are compactly arranged which ensure minimal resistance during dissection and almost nil chances of stromal bridges, consistently repeatable superior quality flaps with smooth interfaces, and advanced software patterns for the creation of elliptical flaps and flaps with everted edges for greater mechanical stability.
- Always a well-centered flap on the pupil as the trajectory of the femtolaser can be moved during the vacuum buildup.

- Some femtolasers can create an elliptical flap for high cylindrical powers, which is not possible in microkeratomes.

DISADVANTAGES AND UNIQUE COMPLICATIONS
Some significant complications unique to FS laser are:
- *Opaque bubble layer (OBL):* Gas bubbles that accumulate in the flap interface during FS laser treatment, may dissect into the deep stromal bed and interfere with the laser eye tracker device. The bubbles may also seep into the anterior chamber through the trabecular meshwork. *Can be prevented by using the raster pattern or centripetal pattern and peripheral gutters while selecting the cut.*
- Ocular surface inflammatory mediators and microscopic tissue injury and may cause lamellar keratitis. *Lamellar keratitis after Fs LASIK usually resolves with nil sequelae.*
- *Transient light sensitivity syndrome (TLSS):* Patients present with extreme photophobia due to inflammatory sequelae and good visual acuity with no clinical findings on examination. *Requires aggressive topical steroids for weeks then resolves.*
- *Cost, skill, and learning curve:* A constant debate and an uphill climb for those who wish to diversify.

CONCLUSION
Femtosecond laser fashions custom corneal flaps which have the highest safety margin and uniform thickness predictability. The flaps are planar and uniform in width as compared to manual meniscus flaps made with mechanical keratomes. Additionally, the flap adheres better and not affected by trauma in most cases the flap adherence is stronger and less influenced by trauma; among other advantages, it has minimal chances of epithelial ingrowth and dry eyes, and better contrast sensitivity. Incidence of short flaps, epithelial injuries, buttonhole flaps is almost nil. With newer femtolasers and the technique of small incision lenticular extraction, with a cap of 130 µm is widely documented to have a lesser incidence of dry eyes and no risk of flap complications such as striae or folds. This will truly stand the test of time.

Though it is associated with more chances of developing photosensitivity, diffuse keratitis, etc., given the choice of modern steroid eye drops exceptional results with femto LASIK will give a tough time to its rivals.

Upcoming research will reveal whether modern flapless lenticule technology is capable of overtaking flap LASIK in refractive surgery.

REFERENCES
1. Soong HK, Malta JB. Femtosecond lasers in ophthalmology. Am J Ophthalmol. 2009;147(2):189-97.
2. Binder PS. One thousand consecutive IntraLase laser in situ keratomileusis flaps. J Cataract Refract Surg. 2006;32(6):962-9.

5.6 Femtosecond Lasers for Flap Making

Mahipal Sachdev, Charu Khurana, Raghav Malik
Centre for Sight, New Delhi
drmahipal@gmail.com

INTRODUCTION
The microkeratome has been the standard instrument to create a laser-assisted in situ keratomileusis (LASIK) flap for many years. However, with the introduction of femtosecond lasers in refractive surgery, flap making has undergone a sea change and now the majority of LASIK flaps are being created with a femtosecond laser.[1]

SECTION 5: Refractive Surgery

TABLE 5.6.1: Comparison of newer femtolaser systems.

Feature	VisuMax 500 (Zeiss)	VisuMax 800 (Zeiss)	Femto LDV Z8 (Ziemer)	ATOS (Schwind)	EUTA (JJSV)	iFS (JJSV)
Source laser wavelength	1,043 nm	1,043 nm	1,030 nm	1,030 nm	1,040 nm	1,053 nm
Laser pulse repetition rate	500 kHz	2 MHz	Up to 20 MHz	Up to 4 MHz	10 MHz	150 kHz
Energy per pulse	11–150 nJ	110–150 nJ	<<100 nJ	75–135 nJ	50–70 nJ	0.75 µJ
Laser cut time	About 30 seconds	About 10 seconds	About 30 seconds	About 30–40 seconds	About 16 seconds	9 seconds (flap)
Patient interface	Curved	Curved	Flat	Curved	Flat	Flat
Cyclotorsion compensation	No	Yes	Yes	Yes	Yes	No
Inbuilt centration system	No	Yes	Yes	Yes	Yes	Yes
Lenticule extraction option	+	+	+	+	+	–

Various studies have been performed which list the advantages of femtosecond laser flaps compared to microkeratome flaps including greater accuracy in flap thickness, configuration, and depth. In addition, microkeratome-related complications such as free caps, button holes, and incomplete flaps are not seen with the femtolaser increasing the overall safety and efficiency of the refractive procedure.

Multiple femtolaser platforms are available commercially for refractive surgery, chiefly (1) IntraLase (Abbott Medical Optics Inc., Santa Ana, California), (2) VisuMax 500 and VisuMax 800 (Carl Zeiss Meditec AG, Jena, Germany), (3) WaveLight FS200 (Alcon Laboratories Inc., Ft Worth, Texas), (4) Femto LDV (Ziemer Ophthalmic Systems, Port, Switzerland), (5) FemTec (20/10 Perfect Vision, Heidelberg, Germany), (6) ATOS (Schwind). Another femtolaser platform by JJSV, Elita is in its Limited Market Release phase, capable of creating flaps and lenticules both. A comparison of the various newer femtolaser systems is given in **Table 5.6.1**.

■ TECHNICAL ASPECTS

The femtosecond laser with a wavelength of 1,053 nm is an infrared laser with a very short pulse duration of 10–15 seconds. A solid state Nd:Glass laser, it operates on the principle of photoionization and photodisruption resulting in a rapidly expanding cloud of free electrons and ionized molecules or plasma. As small amounts of tissue are vaporized, carbon dioxide and water are released which coalesce to form cavitation gas bubbles which dissipate into surrounding tissues with minimum collateral damage. The laser wavelength has a diameter of 0.001 mm and can be focused to a 1.8 µm spot with an accuracy of 5 µm. This allows the laser to be focused to a very precise location and depth with minimal trauma to adjacent tissue **(Fig. 5.6.1)**. This property of the femtosecond laser enables it to be used for corneal surgery as there is minimal damage to surrounding tissues and tissue cleavage planes can be created with precision and accuracy. The earlier generation of femtolasers began with a frequency of 10 kHz while the newest ones have

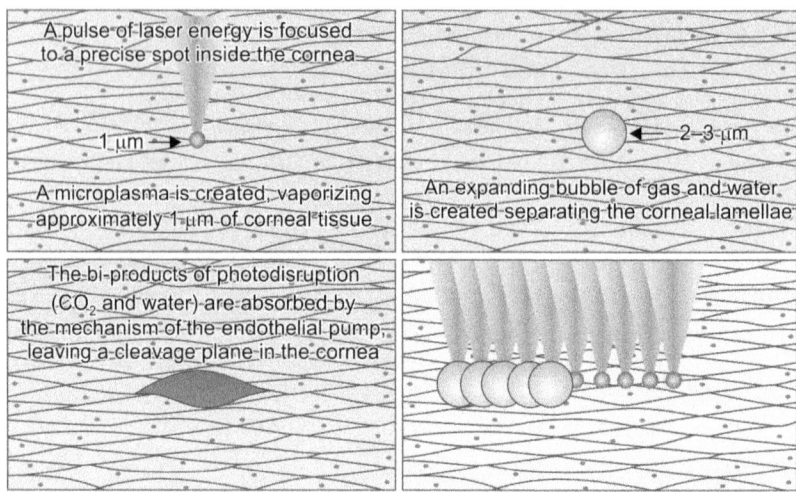

Fig. 5.6.1: *Mechanism of femtosecond laser action:* The focused laser pulse creates a microplasma bubble which join together to form a cleavage plane of separation without damage to surrounding tissue.

a frequency as high as 20 MHz in the Femto LDV platform. The higher frequency and low pulse energy in the latest generation of femtolaser platforms reduce the time needed to create a flap and create smooth stromal beds, respectively.

Mechanism

We will be discussing the IntraLase femtosecond laser as the prototype femtosecond laser for discussion. The basic principles remain the same but every femtosecond laser platform has its own unique features **(Table 5.6.1)**. Essentially, all femtosecond lasers increase the overall safety, precision, and accuracy of a corneal flap and eliminate the use and risk of a microkeratome and blade.

The femtosecond laser is aimed at a specific depth and position in the cornea where each laser pulse forms a microscopic plasma bubble. As the laser is fired these plasma bubbles connect to form a cleavage plane of separation without any damage to the surrounding tissue **(Fig. 5.6.1)**. The flap is then separated across this cleavage plane by the surgeon without use of any microkeratome or blade and the excimer laser is then fired to obtain the refractive correction.

■ CLINICAL ASPECTS

Steps of the Femtosecond Laser Flap Making Procedure

1. Name and refractive error and surgery plan of the patient are confirmed.
2. Topical anesthetic drops are administered and the eyes are prepared and cleaned with betadine solution.
3. The patient is made to lie on the operating table and the head fixed.
4. Surgical LASIK drapes which are lint and fiber-free are placed and appropriately opened at the eye. The patient is instructed not to make any sudden movements.
5. A thin wire speculum which opens the eye wide is applied. Topical anesthetic may be supplemented and any excess needs to be wiped off as any fluid accumulations may interfere with suction.
6. Watch for a prominent brow and nose and tilt the head accordingly toward the opposite side so that it does not obstruct during docking.
7. A suction ring is applied and centration is checked.

8. Docking is initiated to applanate the cornea.
9. Once the applanation is complete and stable, the femtosecond laser is fired.
10. First the pocket is created then the flap followed by side cuts, the entire procedure taking around 20 seconds **(Figs. 5.6.2 to 5.6.7)**. The plasma bubbles join to form an OBL (opaque bubble layer) which acts to create a cleavage plane of separation.
11. The procedure is repeated on the other eye in bilateral cases before the excimer laser is carried out to allow the OBL to dissipate to some extent.
12. The patient is then moved to the microscope where the surgeon then lifts the flap edge and dissects the cleavage plane between the flap and the stromal bed to allow treatment by excimer laser **(Figs. 5.6.8 to 5.6.11)**.
13. The excimer laser is performed according to the refractive error of the patient.
14. The flap is repositioned and washed as for a routine LASIK procedure.
15. Antibiotic and anti-inflammatory drops are instilled.

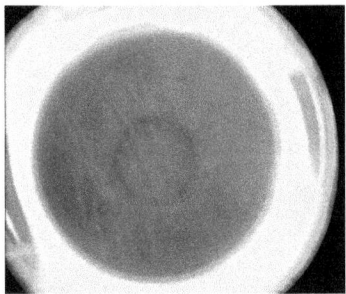

Fig. 5.6.2: Applanation of the corneal surface.

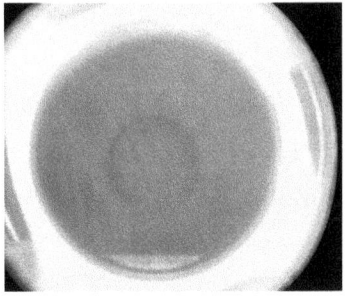

Fig. 5.6.3: Creation of laser pocket at a deeper depth.

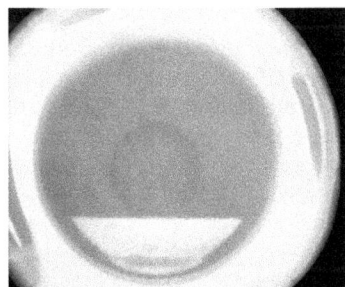

Fig. 5.6.4: Laser beam traveling forward creating a tissue plane.

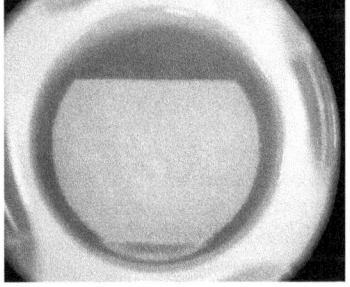

Fig. 5.6.5: Femtolaser-assisted flap almost 80% complete.

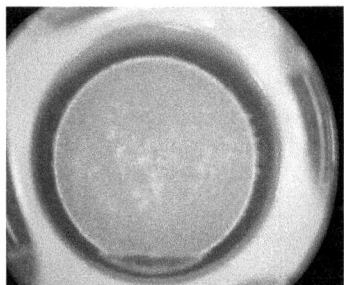

Fig. 5.6.6: Flap complete, side cut being delivered.

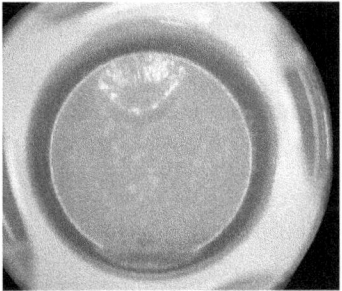

Fig. 5.6.7: "Burp" where a condensed water bubble appears at the cleavage plane.

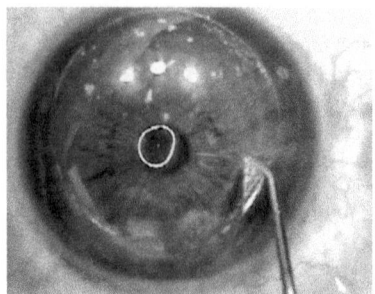

Fig. 5.6.8: Lifting the flap by delineating the edge.

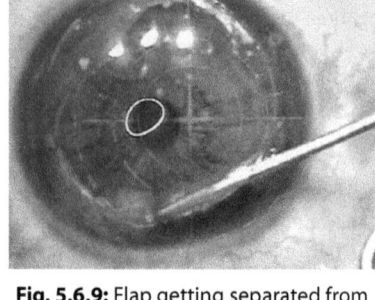

Fig. 5.6.9: Flap getting separated from the stromal bed.

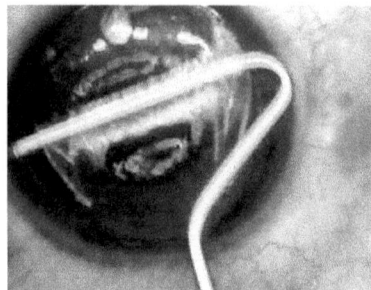

Fig. 5.6.10: Flap completely separated.

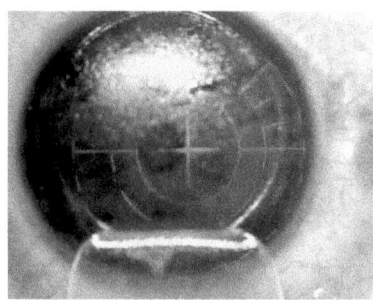

Fig. 5.6.11: Excimer ablation being performed on the stromal bed with the flap deflected back.

Advantages of a Femtolaser Flap

The femtolaser allows the surgeon not only a blade-free procedure but also the freedom to create a customized flap according to the requirements of the patient. Laser specifications which can be modified to meet individual patient's needs include flap diameter, depth, hinge location and width, and side-cut architecture. The IntraLase laser also creates a distinctive beveled edge flap which allows for precise repositioning and alignment after LASIK is completed. The various advantages of a femtosecond laser flap are listed below.

- Reduced incidence of blade-related complications such as free caps, button holes, and irregular flaps.
- Ability to customize flaps according to patient need with 0.1 mm precision and accuracy for flap diameter, flap shape (circular or elliptical), flap thickness, hinge location and length, and edge contour or side-cut angle.
- Stable flap because of the inverted bevel-in side cut up to 150°.
- Ability to make thinner flaps with stable flap architecture, up to 90 µm also known as sub-Bowman keratomileusis or SBK which in turn allows you to treat thinner corneas and higher powers.
- Uniform flap thickness with planar shape.
- Flap adherence is higher with femtolaser and hence these flaps are less prone to be displaced with trauma giving an edge over the microkeratome in long-term safety.
- Visual outcomes are better as lesser higher order aberrations are induced.
- Better contrast sensitivity.
- Lesser dry eye as compared to microkeratome as corneal nerves are not cut.

Various studies have compared the differences in flap architecture among the multiple femtolaser platforms and the microkeratome. In a study by Ahn and Kim et al., flap thickness and side-cut angle were compared between four groups: IntraLase (group 1), VisuMax (group 2), Femto LDV (group 3), and M2 microkeratome (group 4).

They found that groups 1 and 2 (IntraLase and VisuMax) had even-configuration flaps while groups 3 and 4 (Femto LDV and M2 microkeratome) had meniscus-shaped flaps. Also, flaps in group 1 (IntraLase) had least difference between mean central and peripheral flap thickness ($p < 0.001$) and side-cut angle was closest to 90° ($p < 0.001$). The greatest flap thickness predictability (measured versus intended thickness) was in femtosecond group 3 ($p < 0.001$). They concluded that though flap morphology differed according to the system used, the 3-femtosecond laser systems appeared to be superior to the microkeratome system generally.

Another study was performed by Pajic et al. where patients scheduled for bilateral LASIK underwent flap creation using microkeratome in one eye and femtolaser in the other eye. They found that femtosecond laser was superior to microkeratome-assisted LASIK in terms of flap thickness predictability and the speed of visual acuity recovery. In this study, one eye from each patient was randomly selected for Femto LDV-assisted LASIK treatment, while the fellow eye was operated using the Amadeus II microkeratome (Amadeus; Ziemer Ophthalmic Systems AG). All flaps created using the femtosecond laser deviated significantly less from the intended flap thickness, as evaluated by confocal microscopy and optical coherence pachymetry (OCP) (Technolas Perfect Vision GmbH) in comparison to the microkeratome group. Furthermore, the increased precision of the femtosecond laser seemed to have a direct effect on uncorrected distance visual acuity (UDVA), since less deviation in terms of flap thickness from the intended value correlated with the UDVA postoperatively.

Newer advancements in the femtosecond lasers such as the reverse side-cut architecture causes better flap apposition and stability, faster return of corneal sensation, and faster recovery from dry eye. In addition to eliminating irregular cuts and trauma induced by manipulation, the thickness of a femtolaser flap has been found to be highly predictable which protects against ectasia as well. A study by Kanellopoulos et al. studied the variability in flap thickness between a microkeratome and femtolaser using anterior segment optical coherence tomography. They found that some of the microkeratome flaps which were thought to be 130–150 µm were actually 200 µm which reduced the predicted stromal bed calculation while femtolaser flaps showed a variability consistently <10 µm **(Table 5.6.2)**.

TABLE 5.6.2: Comparison between femtolaser flap and microkeratome flap.

Parameter	Femtolaser flap	Microkeratome flap
Flap architecture	Uniform thickness	Meniscus shaped, thinner in center, thicker periphery
Flap diameter	Can be customized with precision up to 0.1 mm	Fixed depending on ring size
Flap shape	Round or elliptical	Round only
Hinge location	Customized	Fixed by microkeratome
Side-cut angle	90°/obtuse/variable according to surgeon preference	Fixed
Stability of thinner flaps	Good even up to 90 µm	Lesser
Flap adherence	Higher	Lower
Predictability	High	Moderate
Complications	Opaque bubble layer, vertical gas breakthrough, transient light sensitivity (not seen with latest versions)	Button hole/free cap

COMPLICATIONS

- *Opaque bubble layer:* The cavitation bubbles released may interfere with visualization and tracking of the pupil and registration of the iris which may come in the way of the excimer laser.
- Transient light sensitivity was reported with earlier models but is rarely seen these days. It is characterized by photophobia with good vision and no clinical findings, responds to topical corticosteroids.
- Rainbow glare also reported earlier occurred due to light scattering from the laser spots on the back surface of the flap and is inconsequent visually.
- Diffuse lamellar keratitis (DLK) is usually mild and transient, more common in the periphery due to the higher energy used to make side cuts. Usually responds to increased topical steroids.
- Vertical breakthrough can occur in areas of a corneal opacity or thinning similar to button hole in a microkeratome.
- Suction loss resulting in incomplete flap is usually not a problem as the laser can be redocked and the flap completed.
- Subconjunctival hemorrhage due to the suction rings may be seen in initial cases and usually fade away within a week.

Tips to Avoid and Manage Complications

In order to understand how to make better femtoflaps, it is important to understand where common problems are encountered.

- *Docking problems:* Patients with a prominent nose, high brows, and deep set eyes need to be docked by tilting their head opposite to the eye being docked. The assistant should help position the head while the surgeon performs the docking.
- Suction loss will commonly occur in the following situations:
  - Patients with narrow apertures or tight lids.
  - Patients who squeeze their eyes or have a hyperactive Bell's phenomena or anxious patients.
  - Patients with flat corneas.

  Instill an extra drop of anesthetic, reassure the patient and try again. Inform the patient to look at the fixation light and keep the other eye open to prevent the eyeball from rolling upward. Make sure there is no loose conjunctiva or fluid which will interfere with the maintenance of suction. Clean any debris or eyelashes that may be coming in the way. Retract the lids properly, push back any redundant conjunctiva into the fornices and hold down the suction ring on the globe with a little pressure when applanating. Sometimes the suction ring may be defective and need to be replaced. As a last resort, if repeated suction losses occur, reduce the flap diameter to complete the procedure faster.

  Once a suction loss has occurred, further management will depend on the stage at which it occurred. If it occurs before initiating the side cut, you can repeat the laser with the same diameter and pocket off. If it occurs during the side cut, skip the raster stage and only perform the side cut with a smaller diameter.
- Extensive OBL can be minimized by using less energy and smaller spot separation and minimizing suction. Wait 3–8 minutes before you attempt to lift the flap when the OBL is more than usual. That is why it is better to complete the femtolaser flap creation in both eyes before you move to excimer so that by the time the second eye femto laser flap is completed, the first eye OBL has dissipated and is ready for excimer.
- *Vertical gas breakthrough:* Look carefully for any corneal opacities which are common especially paracentrally in contact lens users. If present assess the thickness and try and go below the scar or opacity by creating a thicker flap instead of the usual 100 µm or 110 µm flap. In case you have missed the opacity and a breakthrough occurs, assess the size and location. If it is small and paracentral, i.e., beyond the 6 mm zone,

lift the flap and proceed and place a bandage contact lens at the end of the procedure. If it is larger than 0.5 mm × 0.5 mm, postpone the procedure and plan later either with a thicker flap or perform a photorefractive keratectomy.

NEWER PLATFORMS

The VisuMax 500 operates at 500 kHz. Using it, flap creation takes under 20 seconds and a lenticule creation for SMILE takes under 30 seconds. With the VisuMax 800, flaps are created in under 7 seconds and a lenticule takes <10 seconds. The difference in the time for lenticule creation is especially noteworthy because docking time is probably the most critical and stressful time for both patients and surgeons during a procedure. The VisuMax 800 does not change the basic steps of this time-proven procedure, but it raises the experience to a new level for patients and surgeons.

The Femto LDV Z8 includes a new Z-LASIK method that performs the resection in a three-dimensional mode. Each flap can be customized to accommodate the desired geometry. It provides round and oval flaps with angled edges, as desired by surgeon. It also includes a built-in OCT system, giving a clear visualization of the ocular surfaces—before, during and after the procedure.

The ELITA femtosecond laser by JJSV **(Fig. 5.6.12)** is designed for use in the creation of a corneal lenticule in patients undergoing a flapless lenticule removal refractive correction procedure, as well as flap-based procedures. It delivers low energy treatment with no spot separation through combination of ultrashort pulse duration, ultrafast pulse frequency, and small focus spot size. Induces minimal tissue disruption in the stroma. Pilot studies, with the purpose of evaluating the accuracy of flap thickness for Laser In-situ Keratomileusis (LASIK) with a new femtosecond laser compared to iFS on this machine demonstrated excellent accuracy when compared to iFS in creating flaps for LASIK. Both systems were able to achieve consistent flap thicknesses with similar variability.

CONCLUSION

With continued advancements in femtosecond laser technology, the innovations and applications of the femtosecond laser are increasing day-by-day leading to refinements in vision correction with a much better safety profile making it an indispensable tool for refractive surgery in years to come.

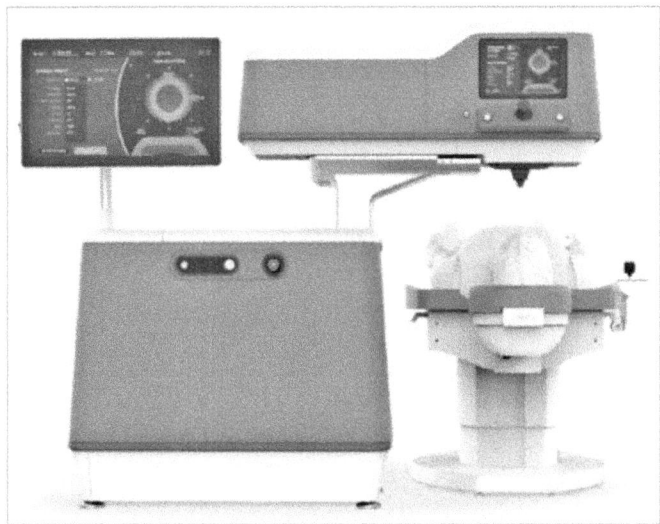

Fig. 5.6.12: ELITA femtosecond laser.

SUMMARY

The femtosecond laser creates a corneal flap of precise size, shape, and depth to micron-level accuracy 100% greater than that of blade-keratome and markedly reduces the risk of blade-related flap complications such as free caps, button holes, incomplete or decentered flaps. Not only is the visual acuity better but the incidence of postoperative dry eye symptoms is reduced. It also creates fewer high-order and low-order aberrations which may cause glare and haloes at night. The precision of the flap also reduces the incidence of induced postoperative astigmatism as compared with microkeratome-created flap. Complications include suction loss, transient DLK, and vertical breakthrough but none of them has serious sequelae unlike a microkeratome where flap complications such as button hole, flap folds, and flap displacements can be difficult to manage.

REFERENCE

1. Binder PS. Femtosecond applications for anterior segment surgery. Eye Contact Lens. 2010;36(5):282-5.

5.7 Intraocular Lens Power Calculation Postrefractive Surgery

Anagha Heroor, Vikram Vaidee
Anil Eye Hospital, Dombivli
aaheroor@gmail.com

INTRODUCTION

Refractive surgery techniques are popular, widely accepted and have been developing rapidly. Patients undergoing refractive surgery usually have higher requirements for vision. As a result, they also have high expectations for visual acuity after cataract surgery. Patients presenting with cataract after refractive corneal surgery have been increasing over the years. Intraocular lens (IOL) calculation remains a challenge, although the issues in these eyes are well understood. Over the years with advances in technique, technology, and patient demands, the margin for postoperative refraction has reduced and falls within ±0.75 D of target refraction.

PITFALLS

After refractive surgery, if eyes are treated as normal eyes by utilizing the erroneous postoperative K-reading into standard IOL power calculation formulas, high hyperopic errors can occur in previously myopic eyes and moderate myopic errors in formerly hyperopic eyes.

EFFECT OF RADIAL KERATOTOMY ON THE CORNEA (FIG. 5.7.1A)

Radial keratotomy (RK) leads to extreme variation in corneal power between center and periphery. Scheimpflug imaging has shown that the posterior corneal surface undergoes more flattening than the anterior making the keratometric index no longer valid. The ratio between the posterior/anterior corneal radii is increased. This produces an overestimation of the corneal power, underestimation of the

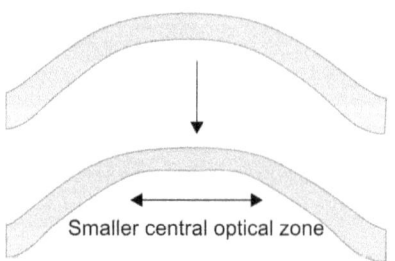

Fig. 5.7.1A: Effect of radial keratotomy on the cornea.

IOL power, and postoperative hyperopia. The mechanical instability of the cornea may lead to opening of the RK incisions postsurgery which may exacerbate central flattening and peripheral bulging and lead to residual flattening of the cornea.

EFFECT OF LASER VISION CORRECTION ON THE CORNEA (FIG. 5.7.1B)

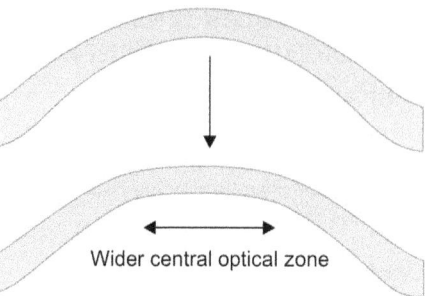

Fig. 5.7.1B: Effect of laser vision correction on the cornea.

In myopic keratorefractive surgeries [laser-assisted in situ keratomileusis (LASIK) and photorefractive keratectomy (PRK)] the ratio between the posterior-anterior corneal radii is decreased.

INTRAOCULAR LENS CALCULATION ERROR SOURCES

Essentially, there are three main sources of errors in IOL calculation after refractive surgery—the radius measurement error, the keratometer index error, and the IOL formula error.

RADIUS MEASUREMENT ERROR

Corneal power (K) cannot be measured directly in diopters by any of the currently available instruments. Keratometry or topography derives corneal power from the radius of corneal curvature away from the optical axis. Depending on the optical zone of the ablation, there is a high probability of measuring a steeper radius than is actually effective at the center. Therefore, the corneal power will be overestimated, the IOL power underestimated and the patient left hyperopic. This radius measurement error is relevant when patients have had laser surgery for myopia.

KERATOMETRIC INDEX ERROR

The keratometer index error is seen as classical keratometry or corneal topography measures the corneal power from the anterior surface without taking into account the posterior corneal surface. This does not work as refractive surgery alters both the anterior and posterior surface of the cornea. Consequently, the keratometer index is no longer constant and will lead to faulty K values in these cases.

INTRAOCULAR LENS FORMULA ERROR IN EFFECTIVE LENS POSITION

The IOL formula error is seen with formulas (Hoffer Q, Holladay-1, SRK/T), all of which use Ks to predict the effective lens position (ELP). Refractive surgery changes only the corneal radii and not the depth of the lens. As a result, postrefractive surgery, the flat corneal radii lead to a falsely shallow ELPs, causing a hyperopic refractive shift in patients after laser surgery for myopia and a myopic shift after preceding laser vision correction (LVC) for hyperopia.

The radius error depends on the measurement area of the keratometry instrument and on the optical zone affected by the laser. Typical diameters of keratometer measurement areas are 3.4 mm for the Haag-Streit and 2.5 mm for the Zeiss keratometers. Modern lasers use wider optical zones which lead to a minor radius error. The keratometer index and the IOL formula errors contribute the most for the postoperative refractive surprise in refractive surgery patients undergoing cataract surgery.

INTRAOCULAR LENS CALCULATION METHODS TO OBTAIN TRUE CORNEAL POWER

Clinical History

This was described by Eiferman and Holladay. With this method the value is calculated by subtracting the change in refraction, induced by the treatment, to the mean preoperative corneal power. This method was considered to be the gold standard, but today it is considered outdated.

Contact Lens Over Refraction

The contact lens method was first described by Ridley in 1948. Corneal power is calculated as the sum of the contact lens base curve, power, and over-refraction minus the spherical equivalent of the manifest refraction without a contact lens. This method was not suitable for dense cataracts.

Topography-based post-LASIK Adjustment

The corneal topography central Ks are used by these regression formulas to get the true corneal power. They are based on LASIK data and are not suitable for post-RK cases. These include the Koch and Wang Formula and the Shammas Formula.

True Corneal Power Measurement

Scheimpflug, slit scanning, and optical coherence tomography (OCT) based instruments such as the Orbscan, Galilei, Sirius, and the Pentacam can directly measure both anterior and posterior corneal curvature and thereby calculate the net corneal power. Pentacam (Oculus, Germany) system generates the central corneal power in diopters using data from the anterior and the posterior cornea. It also calculates the equivalent K-reading (EKR) **(Fig. 5.7.2)** at the 4.5 mm zone which is an accurate measure of the true corneal power in the Holladay report that can be used for IOL power calculation.

Intraocular Lens Power Calculation by Ray-tracing

Ray-tracing has the advantage of not being subject to the above discussed errors. It is based on real curvature data from both corneal surfaces, can be calculated over any corneal diameter, and the IOL position can be estimated without relying on the anterior

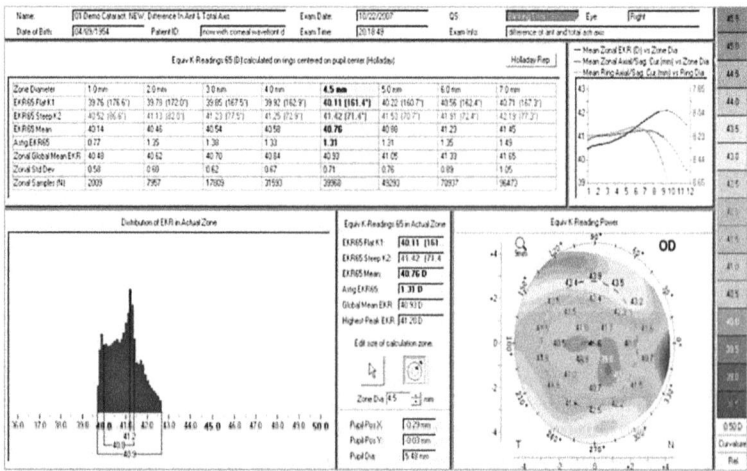

Fig. 5.7.2: Pentacam EKR report. (EKR: equivalent K-reading)

corneal curvature. Different solutions are commercially available which include Okulix, PhacoOptics, and RTVue spectral-domain OCT.

Intraocular Lens Power Formulas for Postrefractive Surgery Eyes

Intraocular lens calculation methods for eyes after refractive surgery differ most in whether they require historic patient data or whether they rely only on current measurements. In the Aramberri's double-K IOL formula, the postrefractive surgery corneal power reading is used in the vergence calculation while the prerefractive surgery corneal power is used in the ELP prediction formula. This reduces the error in ELP calculation. The Hoffer Q formula is less sensitive to corneal power variation in estimating ELP, thereby inducing fewer errors in postrefractive surgery eyes than other single-K formulas. The Shammas and Haigis formulas for the IOL master do not use the corneal curvature as an ELP predictor. Haigis-L formula is based on the regular Haigis formula, uses a correlation curve to compensate for the radius and keratometric index errors in the keratometry module of the IOLMaster.

ASCRS Online Calculator (Fig. 5.7.3)

Intraocular lens power calculation in eyes that have undergone LASIK/PRK/RK. This website provides three calculator tools.
1. IOL Calculator for Eyes with Prior Myopic LASIK/PRK
2. IOL Calculator for Eye with Prior Hyperopic LASIK/PRK
3. IOL Calculator for Eyes with Prior RK

Barrett True-K Formula

It is available online on the websites of the Asia-Pacific Association of Cataract and Refractive Surgeons (www.apacrs.org) and the American Society of Cataract and Refractive Surgery (www.ascrs.org). It is based on the Barrett Universal II formula, uses a modified

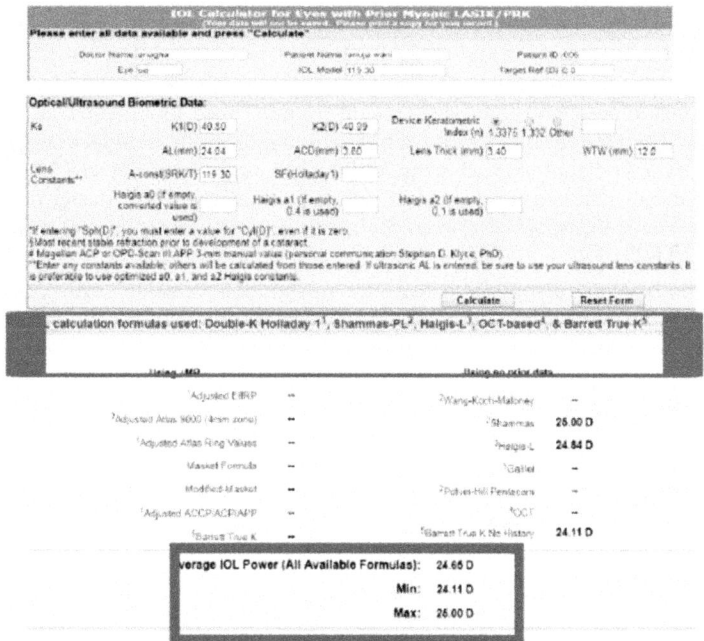

Fig. 5.7.3: ASCRS online calculator report. (LASIK: laser-assisted in situ keratomileusis; PRK: photorefractive keratectomy)

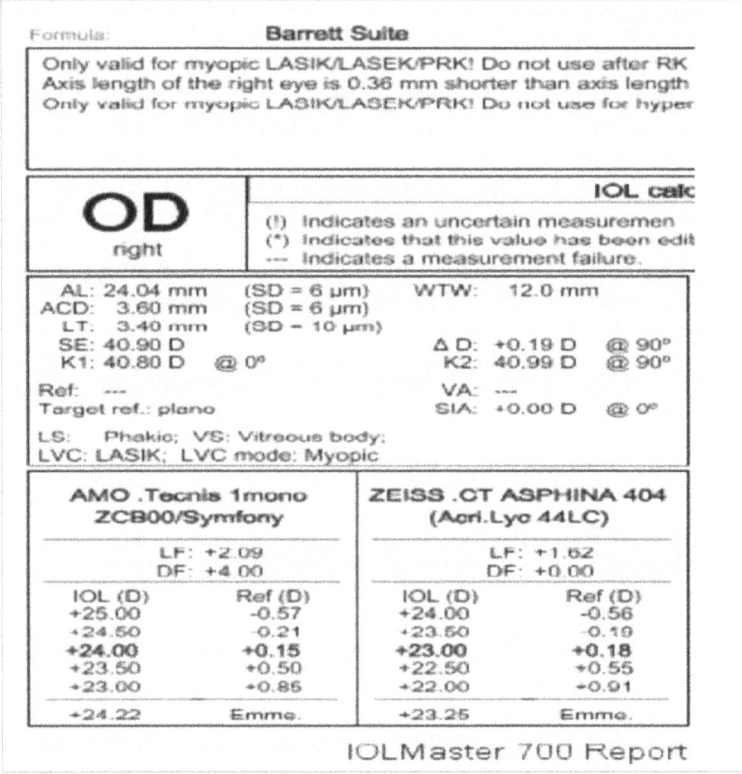

Fig. 5.7.4: IOLMaster 700 Barrett Suite calculation.
(LASIK: laser-assisted in situ keratomileusis; PRK: photorefractive keratectomy)

keratometry value and uses a double K solution to accurately calculate the corneal height. It is now considered as one of the most reliable options both after myopic and hyperopic PRK/LASIK. The Barrett True-K formula built into the biometer is equal or noninferior to the multiple method approach using the ASCRS online calculator. **Figures 5.7.3 and 5.7.4** show the IOL calculation using the ASCRS online calculator and IOL Master 700.

■ BIOMETRY

Patients who have undergone refractive surgery should have axial length measurement using optical biometry (or immersion ultrasound) rather than contact ultrasound. In cases of decentered ablations, aphakic refraction formulas may need to be used.

■ CHOICE OF INTRAOCULAR LENS

Negative aspheric IOLs are preferred for postmyopic refractive surgery patients as they usually have higher positive corneal spherical aberrations. Regular, symmetric corneas without excessive higher order aberrations can be considered for premium IOLs; toric IOLs and multifocal IOLs to be used with caution.

■ CONCLUSION

Dry eye is common post-Lasik which can affect visual outcome post-IOL surgery. Clinical evaluation is essential to assess if the ocular surface is smooth and well lubricated. It is useful to obtain an average recommended IOL power using several methods. While using multiple methods it is advisable to select the flattest K for central corneal power, choose the highest IOL power, and to hedge toward myopic results. In post-RK eyes a scleral tunnel is preferred, counsel patients about diurnal fluctuations, hyperopic progression, and gradual stabilization of refraction postsurgery. The predictability of outcomes postrefractive cataract surgery is still not as good as in virgin eyes even with the use of various methods to eliminate errors. Thus, patients who had previous refractive surgery should be warned about the potential need for refractive correction after their cataract surgery.

SUGGESTED READING

1. Hoffer KJ. Intraocular lens power calculation after previous laser refractive surgery. J Cataract Refract Surg. 2009;35:759-65.
2. Savini G, Hoffer KJ. Intraocular lens power calculation in eyes with previous corneal refractive surgery. Eye Vis (Lond). 2018;5:18.

5.8 Phakic Intraocular Lens: Indications and Preoperative Evaluation

Shreesha Kumar Kodavoor, Ashalyne James
The Eye Foundation, Coimbatore
eskay_03@rediffmail.com, ashalyne.james@gmail.com

INTRODUCTION

Phakic intraocular lens (IOL) is an artificial lens implanted in the anterior or posterior chamber of eye, in the presence of a natural crystalline lens. It is a solution for all refractive errors today. It is the procedure of choice as it is inert, has the best optical quality, has the largest optic zone and also has the highest efficacy and stability. It also leaves the cornea untouched and it is reversible.

HISTORY

The first phakic IOL used was placed in the anterior chamber by Dr Strampelli in 1953. Posterior chamber phakic IOLs were first developed by Dr Fyodorov in 1986. Current models that are commonly used include STAAR Surgical, the Visian implantable collamer lens (ICL). It is made of collamer, which is a copolymer of hydroxyethyl methacrylate and porcine collagen. Other lenses available are implantable phakic contact lens (IPCL) from Care Group, Eyecryl from Biotech, and refractive implantable lens (RIL) from Appasamy Associates.

CLASSIFICATION

Classification of phakic IOLs is as shown in flowchart below:

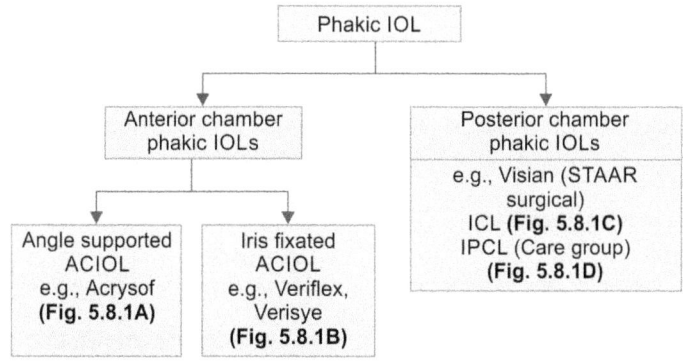

SECTION 5: Refractive Surgery

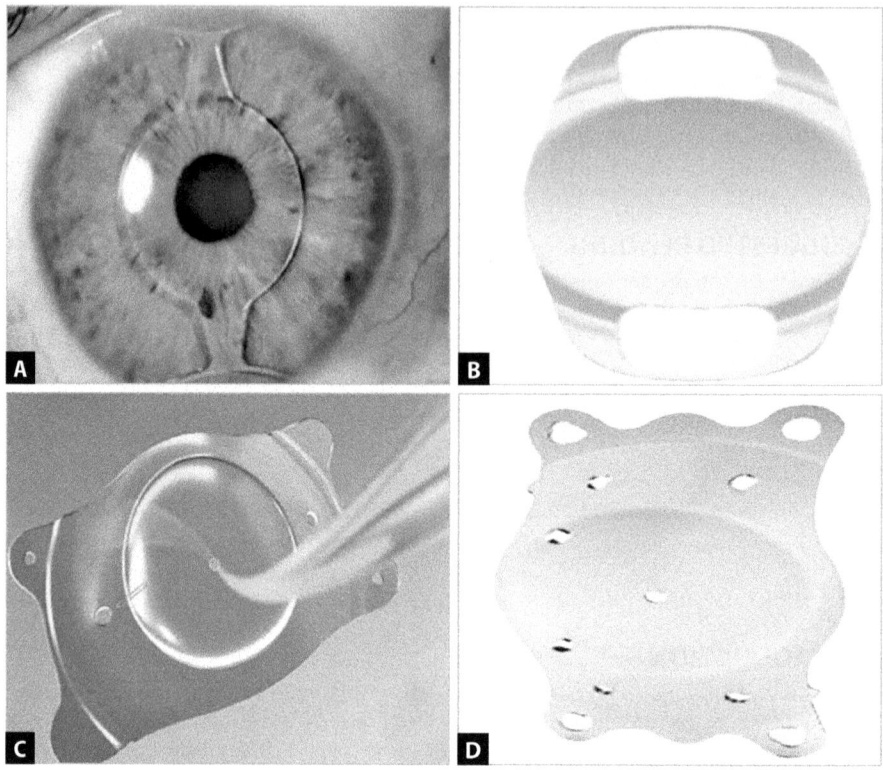

Figs. 5.8.1A to D: Types of phakic IOLs.

1. AcrySof angle-supported AC phakic IOL
2. Verisyse iris fixated AC phakic IOL
3. ICL
4. IPCL

IMPLANTABLE COLLAMER LENS

It is made of collamer, which is a combination of 0.2% porcine collagen and 60% hydroxyethylmethacrylate copolymer. It is fixated to sulcus and is not mobile. It is used for both spherical and cylindrical power correction.

COMPARISON OF IMPLANTABLE COLLAMER LENS AND IMPLANTABLE PHAKIC CONTACT LENS

Implantable collamer lens	*Implantable phakic contact lens*
• Imported version • Made of collamer; more biocompatible	• Indian version • Made of hybrid hydrophilic material; less biocompatible
• Optic size 5.5–6.5 mm	• Optic—6.6 mm (upto 7.5)
Manufacturers give only one lens	Manufacturers give two lenses
• Higher price • Comparatively lesser range of refractive correction, customized lens • Requires rotation after implantation	• Lower price • Comparatively more range of refractive correction • Has to be just aligned at 0–180°

INDICATIONS OF PHAKIC INTRAOCULAR LENSES
- Typically recommended for more severe degrees of refractive error. Phakic IOLs are available for mild-severe ametropia.
  - *Myopia:* -23 D to -3 D
  - *Hypermetropia:* +3 D to +12 D
  - *Astigmatism:* 1 D to 6 D
- Age >21 years
- Patients with stable refraction for at least 1 year (change in power not >0.25 D)
- Patients with poor tolerance for glasses or contact lens
- Patients who are poor candidates for laser vision correction
- Thinnest pachymetry <475 μm.
- Residual stromal bed <280 μm
- *Corneal ectatic disorders:* Stable/postcollagen cross linking cases of keratoconus with centered cone and good visual potential.
- Iridocorneal angle >30°
- Central endothelial cell count >2,300 cells/mm^2
  OR
  Endothelial cell count >2,500 cells/mm^2 if age >21 years and endothelial cell count >2,000 cells/mm^2 if age >40 years.
- Mesopic pupil size <6 mm; to avoid glare or haloes.
- Anterior chamber depth >2.8 mm
- Absence of other major ocular comorbidities such as cataract, uveitis, glaucoma, retinal disorders.

CONTRAINDICATIONS OF PHAKIC INTRAOCULAR LENSES
- Active anterior segment disease
- Anterior chamber depth (ACD) <2.8 mm
- Glaucoma/intraocular pressure (IOP) >21 mm Hg
- Recurrent or chronic uveitis
- Cataract
- Retinal disorders
- Anomalous iris/pupil
- History of retinal detachment
- Untreated peripheral retinal degeneration

PHAKIC INTRAOCULAR LENS AND KERATOCONUS
In early and stable keratoconus with centered cone, phakic IOL is highly safe and efficacious. In more advanced keratoconus, initially collagen cross-linking combined with topography-guided photorefractive keratectomy (PRK) or Intacs to regularize the central cornea can be done. Collagen cross-linking itself can lead to a hyperopic shift. Hence, we should wait for an adequate time of at least 6 months and then proceed with phakic IOL implantation.

PREOPERATIVE EVALUATION
The following are to be included for preoperative evaluation for a candidate of phakic IOL:
- *History:*
  - Presenting complaint
  - History of previous ocular procedures
- *Visual acuity:* Both uncorrected and best corrected visual acuity is recorded.
- *Refraction:* Both objective and subjective acceptances are recorded.
- *Slit lamp evaluation:* Detailed examination of anterior segment is done.
- *Fundus evaluation:* After dilatation, fundus examination will be done with a 90 D lens and slit lamp to look for any evidence of glaucoma or any macular pathologies.

Peripheral retinal examination will be done using indirect ophthalmoscope and 20 D lens to look for any treatable peripheral retinal degeneration. If present, the same should be treated with barrage laser 2-3 weeks prior to phakic IOL implantation.
- *Intraocular pressure:* It is measured using applanation tonometry.
- *Specular microscopy:* It is done to assess the corneal endothelial cell count.
- *Keratometry:* Flat K (K1) and Steep K (K2) can be recorded using manual/automated keratometry.
- *Topography:* It can be done with devices such as Pentacam/Orbscan. Parameters such as keratometry reading, pupil size, and anterior chamber depth are recorded.
- *Anterior chamber depth assessment:* Using anterior segment optical coherence tomography (OCT)/ultrasound biomicroscopy/Pentacam/IOLMaster/Orbscan. It is measured from corneal endothelium to the anterior surface of the crystalline lens. A minimum anterior chamber depth of 2.8 mm is required for safe phakic IOL implantation.
- *White-to-white measurements:* It is a very important measure, especially for estimating the size of the phakic IOL.

  It can be measured in different ways:
  a. *Digital calipers/Vernier calipers:* Horizontal white-to-white is measured from middle of the limbus.
  b. IOL Master/Pentacam/Orbscan/Topolyzer/Ultrasound biomicroscopy Orbscan/Topolyzer—measures from limbus to limbus

  IOLMaster measures from sclera to sclera—it gives a higher value ultrasound biomicroscopy—measures from sulcus to sulcus Pentacam—measures the corneal diameter.

INTRAOCULAR LENS POWER CALCULATION

Parameters Required for Phakic Intraocular Lens Power Calculation

Various parameters are required to calculate the phakic IOL power to get the best outcomes. These include the following:
- *Refraction:* Subjective refraction is used for calculation.
- *Keratometry:* Flat K and Steep K
- Internal anterior chamber depth
- Pachymetry
- Axial length
- *White-to-white:* Digital and optical

Power Calculation

Various software are provided by different lens companies to calculate phakic IOL power. Various measurements of the patient are entered into the software. These software use formulas that are proprietary to the manufacturers. They then provide a phakic IOL power that is ideally within 0.5 D–1.0 D of emmetropia, such that vision closed to 20/20 can be attained.

Anterior chamber phakic IOL power is calculated using a Van Der Heijde nomogram. This requires the patient's keratometry, refraction, and anterior chamber depth.

Posterior chamber phakic IOL power is calculated using a Binkhorst nomogram. This requires data including the patient's corneal power, spectacle plane refraction, and anterior chamber depth.

Accurate measurement of white-to-white is required for appropriate sizing of lens. If the anterior chamber depth is <3.5 mm, we should add 0.5 mm to the horizontal white-to-white. If the anterior chamber depth is >3.5 mm, we should add 1.0 mm to the horizontal white-to-white.

If the posterior chamber phakic IOL is too long, it can lead to complications such as secondary angle closure glaucoma, pigment dispersion syndrome, and pupillary block.

If the posterior chamber phakic IOL is too short, it can lead to complications such as anterior subcapsular cataract and rotation and subluxation of phakic lens.

LENS VAULT

It is the distance between the posterior surface of the phakic IOL and the anterior surface of the crystalline lens. The ideal lens vault should be 250–750 μm, which is approximately half to 1.5 times the corneal thickness. Inaccurate measurements had led to a high or low vault. Patients with low vault are at risk of developing anterior subcapsular cataract.

Patients with high vault are at risk of developing angle closure, peripheral anterior synechiae, iris chaffing, pigment dispersion, and pigmentary glaucoma.

ADVANTAGES OF USING PHAKIC INTRAOCULAR LENSES IN HIGH REFRACTIVE ERRORS

The following are the advantages of using phakic IOLs in high refractive errors:
- Preservation of corneal architecture
- Preservation of accommodation
- Predictable refractive results
- Predictable healing
- Rapid visual recovery
- Stable postoperative refraction
- Reversible and adjustable
- No extra equipment is required; cheaper than laser vision correction.

PRESBYOPIC PHAKIC INTRAOCULAR LENSES

Presbyopia can be associated with myopia, hyperopia, and astigmatism. When a presbyopic patient selects refractive surgery, the choices are limited. Phakic IOLs with diffractive structure can correct both distance and near refraction. Presbyopic phakic IOLs provide good outcomes of safety, predictability, stability, and efficacy to correct moderate to high levels of myopia, hyperopia, and astigmatism along with presbyopia. Thus, it can correct and provide spectacle independence for distance and near vision.

SUGGESTED READING

1. Roberto Pineda II, Chauhan T. Phakic intraocular lenses and their special indications. Journal of Ophthalmic & Vision Research. 2016;11(4):422.
2. Stodulka P, Slovak M, Sramka M, Polisensky J, Liska K. Posterior chamber phakic intraocular lens for the correction of presbyopia in highly myopic patients. Journal of Cataract and Refractive Surgery. 2020;46(1):40-4.

5.9 Phakic Intraocular Lens: An Overview

Partha Biswas
Trenetralaya, Kolkata
drpartha_biswas07@yahoo.co.in

(Lt Col) Billal Hossain
CMH, Dhaka
drbillalhossain@gmail.com

Sneha Batra
The Himalayan Eye Institute, Siliguri
snehabatra89@gmail.com

INTRODUCTION

Phakic intraocular lens (IOL) surgery has developed significantly in the past few years to produce optimum results with minimum complications in refractive error correction. It started with anterior chamber phakic IOL (PIOL) and the iris fixated variety, but over the last decade, the posterior chamber PIOL has given efficacy, safety, and satisfactory long-term results.

TYPES

Phakic IOL can be classified according to their site of implantation in the eye:
- Anterior chamber PIOLs were prone to a number of complications, such as glaucoma and an accelerated corneal endothelial cell loss, thus they went out of practice.
- Iris-fixated PIOLs had problems of progressive endothelial cell loss, pigment dispersion, and iritis which led to their decrease in popularity.
- Posterior chamber PIOLs are used most commonly and ICL (implantable collamer lens), Eyecryl Phakic IOL, implantable phakic contact lens (IPCL), and RIL (refractive implantable lens) are the prototypes of this generation.

Implantable Collamer Lens (STAAR Surgical) (Fig. 5.9.1)
- The ICL (STAAR Surgical Company, Monrovia, CA, USA), also known as implantable collamer lens or Visian ICL, is a single-piece plate lens made of collamer.
- The posterior surface of the lens is concave, providing a space between the anterior capsule of the crystalline lens and the posterior surface of the PIOL (vault).
- The newest version, EVO+ ICL has an expanded optic for myopes with larger pupillary aperture.

Eyecryl Phakic Intraocular Lens (Biotech)
- Monofocal hydrophilic acrylic foldable single piece posterior chamber phakic lenses
- Available from +10 D to -25 D.

Implantable Phakic Contact Lens (Care Group)
- Implantable phakic contact lens made from reinforced hybrid acrylic material.
- Power correction ranges from +15 D to -30 D with cylindrical power up to 8 D.

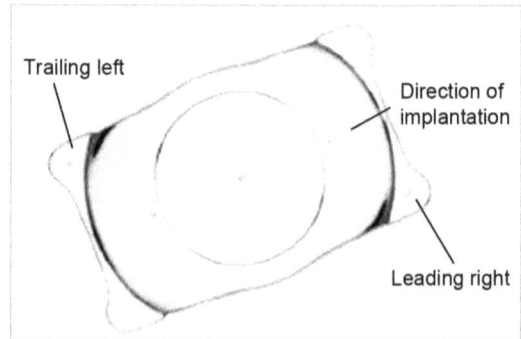

Fig. 5.9.1: Implantable collamer lens with CentraFlow technology.

Refractive Implantable Lens (Appasamy Associates)
- Refractive implantable lens is an implantable IOL made up of biocompatible hydrophilic acrylic material.
- Range of myopic correction is between −1.0 D and −21.0 D.
- Four peripheral holes for aqueous humor circulation.
- Peripheral iridectomy is required.

INDICATIONS
The PIOL is indicated for adults 21–45 years of age:
- To correct myopia ranging from −3.0 D to −18.0 D with or without less than or equal to 5.50 D of astigmatism at the spectacle plane
- To reduce myopia >−18.0 D which may be corrected by bioptics.

CONTRAINDICATIONS
- An anterior chamber depth (ACD) <2.80 mm
- Anterior chamber angle less than grade II by gonioscopy
- Pregnant or nursing mother
- *Less than minimum endothelial cell density according to age:*
  - ≤3,500 cells/mm^2 at 21 years of age
  - ≤2,800 cells/mm^2 at 31 years of age
  - ≤2,200 cells/mm^2 at 41 years of age
- Significant myopic degeneration causing impaired vision
- Any lenticular change which could progress.

ROUTINE PREOPERATIVE INVESTIGATIONS
- A thorough examination of the eye to rule out any pathology
- Intraocular pressure (IOP)
- Stability of refraction over 1 year
- Anterior chamber depth from endothelium
- Corneal topography
- Specular microscopy
- Pachymetry
- White-to-white measurement
- Gonioscopy
- Dilated retinal evaluation with scleral indentation

COUNSELING
- This procedure does not treat presbyopia.
- Glasses may still be required for sharpest vision for distance, for night driving or other activities performed in low light, for reading or for all of these activities.
- Long-term effects on the corneal endothelium are uncertain.
- Cataract is bound to develop with increasing age. Whenever cataract surgery is required, the PIOL would have to be removed and cataract surgery with IOL implantation would be required.
- The potential of the lens to alter IOP and the long-term risks of glaucoma, peripheral anterior synechiae, and pigment dispersion.
- Patients with higher degrees of myopia experience lower efficacy and higher rates of adverse events and complications such as retinal detachment.

WHITE-TO-WHITE MEASUREMENTS
It is an indirect measurement and is supposed to correlate with sulcus measurements. This can be done by:

- Orbscan
- *Digital slide calipers:*
  - Implantable collamer lens too short—lens vault smaller, more risk of anterior capsular cataract.
  - Implantable collamer lens too long—excessive lens vault, angle crowding, increased possibility of closed angle glaucoma.

VAULT
- Ideally should be 500 μ = one corneal thickness.
- *High vault:* Iris chafing and subsequently pigment dispersion glaucoma.
- *Low vault:* ICL contact with crystalline lens, cataract formation.

IMPLANTABLE COLLAMER LENS LENGTH DETERMINATION
- Sizing of the ICL myopic lenses (12.1–13.7 mm) was determined by the horizontal white-to-white and the ACD measurements.
- For eyes with ACD measurement less than or equal to 3.5 mm, the lens size was calculated by adding 1.1 mm to the horizontal white-to-white measurement.
- Eyes exhibiting an ACD >3.5 mm required the addition of up to 1.6 mm to the white-to-white measurement, up to a maximum length of 13.7 mm.
- Calculated lens sizes between the available lens diameters (in 0.5 mm steps) were generally rounded down if the ACD was less than or equal to 3.5 mm and rounded up if the ACD was >3.5 mm.

AXIS MARKING FOR TORIC PHAKIC INTRAOCULAR LENS
- Manual axis marker
- Digital microscope mounted toric marking device.
- AXsys™ electronic toric marking device.

ADVANTAGES
- The procedure is reversible unlike laser-assisted in situ keratomileusis (LASIK).
- Preserves accommodation
- It creates a small corneal incision thus astigmatism is minimum.
- Corneal tissue is not removed, thus retaining corneal asphericity and tear film integrity.
- Reduction of risk of optical distortions and higher order aberrations.

PHAKIC INTRAOCULAR LENS IMPLANTATION (FIGS. 5.9.2 TO 5.9.9)

Loading
- Careful loading of ICL from vial into the injector with methylcellulose mixed with balanced salt solution.
- Place lens into cartridge ensuring that the whole lens is seated in the groove created by the open wings of the cartridge.
- Align the back of the cartridge with the injector mouth and press in firmly.
- Press the plunger in one smooth slow motion till the lens is inside the lumen. Check during this step that no excessive force is required as this may be an indication of the lens being trapped between the wings, or the plunger tip has overridden the lens.

Implantation in Eye
- Under topical anesthesia, two 0.6 mm side ports and a 2.8–3.2 mm clear corneal temporal incision are made.
- Lens is implanted temporally and gently rotated to align the axis with the cylindrical axis, if required and tucked under the iris.
- It vaults over the crystalline lens.

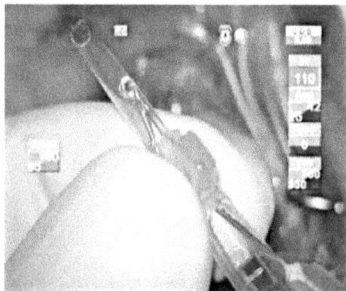

Fig. 5.9.2: Mixture of methylcellulose with balanced salt solution in cartridge.

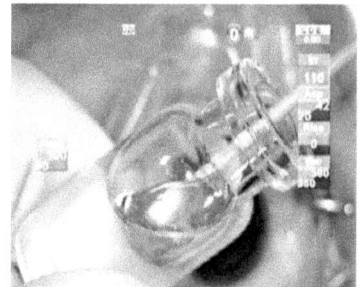

Fig. 5.9.3: Implantable collamer lens is taken from glass vial with special applicator.

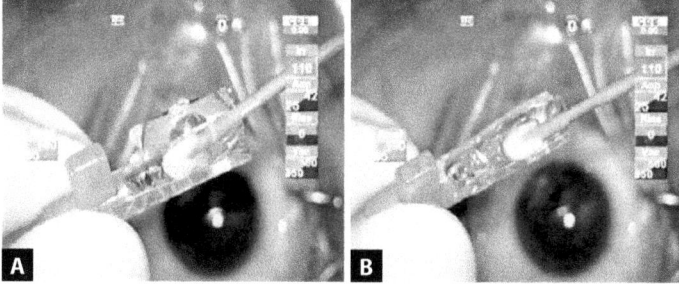

Figs. 5.9.4A and B: Implantable collamer lens is set properly in the groove of cartridge.

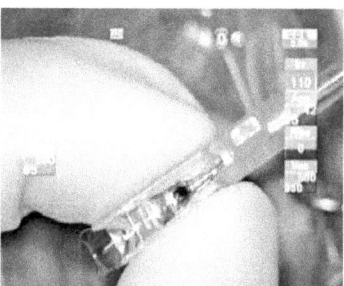

Fig. 5.9.5: Implantable collamer lens is held with aus de aur forceps and gently moved forward to the nozzle of the cartridge.

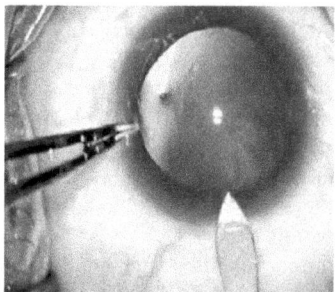

Fig. 5.9.6: Main port is made temporally and implantable collamer lens is injected through it.

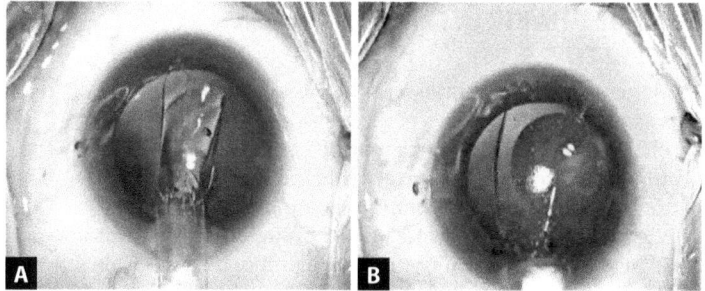

Figs. 5.9.7A and B: Slow gradual dislodging of implantable collamer lens in anterior chamber.

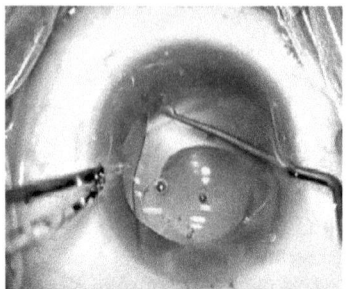 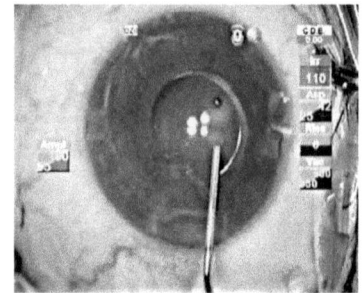

Fig. 5.9.8: Injecting gel over the implantable collamer lens and tucking it under the iris.

Fig. 5.9.9: Anterior chamber is washed properly and incision is closed by hydration.

- Complete removal of viscoelastic material, aided by holding the infusion flow over the central port in the V4c ICL model.
- Miotic agent may be injected and washed out meticulously.
- Incision closed by hydration.

PERIPHERAL IRIDOTOMY

With ICL with the central port (360 µm), peripheral iridotomy (PI) is not necessary. However, with ICL correcting hypermetropia, preoperatively iridotomy may be done with Nd:YAG laser or intraoperatively with Vannas scissors or vitrectomy cutter. The PI should be sufficiently wide, positioned superiorly, well away from the haptics—to provide outlet for aqueous flow around lens.

Postoperative Evaluation
- Complete ophthalmic evaluation
- Anterior segment optical coherence tomography (**Figs. 5.9.10 and 5.9.11**)
- Intraocular pressure
- Specular microscopy if necessary.

Complications
- Corneal decompensation—very rare in an uneventful surgery.
- Glaucoma—central flow technology has prevented this complication in the newer version.
- Chronic uveitis is rare and the cause is to be treated.
- Cataract—removal of ICL with cataract surgery and IOL implantation.
- Displacement of PIOL needs repositioning and in case of recurrent displacement, removal, and replacement of appropriate size ICL.
- Undercorrection or overcorrection of refractive error can be treated with photorefractive keratectomy or LASIK.

REMOVAL OF PHAKIC INTRAOCULAR LENS (FIGS. 5.9.12 TO 5.9.14)

- After proper counseling and preoperative measurement with full dilated pupil, two side ports are made with injection of viscoelastics.
- Anterior chamber is entered through main 2.8–3.2 mm ports.
- A small amount of viscoelastic is injected behind the PIOL.
- Haptics are lifted to the anterior chamber by a spatula.
- The ICL is held with lens holding forceps and brought gently into the anterior chamber.
- The ICL is held at the junction of the haptic and optic, then pulled out through an adequate incision. The incision may need to be extended.

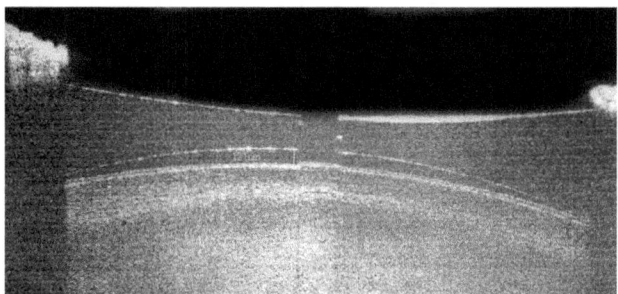

Fig. 5.9.10: Anterior segment optical coherence tomography 1 month after implantable collamer lens implantation with V4c model, CentraFlow technology—low vault (121 μm).

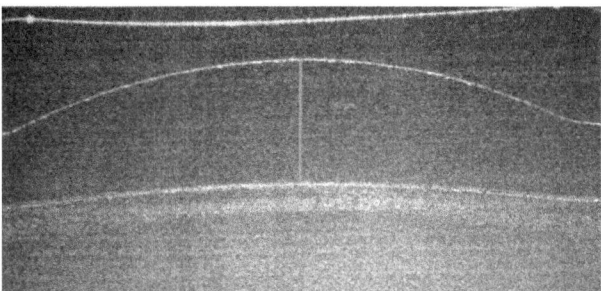

Fig. 5.9.11: Anterior segment optical coherence tomography 1 month after implantable collamer lens implantation—high vault (746 μm).

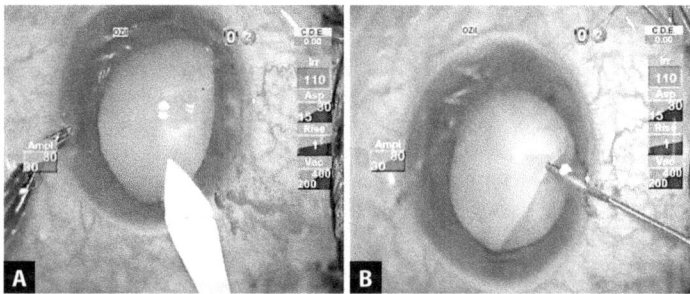

Figs. 5.9.12A and B: Main incision for implantable collamer lens explanation and injecting visco behind the lens to lift up the implantable collamer lens.

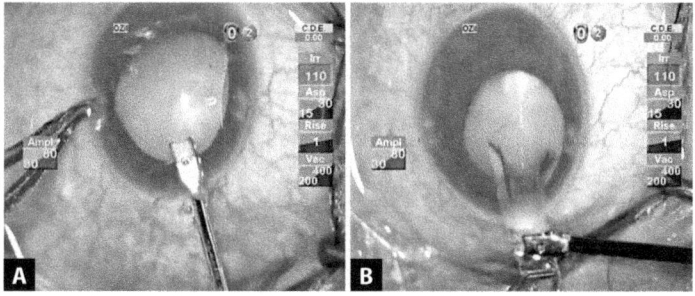

Figs. 5.9.13A and B: Holding the lens with forceps at the junction of haptic and optic and gently pulling it out of the anterior chamber.

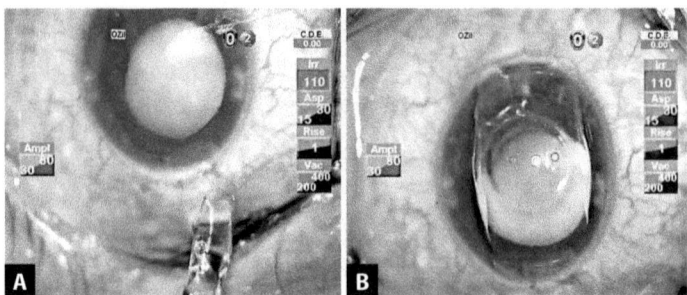

Figs. 5.9.14A and B: Explanted implantable collamer lens should be checked to ensure total removal.

■ HANDLING THE UPSIDE DOWN PHAKIC INTRAOCULAR LENS

Upside down PIOL may occur due to faulty loading, quick injection of the ICL, or faulty disengagement. This may result in anterior subcapsular cataract, extreme rise of IOP, or excessive pigment dispersion. This condition needs:
- Removal of the PIOL and then reimplantation of the same IOL.

■ CLINICAL RESULTS

Multiple published literatures as well as reports from Food and Drug Administration (FDA) studies proved impressive results, including a high predictability, safety, efficacy, stability, as well as very high level of patient satisfaction after ICL implantation. Another long-term follow-up on a large series demonstrated the safety of spherical ICL. It provides an excellent visual and refractive outcome with very minimum number of complications.

■ CONCLUSION

Phakic IOL is an excellent tool for the correction of refractive errors, especially in those in whom laser refractive correction is not possible. It may also be combined with a laser procedure to achieve higher levels of refractive correction (bioptics). Appropriate preoperative evaluation and proper patient selection are essential for excellent outcome of phakic IOL.

■ SUGGESTED READING

1. Sanders DR, Doney K, Poco M, et al. United States Food and Drug Administration clinical trial of the implantable collamer lens for moderate to high myopia: three-year follow-up. Ophthalmology. 2004;111:1683-92.

5.10 Wavefront-guided and Optimized Ablations: What We Need to Know?

Ananth D
Lotus Eye Hospital and Institute, Coimbatore
doctorananth@gmail.com

■ ABERRATIONS

Optical aberrations are discrepancy in the refracting system of the eye. The eye is by no means optically perfect—the lapses from perfection are called aberrations. Each image point receives light predominantly from one object point but also receives some light from neighboring object points. The image point resembles, but does not

SECTION 5: Refractive Surgery

duplicate, the object point. Because rays do not focus perfectly stigmatically, the image does not contain as much detail as the original object. This discrepancy is referred to in general as the aberration of an optical system.

Aberrations may be monochromatic or chromatic. Monochromatic aberrations occur when light is reflected or refracted; they are not a function of the wavelength of light and may be observed with monochromatic light as well. They may be further classified as lower-order aberrations (LOAs) or higher-order aberrations (HOAs) **(Tables 5.10.1 and 5.10.2)**.

TABLE 5.10.1: Monochromatic aberrations of the human eye.

Order of aberrations	Types	Clinical significance	Management
Zero order	Piston	Lower order aberrations—80–90% of total aberrations	• Piston-perfect optical system • Easily corrected with spectacles, contact lenses or refractive surgeries
First order	Tilt (prism)		
Second order	• Defocus (myopia, hyperopia) • Astigmatism		
Third order	• Coma • Trefoil	• Higher order aberrations—15% of total aberrations • Impact visual quality-lead to night vision disturbances, glare and halos	• Wavefront optimized ablation—prevent induction of new HOAs • Wavefront-guided ablation—correct pre-existing HOAs
Fourth order	• Spherical aberration • Tetrafoil • Secondary astigmatism		
Fifth order	• Pentafoil • Secondary trefoil • Secondary coma		
Sixth order	• Hexafoil • Secondary tetrafoil • Tertiary astigmatism		

(HOA: higher order aberration)

TABLE 5.10.2: Clinically significant higher order aberrations (HOAs).

Higher order aberration	Order	Mechanism	Clinical significance
Coma	Third order	Light rays from one edge of the pupil come into focus before light rays from the opposite edge	• "Comet tail" appearance—zone of sharp focus at one edge of image and fuzzy focus at the other edge • Create effect of "smearing" an image • Observed after decentered ablations
Trefoil	Third order	Point of light is received by the eye as a "Mercedes Benz" symbol or "trifoliate clover leaf pattern"	• Triangular astigmatism • Peripheral vision affected more than central vision • Less degradation of image quality than coma
Spherical aberration	Fourth order	Light rays from the peripheral cornea or lens focus in front those from the central cornea	• Night myopia • Halos around point light sources • Increases depth of focus • Decreases contrast sensitivity • Most visually significant HOA after corneal ablation

These aberrations are typically evaluated by wavefront (WF)-sensing systems and are amenable to correction by laser refractive surgeries. Aberrometers are instruments devised to analyze the WF of the human eye to provide detailed information regarding lower- and higher-order aberrations.

IMPORTANCE IN REFRACTIVE SURGERY

Keratorefractive surgery involves altering the refractive state of the eye by modifications to the corneal curvature and thus, the corneal refractive power. As clinicians, we must know how aberrations affect the visual quality to make good clinical decisions with proper patient selection and knowing what to expect after a refractive procedure **(Table 5.10.3)**. High magnitude of aberrations in patients with a small mesopic pupil diameter has a greater impact on visual quality, and the aberrations further increase with dilatation of the pupil.

Conventional refractive surgical procedures correct lower order aberrations. In contrast, higher order aberrations, especially spherical aberration and coma, may increase after conventional surface ablation or laser in situ keratomileusis (LASIK) and lead to unpleasant dysphotic symptoms including night vision disturbances, glare, haloes, and starbursts. This increase in HOAs correlates with the degree of preoperative myopia in case of LASIK.

Wavefront optimized corneal ablative procedures minimize the induction of new HOAs after refractive surgery; however, they do not correct preexisting HOAs. Wavefront-guided LASIK takes in to account the preoperative WF of the optical system and has the distinct advantage of correction of preexisting higher-order aberrations. Compared with myopic eyes, hyperopic eyes undergoing a laser refractive procedure experience a higher increase in the postoperative HOAs.

Newer modalities such as small incision lenticule extraction (SMILE) lead to lesser induction of aberrations as compared with conventional femtosecond LASIK (FS-LASIK). This may be attributed to the absence of a flap with a better preservation of corneal integrity in SMILE as compared with a circumferential LASIK flap. Moreover, more energy is delivered to the cornea with FS-LASIK in higher attempted corrections, while energy levels are constant in SMILE and independent of the attempted correction.

WAVEFRONT-OPTIMIZED ABLATION

Wavefront-optimized (WO) ablation is an aspheric ablation profile that aims to pre-compensate for spherical aberrations, which would otherwise be induced after classical ablation. It does not correct preexisting HOAs. It is designed to preserve the physiologic prolate state of the cornea postsurgery by applying more laser pulses in the periphery and involves the removal of more peripheral stromal tissue. Mrochen et al. described a model of WF-optimized ablation algorithm where the subjective refraction of the patient and the amount of spherical aberrations induced by the classic aberration profiles were used to create a nomogram to modify the existing ablation profile.

TABLE 5.10.3: Clinical applications of wavefront sensing in refractive surgeries.

Preoperative	Intraoperative	Postoperative
• Decision making—>0.40 microns HOA better suited for wavefront-guided ablations • Increased lenticular aberrations—may not be ideal candidate for cornea-based refractive procedures	Wavefront maps used as a guide for wavefront-guided ablations	Objective assessment of visual quality—correlate with visual complaints such as blur, glare, and halos

(HOA: higher order aberration)

The WO profiles lead to more aspheric shape without a substantial increase in the central ablation depth; however, the depth of peripheral ablation is 35% more than that seen with the classical profiles.

Advantages
The WO treatment algorithm predicts the precompensation required based on patient's subjective refraction alone, without requiring any preoperative aberrometry or topography measurements. It allows the creation of larger optical zones with more realistic dimensions and takes average epithelial remodeling into account while planning treatments.

Disadvantages
The assumptions on precompensation for the HOAs are applicable to an average eye only. Better results may be obtained, if each surgeon creates his own nomogram for WF-optimized treatments based on his patients' outcomes. In addition, precompensation is performed only for rotationally symmetrical aberrations. Preexisting HOAs are not corrected. Spherical and cylindrical errors are treated in two steps, one following the other. Lastly, more tissue is ablated per diopter of refractive error with a greater amount of tissue ablated in the periphery.

■ WAVEFRONT-GUIDED ABLATION
Ocular WF-guided ablation profile aims to treat both the preexisting higher order aberrations and minimize the induction of new HOAs in order to improve the visual quality and contrast sensitivity as compared with conventional and aspheric treatment profiles. The ocular aberration data of the patient obtained by a WF sensor is fed electronically in to the treating laser and used to program the pattern of laser ablation.

Wavefront-guided LASIK is indicated for patients who suffer from high preexisting ocular HOAs (>0.4 microns) and associated visual disturbances such as glare, haloes, and starbursts. In addition, patients with larger mesopic and scotopic pupil size may benefit from WF-guided (WG) LASIK as lower postoperative HOAs will result in better visual quality in low light conditions.

Wavefront-guided LASIK should be avoided in cases where repeatable ocular WF measurements cannot be acquired successfully.

Advantages
Wavefront-guided ablation aims to correct all preexisting HOAs in addition to sphere and astigmatism by taking into account the entire eye's HOAs. Postoperative induction of new HOAs is lesser as compared with WO treatments.

Disadvantages
The WF measurements are acquired at a single time point preoperatively and are thus static, while the ocular optical system and its WF are dynamic in nature, being affected by various other factors such as ambient lighting and accommodative status of the eye. It considers only monochromatic aberrations and precompensates for rotationally symmetrical aberrations alone.

■ SUGGESTED READING
1. Brodie SE, Ang M, Irsch K, Jackson ML, Mauger TF, Oostra T, Riaz KM, Young JA. Aberrations. In: Clinical Optics and Vision Rehabilitation by American Academy Of Ophthalmology, 2022–2023 Basic and Clinical Science Course.
2. Titiyal JS, Kaur M, Nair S. Aberrometry and Wavefront Analysis. In: Current concepts in Refractive Surgery. Comprehensive Guide for Decision Making and Surgical Techniques, First Edition, 2022.

3. Titiyal JS, Kaur M, Nair S. Customized Corneal Ablation. In: Current Concepts in Refractive Surgery. Comprehensive Guide for Decision Making and Surgical Techniques, First Edition, 2022.

5.11 | Contoura Vision

Shreesha Kumar Kodavoor, Neha K Rathi, Gopal R
The Eye Foundation, Coimbatore
eskay_03@rediffmail.com, rathineha1987@gmail.com, dr.gopal@yahoo.com

■ INTRODUCTION

Astigmatism correction with femtosecond-laser assisted in situ keratomileusis (LASIK) is challenging because as small as 1° deviation in astigmatic axis results in a loss of correction of 3.3%.[1] The conventional treatment with wavefront-guided LASIK corrects aberrations from entire eye, with the outcomes not proven to be significantly better. Topography-guided LASIK corrects irregular astigmatism of cornea providing regular corneal surface along with reduction in higher order aberrations (HOAs). This customization of ablation pattern by utilizing topography data has been reported to provide excellent refractive data. Recently, Alcon presented the innovative Contoura Vision (CV) technique based on the WaveLight Refractive Suite which has been US Food and Drug Administration (FDA) approved for correction on normal corneas without irregular astigmatism.[1] The final selection of astigmatism magnitude and axis is surgeon dependent; some consider only topography and others combine both manifest and topography values. However, considering only manifest refraction is the best option according to studies. The topography-guided treatment profile is fixed by the Contoura software, designed to treat all corneal topographic aberrations.

■ PATIENT SELECTION AND TREATMENT PLANNING

Preoperatively regular LASIK work-up is planned including dry and wet refraction, topography, pupillometry, wavefront analysis, dry eye work-up, slit lamp examination, and fundus examination. Patients with myopia up to −8 D and cylinder up to −6 D with preferably some inferior-superior asymmetry on corneal topography were selected; also patients with high and mixed astigmatism are good candidates for Contoura Vision correction. A patient with manifest refractive power of −1.50 D sphere and −1.75 D cylinder at 5° in right eye and −1.75 D sphere and −1.00 D cylinder at 180° along with topography as shown in **Figures 5.11.1A and B** with slight Inferior-Superior (I-S) asymmetry in left eye appears good candidate for Contoura Vision correction.

The first line of data on the treatment planning is the clinical refraction data on software window shown in **Figure 5.11.2**. A patient's example is shown in the figure with the clinical refraction on the top, of −2.00 D of sphere and −1.25 D of cylinder at 175°. The topography software-recommended cylindrical refraction is shown in the middle line of refraction in the figure. While planning this case, the sphere is −0.59 D (since axial length cannot be calculated with the topography software and cannot calculate myopia), and the cylinder of −1.44 D at 10° is derived from several consistent Vario, Topolyzer (Alcon, Fort Worth, TX, USA). The surgeon modifies the lower third refraction. The topography-guided software correction will reveal the ablation required in order to normalize this cornea with regard to corneal vertex by putting all refraction data on purpose to 0°. The trefoil-like ablation in correlation with the pupillary aperture is obtained, also has decentration to the trefoil-like normalization ablation, for angle-kappa compensation by the topography software. Since this ablation pattern induces some myopia and which is calculated to keep it neutral there is a need to add −0.25 D of

SECTION 5: Refractive Surgery

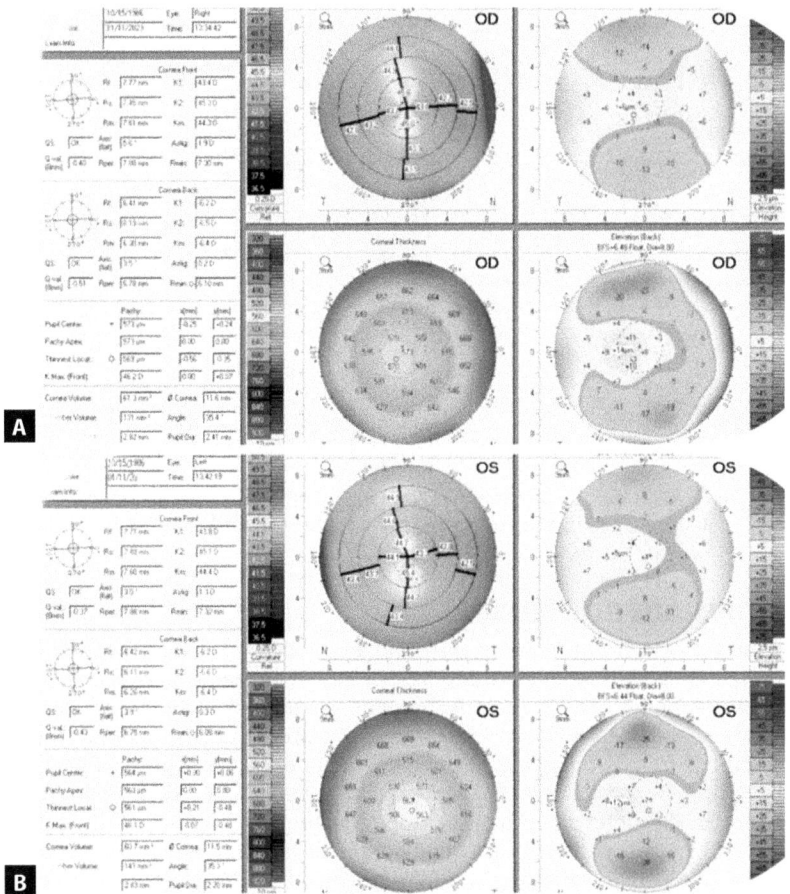

Figs. 5.11.1A and B: Corneal topography. (A) Right eye; (B) Left eye showing minimal Inferior-Superior asymmetry.

myopia to the clinical refraction sphere, so the total sphere calculated should be −2.25 D. The cylinder suggested is higher and of different axis as suggested by the software (middle refraction): 10° instead of 175°. The clinical-suggested cylinder is then entered into the third lower "modified" refraction −1.25 D at 175°. After nomogram correction the modified spherical refraction is corrected as −2.25 D. One thing to keep in mind is that if the corrected cylinder chosen is higher from Topolyzer then the same amount is deducted from clinical sphere in order to keep the same spherical equivalent.

■ PROCEDURE

The VisuMax platform (Carl Zeiss Meditec) is used to create the corneal flap with a depth of 100 μm and diameter of 8.5 mm. The corneal flap hinge is located 90° superiorly. The diameter of optical zone ablation is kept 6.5 mm. All the patients then undergo topography-guided keratomileusis in the EX500. Appropriate diopter compensation is considered for the spherical aberration that may be caused by elimination of HOAs. After the surgical design was completed, corneal ablation was performed using the automatic iris tracking system. Postoperatively patients are started on topical antibiotics, steroids which are tapered subsequently and lubricants.

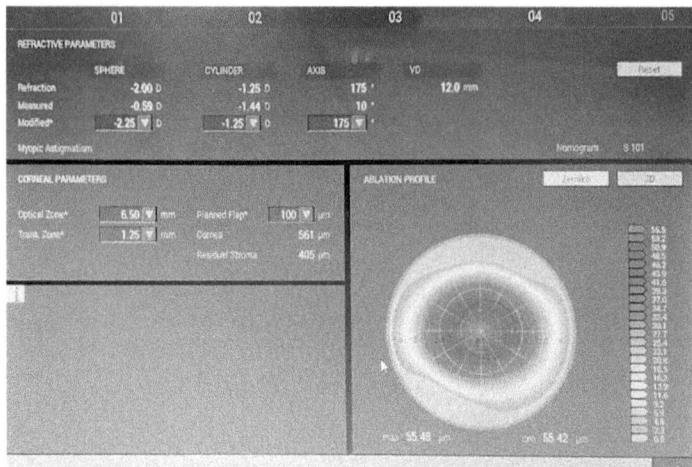

Fig. 5.11.2: Topography treatment pattern after the refraction has been adjusted by the user to the desired sphere and cylinder.

◼ POSTOPERATIVE OUTCOME

Conventional LASIK produces more spherical and coma aberrations postoperatively causing increased incidence of glare and haloes. The root mean square is increased 1.9 fold after conventional LASIK,[1] such decrease in visual quality is unacceptable which lead to more customized ablation techniques. Wavefront-guided treatment includes optic aberrations from entire eye neglecting the major causative aspects of aberrations such as tear film, pupil, and lens adjustment on aberrations, hence does not prove to be superior. On the other hand, corneal topography-guided LASIK works primarily on corneal surface and proves to be a good option for highly irregular and asymmetric corneas. The automatic iris tracking system is designed according to the iris texture and can detect pupil size from 1.5 to 8 mm^2. The three-dimensional tracking mode effectively reduces the eye rotation caused by the position change of the subject providing superior outcomes.

It has been observed that corneal parameters such as index of corneal variance and index of vertical asymmetry obtained from Oculyzer are decreased after 3 months of surgery which describes increased improvement in regularity of cornea. Also, C7 on Topolyzer is decreased after Contoura Vision correction amounting to decreased vertical coma and spherical aberrations postsurgery. The spatial frequencies of contrast sensitivity are found to be greatly increased after Contoura Vision correction. This notion of Contoura describes corneal topography-guided customized ablations to subjects with normal cornea. It corrects both low-order aberrations such as myopia and astigmatism and also subject's own higher order aberrations. Elimination of higher-order phase difference can improve visual quality. All in all, Contoura eliminates aberrations from anterior corneal surface to achieve stable corrected distance visual acuity in subjects.

◼ REFERENCES

1. Lin Y, Su HJ, Yuan MZ, Zhang Y. Vector analysis of Contoura Vision for the correction of myopia and myopic astigmatism. Int J Ophthalmol. 2022;15(6):983-89.
2. Kanellopoulos AJ. Topography-modified refraction (TMR): adjustment of treated cylinder amount and axis to the topography versus standard clinical refraction in myopic topography-guided LASIK. Clin Ophthalmol. 2016;10:2213-21.

5.12 Topography-guided Ablations in Normal and Abnormal Corneas

Jagadesh C Reddy
Pristine Eye Hospitals, Hyderabad
drcjagadeeshreddy@gmail.com

INTRODUCTION

Topography-guided (TG) ablation is a surgical technique that uses excimer laser to reshape the cornea based on a detailed map of its surface shape. This procedure is used to correct refractive error in normal cornea and correct visual impairments caused by irregular corneal shapes, such as keratoconus and post-LASIK (laser-assisted in situ keratomileusis) ectasia.

The first step in a topography-guided ablation procedure is to create a detailed map of the patient's cornea using topographer or Topolyzer. This device uses a series of light beams and cameras to create a three-dimensional map of the cornea's surface. This map is then used to guide the laser ablation process, ensuring that the laser is used to reshape the cornea in a precise and controlled manner. One of the advantages of TG ablation over traditional laser ablation techniques or lenticular extraction procedures is that it allows for the correction of a wider range of corneal irregularities thus leading to accurate postoperative refraction predictability and less surgically induced higher order aberrations (HOAs) and improved quality of vision.

TOPOGRAPHY-GUIDED ABLATION VERSUS OTHER ABLATION PATTERNS

The basic differences in the ablation pattern between TG ablation and other ablation patterns are:
- TG ablation measures and treats the aberration profile on the anterior surface of the cornea.
- TG ablation is centered on the apex of the cornea and not the center of the pupil.
- TG ablations allow the new regular shape of each cornea by the placement of extra-peripheral pulses to blend out the treatment and minimize peripheral corneal aberrations.

TOPOGRAPHY-GUIDED ABLATION (CONTOURA) IN NORMAL/VIRGIN CORNEA

Patient Selection Criteria
- The selection criteria are like any other keratorefractive surgery.
- According to FDA the range of correction is myopia up to −8.00 D with astigmatism of −3.00 D or less.

Contoura Work-up
- Apart from complete ocular examination, precise manifest refraction and highly repeatable Topolyzer maps.
- At least four high-quality scans with appropriate iris registration and complete data are needed to proceed in surgical planning.
- In case of discrepancy in the manifest and measured cylinder a customized nomogram [personal, Phorcides Analytic Engine, Layer Yolked Reduction of Astigmatism (LYRA) Protocol, etc.] can be considered.

Contoura Planning

- Appropriate planning is the most crucial step for good outcomes.
- Each of the four selected maps is within 0.50 D of each other across the entire difference map.
- When there is a match between the measured and manifest astigmatism, we can proceed further with the completing of the planning process. In case of discrepancy in the magnitude and/or astigmatism we can use one of the following planning methods.
- Phorcides Analytical Engine (https://phorcides.com/) was developed based on a combination of geographic imaging software (GIS, evaluate the topography of Earth's terrain) and optics. The GIS allows more precise characterization of irregularities on the corneal surface and then allows the expected optical effect of "smoothing" these irregularities to be determined. Modifications to the treatment profile can then be made based on eliminating any number of identified irregularities. Recent research has indicated that results obtained when Contoura surgery is planned with the Phorcides Analytical Engine are comparable or superior to those achieved when planned with the manifest refraction, based on theoretical and actual clinical outcomes.
- In the LYRA protocol aberration removal layer is linked to the refraction correction layer. Contoura calculates the results of that linkage. The protocol is as follows:
  - Manifest refraction is entered into presurgical Contoura planning page.
  - The astigmatism and sphere are zeroed to see ablation pattern for the aberration correction layer.
  - The Topolyzer measured astigmatism and axis are entered for the final correction. The ablation map is compared with Pentacam anterior elevation map for understanding the ablation when there is a significant discrepancy between manifest versus measured magnitude of astigmatism and axis.
  - The spherical error is entered after adjustment for the spherical equivalent of the change in the magnitude of astigmatism.

■ OUTCOMES

Topography-guided ablation in normal cornea produced more accurate postoperative refraction predictability and less surgically induced HOAs compared to wavefront optimized or guided ablation. The only limitation of the research has been a variable method used by surgeons in adjusting the astigmatism magnitude and axis inputs, on the excimer laser planning software. The FDA trial did show that about 65% of eyes treated with TG ablation experienced 20/16 vision or better.

■ TOPOGRAPHY-GUIDED ABLATION IN KERATOCONUS

Keratoconus, a condition in which the cornea becomes thin and cone-shaped, traditional laser ablation techniques can only correct a limited amount of the irregularity. TG ablation, on the other hand, can correct a greater amount of the irregularity, resulting in improvement in the patient's quality of vision and achieve better contact lens fit. The aim of the procedure is not to give a complete refractive correction. Another advantage of TG ablation is that it can be used to correct visual impairments caused by previous refractive surgeries, such as LASIK.

It is important to note that TG custom ablation is not suitable for all patients with keratoconus. It is most effective for patients with mild to moderate cases of the condition. Additionally, the procedure may not be suitable for patients with other eye conditions such as cataracts or glaucoma.

Planning for TG custom ablation for the treatment of keratoconus involves a series of steps to ensure that the procedure is safe and effective for the patient. The first step in planning for the procedure is a comprehensive examination of the patient's eyes to determine the severity of their keratoconus and to ensure that they are a suitable candidate for the procedure.

SELECTION CRITERIA
- Mild-to-moderate keratoconus
- Thinnest pachymetry >450 μm/predicted postoperative thinnest pachymetry of at least 400 μm after TG ablation
- Poor contact lens fit/unhappy with vision
- No active eye disease
- No corneal scarring

The next step is to create a detailed map of the patient's cornea using advanced technology such as corneal topographer or Topolyzer or wavefront analyzer. This map is used to create a customized treatment plan that addresses the specific areas of the cornea affected by the condition.

Once the map has been created, a specialized planning software from Excimer Laser System (WaveLight Laser Technologie AG) is used to design the laser treatment plan. This plan considers the patient's specific needs and goals for the procedure, such as regularizing the asymmetry or/and correcting the refractive error. The approach varies based on the final goal. The procedure can also be done as two-stage procedure wherein the first stage can address the irregularity using the TG ablation and the second stage can address the correction of refractive error after 4–6 weeks.

TIPS FOR PLANNING
- Do not address Q value if it is in the accepted range of –1 to 0.
- To consider making sphere and cylinder as 0 in the modified column. Select Zernike table for C4 compensation. To make C4 (defocus) value equal to C12 (spherical aberration) by means of adding sphere value. This method addresses the regularizing the cornea.
- In situations where the regularization and correction of some refractive error is intended, we need to consider adding the C4 compensation value to the clinical refraction. While correcting the cylinder the axis of the Topolyzer and the manifest cylinder should be within 15°. If not better to avoid correcting the cylindrical error.

In conclusion, planning for topography-guided custom ablation for the treatment of keratoconus involves a series of steps to ensure that the procedure is safe and effective for the patient.

SUGGESTED READING
1. Cheng SM, Tu RX, Li X, Zhang JS, Tian Z, Zha ZW, Ruan KW, Yu AY. Topography-guided versus wavefront-optimized LASIK for myopia with and without astigmatism: a meta-analysis. J Refract Surg. 2021;37(10):707-14.
2. Kang EM, Ryu IH, Lee IS, Kim JK, Kim SW, Ji YW. Comparison of corneal higher-order aberrations following topography-guided LASIK and SMILE for myopic correction: a propensity score matching analysis. J Clin Med. 2022;11(20):6171.

5.13 Complications of Small Incision Lenticule Extraction

Neha K Rathi, Shreesha Kumar Kodavoor, Ramamurthy Dandapani
The Eye Foundation, Coimbatore
rathineha1987@gmail.com, eskay_03@rediffmail.com, drramamurthy@theeyefoundation.in

INTRODUCTION
Small incision lenticule extraction (SMILE) is a femtosecond-assisted flapless refractive procedure which involves extraction of a carved lenticule through a small incision for correction of refractive errors. Ever since its introduction in 2011, it has opened advanced channels in the field of refractive surgery. It alleviates multiple unwanted

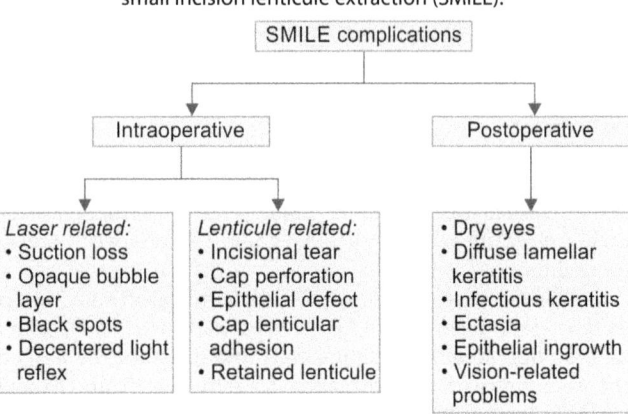

Flowchart 5.13.1: Categorical chart of complications of small incision lenticule extraction (SMILE).

obstacles occurring due to flap in FS-LASIK (femtosecond-laser in situ keratomileusis), in overcoming dry eyes postrefractive surgeries along with better biomechanical stability. However, the main challenge is to perform the procedure which has a steep learning curve initially and so comes with various complications. These complications even though are new to arise, can be managed effectively. These can be divided into intraoperative and postoperative which will be discussed intently in the following sections **(Flowchart 5.13.1)**.

INTRAOPERATIVE COMPLICATIONS

Multiple intraoperative complications arise during the procedure which is either due to laser or lenticule dissection and extraction related are discussed below.

Suction Loss

Incidence of suction loss during the procedure is highly variable and it ranges from 0.17 to 0.93% depending upon the surgeon's experience. Risk factors include patient related such as small palpebral fissure, deep set eyes, smaller corneas, inappropriate eye fixation, forcible eye squeezing, head movement, anxiety or procedure related such as fluid ingress through conjunctival sac, inadvertent conjunctival entrapment, conjunctivochalasis, incompatibility of cone shape, and due to low docking pressure system in SMILE. In an event of suction loss management depends according to stage at which it has occurred, suction loss when <10% of lenticule is dissected needs redocking with same parameters however suction loss occurring after >10% of lenticule dissection requires conversion into flap-LASIK which is already in-built in VisuMax platform or conversion into transepithelial photorefractive keratectomy (PRK) to avoid irregular lenticule cut **(Fig. 5.13.1B)**; suction loss during lenticular side cut is managed by reducing the diameter by 0.2 mm along with 10 μ deeper cut; if suction loss occurs during cap cut redocking with same parameters is advised. It can even happen during incision cut and may be noted after suction release and manual incision with an 11 number surgical blade at approximately one-fourth the depth of cornea will help in completion of the procedure. Its prevention includes drying of conjunctival surface with Merocel sponge before docking along with efficient preoperative counseling to release patient's anxiety.

Opaque Bubble Layer

Excessive entrapment of gas bubbles at the interface due to blockage of its dissipation in surrounding stroma results into opaque bubble layer (OBL) formation which hinders

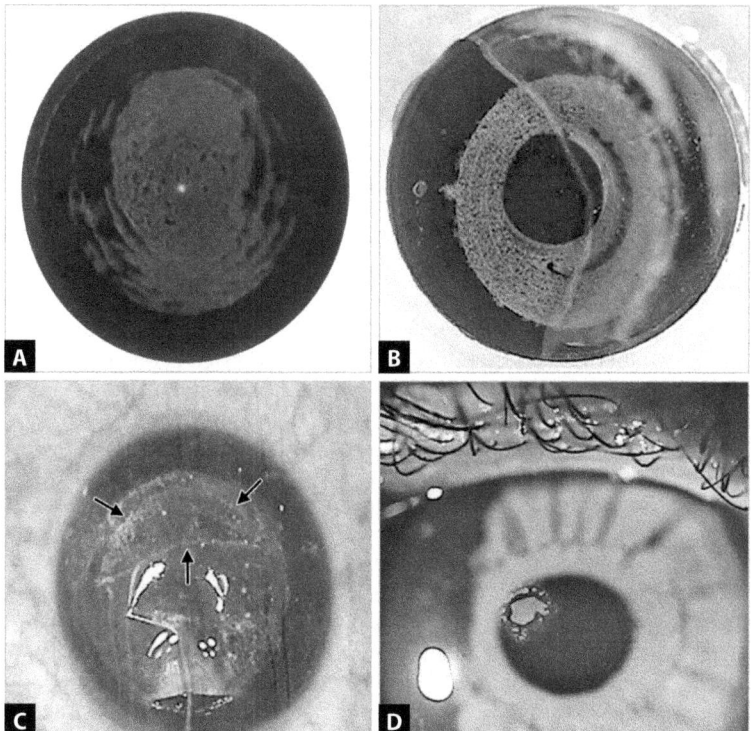

Figs. 5.13.1A to D: (A) Black spots; (B) Suction loss; (C) Retained lenticule stained with triamcinolone acetate highlighting the edge of lenticule (marked with arrow); (D) Epithelial ingrowth.

in smooth lenticular dissection and subsequently leading to complications such as cap tear and false plane formation. Its incidence is around 0.73% and risk factors include high energy delivery, thick corneas, thin lenticule (low correction), and stiffer corneas (old age). It can be managed with push up or push down techniques along with delivering lower laser energy.

Black Spots

Inability of the femtosecond laser to pass through the corneal tissue due to entrapment of meibomian gland secretion, debris, water droplets in between the suction cone and corneal surface results into black spots and incomplete lenticule dissection **(Fig. 5.13.1A)**. Its incidence ranges from 0.33 to 11% and can be well managed by manual dissection in cases of small spots; however in larger black islands abandonment of the procedure is preferred. Meibomian gland disease management and adequate conjunctival surface cleaning prior to surgery is desirable.

Decentered Light Reflex

Coaxial corneal light reflex is considered closest to visual axis and is preferred as ablation center in order to avoid issues arising from decentered ablation such as increase in spherical aberrations and coma. Myopic astigmatism and hyperopia are refractive errors more sensitive in a case of decentered ablation. In such an event it is preferred to undock and recenter however in patients with large angle kappa it might appear that the fixation light is decentered in relation to pupillary center but it is unnecessary to undock and recenter.

Lenticule Dissection-related Problems

Incisional Tear, Cap Perforation, and Epithelial Defect
Its incidence is dependent on the experience of surgeon; novice surgeon can cause inadvertent manipulation during dissection which can lead to incisional tear, cap perforation, and sloughing of the adjacent epithelium. It can be managed effectively with bandage contact lens and lubricants without hampering the visual outcome.

Cap Lenticular Adhesion
Inadvertent dissection of posterior plane first causes the lenticule to adhere with cap anteriorly which causes impossible dissection leading to complications such as lenticule remnant and cap perforation during manipulation. Its incidence varies from 0.33 to 7% and reduces with increasing experience of surgeon. Stop sign is one of the convenient ways to delineate both the planes separately; this describes the resistance noted at the junction between the dissected and undissected halves, interfering with subsequent lateral movement of the instrument. Also, in recent times use of intraoperative anterior segment-optical coherence tomography (OCT) appears promising in identifying the anterior plane along with its guided dissection.

Retained Lenticule
Incomplete dissection and manipulation during lenticule removal can cause its retention which can give rise to irregular astigmatism and interface haze in the postoperative period (**Figs. 5.13.1A to D**). Its incidences range from 2.16 to 9% and can be identified on topography, anterior segment OCT and on slit lamp using retro-illumination after full dilatation. Its management includes immediate removal of remnant lenticule for optimal outcome, in rare cases of complete lenticule remnant PRK or LASIK is performed (**Figs. 5.13.2A to D**). The CIRCLE software present on VisuMax platform provides an advantage of cap conversion into a flap for lenticule removal.

■ POSTOPERATIVE COMPLICATIONS
Small incision lenticule extraction is considered superior to other refractive procedure as being a flapless procedure which alleviates major complications occurring post-LASIK/PRK, nonetheless these complications are still present in lower intensity. Various postoperative complications are as follows.

Dry Eyes
Dry eyes postrefractive surgery occurs due to transection of corneal nerves leading to reduced tear production; it is much reduced in SMILE due to factors such as small incision, lower docking system pressure causing lesser damage to ocular surface which promotes quicker healing. Postoperative symptoms and tear film instability return to baseline levels within 3 months of the procedure as opposed to flap-LASIK and PRK which becomes a determining factor in patient satisfaction. Patients with mild dry eye symptoms can be preferred for SMILE procedure over other refractive surgeries, also postoperatively preservative free lubricating drops is indispensable.

Diffuse Lamellar Keratitis
Diffuse accumulation of sterile, inflammatory cells under cap in the postoperative period is called diffuse lamellar keratitis (DLK) which is a dreadful complication if not treated efficiently. It appears within 24–48 hours postprocedure however late onset cases are also observed. Its risk factors are glove talc, marking pen, high energy femtosecond laser, atopy, epithelial defects, chemical toxin, bacterial endotoxin on instruments, meibomian gland secretions, thinner lenticule, and larger corneal diameter. However as with other complications its incidence is around 1.6% which is lower than other flap-based

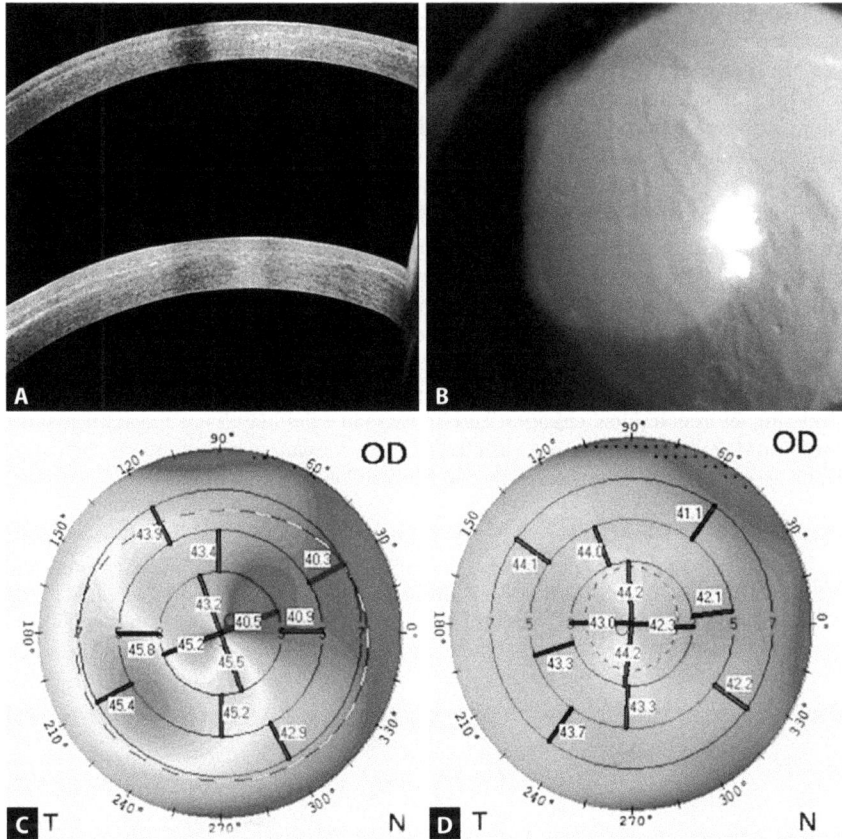

Figs. 5.13.2A to D: (A) Retained lenticule on AS-OCT (marked with arrow); (B) Retained lenticule delineated on retroillumination; (C) Corneal topography showing localized elevation due to retained lenticule; (D) Corneal topography of same patient after removal of the lenticule showing regular corneal surface.

procedures because of factors such as high pulse frequency and lower pulse energy use in SMILE which incites lower inflammation and less keratocyte apoptosis, proliferation, and inflammation. Mild to moderate cases can be well managed with topical corticosteroids and followed within 24–48 hours but severe cases require interface irrigation along with intensive topical steroid regimen.

Infectious Keratitis

Infectious keratitis post-SMILE is a rare occurrence but is a sight-threatening complication which requires prompt treatment. Its incidence is low with few reported cases and risk factors include dry eye, blepharitis, immunocompromised state, contamination of surgical instruments or surroundings, intraoperative epithelial defect, use of contact lens, retreatment, and trauma. Respecting all aseptic precautions becomes mandatory in its avoidance. Management involves thorough interface wash with bactericidal povidone-iodine and antibiotic solution along with aggressive topical antibiotics.

Ectasia

Small incision lenticule extraction procedure is performed in deeper stromal plane sparing anterior corneal stroma which is physiologically stronger due to strongly interwoven, increased density and steeper angles of the collagen bundles which provide better biomechanical stability postprocedure. However, though very few but post-SMILE ectasia cases are reported. It is wise to avoid performing SMILE in patients with abnormal topography or subclinical keratoconus. These cases are managed with collagen cross-linking and visual rehabilitation can be achieved with rigid gas permeable contact lens and intrastromal ring segments if indicated.

Vision-related Problems

Increase in residual error and higher order aberration is noticed in patients with astigmatism >0.75 D due to absence of cyclotorsion correction in SMILE machine which can be overcome by three-point technique in which 0–180° is marked on slit lamp before procedure and after docking the eye is aligned accordingly for optimal outcome.

Myopic regression is also observed after SMILE in patients with high myopia and astigmatism, even though the incidence is comparatively less than FS-LASIK; corneal remodeling, biomechanical changes, and increase in axial length are mechanisms for its cause. VisuMax platform provides with the CIRCLE software which converts the cap into a flap to assess corneal stroma for regression correction using excimer laser.

■ SUGGESTED READING

1. Asif MI, Bafna RK, Mehta JS, Reddy J, Titiyal JS, Maharana PK, Sharma N. Complications of small incision lenticule extraction. Indian J Ophthalmol. 2020;68(12):2711-22.
2. Krueger RR, Meister CS. A review of small incision lenticule extraction complications. Curr Opin Ophthalmol. 2018;29(4):292-8.

5.14 | Small Incision Lenticule Extraction

Krishana Prasad Kudlu, Aparna Nayak N
Prasad Netralaya, Udupi, Karnataka
krishprasadk73@yahoo.com, meandyoureyes@gmail.com

■ INTRODUCTION

Refractive lenticule extraction has made a major breakthrough in the field of refractive surgery where it has become a successful alteration to a femtosecond laser-assisted in situ keratomileusis (FS-LASIK) which is a flap-based procedure, thereby circumventing the need of photoablation using the excimer laser. More than 7 million SMILE (small incision lenticule extraction) procedures have been performed till date by >2,500 surgeons in 80 different countries (Carl Zeiss, Meditec).[1]

The first lenticule-based procedure named RELEx (refractive lenticule extraction) was introduced in 1996 where the lenticule was created using picosecond laser and was removed after creating and lifting a flap.[2] Thorough manual dissection was required which resulted in irregular surface. A shift to femtosecond laser improved its accuracy. In 2000, Food and Drug Administration (FDA) approved femtosecond laser use in ophthalmology as intralaser pulsion. It was initially used in corneal lamellar surgery and in 2001 became commercially available for the creation of corneal flap. In 2008, FDA approval was obtained for femtosecond LASIK. In the same year, Sekundo et al. described a method of creating intrastromal femto-based lenticule and its extraction by lifting a flap similar to that of LASIK flap (FLEX)[3] and this technique further evolved to the present-day SMILE in 2010 where the refractive lenticule is extracted through a small side cut incision (2–5 mm). Initially Sekundo described extraction of intrastromal refractive lenticule via two small cut incisions of 80°, placed 180° apart. The entire procedure of lenticule dissection and extraction is challenging, but the incidence of micro striae and dry eyes are minimal, owing to excellent structural stability. SMILE was commercially introduced in 2011 which used a frequency of 200 kHz. VisuMax femtosecond laser received FDA approval for SMILE in September 2016. SMILE is approved to treat myopia up to -10 D astigmatism up to -5.00 D.[1] SMILE is said to have similar effects as that of FS-LASIK with more beneficial effects such as better biomechanical stability, faster recovery of postoperative dry eye, faster healing, and reinnervation of corneal nerves.[4]

Small incision lenticule extraction is comparable with femto-LASIK in terms of safety, predictability, and efficacy. SMILE is said to be biomechanically stable and maintains good ocular surface health compared to femto-LASIK. It provides excellent visual acuity and quality and is increasingly being preferred for the treatment of myopia and myopic astigmatism. Compared to femto-LASIK, learning curve of SMILE is more and might be challenging for beginners. Hence, observation, training in wet laboratory, and even flap-based lenticule extraction may help the beginner to get familiarized with the procedure. Incidence of complication may be high in the initial learning period mainly while dealing with lenticule extraction and dissection. Work-up and planning is similar to that of femto-LASIK.

CHANGES AFTER SMALL INCISION LENTICULE EXTRACTION

Biomechanical Changes

Flap-based procedures result in vertical transection of the collagen lamellae in the anterior and peripheral stroma which is less stable biomechanically. SMILE on the other hand causes transection of the anterior collagen lamellae only in localized region of cap cut, thereby preserving major anterior and peripheral collagen after the procedure.[5] There has been noted to have decreased corneal hysteresis and corneal resistance factor post-SMILE surgery.[6,7] These changes are lesser compared to that of flap-based procedures. Intraocular pressure (IOP) measurements are said to be more stable after SMILE than flap-based procedures due to good biomechanical stability.[8]

Functional Changes

Transection of the sub-basal corneal nerves results in reduced corneal sensation, affects the tear secretion as well as reduces the blinking frequency. These factors contribute to postoperative dry eye leading to poor ocular surface health. Central cornea showed reduced corneal sensation after SMILE, they begin to recover in the first month and gradually return to normal values by 6-12 months.[9,10] When compared to flap-based procedures, the nerve damage is relatively lesser in SMILE and has lesser effect on postoperative dry eyes.[4] Ocular surface symptoms appear post-SMILE using the Ocular Surface Disease Index (OSDI). The OSDI returns to baseline in majority of patients by the end of 1 month. Ocular surface instability is observed after SMILE and showed decreased tear breakup time (TBUT) and increased FS staining of corneal surfaces, overall symptoms are lesser in SMILE compared to LASIK.[11]

MACHINE PRINCIPLE

The VisuMax machine works on the principle of photo-disruption where femtosecond laser machines use near infrared lasers which use pulses of duration to the order of 10-15 seconds which has minimal collateral tissue damage. These laser pulses form a plasma of free electrons and ionized molecules and this phenomenon is called laser-induced optical breakdown (LIOB). This plasma expansion results in cavitation bubbles which increase in size and coalesce, which allows separation of tissue with minimal damage to the surrounding.

Components of the VisuMax Machine

- *Computer unit:* Mainly to feed the treatment data. Left screen is for treatment planning and live monitoring and right-hand screen displays progression of treatment.

- *Laser arm and vacuum system:* Laser arm directs the laser from the laser unit to the exit aperture. The vacuum system provides attachment for contact lens onto the laser aperture and fixes the eye on the contact lens of the treatment pack.
- *Microscope:* Different illumination systems are incorporated in the machine including diffuse, infrared, and slit system. There is a patient interface consisting of a disposable contact lens with an attached tubing system that forms an interface between the patient's cornea and the machine and is called the treatment pack.
- *Treatment pack:* The size depends on white-to-white (WTW) diameter of the patient. In standard cases WTW around 10–12 mm the size is usually small (S). To ensure a good suction, choosing the right treatment pack is of utmost importance.
- *Foot switch:* It controls femto-laser delivery.

MACHINE AND LASER SETTINGS

The VisuMax laser system delivers a frequency of 500 kHz and a wavelength of 1,043 nm in a spiral pattern creating an intrastromal refractive lenticule with a calculated depth and precision. It also has an in-built application for Flex, circle software, flap, keratoplasty, Intacs along with Relex SMILE. Accurate entry of data into the system is important in treatment planning.

There are three modes of laser settings:
1. *The standard mode:* Programmed by the manufactures as the default setting.
2. *The fast mode:* This mode is customized according to the geographic region and can be altered only by application specialists.
3. *The expert mode:* This can be altered by the surgeon as and when required as per the surgeons need and patients' response. It is recommended to contact the application specialist in the initial learning phase.

Laser Setting Selection

- *Spot spacing:* Distance between two adjacent laser spots. It ranges from 1 to 4.5 μm.
- *Track spacing:* Distance between two laser spots in adjacent tracks. It ranges from 2 to 4.5 μm.
- *Pulse energy:* Defines the size of the cavitation bubbles during the femtosecond laser cuts. Ranges from 100 to 160 nJ.

Lenticule Parameters

- *Optical zone:* It usually ranges from 5 to 8 mm. It is selected based on pupil size and usually kept at 6–6.5 mm for average corneal diameters of 10–12 mm.
- *Transition zone:* It is inbuilt and depends on refraction. In pure spherical errors it is zero and any refractive error with cylinder it is 0.1 mm.
- *Lenticule diameter:* It is the additional sum of optical zone and the transition zone.
- *Minimum lenticule thickness:* It refers to the peripheral edge of the lenticule. This can be preset while the central thickness varies with refractive error.
- *Total lenticule thickness:* It is the sum of minimum thickness of the lenticule and the amount of tissue that will be removed based on the amount if refractive error.

Cap Parameters

- *Cap thickness:* 120 μm
- *Cap diameter:* 7–8 mm (1 mm over the lenticule diameter)
- *Lenticule diameter:* 6–7 mm (based on mesopic pupil size)
- *Cap side cut (entry):* 4–5 mm (two side cuts can be used instead of one)
- *Minimum thickness of the lenticule:* 10–15 μm for higher refractive errors and 25–30 μm for low refractive errors.

SURGICAL TECHNIQUES

- *Counseling and informed consent:* A thorough counseling is mandatory and delivery of realistic expectations to the patient has to be planned. Detailed information is conveyed about the pros and cons of the surgery. Informed consent should be documented in a written format. Explain the procedure in detail and address in detail.
- *Preoperative preparation:* Topical antibiotic/betadine is instilled before the surgery.
- *Patient positioning:* The patient is placed in supine position with a right positioning of the head, in the head ring to avoid inadvertent movement during docking resulting in suction loss. In patients having deep nose and a narrow palpebral aperture it might be challenging **(Fig. 5.14.1)**.
- *Docking:* The patient is initially asked to look at a yellow/white light and asked to fixate on it. The conjunctiva is dried using the Merocel sponge and the cornea is made semimoist with no pooling fluid or any dry spots. Then it is shifted to the docking station where the patient is advised to look at a green blinking light. Once the patient interface and cornea comes in contact a tear film is formed, the green light appears clearer. Always check for centration. Once confirmed then suction is activated. One can use infrared light to confirm the docking centration. This is a soft suction created by VisuMax raises IOP only by 35 mm Hg, which is safe. In case of high astigmatism manual cyclotorsion compensation is preferred.
- *Laser application:* The femtosecond laser settings can be modified in expert mode as and when required. The anterior cap thickness is kept at 120 µm (100–160 µm) with minimal lenticule thickness (lenticule edge thickness) of 15 µm (10–30 µm) along with a side cut of 2–5 µm based on surgeons' comfort. An optical zone of 6.5 mm is kept with no transition zone in pure spherical errors and 0.1 in associated astigmatism. Pulse energy is varying at a range of 100–160 µm and it changes from surgeon to surgeon.

    Femtosecond laser creates a refractive intrastromal lenticule. The first lenticule cut **(Fig. 5.14.2)** is from an outside in manner, followed by lenticule side cut **(Fig. 5.14.3)**, and cap cut **(Fig. 5.14.4)** in inside out pattern. In the end the incision cut is made which is around 2–5 mm **(Fig. 5.14.5)**.
- *Dissection and extraction of the lenticule:* Once the femtosecond laser is delivered, a uniform bubble layer is observed in the corneal stroma. Two silver rings appear corresponding to the diameter of the cap cut and lenticule cut which acts as a guide to perform further dissection **(Fig. 5.14.6:** Yellow arrow-outer ring, white arrow, and inner ring). The cap incision is opened using a thin hooked instrument lifting the cap to make sure of being in the anterior plane. The lenticule cut is then identified by an inner silver circle and is dissected by its entire depth to create a small pocket on the periphery of the incision **(Fig. 5.14.7)**. These two channels are created so as to avoid inadvertent mis-dissection of the planes. A blunt dissection is then performed in the anterior plane using the long end of the dissector **(Fig. 5.14.8)**. The posterior plane is approached from the small pocket created earlier and dissected carefully from side wavefront-optimized (WO) side in a windshield wiper fashion equally from both the sides so as not to fold the lenticule over itself **(Fig. 5.14.9)**.

    Once the dissection is complete, the lenticule is extracted by using a lenticule holding forceps and placed on the cornea to look for its integrity. The interface is then irrigated with balanced salt solution and ironed out to avoid any micro-distortions or striae.

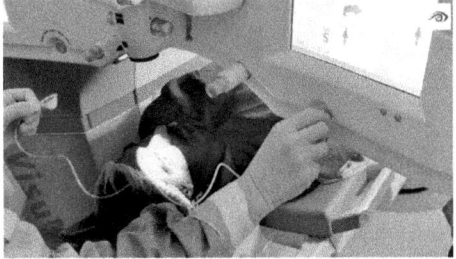

Fig. 5.14.1: VisuMax 500 platform.

SECTION 5: Refractive Surgery

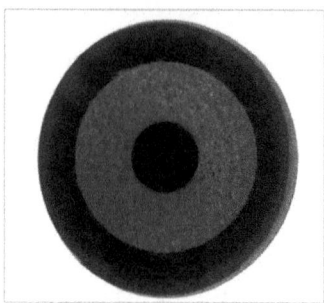

Fig. 5.14.2: Lenticule cut.

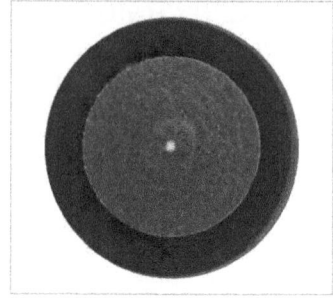

Fig. 5.14.3: Side cut.

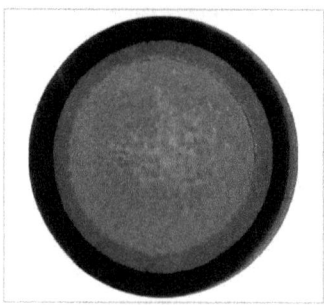

Fig. 5.14.4: Cap cut.

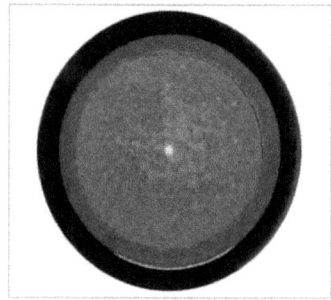

Fig. 5.14.5: Incision.

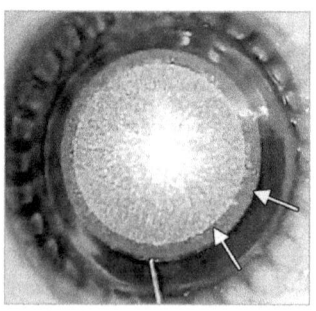

Fig. 5.14.6: Yellow arrow—outer ring—cap cut; White arrow—inner ring—lenticule cut.

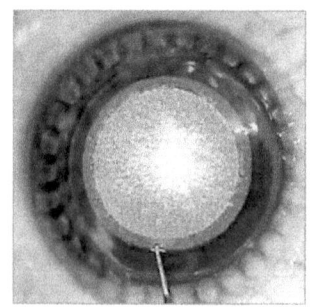

Fig. 5.14.7: Entry

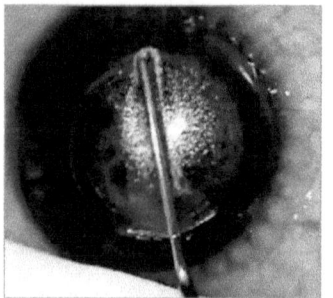

Fig. 5.14.8: Anterior plane dissection.

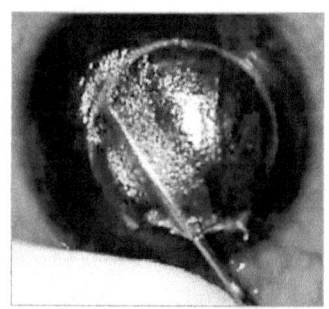

Fig. 5.14.9: Posterior plane dissection.

Using a Merocel sponge the surface of the cap is ironed out from end-to-end to avoid any mismatch between cap and stromal bed.

Complications
Small incision lenticule extraction has comparatively lesser complications than FS-LASIK which has flap-related complications. During the learning phase, one might face difficulties during lenticule dissection and handling. Intraoperative suction loss, difficult extraction of the lenticule, tearing of the lenticule, extension of the side cut has been noted in the initial phase.

Complications that are common to all the refractive procedures include undertreatment, overtreatment, regression, and epithelial erosion. SMILE has greater biomechanical stability and has a lower risk of ectasia.

Advancements
Small incision lenticule extraction VisuMax 800, launched in 2021, is a second generation femtosecond laser with the same laser head and optics as VisuMax (500 kHz). It has a main hardware difference in the femtosecond laser head with an increased pulse frequency of 2,000 kHz, which has reduced the lenticule delineation time from 30 seconds to <10 seconds. Another valuable addition is computerized centration more useful in hyperopic corrections. VisuMax 800 incorporates Centralign and OcuLign software which helps in centration and cyclotorsion compensation. This enables more efficient treatment with 85% of eyes with postoperative cylinder of 0.50 D or less and 19% of eyes with angle of error within ±15° for the VisuMax 800, compared to VisuMax 500, which showed 91% of eyes with postoperative cylinder of 0.50 D or less and 15% of eyes with angle of error within ±15° .5[1]. A study by Dan Rienstien et al. in their study have performed SMILE using the VisuMax 800 with 3 months follow-up in myopes and myopic astigmatism and concluded that VisuMax 800 is safe and an efficacious platform. The results are equivalent to that of VisuMax 500 and a data of large scale with 1 year follow-up will be needed.[1]

CONCLUSION
Small incision lenticule extraction is an efficacious, safe, and predictable surgical procedure. It has excellent visual outcomes and reduced risk of complications and also maintains the ocular surface health and biomechanical stability of the cornea. SMILE has a significant learning curve but is a promising technique once mastered.

REFERENCES
1. Reinstein DZ, Archer TJ, Potter JG, Gupta R, Wiltfang R. Refractive and visual outcomes of SMILE for compound myopic astigmatism with the VISUMAX 800. J Refract Surg. 2023; 39(5):294-301.
2. Ito M, Quantock AJ, Malhan S, Schanzlin DJ, Krueger RR. Picosecond laser in situ keratomileusis with a 1053-nm Nd:YLF laser. J Refract Surg. 1996;12(6):721-28.
3. Sekundo W, Kunert K, Russmann C, Gille A, Bissmann W, Stobrawa G, et al. First efficacy and safety study of femtosecond lenticule extraction for the correction of myopia: six-month results. J Cataract Refract Surg. 2008;34(9):1513-20.
4. Li M, Zhao J, Shen Y, Li T, He L, Xu H, et al. Comparison of Dry Eye and Corneal Sensitivity between Small Incision Lenticule Extraction and Femtosecond LASIK for Myopia. PLoS ONE. 2013;8(10):e77797.
5. Reinstein DZ, Archer TJ, Randleman JB. Mathematical model to compare the relative tensile strength of the cornea after PRK, LASIK, and small incision lenticule extraction. J Refract Surg. 2013;29(7):454-60.
6. Osman IM, Helaly HA, Abdalla M, Shousha MA. Corneal biomechanical changes in eyes with small incision lenticule extraction and laser assisted in situ keratomileusis. BMC Ophthalmol. 2016;16:123.

7. Wu D, Wang Y, Zhang L, Wei S, Tang X. Corneal biomechanical effects: small-incision lenticule extraction versus femtosecond laser-assisted laser in situ keratomileusis. J Cataract Refract Surg. 2014;40(6):954-62.
8. Li H, Wang Y, Dou R, Wei P, Zhang J, Zhao W, et al. Intraocular pressure changes and relationship with corneal biomechanics after SMILE and FS-LASIK. Invest Ophthalmol Vis Sci. 2016;57(10):4180-6.
9. Cai WT, Liu QY, Ren CD, Wei QQ, Liu JL, Wang QY, et al. Dry eye and corneal sensitivity after small incision lenticule extraction and femtosecond laser-assisted in situ keratomileusis: a meta-analysis. Int J Ophthalmol. 2017;10(4):632-8.
10. Shen Z, Zhu Y, Song X, Yan J, Yao K. Dry Eye after Small Incision Lenticule Extraction (SMILE) versus Femtosecond Laser-Assisted in Situ Keratomileusis (FS-LASIK) for myopia: a meta-analysis. PloS One. 2016;11(12):e0168081.
11. Denoyer A, Landman E, Trinh L, Faure JF, Auclin F, Baudouin C. Dry eye disease after refractive surgery: comparative outcomes of small incision lenticule extraction versus LASIK. Ophthalmology. 2015;122(4):669-76.

5.15 Refractive Lens Exchange: Current Perspective

Ritika Sachdev, Kanika Bhardwaj
Centre for Sight
ritikasachdev@gmail.com, drkanikabhardwaj1@gmail.com

INTRODUCTION

Refractive lens exchange (RLE) or clear lens extraction (CLE) or refractive lensectomy has gained immense popularity in the recent years for people with high myopia, high hyperopia, astigmatism, and even presbyopia, who are otherwise unsuitable for laser vision correction (LVC). The procedure involves removal of clear crystalline lens along with replacement by an appropriate power intraocular lens (IOL) and thus is considered under the umbrella of modern-day refractive surgery procedures.

The various indications for RLE in present times are:
- High refractive errors unsuitable for LVC
- High myopes SANS retinal pathologies.
- Moderate to high hyperopes with shallow chambers
- Presbyopes with reduced accommodative capacity (age 40 years and above).
- Children with severe anisometropia or bilateral ametropia.
- Postrefractive surgery residual errors.
- *Dysfunctional lens syndrome (DLS):* It is a broad categorization of the aging changes in the crystalline lens and a comparatively newer indication for RLE.
- *Myopia associated with early-stage keratoconus:* RLE can be offered with customized toric IOL implantation or even in combination with intracorneal rings in patients with stable keratoconus nearing presbyopia.

CONTRAINDICATIONS

Certain ocular pathologies can degrade the quality of the image formed and result in poor vision postoperatively such as:
- Corneal diseases
- Age-related macular degeneration
- Diabetic retinopathy
- Uncontrolled glaucoma
- Risk factors for retinal detachment (advanced peripheral lattice degenerations, lacquer cracks) and ocular inflammatory diseases.

COUNSELING OF A PATIENT UNDERGOING REFRACTIVE LENS EXCHANGE

A detailed discussion needs to be done about the side effects and risks involved in the surgery. In particular, we believe one should discuss with patient about chances of endophthalmitis, chances of retinal detachment and posterior capsule opacification (PCO) formation. The patient undergoing a multifocal IOL should be explained about chances of glare, halos, and other visual phenomenon postsurgery. The patient should also be counseled and assessed preoperatively for a possible need of LVC for minor refractive errors warranting correction post-RLE.

PLANNING A PATIENT FOR REFRACTIVE LENS EXCHANGE

The advancement in surgical technique of cataract extraction as well as the availability of wide array of intraocular lenses including odd power minus lenses, multifocal lenses, accommodative lenses and EDOF (extended depth of focus) lenses has enabled surgeons to provide their patients with good quality vision and independence from glasses. Refer to **Table 5.15.1** for details about various multifocal lenses available.

Detailed lifestyle habits of patient should be taken into account while choosing the type of multifocal IOL implant for the patient. For instance, a patient who is not an avid reader but uses laptop or a desktop screen more for his/her daily activities, an EDOF lens such as Tecnis Symfony may be the preferred choice.

A patient who loves to drive at night and willing to wear reading glasses for some of his daily tasks may be a good candidate for EDOF monofocal IOLs such as Tecnis Eyhance. A patient who does not drive much and is indoor most of the daily routine, fond of reading and is an active user of laptop/desktop screen, may be a good candidate for trifocal lenses such as Carl Zeiss AT Lisa Tri or Alcon PanOptix.

PREOPERATIVE CONSIDERATIONS FOR REFRACTIVE LENS EXCHANGE

The surgical technique of RLE is a variation of standard cataract surgery, the only difference being younger age and presence of clear crystalline lens along with anatomical variation causing high refractive error.

- *Angle kappa:* It is the difference between the pupillary and visual axis. Angle kappa should be part of routine preoperative assessment while planning a patient for multifocal intraocular lens (MFIOL) to reduce incidence of photic phenomenon post-MFIOL implantation. Angle kappa can be measured clinically as well as with help of devices such as synoptophore, *ORBSCAN II*®, *iTrace*®, *LENSTAR*®, and *Pentacam*®.
- *Intraocular lens power calculations:* The most important assessment for successful multifocal lens use requires precise preoperative measurements of axial length and accurate lens power calculations. Optical and immersion ultrasound biometry techniques in combination with the Holladay 2 formula can yield accurate and consistent results. As a final check in the lens power assessment, the SRK-T and the SRK II formulas can also be used or, Hoffer Q formula should be utilized for eyes with axial length <22.0 mm **(Table 5.15.2)**.
- *Special case of irregular corneas:* Accurate estimation of the central corneal refractive power in irregular corneas, such as those that have undergone prior keratorefractive surgery, is difficult and requires adjustments.
  - *Post-RK (radial keratotomy) patients:* Standard keratometers assume a certain relationship between anterior and posterior corneal curvature and take measurements for a larger optical zone. This leads to falsely high corneal power results which in turn lead to falsely low IOL power results. Thus, it is important to correct for the errors in true corneal power measurements by using EK readings from Pentacam maps.

TABLE 5.15.1: Properties of various types of multifocal IOLs available.

Company	Type of model MFIOL		Addition (D)/ DOF (IOL plane)	Material	Spherical aberration (μm)
			Bifocal		
J&J	Diffractive	Tecnis	2.75, 3.25, 4.00	Hydrophobic acrylic	−0.27
Alcon	Diffractive	AcrySof Restot	2.50	Hydrophobic acrylic	−0.20
Alcon	Diffractive	AcrySof Restot	3.00, 4.00	Hydrophobic acrylic	−0.10
Zeiss	Diffractive	AT LISA 809	3.75	Hydrophilic acrylic with hydrophobic surface	−0.18
			Trifocal		
Alcon	Diffractive	AcrySof PanOptix	3.25 (N)–2.75 (I)	Hydrophobic acrylic	−0.10
Zeiss	Diffractive	AT LISA Tri 839MP	3.33 (N)–1.66 (I)	Hydrophilic acrylic with hydrophobic surface	−0.18
			EDOF		
Zeiss	Diffractive	AT LISA	2.00, 2.25*	Hydrophilic acrylic with hydrophobic surface	0.0
J&J	Diffractive	Symfony	1.25 to 2.50*	Hydrophobic acrylic	N/A
J&J	Diffractive	Synergy	0.00 to 3.75*	Hydrophobic acrylic	N/A
Alcon	Non-diffractive	AcrySof Vivity	2.00*	Hydrophobic acrylate/ Methacrylate Copolymer	−0.20
			Pseudo-EDOF Monofocal		
J&J	Refractive	Eyhance	1.5*	Hydrophobic acrylic	N/A

TABLE 5.15.2: IOL calculation criteria depending upon axial length.

Criteria	Axial length <22.0 mm	Axial length 22.0 mm	Axial length 24.5 mm	Axial length >26.0 mm
1st choice formula	HOFFER-Q, HAIGIS	SRK-T, HAIGIS	SRK-T, HAIGIS	SRK-T, HAIGIS
2nd choice formula	HOLLADAY II	HOLLADAY	HOLLADAY	—

- *Post-LVC patients:* Unlike RK surgery, LVC surgeries alter only the anterior corneal curvature. This leads to an alteration in the ratio of anterior-posterior corneal curvature. The standard keratometers, measure only the anterior corneal curvature and presume the posterior corneal curvature to be of standard normal value. This leads to false estimation of the anterior-posterior corneal curvature ratio and therefore, inaccurate true corneal power measurement. Thus, it is important to use instruments which actually measure both anterior and posterior curvature independently (like Pentacam, IOL master 700) and thus, will be able to give an actual true net power in such cases.

Intraoperative considerations for a patient undergoing RLE with MFIOL implantation:
- *Incision:* The aim is to minimize surgically induced astigmatism, which can be achieved by decreasing the size of incision. With the advent of minimal incision cataract surgery (MICS), the incision size has been reduced to <2 mm. The foldable MFIOLs available can be implanted through incision as small as 1.8 mm. One should always prefer a clear corneal incision with a tunnel of at least 2 mm length to reduce chances of postoperative hypotony, endophthalmitis, etc. Posterior limbal incision or scleral incision is preferred particularly in post-RK patients to prevent opening of RK scars during surgery. One should aim to keep the width of incision <3 mm to ensure SIA <0.5 D.
- *Capsulorhexis:* The ideal size of capsulorhexis is 5 mm, to ensure adequate overlap of capsulorhexis around IOL optic edge. In addition, capsulorhexis should be well centered. This helps in ensuring the IOL is well centered and to avoid IOL tilt. Tilting of IOL in such cases can lead to higher incidence of glare and halos and in certain cases can lead to loss of multifocality as well.
- *Hydrodissection and hydrodelineation:* Careful and gentle hydrodissection is important in these cases to ensure better cortical removal and thus decrease the incidence of PCO formation.
- *Phacoemulsification:* Myopia is more commonly corrected refractive error than hyperopia. Myopic eyes are known to have deep AC, vitreous liquification, weak zonular support and increased lens thickness. At the start of phacoemulsification, there can be sudden deepening of AC on inserting the phacoemulsification probe because of weak zonular support and vitreous liquefaction. In such a situation, the surgeon should consider decreasing the bottle height. During phacoemulsification, the surgeon can expect increased surge and fluttering movement of the posterior capsule due to poor support from the vitreous jelly. Thus, it is advisable to perform phacoemulsification at low vacuum parameters and ensuring a maintained AC during surgery in such cases. After the emulsification of the nuclear fragments, it is important to perform a meticulous cortical clean up and polishing of the posterior capsule in such cases. Due to increased lens thickness and higher volume of the capsular bag, the incidence of PCO formation is higher in myopic eyes. In addition, any residual posterior capsular plaque can cause increased incidence of glare, halos, and other visual phenomena.
- *Intraocular lens implantation:* To achieve best results, it is important to ensure centration of the IOL. After implanting the IOL, one should always make sure the optic as well as both haptic are in the bag and the optic edges are covered well with the capsulorhexis margin, so that IOL does not get tilted.

RECENT ADVANCES IN CATARACT SURGERY TECHNIQUE
- *Femto laser-assisted cataract surgery (FLACS)* can provide excellent outcomes with augmented safety in RLE. Precise incisions with desired size and position, well centered regular capsulorhexis, intraoperative anterior segment optical coherence tomography (ASOCT) guided nuclear fragmentation, astigmatic corrections with limbal relaxing incisions, and toric alignment marking can be achieved flawlessly in a matter for few seconds (<30 seconds) with the use of FLACS.

- *Toric intraocular lenses:* These can correct astigmatic errors and even can be customized to correct irregular astigmatism. Preoperative corneal marking of implantation axes can be achieved using manual markers on slit lamp, bubble marker as well as intraoperative alignment systems such as *Verion* (Alcon) and *Callisto* (Zeiss).
- *Active Fluidics system (AFS):* This system in a phacoemulsification machine is said to provide stable anterior chamber parameters intraoperatively. It monitors intraocular pressure (IOP) at all times and compresses or decompresses the balanced salt solution (BSS) fluid bag with two metal plates and adjusts the perfusion flow in time to maintain IOP.

CONCLUSION

To summarize, we can safely pronounce that refractive lens exchange (RLE) can serve as an enhanced and sophisticated method of refractive surgery in a myriad of indications and despairing candidates who have been deemed unfit for other methods of refractive correction procedures. However, the most important role here to play is of the surgeons, for their planning and patient selection must be meticulous keeping in mind the risk versus benefit ratio. The role of good preoperative counseling can never be undermined. While modern day procedures are highly effective and safe, but the cognizance of possible complications should always be at the back of the surgeon's mind and help in making informed decisions.

SUGGESTED READING

1. Alió JL, Grzybowski A, Romaniuk D. Refractive lens exchange in modern practice: when and when not to do it? Eye Vis (Lond). 2014;1:10.
2. Kaweri L, Wavikar C, James E, Pandit P, Bhuta N. Review of current status of refractive lens exchange and role of dysfunctional lens index as its new indication. Indian J Ophthalmol. 2020;68(12):2797-803.

5.16 Retreatment Options Following Refractive Surgery

Chitra Ramamurthy, Soundarya B
The Eye Foundation
drchitra@theeyefoundation.com, soundslikeme@gmail.com

INTRODUCTION

Regression following refractive surgery is a multifactorial entity with risk factors ranging from high refractive errors, thin residual stromal beds, small optic zones, higher astigmatism, older age group, presence of dry eye disease to progression of axial length with myopic shift, latent hyperopia unravelling postprocedure, and lenticular myopic shifts.

The incidence of regression tends to be slightly higher with microkeratome laser in situ keratomileusis (LASIK) when compared to femtosecond LASIK which could be due to the meniscus configuration of the flaps when compared to the planar configuration in femtosecond flaps. When compared to flap-based procedures, some studies have shown a lower incidence of regression following small incision lenticule extraction (SMILE).

PATHOPHYSIOLOGY

The pathophysiological responses of the epithelium and stroma play an important role in regression, which include epithelial hyperplasia and remodeling with inflammatory cascades and altered reinnervation patterns increasing these epithelial changes, as does the creation of steeper surface gradients resulting from high myopic/astigmatic and hyperopic corrections. Stromal biomechanical response and a reduced tensile strength are other contributing responses.

▪ EVALUATION

Patient evaluation begins with a thorough slit lamp examination to note the flap architecture, centration, hinge characteristics, flap edge definition, presence of fibrosis, etc. Corneal topography is mandatory to estimate pachymetry and keratometry values, to look for an irregular surface and to rule out ectasia. Other investigative modalities that are useful are aberrometry to note the higher order aberrations and anterior segment optical coherence tomography (ASOCT) to measure flap thickness.

Epithelial thickness mapping is particularly useful to look at the remodeling patterns and to assess the amount of epithelium to be removed in cases planned for enhancement by surface ablation. Biometry can be done to rule out progression seen as an elongation in axial length. Dry eye evaluation also becomes an integral part of work-up in these patients, which helps in adequately treating it before planning for an enhancement procedure.

▪ RETREATMENT OPTIONS

Options for treating regression depend on factors such as type of primary procedure, presence of significant epithelial hyperplasia or corneal surface irregularities, thickness of cornea available for recorrection, and duration of presentation following primary procedure.

The various available procedures include:
- Flap lift
- Flap recut
- Surface ablations which can be done post LASIK/SMILE/surface ablation/radial keratotomy
- Surface ablations in combination with corneal collagen cross-linking (CXL)
- Cap to flap conversion following SMILE
- Thin flap LASIK over the cap of SMILE
- SMILE over SMILE
- Phakic intraocular lens implantation

Flap Lift

Flap lift is generally advised when the duration from primary procedure is within 3 years. Although a flap lift can be done even beyond this cut off point, the higher incidence of epithelial ingrowth has to be kept in mind. Defining the flap edges preoperatively with the help of marking aids in the smooth lift of flap without surrounding epithelial disruption, that reduces the chances of epithelial in growth. If flap lift considered beyond 3 years interval, it may be prudent to debride epithelium beyond the flap margin all around. It is advisable to avoid lifting very thin, button holed or irregular flaps with low hinges.

Flap Recut

Flap recut is done if the original flap is decentered or small. A deeper and larger diameter flap is the ideal. The presence of different planes can result in flap fragmentation and also irregular astigmatism and loss of best corrected vision, thus it is usually not a preferred option.

Surface Ablation

Surface ablation has been a reliable and safe option in all situations. It can be carried out using the wavefront optimized or topography-guided approach. Mitomycin can be used in order to address the haze resulting from the migratory fibroblast proliferation. It can also be combined with low or half fluence CXL in eyes with borderline corneal thickness to prevent ectasia and in cases of hyperopic ablations to prevent further regression.

Retreatment Options Following SMILE

The choice of approach depends on the degree of enhancement required, the depth of anterior cap, residual stromal thickness following primary SMILE and also the patient's desire to maintain flaplessness.

The various options for retreatment following SMILE include:
- Surface ablation
- Thin flap LASIK
- Secondary SMILE
- Sub-cap lenticule extraction
- Circle software—cap to flap
- Phakic intraocular lens

Surface Ablation

Surface ablation in the form of photorefractive keratectomy (PRK) is currently the most commonly preferred option due to the ease at which it can be done. Wavefront optimized or topography-guided approaches can be used as mentioned before. In eyes with irregular astigmatism, a topography-guided treatment provides desirable outcomes by regularizing the corneal surface thus reducing the higher order aberrations and improving visual quality. It can be either combined with or followed sequentially by a wavefront optimized PRK at a later date to address the residual refractive error once the cornea is stabilized.

Photorefractive keratectomy carries the advantage of being flapless and it also preserves corneal biomechanical stability. The drawbacks of PRK include a slower visual recovery, patient discomfort in terms of pain and chances of haze formation.

Thin Flap LASIK

This procedure needs a minimum cap thickness of 120–130 µ. Care has to be taken while planning in order to not impinge on the original interface, which can end up with irregular astigmatism and a loss in best corrected visual acuity. If the space between the respective cleavage planes, that the enhancement flap and the original cap is too small, the bubbles may create punctures in the corneal stroma during migration. Thus gas bubble breakthroughs and buttonholes need to be avoided.

Secondary SMILE

There is limited experience with this option till date. It can be done anterior or posterior to the primary SMILE. When planned anteriorly, the primary SMILE should have had a thicker cap than the correction planned for the retreatment.

SMILE to FLAP—The CIRCLE Software

Here, three new cuts are created as follows:
1. An incision plane encircling the original cap cut as a lamellar ring.
2. A side cut with a hinge around the new incision plane.
3. A junction cut, which allows the original cap and the new incision plane to be part of one larger surface **(Fig. 5.16.1)**.

The major drawback involved in this procedure is the higher cost involved and also the loss of the flapless advantage of SMILE.

Phakic Intraocular Lens Implantation

This procedure is preferred in cases with larger residual errors, which cannot be corrected using keratorefractive options that would either lead to a corneal biomechanical instability or end up with further regression postoperatively. It can also be done in

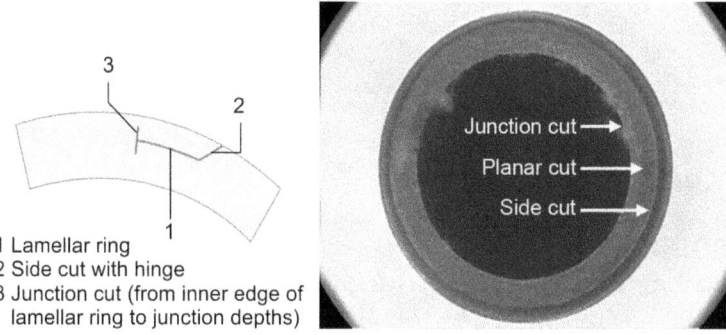

1 Lamellar ring
2 Side cut with hinge
3 Junction cut (from inner edge of lamellar ring to junction depths)

Fig. 5.16.1: Cuts used in SMILE.

cases of progression of myopia, provided that the error has remained stable for at least 6 months–1 year.

Phakic intraocular lenses obviate all challenges associated with flap and cap management. The major disadvantages include the fact that it is a surgical intraocular procedure and it carries its own set of complications such as the risk of development of cataract, glaucoma, etc.

COMPLICATIONS OF RETREATMENTS

Each of the above-mentioned methods carries its own set of unique complications.
- It is important to anticipate *epithelial ingrowth* in cases of flap lifts and to strategize appropriate treatment protocols.
- *Haze* in cases of PRK has to be prevented and managed adequately.
- The risk of *ectasia* increases postretreatments and this has to be kept in mind by the surgeon and has to be informed to the patient as well. Thus the need for periodic follow-up has to be emphasized.
- The risk of *diffuse lamellar keratitis (DLK)* also may be higher following retreatments and has to be anticipated. Even in PRK following SMILE DLK can be expected in the primary interface.
- As with any ocular procedures, the rare occurrence of *infections* is always a possibility, especially in cases of surface ablations. Timely management and evaluation can help in preventing any vision threatening complications.
- The chances of *dry eye* may also be higher following retreatments and patient comfort has to be kept in mind while managing.

CONCLUSION

It is important to adequately assess the patients before taking them up for retreatments and also to make sure that the refractive error is stable. Proper choice of method becomes very important in providing a good visual outcome in these patients.

SUGGESTED READING

1. Chansue E, Tanehsakdi M, Swasdibutra S, McAlinden C. Safety and efficacy of VisuMax® circle patterns for flap creation and enhancement following small incision lenticule extraction. Eye Vis (Lond). 2015;2:21.
2. Liu YC, Rosman M, Mehta JS. Enhancement after small-incision lenticule extraction: incidence, risk factors, and outcomes. Ophthalmology. 2017;124(6):813-21.
3. Lyle WA, Jin GJ. Retreatment after initial laser in situ keratomileusis. J Cataract Refract Surg. 2000;26(5):650-9.

5.17 Corneal Procedures for Correction of Presbyopia

Sri Ganesh, Sheetal Brar
Nethradhama Superspeciality Eye Hospital, Bengaluru
chairman@nethradhama.org

■ INTRODUCTION

Presbyopia correction is the holy grail of refractive surgery. An ideal presbyopia correcting procedure should be able to improve functional near vision to adequate levels without causing a drop in distant vision or inducing collateral symptoms. It should be minimally invasive, easy to perform, stable over time, and be reversible or adjustable.

Presbyopia procedures can be broadly classified into:
- *Cornea-based procedures:*
  - Additive procedures—corneal inlays, tissue addition
  - Subtractive procedures—laser-assisted in situ keratomileusis (LASIK) procedures including monovision, multifocal LASIK, and laser blended vision (Presbyond)
  - Molding techniques—LTK and CK
- *Lens-based procedures:*
  - Refractive lens exchange with multifocal/EDOF intraocular lenses (IOLs)
  - Presbyopic phakic IOLs
- *Sclera-based procedures:*
  - Scleral incision
  - Scleral expansion

In this chapter, we will discuss the most performed and popular cornea-based procedures for correction of presbyopia.

Most of the presbyopia correcting corneal procedures work by increasing the depth of focus which improves the defocus tolerance mechanism of the eye. For a given setting of an optical system (or a steady state of accommodation) it is the range distance in the retinal field, over which the image of an improperly focused object is acceptably sharp. Depth of field, however, is the distance over which an object may be moved without causing a reduction in sharpness beyond a certain tolerable amount. Depth of field and depth of focus can also be used interchangeably while describing the defocus tolerance of the eye.

Depth of focus serves an important function of defocus tolerance and can effectively reduce the required amount of accommodative effort to focus on targets moving through a range of distances without causing the perception of blur.

■ CORNEAL INLAYS

Jose Barraquer first introduced corneal inlay for the treatment of high myopia using polymethyl methacrylate (PMMA).[1] With newer designs, materials, and femtosecond

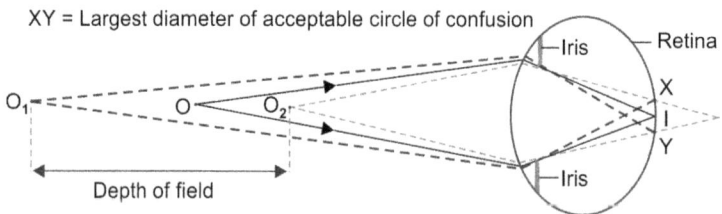

Fig. 5.17.1: DOField relates to the object plane and DOFocus images formed in the retinal plane (DOF).

TABLE 5.17.1: Comparison of three corneal inlays.

	Diameter	Thickness	Flap, pocket placement	Mechanism of action	Centration	Material
Raindrop	2 mm	32 μm	120–200 μm	Increase central radius of curvature of overlying cornea	Central overlight constricted pupil	Hydrogel
Flexivue Microlens	3 mm	15–20 μm	280–300 μm	Corneal multifocality (distance vision through a piano central zone surrounded by rings of varying additional power)	Placement over the first Purkinje image	Hydroxyethyl methacrylate and methyl methacrylate
KAMRA	3.8 mm with 1.6 mm central aperture	5 μm	200–250 μm	Increase depth of focus with pinhole principle	Placement over the first Purkinje image	Polyvinylidene fluoride

Source: Reproduced from—Moarefi MA, Bafna S, Wiley W. A review of presbyopia treatment with corneal inlays. Ophthalmol Ther. 2017; 6(1):55-65.[2]

lasers to aid in creating flap/pocket, the success rate of treating presbyopia with corneal inlays has greatly increased. The advantage of corneal inlays is the fact that they do not remove corneal tissue and hence are reversible. Currently corneal inlays are implanted in the nondominant eye of a patient with emmetropia producing a modified monovision effect. Majority of patients lose only one or no lines of distance vision for about a 5-6-line improvement in near vision **(Table 5.17.1)**.

Some of the intrinsic drawbacks faced by small aperture optics are only about 20% of the incident light passes through the disc's central aperture, as much as 5% of incident light is diffracted by the disc's micro holes and there is reduced binocular symmetry and stereoacuity. Though KAMRA has a good efficacy, the explantation in the literature ranges from 1.5 to 10%. In the original FDA trial, the vast majority of explantations were due to refractive shifts mostly hyperopic or dissatisfaction with visual outcomes.

ALLOGENIC CORNEAL IMPLANTS

Recently, the TransForm Corneal Allografts, which are allogenic lenticules obtained from eye bank and processed by Allotex into 2.50 D add lenses with a diameter of 2.65 mm and a central thickness of around 29 μm have been investigated for potential management of presbyopia.

In addition, the presbyopic allogenic refractive lenticule (PEARL) implantation procedure using a lenticule of suitable thickness obtained from a myopic patient undergoing small incision lenticule extraction (SMILE) procedure has also shown to provide promising results.

Presbyopic LASIK

Presbyopic LASIK using an aspheric ablation profile, increases the depth of field of the eye and allows monovision to treat presbyopia in combination with myopia, hyperopia, and emmetropia.

There are three main types of multifocal corneal excimer laser profiles: Multifocal transition profile.

This technique created a transitional vertical multifocal ablation based on an intentional decentration of a hyperopic ablation profile. There are very few reports on this technique, and it was not well accepted by surgeons because it induced significant levels of vertical coma.

Peripheral PresbyLASIK

In peripheral presbyLASIK, peripheral cornea is ablated for near, and the center is left for distance **(Fig. 5.17.2A)**. In myopes undergoing peripheral presbyLASIK, a significant amount of corneal tissue must be removed to create a hypernegative ablation profile. Thus, peripheral presbyLASIK is typically performed in presbyopic hyperopes or presbyopic low myopes.

Central PresbyLASIK

This technique creates a hyperpositive area for the near vision at the center, and the periphery is left for far vision **(Fig. 5.17.2B)**. An advantage is that it can be performed in the corneal center in myopic and hyperopic profiles, and in emmetropes with minimal excision. Main limitation is the lack of adequate alignment among the line of sight, the central pupil, and the corneal vertex, inducing coma aberrations.

Supracor

The Supracor (Bausch and Lomb Technolas, Germany) algorithm creates topographic profiles wherein there is an elevation in the center of the cornea for good reading vision (center-near) and flatter topography toward the periphery for good intermediate and distance vision. Thus, it creates a varifocal cornea where there is a 12-µm elevation in the central 3 mm of the cornea to give a near addition of approximately two diopters (D). Currently, the treatment is CE marked for use in correction of moderate hyperopia.

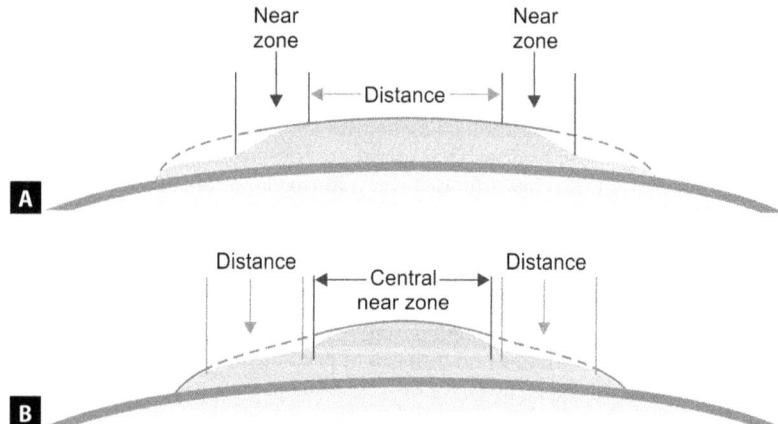

Figs. 5.17.2A and B: (A) In peripheral presbyLASIK, the center of the cornea is treated for distance vision and the periphery for near; (B) In central presbyLASIK, the center of the cornea is treated for near vision and the periphery for distance vision.

Supracor being a LASIK-based algorithm, has the advantage of correcting refractive error and presbyopia in a single procedure.

PresbyMAX

PresbyMAX (SCHWIND eye-tech-solutions GmbH, Kleinostheim, Germany) is based on the creation of a biaspheric multifocal corneal surface with a central hyperpositive area to achieve +0.75 to +2.50 D of near vision correction, surrounded by an area in which the ablation is calculated to correct the distance refractive error **(Fig. 5.17.3)**. Luger et al. reported using PresbyMAX treatment in myopes and hyperopes with or without astigmatism and published the outcomes of a year follow-up. 70% of patients had UDVA of 0.1 logMAR or better, 84% had UNVA of 0.1 logRAD or better, and 85% of patients had UDVA of 0.2 logMAR and UNVA of 0.2 logRAD or better. 3% of the eyes lost two lines of CDVA and 8% of the eyes lost two lines of corrected near visual acuity (CNVA).

Presbyond Laser Blended Vision

Traditional LASIK monovision was shown to be associated with side effects such as poor intermediate vision, reduced contrast sensitivity, loss of stereopsis, increased photic phenomena, and longer adaptation time; all factors potentially reducing patient satisfaction.

Presbyond Laser Blended Vision (LBV),[3] performed with MEL 80 excimer laser and the CRS-Master successfully combines monovision with extended depth of field achieved by aspheric laser ablation profile using a micro-monovision protocol to treat presbyopia.

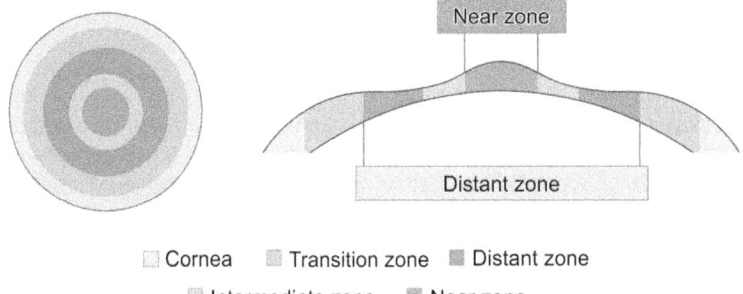

Fig. 5.17.3: Schematic diagram and cross-section of the cornea showing distant, intermediate, and near vision zone after PresbyMax treatment.

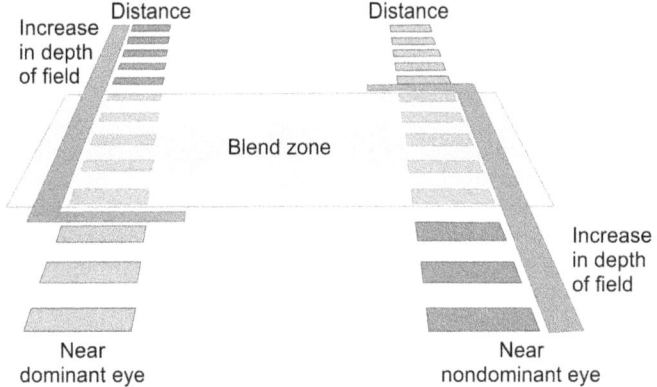

Fig. 5.17.4: Principle of laser blended vision/Presbyond.

LBV involves a combination of controlled induced corneal spherical aberrations and a micro-monovision protocol. In Presbyond LBV, the software targets a micro-monovision with mild myopia of −1.50 D or less for the near eye, irrespective of age. In addition, the optimized aspheric ablation profile is intended to increase the depth of field of each eye, within the safe limits of up to 1.50 D by inducing a controlled amount of spherical aberration, and as a result provides a blend zone to enable continuous distance to intermediate to near vision between the two eyes.

This procedure has been shown to be safe and effective across all types for ametropia, without a significant loss of contrast sensitivity.[3,4]

MOLDING PROCEDURES

These procedures are obsolete now for presbyopia correction, however, are discussed briefly here.

Sclera Based

The idea behind the scleral approaches is that radial slits in the sclera (radial sclerotomy) or PMMA scleral expansion bands inserted into four scleral tunnel incisions overlying the ciliary muscle will expand the diameter of the sclera over the ciliary muscle. These scleral surgical procedures are, however, prone to complications, such as thin scleral pockets and extrusion of the bands, anterior chamber perforation, ischemia, scleral thinning, and axial myopia, due to which these procedures have gone into disrepute.

Cornea Based

Many corneal surgical procedures are being used to alleviate the symptoms of presbyopia. These include thermal keratoplasty and conductive keratoplasty.

Thermal Keratoplasty

The idea of thermokeratoplasty, the refractive reshaping of the cornea from the application of heat, has been attempted in several ways. S Fyodorov, used a nichrome wire probe heated to 600°C for 0.3 seconds, the depth of which was set by ultrasonic pachymetry to 90% of corneal thickness. Applications were made in a series of radial spots in the corneal midperiphery in a surgical strategy they termed *radial thermal keratoplasty*. However, the technique was confounded by lack of predictability and regression of effect. In a series by these same investigators, there was an 80% regression in effect at 1 year. Various lasers such as holmium:YAG (Ho:YAG), CO_2 lasers and diode lasers have been used for this purpose, all of these suffering from common pitfalls of unpredictability and regression of results.

Conductive Keratoplasty

Conductive keratoplasty consists of application of high-frequency, low-energy electric current to shrink corneal collagen. In the CK procedure, radio frequency energy is produced at a fundamental frequency of 350 kHz.

Postoperatively at 1 year, 35% (37 eyes) were J1 or better and 77% were J3 (82 eyes) or better. Measuring binocular near visual acuity, 42% (45 patients) were J1 or better and 80% (85 patients) were J3 or better.

The authors concluded that near visual function improved without loss of distance function in many patients, possibly potentiated by the changes in corneal optics. However, a perceived loss of binocularity and depth perception may lead to patient dissatisfaction.

TAKE HOME MESSAGE

Presbyopic treatments are still evolving, and successful management of presbyopia is still a challenge. However, various technological advancements in this field have resulted in improved safety, efficacy, and stability of results and improved patient satisfaction.

REFERENCES

1. Barraquer JI. Modification of refraction by means of intracorneal inclusions. Int Ophthalmol Clin. 1966;6(1):53-78.
2. Moarefi MA, Bafna S, Wiley W. A review of presbyopia treatment with corneal inlays. Ophthalmol Ther. 2017; 6(1):55-65.
3. Reinstein DZ, Couch DG, Archer TJ. LASIK for hyperopic astigmatism and presbyopia using micro-monovision with the Carl Zeiss Meditec MEL80 platform. J Refract Surg. 2009;25(1):37-58.
4. Ganesh S, Brar S, Gautam M, Sriprakash K. Visual and refractive outcomes following laser blended vision using non-linear aspheric micro-monovision. J Refract Surg. 2020; 36(5):300-07.

5.18 | Surface Ablation

Komal B Patekar, Shreesha Kumar Kodavoor
The Eye Foundation, Coimbatore
komalbpatekarsss@gmail.com, eskay_03@rediffmail.com

INTRODUCTION

Surface ablation is a procedure in which excimer laser is directly applied to the anterior stromal surface after the removal of epithelium. The surface ablation technique includes photorefractive keratectomy (PRK), transepithelial PRK, laser-assisted subepithelial keratomileusis (LASEK), epithelial laser-assisted in situ keratomileusis (epi-LASIK), and topo-guided PRK (TG-PRK). Corneal surface ablation in the form of PRK is the oldest technique of laser vision correction. Recently, there is an increase in the number of surface ablation procedure due to their utility in thin corneas and no risk of flap-related complications such as epithelial ingrowth, diffuse lamellar keratitis, free flap, and buttonhole.

INDICATIONS

- To correct myopia up to −10 D, hypermetropia up to +6 D and astigmatism up to 4 D.
- For residual refractive correction, postcataract surgery, post-LASIK or post-SMILE. Enhancement can be done even after 10 years of refractive surgery.
- Preferred procedure when LASIK is contraindicated, e.g., flat cornea, steep cornea, thin cornea, deep set eyes, epithelial basement membrane dystrophy, and superficial corneal opacity.
- In special situations such as army personnel, pilots, and athletes where there is a risk of LASIK flap complications.

CONTRAINDICATIONS

- *Absolute contraindications:* Keratoconus, corneal edema, neurotrophic keratitis, previous HZO infection, severe dry eyes, significant cataract, and unstable glaucoma.
- *Relative contraindications:* Unstable progressive myopia, herpes simplex keratitis, corneal scar, uveitis, irregular astigmatism, uncontrolled diabetes, pregnancy or breastfeeding as hormonal influence may lead to refractive changes. Active systemic connective tissue diseases such as SLE and RA, as there is increased risk of corneal melt.

PREOPERATIVE ASSESSMENT

Patient's medical and ophthalmic history should be taken and complete ophthalmological examination should be carried out prior to surgery.

Refraction, tonometry, slit lamp examination, fundus to rule out retinal hole and lattice degeneration, corneal topography for the detection of irregular astigmatism and keratoconus, pupillometry, aberrometry, and Schirmer's test should be done. Patients must be informed to discontinue soft contact lenses for 3 days and hard contact lenses for 2 weeks prior to surgery in order to avoid corneal warpage. Topical fluoroquinolone such as moxifloxacin is given to reduce the chance of infection.

Pupil fixation: Patient is asked to focus on a target light in order to avoid decentration. Built-in tracking system is available in new excimer lasers that stop firing if there is significant amount of eye deviation. Surgeon should communicate with the patient throughout the entire procedure and encourage them to look at the target light and inform the patient when their vision will be blur.

▰ SURFACE ABLATION TECHNIQUES

a. *Photorefractive keratectomy:* In PRK, epithelium and Bowman's membrane is completely removed either by mechanical debridement, alcohol-assisted removal or by PTK and anterior corneal stroma is photo-ablated with 193 nm argon-fluoride excimer laser.
   i. *Mechanical epithelial debridement:* Epithelium is removed mechanically with a spatula, blade or a specialized brush.
   ii. *Alcohol-assisted epithelial debridement:* The cornea is exposed to 20% ethyl alcohol for 15-20 seconds in a 7-9.5 mm central corneal well. The alcohol is adsorbed with a Merocel sponge and excess alcohol is washed out with balanced salt solution (BSS). The loosened epithelium is then removed from the surface using a dry sponge, blade or an epithelial scrape.
   iii. *Transepithelial PRK:* Epithelium is removed within a fixed diameter using excimer laser in PTK mode, followed by application of laser to the stroma in PRK mode.
   Ablation zone is kept to 6.5 mm as it is ideal for myopic correction. Iris registration and pupil tracking are present in excimer laser for proper centration of ablation. In order to correct myopia, larger number of pulses is placed centrally and fewer pulses in the periphery of optical zone to flatten the natural arc of cornea; whereas, for hyperopia correction, large number of pulses is placed in the periphery to steepen the corneal arc.
b. *Laser-assisted subepithelial keratectomy (LASEK):* A partial incision is made on the edges of cornea with the help of trephine blade and ethanol solution is used to detach the epithelium from one side. Corneal stromal ablation is then done with the help of excimer laser and the corneal epithelial flap is repositioned to its original position.
c. *EPI-LASIK:* Epithelial flap is created with the help of an epikeratome and a vacuum suction ring and stromal ablation is done with an excimer laser. Epithelial flap is then reposited after irrigating the stromal bed with BSS.
d. *Topo-guided PRK (TG-PRK):* TG-PRK is a treatment for mild-to-moderate keratoconus in an attempt to regularize the cornea. It flattens the cone peak by providing myopic ablation to the cone and hyperopic ablation to mid-periphery. Minimum corneal thickness of 450 µ is necessary prior to the treatment. Here epithelium can be removed in PTK mode and maximum 50–60 µ of tissue is ablated in 5.5–6 mm optic zone depending upon the tissue availability. Residual stroma of >350 µ is must postsurgery.

▰ ROLE OF MITOMYCIN C IN SURFACE ABLATION

Mitomycin-C (MMC) is an antimetabolite which prevents cell proliferation by inhibiting deoxyribonucleic acid (DNA) synthesis. 0.02% of MMC is applied with a soaked pledget for a period of 30 seconds in order to reduce the corneal haze and regression. The cornea is then irrigated with BSS and bandage contact lens (BCL) is placed for a period of 3-5 days for faster epithelial healing.

POSTOPERATIVE MANAGEMENT

Topical corticosteroid is used in a tapering manner to modify the inflammatory response. Moxifloxacin drops help to decrease the risk of infection with the use of BCL over a healing epithelial defect. Tear substitutes are used to reduce the dry eye symptoms.

COMPLICATIONS OF SURFACE ABLATION TECHNIQUES

Pain: Exposure of nerve endings due to epithelium removal results in severe pain and dry eyes.

Corneal haze: It occurs following high myopia correction (>6 D) due to increased number of activated keratocytes which transforms into myofibroblast and deposits new collagen and proteoglycans. Corneal haze begins 4-6 weeks after surgery and resolves by 6-12 months.

Decentration of ablation zone: It occurs due to poor fixation or due to eye movements during surgery.

Night glare and haloes: Seen with small ablated zones, as during scotopic condition, light rays passes through mid-peripheral cornea to reach the posterior pole.

Corneal infiltration: Sterile infiltrates are usually focal and appear days to weeks after surgery. If they are central, they may hamper the visual acuity. Corneal infection must be treated with hourly fluoroquinolone drops and tapering should be done following clinical improvement.

Ectasia: It is rare after PRK. The use of collagen cross-linking in patients with keratoconus undergoing TG PRK halts the progression of disease and prevents further ectasia.

SUGGESTED READING

1. Reynolds A, Moore JE, Naroo SA, Moore CB, Shah S. Excimer laser surface ablation: a review. Clin Exp Ophthalmol. 2010;38(2):168-82.
2. Taneri Suphi, Weisberg Michael, Azar Dimitri T. Surface ablation techniques. Journal of Cataract and Refractive Surgery. 2011;37(2):392-408.

5.19 Corneal Collagen Cross-linking in Refractive Surgery

Pooja Khamar, Sailie Shirodkar, Ritica Mukherji
Narayana Nethralaya, Bengaluru
dr.poojakhamar@gmail.com

INTRODUCTION

Corneal collagen cross-linking (CXL) has been found to stabilize weaker corneas in patients with keratoconus and those with iatrogenic keratectasia by virtue of formation of covalent bonds between the amino groups of collagen molecules, thus making the anterior corneal stroma stiffer. Studies have also established that CXL leads to minor flattening of the cornea, thereby contributing to the refractive outcome in eyes with keratoconus. Postrefractive surgery ectasia is a fairly uncommon yet dreaded occurrence of refractive surgery. It may be driven by patient-related factors, type of refractive procedure, and postoperative changes in the corneal collagen structure. In recent years, many refractive surgeons are performing refractive procedures in tandem with a corneal strengthening procedure to circumvent these risk factors upon identification.

FUNDAMENTAL CONCEPT

While the essential requirements for collagen cross-linking with respect to refractive surgery more or less remain the same, i.e., role of O_2, photosensitizer and UV-A light;

we need to especially consider differences in fluence rates, riboflavin soaking time, effect of flap or lenticule as well as the standardization protocol for selecting candidates for such combined procedures.

■ PATIENT SELECTION

- Refractive error of >6 D with other contributory factors.
- Suspicious topography but no keratoconus, i.e., forme fruste keratoconus
- Thin corneas with central pachymetry <480 μ
- Residual stromal bed between 250 and 280 μ
- BAD-D >1.65
- CBI >0.5
- TBI >0.29
- History of eye rubbing, allergic conjunctivitis
- Randleman's ectasia scoring >3

Three or more of these risk factors should be considered as an indication for an Xtra procedure. Ultimately, the choice of surgery rests on surgeon and patient preference.

■ TYPES OF XTRA PROCEDURES

LASIK Xtra

The main goal of a combining laser-assisted in situ keratomileusis (LASIK) with crosslinking is to compensate for the mechanical corneal weakness induced by the vertical laser cut for creation of the flap as well as the tissue ablation. A possible disadvantage to this would be unexpected change in refractive outcome induced by the crosslinking procedure; however, a finite element model study conducted by Seven et al. provided a theoretical basis for LASIK Xtra and showed that there was an increase in corneal stiffness without concurrent change in refractive outcome.

- *Variation in riboflavin:* VibeX Xtra 0.22% (Avedro, Waltham, Massachusetts, USA) was created especially for this procedure. It is a dextran-free isotonic riboflavin which has faster diffusion through corneal stroma allowing for a shorter soak time and allows the solution to reach the adequate depth in time.
- *Variation in UV exposure:* This varies according to surgeon preference but a total exposure dose of 2.7 J/cm^2 should be maintained according to the manufacturer. A common practice is to allow the riboflavin to soak the corneal bed for 45–90 seconds and allow UV exposure of 30 mW/cm^2 over the repositioned flap for up to 90 seconds for adequate cross-linking. This allows for faster diffusion of the riboflavin at a concentration which is not toxic to the corneal endothelium.
- *Efficacy and safety:* Many studies have that there was no significant difference in the refractive outcome, i.e., UCVA, BCVA, MRSE, K mean between LASIK and LASIK Xtra but not many have proven that the added procedure in fact led to a decreased incidence of postrefractive ectasia. A study by Dong et al. showed 76% eyes undergoing LASIK Xtra developed a mild haze that was seen for up to 6 months after surgery.

PRK Xtra

Photorefractive keratectomy (PRK) Xtra should be reserved for candidates with suspicious topographies, thin corneas who are highly motivated to under a refractive error corrective procedure. With respect to ectasia post-PRK, they often have a late-onset making them difficult to diagnose. A possible cause for this may be injury to the Bowman's layer. So, an added corneal strengthening procedure should theoretically make PRK surgery possible for such candidates. A major consideration is the timing of the CXL procedure, as CXL followed by PRK will lead to loss of cross-linked collagen and surprise in refractive outcomes. Simultaneous PRK with crosslinking with or without MMC application will prevent this.

- *Variation in riboflavin:* VibeX Xtra 0.22% (Avedro, Waltham, Massachusetts, USA) may be used for PRK Xtra similar to LASIK Xtra as the riboflavin properties allow for adequate tissue penetration after corneal epithelial removal. Kymionis et al. have also described a technique using 0.1% riboflavin instilled on the stromal bed every 3 minutes for 15 minutes.
- *Variation in UV exposure:* Epithelial removal may be done in single step via laser-based PRK or in a two-step process using PTK mode set at a depth of 50 μ as described by Sachdev et al. Fluence may vary according to surgeon preference and concentration of riboflavin used. For 0.2% riboflavin a total dose of 2.7 J/cm^2 should be targeted and for 0.1% a target of 5.4 J/cm^2.
- *Efficacy and safety:* Kymionis et al. reported corneal stability in suspect keratoconus patients after PRK Xtra with a follow-up of 5 years. Similar safety profiles were demonstrated by Lee et al. and Sachdev et al. based on endothelial cell counts. All long-term and short-term studies on the subject have reported either similar or better efficacy after treatment as compared to PRK alone.
- *Role of MMC:* While cross-linking in itself causes keratocyte apoptosis thereby eliminating risk of haze in patients with PRK Xtra, however, cases of haze have been reported in literature not lasting beyond 6 months postprocedure. Sachdev et al. based on their study have recommended use of 0.02% MMC to counter development of haze. They postulate that the reduced fluence time may not be sufficient to cause adequate apoptosis of keratocytes in the anterior stroma.

SMILE Xtra

Although many studies have shown SMILE to induce the least amount of biomechanical instability as compared to LASIK and PRK, cases of ectasia have been reported to occur after SMILE surgery. This could be attributed to a preoperative weaker cornea or genetic factors affecting collagen structure.
- *Variation in riboflavin:* Most long-term studies on SMILE Xtra have used 0.2% riboflavin solutions for cross-linking with an exposure of 3 minutes in the corneal pocket. One author has also used 0.1% solution with dextran for 15 minutes. Using solutions without dextran will ensure faster diffusion of riboflavin to the desired level.
- *Variation in UV exposure:* A total energy dose of 3.2–3.7 J/cm^2 may be used to determine duration of UV exposure; 45 mW/cm^2 for 90 seconds or 18 mW/cm^2 for 3 minutes.
- *Efficacy and safety:* Long-term studies have shown a similar safety and efficacy profile with SMILE Xtra as compared to SMILE and little to no haze.
- *LASIK Xtra versus SMILE Xtra:* SMILE is a flap-less procedure thereby bypassing flap-related complications that may occur with LASIK surgery. In LASIK Xtra, contact of flap with riboflavin is meticulously avoided to prevent cross-linking of the flap as it may lead to irregular interface, micro striae, making it difficult to lift the flap in case of re-surgery at a later date. This is not the case in SMILE Xtra, wherein riboflavin diffuses into the cap as well as the underlying residual bed thereby exerting the stiffening effect on both.

FUTURE DIRECTION

While most of the literatures with regard to corneal strengthening procedures combined with refractive procedures have attempted to establish safety and efficacy, not many have proven a quantifiable stiffening effect on corneal stroma. This is necessary as the protocols used for cross-linking are variable to those used in patients with keratoconus. Further, it may be useful to understand role of oxygen as it is an integral component of the cross-linking reaction and the level of O_2 diffusion beneath the flap or at the cap level should be analyzed.

SUGGESTED READING

1. Brar S, Gautam M, Sute SS, Ganesh S. Refractive surgery with simultaneous collagen cross-linking for borderline corneas: a review of different techniques, their protocols and clinical outcomes. Indian J Ophthalmol. 2020;68(12):2744-56.
2. Dong R, Zhang Y, Yuan Y, Liu Y, Wang Y, Chen Y. A prospective randomized self-controlled study of LASIK combined with accelerated cross-linking for high myopia in Chinese: 24-month follow-up. BMC Ophthalmol. 2022;22(1):280.
3. Juthani VV, Chuck RS. Corneal crosslinking in refractive corrections. Transl Vis Sci Technol. 2021;10(5):4.
4. Kymionis G, Kontadakis G, Grentzelos M, Petrelli M. Long-term follow-up of combined photorefractive keratectomy and corneal crosslinking in keratoconus suspects. Clin Ophthalmol. 2021;15:2403-10.

5.20 | Complications of Collagen Cross-linking

Ashalyne James, Shreesha Kumar Kodavoor
The Eye Foundation, Coimbatore
ashalyne.james@gmail.com, eskay_03@rediffmail.com

INTRODUCTION

Keratoconus is a bilateral, progressive, often asymmetrical, and noninflammatory corneal ectasia. Collagen cross-linking (CXL) is based on the combined use of the photosensitizer riboflavin and ultraviolet A (UV-A) light of 370 nm. It was first introduced by Wollensak et al. from Germany in 2003. CXL is the only available treatment which corrects the underlying pathology in keratoconic cornea. It helps in the formation of new covalent bonds in the stromal collagen. This helps to increase the stromal biomechanical and structural stability, thus halting the progression of ectasia. It is minimally invasive and relatively safe, but not without complications.

INDICATIONS OF COLLAGEN CROSS-LINKING

- To halt progression of progressive ectatic diseases of cornea.
  - Keratoconus
  - Pellucid marginal degeneration
  - Postrefractive surgery ectasia
- Infectious keratitis—cases which are recalcitrant to medical therapy.

PROTOCOLS IN PRACTICE

The various CXL protocols in practice are summarized in **Table 5.20.1**.

TABLE 5.20.1: CXL protocols in practice.

Types of CXL	Total energy	Time	Power	Wavelength of UV light	Riboflavin %	Soaking time
Dresden protocol	5.4 J	30 minute	3 mW/cm²	370 nm	0.1%	30 minute
Accelerated	5.4 J	10 minute	9 mW/cm²	370 nm	0.1%	10 minute
Topoguided PRX+ CXL	5.4 J	10 minute	9 mW/cm²	370 nm	0.1%	10 minute
LASIK/PRK/SMILE XTRA	2.7 J	90 seconds	30 mW/cm²	370 nm	0.25%	90 minute
Hypotonic accelerated CXL	5.4 J	10 minute	9 mW/cm²	370 nm	0.1% Dextran-free	10 minute

RISK FACTORS FOR DEVELOPING COMPLICATIONS AFTER COLLAGEN CROSS-LINKING

Collagen cross-linking is a relatively safe procedure with a low complication rate. Most of the complications occur due to debridement of epithelium. Preexisting medical conditions that can increase the risk of complications in CXL include the following:
- Atopy
- Vernal keratoconjunctivitis
- Herpetic eye disease
- Diabetes
- Prior laser-assisted in situ keratomileusis (LASIK)
- Autoimmune conditions

The risk factors should be treated and well controlled prior to CXL to minimize the complications rate. Patients with history of herpetic eye disease can be put on prophylactic acyclovir.

COMPLICATIONS OF COLLAGEN CROSS-LINKING

Commonly encountered complications after CXL are as follows:
- Keratitis:
  - Infectious
  - Sterile
- Corneal haze
- Endothelial damage
- Progression after CXL
- Stromal degeneration
- Persistent epithelial defect
- Corneal melt
- Corneal perforation
- Complications in post-LASIK patients
- Reduced postoperative visual acuity

Keratitis

This mainly occurs due to epithelial removal during CXL. It can be broadly divided into two types—infectious and sterile keratitis.

Infectious keratitis **(Figs. 5.20.1A to D)** is a sight-threatening complication of CXL. Causative organisms reported include *Staphylococcus aureus* (which is a part of the normal microbial flora of the ocular surface), *Pseudomonas aeruginosa, Escherichia coli, Microsporidia*, etc.

They are usually first treated with fourth generation fluoroquinolones. Cases of antibiotic resistance have been reported. This mainly occurs due to the widespread use of fluoroquinolones as the initial drug for any infectious keratitis. In resistant cases, fortified antibiotics (e.g., fortified cefazolin 5%) are required.

Herpetic reactivation post-CXL has also been reported. This can occur due to exposure to UVA light, mechanical trauma and prolonged use of topical steroids. Prophylactic systemic antiviral therapy helps to prevent reactivation of herpetic infection.

The exact mechanism of sterile keratitis **(Figs. 5.20.2A to D)** is not known. The proposed mechanism includes antigenic alterations in patient's native proteins and development of an immune response against it. Another proposed mechanism is a sterile immune response to staphylococcal antigens in the tear pooling beneath the BCL.

Risk factors for development of sterile keratitis include history of atopy, thinnest pachymetry <400 μm and high corneal curvature (K_{max} >58 D). They usually respond well with a topical steroid alone.

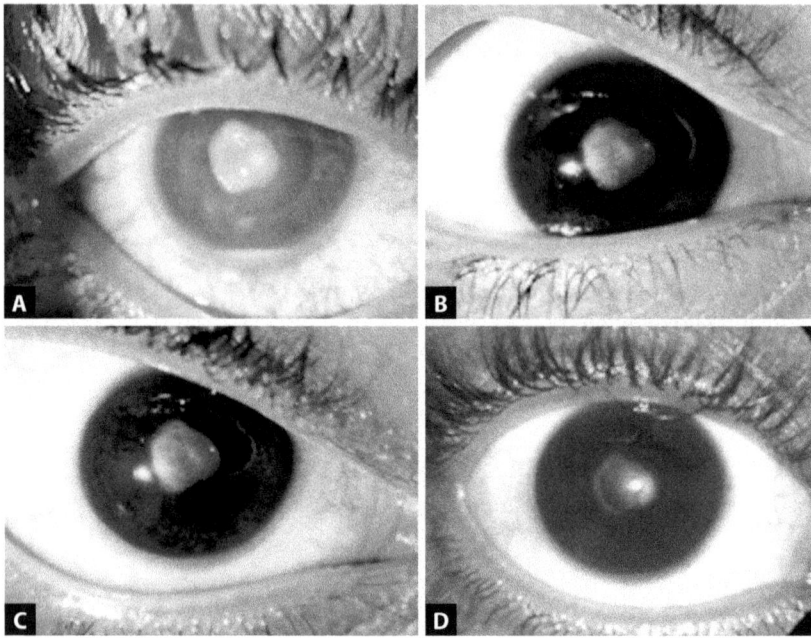

Figs. 5.20.1A to D: (A) Case of post-accelerated corneal collagen cross-linking staphylococcal keratitis with central infiltrate; (B) After 2 weeks of treatment with moxifloxacin and tobramycin, prednisolone acetate; (C) After 1 month of treatment; (D) At 6 months follow-up with nebular-macular scar.

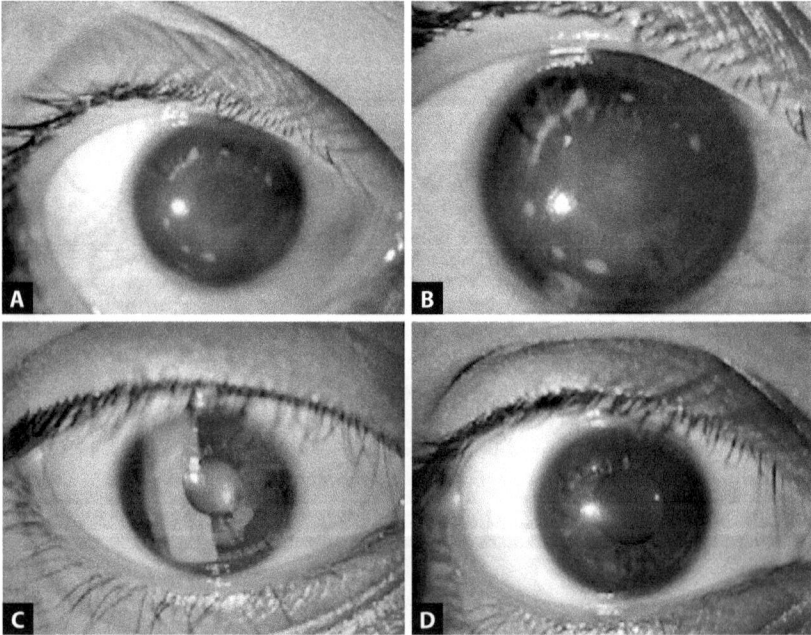

Figs. 5.20.2A to D: (A) Case of post-accelerated corneal collagen cross-linking sterile infiltrate in mid-periphery; (B) After 1 week of treatment with topical steroids; (C) After 4 weeks of treatment; (D) At 3-month, follow-up with very faint scar in mid-periphery.

Corneal Haze

It is a transient finding commonly observed after CXL. Postoperative topical steroid application helps to reduce the occurrence of corneal haze. Stromal haze after CXL is deeper (approximately 300 μm) than the subepithelial haze of photorefractive keratectomy (PRK). Haze occurs due to keratocyte loss and corneal edema. Dense persistent haze should be treated with intensive topical steroid regimen to avoid visually significant haze (**Fig. 5.20.3**).

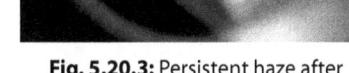

Fig. 5.20.3: Persistent haze after 3 years of CXL.

Corneal haze can be graded as given below:
- Grade 0: Clear with no opacity seen by any method of microscopic slit-lamp examination
- Grade 1: Haze of minimal density seen with difficulty with direct or diffuse examination
- Grade 2: Mild haze easily visible with direct focal slit lamp illumination
- Grade 3: Moderate opacity that partially obscured details of iris
- Grade 4: Severe opacity that completely obscured the details of intraocular structures

Endothelial Damage

It can occur due to the toxic effect of UVA on the endothelium. Patients with thinner cornea and patients undergoing conventional CXL are at higher risk of developing this. Normally an irradiance of 0.18 mW/cm^2 reaches the endothelium with standard Dresden protocol. The endothelial damage threshold was shown to be at an irradiance of 0.35 mW/cm^2. The risk is lower in patients with thicker cornea and patients undergoing accelerated CXL. This is due to the prolonged UV irradiation in conventional CXL.

Endothelial damage can lead to corneal edema which may be temporary or permanent. Patients with permanent corneal edema require endothelial keratoplasty.

Progression after Collagen Cross-linking

An increase in K_{max} of >1.0 D is known as progression after CXL. Progression of keratoconus after CXL leads to failure of CXL.

Risk factors for progression after CXL include:
- Very steep cornea; $K_{max} \geq 58.0$ D
- History of eye rubbing and allergic conjunctivitis
- Thin cornea; thickness <400 μm—to prevent this hypotonic CXL is done
- Pediatric age group
- Eccentric and thin cones
- Female gender

Patients with severe progression might require deep anterior lamellar keratoplasty later.

Stromal Degeneration

It is a late and rare complication on CXL. It occurs due to severe stromal thinning. The etiology is related to the exposure to UV-A irradiation. UV-A exposure can lead to fibroblastic transformation of keratocytes in the deep stroma. This can reduce the nutrition supply to superficial cornea.

This complication can be prevented by optimizing the exposure time and dosage of UV-A exposure. Surgical treatment is done with deep anterior lamellar keratoplasty.

Persistent Epithelial Defect

Epithelial regrowth usually completes within 4–5 days post-CXL. However, keratocyte damage and apoptosis post-CXL may retard the epithelium regrowth leading to persistent epithelial defects. Such patients are at a higher risk of developing complications such as infectious keratitis and corneal melt.

Risk factors include thin cornea, unregulated UV exposure, prolonged topical NSAID use, presence of lagophthalmos. Patients are treated with frequent lubrication and antibiotics.

Corneal Melt

Patients with persistent epithelial defects are at risk of developing corneal melts. Various mechanisms leading to melt are (a) increased proinflammatory activity, (b) mismatch between BCL and cornea, (c) UV light-induced hypoxia and keratocyte apoptosis and (d) *Staphylococcal* antigens. Patients are started on topical antibiotics, steroids, and eye patching or BCL placement is done. Temporary tarsorrhaphy can also be done.

Corneal Perforation

Patients with persistent epithelial defects and corneal melt are at high risk of developing corneal perforation. Small perforations can be sealed with cyanoacrylate glue. Larger perforations are treated with tectonic penetrating keratoplasty.

Dry Eyes

Corneal nerve fiber regeneration starts as early as 1 month and is usually fully restored within 6 months post-CXL. However abnormal nerve migration can occur in some cases leading to corneal denervation and dry eyes.

Complications in Post-LASIK Patients

Epithelial ingrowth and diffuse lamellar keratitis can occur in post-LASIK patients undergoing CXL.

Reduced Postoperative Visual Acuity

This can occur due to any of the complications mentioned above. The etiology should be identified and corrected accordingly.

■ CONCLUSION

Collagen cross-linking is a relatively safe and noninvasive procedure which helps to halt corneal ectasia. Preexisting medical conditions should be treated prior to the procedure. Treatment of preexisting risk factors and careful case selection can help to prevent complications in CXL. Newer treatment protocols help to prevent the development of complications post-CXL.

■ SUGGESTED READING

1. Agarwal R, Jain P, Arora R. Complications of corneal collagen cross-linking. Indian J Ophthalmol. 2022;70:1466-74.
2. Kodavoor SK, Sarwate NJ, Ramamurthy D. Microbial keratitis following accelerated corneal collagen cross-linking. Oman Journal of Ophthalmology. 2015;8(2):111-3.
3. Kodavoor SK, Tiwari NN, Ramamurthy D. Profile of infectious and sterile keratitis after accelerated corneal collagen cross-linking for keratoconus. Oman J Ophthalmol. 2018;13:18-23.

5.21 Newer Procedures in Refractive Surgery

Rupal Shah
Centre for Sight
rupal@newvisionindia.com

◼ INTRODUCTION

In the last 30 years, refractive surgery has come a long way. The advent of the ophthalmic excimer laser in the late 1980s led to a dramatic improvement in the safety, predictability, and accuracy of refractive surgery. The development of laser-assisted in situ keratomileusis (LASIK) made excimer laser procedures a lot more acceptable by a dramatic reduction in the pain experienced by patients after the procedure and a huge improvement in the visual recovery immediately after the procedure. The introduction of the femtosecond laser improved the safety and reliability of the LASIK procedure, and eventually led to the development of all femtosecond procedures like small incision lenticule extraction (SMILE). All of this has led to refractive surgery becoming a mainstream ophthalmic procedure, and enormous popularity of refractive surgery, both amongst the general populace, as well as amongst ophthalmologists.

In the last decade, the pace of improvements and advances in refractive surgery has slackened somewhat. Rather than a paradigm shift, what we have experienced are incremental improvements, which have led to the procedures becoming easier to perform. There has also been an improvement in how we can customize the treatments to individual eyes. Machines have become more reliable, and the choices before ophthalmologists in terms of technology have become more diverse.

Of particular note is the increasing acceptance of SMILE amongst both physicians and patients. While earlier, SMILE was only possible with the VisuMax femtosecond laser (Carl Zeiss Meditec), lately there are also other possibilities, including the CLEAR (Ziemer) and another machine from Johnson and Johnson (SILK). We shall discuss SMILE in more detail below.

Another procedure which has got increased acceptance is a form of topographically linked LASIK, called Contoura Vision Technology. We shall discuss this in more detail below.

There have been other possibilities that have emerged in the last decade. There is increased use of the Intraocular Contact Lens (ICL) technology, particularly for those individuals whose refractive power exceeds what can be safely achieved with the excimer or femtosecond laser. This includes those patients who have high myopia exceeding –10 diopters spherical error, or those patients who have thin but stable corneas.

There have also been improvements in diagnostic instruments. Epithelial mapping (e.g., RTVue XR), dynamic corneal response analysis (e.g., Corvis), the Optical Quality Analysis System (OQAS II) have also become mainstream in the last decade.

Mapping the corneal epithelium with layered tomographic imaging can be useful in determining whether refractive surgery candidates are at risk of postoperative ectasia. In eyes with keratoconus, the corneal epithelium gets thinner at the cone but thickens around the cone. The result is that epithelial mapping will show a donut pattern that is highly characteristic of the condition.

The Corvis ST records the reaction of the cornea to a defined air pulse using a newly developed high-speed Scheimpflug camera. Based on a video of 140 images, taken within 31 ms after onset of the air pulse, the Corvis® ST provides a detailed assessment of corneal biomechanical properties.

The information obtained on the biomechanical response of the cornea is used to calculate a biomechanically corrected IOP (bIOP). Furthermore, it allows ectatic diseases such as keratoconus to be detected at a very early stage.

OQAS™ II is based on the double-pass technique and provides an objective measurement of the optical quality of the eye. A punctate light source is imaged on the retina. The size and the shape of the light spot (light passes twice through ocular media) is analyzed by OQAS II. OQAS™ II images contain all the information about the optical quality of the eye including all the higher order aberrations and scattered light. This is very useful for an objective evaluation of the eye's visual quality.

■ SMALL INCISION LENTICULE EXTRACTION

Small incision lenticule extraction (SMILE), a relatively new technique of performing refractive surgery, uses a femtosecond laser for all steps of the keratomileusis procedure. SMILE involves the creation of a refractive lenticule within the cornea using a femtosecond laser, and subsequent extraction of the refractive lenticule from within the cornea. The refractive error that needs to be treated defines the shape of the refractive lenticule to be created. SMILE is, therefore, a refractive surgery technique which uses only a femtosecond laser to perform the whole refractive surgery procedure. No excimer laser is needed for the whole procedure.

Currently, SMILE is available to treat myopic errors up to -12.5 diopters spherical equivalent, with or without astigmatism of up to -5 diopters. Clinical trials are underway for the treatment of hyperopia or hyperopic astigmatism of up to +8 diopters spherical equivalent. Patient selection criteria are like LASIK.

There are economic, clinical, and work-flow advantages of an only femtosecond laser procedure like SMILE over performing Femto-LASIK or conventional LASIK or photorefractive keratectomy (PRK).

The economic advantages of using an all Femto procedure over Femto-LASIK are obvious. You require only one laser to perform the entire refractive surgery procedure, instead of two. This means saving on capital costs, maintenance costs, and consumable costs.

The clinical benefits are critical too. An excimer laser ablates the lenticule required to correct the refractive error. In SMILE, the lenticule is carved out within the cornea by a cutting action. This difference between cuttings with the femtosecond laser, as opposed to ablation with the excimer laser is significant. Excimer laser ablation rates are dependent on corneal hydration levels, environmental conditions such as humidity and temperature, and on the depth in the stroma at which ablation occurs. The scatter in ablation rates is particularly high, when the ablation depth is large, which explains the greater scatter in the results of treatment of larger refractive errors. The femtosecond laser's cutting action is not dependent on any of the above factors. The scatter in the thickness of the lenticule is minimized, and it is also independent of the refractive error being treated. For all these reasons, several studies have shown that the refractive predictability with the SMILE procedure is higher than with an excimer laser, particularly for higher amounts of refractive errors.

Several studies have also shown that SMILE preserves the tear function and corneal sensitivity more than Femto-LASIK, which is to be expected considering the smaller incision. There are also biomechanical advantages of SMILE over Femto-LASIK.

■ CONTOURA VISION TECHNOLOGY

Contoura Vision is a type of topographically linked excimer laser treatment offered by the Alcon Platform. It uses a highly accurate topography device (the Vario), and then uses T-CAT software to customize the patient treatment while treating the refractive errors.

Primarily, there are three differences between conventional LASIK and such topographically guided procedures. First, it treats the aberration profile on the corneal surface. Second, the treatment is centered on the corneal apex, rather than on the pupil center. Third, the ablation is guided by the unique topographic features of the cornea, allowing for better control on the spherical aberration post the procedure.

There are challenges to such topography-guided ablations, including at times when there is a large difference between refractive astigmatism and topographically determined astigmatism. However, the unique features of the topographically guided procedures allow for very good control over corneal asphericity and excellent visual outcomes.

5.22 Phototherapeutic Keratectomy

JK Reddy
Sankara Eye Hospital, Coimbatore
reddyjk@yahoo.com

■ INTRODUCTION

Phototherapeutic keratectomy (PTK) involves treating anterior corneal lesions with an excimer laser (193 nm). This is based on the principle of photoablation/photoevaporation which is characterized by breaking of bonds between the molecules by picosecond laser of 6–8 picoseconds. Each pulse of laser removes precise volume of corneal tissue making it very accurate, precise with smooth and regular surface. PTK is most effective when the lesions are confined to the anterior 10–20% of the cornea involving the Bowman's membrane and anterior stroma. The common indications are recurrent corneal epithelial erosions (RCE), anterior corneal dystrophies, spheroidal degeneration, keratoconus, and corneal scars.

Preoperative evaluation includes corneal topography which documents irregular astigmatism if any along with pachymetry and other measurements. Anterior segment optical coherence tomography helps in assessment of depth of corneal scar, epithelial mapping, and pachymetry analysis. Both the above investigations help in pre- and postoperative follow-up as well.

■ COMMON INDICATIONS

- *Recurrent corneal erosions:* RCE is often seen post-trauma or in cases of epithelial basement membrane dystrophies. Hemidesmosomes, the key for attachment of epithelium to basement membrane are hypothesized to be weak as the cause of epithelial erosions. Under topical anesthesia the loose corneal epithelium is removed by manual debridement. A large area PTK (7 mm) is done with ablation depth of 10–15 μm followed by placement of a bandage contact lens. The depth of stromal ablation is less, so the use of topical perioperative mitomycin C to prevent postoperative haze is not necessary. Ablation depth over 25–30 μm causes postoperative haze and hyperopic shift. The principle is to form adhesion complexes between the epithelium and basement membrane by photoablation of the Bowman's layer which is established with PTK.
- *Corneal dystrophies:* PTK is indicated for anterior basement membrane dystrophies and stromal dystrophies to treat RCE, decrease the stromal opacities and there improving visual outcome. Intraoperative application of MitoMycin C (MMC) helps prevent recurrences. Some of the dystrophies treated include map-dot-fingerprint dystrophy, granular dystrophy, and lattice dystrophy.
- *Corneal scars:* Post-traumatic, postinfectious keratitis, and postpterygium excision scars up to a depth of 100 μm can be treated with PTK. Transepithelial PTK and topography-guided treatments can be done in these cases. The aim is to reduce the scar rather than removing it completely.
- *Spheroidal degeneration or climatic droplet keratopathy:* Spheroidal degeneration of cornea can be either "smooth" or "irregular" type or mixed type. Smooth type of spheroidal degeneration is more likely to have clearer cornea than irregular type.

Irregular type is also associated with postablation irregular surface delayed epithelial healing. 1% methylcellulose can be used as masking fluid to get a better surface in irregular type.
- *Band-shaped keratopathy:* The calcific deposits can be ablated with PTK thereby resulting in a clearer, smooth cornea with improvement in vision. In smooth BSK, transepithelial PTK can be done. In cases with rough BSK, masking fluid is needed to get a smoother surface after PTK.
- *Keratoconus:* As per Cretan protocol, transepithelial PTK of up to 50 μm depth in a 6.5–7.0 mm ablation zone is done followed by mechanical removal of surrounding epithelium to enlarge the de-epithelialized area to an 8.0–9.0 mm. It is followed by conventional or rapid collagen cross-linking (CXL) with riboflavin and ultraviolet A (UVA). This results in visual and topographical improvement in keratoconus. Topography-guided removal of epithelium has also been reported in treatment of keratoconus (TREK). PTK can be centered on the cone apex in keratoconus, which helps in reducing the height of the cone.
- *Postrefractive surgery complications:* Post-PRK haze can be successfully treated with TRANS PTK with MMC.
- Other indications of PTK include Salzmann's nodular degeneration and keratoconus nodules.

POSTOPERATIVE COMPLICATIONS
- *Disease recurrence:* The fastest recurrence within a few years has been noted with Thiel-Behnke and Reis–Bücklers corneal dystrophies. Recurrence is common with granular and lattice corneal dystrophies over 3–6 years. In case of Schneider corneal dystrophy takes long time of more than a decade to recur. But in recurrences the opacities are often in the anterior stroma, making retreatment possible in most cases. MMC also helps in preventing recurrences and corneal haze with deep ablations.
- *Induced refractive error:* Most commonly include hyperopia and irregular astigmatism. Induced refractive error/irregular surface can be decreased with the use of 1% methylcellulose as masking agent, adoption of large ablation zone, and transition zone. A masking agent is a high viscosity fluid that helps in preferential ablation by filling the gaps between irregular surfaces and covering the deeper tissues and leaving the elevated peaks exposed for photoablation. Examples include sodium hyaluronate, 1% methylcellulose, and dextran 0.1%.

CONCLUSION
Phototherapeutic keratectomy is a safe, less invasive, and effective surgical procedure for treating anterior corneal pathologies. It has a faster visual recovery and repeatability when compared to keratoplasty.

5.23 | Refractive Surprise after Cataract Surgery

Rishi Swarup
Swarup Eye Centre, Hyderabad
rishiswarup@yahoo.com

Samita Moolani
Moolani's Eye Care Centre, Pune

INTRODUCTION
Refractive surprise is a disappointing outcome for both patient and surgeon. Even though it is less common, dealing with patients who present with refractive surprise can be daunting and cumbersome.

The most important step to take once you are challenged with these cases is the management and hand holding of the patient to achieve a satisfactory outcome.

In this chapter, we will talk about the evaluation of a patient with refractive surprise after cataract surgery, as well as discuss the causes and management. We will highlight the ways to prevent refractive surprise after cataract surgery.

■ CAUSES OF REFRACTIVE SURPRISE AFTER CATARACT SURGERY

Preoperative causes	Operative causes	Postoperative causes
Errors in Biometry—keratometry, Axial length	Surgically induced astigmatism	Anterior movement of lens
Wrong A constant value of IOL	Misalignment of toric IOL	Capsular bag distension
• Improper IOL selection Inappropriate IOL power formula • Uncorrected and overlooked preoperative corneal astigmatism • Overlooked pathology such as dry eye disease, keratoconus	• Inverted/Upside down implantation of IOL • Malposition of the IOL • Wrong lens inserted	• Lens tilt • Capsular phimosis • Posterior capsular opacification or wrinkling of the capsule

■ EVALUATION OF THE PATIENT AND OPERATED EYE

Refraction

Autorefractometry

This reading is often the first clue that one may be dealing with a case of postoperative refractive surprise. Subjective refraction is more important to consider in these patients.

The acceptance of refractive correction will give an idea of how large the postoperative error is. Small myopic errors are acceptable by most patients however hyperopic errors create a lot of dissatisfaction.

Evaluation of the Intraocular Lens

- Check for lens position; look for any subluxation, or tilt.
- Evaluate the intraocular lens condition, any cracks, or indentation by any instrumentation.

Position of toric intraocular lens (IOLs): Recheck the toric marking alignment with the intended axis.

Look for trapped ophthalmic viscoelastic device (OVD) in the bag causing distension syndrome which will cause a myopic surprise.

Evaluation of the Posterior Capsule

Look for wrinkling of the posterior capsule and posterior capsular plaques.

Evaluation of the Ocular Surface and Anterior Chamber

- Look for dry ocular surface and meibomian gland dysfunction, cornea evaluation for edema, and Descemet folds.
- Keratoconic eyes may cause a hyperopic shift due to an error in the estimated lens position.

Posterior Segment Evaluation

Evaluation of the macula, cystoid macular edema may lead to a hypermetropic shift.
Rule out vitritis or any retinal detachment.

Retrospective Evaluation

The key to managing refractive surprise is to perform a self-analysis.
- Is the ocular surface unhealthy or irregular?
- Was the eye a high myopic or hypermetropic eye preoperatively?
- Was there a keratoconus which was missed?
- Has any refractive surgery been done in the past?
- Is there a residual astigmatism which was not corrected with an appropriate toric IOL or procedure?
- Is there any silicon oil in the eye or has vitrectomy been done?

PREOPERATIVE BIOMETRY, KERATOMETRY, AND LENS POWER CALCULATION ERRORS

Error in optical biometry or immersion biometry scanning may occur. Thick subcapsular cataracts show errors in axial length readings during ultrasound biometry. Crosscheck axial length readings using two forms of biometry such as optical as well as immersion.

Was the wrong formula used to calculate the IOL power?

In shorter and longer eyes specific formulae are more accurate. In postrefractive eyes it is tricky to get the appropriate values.

SRK-T and Barrett's Universal II formulae work well in most eyes however in short eyes with axial length of <22 mm Hoffer Q is preferred and in longer eye with axial length of >26 mm Holladay II formula is preferred.

In postrefractive eyes, Shammas formula helps as done Barrett postrefractive formula.

Was all the data entered correctly if a manual input machine was used to calculate the power?

Repeat the biometry in pseudophakia mode to crosscheck all the parameters.

Errors in Surgical Technique

Was the correct side eye of patient operated which corresponds to the biometry in question?

Is the incision position appropriate with regard to position and size?

Error in Labeling

Recheck the marking on the lens pack both inside and outside. Confirm that the correct lens was indeed inserted.

Human Errors

Recheck the right lens was put in the right eye.

MANAGEMENT

Intraocular Lens Exchange

The most common cause for IOL exchange has been described as decentration or dislocation (85.3%). IOL exchange is best done as soon as possible before fibrous adhesions form between the capsule and the haptics.

Intraocular lens exchange comes with possible complications such as vitreous loss, zonular dialysis, and a repeat refractive surprise. Corneal endothelial count should also be considered. IOL exchange may not be avoided in small residual errors due to the risk that is associated with the procedure.

The IOL can be explanted by bisecting the lens with a lens cutting scissor, and removing the lens from the same incision, or by partial transection and hinging it at the incision site, alternately a scleral frown incision has been described to remove the lens.

In late postoperative IOL exchange, a technique of cutting the haptics and leaving them in the bag has been described as well.

The importance of correct lens calculation, and using the correct formula for calculation based on axial length, refractive surgery status cannot be emphasized enough.

Piggyback Intraocular Lens

This is a safer option to IOL exchange however long-term complications such as pigment dispersion, uveitis, and glaucoma may arise.

It is important that the primary lens is properly in the bag and the anterior chamber is deep with open angles.

The lenses which can be used for Piggyback IOL implantation are Sulcoflex from Rayner (**Fig. 5.23.1**).

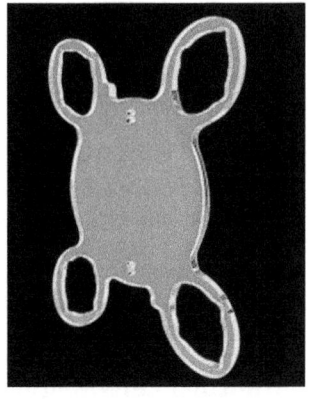

Fig. 5.23.1: Add-on Sulcoflex lens by IOCare.

Piggyback IOL calculation:
Hyperopic error (spherical equivalent)
Multiplied by 1.5
Example: + 4.0 D (4 × 1.5) = + 6.0 D

Myopic error (spherical equivalent)
Multiplied by 1.2
Example: –4.0 D (4 × 1.2) = – 4.8 D

Ideal candidates for piggyback IOL:
- Primary IOL in intact capsular bag
- Normal or deep anterior chamber
- No glaucoma, pigment dispersion
- Intact pupil and iris
- Normal corneal endothelial cell count
- This is the surgery of choice for hyperopic errors.
- Preferred surgery for patients who present late and have significant high order aberrations and cannot undergo laser correction.

Cornea-based Procedures

- Photorefractive keratectomy (PRK) or laser in-situ keratomileusis (LASIK) are often used to correct residual errors. This procedure is referred to unplanned bioptics.
- LASIK can be done after 3 months, and the correction should be based on the subjective refraction.
- Photorefractive keratectomy is more predictable and can be done earlier about 1 month postoperatively.
- In both cases corneal thickness, ocular surface health should be considered prior to planning the surgery.
- Limbal relaxing incisions can also be done using Femto or with guarded blades however the predictability is lower than PRK or LASIK.

Depending on the Type of Intraocular Lens Implanted

In eyes with multifocal IOL implant: If the patient presents 2–4 weeks after surgery IOL exchange is best option. When the patient presents months after the surgery then piggyback lens is the best option or PRK can be considered.

In eyes with monofocal IOL implant: If patient presents 2–4 weeks after surgery IOL exchange is best option. PRK or piggyback lens can be tried; when the patient presents months after the surgery. Piggyback lens is the best option or LASIK with the hinge near the incision if performing Femto-LASIK.

In eyes with toric intraocular lens: If IOL is rotated or misaligned; then rotate it back to original axis from original calculation. It is better to recalculate the position based on online resources such as www.astigmatismfix.com or use iTrace.

Excimer wavefront-guided procedure, IOL exchange if there is a large error remaining.

■ TREAT THE CAUSE

Capsular distension syndrome: When there is a trapping of OVD between the IOL and posterior capsule a hyperopic shift is seen.

One can plan a YAG capsulotomy to the peripheral anterior capsule as shown in **Figure 5.23.2**.

YAG capsulotomy can also be planned in the posterior capsule. Alternatively capsular bag wash can be done.

Intraocular Lens Malposition

The patient can be taken up for IOL repositioning if the cause of the refractive error is due to rotated toric IOL. This should be done within 1–2 weeks of surgery before the capsular adhesions form between the IOL.

Posterior capsular plaques if present are more safely dealt with a YAG Cap done preferably after 6 months of surgery (**Fig. 5.23.3**).

Spectacle or Contact Lens Rehabilitation

Counsel the patient well, and most patients will be amicable to using spectacles or contact lenses postoperatively when the error is smaller.

Plan the Fellow Eye

If the refractive error is below −1.5 and myopic, and the other eye is still unoperated, one can plan the other eye to be emmetropic and create a blended vision or mono vision which works well for most patients.

The challenge of these cases is convincing the patient to go ahead with the other eye when one is already dissatisfied with the vision of the first eye.

Keep in mind if the issue of refractive surprise is because of wrong calculation of effective lens position (ELP) then the same refractive surprise is likely to occur in the other eye.

■ FUTURE CONSIDERATIONS

- Newer optical biometry machines using laser partial coherence interferometry or low-coherence optical reflectometry are more accurate.

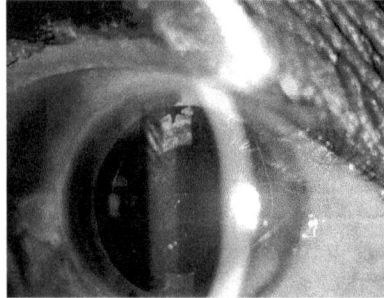

Fig. 5.23.2: Peripheral anterior capsule Nd:YAG opening made to create a drainage for the trapped OVD.

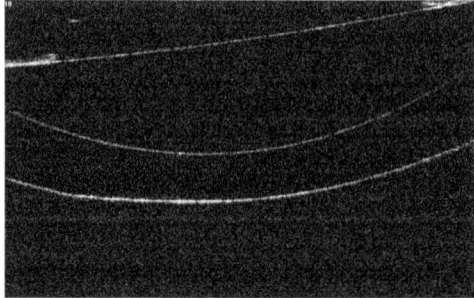

Fig. 5.23.3: Malposition of IOL is the most common cause reported of postcataract surgery refractive surprise. Photographed is an eye on postoperative day 1 with a "sunrise IOL" position.

- Toric marking technologies have made calculation of lens powers easier and more reliable.
- New formulae are available online and on these machines which improve accuracy.
- Light adjustable lenses are an exciting proposition particularly in those individuals who appear at risk for refractive surprise.

TAKE HOME MESSAGE

Prevention is better than cure; the following guidelines can help avoid postcataract refractive surprise:
- Treat the ocular surface preoperatively for dryness.
- Calculators and formulae should always be customized to the correct size of the eye.
- Check lens label inside box as well as on the packet.
- Always do a time out before every surgery to verify that the scanning biometry information, eye, patient, and lens type all match.
- Constant maintenance of machines, biometers, and calibration is very important. If one has access to two types of biometers, then it is better to perform both and crosscheck readings.
- Always under promise and over deliver.

SUGGESTED READING

1. Marques FF, Marques DM, Osher RH, et al. Longitudinal study of intraocular lens exchange. J Cataract Refract Surg. 2007;33:254-7.
2. Shalchi Z, Restori M, Flanagan D, Watson M. Managing refractive surprise. Focus; 2018.

5.24 Complications in Laser-assisted In Situ Keratomileusis

Madhuvanthi Mohan, Sujatha Mohan
Rajan Eye Care Hospital Pvt Ltd, Chennai
mohan_sujatha@hotmail.com

INTRAOPERATIVE COMPLICATIONS

Usually flap-related, which can occur either with a microkeratome or a femtosecond laser.

Microkeratome-related Flap Complications

Incomplete Cut

It can occur if the microkeratome head stops prematurely or even due to suction loss in a femtosecond laser.

Reasons for an incomplete/irregular flap include loss of suction, flat corneas, low intraocular pressure (IOP), inadequate globe exposure, electrical failure or motor breakdown, blockage or premature release of foot pedal.

Tips for prevention include testing the movement of the microkeratome blade before start of the procedure, good exposure, and draping of the eye and checking the IOP prior to the procedure.

Management
- *If the irregular flap is in the periphery:* Can proceed with ablation by reducing the optical zone or by shielding the flap hinge.
- *If it is paracentral or central in nature:* Abort the procedure and reposition the flap. Retreatment can be done after 2-3 months.

Irregular Cut

It can be due to uneven movement of the microkeratome, irregularity of the blade, displacement of the suction ring, loss of suction, and obstruction during the microkeratome pass.

Tips for prevention include testing the movement of the microkeratome blade before start of the procedure, good exposure and draping of the eye, adequate tear status, smooth conjunctiva and checking the blade edge prior to procedure.

Management
- Realignment of the flap
- Adequate drying time
- Placement of bandage contact lens
- And repeat of procedure after 4–6 months.

Free Cap

This is when the entire flap is dislodged from the cornea.

It is more common with a microkeratome flap and occurs due to failure of stop mechanism of microkeratome.

Predisposing factors
- Loss of suction
- Flat cornea
- Defective microkeratome blades
- Insufficient exposure of cornea
- Poor positioning/surgeon torqueing
- Failure of stop mechanism
- ↓ intraoperative IOP
- Tearing of the dehydrated flap

Management: Reposition cap after ablation and place BCL on top.

Buttonholes

Due to superficial pass of microkeratome

Predisposing factors
- Loss of suction
- Obstruction of tubing and suction ring
- Presence of a corneal scar
- Steep cornea
- Faulty microkeratome blade
- Preoperative dry eye

Management
- Do not lift the flap. Abort ablation.
- Careful cleaning of interface to remove infiltrating epithelial cells
- Complete flap removal with PTK
- Placement of BCL

■ FEMTOSECOND LASER-RELATED FLAP COMPLICATIONS

Suction Loss

Predisposing Factors
- Sudden head movement
- Excessive lid squeezing
- *Anatomical factors:* Deep set eyes, small palpebral fissure, and flat cornea
- Improper placement of suction ring

Management
- Proper preoperative counseling is of utmost importance.
- *If it occurs at the start of the procedure:* Redock suction ring and restart.
- *If it occurs during the procedure:* Abort ablation if involving visual axis.

Vertical Gas Breakthrough
Escape of gas bubbles from dissection plane into subepithelial space.

Predisposing Factors
- Localized areas of stromal weakening/scars at the dissection level
- Thin flaps
- Focal defect in Bowman's layer
- Basement membrane dystrophy

Management
- Preoperatively assessment of corneal scar with anterior segment optical coherence tomography (AS OCT) to rule out thinning/irregularities.
- *Small peripheral breakthrough:* Lift the flap carefully and proceed with laser ablation.
- *Large breakthrough:* Abandon procedure.

Intracameral Gas Bubbles
Gas bubbles escape from the dissection plane into the trabecular meshwork, and then into the anterior chamber. These bubbles can interfere with pupil tracking.

Predisposing Factors
- Large diameter flaps
- Small corneal diameter
- High IOP

Management
- Wait for gas resorption.
- Manual pupil tracking

Opaque Bubble Layer
Escape of gas bubbles from dissection plane into stromal bed.

Predisposing Factors
- Steep corneas
- Smaller white to white diameter (WTW)
- Smaller flaps
- Decentered flaps

Management
- *Peripheral OBL:* Can proceed with ablation after careful lifting of flap.
- *Central OBL:* Wait for resorption of bubbles and then proceed.

■ MICROKERATOME AND FS-RELATED FLAP COMPLICATIONS
Limbal Bleed
Predisposing Factors
- Large diameter flaps
- Hyperopia

- Inappropriately sized/improperly positioned suction rings
- Corneal pannus
- Associated with delayed wound healing, sterile interface keratitis, and decreased contrast sensitivity and glare acuity.

Management
- Gentle pressure on bleeding vessels with help of wexcel sponge
- Thorough washing of interface before flap repositioning

Flap Tears

Predisposing Factors
- Thin flaps
- Underlying tissue adhesions
- Head movement
- Improper flap dissection

Management
- *Small, peripheral tears:* Continue dissection gently and careful lifting of flap.
- *Large tears involving visual axis:* Reposit flap and abandon procedure.

Corneal Epithelial Defect

Predisposing Factors
- Older age
- Steep cornea
- Prior corneal trauma
- Hyperope
- Diabetes/systemic immunosuppression
- History of contact lens use
- Increased corneal thickness
- Basement membrane dystrophy
- Faulty microkeratome

Epithelial defect can predispose to:
- Delayed healing
- DLK
- Epithelial ingrowth
- Flap striae
- Infectious keratitis

Prevention
- Limit toxic topical medications
- Minimize use of topical anesthetics
- Frequent use of lubricating drops
- Preoperative blade inspection and microkeratome maintenance

Management
- Frequent lubricants
- Adequate hygiene
- Placement of BCL on top of defect

Interface Debris

While creating and lifting the flap, debris can accumulate within the interface.

Predisposing Factors
- Preoperative lid disease
- Bleeding from limbus
- Epithelial cells and debris from tear film
- Unsterile instruments

Prevention
- Use an aspirating speculum
- Operate in a lint-free environment
- Drape the lashes and eyelids.

Management
Thorough irrigation of flap and bed before positioning the flap

ABLATION COMPLICATIONS
Central Islands
- Small central elevations in the corneal topography that occur due to beam profile abnormalities, increased hydration of corneal stroma, or particulate material falling onto the cornea may block subsequent laser pulses.
- Resolve with time due to epithelial remodeling.

Decentration
- Due to poor fixation, asymmetrical hydration of the cornea.
- The higher the myopia, the greater is the risk of a decentered ablation, which can cause glare, irregular astigmatism, and a decrease in visual acuity.
- Prevented by incorporating eye-tracking systems and iris registration.
- If decentration >1 mm, the irregular astigmatism that occurs is symptomatic.
- Management of decentration by treatment based on wavefront or topographical information may decrease symptoms.

POSTOPERATIVE COMPLICATIONS
Flap Striae
Predisposing Factors
- Excessive irrigation of flap during LASIK
- Improper repositioning of the flap at the end of procedure
- Thin flaps
- Poor flap handling
- Free caps
- Microkeratome flaps
- Deep and highly myopic ablation
- Postoperative rubbing/squeezing

Flap folds may be classified into macrostriae and microstriae.

Macrostriae
Full thickness, stromal folds, due to flap malposition or slippage.

Management
- *Early postoperative period:* Flap should be immediately lifted, irrigated, and repositioned with BCL on top.
- *After 24 hours:* De-epithelialization, hydration and suturing.
- *If asymptomatic and not involving the visual axis:* Can be left alone.

Microstriae
- Fine folds in Bowman's layer, due to mismatch of flap to new bed.
- Usually visually insignificant.

Management
- Observation
- *If visually significant:* Refloating and suturing.

Flap Dislocation

Movement of the flap from its previous reposited position. It can occur years after procedure.

Predisposing Factors
- Excessive lid squeezing or eye rubbing
- Trauma
- Severe dry eye
- Epithelial abrasions
- Poor intraoperative repositioning
- Excessive irrigation of flap during procedure

Prevention
- Proper preoperative counseling of patient regarding postoperative behavior.
- Remind the patient not to squeeze or rub the eyes.
- Check adhesion of flap at the end of procedure.
- To wear eye shield for the first 24 hours and every night for the first week.

Management
- Reposition the flap.
- Suture the flap in the event of persistent fold.
- Lubricants.

Epithelial Ingrowth

- Aberrant epithelial cells within the flap interface
- *Sources of cells:* Intraoperative epithelial cell implantation/postoperative migration of cells through flap edge

Predisposing Factors
- Intraoperative loose epithelium
- Poor flap adhesion
- Epithelial abrasions/irregularity at the flap margin
- Flap buttonhole
- Free cap
- Flap relifting
- Introduction of epithelial cells during the cut or insertion of instruments
- Inadequate irrigation
- Previous DLK

Prevention
- Avoid epithelial defects.
- Remove epithelial cells and debris from the interface.
- Avoid wide ablation zone.

Management
- *Grade 1:* Thin ingrowth limited to 2 mm of flap edge—No treatment.
- *Grade 2:* Thicker ingrowth, 2 mm from flap edge, progressive—Topical steroids.
- *Grade 3:* Pronounced ingrowth, >2 mm from flap edge, quick progression—Flap lifting and scraping of epithelial cells followed by BCL.

Diffuse Lamellar Keratitis (DLK)
- Accumulation of fine granular appearing infiltrates giving a grainy corneal opacification in the early postoperative period after LASIK.
- Also known as "Sands of Sahara syndrome"

Predisposing Factors
- Intraoperative exposure to red blood cells, fine sponge fibers, or meibomian gland secretions
- Perioperative epithelial defect
- Flap manipulation
- Trauma

Management
- Topical corticosteroids.
- *Nonresponding cases:* Irrigation beneath the flap and repositioning of the flap.

Infectious Keratitis
Predisposing Factors
- Previous ocular surface disease
- Diabetes/systemic immunosuppression
- Surface/interface contamination
- Epithelial defect
- Multiple use of same MK blade
- Delayed epithelial healing
- Prolonged topical steroid use

Prevention
- Adequate sterilization of the instruments
- Preoperative treatment of lid disease/ocular surface disease/dry eye disease
- Use of sterile surgical technique

Management
- Lift flap, scrape and culture the organism
- Fortified antibiotics
- Interface irrigation with antibiotics

Pressure-induced Stromal Keratitis (PISK)
Late-onset interface opacity with a visible fluid cleft in the interface due to elevated IOP because of prolonged corticosteroid treatment.

Management
- Discontinue/taper steroids
- Antiglaucoma medications if required to reduce the IOP.

Central Toxic Keratitis (CTK)

Predisposing Factors

Keratocyte apoptosis/enzymatic degradation

Management
- Spontaneous resolution
- Oral doxycycline/vitamin C/topical hyperosmotics

Dry Eye

Predisposing Factors
- Preoperative dry eye disease
- Chronic CL use
- Diabetes/underlying collagen vascular disorder

Management
- Artificial tears—preservative free
- Anti-inflammatory therapy
- Punctal occlusion
- Treatment of underlying systemic disease

Overcorrection and Undercorrection/Regression
- Result from high refractive errors, improper surgical ablation, malfunction of the laser, abnormal corneal hydration status, and inadequate wound-healing response.
- Crucial to maintain consistent hydration of the cornea, because excessive fluid on the cornea results in an undercorrection.
- If desiccation of the corneal stroma is present, then overcorrection and haze may occur.

Management
- Glasses
- Contact lens
- Repeat ablation

Ectasia

Predisposing Factors
- Abnormal preoperative topography
- Preoperative forme fruste keratoconus
- Low preoperative pachymetry (<500 μm)
- Low residual stromal bed thickness (<250 μm)
- Percentage tissue altered >40%
- High preoperative refractive error

Management
- Assess stability of ectasia
- Contact lens
- CXL
- DALK/PK in progressive cases

SUGGESTED READING

1. Melki SA, Azar DT. LASIK complications: etiology, management, and prevention. Surv Ophthalmol. 2001;46(2):95-116. doi: 10.1016/s0039-6257(01)00254-5. PMID: 11578645.

2. Sahay P, Bafna RK, Reddy JC, Vajpayee RB, Sharma N. Complications of laser-assisted in situkeratomileusis. Indian J Ophthalmol. 2021;69(7):1658-69.
3. Schallhorn SC, Amesbury EC, Tanzer DJ. Avoidance, recognition, and management of LASIK complications. Am J Ophthalmol. 2006;141(4):733-9.

5.25 Posterior Segment Complications after Refractive Surgeries

Shrinivas Joshi, Giriraj Vibhute, Rajashree Salvi
MM Joshi Eye Institute
shrinivasmjoshi@gmail.com

■ INTRODUCTION

As we move forward in the decade, with boom in social media; awareness regarding refractive surgeries in increasing. As the numbers and follow-ups of these patients increase it becomes more and more important for general ophthalmologists to know about these procedures, their merits and possible complications. It is important to remember that in handling refractive surgery patients *"An ounce of prevention is better than a pound of cure."*

Refractive surgeries are meant to improve the refractive status of the eye such as myopia, hypermetropia, presbyopia as well as in cases of stable keratoconus, thus reducing the dependency on spectacles or contact lenses which is the need in younger generation. This includes surgical remodeling and thus is divided into:

■ CORNEA-BASED SURGERIES/KERATOREFRACTIVE PROCEDURES

- LASIK/FEMTO LASIK (Femtosecond-assisted laser in-situ keratomileusis)
- SMILE (small incision lenticule extraction)
- *Surface ablation:*
  - PRK
  - LASEK (laser subepithelial keratomileusis)
  - Epi-LASIK (epithelial laser in situ keratomileusis)
  - CONTURA
- Corneal inlays/rings
- RK

■ LENS-BASED SURGERIES

- Clear lens extraction with intraocular lens (IOL) implantation
- Phakic IOL

■ COMBINED

A detailed preoperative evaluation including peripheral examination of retina is mandatory before going ahead with refractive surgery. If preoperative evaluation is suggestive of retinal holes/breaks, these are managed first by laser photocoagulation after which refractive surgery is done.

Irrespective of all the precautionary measures, posterior segment complications are known to occur postrefractive surgery.
- *Keratorefractive procedures:* The exact relationship is difficult to establish between keratorefractive procedures and retinal complications. Following are the common vitreoretinal complications noted:
  - *Posterior vitreous detachment (PVD):* Suction applied during LASIK, which can be as high as 90 mm Hg, results in increase in the anteroposterior diameter of

the eye thus resulting in reduction of horizontal diameter. This causes the lens to be pushed anteriorly resulting in traction over the vitreous base and posterior pole as well thus leading to PVD.

Using femtosecond instead of microkeratome for the flap requires lesser suction but is more prolonged and so is Epi-LASIK, thus resulting in other rare complications such as optic disc edema and vascular insult.

- *Retinal detachment (RD):* A study by Arevalo JF et al. has shown that the incidence of RD was 0.06% in post-LASIK eyes. Similar study carried out by Qin B et al. suggested incidence of RD to be even less of 0.03% 9 months post-LASIK. These two major studies show that RD cannot be directly linked to refractive procedure and can also be secondary to preexisting refractive error, thus suggesting a temporal though not necessarily a causal relationship. In case series by Ruiz Moreno JM et al. 11 RD cases were noted postphotorefractive keratectomy (PRK) although the exact incidence is not known.
- *Macular hemorrhage:* This has been noted in eyes with preexisting break in Bruch's membrane and thus should not be taken up for refractive surgery.
- *Epiretinal membrane (ERM):* Preexisting breaks in BM or new breaks developed secondary to suction used during LASIK releases the glial cells, which after PVD results in ERM formation.
- *Other rare complications:* This includes choroidal neovascular membrane (CNVM), optic disc edema, Valsalva such as retinopathy (as early as 15 hours post-hyperopic LASIK), cystoid macular edema (CME), full thickness macular hole (FTMH), peripheral retinal tears, uveal effusion (mainly after hyperopic LASIK), central serous chorioretinopathy (CSCR), toxoplasmosis reactivation, etc.

■ *Lens-based procedures:* This can be differentiated into:
- *Clear lens extraction with IOL implantation:*
  - Globe perforation (due to peribulbar anesthesia)
  - Suprachoroidal hemorrhage (intraoperative or postoperative)
  - Dropped nucleus
  - Posterior capsular opacification (PCO)
  - RD
  - CME
  - Macular phototoxicity (due to UV radiation from the operating microscope)
  - Macular infarction
  - Endophthalmitis
  - Postoperative difficult retinal evaluation and management if required (after MFIOL insertion), etc.
- *Phakic IOL implantation:* This includes complications such as RD, CME, endophthalmitis, difficulty in peripheral retinal evaluation, optic neuropathy, etc.

The most common of all the complications listed above is:

Retinal detachment: The rate of retinal detachments after lens-based refractive surgery is significantly higher than it is after corneal refractive surgery.

- Neuhann et al. studied 2,356 eyes in 1,500 myopic patients and found an incidence of retinal detachment between 1.5% and 2.2%, which was significantly higher than that noted after keratorefractive surgeries.
- Similarly, Alió et al. studied 439 eyes of 274 myopic patients and found a slightly higher rate of retinal detachment at 2.7%. Alió's study also pointed to an increased risk of retinal detachment in the long term. The rate of detachment was only 0.47% at 3 months; however, it increased to 3.28% at 5 years.
- An incidence of 4.8% of retinal detachment was reported following the implantation of phakic intraocular lenses to correct severe myopia by Ruiz-Moreno JM et al. This can be attributable to preexisting myopia as well as fluidics during phakic IOL surgery.

- Incidence of RD post-CLE without IOL implantation was found to be 7.3% by Barraquer et al. This can be attributed to myopia, surgical trauma and aphakia as well.

Thus, thorough preoperative counseling becomes a must to avoid untoward consequences. Preoperative consent from the patient should be taken by anterior segment surgeon which includes risk of retinal complications for which further treatment may be required. Also an urgent referral to vitreoretinal surgeon should be done if a patient complains of sudden onset of floaters, flashes of light or significant decrease in vision at any point of time after refractive surgery.

Few points to be remembered with respect to the management of RD:
1. If Scleral Buckling is planned for RD postrefractive surgery, patient may have induced myopia or rarely may develop hyperopia and would not be happy about it, for which LASIK enhancement/another refractive procedure might be required. Hence conjunctival scarring or anterior placement of encerclage should be avoided by VR surgeons as far as possible.
2. In eyes with phakic IOLs if vitrectomy is planned, then the tamponading agents sometimes might cause shallowing of anterior chamber thus resulting in endothelial touch by the phakic IOL. This is not the case with cornea-based refractive procedures.
3. In post-Lasik patients if epithelial debridement is required during vitrectomy, then care should be taken to protect the flap. Complications may include complete loss of flap, epithelial ingrowth, interface particles and striae in the flap. Hence it is always helpful to know the location of hinge in LASIK eyes, and if not known then to proceed with epithelial debridement from nasal to temporal aspect.
4. In eyes that have underwent PRK, corneal haze may hamper retinal visualization.
5. There can be difficulty in visualization of peripheral retina in eyes with phakic IOL.

Thus every ophthalmologist should remember that *"An ametropic eye that has undergone refractive correction always remains ametropic with regard to the retina".*

SECTION 6
Uveitis and Ophthalmic Pathology

Editor: *Jyotirmay Biswas*

A. Uveitis

6.1 **Anterior Uveitis** 412
Amala E George

6.2 **Intermediate Uveitis** 415
SR Rathinam, Rajshree E

6.3 **Posterior Uveitis** 420
S Sudharshan, Nivedita Nair

6.4 **Panuveitis** 424
Vishali Gupta

6.5 **Retinal Vasculitis** 425
Reema Bansal, Vishali Gupta, Amod Gupta

6.6 **Viral Retinitis** 429
Suchitra Pradeep

6.7 **Coronavirus Disease 2019 and Eye** 430
Aditya Patil, Ankush Kawali, Srinivasan Sanjay, Sai Bhakti Mishra, Padmamalini Mahendradas

6.8 **Uveitic Pathology** 434
Jyotirmay Biswas, Dipankar Das

6.9 **Immunosuppressives in Uveitis** 435
Namita Dave, Somasheila I Murthy

B. Ocular Pathology

6.10 **Pathology of the Eyelid** 441
Dipankar Das, Bidhan Chandra Das, Obaidur Rehman, Apurba Deka

6.11 **Ocular Pathology: Laboratory Procedures** 445
Jyotirmay Biswas, Dipankar Das

6.12 **Intraocular Tumors** 450
S Krishnakumar, Jyotirmay Biswas

6.13 **Orbital Tumors** 453
Jyotirmay Biswas, Dipankar Das

A. UVEITIS

6.1 Anterior Uveitis

Amala E George
Sankara Nethralaya, Chennai
amalaelizabeth@gmail.com

■ ANTERIOR UVEITIS AND RELEVANT HISTORY

Anterior uveitis refers to inflammation of the anterior part of the uveal tract, viz., iris and ciliary body.

History

Age and Sex of the Patient
- *Children:* Juvenile idiopathic arthritis (JIA) associated anterior uveitis, Blau syndrome, granulomatous anterior uveitis associated with tuberculosis (TB)
- *Young adults:* Human leukocyte antigen (HLA)-B27-related anterior uveitis, JIA-associated anterior uveitis, granulomatous anterior uveitis associated with TB/sarcoidosis
- *Middle age:* Sarcoidosis, HLA-B27-related anterior uveitis
- *Elderly:* Infectious uveitis, Masquerade syndromes, postoperative, drug-induced
- *Any age:* Infections, post-trauma, surgery.

Symptoms
- *Pain, redness, decrease in vision:* Present/absent; severity
- *Type of onset of the problem* Sudden, gradual
- *Associated symptoms:* Ocular, systemic.

Systems Review
Specific questions related to other systems: Arthritis, central nervous system (CNS) symptoms gastrointestinal tract (GIT)/genitourinary tract (GUT), skin involvement/recent dental procedures.

Family History
History of uveitis in the family: HLA-B27-related uveitis, Blau syndrome (early onset of granulomatous anterior uveitis progressing to panuveitis).

Past Ocular History
- *Number of attacks:* Date of first attack, latest attack; interval between attacks
- Unilateral/bilateral involvement
- History of ocular trauma/surgery.

Treatment History
- *Use of steroids:* Topical, periocular, intravitreal, systemic
- If periocular steroids have been used—when was the last injection given?
- Use of immunosuppressive agents—type
- Use of biologics—type
- *Complications of past treatment:* Ocular/systemic side effects (cataract, glaucoma, Cushing's syndrome)
- Treatment of complications—any glaucoma medication/cataract surgery
- Current medication—drug-induced uveitis (prostaglandins, bisphosphonates, biologics such as etanercept).

Ocular Surgery
- *Cataract surgery:* Type of surgery, intraocular lens (IOL), history of uveitis prior to surgery, postoperative complications, adequate steroid cover given perioperatively in preexisting uveitis cases or possibility of infection
- Any other ocular surgery—glaucoma, vitreoretinal surgery.

■ EXAMINATION OF A CASE OF ANTERIOR UVEITIS
External Examination
- *Face:* Any scars of herpes zoster ophthalmicus (HZO); Hansen's disease
- *Hand:* Rheumatoid arthritis; Hansen's disease
- *Posture:* Ankylosing spondylitis; JIA.

Ocular Examination
Torch Light Examination
Extent, color, and pattern of congestion: Scleritis versus circumciliary congestion.

Slit-lamp Examination
- *Conjunctiva:* Congestion, nodules, necrosis
- *Sclera:* Congestion, nodules, necrosis
- *Cornea:* Band-shaped keratopathy; scars of viral keratitis—active/healed; corneal edema
- *Keratic precipitates:* Fresh/old; size—fine, small, medium, large, mutton fat; distribution—Arlt's triangle—diffuse and localized
- *Anterior chamber:* Grading of cells, flare; hypopyon—type, color, thickness in mm; hyphema; fibrin
- *Iris*—atrophy—sectoral/diffuse; nodules—Koeppe-Busacca nodules; posterior synechiae—localized—number of clock hours; 360°; peripheral anterior synechiae—number of clock hours; iris bombe
- *Lens*—clear/cataractous; type of cataract—posterior subcapsular, nuclear, total; synechiae
- *IOL*—in postoperative uveitis—type of IOL, fixation of haptics, deposits on IOL
- Intraocular pressure (IOP)
- Gonioscopy—keratic precipitates in the angle, inflammatory synechiae—number of clock hours
- Anterior vitreous—grading of anterior vitreous cells
- Fundus examination (slit-lamp biomicroscopy/indirect ophthalmoscopy) to look for any posterior segment pathology especially pars planitis and cystoid macular edema.

■ GRADING OF AQUEOUS FLARE AND CELLS IN ANTERIOR UVEITIS (STANDARDIZATION OF UVEITIS NOMENCLATURE WORKING GROUP CLASSIFICATION)
Standardization of uveitis nomenclature (SUN) working group classification (field 1 × 1 mm slit beam) is shown in **Tables 6.1.1 and 6.1.2**.

■ INVESTIGATIONS NEEDED IN A CASE OF NONGRANULOMATOUS ANTERIOR UVEITIS
- In patients with inflammatory arthritis—rheumatoid factor, antinuclear antibody levels, erythrocyte sedimentation rates
- In spondyloarthropathies and severe anterior uveitis—HLA-B27 typing; sacroiliac joint X-ray

TABLE 6.1.1: Anterior chamber cells.

Grades	Cells in field
0	<1
0.5+	1–5
1+	6–15
2+	16–25
3+	26–50
4+	>50

TABLE 6.1.2: Anterior chamber flare.

Grades	Descriptions
0	None
1+	Faint
2+	Moderate (iris and lens details clear)
3+	Marked (iris and lens details hazy)
4+	Intense (fibrin or plastic aqueous)

INVESTIGATIONS NEEDED IN A CASE OF GRANULOMATOUS ANTERIOR UVEITIS

- Investigations to rule out TB, syphilis and sarcoidosis
- Chest X-ray or computed tomography (CT) chest
- Mantoux test
- Erythrocyte sedimentation rate
- QuantiFERON test
- Rapid plasma reagin test and *Treponema pallidum* hemagglutination tests
- Serum angiotensin-converting enzyme levels, serum lysozyme levels
- Serum calcium, phosphorus levels
- In cases with features and family history suggestive of Blau syndrome gene sequencing (NOD2 mutations).

ANTERIOR CHAMBER PARACENTESIS

- In cases of suspected viral anterior uveitis (raised IOP/corneal opacities)—varicella zoster virus (VZV), herpes simplex virus (HSV)
- Granulomatous uveitis suggestive of TB.

TREATMENT OF ANTERIOR UVEITIS

Local Therapy

The mainstay of treatment in anterior uveitis is topical steroids and cycloplegic agents.

Topical steroids: Reduces the inflammation; frequency of application can be varied according to the severity of inflammation. The preferred topical steroid is often prednisolone acetate eye drop. In severe anterior uveitis topical steroids can be applied as frequently as 1 drop every 5–10 minutes along with strong cycloplegics.

The most commonly used cycloplegic is homatropine eye drops taken 2–4 times per day. In severe anterior uveitis with posterior synechiae of recent origin atropine eye drops can be used to break the synechiae. Once the synechiae are broken, homatropine drops can be used. With control in inflammation the topical steroids can be tapered gradually.

Systemic Therapy

Viral uveitis: Anti-viral therapy—oral acyclovir or valaciclovir in VZV- or HSV- related cases; oral valganciclovir in cytomegalovirus (CMV)-associated anterior uveitis; ganciclovir gel is a useful addition in CMV-related cases; the epithelial toxicity of acyclovir ointment limits its use to situations when dendritic lesions are present.

HLA-B27 uveitis and JIA-related uveitis: Periocular or oral steroids may be required in severe cases. Immunosuppressives/biologics may be required in chronic recurrent HLA-B27-related anterior uveitis and for the long-term management of JIA-related uveitis.

MANAGEMENT OF COMPLICATIONS

It is important to make sure that complications if present are managed simultaneously.
- *Raised IOP:* Addition of antiglaucoma agents, yttrium–aluminum–garnet (YAG) peripheral iridotomy (PI) if iris bombe/relative pupillary block is present
- Band-shaped keratopathy (BSK) removal
- Cataract surgery.

CONCLUSION

Anterior uveitis is the most common type of uveitis encountered in the general population. Prompt recognition and treatment with topical steroids and cycloplegics preserve vision and avoid long-term sight-threatening complications.

6.2 Intermediate Uveitis

SR Rathinam, Rajshree E
Aravind Eye Hospital and PG Institute of Ophthalmology, Madurai
rathinam@aravind.org

INTRODUCTION

Standardization of Uveitis Nomenclature (SUN) defines intermediate uveitis (IU) as a subset of uveitis where the vitreous is the major site of inflammation in the absence of choroiditis or retinitis.[1] The overall prevalence of IU in various parts of India is 10.66% (North India),[2] 11.3% (Himalayan belt region),[3] 23.61% (Northeast India),[4] 31.9% (Central India),[5] 16.7% (Western India),[6] and 13.33% (Southern India).[7]

Large-scale studies have shown that the cause is unknown (idiopathic) in majority of IU in all age groups. Tuberculosis was found to be the major cause of infectious uveitis.

ETIOLOGY

Etiology of intermediate uveitis is diverse **(Table 6.2.1)**:
- *Intermediate uveitis:* This entity includes vitritis and an associated systemic etiology. It may be either infectious or noninfectious causes.
- *Pars planitis:* It presents with snowballs and snowbanking. It is usually eye-limited and immune-mediated without any specific systemic etiology **(Table 6.2.2)**.
- *Intermediate uveitis:* It is of non-pars planitis type. Recently, SUN working group (2021) has introduced this entity, which does not have features of pars planitis like snowbanking but it is still eye-limited and immune-mediated and does not have a systemic etiology **(Table 6.2.3)**.

TABLE 6.2.1: Intermediate uveitis.

Infectious	Noninfectious
• Tuberculosis	• Sarcoidosis
• Leptospirosis	• Multiple sclerosis
• Toxoplasmosis	• Pars planitis
• Toxocariasis	• Masquerade
• Lyme disease	• Amyloidosis
• Cat scratch disease	
• Immune recovery vitritis	

SYMPTOMS

- Floaters
- Blurred vision
- Redness and pain—usually absent unless there is spill over anterior uveitis
- Sudden deterioration of vision—in vitreous hemorrhage or retinal detachment
- Scotoma—in case of macular edema

TABLE 6.2.2: Classification criteria for pars planitis.[8]

Criteria	Exclusions

• Evidence of intermediate uveitis:
  – Vitreous cells AND/OR vitreous haze
  – If anterior chamber cells are present, anterior chamber inflammation severity less than vitreous severity
  – No evidence of retinitis or choroiditis
  – No retinal vascular occlusion in posterior pole and mid-periphery*
• Evidence of pars planitis:
  – Vitreous snowballs
  – Pars plana snowbanks
	• Multiple sclerosis, defined by the McDonald criteria
	• Positive serology test result for syphilis using a treponemal test
	• Evidence of sarcoidosis (either bilateral hilaradenopathy on chest imaging or tissue biopsy demonstrating noncaseating granulomata)
	• Positive serology for Lyme disease, either IgG or IgM (e.g. positive ELISA AND Western blot with requisite number of bands for assay used)

*Peripheral retinal nonperfusion on wide-field angiography is compatible with pars planitis diagnosis
(ELISA: enzyme-linked immunosorbent assay; IgG: immunoglobulin G)

TABLE 6.2.3: Classification criteria for intermediate uveitis, non-pars planitis type.[8]

Criteria	Exclusions

• Evidence of intermediate uveitis:
  – Vitreous cells AND/OR vitreous haze
  – If anterior chamber cells are present, anterior chamber inflammation less than vitreous humor
  – No evidence of retinitis
• No evidence of pars planitis:
  – No vitreous snowballs
  – No pars plana snowbanks
	• Multiple sclerosis, defined by the McDonald criteria
	• Positive serology test result for syphilis using a treponemal test
	• Evidence of sarcoidosis (either bilateral hilaradenopathy on chest imaging or tissue biopsy demonstrating noncaseating granulomata)
	• Positive serology for Lyme disease, either IgG or IgM (e.g. positive ELISA AND Western blot with requisite number of bands for assay used)
	• Evidence of intraocular lymphoma on diagnostic vitrectomy

(ELISA: enzyme-linked immunosorbent assay; IgG: immunoglobulin G)

EXAMINATION

Slit lamp biomicroscopy with +90 D or +78 D lens is very important in the evaluation of vitreous inflammation, status of the macula, and optic nerve head in case of IU. A thorough indirect ophthalmoscopy with scleral indentation with +20 D lens is a must for identifying snowbanking in a case of pars planitis.

SIGNS

Anterior Segment
- Minimal anterior chamber cells may be present (spill over)
- Keratic precipitates (granulomatous or nongranulomatous)
- Band-shaped keratopathy in long-standing cases, especially in children
- Complicated cataract.

Posterior Segment
- Vitreous cells are the most important feature in active IU. Uniform and coarse vitreous cells in elderly patients point more towards lymphoma
- Fluffy, yellowish white vitreous aggregates called snowballs are seen in the inferior periphery
- Snowbanking occurs when the exudates (fibroinflammatory material) get deposited over the pars plana and is usually seen through indirect ophthalmoscopy by scleral depression. In chronic cases, fibrosis of pars plana can occur
- Peripheral vasculitis and neovascularization
- Cystoid macular edema.

SPECIFIC CLINICAL ENTITIES

Tuberculosis
Tuberculosis is the common infectious cause of IU in developing countries like India. History, systemic and ocular examination with appropriate investigations, and imaging will help in diagnosing a case of TB IU. Presence of chorioretinal scar along the vascular arcade is a typical feature of TB uveitis.

Leptospirosis
Leptospirosis is one of the causes of IU in agricultural countries like India, where exposure to cattle excreta, which is the common source of the spirochete is common. Presence of veil-like vitreous membrane is the pathognomonic feature of leptospiral uveitis. Rapid maturation of unilateral cataract is another feature suggestive of ocular leptospirosis.

Sarcoidosis
Sarcoidosis is being identified as one of the common causes of IU in the recent years even in developing countries where TB is endemic. Though ocular and systemic clinical picture may mimic tuberculosis in certain cases, there are few signs which are specific for sarcoidosis. Presence of focal candle wax retinal vasculitis in a patient with hilar lymphadenopathy without calcified nodes is more in favor of sarcoidosis.

Multiple Sclerosis
Though multiple sclerosis (MS) is portrayed as the common cause of IU in western population, the incidence and diagnosis has also increased in our country due to the affordability and availability of imaging techniques. Hence MS should also be considered as a differential while evaluating a patient with IU.

INVESTIGATIONS

TABLE 6.2.4: Ocular investigations and significance.

Ocular investigations	Significance
B scan	Done when there is cataract or dense vitritis obscuring the fundus view; it is done to document vitritis; retinal detachment
Fundus fluorescein angiography	Done for identifying the extent and severity of vasculitis, neovascularization, capillary non perfusion areas
Ultrasound biomicroscopy	• To detect the cause of hypotony (ciliary body atrophy or detachment) • Presence of exudates or cyclitic membrane over pars plana
Optical coherence tomography	To quantify macular edema and to monitor its response for the treatment

TABLE 6.2.5: Systemic diseases and investigations.

Systemic diseases	Investigations
Tuberculosis	• Mantoux, Chest X-ray/High resolution CT chest and abdomen • QuantiFERON TB • Lymph node examination biopsy • Sputum for culture
Sarcoidosis	• High resolution CT • Angiotensin converting enzyme • Lysozyme • Gallium scan • Biopsy • Bronchoalveolar lavage
Syphilis	TPHA, VDRL
Multiple sclerosis	MRI brain
Intraocular lymphoma	• Vitreous biopsy • CSF analysis • MRI brain
Cat scratch disease	*Bartonella henselae* immunofluorescence assay (IFA)
HIV, Lyme's disease	ELISA

(CT: computed tomography; ELISA: enzyme-linked immunosorbent assay; HIV: human immunodeficiency virus; MRI: magnetic resonance imaging; TPHA: *Treponema pallidum* hemagglutination; VDRL: venereal disease research laboratory)

■ TREATMENT

Active inflammation requires immediate treatment. Though some of the literature indicates treatment for visual acuity equal to or <6/12, and long-standing inflammation could be a potential threat to the visual prognosis. Therefore even a patient with 6/6 visual acuity with significant complaint of floaters is eligible for treatment in IU.

Treatment for Infectious Intermediate Uveitis

Even the infectious type will need steroid for control of associated inflammation, but under antimicrobial cover.

Tuberculosis

Antitubercular therapy (ATT) is prescribed for 7–9 months depending on associated systemic picture in patients with tubercular uveitis.

Toxoplasmosis

Four-drug regimen is commonly used in ocular toxoplasmosis. Oral azithromycin 500 mg OD for 7–10 days along with cotrimoxazole (trimethoprim 160 mg/sulfamethoxazole 800 mg) for up to 21 days along with oral steroid are used in suspected cases.

Toxocariasis

Steroid therapy is recommended in cases where there is active inflammation. Role of antihelminthic therapy is controversial. Oral albendazole 400 mg twice daily is the recommended standard drug regimen.

■ TREATMENT FOR NONINFECTIOUS INTERMEDIATE UVEITIS

- Corticosteroids remain to be the mainstay of treatment in noninfectious IU. Oral steroids (prednisolone 1–2 mg/kg bodyweight) and periocular steroids

- (injection triamcinolone acetonide 2–4 mg/0.1 mL by posterior sub-Tenon's route) are preferred
- Intravitreal triamcinolone acetonide is preferred in severe macular edema, whereas intravitreal Ozurdex implant is preferred for macular edema in post-vitrectomized eyes
- Uveitis which is refractory to steroids or in conditions where steroids are contraindicated are treated with immunosuppressants such as methotrexate, mycophenolate mofetil, azathioprine, or cyclophosphamide
- Severe cases require newer biologic agents like tumor necrosis factor alpha (TNF-α) inhibitors—adalimumab(40 mg) and infliximab injection 5 mg/kg (3–10 mg/kg). Studies have shown that noninfectious uveitis attained quiescence when treated with adalimumab with minimal corticosteroid support and also achieved improvement in the mean best corrected visual acuity[9]
- Pediatric uveitis needs aggressive and long-term treatment than adult onset uveitis as the presentation is usually bilateral and severe
- Nonselective TNF-α inhibitors are avoided in MS as central nervous system (CNS) demyelination is a potential adverse effect[10]
- Presence of vitreous opacification, vitreous hemorrhage, retinal detachment, and dense epiretinal membrane warrant pars plana vitrectomy. Diagnostic vitrectomy is essential to rule out lymphoma, amyloidosis, and masquerade
- Laser photocoagulation is done in patients with capillary nonperfusion areas secondary to neovascularization caused by vasculitis
- Cryotherapy is not preferred these days due to its high complication rate
- Cataract surgery is planned only after a quiescence period of 3 months, under steroid cover with or without immunosuppressives
- Interferon alpha is an effective drug in treating refractory post-uveitic macular edema.[11]

COMPLICATIONS

The common complications seen in IU include:
- Cataract
- Glaucoma
- Cystoid macular edema
- Ocular hypotony
- Cyclitic membrane
- Band-shaped keratopathy
- Exudative or rhegmatogenous retinal detachment
- Retinal and choroidal neovascularization.

PROGNOSIS

Intermediate uveitis is considered as a benign disease which can attain remission with proper immunomodulatory therapy. But the chronicity, recurrence rate, and vision-threatening complications worsen the visual prognosis. Hence prompt diagnosis, treatment, and regular follow-ups are extremely important for successful remission of the disease.

REFERENCES

1. Jabs DA, Nussenblatt RB, Rosenbaum JT; Standardization of Uveitis Nomenclature (SUN) Working Group. Standardization of uveitis nomenclature for reporting clinical data. Results of the First International Workshop. Am J Ophthalmol. 2005;140(3):509-16.
2. Dogra M, Singh R, Agarwal A, Sharma A, Singh SR, Gautam N, et al. Epidemiology of Uveitis in a Tertiary-care Referral Institute in North India. Ocul Immunol Inflamm. 2017;25(sup1):S46-53.

3. Pandurangan S, Samanta R, Kumawat D, Sood G, Devi TS, Agrawal A. Pattern of uveitis from a tertiary eye care center in Himalayan belt of North India. Indian J Ophthalmol. 2022;70(5):1642-7.
4. Das D, Bhattacharjee H, Das K, Tahiliani PS, Bhattacharyya P, Bharali G, et al. The changing patterns of uveitis in a tertiary institute of Northeast India. Indian J Ophthalmol. 2015;63:735-7.
5. Borde P; Priyanka, Kumar K, Takkar B, Sharma B. Pattern of uveitis in a tertiary eye care center of central India: Results of a prospective patient database over a period of two years. Indian J Ophthalmol. 2020;68(3):476-81.
6. Palsule AC, Jande V, Kulkari AA, Beke NN. Pattern of uveitis in tertiary care center in Western India. J Clin Ophthalmol Res. 2017;5:127-31.
7. Tyagi M, Das AV, Kaza H, Basu S, Pappuru RR, Pathengay A, et al. LV Prasad Eye Institute Eye Smart electronic medical record-based analytics of big data: LEAD-Uveitis Report 1: Demographics and clinical features of uveitis in a multi-tier hospital based network in Southern India. Indian J Ophthalmol. 2022;70(4):1260-7.
8. Standardization of Uveitis Nomenclature (SUN) Working Group. Classification Criteria for Pars Planitis. Am J Ophthalmol. 2021;228:268-74.
9. Suhler EB, Adán A, Brézin AP, Fortin E, Goto H, Jaffe GJ, et al. Safety and Efficacy of Adalimumab in Patients with Noninfectious Uveitis in an Ongoing Open-Label Study: VISUAL III. Ophthalmology. 2018;125(7):1075-87.
10. Fresegna D, Bullitta S, Musella A, Rizzo FR, De Vito F, Guadalupi L, et al. Re-Examining the Role of TNF in MS Pathogenesis and Therapy. Cells. 2020;9(10):2290.
11. Dimopoulos S, Deuter CME, Blumenstock G, Zierhut M, Dimopoulou A, Voykov B, et al. Interferon Alpha for Refractory Pseudophakic Cystoid Macular Edema (Irvine-Gass Syndrome). Ocul Immunol Inflamm. 2020;28(2):315-21.

6.3 Posterior Uveitis

S Sudharshan
Sankara Nethralaya, Chennai
drdharshan@gmail.com

Nivedita Nair
KIMS Health Hospital, Bahrain
nivedita33@gmail.com

■ COMMON TYPES

Posterior uveitic entities can be varied and can be classified based on:

Etiology

- *Infective causes:* These include toxoplasmosis, toxocariasis, tuberculosis (TB), syphilis, viral [herpes simplex, varicella zoster, cytomegalovirus, dengue, chikungunya, West Nile, coronavirus disease 2019 (COVID-19) and human immunodeficiency virus (HIV)], *Bartonella*, and others.
- *Noninfective causes:* These include sarcoidosis, white dot syndromes (WDSs) such as acute posterior multifocal placoid pigment epitheliopathy (APMPPE), multiple evanescent white dot syndrome (MEWDS), serpiginous choroiditis, multifocal choroiditis (MFC), punctate inner choroidopathy (PIC), birdshot choroidopathy, presumed ocular histoplasmosis syndrome (POHS), subretinal fibrosis and uveitis syndrome, diffuse unilateral subacute neuroretinitis (DUSN), and retinal pigment epithelitis (Krill's disease).

Clinical Characteristics of a Lesion

Clinical characteristics include choroiditis, retinochoroiditis/chorioretinitis, retinitis, neuroretinitis, retinal vasculitis, granuloma, exudative retinal detachment/subretinal fluid pockets, optic neuritis, optic nerve head (ONH) granuloma, and uveitic mass lesions or those masquerading as uveitis.

COMMON COMPLAINTS

Common complaints include floaters due to vitritis, metamorphopsia, and diminution of vision due to intense vitritis and lesions adjacent to and/or involving the macula, fovea, and/or ONH. Peripheral lesions can even be asymptomatic.

EXAMINATION OF A CASE

Slit-lamp biomicroscopy with +90 D or +78 D lens is very important in the evaluation of vitreous inflammation, status of the macula, and ONH in case of posterior uveitis. A thorough indirect ophthalmoscopy with scleral indentation with +20 D is a MUST in every case of posterior uveitis.

ANCILLARY TESTS

- *Color fundus photography:* This test is done for serial documentation of lesions. Fundus photography helps in serially documenting the retinal lesion. A typical camera views 30°–50° of retinal area, with a magnification of 2.5x. Newer widefield and ultra-widefield fundus photography instruments [Optos® camera (Optos PLC, Dunfermline, UK), Clarus® 500 (Carl Zeiss Meditec)] view around 200° of retinal area and helps in documentation and follow-up of peripheral lesions. The newer camera and widefield imaging systems can give high-quality images even with small and/or undilated pupils
- *Fundus autofluorescence:* This is a noninvasive procedure depicting the status of metabolic activity of the retinal pigment epithelium. It helps in diagnosis and monitoring of lesions during follow-up with treatment. Healed and active lesions have very characteristic patterns
- *Fundus fluorescein angiography (FFA):*
  - Confirms activity of choroiditis/retinitis
  - Detects disease sequelae such as neovascularization of disc (NVD) and neovascularization elsewhere (NVE), capillary nonperfusion (CNP) areas and vascular leakage and staining in cases of retinal vasculitis
  - Reveals atypical flower petal pattern in cystoid macular edema (CME)
  - Typical pinpoint hyperfluorescence in case of Vogt–Koyanagi–Haradagi (VKH) disease, sympathetic ophthalmia (SO), or posterior scleritis
  - Pooling of dye in late phase in subretinal fluid in VKH, SO, etc.
  - Most useful to detect the presence, type, and activity of choroidal neovascularization (CNV).

Widefield and ultra-widefield FFA are helpful even in small pupils to have a wider field of retinal vasculature especially in conditions such as retinal vasculitis.
- *Indocyanine green angiography (ICG):* It is useful in deeper choroidal lesions, CNV, and in presence of hemorrhages. It helps in detection, identification, and follow-up of WDSs. It is used nowadays in detecting early posterior segment activity in convalescent and chronic recurrent phases of VKH
- *Optical coherence tomography (OCT):* OCT is categorized into time-domain and spectral-domain OCT. Spectral-domain gives a higher resolution imaging and is useful in detecting and monitoring posterior pole pathologies such as CME, epiretinal membrane (ERM), choroidal neovascular membrane (CNVM), and macular hole. Newer enhanced-depth imaging like swept source OCT (SS–OCT) can help in detecting the choroidal thickness and changes in the choroid such as stromal choroiditis, and subfoveal choroidal thickening, which as a noninvasive technique is helpful in diagnosis and follow-up of patients with VKH and sympathetic ophthalmia

- *OCT angiography (OCTA):* This is noninvasive, depth-resolution imaging tool which gives qualitative and quantitative information about the status of retinal and choroidal vessels
  - Helpful in detecting CNVMs
  - Demonstrates neovascularization and capillary nonperfusion areas in retinal vasculitis
  - Full-thickness granulomas can be visible in the form of hyporeflectivity, corresponding to reduced flow on OCTA
- Visual field testing as function of ONH and in select WDS and retinopathies
- *Ultrasonography:*
  - Rules out intraocular tumors in case of elevated mass-like lesions such as tuberculous subretinal abscess
  - To detect choroidal thickness, *T* sign and retinal detachments in case of no view of fundus
- *Ultrasound biomicroscopy:*
  - Useful in detecting status of pars plana, peripheral toxocara granuloma, etc.
  - Especially useful in case of hypotony for detecting the cause and decide medical or surgical management of the same
  - Supraciliary effusion, foreign bodies, etc.
- *Electroretinogram (ERG)/multifocal ERG:*
  - Useful in WDSs—for follow-up of activity
  - Acute zonal occult outer retinopathy (AZOOR), autoimmune retinopathy and other WDS.

COMMON LABORATORY TESTS

Hemogram is done in most cases. Other specific tests commonly done include:
- *TB:* Chest X-ray/high-resolution computed tomography (CT) scan of chest, Mantoux test, QuantiFERON-TB gold tests in selected cases, polymerase chain reaction (PCR) from ocular fluid, bronchoscopy, bronchial lavage and biopsy from mediastinal lymph nodes
- *Toxoplasmosis:* ELISA (enzyme-linked immunosorbent assay) for *toxoplasma* antibodies [immunoglobulin G (IgG)/IgM], PCR from aqueous tap. Aqueous antibody is also useful with Goldman–Witmer coefficient calculation
- *Toxocara:* ELISA for *toxocara* antibodies
- *Syphilis:* Venereal diseases research laboratory test (VDRL) rapid plasma reagin test, *Treponema pallidum* hemagglutination test
- *HIV:* ELISA
- *Viral:* PCR from aqueous or vitreous in selected cases with when there is diagnostic dilemma
- *Sarcoidosis:* Chest X-ray/high-resolution CT scan of chest, Mantoux test, serum angiotensin-converting enzyme (ACE), serum calcium and inorganic phosphorous, bronchoscopy, bronchial lavage, and biopsy from mediastinal lymph nodes in necessary cases.

In patients on systemic steroids and immunosuppressives, blood sugar, blood counts, and liver and renal function tests to monitor for side effects as the case maybe.

MANAGEMENT

A Case of Noninfective Posterior Uveitis
- Systemic steroids are the mainstay of noninfective posterior uveitis
- Intravenous methylprednisolone (IVMP) therapy 1 g daily in 3 consecutive days under monitoring in acute vision-threatening lesions
- *Oral steroids:* Prednisolone 1–1.5 mg/kg/day tapered 5–10 mg per week and based on the response may have to continue low maintenance dose of oral steroids for longer duration

- Monitor blood pressure (BP), blood sugar, and for other side effects
- Use immunosuppressives, with caution, in recalcitrant cases
- Monitor blood counts and liver and renal function tests as and when required
- Common immunomodulators used are azathioprine, mycophenolate mofetil, methotrexate (more commonly in children), cyclophosphamide, and cyclosporine
- *Biologicals:* Infliximab, adalimumab, daclizumab—in case of Behçet's disease, JIA, and refractory posterior uveitis
- *Intravitreal steroids:*
  - Ozurdex can be helpful in recalcitrant macular edema. It can be planned at an interval of 3 months under monitoring of intraocular pressure (IOP), and can be helpful in cases where systemic steroids are contraindicated or in special situations like pregnancy
  - Fluocinolone acetonide is used as an intravitreal implant in recalcitrant CME and has long duration of action of 3 years.

A Case of Infective Posterior Uveitis

Principles of Treatment

- To treat the infection primarily
- Additional low-dose systemic steroids to prevent side effects of inflammation
  - *Toxoplasmosis:* Clindamycin 300 mg QID or cotrimoxazole (if no sulfa allergy) for 6 weeks to 3 months; in case of allergy to sulfonamides, azithromycin 500 mg OD is the best alternative. Spiramycin is used in pregnancy and atovaquone is the only sporicidal drug, though not easily available in India. Intravitreal clindamycin - 1 mg/0.1 mL is an effective add-on drug in case of lesions threatening the macula. Oral prednisolone 1–1.5 mg/kg is added under the cover of anti-toxoplasma therapy to minimize the effects due to inflammation, 48–72 hours after initiation of anti-toxoplasma therapy
  - *Toxocariasis:* Systemic steroids + antihelminthic therapy (albendazole—role not proven)
  - *TB:* Full-dose antitubercular therapy (ATT) for 9–12 months under care of internist
  - *Syphilis:* To treat on the same lines as neurosyphilis; drug of choice is IV crystalline penicillin G 12–18 million units/day for 10–14 days, followed by intramuscular penicillin G 2.4 million units weekly for 3–4 weeks. Alternative options are procaine penicillin G: 2.4 million units intramuscular (IM)/day PLUS probenecid 500 mg orally four times a day, both for 10–14 day. In case of penicillin allergy: injection ceftriaxone 2 g daily either intramuscularly or intravenously for 10–14 days or oral doxycycline 100 mg twice daily for 4–6 weeks is a good alternative
  - *Bartonella neuroretinitis:* Oral doxycycline 100 mg twice a day for 2–4 weeks
  - *Herpetic retinitis:* Induction—IV acyclovir 500 mg 8th hourly for 2–3 weeks followed by ones valacyclovir 1g TDS and long, slow taper. Close watch, laser barrage (although not proven and not routinely done) has been attempted to reduce the chance of retinal detachment and is advocated by some in select situations of acute retinal necrosis (ARN)
  - *Cytomegalovirus retinitis:* Induction—IV ganciclovir: 5 mg/kg twice daily for 14–21 days
- *Alternate options are* foscarnet (IV)—90 mg/kg twice daily for 14 days, followed by oral valganciclovir—900 mg twice daily 6–8 weeks
  - Maintenance IV ganciclovir—5 mg/kg/day to continue or foscarnet—120 mg/kg/day or oral valganciclovir—900 mg once daily to continue
  - Intravitreal ganciclovir: induction—2 mg/0.1 mL, twice weekly, maintenance—2 mg/0.1 mL weekly
- *Post-fever retinitis (PFR):* This is caused by rickettsial, typhoid, dengue, West Nile, chikungunya, and Zika virus infections. Serological investigations and molecular

diagnostics are required to pinpoint exact etiological agent. In most cases, the course of the disease is self-limiting with good visual outcomes without any recurrences. They are treated with anti-infective agents along with anti-inflammatory therapy in the form of steroids
- *Diffuse unilateral subacute neuroretinitis (DUSN):* This can be confirmed or presumed and can lead to severe visual impairment and blindness. In confirmed DUSN, the classic treatment is directly photocoagulation of the worm; however, it can only be visualized in 30% (to 40%) of cases. Treatment of presumed DUSN cases is with high-dose oral albendazole and anti-inflammatory therapy in the form of steroids.

6.4 Panuveitis

Vishali Gupta
PGIMER, Chandigarh
vishalisara@yahoo.co.in

COMMON PANUVEITIS CONDITIONS

Conditions causing panuveitis show variations in different populations based on diverse geographical, racial, nutritional, and socioeconomic differences. Those with specific causes can be differentiated into noninfectious and infectious **(Table 6.4.1)**.

The less common causes of panuveitis are **(Table 6.4.2)**.

The common causes of panuveitis in Asian populations include tuberculosis (TB), Vogt–Koyanagi–Harada (VKH) syndrome, sympathetic ophthalmia, Behçet's disease, and sarcoidosis.

TABLE 6.4.1: Specific causes of panuveitis.

Noninfectious	Infectious
• Vogt–Koyanagi–Harada (VKH) disease	• Tuberculosis
• Sympathetic ophthalmia	• Toxoplasmosis
• Behçet's disease	• Syphilis
• Sarcoidosis	• Leprosy

COMMON OCULAR SYMPTOMS

Although pain, redness, and photophobia are typical symptoms of anterior uveitis, they may be present in varying degrees in panuveitis.

More disturbing complaints of floaters and decreased vision because of concurrent posterior segment involvement often dominate these symptoms.

TABLE 6.4.2: Common causes of panuveitis.

Noninfectious	Infectious
• Ankylosing spondylitis	• Coxsackievirus B infection
• Nonpenetrating ocular trauma	• Candidiasis
• Masquerade syndrome	• Borreliosis
• Multifocal choroiditis with panuveitis	• Herpes zoster viral infection
• Rheumatoid arthritis	• Streptococcal
• Systemic lupus erythematosus	• Aspergillosis
• Actinomycosis	

ANCILLARY TESTS

A thorough history and complete ophthalmic evaluation can eliminate many specific causes. Baseline and follow-up photographic documentation of the anterior segment and color fundus photography, in spite of vitritis, is helpful in monitoring the course of the disease.

Fundus fluorescein angiography (FA): It is useful in diagnosing cystoid macular edema (CME), choroidal neovascular membrane (CNVM), VKH, sympathetic ophthalmia, posterior scleritis, and retinal vascular diseases.

Ultrasound: Extremely valuable in panuveitis with poor media clarity due to widespread, severe inflammation, and/or cataract. It is mandatory in all cases of VKH or sympathetic ophthalmia for detecting choroidal thickening which corroborate the diagnosis of these diseases.

Ultrasound biomicroscopy (UBM): This is useful for ciliary body evaluation, granulomas of the ciliary body in TB or sarcoidosis, to detect structural abnormalities of ciliary body in ocular hypotony, and monitoring the ciliary body status during the course of disease causing extensive inflammation of the ciliary body.

Optical coherence tomography (OCT): Although hazy media may restrict its use in panuveitis, the use of spectral-domain OCT (SD-OCT), (Cirrus HD-OCT; Carl Zeiss, Dublin, California, USA) provides distinct benefits in comparison to the time-domain OCT (TD-OCT) (Stratus version 4; Carl Zeiss). It captures detailed images of the macula in patients of uveitis with poor media clarity, thereby allowing identification of normal and pathologic structures.

MANAGEMENT

A Case of Tuberculous Panuveitis

Tuberculosis is the most common cause of panuveitis in India. Upon establishment of TB as the underlying cause of panuveitis, the initial treatment involves a first-line regimen consisting of four drugs. These drugs include isoniazid at a daily dosage of 5 mg/kg, rifampicin at a daily dosage of 450 mg (for individuals with body weight <50 kg) or 600 mg (for body weight >50 kg), ethambutol at a daily dosage of 15 mg/kg, and pyrazinamide at a daily dosage of 25–30 mg/kg. This therapeutic regimen is initiated and supervised by an internist, and it typically continues for a duration of 3–4 months. Subsequently, a combination of rifampicin and isoniazid is continued for a duration of 9–14 months. Oral corticosteroids are prescribed at a dosage of 1 mg/kg body weight per day, and subsequently tapered based on the patient's clinical response. Close monitoring for potential liver toxicity is mandatory. Additionally, all patients undergoing antitubercular therapy (ATT) are provided with pyridoxine supplementation until the completion of therapy.

A Case of Noninfective Panuveitis

Corticosteroids are the mainstay of treatment of noninfective panuveitis. Anterior segment inflammation is treated with topical steroids and cycloplegics. Periocular injection of depot corticosteroids by posterior sub-Tenon's route may be tried in unilateral panuveitis. Those unresponsive or intolerant to periocular injections or bilateral cases are given oral corticosteroids in a daily dose of 1–1.5 mg/kg/day. As the inflammation subsides, corticosteroids are tapered gradually and maintained on a low dose without stopping it abruptly depending upon the disease entity like VKH or sympathetic ophthalmia.

Recurrences are treated with repeat courses of systemic steroids or immunosuppressive. Appropriate blood tests for monitoring their side effects need to be done periodically. Recalcitrant Behçet's disease has been found to benefit from immunomodulating agents and biologicals. Vitrectomy in panuveitis may be indicated for diagnostic or therapeutic purpose.

6.5 Retinal Vasculitis

Reema Bansal, Vishali Gupta, Amod Gupta
PGIMER, Chandigarh
dramodgupta@gmail.com

COMMON CAUSES

Classically, retinal vasculitis is divided into entities localized to the retina and into systemic diseases involving the eye. Common causes of retinal vasculitis are mentioned below.

Primary Vasculitis

Primary (ocular) vasculitis is where vessel is the primary target of the inflammatory process.

Localized to the Eye
- Idiopathic
- Intermediate uveitis of the pars planitis type
- Frosted branch angiitis
- Idiopathic retinal vasculitis, aneurysms, and neuroretinitis (IRVAN)
- Acute multifocal hemorrhagic retinal vasculitis

Involving the Eye and Other Organs (Primary Systemic Vasculitides)
- Giant cell arteritis
- Takayasu arteritis
- Polyarteritis nodosa
- Wegener's granulomatosis

Rare Causes
- Churg–Strauss syndrome*
- Essential cryoglobulinemic vasculitis*
- Cutaneous leukocytoclastic angiitis*

Secondary Vasculitis

Secondary (ocular) vasculitis is where vasculitis is a prominent feature but is secondary to an inflammatory process not primarily directed against the vessel.

Localized to the Eye
Immune-mediated:
- Ocular sarcoidosis
- Birdshot chorioretinopathy retinal vasculitis*

Infectious:
- Necrotic herpetic retinopathies (herpes simplex, varicella zoster virus)
- Toxoplasmic retinochoroiditis
- Tuberculosis
- Diffuse unilateral subacute neuroretinitis (DUSN)

*Neoplasms:** Primary intraocular lymphoma

Associated with Systemic Involvement
Immune-mediated:
- Sarcoidosis
- Behçet's disease
- Multiple sclerosis
- Systemic lupus erythematosus (SLE)
- Spondyloarthritis with human leukocyte antigen (HLA)-associated uveitis
- Inflammatory bowel diseases
- Relapsing polychondritis
- Susac's syndrome*
- Sjogren's syndrome*
- Rheumatoid arthritis*
- Juvenile idiopathic arthritis*

---
*Rare causes

Infectious:
- Tuberculosis
- Syphilis
- Lyme's disease
- Viral [cytomegalovirus, human immunodeficiency virus (HIV), West Nile*]
- Toxocara canis
- Bartonella henselae viral (cytomegalovirus, HIV, West Nile*)
- Whipple's disease*
- Rickettsial diseases*

*Drug-induced:**
- Intravenous immunoglobulins
- Inhalation of methamphetamine

*Secondary to malignancies:**
- Cancer-associated retinopathy
- Oculocerebral lymphoma

INVESTIGATIONS

Investigating a case of retinal vasculitis involves a tailored approach.

Ancillary tests required include:
- Fundus photography, fundus fluorescein angiography
- Optical coherence tomography
- Ultrasonography
- Indocyanine green angiography
- Ultrasound biomicroscopy

The routinely ordered laboratory tests in all our patients of retinal vasculitis include:
- Full blood counts
- Erythrocyte sedimentation rate
- Mantoux test
- Computed tomography (CT) chest (contrast enhanced)
- Syphilis serology (*Treponema pallidum* hemagglutination test)

When strongly suspecting a specific etiology, the following tests are ordered in relevance to the particular disorder:
- Toxoplasmosis serology
- HIV
- Lyme disease serology
- X-ray of sacroiliac joint
- C-reactive protein
- Serum angiotensin-converting enzyme
- HLA-typing (B51 for Behçet's disease, DR3 for systemic lupus erythematosus (SLE) and A29 for birdshot retinochoroidopathy)
- Rheumatoid factor (RA)
- Antinuclear antibody (ANA) for juvenile idiopathic arthritis and SLE
- Antineutrophil cytoplasmic antibody (ANCA)
- Polymerase chain reaction (PCR) of intraocular fluids (suspected tubercular or viral etiology)
- Vitreous biopsy (suspected intraocular lymphoma)
- Magnetic resonance imaging
- Cerebrospinal fluid analysis—cytology and cell count

---
*Rare causes

In case of occlusive vasculopathies:
- Coagulation profile
- Homocysteine levels
- Antiphospholipid antibodies

▎TREATMENT

Treatment of retinal vasculitis can be divided into following steps:
- Suppression of inflammation
- Treatment of specific disease, if identified
- Treatment of complications.

Suppression of Inflammation

Corticosteroids

Corticosteroids are the mainstay of treatment in primary retinal vasculitis or those with underlying systemic vascular disease. Posterior sub-Tenon's injection of periocular depot steroids is also helpful in unilateral disease and in case of associated cystoid macular edema (CME).

Immunosuppressive Agents

Immunosuppressive agents are given as second-line therapy in patients showing poor response to conventional corticosteroids or developing adverse effects of corticosteroids. They are especially necessary in sight-threatening occlusive noninfective vasculitis such as Behçet's disease.

Treatment of Specific Disease

Identification of noninfectious systemic associations warrants initiation of specific therapy including systemic steroids and immunosuppressive agents.

Infective Retinal Vasculitis

Retinal vasculitis caused by infectious agents needs to be managed with specific antimicrobial therapy along with systemic steroids.

Tuberculosis: This is the most common etiology of infective retinal vasculitis. Along with oral corticosteroids, first-line four-drug antituberculosis therapy (ATT) is initiated under the supervision of an internist for initial 2–3 months, followed by two-drug regimen for 9–10 months with pyridoxine supplementation. Liver function tests are regularly monitored to detect any hepatotoxicity.

Toxoplasmosis: Appropriate antitoxoplasma therapy along with systemic steroids is the treatment of choice. A more recent approach involves the administration of intravitreal clindamycin with dexamethasone to avoid systemic side effects of oral clindamycin.

Syphilis: Penicillin remains the standard treatment for ocular syphilis. Recommended regimen for treatment of ocular syphilis is the same as that for neurosyphilis, i.e., intravenous crystal penicillin G 12–18 million units/day for 10–14 days, followed by supplementary intramuscular penicillin G 2.4 million units weekly for 3–4 weeks. If the patient is allergic to penicillin, then oral tetracycline 500 mg four times a day for 4–6 weeks is a good alternative.

Lyme's disease: It greatly mimics syphilis and should be considered in endemic areas. It is treated as neuroborreliosis with intravenous ceftriaxone, 2 g daily for adults (50–100 mg/kg/day for children) for 21 days; or penicillin G, 20 million units daily, or 0.25–0.5 million units/kg/daily for children. Doxycycline, 100 mg twice daily, is a good alternative in adults with less severe infection but contraindicated in children, pregnant or breastfeeding women. Some patients with severe ocular inflammation may require concomitant oral prednisolone (0.5–1.0 mg/ kg/day) because of the possibility of paradoxical worsening (Jarisch–Herxheimer reaction). But steroids should not be used without appropriate antibiotic cover.

Treatment of Complications

Scatter laser photocoagulation is indicated in areas of capillary nonperfusion or if there is retinal neovascularization. Pars plana vitrectomy is indicated for treating complications such as nonresolving or recurrent vitreous hemorrhage, epiretinal membrane, tractional retinal detachment threatening the macula, combined-tractional and rhegmatogenous retinal detachment, and a densely-opacified vitreous. Oral corticosteroids are effective for bilateral CME. Intravitreal steroids (Ozurdex/triamcinolone acetate) are a good option for unilateral CME.

6.6 Viral Retinitis

Suchitra Pradeep
Sankara Nethralaya, Chennai
drspd@snmail.org

■ ETIOLOGY

- *Human herpes viruses (HHVs):* Herpes simplex virus (HSV), varicella zoster virus (VZV), cytomegalovirus (CMV)
- *Arboviruses:* Chikungunya and dengue virus
- *Other rare causes:* Rubella, measles, West Nile virus, etc.

Immunocompetent patients: Acute retinal necrosis (ARN) and posterior pole retinitis.

Immunocompromised patients: CMV is the most common cause of viral retinitis. VZV causes progressive outer retinal necrosis (PORN).

■ ACUTE RETINAL NECROSIS

Acute retinal necrosis (ARN) is a severe, sight-threatening ocular emergency presenting with acute unilateral panuveitis with retinal periarteritis progressing to diffuse necrotizing retinitis with retinal detachment.

Etiology:
- VZV—leading cause
- HSV 1 and HSV 2
- Epstein–Barr virus (EBV)
- CMV

Symptoms: Redness, blurring of vision, photophobia, floaters, ocular pain.

Clinical signs: Anterior chamber reaction, vitritis, peripheral necrotizing retinitis, and occlusive vasculitis with arteriolar narrowing.

Diagnosis: Polymerase chain reaction of aqueous or vitreous aspirate confirms the etiological agent.

Treatment:
- The standard of care is inpatient hospitalization and induction with intravenous (IV) acyclovir 10 mg/kg every 8 hours or 1,500 mg/m^2 per day for 7–10 days, followed by maintenance with oral acyclovir 800 mg five times daily for at least next 6 weeks
- Oral valacyclovir 1 g three times daily for 6–8 weeks achieves same results as IV acyclovir therapy
- Intravitreal ganciclovir 4 mg/0.1 mL can be used as adjuvant for oral antiviral therapy

- Systemic and topical corticosteroids are used to suppress the local inflammatory response
- Prophylactic photocoagulation in selected cases
- Vitreoretinal surgery for the eyes that develop retinal detachment.

Outcomes: ARN is a blinding disease with poor visual outcomes despite adequate treatment.

Complications: Involvement of the second eye is seen in at least one-third of untreated cases, retinal detachment in at least 75% of untreated eyes. Other complications are optic atrophy, epiretinal membrane, hypotony, and phthisis bulbi.

PROGRESSIVE OUTER RETINAL NECROSIS

Progressive outer retinal necrosis is a rapidly progressing and highly destructive form of retinal necrosis seen in immunocompromised patients caused by VZV. Extensive multifocal retinitis begins at posterior pole and spreads to periphery. It is distinct from ARN in not having vitritis and vascular inflammation. Treatment is with IV ganciclovir 5 mg/kg/day along with intravitreal ganciclovir 4 mg/0.1 mL. PORN has very poor visual prognosis compared to ARN as it is resistant to antiviral therapy.

CYTOMEGALOVIRUS RETINITIS

Cytomegalovirus retinitis is an opportunistic infection seen in immunocompromised AIDS patients (CD4 counts <50 cells/μL) and in secondary immunosuppressed patients due to organ transplantation and systemic corticosteroid therapy. The classical feature is a single focus of full-thickness, yellow-white necrotizing granular retinitis in the peripheral retina with a perivascular distribution that expands centrifugally along with retinal hemorrhages. It is described as a "pizza pie retinopathy". Treatment is with systemic ganciclovir with intravitreal ganciclovir injections.

ARBOVIRAL RETINITIS

Dengue and Chikungunya retinitis are morphologically similar to herpetic posterior pole retinitis. History of fever, joint pain, rash, and arthralgia before the onset of ocular lesions gives the clue. Treatment is supportive. Oral and topical steroids help in selected cases.

6.7 | Coronavirus Disease 2019 and Eye

Aditya Patil, Ankush Kawali, Srinivasan Sanjay, Sai Bhakti Mishra, *Padmamalini Mahendradas*
Narayana Nethralaya, Bengaluru
ikor117@gmail.com, akawali332@gmail.com, sanjay.srinivasan@gmail.com
drsaibhakti@gmail.com, m.padmamalini@gmail.com

INTRODUCTION

Severe acute respiratory syndrome coronavirus 2 (SARS-CoV-2) is a novel enveloped, positive single-stranded RNA belonging to the coronaviridae family. Like other respiratory viruses, SARS-CoV-2 spreads via infected body fluids and respiratory droplets through inhalation, fomites, and via direct contact with the face, mucous membranes of the mouth, and the eyes of the infected person. Whether the exposed ocular surface is a route for transmission of the virus is a matter of controversy.

Ocular manifestations of coronavirus disease 2019 (COVID-19) are due to any of the following mechanisms:
- Direct invasion of virus into ocular tissues
- Hypersensitivity reaction to viral antigens

- Hypercoagulable state causing vascular insults
- Various opportunistic infections due to compromised immunity

CLINICAL FEATURES
Following are the various ocular manifestations in association with COVID-19:

Eyelid Manifestations
Meibomian orifice abnormalities, lid margin hyperemia/telangiectasia were found in 11/27 (38%) of the patients in a study by Meduri et al.[1] in Italy. Blepharitis has also been reported.

Anterior Segment Manifestations
Conjunctivitis is the initial and most prevalent ocular manifestation in patients with COVID-19. It may be follicular or hemorrhagic and pseudomembranous. In a large series of cases of mild COVID-19, Sindhuja et al.[2] reported that 11/127 (8.66%) cases had conjunctivitis. Presence of respiratory tract symptoms was associated with conjunctival congestion. It has been proposed that the virus may get transferred from ocular surface via lacrimal passage to the lower respiratory tract. Keratoconjunctivitis, episcleritis, and anterior uveitis have also been described. Other reported symptoms include: dryness, foreign body sensation, tearing, itching, and discharge.

Kawasaki-like disease has been reported in children in association with COVID-19. It is an atypical presentation known as multisystemic inflammatory syndrome in children (MIS-C). Kawasaki disease is a form of self-limiting vasculitis associated with anterior uveitis, punctate keratitis, vitreous opacities, papilledema, subconjunctival hemorrhage, and conjunctival injection.

Posterior Segment Manifestations
Posterior segment involvement in COVID-19 may be benign and self-limiting like cotton-wool spots, dot hemorrhages or may be vision-threatening such as retinal vascular occlusions, retinitis, acute retinal necrosis, endophthalmitis, choroiditis, panuveitis, optic neuritis, and eventually optic atrophy.

SARS-CoV-2 has an affinity for vascular endothelial cell angiotensin converting enzyme 2 (ACE2) receptors which initiate the apoptotic pathway signaling and prothrombotic cascade. There have been numerous reports of post-COVID-19 central retinal vein occlusion (CRVO), central retinal artery occlusion (CRAO), and even combined vessel occlusions.

Acute macular neuroretinopathy (AMN) and paracentral acute middle maculopathy (PAMM) have been reported. Ischemic mechanism involving the deep capillary plexus secondary to COVID-related alteration in hemodynamic state has been proposed. AMN/PAMM present as faint paracentral scotomas and painless diminution of vision.

Immune suppression and use of aggressive immunosuppressives have increased the risk for opportunistic infections in COVID-19 patients. Candida retinitis cases have been reported and treated with intravitreal, intravenous, and systemic antifungal agents. Roth spots and infectious endocarditis in patients with COVID-19 has been reported.

Neuro-ophthalmic Manifestations
Papillophlebitis is a rare, idiopathic entity that occurs due to inflammation of the retinal vessels and capillaries at the optic disc. It is considered as a clinical variant of CRVO and has been reported in patients who have recovered from COVID-19.

Optic neuritis may occur secondary to autoimmune inflammatory condition which presents as a sudden drop in vision with painful ocular movements. Ischemic stroke has also been reported secondary to various mechanisms such as hypercoagulable state, intracranial cytokine storm-induced vasculitis, and atrial fibrillation. A case of bilateral visual loss secondary to ischemic stroke has been reported by Atum et al.[3]

Uveitis in Coronavirus Disease 2019

Coronavirus disease 2019 can trigger autoimmune and autoinflammatory responses mainly via molecular mimicry and can play a primary role in the development of ocular inflammation.

Recurrent bilateral idiopathic anterior uveitis has been reported in a COVID-19 recovered patient. Liu et al.[4] reported a case of severe panuveitis associated with monocular blindness in a patient who recovered from COVID-19.

Reactivation of serpiginous choroiditis following COVID-19 infection has been reported by Providencia et al.[5] There are unpublished reports of multifocal or serpiginous choroiditis presenting in patients with history of COVID-19 infection. SARS-CoV-2 causing reactivation of autoimmune process has been proposed to play a role. It is necessary to rule out other causes of serpiginous and multifocal choroiditis in these patients, namely tuberculosis, syphilis, and other viral etiologies.

Ocular inflammation has been reported post-COVID-19 vaccination. Reactivation of tubercular choroiditis and uveitis are most commonly reported manifestations post-COVID-19 vaccination. There are reports of scleritis, varicella zoster virus reactivation, optic neuritis, AMN, Vogt–Koyanagi–Harada-like syndrome, uveitis, choroiditis, central serous chorioretinopathy, retinal vascular occlusions, optic neuritis, and abducens nerve palsy following COVID-19 vaccination. The reactivation of ocular inflammation has thought to be due to an immune reaction process to mRNA vaccines in general, although the exact mechanism is not known.

Orbital Manifestations

The most common and fatal orbital manifestation of COVID-19 is rhino-orbital mucormycosis, which is an angioinvasive disease caused by mold fungi. It affects patients with moderate-to-severe COVID-19 with reduced $CD4^+$ and $CD8^+$ counts.[6] Risk factors include diabetes, hypertension, underlying autoimmune condition, and use of systemic steroids and immunosuppressive therapy. Clinical diagnosis is based on presence of black, necrotic nasal mucosa, blood-tinged nasal discharge, facial or orbital swelling, ptosis, proptosis, diplopia, ophthalmoplegia.

Orbital myositis has been reported by Armstrong et al.[7] and Eleiwa et al.[8] in cases of COVID-19. Other orbital manifestations include orbital cellulitis, sinusitis, dacryoadenitis, and retro-orbital pain. All these conditions have favorable outcomes except for some cases of mucormycosis.

■ INVESTIGATIONS

Investigations can be divided into systemic, ocular, and radiological.

Systemic Investigations

Basic investigations such as complete blood count, blood glucose tests, urine analysis, erythrocyte sedimentation rate can be ordered as part of routine investigations. D-dimer, C-reactive protein, serum ferritin, serum fibrinogen, prothrombin time (PT), and activated partial thromboplastin time (aPTT) can be ordered to rule out any hypercoagulable state. Wherever indicated, lipid profile, serum homocysteine, anticardiolipin immunoglobulin G (IgG) and IgM antibodies and screening for genetic thrombophilia can be carried out.

Ocular Investigations

In cases of CRVO, investigations such as fundus fluorescein angiography (FFA), OCT demonstrate features not different from non-COVID-19 related causes. However, in patients with COVID-19 or post-COVID recovery, it is important to order investigations to monitor the inflammatory parameters and rule out any hypercoagulable state.

Radiological Investigations

In cases of optic neuritis, magnetic resonance imaging (MRI) is advisable to detect any optic nerve swelling. A case of cavernous sinus thrombosis has been reported where MRI revealed diffuse preseptal and retro-orbital edema with swollen optic nerve sheath.

Computed tomography (CT) scan and MRI scans are ordered in cases of suspected mucormycosis to look for involvement of the orbit, paranasal sinuses, cavernous sinus, and to rule out any intracranial extension of the disease.

■ MANAGEMENT

Management depends on the type of ocular manifestation.

Conjunctivitis and episcleritis has been managed with topical steroids and lubricating eye drops. Ribavirin has been used in some cases. Hemorrhagic and pseudomembranous conjunctivitis has been treated with azithromycin and dexamethasone drops and daily debridement of the membrane. In case of Kawasaki disease-like presentation, treatment is directed toward suppressing the inflammation by using corticosteroids, intravenous immunoglobulin (IVIg), and aspirin.

Cases of CRVO have been managed with oral corticosteroids and intravitreal anti-vascular endothelial growth factor (VEGF) agents, along with management of systemic hypercoagulable state. A case of papillophlebitis was treated with intravitreal dexamethasone implant for macular edema, resulting in significant improvement. Optic neuritis has been treated with 1g intravenous methylprednisolone for 3 days followed by 1 mg/kg oral prednisolone in tapering doses. Mucormycosis management is challenging and requires aggressive antifungal treatment and surgical removal of necrotic tissue, even exenteration of orbit in case of severe life-threatening cases.

In patients with severe systemic COVID-19 infection, early anticoagulant prophylaxis should be considered, along with systemic corticosteroids to suppress the inflammation. In case of a deranged coagulation profile, hematologist consultation should be sought to prevent vascular insults.[9]

■ CONCLUSION

Ophthalmic manifestations of COVID-19 have a varied presentation as elucidated. Eye care professionals should be aware of the vision-threatening entities and their treatment following COVID-19 infection.

■ REFERENCES

1. Meduri A, Oliverio GW, Mancuso G, et al. Ocular surface manifestation of COVID-19 and tear film analysis. Sci Rep. 2020;10(1).
2. Sindhuja K, Lomi N, Asif M, Tandon R. Clinical profile and prevalence of conjunctivitis in mild COVID-19 patients in a tertiary care COVID-19 hospital: A retrospective cross-sectional study. Indian J Ophthalmol. 2020;68(8):1546-50.
3. Atum M, Demiryüre BE. Sudden bilateral vision loss in a COVID-19 patient: A case report. Indian J Ophthalmol. 2021;69(8):2227-8.
4. Liu L, Cai D, Huang X, Shen Y. COVID-2019 Associated with Acquired Monocular Blindness. Curr Eye Res. 2021;46(8):1247-50.
5. Providência J, Fonseca C, Henriques F, Proença R. Serpiginous choroiditis presenting after SARS-CoV-2 infection: A new immunological trigger? Eur J Ophthalmol. 2022; 32(1):NP97-NP101.
6. Sen M, Honavar SG, Sharma N, Sachdev MS. COVID-19 and Eye: A Review of Ophthalmic Manifestations of COVID-19. Indian J Ophthalmol. 2021;69(3):488-509.
7. Armstrong BK, Murchison AP, Bilyk JR. Suspected orbital myositis associated with COVID-19. Orbit. 2021;40(6):532-5.
8. Eleiwa T, Abdelrahman SN, ElSheikh RH, Elhusseiny AM. Orbital inflammatory disease associated with COVID-19 infection. J AAPOS. 2021;25(4):232-4.
9. Dutta R, Sadhu S, Biswas J. The ocular manifestations of novel coronavirus: A literature review. Indian Journal of Inflammation Research. 2022;(6)1:R2.

6.8 Uveitic Pathology

Jyotirmay Biswas
Sankara Nethralaya, Chennai
drjb@snmail.org

Dipankar Das
Sri Sankaradeva Nethralaya, Guwahati
dr_dasdipankar@yahoo.com

■ PATHOLOGY OF SYMPATHETIC OPHTHALMIA

Grossly, most of the enucleated eyeballs are phthisical with disorganized internal structure and increased in retino-choroidal thickness. Histopathologically, there is panuveitis or diffuse uveitis. Following features are seen in sympathetic ophthalmia (SO):
- Diffuse lymphocytic infiltration of the choroidal layers with epithelioid cells and occasional giant cells infiltrations
- Focal chorioretinal scar with retinal pigment epithelial cells undulation
- Pigment migration in disorganized retina
- Pigment phagocytosis of epithelioid cells
- *Dalen-Fuch's nodules:* Focal collection of epithelioid cells, macrophages, and lymphocytes between the retinal pigment epithelium and Bruch's membrane. Dalen-Fuch's nodule is seen in acute active stage of SO
- Neutrophils, plasma cells and eosinophils are seen occasionally
  Sparing of choriocapillaries was seen in acute stage of SO **(Fig. 6.8.1)**.

■ PATHOLOGY OF VOGT–KOYANAGI–HARADA'S DISEASE

Histopathological features VKH depend on the stages of the disease. The features include:
- Diffuse thickening of the uveal tract particularly juxtapapillary choroid
- In acute uveitic stage, there is a granulomatous reaction and diffuse lymphocytic infiltration with focal aggregates of epithelioid and multinucleated giant cells without any necrosis
- Subretinal fluid is seen in exudative retinal detachment containing eosinophilic proteinaceous material
- Retinal pigment epithelium and choriocapillaries in active disease are not spared unlike SO **(Fig. 6.8.2)**
- Dalen Fuch's nodule are seen in VKH-like SO in acute phase of the disease
- In convalescent stage, nongranulomatous inflammation sets in and there is gradual loss of melanin granules in melanocytes. This is the cause of sunset glow fundus
- In chronic recurrent stage, there may be resurgence of granulomatous choroiditis but there is extensive damage to the choriocapillaries. Later, there may be thinning of the choroid with choroidal adhesion, sclerosis, and atrophies.

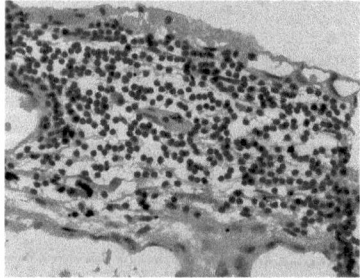

Fig. 6.8.1: Diffuse lymphocytic infiltration in choriocapillaris.

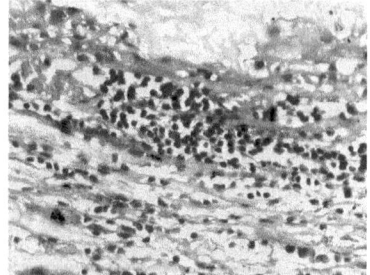

Fig. 6.8.2: Diffuse lymphocytic infiltration in VKH.

PATHOLOGY OF LENS-INDUCED UVEITIS

Phacoanaphylactic lens-induced uveitis is a rare, unilateral, autoimmune, and zonal granulomatous inflammation centered on the damaged lens capsule **(Fig. 6.8.3)**. Histopathologically, neutrophils surround and dissolved the lens material. Plasma cells, epithelioid, multinucleated giant cells, fibroblasts, and blood vessels form a granulation tissue around the lens.

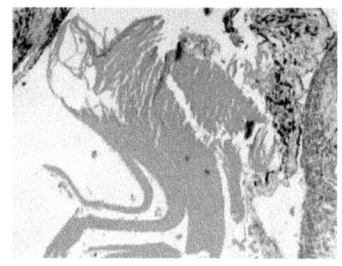

Fig. 6.8.3: Ruptured lens capsule with granulomatous reaction.

PATHOLOGY OF TUBERCULOUS UVEITIS

Tuberculous uveitis can present as anterior, intermediate, posterior, and pan uveitis. Choroidal tubercles can have varied pathological presentations and can be seen in miliary tuberculosis or accompanied with tuberculous meningitis. Choroidal tubercles may present as a white or grayish yellow lesion accompanied with hemorrhage and exudation. There may be associated edema seen in the choroidal layers and adjoining retina. They can be multiple and can be present with serpiginous like choroiditis spreading to the periphery of the lesion. These lesion regresses with antituberculous medication and oral steroids and often residual chorioretinal scar forms. Retina is also involved in many of the cases which can be focal or diffuse retinitis. Lymphocyte, plasma cells, and epithelioid cells form the granuloma in the choroid and retina. Tuberculous chorio-retinal abscess can harbor acid-fast bacilli in the caseating necrosis. Retinal vasculitis had been found associated with tuberculosis. Retinal vasculitis which is usually due to immune reaction to the mycobacterium. Eales disease is a form of retinal perivasculitis which affect peripheral retina mostly. Tuberculous DNA tested by polymerase chain reaction has been reported from anterior chamber, vitreous and epiretinal membranes in tuberculous uveitic patients.

SUGGESTED READING

1. Das D, Krishnakumar S, Biswas J. Sympathetic ophthalmia with incidental finding of chicken pox supported by histopathology and immunohistochemistry. Indian J Pathol Microbiol. 2019;62:592-4.
2. Das D, Boddepalli A, Biswas J. Clinicopathological and immunohistochemistry correlation in a case of Vogt-Koyanagi-Harada disease. Indian J Ophthalmol. 2019;67:1217-9.
3. Gupta A, Sharma A, Bansal R, Sharma K. Classification of intraocular tuberculosis. Ocul Immunol Inflamm. 2015;23:7-13.

6.9 Immunosuppressives in Uveitis

Namita Dave
Narayana Netralaya, Bengaluru
LV Prasad Eye Institute, Hyderabad
davenamita1@gmail.com

Somasheila I Murthy
LV Prasad Eye Institute, Hyderabad
smurthy@lvpei.org

COMMON IMMUNOSUPPRESSIVE AGENTS

Antimetabolites, calcineurin (T-cell) inhibitors, and alkylating agents are the most commonly used drugs for patients whose uveitis is unresponsive or intolerant to oral corticosteroids.

Antimetabolites
- Azathioprine
- Methotrexate (MTX)
- Mycophenolate mofetil
- Leflunomide

Calcineurin Inhibitors
- Cyclosporine
- Tacrolimus
- Sirolimus
- Voclosporin
- Colchicine

Alkylating Agents
- Cyclophosphamide
- Chlorambucil

INDICATIONS

Immunosuppressive agents are usually used as corticosteroid-sparing agents and/or as agents able to control refractory uveitis in sight-threatening uveitis. Early and aggressive use of immunosuppressive therapy can be invaluable in preventing irreversible visual loss. In cases of severe disease, these agents are used in conjunction with steroids as the primary mode of immunosuppression.

Informed consent from the patient and physician's clearance for fitness for immunosuppressive usage are a must.

Indications of Primary Immunosuppressive Therapy
- Behçet's disease
- Vogt–Koyanagi–Harada's (VKH) disease
- Sympathetic ophthalmia
- Juvenile idiopathic arthritis (JIA)-associated uveitis
- Human leukocyte antigen (HLA)-associated diseases

Other Common Indications
- Recurrent intermediate uveitis
- Noninflammatory choroiditis involving or threatening the macula
- Optic-nerve head involvement
- As steroid-sparing agents

Examples of immunosuppressive agents are as follows:

MTX: It has been used to treat a variety of uveitis in both children and adults.

Common indications:
- HLA-B27 uveitis
- JIA-associated uveitis
- Par planitis in children
- Sarcoidosis

Azathioprine: It is used most often as a corticosteroid-sparing agent in chronic inflammatory disease especially in adults and elderly.
- Anterior uveitis in autoimmune diseases
- Pars planitis
- VKH disease
- Sympathetic ophthalmia
- Behçet's disease

- Retinal vasculitis
- In combination therapy in serpiginous choroiditis

Cyclosporine: Common indications:
- Sympathetic ophthalmia and VKH
- Behçet's disease

Cyclophosphamide: Common indications:
- Behçet's disease
- Wegener's granulomatosis

DOSES OF COMMONLY USED IMMUNOSUPPRESSIVE AGENTS
- *Methotrexate:* Once-a-week dose—oral, intramuscular, or subcutaneous—7.5-25 mg given along with folate supplements (folic acid or folinic acid, 5 mg oral tablet given 3-5 days a week)
- *Azathioprine:* 1-2.5 mg/kg/day in a single or two divided doses—oral
- *Mycophenolate mofetil:* 1,000-2,000 mg/day—oral
- *Cyclosporine A:* 5 mg/kg/day up to a maximum of 7 mg/kg/day in a single or two divided doses—oral
- *Cyclophosphamide:* 1-3 mg/kg/day oral in divided doses, 500-750 mg as intravenous (IV) pulse therapy.

Common Side Effects
In using these agents, one must be aware of their adverse reactions, side effects and toxicity. It is often prudent for the treating ophthalmologist to team with a rheumatologist, pulmonologist, and/or an internist in order to monitor the side effects of these agents.

Methotrexate
- *Gastrointestinal:* Nausea, stomatitis, anorexia (25%)
- Alopecia, rash
- *Bone marrow suppression:* Lymphocytopenia and thrombocytopenia
- *Reversible hepatotoxicity:* Elevation of liver enzymes in 15%
- *Cirrhosis:* 0.1%
- *Acute pneumonitis:* Occurs due to drug hypersensitivity reaction
- Teratogenicity

Azathioprine
Azathioprine is avoided in very young patients due to increased risk of hematological malignancy and bone marrow toxicity. Other side effects include:
- Nausea, vomiting (25%)
- Hepatotoxicity (<2%)
- Reversible bone marrow suppression
- Possibly increases risk of neoplasia such as non-Hodgkin's lymphoma.

Mycophenolate Mofetil
- Gastrointestinal intolerance
- Bone marrow suppression
- Opportunistic infections [cytomegalovirus (CMV), herpes simplex virus (HSV)]
- Secondary malignancy.

Cyclosporine A
- Fatigue
- Anemia
- Gingivitis
- Paresthesia

- Epigastric burning
- Decreased appetite
- Hypertrichoism
- Hidradenitis
- Fibroadenoma
- Hypertension
- *Renal toxicity:* Renal tubular atrophy and interstitial fibrosis: 75–100% in 5 years
- *Metabolic abnormalities:* Hyperuricemia, abnormal liver function tests, increased *erythrocyte sedimentation rate* (ESR).

Cyclophosphamide
- Nausea, vomiting
- Alopecia
- Secondary infections
- Visual disturbances
- Bone marrow suppression
- Hemorrhagic cystitis
- Malignancy (leukemia, bladder)
- Irreversible gonadal atrophy
- Interstitial fibrosis of lungs.

Biologics

Drugs directed against specific cytokines or their receptors by molecular biologic techniques are collectively called biologics. They are manufactured by recombinant DNA-technology and include different drugs, such as monoclonal antibodies, soluble receptors, cytokines themselves, and natural cytokine antagonists.

Biologics currently in use for uveitis are as follows:
Drugs against cytokine tumor necrosis factor (TNF) alpha

Anti-TNF-α agents used in uveitis include:
- Infliximab
- Adalimumab
- Etanercept

Of these, both adalimumab and Infliximab have a better efficacy as compared to etanercept for ocular use.

Reactivation of tuberculosis is a serious complication of anti-TNF therapy.

Method of dosing: IV route is required, with the dose ranging from 3–10 mg/kg (in most cases) to 10–20 mg/kg (high doses) of infliximab. At these dosages, there is adequate efficacy with few adverse effects. The dose must be repeated to sustain the effectiveness. Several infusions need to be administered over 1–2 months apart, and this needs to be repeated for a few months to help achieve stability and even remission. In to account for the antibody-forming tendency toward the nonhuman (murine) part of the molecule, additional immunosuppressants such as antimetabolites are necessary. MTX is commonly used for this purpose. For this reason, we need to use concomitant therapy with an antimetabolite or glucocorticoid to suppress antibody production. Adalimumab, a recombinant immunoglobulin G1 (IgG1) monoclonal antibody targeting TNF-α, is effective either as stand-alone therapy or when combined with combination with a certain group of drugs called disease-modifying antirheumatic drugs (DMARDs). These drugs can also be administered subcutaneous by the patient at a dose of 40 mg every 2 weeks.

Table 6.9.1: The biologics that are being presently used in uveitis therapy.

Anti-interleukin Therapies: Anti-IL-1, Anti-IL-2
- A monoclonal antibody which is humanized and is effective against interleukin (IL)-2 receptors is daclizumab. It is indicated in severe sight-threatening noninfectious uveitis

TABLE 6.9.1: Biological therapies to treat chronic systemic immunological-based diseases related to uveitis.

Biologics (FDA initial approval date)	Brand name	Mechanism of action	Principal indications
Proinflammatory cytokine inhibitors TNF blockers:			
Infliximab (1998)	Remicade	Anti-TNF-α	CD, UC, RA, PA, AS, Ps
Etanercept (1998)	Enbrel	Anti-TNF-α-β	RA, PJIA, PA, AS, Ps
Adalimumab (2002)	Humira	Anti TNF-α	RA, PJIA, PA, AS, CD, Ps
Certolizumab (2008)	Cimzia	Anti TNF-α	CD, UC, RA
Golimumab (2009)	Simponi	Anti TNF-α	RA, PA, AS
Specific receptor antagonists:			
Gevokizumab	Eyeguard	Anti-IL-6R	BD, NIU
Tocilizumab (2010)	Actemra	IL-17A	RA, PJIA, BD
Secukinumab (2015)	Cosentyx	Anti-CD11a	AS, PA, MS, BSR
Canakinumab (2009)	Ilaris	IL-1β	JIA, BD
Anakinra	Kineret	IL-1 receptor	RA, BD
Efalizumab	Raptiva	CD11a receptor	Withdrawn from market
Alefacept	Amevive	CD2 receptor	
T-cells inhibitors:			
Daclizumab (1997)	Zenapax	Anti-CD25 (IL-2R)	PRR, NIU, BSR, JIA
Abatacept	Orencia	CTLA-4	IU, VKH
Basiliximab	Simulect	Anti-CD25 (IL-2Rα)	RA, JIA Not used for uveitis
B-cells inhibitors:			
Rituximab (1997)	Rituxan	Anti-CD 20	RA, CLL, n-HL
Alemtuzumab (2001)	Campath	Anti-CD 52	CLL
VEGF inhibitors:			
Bevacizumab (2004)	Avastin	Anti-VEGF	MCC
Other:			
Interferon α-2a	Roferon-A	Nonspecific	BD, MS
Intravenous immunoglobulin		Nonspecific	

(AS: ankylosing spondylitis; BD: Behçet's disease; BSR: birdshot retinopathy; CD: Crohn's disease; CLL: chronic lymphocytic leukemia; FDA: Food and Drug Administration; IU: intermediate uveitis; MCC: metastatic colorectal cancer; MS: multiple sclerosis; n-HL: non-Hodgkin's lymphoma; NIU: noninfectious uveitis; PA: psoriatic arthritis; PG: pyoderma gangrenosum; PJIA: polyarticular juvenile idiopathic arthritis; PRR: prophylaxis of renal rejection; Ps: psoriasis; RA: rheumatoid arthritis; TNF: tumor necrosis factor; UC: ulcerative colitis; VKH: Vogt–Koyanagi–Harada)

- IL-1 receptor antagonist (IL-1RA) is a naturally-occurring inhibitor of IL-1
- A recombinant form of human IL-1RA, anakinra can be given as a daily dose of 100 mg in adults by the subcutaneous route.

Interferons

Recombinant interferons-alpha (INFs-α) 2a and INF-α 2b.

A cytokine that occurs naturally is IFN-α. It is known to be produced in nature as a response to viral stimuli such as in viral infections. Its mechanism of action includes upregulation of suppressor-T cells, downregulation of proinflammatory cytokines and increased activity of phagocytes. It is administered subcutaneously with a dose of 6 million units every day and then decreased 3 million units either thrice or twice in a week.

Lymphocytes

- *All lymphocyte subsets (alemtuzumab):* Alemtuzumab, humanized B monoclonal antibody against the pan lymphocyte antigen CD52; by IV infusion, it is an effective treatment for uveitis
- *B-cells (Rituximab):* Rituximab is a mouse-human chimeric monoclonal IgG1 antibody against CD20, expressed by B-cells. It is effective against predominantly T-cell-mediated autoimmune diseases
- *Intravenous immunoglobulin (IVIg):* This acts through several pathways to upregulate immunity. As it does not cause systemic immunosuppression, this is of specific utility in many conditions. The dosage schedule is 1–2.5 g/kg/cycle per 2 or 4 weeks; till resolution of the condition is noted.

■ INDICATIONS FOR BIOLOGICALS IN UVEITIS

These agents are considered as third line of therapy in refractory disease, after systemic corticosteroids and immunomodulators in chronic sight-threatening noninfectious uveitis. The more frequent indications of use are mentioned here.

Anti-TNF-α Agents and Anti-interleukins

- Behçet's disease (infliximab, adalimumab)
- Chronic macular edema (infliximab)
- JIA-associated uveitis (infliximab, adalimumab, rituximab)
- Sarcoidosis (infliximab, daclizumab)
- Multifocal choroiditis (infliximab, daclizumab)
- Idiopathic panuveitis (infliximab, daclizumab)
- VKH syndrome (infliximab, daclizumab).

Interferon Alpha

- Behçet's disease
- Idiopathic panuveitis
- Intermediate uveitis
- Serpiginous choroiditis
- Birdshot chorioretinopathy
- VKH and sympathetic ophthalmia.

Dosages Used

Infliximab: 3–5 mg/kg loading at week 0, 2, 6 then maintenance 3–10 mg/kg every 4–8 weeks

Adalimumab: 40 mg every 1–2 weeks [if body weight (BW) <30 kg: 20 mg every two weeks]

Etanercept: Adults 25 mg twice a week or 50 mg once a week; children 0.8 mg/kg/week

Certolizumab: 400 mg at week 0, two, four then every four weeks

Golimumab: 50 mg monthly

Daclizumab: 1–2 mg/kg every 2–4 weeks

Rituximab: 500 or 1,000 mg at week 0 and 2

Abatacept: 500 or 1,000 mg at week 0, 2, 4 then every 4 weeks

Basiliximab: 40 mg at week 0, two, four, eight and 12

Anakinra: 100 mg daily

Efalizumab: 0.7 mg/kg first dose, then 1 mg/kg weekly

Alefacept: 15 mg IM or 7.5 mg IV weekly for 12 weeks

Interferon α-2a: 3–6 million IU/day

IVIg: 0.4 g/kg for 5 days/month, or 0.5 g/kg for 3 days/month

Common Side Effects of Biologicals in Uveitis

Anti-TNF-α

Risk of malignancy, reactivation of latent tuberculosis, multiple sclerosis and lupus-like reaction, congestive cardiac failure, thrombotic events, hypersensitivity, hepatotoxicity, pancytopenia, opportunistic infections on long-term use.

Anti-interleukin Therapy

Increased risk of cellulitis, wound infections, hives and dermatitis, lower extremity edema.

Interferons

Flu-like symptoms (100%), depression, neutropenia, alopecia, elevated liver enzymes, epilepsy, reaction at injection site, thrombocytopenia, and severe depression. Ocular side effects are typical cotton wool spots and retinal hemorrhage seen in the posterior fundus.

All of these agents are extremely expensive and availability is restricted. They need close systemic monitoring to look for side-effects. The availability of biosimilars in our country has made the use of these targeted therapies possible due to decreased cost. "Similar biologics" approved and marketed in India since 2014 include biosimilars of adalimumab, rituximab, infliximab, and IFN.

B. OCULAR PATHOLOGY

6.10 Pathology of the Eyelid

Dipankar Das, Bidhan Chandra Das, Obaidur Rehman, Apurba Deka

Sri Sankaradeva Nethralaya, Guwahati

dr_dasdipankar@yahoo.com, bdhn.ds@gmail.com, obaid.rehmann@gmail.com, dekaapurba10@gmail.com

■ XANTHELASMA

Xanthelasma is a common kind lesion of eyelid found in elderly population, which presents with yellowish subcutaneous plaques located at the medial aspect of eyelids **(Fig. 6.10.1A)**. There can be associated increased levels of serum lipid and cholesterols especially in younger individuals.

Microscopically, the lesion shows lipid laden histiocytes in the dermis **(Fig. 6.10.1B)**.

■ CHALAZION

A chalazion is a chronic lipogranulomatous inflammatory lesion caused by blockage of gland orifices and stagnation of sebaceous secretion which presents with painless nodule

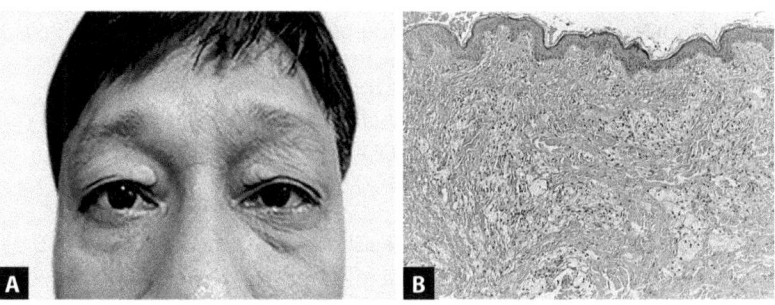

Figs. 6.10.1A and B: (A) Xanthelasma; (B) Lipid laden dermal histiocytes.

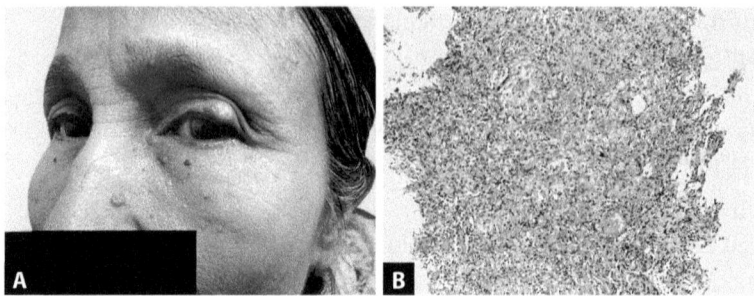

Figs. 6.10.2A and B: (A) Chalazion of upper lid; (B) Lipogranulomatous inflammation.

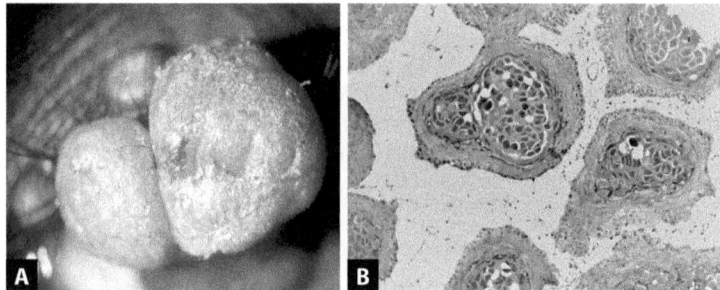

Figs. 6.10.3A and B: Molluscum contagiosum.

in the lid **(Fig. 6.10.2A)**. Microscopic examination shows formation of focal granuloma with small microabscesses, each centered on lipid globule discharged from sebaceous gland with a granulomatous reaction containing multinucleated giant cells and epithelioid cells intermixed with neutrophils, lymphocytes and plasma cells **(Fig. 6.10.2B)**.

MOLLUSCUM CONTAGIOSUM

Molluscum contagiosum is an uncommon skin infection caused by the poxvirus group and presents with single or multiple, small, raised, pale, waxy, pearly, and umbilicated nodules in the lid or other parts of the body **(Fig. 6.10.3A)**.

Microscopic examination reveals the epithelium with pear-shaped lobules of acanthotic cells that open into central crater containing characteristic inclusion bodies called molluscum bodies. These are small eosinophilic bodies in deeper layer of epidermis, becoming larger and basophilic superficially before being extruded. As the inclusions increase in size, they displace and compress the nuclei of infected cells **(Fig. 6.10.3B)**.

PYOGENIC GRANULOMA

Pyogenic granuloma is a fast-growing pseudo-granulomatous hemangiomatous lesion which is usually antedated by surgery, infection, or trauma. It usually presented with pinkish pedunculated or sessile mass **(Fig. 6.10.4A)**.

Microscopically, the lesion is composed of mass of granulation tissue with capillary proliferation, acute inflammation, and surface ulceration **(Fig. 6.10.4B)**.

SQUAMOUS PAPILLOMA

Squamous cell papilloma (viral wart) is the most common benign tumor of the eyelid which is usually found in adults and presents with pedunculated or broad-based (sessile) lesion with characteristic raspberry-like surface **(Fig. 6.10.5A)**.

Microscopically, papillomas are made up of finger-like projections of hyperplastic epithelium with a fibrovascular core. In addition, the epithelium shows acanthosis, parakeratosis, hyperkeratosis, and elongation of the rete ridges **(Fig. 6.10.5B)**.

■ BASAL CELL CARCINOMA

Basal cell carcinoma (BCC) is the most common malignant neoplasm of the eyelids, accounting for >90% of all eyelid malignancies. Lesions typically occur on the face, lower lid more than upper lid **(Fig. 6.10.6A)**. The classical description is that of a "rodent" ulcer which is slowly enlarging ulcer with pearly, raised, rolled edges. Other types are nodular, nodulo-ulcerative, sclerosing (morphoeic), and cystic.

Microscopically, the tumor shows nest of uniform basaloid cells with high nuclear cytoplasmic ratio, characteristic palisading of cells around outer edge of tumor, and artifactitious separation between the nest of tumor cells and the dermis (cracking artifact shown with arrow) **(Fig. 6.10.6B)**.

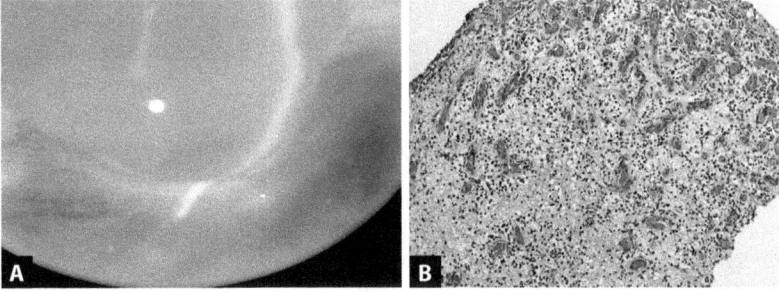

Figs. 6.10.4A and B: Pyogenic granuloma.

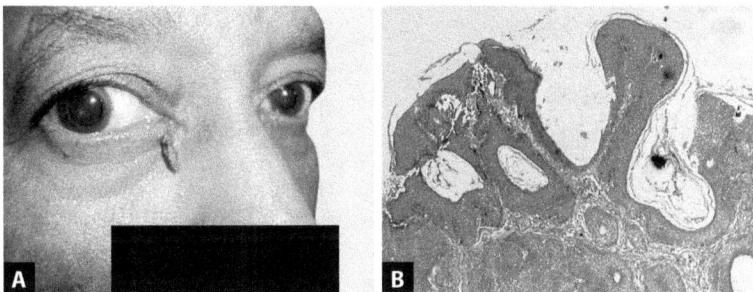

Figs. 6.10.5A and B: Squamous papilloma.

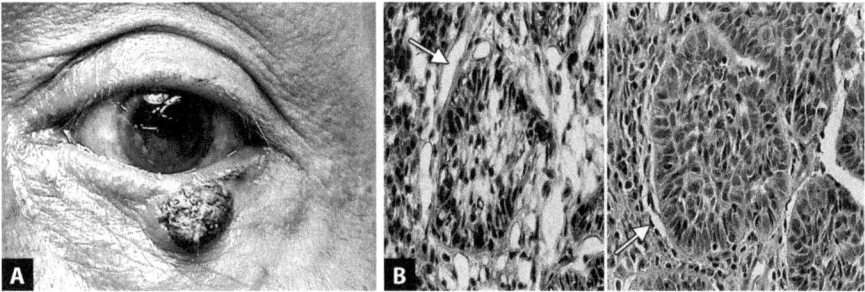

Figs. 6.10.6A and B: Basal cell carcinoma.

■ SQUAMOUS CELL CARCINOMA

Squamous cell carcinoma (SCC) may arise from preexisting lesion such as actinic keratoses or Bowen's disease. Lower eyelid is more commonly affected than upper lid **(Fig. 6.10.7A)**.

Microscopically tumor shows atypical squamous cells forming nests (epithelial pearl) and strands, extending beyond epidermal basement membrane, infiltrating the dermis, and inciting a desmoplastic fibrous tissue reaction **(Fig. 6.10.7B)**.

Tumor can be well (keratin pearl), moderately, and poorly differentiated. Regional lymph node metastasis is reported to occur in 1–21% of the patients with SCC.

■ SEBACEOUS GLAND CARCINOMA

Sebaceous gland carcinoma (SGC) most commonly involves the upper eyelid of elderly person **(Fig. 6.10.8A)**. It may originate in the meibomian gland of the tarsus, the gland of Zeis in the skin of the eyelid, or sebaceous gland of the caruncle. Clinical diagnosis is often missed or delayed because of the lesion propensity to mimic a chalazion or chronic blepharoconjunctivitis with history of loss of eyelashes. The three main types are nodular meibomian gland carcinoma, spreading (pagetoid) meibomian gland carcinoma, and gland of Zeis carcinoma.

Histologically, SGC can be classified by degree of differentiation into three groups. Well differentiated tumors contain many neoplastic cells exhibiting sebaceous differentiation. These cells have an abundant, finely vacuolated cytoplasm that appears foamy or frothy **(Fig. 6.10.8B)**. Moderately differentiated tumors may exhibit some degree of sebaceous differentiation. Poorly differentiated tumors, however, may be difficult to distinguish from the other, more commonly epithelial malignancy.

The demonstration of lipid within cytoplasm of tumor cells by special stains, such as oil red O or Sudan black, is diagnostic, but it must be performed on tissue prior to processing and paraffin embedding. Alternatively, osmium staining of tissue processed for electron microscopy will highlight intracytoplasmic lipid.

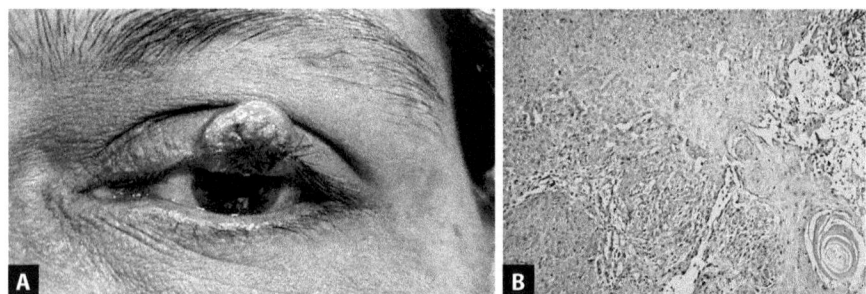

Figs. 6.10.7A and B: Squamous cell carcinoma.

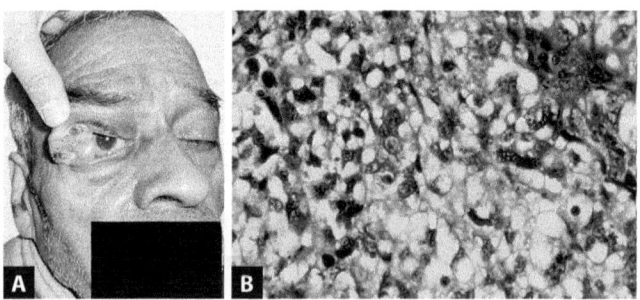

Figs. 6.10.8A and B: Sebaceous gland carcinoma.

6.11 Ocular Pathology: Laboratory Procedures

Jyotirmay Biswas
Sankara Nethralaya, Chennai
drjb@snmail.org

Dipankar Das
Sri Sankaradeva Nethralaya, Guwahati
dr_dasdipankar@yahoo.com

HOW TO SEND A SPECIMEN FOR HISTOPATHOLOGICAL EXAMINATION?

Specimens have to be documented and immersed in a proper fixative and sent to histopathological laboratory.[1,2] Identifying information includes name of the patient, age, medical records department (MRD) number, address, gender, and surgeon's name. Precise location from the surgical site and mention of eye in a destructive surgery is very important. Pertinent clinical note, duration of the lesion, history of previous surgery, medicine used etc. should be there. Note of previous pathology slides sometimes gives lot of information. Preoperative photographs, ultrasound, computed tomography (CT) scan or magnetic resonance imaging (MRI) scan report or picture can help the pathologist. If malignancy is suspected, margin should be identified by different color suture etc. and same diagram can be drawn in the grossing form or additional paper. For frozen sections, surgeon can discuss with the pathologist before the surgery and draw a plan for the procedure and demarcate the margins with identification tag. While handling the conjunctival tissue(s) which have tendency to curl, spreading of the tissue in flattened absorbent surface such as paper wrapping for gloves. Allow the fragile conjunctival tissue to become adherent to the surface for 30 seconds. When the tissue is adherent to its support, float the supporting surface and tissue on to 10% neutral buffered formalin with the tissue surface facing up. Avoid pinning the specimen to the surface as pin may rust and deposit iron on the specimen creating confusion while permanent section reporting is done. Also avoid smearing the specimen.

Fixative used in the histopathology laboratory includes 10% neutral buffered formalin and this is being satisfactory for most of the specimens in ophthalmic pathology. The recommended volume of tissue fixative is 1 (specimen): 10 (formalin). The tissue need to be submerged in the solution completely. Formalin need not be injected in the enucleated specimen. Crystals such as urate etc. need to be fixed in absolute alcohol. Cytology can be fixed with methanol or ethanol. Live parasites retrieved after surgeries can be transported in normal saline to the laboratory. For electron microscopy, fixative used is 2% glutaraldehyde. For frozen section, fresh tissues are required without any fixative and shifted immediately to the laboratory. Please remember, if surgeons have any doubt about the fixatives, they can consult the pathologist **(Table 6.11.1)**.

Types of specimen received in ocular pathology department are varied. They include conjunctival tissues, corneal scrapings, corneal buttons, sclerocorneal rim, skin and lid biopsies, orbit, lacrimal glands, iris, ciliary body, retinal tissues, enucleated globes, eviscerated specimen, exenterated specimens, optic nerve lesions, explanted intraocular lens, cytology from aqueous, vitreous etc., and fine needle aspiration biopsy.

Cytological studies of vitreous biopsies remain the first line of investigation in morphological diagnosis of primary intraocular lymphoma. Preparation of vitreous specimen for cytological evaluation varies from in different laboratories. Cytospin preparation technique can be used for both unfixed and fixed specimen. Fixed specimen can be transported in the lab quickly in CytoLyt. A similar procedure had been described by Mulay et al. where ethanol, methanol, and propranolol fixative can be used in an 8:1:1 ratio.[4]

TABLE 6.11.1: Fixatives used in ocular pathology.

Fixative	Color	Examples of used
10% neutral-buffered formalin	Clear	Routine fixation of all tissues
Bouin solution	Yellow	Small biopsy specimens such as conjunctival tissues, lymphoma specimens etc.
Absolute ethanol or methanol	Clear	Crystals such as corneal urate crystals etc.
Cytology fixatives (ethanol or methanol)	Clear	Liquid specimens or smears (aqueous humor, vitreous, fine needle aspirates or corneal smears etc.
2% glutaraldehyde	Clear	Electron microscopy specimen
Zeus transport media	Clear	Immunofluorescence (e.g.: Conjunctival biopsy in mucocele pemphigoid
Roswell Park Memorial Institute (RPMI) tissue culture media	Pink, Salmon	For cytogenetic studies, flow cytometry or transport media for molecular pathologic studies

Source: Adapted from Syed NA. 2022-2023 Basic and Clinical Science Course™, Section 04: Ophthalmic Pathology and Intraocular Tumors; 2022. American Academy of Ophthalmology. p. 21. ISBN 978-1-68104-544-3.[3]

■ HISTOPATHOLOGICAL STAINS

Microscopic slides in ocular pathology are mostly stained by hematoxylin eosin stain. The tissue section is deparaffinized and rehydrated before the stain is carried out. This is done by immersing the slides in successive bath of xylene and alcohol and then in decreasing concentration of alcohol and water. After staining for conventional 8–10 minutes, these slides are dehydrated and cover slips are put over it. Hematoxylin is a basic dye and binds with acidic components including deoxyribonucleic acid (DNA) in the nuclei of the cells and stain blue whereas eosin is acidic and binds with basic components of tissue such as protein and colors pink.

The Periodic acid-Schiff (PAS) stain is used routinely in ocular pathology because it stains the basement membrane such as lens capsule, Descemet's membrane. Additionally it is stains guttae, cuticular drusens, glycogen mucin, and few fungal hyphae. List of special stains is given in **Table 6.11.2**.

The Ziehl–Neelsen stain, also known as acid fast stain, is done for mycobacteria. Modification of this stain can also be done to stain *Nocardia* and *Brucella*. The reagent used in this stain is carbol fuchsin, acid alcohol, and methylene blue. The principle of this stain is based on lipopolysaccharides capsule of the acid fast organisms that take up heated carbol fuchsin and resist decolorization by dilute acid. Acid fast organisms stain red color by this stain.

Alizarin red used for calcium stain is an organic compound derived from prominent dye which is anthraquinone derived from the route of mother plant. Calcium deposits in a tissue are stained as red or orange by this special stain. Von Kossa is another special stain used in histopathology to demonstrate calcium which stains black.

Grocott methenamine silver stain (GMS) is used to stain fungi and *Pneumocystis carinii*. The cell walls of those organisms stain black in green background.

Gram staining or Gram method is a differential stain to demarcate gram-positive and gram-negative organisms. The basic steps of this stain include (1) applying a primary stain (crystal violet) to a heat-fixed smear of bacterial culture, (2) followed by addition of Gram's iodine, (3) rapid decolorization with alcohol or acetone, and (4) counter staining with safranin or basic fuchsin. Gram-positive bacteria stain blue or black while gram-negative bacteria stain red or pink. List of stains to identify microorganisms is given in the **Table 6.11.3**.

TABLE 6.11.2: Special stains in histopathology.

No.	Type of stain	Substance detected	Color of substance	Indicated in
1.	Alcian blue	Acid mucopoly-saccharides	Blue	Macular dystrophy, mucin
2.	Colloidal iron	Acid mucopoly-saccharides	Blue	Macular dystrophy, mucin
3.	Masson trichrome	Hyaline material	Collagen blue, muscle red, nuclei black	Granular dystrophy
4.	Congo red under polarizer or lambda plate	Amyloid	Red apple-green birefringence	Lattice dystrophy
5.	Van Gieson	Elastic fibers	Blackish gray	Elastic tissue
6.	Oil Red O (frozen section)	Lipid	Red	Fat within the cells
7.	Alizarin red	Calcium	Red	Band keratopathy
8.	Von Kossa	Calcium	Black	Band keratopathy
9.	Perls' Prussian blue	Iron	Blue	Iron in the epithelium in keratoconus and iron deposition in foreign body
10.	Fontana–Masson	Melanin and argentaffin cells		Melanin pigments in malignant melanoma and carcinoid tumor
11.	Thioflavin T	Amyloid	Fluorescent yellow-white	Lattice dystrophy

TABLE 6.11.3: Stains used to identify microorganisms in tissues.

No.	Microbe	Stain used	Color
1.	Bacteria	Gram stain	• Purple/blue/black-gram positive • Red-gram negative
2.	Fungi	• Grocott methenamine silver (GMS) • Periodic acid-Schiff (PAS)	Black Pink
3.	Mycobacteria	Ziehl–Neelsen (ZN) using 20% sulfuric acid	Red
4.	Nocardia	ZN using 5% sulfuric acid	Red
5.	Chlamydia	Giemsa	Blue purple inclusion bodies
6.	Acanthamoeba	• PAS • GMS • Calcofluor white	• Purple black • Black • White-green fluorescent
7.	Mycobacterium leprae	Fite–Faraco	Red

IMMUNOHISTOCHEMISTRY

Immunohistochemistry (IHC) is a newer technique that has revolutionized histopathologic diagnostic. Immunohistochemistry uses different antibodies by utilizing the antigen in different cell types. Some of the IHCs markers that are being used in ocular pathology laboratory commonly are given here **(Table 6.11.4)**.

Examples of routine tissue stains, stains for microorganism, and immunohistochemistry are given in **Figures 6.11.1 to 6.11.11**.

TABLE 6.11.4: Immunohistochemistry markers for common ocular tumors/pseudotumors.

No.	Tumors/pseudotumors	Markers
1.	Non-Hodgkin's lymphoma	CD20 (B-cells), CD3 (T-cells), Kappa, Lambda, CD79a, MUM1, MIB1, BCL2, BCl6, Ki-67
2.	Pseudotumor	CD3, CD20, CD45 (LCA), CD138 (plasma cells), IgG4 (for IgG4-related diseases)
3.	Round cell tumors	CD3, CD20, Vimentin, Actin, S100, Desmin, NSE, CD45, Synaptophysin, CK, Neurofilament
4.	Rhabdomyosarcoma	Vimentin, Actin, Desmin, Myogenin, MyoD
5.	Melanoma	HMB45, Melan-A, Ki-67
6.	Squamous cell carcinoma	CK, Ki-67
7.	Schwannoma	Vimentin, S100, CD57
8.	Hemangiopericytoma	Vimentin, S100, CD31, Factor-VIII, CD34
9.	Solitary fibrous tumor	CD34, Vimentin, S100
10.	Leiomyoma/leiomyosarcoma	Vimentin, Actin, Desmin
11.	Retinoblastoma	Neuron specific enolase, Synaptophysin

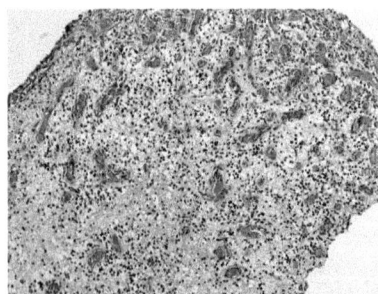

Fig. 6.11.1: Hematoxylin and eosin (H-E) stained slide.

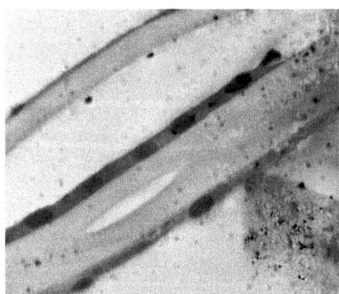

Fig. 6.11.2: Periodic acid-Schiff (PAS) stained slide.

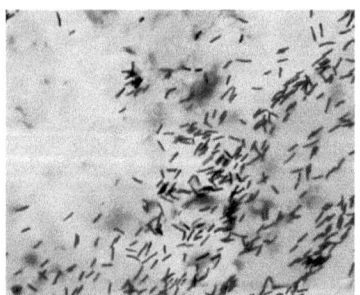

Fig. 6.11.3: Ziehl–Neelsen (ZN) stained slide having red colored acid fast bacilli.

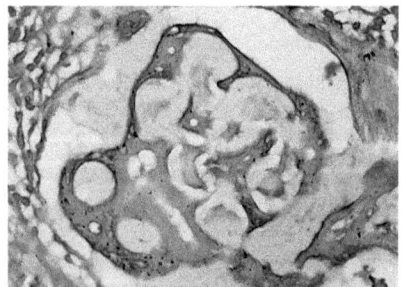

Fig. 6.11.4: Alcian blue stained slide.

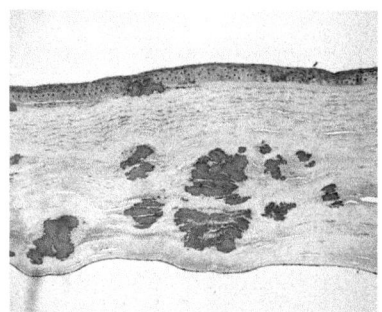

Fig. 6.11.5: Masson trichrome stained slide.

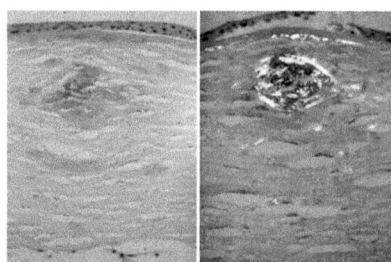

Congo red   Apple green birefringence under polarizer

Fig. 6.11.6: Congo red stained slide. Compared polarizer microscopy picture also seen.

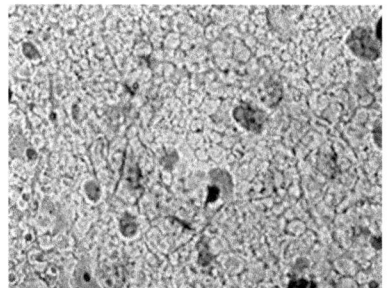

Fig. 6.11.7: Oil Red O stained slide having red colored fat cells in frozen section.

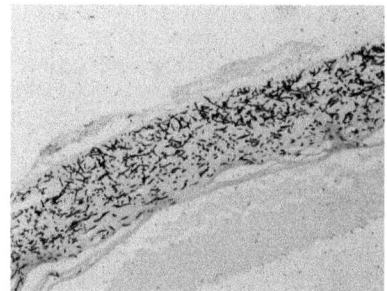

Fig. 6.11.8: Grocott methenamine silver (GMS) stain slide with black colored fungus in corneal button.

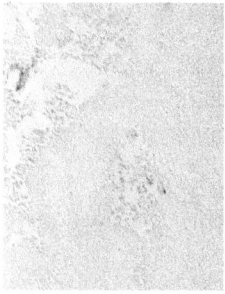

Fig. 6.11.9: Alizarin stain for calcium deposits in retinoblastoma.

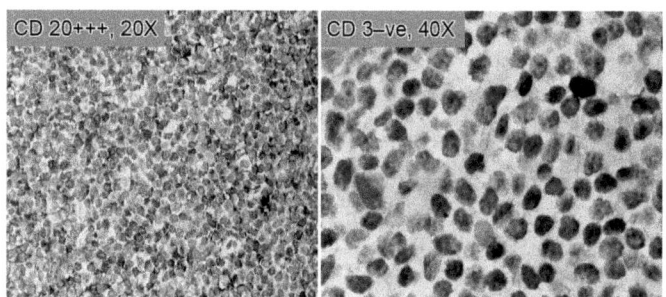

Fig. 6.11.10: Immunohistochemistry slide in non-Hodgkin's lymphoma (CD20 and CD3).

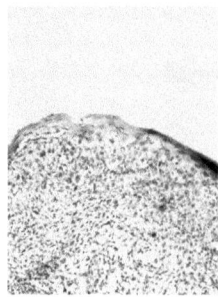

Fig. 6.11.11: Immunohistochemistry slide for cytokeratin (CK) in squamous cell carcinoma.

■ REFERENCES

1. Eagle RC Jr. Eye pathology: An Atlas and Text. 2nd edition. Philadelphia: Wolters Kluwer/Lippincott Williams and Wilkins; 2011.
2. Bancroft JD, Gamble M. Theory and Practice of Histological Techniques. 5th edition. London: Churchill Livingstone; 2002.
3. Syed NA. 2022-2023 Basic and Clinical Science Course™, Section 04: Ophthalmic Pathology and Intraocular Tumors; 2022. American Academy of Ophthalmology. p. 21. ISBN 978-1-68104-544-3.
4. Mulay K, Narula R, Honavar SG. Primary vitreoretinal lymphoma. Indian J Ophthalmol. 2015;63(3):180-6.

6.12 | Intraocular Tumors

S Krishnakumar, Jyotirmay Biswas
Sankara Nethralaya, Chennai
drkk@snmail.org, drjb@snmail.org

1. **What are the nonpigmented malignant intraocular tumors?**
   - Iris leiomyoma
   - Epstein–Barr virus-associated smooth muscle tumor
   - Fuchs' Adenoma of the ciliary nonpigment epithelium
   - Adenoma of the ciliary nonpigment epithelium
   - Ciliary body leiomyoma
   - Ciliary body schwannoma
   - Ciliary adenocarcinoma from nonpigment epithelium
   - Retinoblastoma
   - Vitreoretinal lymphoma
   - Choroidal leiomyoma
   - Choroidal schwannoma
   - Choroidal neurofibroma
   - Primary choroidal lymphoma—part of mucosa-associated lymphoid tissue (MALT) lymphoma.
2. **What are the pigment intraocular tumors?**
   - Iris melanocytic tumors of uncertain malignant potential
   - Iris melanoma
   - Iris pigment epithelial adenocarcinoma
   - Adenoma of the ciliary pigment epithelium
   - Ciliary adenocarcinoma from pigment epithelium
   - Medulloepithelioma
   - Ciliary body melanoma
   - Choroidal melanocytoma

- Choroidal melanoma
- Bilateral diffuse uveal melanocytic proliferation
- Retinal pigment epithelial adenocarcinoma.

3. **What are the common intraocular tumors encountered in pathology laboratory?**
   - *In children:*
     - Retinoblastoma
     - Medulloepithelioma
   - *In adults:*
     - Malignant melanoma of the choroid
     - Metastatic tumor to the choroid
     - Vitreoretinal lymphoma.

4. **What is the gross appearance of the cut section of the globe in malignant melanoma of the choroid?**
   On sectioning the melanoma eye ball characteristic findings are a pigmented mass from iris or the ciliary body and mushroom- or dome-shaped mass arising from the choroid with overlying retinal detachment **(Fig. 6.12.1)**.

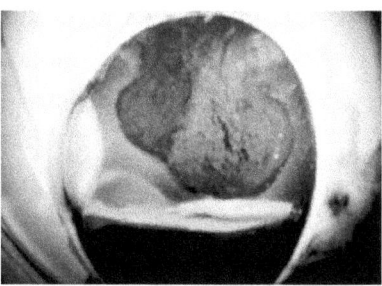

Fig. 6.12.1: Cut section of the globe in malignant melanoma of choroid.

5. **What is the classification of malignant melanoma of the uveal tract?**
   - Spindle cell melanoma
   - Epithelioid cell melanoma
   - Mixed cell melanoma (mixture of spindle and epithelioid cells)
     - Mixed cell melanoma with more spindle cells
     - Mixed cell melanoma with more epithelioid cells.

6. **What is the molecular classification of uveal melanoma?**
   Uveal melanomas are classified into low-grade (low risk for metastasis) (class 1A and class 1B) and high-grade (high risk for metastasis) (class 2) uveal melanoma based on gene expression profiling and clinical outcome.

7. **What are the chromosomal aberrations in uveal melanoma?**
   The chromosomal aberrations in uveal melanoma include loss of 1p, 3, and 6q and gain of 6p and 8q.

8. **Is there one protein marker which can be done by immunohistochemistry on the paraffin sections to predict prognosis in uveal melanoma?**
   Immunohistochemical (IHC) assessment of nuclear BRCA1-associated protein-1 (BAP1) protein loss is associated with increased risk of death in uveal melanoma.

9. **Are there guidelines for retinoblastoma eye ball grossing and how many slides overall are there?**
   There is International Retinoblastoma Staging Working Group has laid protocol for grossing and for reporting. Bread loaf sections of the lateral calotte are taken with anywhere 18–22 slides with serial sections of the globe covering the central and lateral calottes for retinoblastoma reporting. By following this protocol, the pathologist identifies more choroidal invasion.

10. **How does the cut section of the retinoblastoma eye ball appear?**
    On sectioning the retinoblastoma **(Fig. 6.12.2)** eye shows several characteristic

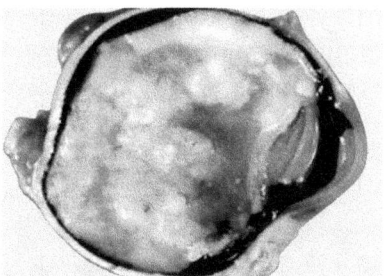

Fig. 6.12.2: Cut section of the eyeball filled with whitish tumor in the posterior segment.

findings are a chalky white mass, often friable seen arising from the retina and there is retinal detachment.

11. **What are the different growth patterns in retinoblastoma?**
    The different patterns of growth patterns are:
    - Exophytic growth pattern
    - Endophytic growth pattern
    - Combined exophytic and endophytic growth pattern
    - Diffuse growth pattern.

12. **What are the high-risk histopathology retinoblastoma?**
    - Choroid invasion >3 mm
    - Diffuse choroidal invasion >3 mm
    - Iris and ciliary body stromal invasion
    - Scleral invasion
    - Post-laminar and surgical end of optic nerve invasion.

13. **What is newest histopathology risk factor that correlates with chromosomal amplification?**
    Retinoblastoma tumor cells, that are large with hyperchromatic nuclei and have a high nucleocytoplasmic ratio, have a rhomboidal shape with tumor cells close to each other are called severe anaplasia and it correlates with gain of chromosome 6p and it correlates with extraocular spread.

14. **What is the newest molecular classification of retinoblastoma to predict aggressiveness?**

    Subtype 1 retinoblastoma-less aggressive: These are heritable tumors, few genetic alterations, well differentiated tumor cells with cone markers, and less aggressive.

    Subtype 2 retinoblastoma: More aggressive and risk for metastasis; these tumors are poorly differentiated tumors and express stem cell markers.

15. **What is the current liquid biopsy research in Retinoblastoma to prognosticate?**
    Cell-free DNA (cfDNA) is analyzed in aqueous humor to study chromosome 6p gain or *MYCN* amplification using a custom hybridization panel to prognosticate without enucleation of the rye with the tumor.

16. **Which is the most common intraocular tumor presenting as masquerade syndrome?**
    Primary vitreoretinal lymphoma commonly presents as masquerading syndromes.

17. **How currently the laboratory diagnosis of intraocular lymphoma is made?**
    - Cytology—gold standard
    - Immunocytochemistry panel including CD20,CD3, Ki-67, and CD68
    - Polymerase chain reaction (PCR) sequencing for *MYD88* L265P mutation
    - Interleukin 10 (IL-10), IL-6, IL-10/IL-6 ratio in the vitreous
    - Flow cytometry immunophenotyping
    - Immunoglobulin heavy chain gene rearrangement.

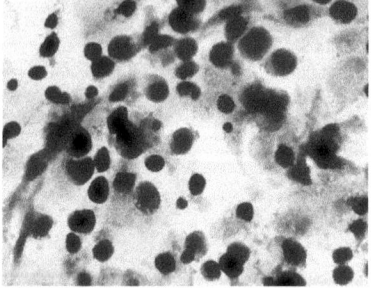

Fig. 6.12.3: Atypical large lymphoid cells with high nucleocytoplasmic ratio in a necrotic background.

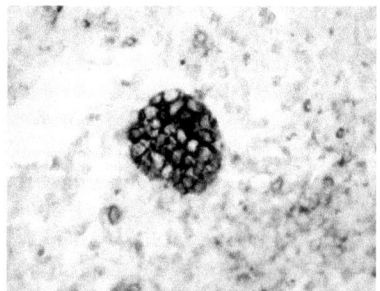

Fig. 6.12.4: Atypical large lymphoid cells with diffuse CD20 membrane positivity in vitreous biopsy cell block preparation.

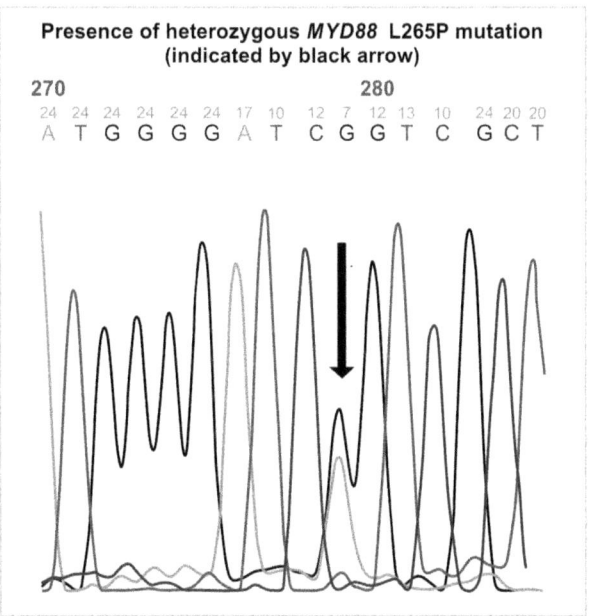

Fig. 6.12.5: Polymerase chain reaction (PCR)-based sequencing for *MYD88* L265P mutation: positive.

18. **How does targeted next generation sequencing useful in the laboratory diagnosis of intraocular lymphoma?**

TABLE 6.12.1: Drugs targeting specific mutations in intraocular lymphoma.

Mutation identified	Drugs available
MYD88 p.L265P mutation	TLR inhibitors
Both p.L265P and p.S243N *MYD88* mutations	Bruton's kinase inhibitor ibrutinib, and IRAK1/4 antagonists
High-level *CDKN2A* loss	Ilorasertib

(TLR: toll-like receptor)

6.13 | Orbital Tumors

Jyotirmay Biswas
Sankara Nethralaya, Chennai
drjb@snmail.org

Dipankar Das
Sri Sankaradeva Nethralaya, Guwahati
dr_dasdipankar@yahoo.com

■ COMMON ORBITAL TUMORS

Primary orbital tumors
- Choristomas
- Hamartomas
- *Vasculogenic tumors:* Cavernous hemangioma or venous malformation, varix, hemangiopericytoma, lymphangioma, capillary hemangioma.

- *Peripheral nerve:* Neurofibroma, schwannoma
  Optic nerve: Optic nerve glioma
- *Lacrimal gland tumors:* Pleomorphic adenoma, adenoid cystic carcinoma
- Lymphoid tumors and leukemia
- Osseous and fibro-osseous tumor
- Cartilaginous tumors
- Rhabdomyoma and rhabdomyosarcoma
- Lipocytic and myxoid tumors
- Primary melanocytic tumors.

Secondary tumors from adjacent structures
- Metastatic

PATHOLOGY OF CAVERNOUS HEMANGIOMA

Gross examination revealed well-circumscribed, encapsulated lesion with dusky red or blackish blue colored mass. Microscopic examination revealed the lesions composed of large dilated blood-filled spaces lined by flattened endothelial cells **(Fig. 6.13.1)**. The stroma contained intervening fibroblasts, smooth muscles, and fat cells and can have hyaline or myxoid changes.

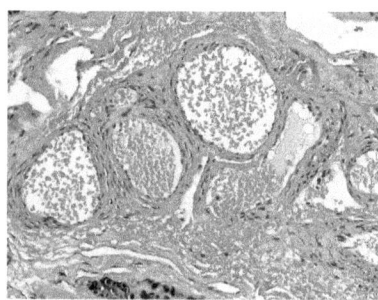

Fig. 6.13.1: Cavernous hemangioma.

PATHOLOGY OF OPTIC NERVE GLIOMA

Grossly, optic nerve glioma is usually a fusiform swelling of the optic nerve. Microscopically, it is composed of proliferation of benign-looking spindle-shaped pilocytic astrocytes. There are eosinophilic cigar-shaped glial filaments seen which are called Rosenthal fibers **(Fig. 6.13.2)**. Mucinous degeneration is sometimes seen in the glioma. Pathologically, optic nerve gliomas are mostly benign. Malignant transformation is seen in posteriorly located optic nerve involvement extending to central nervous system [World Health Organization (WHO) grade-3].

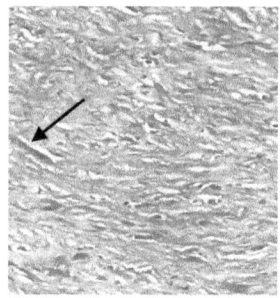

Fig. 6.13.2: Optic nerve glioma.

PATHOLOGY OF ORBITAL MENINGIOMA

Orbital meningioma is a benign tumor arising from meningothelial cells of meninges. It is composed of numerous clusters and whorls of such cells. Intranuclear vacuoles can be seen in this tumor and sometimes numerous calcific bodies called psammoma bodies can be observed **(Fig. 6.13.3)**.

TUMORS OF LACRIMAL GLANDS

Briefly, tumors of lacrimal glands are epithelial and nonepithelial tumors.

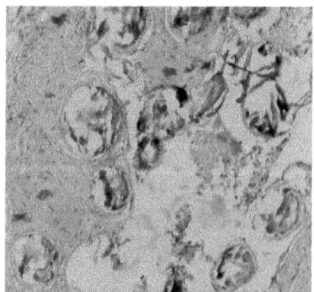

Fig. 6.13.3: Orbital meningioma.

- Epithelial tumors are comprised of following:
  - Pleomorphic adenoma (benign mixed tumor)
  - Malignant mixed tumor
  - Adenoid cystic carcinoma
  - Mucoepidermoid carcinoma
- *Nonepithelial tumors:* Lymphoma and lymphoid tumors

PATHOLOGY OF PLEOMORPHIC ADENOMA OF LACRIMAL GLAND

Pleomorphic adenoma is the most common epithelial tumor of the lacrimal glands. It presents as painless proptosis. Gross examination revealed well-circumscribed, pseudo-encapsulated with surface bosselations. They can sometimes present with expansile mass. Microscopic examination reveals mixture of epithelial and mesenchymal elements **(Fig. 6.13.4)**. Double-layer epithelial ductules and stroma show myxoid tissue, cartilage, fat, and bone.

PATHOLOGY OF ADENOID CYSTIC CARCINOMA

Grossly, adenoid cystic carcinoma can be seen as rounded or globular structures with the margins being irregular. There are five types of adenocystic carcinoma. They are:
- *Cribriform (Swiss cheese pattern):* Cystic spaces are seen within tumor cells in a gland-like pattern and they can have perineural involved **(Fig. 6.13.5)**.
- Basaloid (solid pattern)
- Sclerosing
- Comedo
- Tubular
  Presence of basaloid pattern has been associated with poor prognosis of the tumor.

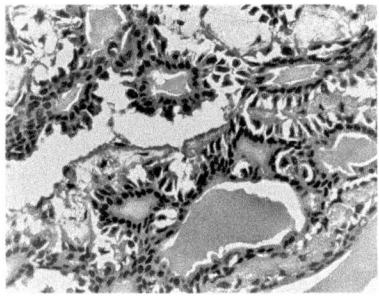

Fig. 6.13.4: Pleomorphic adenoma of lacrimal gland.

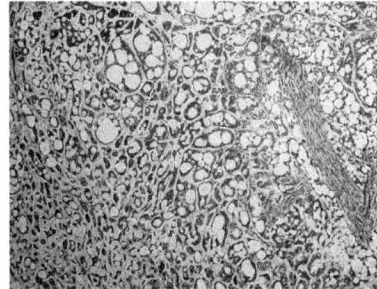

Fig. 6.13.5: Adenoid cystic carcinoma.

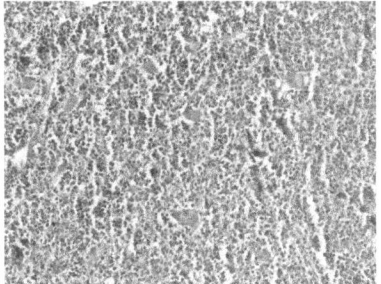

Fig. 6.13.6: Sheets of transformed lymphocytes in orbital lymphoma.

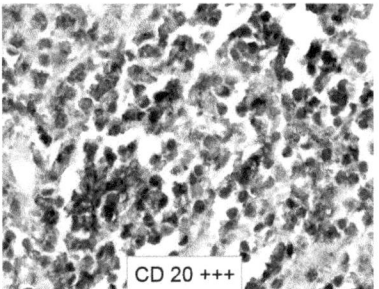

Fig. 6.13.7: Orbital lymphoma B cell type.

ORBITAL LYMPHOMA

Orbital lymphoid tumors include polyclonal reactive lymphoid hyperplasia and malignant lymphomas. Non-Hodgkin's lymphomas of the orbit with B-cell clonal proliferations with low grade are most common malignant tumors seen in orbit and adnexal tumors. They are seen in elderly patients. Grossly, they are seen as grayish white tumors. Microscopically, tumor shows diffuse sheets of transformed lymphocytes **(Fig. 6.13.6)** which can be further differentiated by immunohistochemistry B-cell and T-cell type **(Figs. 6.13.7 and 6.13.8)**.

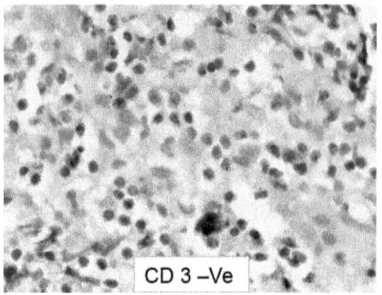

Fig. 6.13.8: Orbital lymphoma T cell type.

SECTION 7

Retina

Editor: Mangat R Dogra

7.1 Rhegmatogenous Retinal Detachment and its Management 459
   Ajay Aurora

7.2 Proliferative Diabetic Retinopathy 463
   Ajit Babu Majji

7.3 Vitreomacular Traction Syndrome 464
   Alay S Banker

7.4 Vitreous Hemorrhage 467
   Alok Sen, Jayanti Singh, Samendra Karkhur

7.5 Management of Posteriorly Dislocated Intraocular Lens 469
   Anand Rajendran, Prabu Bhaskaran

7.6 Pediatric Retinal Imaging 472
   Anand Vinekar

7.7 Branch Retinal Vein Occlusion 478
   Aniruddha Agarwal

7.8 Central Retinal Vein Occlusion 481
   Aniruddha Agarwal

7.9 Management of Neovascular Age-related Macular Degeneration 484
   Aniruddha Agarwal, Deeksha Katoch, Mangat R Dogra

7.10 Understanding Macular Holes 488
   Atul Kumar, Divya Agarwal, Aman Kumar

7.11 Retinitis Pigmentosa and Stem Cell Transplantation 493
   Atul Kumar, Divya Agarwal, Aman Kumar

7.12 Vitrectomy for Diabetic Traction Retinal Detachment 496
   Cyrus Shroff, Charu Gupta

7.13 Fundus Fluorescein Angiography 499
   Deeksha Katoch, Ramanuj Samanta

7.14 Macular Telangiectasia 505
   Dhananjay Shukla, Jay Kalliath

7.15 Polypoidal Choroidal Vasculopathy 510
   Dinesh Talwar, Saurabh Arora

7.16 Wide-angle Viewing Systems 518
   Hemanth Murthy

7.17 Postoperative Cystoid Macular Edema 521
   Jay Chhablani, Komal Agrawal

7.18 Radiation Retinopathy 524
   Karobi Lahiri Coutinho, Samyak V Mulkutkar

7.19 Postoperative Endophthalmitis: An Update 538
   Lalit Verma, Arindam Chakravarti, Anuja Patil

7.20 Retinal Detachment with Proliferative Vitreoretinopathy 548
   Lingam Gopal

7.21 Retinopathy of Prematurity 552
   Anand Vinekar, Gaurav Sanghi, Mangat R Dogra

7.22 Choroidal Melanoma 557
   P Mahesh Shanmugam

7.23 Transconjunctival 25-gauge Vitrectomy 559
   P Mahesh Shanmugam

7.24 Suprachoroidal Hemorrhage 561
   Mallika Goyal

7.25 Submacular Hemorrhage 563
   Manisha Agarwal

7.26 Antivascular Endothelial Growth Factor in Retinal Practice 568
   Mohit Dogra, Simar Rajan Singh

7.27 Fungal Endophthalmitis 571
   Janani Sreenivasan, Muna Bhende

7.28 Exudative Retinal Detachment 578
   Neeraj Sandhuja, Anisha Seth

7.29 Familial Exudative Vitreoretinopathy 581
   Parijat Chandra, Vinod Kumar

7.30 Retained Lens Fragments in Vitreous 583
   Pramod S Bhende

7.31 Management of Myopic Maculopathy 585
   Parveen Sen, Tarun Sharma

7.32 **Cataract Surgery in Diabetic Retinopathy** 591
R Kim, V Muthukrishnan

7.33 **Gene Therapy** 593
Raja Narayanan, Taraprasad Das

7.34 **Diabetic Macular Edema** 595
Rajiv Raman, Chetan Rao, Vikas Khetan

7.35 **Ultrasonography and Ultrasound Biomicroscopy Imaging for Vitreoretinal Diseases** 603
Ramandeep Singh, Mohit Dogra, Simar Rajan Singh

7.36 **Intraocular Foreign Bodies** 606
Ramanuj Samanta, Shalaka Waghamare

7.37 **Optical Coherence Tomography Angiography** 609
Reema Bansal, Simar Rajan Singh, Vinay Patil

7.38 **Photodynamic Therapy** 613
S Natarajan, Alay S Banker, Chinmay Nakhwa

7.39 **Optic Nerve Head Pit with Serous Detachment (Kranenburg Syndrome)** 615
Sangeet Mittal

7.40 **Photic Retinopathy** 617
Saurabh Luthra, Shrutanjoy Mohan Das, Shweta Parakh

7.41 **Hypertensive Retinopathy** 621
Brijesh Thakkar, Soumyava Basu

7.42 **Endogenous Endophthalmitis** 627
Subina Narang, Varsha Jindal

7.43 **Dry Age-related Macular Degeneration** 631
Sunandan Sood, Meenakshi Chandel

7.44 **Retinoblastoma: Current Update—2022** 635
Usha Singh, Khushdeep Abhaypal

7.45 **Retinal Breaks and Vitreoretinal Precursors of Retinal Detachment: Diagnosis and Prophylaxis** 637
Vasumathy Vedantham

7.46 **Optical Coherence Tomography** 639
Vishali Gupta, Mansi Sharma

7.47 **Central Serous Chorioretinopathy** 648
Manpreet Brar

7.48 **Macular Function Tests for Patients Undergoing Cataract Surgery** 652
Lingam Gopal

7.49 **Other Causes of Choroidal Neovascularization** 655
Rohan Chawla, Shakha Gupta

7.50 **Posterior Segment Trauma: Clinical, Surgical Manifestations, and Management** 660
Samendra Karkhur, Baldev Sastya, Sunil Verma, Richa Nyodu, Nikita Yadav

7.51 **Retinal Imaging in Adults** 664
Manish Nagpal

SECTION 7: Retina

7.1 Rhegmatogenous Retinal Detachment and its Management

Ajay Aurora
Vision Plus Eye Centre, Noida and MMR Eye Institute, New Delhi
auroraajay@hotmail.com, auroraeye@gmail.com

■ INTRODUCTION

Rhegmatogenous retinal detachment (RRD) occurs when there is a separation of the neurosensory retina from the retinal pigment epithelium (RPE) with accumulation of subretinal fluid (SRF) in the presence of one or more retinal breaks. The overall incidence of RRD has been estimated to be between 0.0061 and 0.0179% per year.

■ EVALUATION

Evaluation of a patient with RRD involves a complete eye examination with good indirect ophthalmoscopy. The aim is to:
- Find, localize, and document all retinal breaks (Lincoff's rules are helpful)
- Document extent and elevation of retinal detachment (RD) (a subclinical RRD is one in which fluid extends >1 disc diameter (DD) from the break but <2 DD posterior to the equator) **(Fig. 7.1.1)**
- Document macula on or off status or if macula is being threatened (this is an emergency)
- Document presence or absence of posterior vitreous detachment (PVD) and extent/severity of associated proliferative vitreo-retinopathy (PVR)
- Document lens clarity

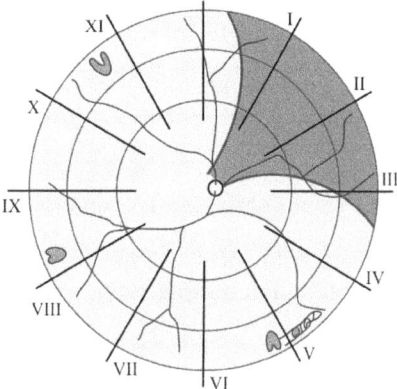

Fig. 7.1.1: Subtotal retinal detachment with three horseshoe tears at 5, 8, and 10.30 o'clock hours, there is a lattice in inferonasal quadrant with an atrophic hole. The red area is of attached retina and the blue area is detached retina.

Localization of Breaks: Lincoff's Rules

- *Detachments that cross the 12 o'clock meridian and total detachment:* In 93% of cases, the hole of origin lies with great frequency within a triangle whose apex is at 12 o'clock position at ora and whose sides intersect the equator one hour to at either side of 12 o'clock **(Fig. 7.1.2A)**.
- *Superior temporal and nasal detachment:* The primary break will be found within 1½ clock hours, of the highest border of the detachment, in 98% cases **(Fig. 7.1.2B)**.
- *Shallow inferior detachment:* The break is mostly inferior. For unequal height of RD, the break lies within 1 o'clock hour of 6 o'clock on the higher side. When the levels are equal, the break is at the 6 o'clock meridian **(Fig. 7.1.2C)**.
- *Bullous inferior detachment:* Mostly caused by a superior break which connects with the detachment by a shallow peripheral sinus.

■ SURGICAL MANAGEMENT

Surgical management of RRD revolves around finding all retinal breaks, sealing them by creating a chorioretinal scar (retinopexy), with or without SRF drainage, and relief of vitreoretinal traction. These goals may be achieved by:
- Scleral buckling (SB)
- Pneumatic retinopexy (PnR)

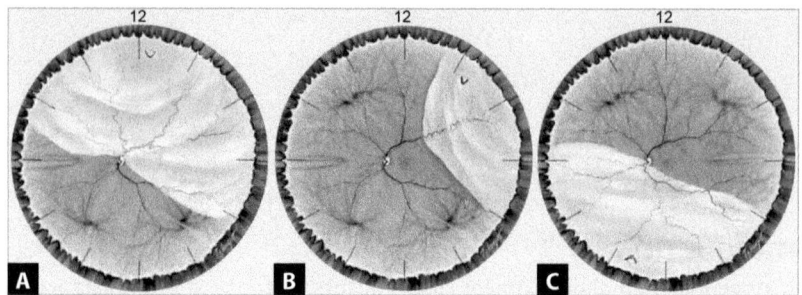

Figs. 7.1.2A to C: Subtotal rhegmatogenous retinal detachment (RRD) and Lincoff's rules.

- Primary pars plana vitrectomy (PPV) with internal tamponade [with gas (SF6, C3F8, or silicon oil)]
- Belt buckle/SB with PPV with internal tamponade in RRD complicated with advanced PVR.

Scleral buckling involves use of segmental buckle alone or buckle with an encircling element. The SB procedure involves: (1) localizing all breaks and sealing them with retinopexy [usually done as an initial step but in some bullous RD after SRF drainage {drain-air-cryotherapy-explant (DACE) procedure}], (2) drainage of SRF (this may be avoided in shallow RRD where after SB the neurosensory retina comes in near apposition to the RPE), (3) placing the buckle (size and extent decided by location of breaks) so that all the breaks preferably fall on its anterior slope. This avoids fish-mouthing. In addition, sterile air/gas can be injected to support the break. This would also avoid fish-mouthing **(Figs. 7.1.3A and B)**. In cases with associated early PVR a 360° laser barrage is done postoperatively posterior to the buckle. The reported success rate of RRD with single SB operation varies from 80 to 96%. Retinopexy in SB may be achieved with cryotherapy, diopexy, and intra-operative laser with laser indirect ophthalmoscope (LIO) or done postoperatively. Cryotherapy is able to "light up" the break and hence is preferred with moderate media opacity where some breaks may be hard to find and treat with laser. Cryotherapy has been shown to cause

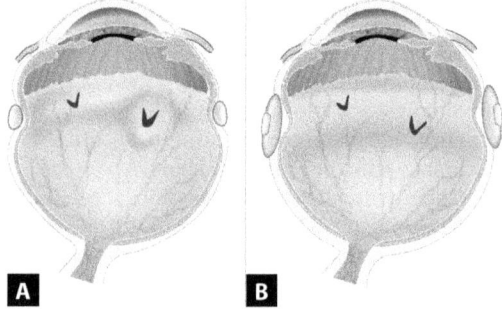

Figs. 7.1.3A and B: (A) Poorly supported break will lead to fish mouthing; (B) Well-supported break with wider buckle prevents fish mouthing.

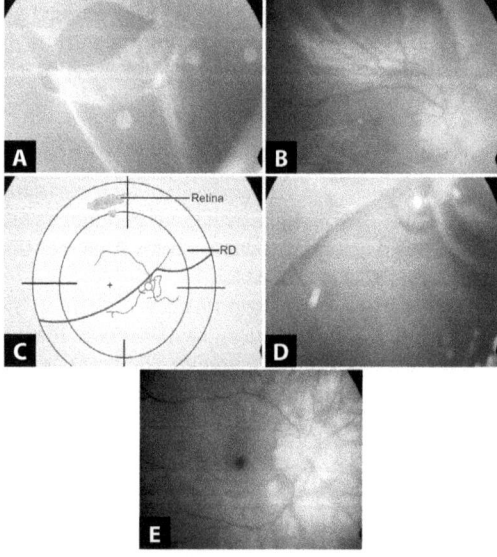

Figs. 7.1.4A to E: Subtotal retinal detachment (RD) treated with scleral buckle and sterile air.

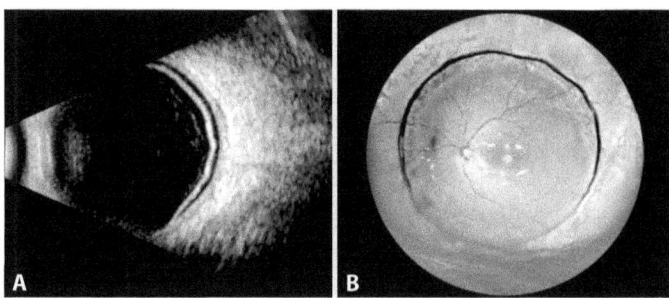

Figs. 7.1.5A and B: Mr AS, 54-year-old, male, total aphakic retinal detachment; BB, PPV, SOI, EL (postoperative VA 6/9). (BB: belt buckle; EL: endolaser; PPV: pars plana vitrectomy; SOI: silicon oil injection; VA: visual acuity)

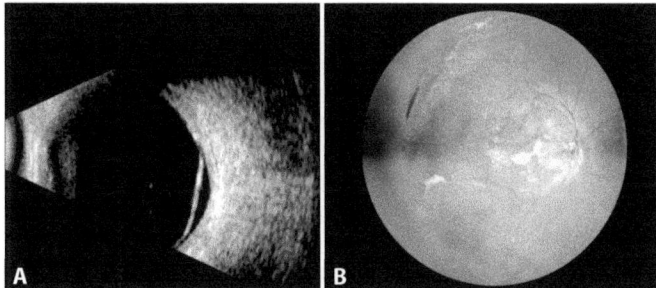

Figs. 7.1.6A and B: Mr AKS, 65-year-old, male: Inf, retinal detachment; BB, PPV, SOI, EL (postoperative VA 6/6). (BB: belt buckle; EL: endolaser; PPV: pars plana vitrectomy; SOI: silicon oil injection; VA: visual acuity)

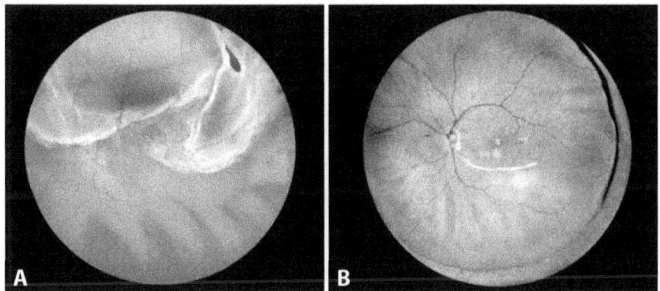

Figs. 7.1.7A and B: Mr VK, 57-year-old, male: LE subtotal bullous RD; BB, PPV, SOI, EL (postoperative VA 6/12). (BB: belt buckle; EL: endolaser; LE: left eye; PPV: pars plana vitrectomy; RD: retinal detachment; SOI: silicon oil injection; VA: visual acuity)

dispersion of live RPE cells and has been implicated in formation of epiretinal membrane though this may also happen with occurrence of PVD in absence of a break.

Primary PPV for uncomplicated RRD is being used increasingly successfully. The reasons cited are greater success in locating small or anterior breaks, more complete resolution of vitreous traction, ability to deal with media opacities and controlled subretinal fluid drainage (SRFD), and availability of microincision vitreous surgery (MIVS). Disadvantages include new iatrogenic retinal breaks and lens damage. The primary reattachment rate of PPV for RRD varies from 64 to 100% across various series.

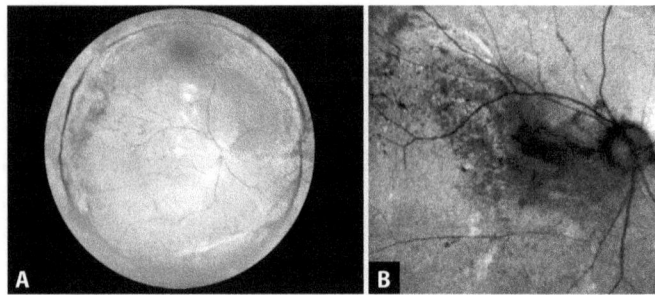

Figs. 7.1.8A and B: Mr AS, 22-year-old, male: RE traumatic old total RD, PVR, and subretinal gliosis. BB, PPV, extensive membrane surgery, SOI, EL (postoperative VA 6/24) awaiting cataract surgery; minimal in torsion of the superotemporal vessels (both color and blue FAF). (BB: belt buckle; EL: endolaser; FAF: fundus autofluorescence; PPV: pars plana vitrectomy; PVR: proliferative vitreoretinopathy; RD: retinal detachment; RE: right eye; SOI: silicon oil injection; VA: visual acuity)

Complications of management of RRD include complications of local anesthesia, complications of the performed procedure (e.g., SB: inadvertent globe perforation, retinal incarceration, dry tap, inadvertent break, intraocular hemorrhage, and excessive cryotherapy).

Scleral Buckling versus Vitrectomy

The SB versus primary vitrectomy in RRD study (SPR study) is a landmark study that compared SB and primary vitrectomy in patients with RRD **(Table 7.1.1)**. The main outcomes of the study were that in patients with RRD of medium complexity, the choice of surgical technique has a significant impact on the results. In phakic patients, better functional success was achieved with SB, whereas in pseudophakic patients, better anatomical outcomes were achieved with PPV. Overall, SB was recommended for phakic eyes with low-to-medium complexity (early PVR), RRD with single break, break extension <1 clock hour, and break with regular edges. In all other conditions, primary vitrectomy with or without scleral buckle was recommended.

Pneumatic retinopexy is used in selected cases of RRD with retinal breaks in the superior 8 clock hours of the retina. A gas bubble (SF6 or C3F8) is injected into the vitreous cavity and the patient's head positioned so that the expanding bubble tamponades the retinal break/breaks, while laser photocoagulation or cryotherapy is used for retinopexy. The reported success rate of RRD with single PnR operation varies from 62 to 73%. It is less effective in aphakic and pseudophakic eyes as compared to phakic eyes. The advantage of PnR is that it is a quick and causes less morbidity than SB or vitrectomy and can be done as an outpatient procedure.

TABLE 7.1.1: Summary of main results from SPR study.

Outcome	SB	PPV
Phakic:		
Improvement in BCVA	−0.71	−0.56
Primary success	63.6%	63.8%
Primary reattachment	73.7%	74.9%
Aphakic/pseudophakic:		
Improvement in BCVA	−0.56	−0.65
Primary success	53.4%	72.0%
Primary reattachment	60.1%	79.5%

(BCVA: best corrected visual acuity; PPV: pars plana vitrectomy; SB: scleral buckling)

Pneumatic Retinopexy versus Vitrectomy

The PIVOT trial was a randomized trial that compared PnR to PPV for the treatment of primary RRD. It demonstrated superior Early Treatment of Diabetic Retinopathy Study (ETDRS) visual acuity outcomes with PnR at all-time points, including the 1-year endpoint. Patients who underwent PnR also experienced less vertical metamorphopsia and had a lower risk of cataract formation. However, patients in the PnR group experienced a 12% lower primary reattachment rate (81% vs. 93% in the PPV group).

A particular case of RRD may be treated differently in different parts of the world or even in the same country depending on the training of the vitreoretinal specialist. The results, to an extent, are expertise dependent. In a recent analysis of nationwide Japanese registry showed that SB but not PPV surgeries require sufficient experience and case numbers to acquire and maintain skills to treat RRDs successfully.

■ SUGGESTED READING

1. Schachat AP, Wilkinson CP, Hinton DR, SriniVas RS, Wiedemann P. Ryan's Retina, 6th edition. Amsterdam, Netherlands: Elsevier; 2018.
2. Schwartz SG, Flynn HW. Primary retinal detachment: scleral buckle or pars plana vitrectomy? Curr Opinion Ophthalmol. 2006;17(3):245-50.
3. Sun Q, Sun T, Xu Y, Yang XL, Xu X, Wang BS, et al. Primary vitrectomy versus scleral buckling for the treatment of rhegmatogenous retinal detachment: a meta-analysis of randomized controlled clinical trials. Curr Eye Res. 2012;37(6):492-9.
4. Yamakiri K, Sakamoto T, Koriyama C, Kawasaki R, Baba T, Nishitsuka K, et al. Effect of surgeon related factors on outcome of retinal detachment surgery: analyses of data in Japan-retinal detachment registry. Sci Rep. 2022;12:4213.

7.2 Proliferative Diabetic Retinopathy

Ajit Babu Majji
Center for Sight, Hyderabad
ajitmajji2012@gmail.com

■ INTRODUCTION

About 422 million are affected by diabetes mellitus worldwide. In India, 77 million are diabetics, this figure is projected to be 125 million by 2045 (WHO data). Diabetic retinopathy is a microvascular complication of diabetes.

Diabetic retinopathy can be classified as nonproliferative diabetic retinopathy (NPDR) and proliferative diabetic retinopathy (PDR). PDR occurs with development of retinal ischemia resulting in growth of new blood vessels on the surface of the retina [neovascularization elsewhere (NVE)] or the optic disc [neovascularization of the disc (NVD)]. The NVE or NVD may bleed resulting in vitreous hemorrhage (VH) and subsequent fibrosis leading to traction retinal detachment (RD), or retinal break formation causing secondary rhegmatogenous RD (RRD). The PDR, subdivided into mild PDR (NVE of less than half disc area), moderate PDR (NVE of more than half disc area, or NVD of less than one-fourth to one-third disc area), high-risk PDR (as defined below), and advanced PDR (fundus partially obscured by VH or RD at the center of the macula).

There is strong evidence to treat PDR with panretinal photocoagulation (PRP), which reduces the risk of severe vision loss by at least 50%. The benefits are more marked in patients with high-risk characteristics (HRC), in whom PRP should be considered without delay. HRC include the presence of more than one-third disc area of NVD or more than half disc of NVE or NVD or NVE of similar size associated with preretinal hemorrhage or VH. Most commonly used wavelengths for PRP are frequency doubled YAG (532 nm) and diode (810 nm). The laser settings for PRP are 500 µ spot size, 0.1-0.2 second duration, and adequate power to achieve a gray white burn. A total of 2,000-3,000 burns, one burn width apart, are placed outside the vascular arcades and 1 disc diameter away from the disc nasally and extend the burns up to the equator and beyond, in two or three separate sittings. These patients need to be followed at 6-8 weeks after PRP for evaluating the response. If good response is observed, one can call the patients at 3-6 monthly intervals depending on the stability of retinopathy. The titration of supplemental laser can be

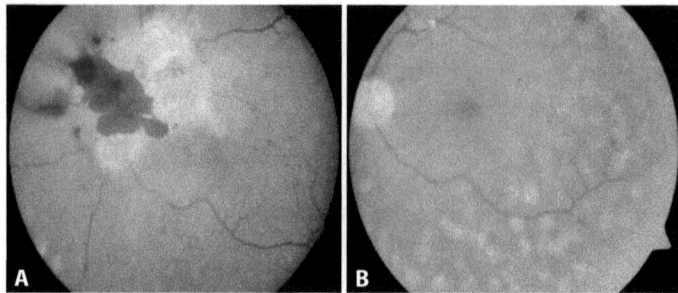

Figs. 7.2.1A and B: (A) A patient of type 2 diabetes mellitus (DM), with fibrovascular proliferation with traction retinal detachment (RD) involving macular center; (B) Relief of traction and stable retinopathy status after pars plana vitrectomy (PPV).

best done by repeating the angiogram and looking for areas of capillary nonperfusion. The complications commonly encountered after PRP are exudative choroidal detachment or RD, subclinical foveal detachment, worsening of macular edema or traction RD, choroidal neovascular membrane (CNVM), transient myopia, photophobia, visual field restriction, impaired accommodation, and dark adaptation.

Protocol S of Diabetic Retinopathy Clinical Research Network (DRCR net), demonstrated that antivascular endothelial growth factor (VEGF) therapy for PDR is not inferior to PRP in terms of visual outcome at 5 years of follow-up and indeed is associated with less visual field loss and lower rates of vision-impairing diabetic macular edema. However, one need to ensure the availability of patient for regular follow-up if planned for anti-VEGF therapy.

Vitrectomy should be considered in patients with persistent VH or when VH prevents other forms of treatment. Other indications include traction RD threatening macula, combined traction and RRD, premacular fibrosis, dense subhyaloid hemorrhage, and persistent neovascularization in spite of maximal laser.

Use of anti-VEGF agents in PDR is restricted to temporary reduction of vascular component of the NVE/NVD prior to PRP or prior to PPV to reduce the incidence of intra- and postoperative bleeding in patients with fibrovascular proliferation.

■ SUGGESTED READING

1. Gross JG, Glassman AR, Liu D, Sun JK, Antoszyk AN, Baker CW, et al. Five-year outcomes of panretinal photocoagulation vs intravitreous ranibizumab for proliferative diabetic retinopathy. A randomized clinical trial. The Diabetic Retinopathy Clinical Research Network. JAMA Ophthalmol. 2018;136(10):1138-48.
2. Mohamed Q, Gillies MC, Wong TY. Management of diabetic retinopathy: a systematic review. JAMA. 2007;298(8):902-16.

7.3 Vitreomacular Traction Syndrome

Alay S Banker
Banker's Retina Clinic and Laser Centre, Ahmedabad
alay.banker@gmail.com

■ CLINICAL FINDINGS

The vitreomacular traction syndrome (VMTS) was first described by Jaffe in 1967. In the classic form of this disorder, the vitreous is separated from the retina throughout the peripheral fundus but remains adherent posteriorly, resulting in anteroposterior traction on a broad, often dumbbell-shaped region encompassing the macular area and optic nerve.

The zone of vitreomacular attachment usually measures several disc areas in size. Associated findings typically include epiretinal membrane and varying degrees of macular edema with fluorescein leakage, macular puckering, and traction macular detachment. Traction on the retina causes retinal distortion and cystoid macular edema (CME) resulting in metamorphopsia and central vision loss. Symptoms and signs tend to progress over time, and full-thickness macular hole (FTMH) development is rare.

TYPES

The International Vitreomacular Traction Study Group in 2013 provided a clinically applicable classification system that is predictive of therapeutic interventions and outcomes.
- Vitreomacular adhesion (VMA) is defined as perifoveal vitreous separation with remaining vitreomacular attachment and unperturbed foveal morphologic features **(Figs. 7.3.1A and B)**.
- Vitreomacular traction (VMT) is characterized by anomalous posterior vitreous detachment (PVD) accompanied by anatomic distortion of the fovea, which may include pseudocysts, macular schisis, CME, and subretinal fluid. VMT is further subclassified by the diameter of vitreous attachment to the macular surface as measured by optical coherence tomography (OCT), with attachment of 1,500 µm or less defined as focal and attachment of >1,500 µm as broad.
- FTMH is defined as a foveal lesion with interruption of all retinal layers from the internal limiting membrane (ILM) to the retinal pigment epithelium.

HISTOPATHOLOGY

The membrane causing traction on the fovea consists of fibrous astrocytes, fibrocytes, myofibrocytes, and extracellular matrix including fragments of ILM and new or old collagen. Although idiopathic epiretinal membrane does not contain ILM, epiretinal membrane in VMTS has fragments of ILM. These histologic characteristics may explain the firm vitreoretinal adhesion in VMTS.

TREATMENT

In eyes with VMT of 1,500 µm or less, patients often have stable visual acuity and incidence of spontaneous release of traction occurs in 23–47% within 1–2 years. Pneumatic vitreolysis (SF6/C3F8 gas) is the best nonsurgical option for cases with focal adhesions **(Figs. 7.3.2A and B)**. Pneumatic vitreolysis is a safe, effective, and minimally invasive and most cost-efficient approach to achieve nonsurgical release of VMT with a high rate of success. Enzymatic vitreolysis (ocriplasmin) is reserved for cases with focal adhesions without ERM, but is very expensive. Pars plana vitrectomy using 23/25/27 G microincision vitrectomy surgery (MIVS) is the best option for cases with ERMs and broader adhesions (>1,500 µm) **(Figs. 7.3.3A and B)**. Various dyes such as indocyanine green (ICG),

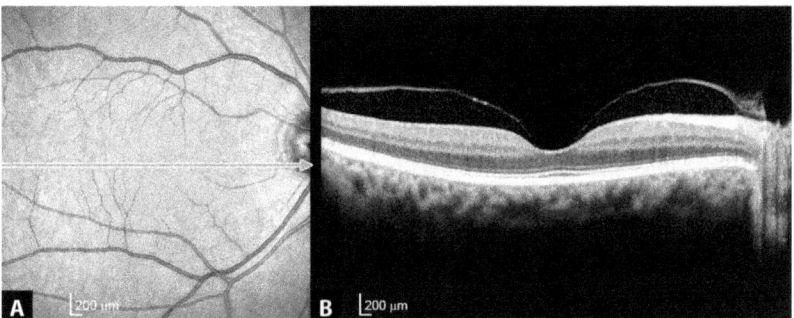

Figs. 7.3.1A and B: Vitreomacular adhesion (VMA).

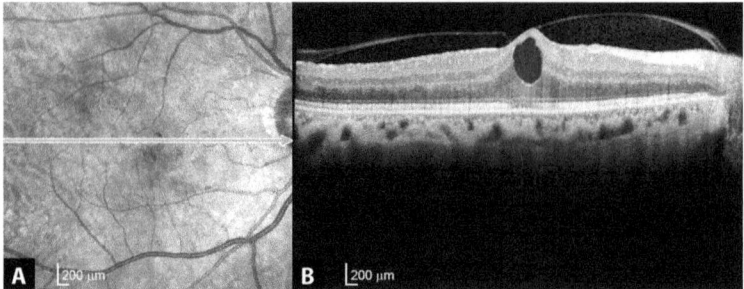

Figs. 7.3.2A and B: Vitreomacular traction (VMT) with focal adhesion.

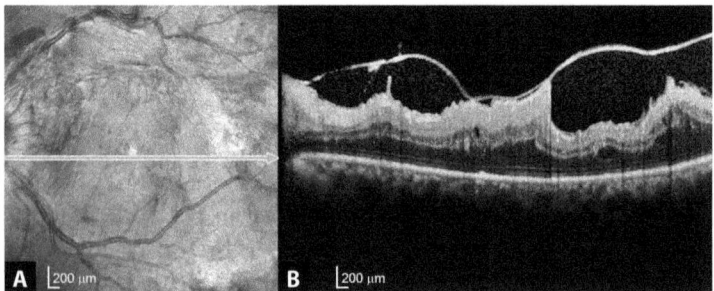

Figs. 7.3.3A and B: Vitreomacular traction (VMT) with broad attachment.

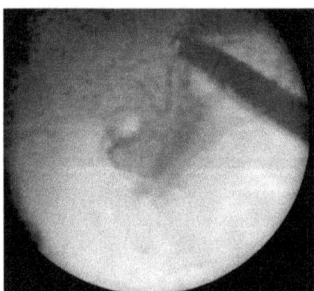

Fig. 7.3.4: Trypan blue staining of vitreomacular traction (VMT).

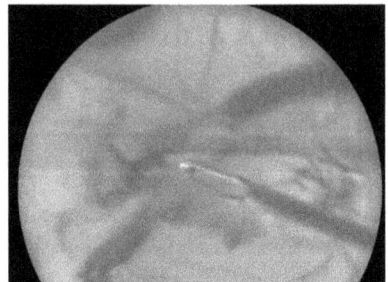

Fig. 7.3.5: Foveal sparing internal limiting membrane (ILM) removal.

trypan blue, brilliant blue G (BBG), and triamcinolone are used to stain the vitreous attachment and the ILM **(Fig. 7.3.4)**. Foveal sparing ILM removal is recommended to prevent deroofing of macula during removal of VMA **(Fig. 7.3.5)**.

■ SUGGESTED READING

1. Duker JS, Kaiser PK, Binder S, de Smet MD, Gaudric A, Reichel E, et al. The International Vitreomacular Traction Study Group classification of vitreomacular adhesion, traction, and macular hole. Ophthalmology. 2013;120(12):2611-9.
2. Flaxel CJ, Adelman RA, Bailey ST, Fawzi A, Lim JI, Vemulakonda GA, et al. Idiopathic Epiretinal Membrane and Vitreomacular Traction Preferred Practice Pattern®. Ophthalmology. 2020;127(2):P145-83.
3. Yu G, Duguay J, Marra KV, Gautam S, Le Guern G, Begum S, et al. Efficacy and safety of treatment options for vitreomacular traction: a case series and meta-analysis. Retina. 2016;36(7):1260-70.

7.4 Vitreous Hemorrhage

Alok Sen, Jayanti Singh, Samendra Karkhur
Sadguru Netra Chikitsalaya, Madhya Pradesh
draloksen@gmail.com

■ INTRODUCTION

Vitreous hemorrhage is one of the most common causes of acute or subacute loss of vision in adults. The reported incidence is 7 per 100,000.[1] Although, the diagnosis of vitreous hemorrhage is straight forward, finding the cause at times could be very difficult. Determining the cause is important since management and treatment outcome of vitreous hemorrhage often depend on the underlying etiology.

■ CAUSES OF VITREOUS HEMORRHAGE

The source of vitreous hemorrhage could be a normal vessel, an abnormal vessel or break through bleed from adjacent source.

The most common cause of *ruptured normal vessel* is an acute posterior vitreous detachment (PVD) with or without retinal tear. In the setting of vitreous hemorrhage with symptomatic PVD, the risk of concurrent retinal break is very high and hence a thorough peripheral retinal examination is warranted in these cases.

Blunt trauma can cause bleeding due to trauma to vessels and is one of the most common causes of vitreous hemorrhage in children.

Abnormal retinal vessels usually result from neovascularization due to retinal ischemia. These vessels are fragile as they lack tight endothelial junction and may bleed either with vitreous traction or even spontaneously. Proliferative diabetic retinopathy (PDR) is one of the leading causes of retinal neovascularization and vitreous hemorrhage in adults. Other common causes include retinal vein occlusions (RVOs) and retinal vasculitis. Vitreous hemorrhage can rarely result from rupture of *retinal arterial macroaneurysm (RAM)* which is an acquired focal dilation of retina artery and seen in elderly hypertensive patients.[2]

Sometimes vitreous hemorrhage can result due to *breakthrough bleed* from a choroidal neovascular membrane, polypoidal choroidal vasculopathy (PCV), or choroidal mass.[3]

Occasionally, bilateral intraocular hemorrhage may be associated with *subdural hemorrhage (Terson's syndrome)*.[4] Although, the exact mechanism of vitreous hemorrhage in these cases is not known, acute rise in intracranial pressure may lead to a rapid rise in intraocular venous pressure and subsequent rupture of peripapillary capillaries leading to vitreous hemorrhage.

■ CLINICAL PRESENTATION AND EVALUATION

Patients usually present with sudden onset floaters or vision loss. The symptoms are generally worse in the morning and improve during the day due to settling of blood inferiorly. Patients with acute PVD may give history of flashes preceding vision loss. History of trauma, hypertension, diabetes, and other risk factors associated with vitreous hemorrhage should be elicited.

Ocular examination must include a proper documentation of visual acuity in both eyes. *Intraocular pressure (IOP)* must be measured in all cases. A low IOP suggests retinal detachment or open globe injury while higher IOP may indicate neovascular glaucoma. Presence of anterior segment reaction would point toward an inflammatory etiology for vitreous hemorrhage. *Gonioscopy* should be performed to rule out anterior segment neovascularization. If *relative afferent pupillary defect (RAPD)* is present, it suggests presence of retinal detachment or retinal vascular occlusion and usually carries a grave prognosis. *Indirect ophthalmoscopy* with *scleral indentation* must be done in all cases (except in cases with open globe injury or suspected posterior globe rupture). Sometimes if the vitreous hemorrhage is not dense, the source and cause of hemorrhage can be determined. The peripheral retina is visible in many cases even in presence of dense vitreous hemorrhage and may provide clue for the cause of hemorrhage. The fundus examination of the contralateral eye is equally important as it may harbor the same disease as the affected eye.

Ultrasonography (B-scan) should be performed in all cases with diffuse dense vitreous hemorrhage. It provides vital information regarding the density of vitreous hemorrhage, location and extent of tractional detachment, presence of retinal detachment, and status of PVD. All these factors help in planning vitreous surgery and predict its outcome.

GRADING OF VITREOUS HEMORRHAGE

Natural History

Rate of clearance of blood from the vitreous cavity is about 1% per day. The clearance is quicker in syneretic vitreous than in well-formed vitreous. Long-standing vitreous hemorrhage may lead to several complications including *hemosiderosis bulbi* that occurs due to break down of hemoglobin in long-standing vitreous hemorrhage and iron deposition in various ocular structures. *Ghost cell glaucoma* is caused by clogging of trabecular meshwork by spherical, rigid, and dehemoglobinized red blood cells (RBCs). *Proliferative vitreoretinopathy* occurs in open globe injury and occurs due to macrophages and chemotactic factors induced fibrovascular proliferation and can lead to fibrosis and subsequent retinal detachment.

TREATMENT

Treatment should be tailored according to etiology and source of hemorrhage. Management options are observation, laser photocoagulation/cryotherapy, and pars plana vitrectomy.

Observation

A fresh vitreous hemorrhage often clears in days or weeks. A fresh vitreous hemorrhage with attached retina should be closely monitored weekly; however, retinal detachment should be ruled out in all patients wherein early intervention is not undertaken.

Laser Photocoagulation

In patients with proliferative retinopathy, laser photocoagulation should be started as soon as any portion of retina is visible. A peripheral retina break if visible should also be treated with prompt laser photocoagulation. *YAG laser hyaloidotomy* facilitates absorption of subhyaloid hemorrhage through drainage into the vitreous.

Pars Plana Vitrectomy

The timing of vitrectomy depends on the underlying etiology. Early vitrectomy is indicated if the vitreous hemorrhage is associated with retinal detachment, presence of anterior segment neovascularization, or if the underlying etiology is likely to progress rapidly if left untreated. In other scenario, vitrectomy may be delayed till good PVD occurs or if the vitreous hemorrhage does not clears for over 2–3 months.

Antivascular endothelial growth factor (anti-VEGF) agents may be considered in patients with proliferative diseases like PDR or neovascularization secondary to RVO. They cause regression of neovascularization and prevent rebleeding. However, they may cause worsening of tractional retinal detachment[5] and hence must be used with caution in patients with extensive fibrovascular proliferation.

Ovine hyaluronidase (Vitrase)[6] facilitates the clearance of vitreous hemorrhage by inducing liquefaction of the vitreous.

CONCLUSION

It is vital to know the cause that led to vitreous hemorrhage. A detailed history, thorough clinical examination and close monitoring can help in establishing the diagnosis. Treatment must then be tailored according to the etiology.

REFERENCES

1. Spraul CW, Grossniklaus HE. Vitreous hemorrhage. Surv Ophthalmol. 1997;42(1):3-39.
2. Asao K, Nakada A, Kawasaki Y. Vitreous hemorrhage caused by ruptured retinal macroaneurysm. Case Rep Ophthalmol. 2014;5(1):44-9.
3. Zhao XY, Luo MY, Meng LH, Zhang WF, Li B, Wang EQ, et al. The incidence, characteristics, management, prognosis, and classification of breakthrough vitreous hemorrhage secondary to polypoidal choroidal vasculopathy. Retina. 2021;41(8):1675-85.
4. Ogawa T, Kitaoka T, Dake Y, Amemiya T. Terson syndrome: a case report suggesting the mechanism of vitreous hemorrhage. Ophthalmology. 2001;108(9):1654-6.
5. Arevalo JF, Maia M, Flynn HW Jr, Saravia M, Avery RL, Wu L, et al. Tractional retinal detachment following intravitreal Bevacizumab (Avastin) in patients with severe proliferative diabetic retinopathy. Br J Ophthalmol. 2008;92:213-6.
6. Kuppermann BD, Thomas EL, de Smet MD, Grillone LR; Vitrase for Vitreous Hemorrhage Study Groups. Safety results of two phase III trials of an intravitreous injection of highly purified ovine Hyaluronidase (Vitrase) for the management of vitreous hemorrhage. Am J Ophthalmol. 2005;140:585-97.

7.5 Management of Posteriorly Dislocated Intraocular Lens

Anand Rajendran, Prabu Bhaskaran
Aravind Eye Hospital, Chennai
anandrjn@gmail.com

INTRODUCTION

Posteriorly dislocated lens may be encountered following intraoperative complications including posterior capsular rupture, trauma, or in pseudoexfoliation. It includes posterior dislocation of crystalline lens, intraocular lens, bag intraocular lens (IOL) complex, and bag IOL complex with capsule tension ring.

DROPPED NUCLEUS/LENS

Dropped cortical matter may be observed if it is minimal and eye is quiet (**Fig. 7.5.1**).

Nucleus fragments have tendency to cause inflammation and raised intraocular pressure, hence should be taken up for surgery early (**Fig. 7.5.2**).

PARS PLANA LENSECTOMY

Three 23 G ports are made and the infusion is checked. Anterior vitrectomy is done to remove any vitreous in the anterior chamber (AC) or in the pupillary plane.

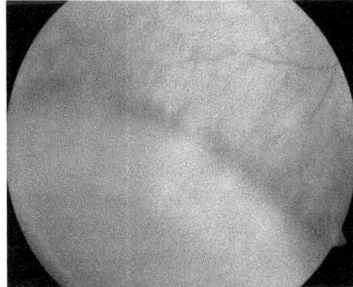

Fig. 7.5.1: Dropped nucleus.

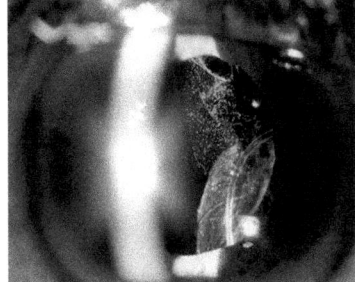

Fig. 7.5.2: Anterior segment photograph of a patient with dropped nucleus and vitreous in the anterior chamber.

Core vitrectomy is done to free the nucleus from vitreous attachments. Intravitreal triamcinolone acetonide can be used to visualize the vitreous. Posterior vitreous detachment (PVD) induction may or may not be done. Soft cortical matter, epinucleus, or soft nucleus can be removed with aspiration alone. Lens matter is removed with lower cut rate (800–1,500 cuts per minute with vacuum 350–450 mm Hg).[1]

For a moderately hard nucleus, the dominant port may be converted to 20 G. 20 G vitrector is used for fragmenting the nucleus using the endoilluminator as a fulcrum. Cut rate is reduced (400–800 cuts per minute) with increased vacuum. Nucleus is fragmented into multiple pieces, each single piece is lifted with vacuum and endoilluminator is used to feed the fragments into the vitrector opening.

For a hard nucleus, fragmatome (20 G) is used. Nucleus is fragmented with ultrasound energy and aspirated. Alternatively it can brought to the pupillary plane by filling the vitreous cavity with perfluorocarbon liquid (PFCL) and manually removed through the tunnel or phacoemulsification.

If two-thirds of the anterior capsule is intact, a three-piece IOL can be placed in sulcus. In case of inadequate support, scleral fixation or iris fixation of IOL is preferred. Scleral fixated IOL is an effective technique for management of dislocated crystalline lens, IOL, or inadequate capsular support in aphakia. It is more physiological than iris fixation of IOL.

■ SUTURED SCLERAL FIXATION OF INTRAOCULAR LENS

Conjunctival peritomies are made nasally and temporally. Triangular incisions 3 × 3 mm are made with blade 180° apart (2 and 8 o'clock). Partial thickness scleral dissections are made up to limbus to create triangular flaps. A superior scleral tunnel is made with the crescent knife.

A straight double armed 10-0 prolene suture is inserted though the base of the temporal triangular flap (for right eye) 1 mm posterior to the surgical limbus till the tip is seen at the center of the eye. A 26 G needle is inserted similarly from the nasal scleral flap. The tip of the prolene suture is inserted the needle and both are withdrawn nasally. A suture holding forceps in introduced through scleral tunnel, the suture is held and externalized through tunnel.[1]

The ends of the suture are cut externally. Each suture is introduced into the eyelet of haptic of IOL and sutured. IOL is introduced into AC. Sutures lying externally below scleral flaps are pulled to center the IOL. Sutures are tied below scleral flaps. Tips of the triangular flaps and finally conjunctiva is sutured.[1]

Other Techniques

Transscleral Suture Fixation of IOL

It can be done in two ways: (1) ab interno methods in which suture is passed from the interior of the eye to the exterior and (2) ab externo methods, in which initially, the suture is introduced from the exterior of the eye.

Conjunctival peritomies are made nasally and temporally. Scleral dissections are made 180° apart (10 and 4 o'clock). 3.0–4.0 mm scleral incision is made 3.0 mm posterior to the surgical limbus at 50% depth and scleral dissection is made up to limbus with crescent. Paracentesis is made inferiorly for placing AC maintainer. Clear corneal or scleral tunnel is made of desired length superiorly.

A 27 G needle is passed through nasal scleral tunnel 1.0 mm posterior to the surgical limbus and inserted into the eye till tip is visible. A double-armed 10-0 prolene is passed through the temporal incision and inserted in the 27 G needle; suture and needle are removed nasally. The other end of the double-armed suture is passed through the IOL haptic eyelet. The 27 G needle is again passed through nasal scleral tunnel 1.0–2.0 mm adjacent to the first pass of the needle. The second arm of the double-armed suture is passed through the clear corneal incision and inserted in the 27 G needle; suture and needle are again removed nasally.

A double-armed 9-0 prolene suture on a curved needle is passed through the superior incision and back through the sclera 1.0 mm posterior to the surgical limbus. The second arm of the suture is passed through the trailing IOL haptic eyelet and similarly passed ab interno through the sclera 1.0-2.0 mm adjacent to the first pass. Sutures are tied and it results in four-point fixation of IOL.

■ SUTURELESS SCLERAL FIXATION OF INTRAOCULAR LENS

Sutureless scleral fixation of intraocular lens (SFIOL) involves introducing the haptics in scleral tunnels made parallel to limbus. A fornix-based conjunctival peritomy is made in superior two-thirds of conjunctiva.

Two partial thickness scleral pockets are made parallel to limbus with a MVR blade at a distance of 1.5 mm from the limbus in a counterclockwise manner taking care that they are exactly 180° to each other. A partial thickness scleral tunnel is constructed superiorly with crescent knife.

Three 23/25 G sclerotomies are made and infusion secured. Pars plana lensectomy (PPL) with pars plana vitrectomy (PPV) is done in cases of dislocated lens. Tunnel entry is made with keratome and extended. Two sclerotomies are made with a 24 G needle or MVR blade 1.5 mm from the limbus exactly 180° from each other at ends of tunnels.

A three-piece IOL is introduced with the leading haptic below the iris and trailing haptic in the tunnel. SFIOL forceps (23 G) are inserted through the sclerotomy, the leading haptic is grasped at the tip with forceps and extruded through the sclerotomy. The haptic is pushed into the tunnel and forceps is then removed. The same technique is applied for the trailing haptic through the second sclerostomy site. Care should be taken that ends of the haptic are in the tunnel to prevent conjunctival erosion, risk of inflammation, or endophthalmitis.

■ GLUED SUTURELESS SCLERAL FIXATION OF INTRAOCULAR LENS

Two partial thicknesses 3 × 3 mm partial thickness limbal-based scleral flaps are made exactly at 180°. Superior scleral tunnel is made. 23/25 G ports are placed and vitrectomy is done.

Sclerotomies are made with 23 G needle 1 mm from the limbus under the scleral flap. Scleral tunnels are made at the edge of the tunnel with a 26 G needle. The haptics are externalized with forceps and introduced into tunnels. Scleral flaps and conjunctiva are fixed with fibrin glue.

X-NIT

X-NIT or extraocular needle-guided haptic insertion technique[2] is relatively a newer technique developed to simplify SFIOL surgeries. Here, a bent 26 G needle is inserted into the sclerotomy site, brought out through the corneoscleral section and the haptic of a three-piece IOL is docked (**Fig. 7.5.3**) into the lumen of the 26 G needle.

Then the leading haptic is exteriorized by simply retracting the 26 G needle. This eliminates the need for any intraocular maneuver which is otherwise needed to transfer the haptic tip from one instrument to another at the level of anterior vitreous face in conventional handshake method. The trailing haptic is then exteriorized in the same manner. Since X-NIT does not involve intraocular maneuvers, it can be easily performed by anterior segment surgeons and novice

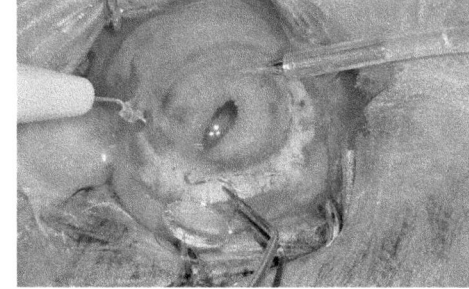

Fig. 7.5.3: Docking of the tip of a three-piece intraocular lens (IOL) into the lumen of 26 G needle (X in X-NIT stands for extraocular docking).

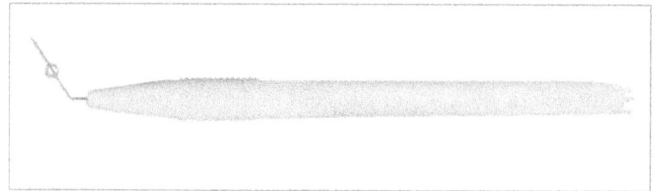

Fig. 7.5.4: Assembly of X-NIT device showing the customized 26 G needle, handle, and sclerotomy markers.

surgeons without any fear of fall of IOL. A small segment of silicone stopper can be inserted into the 26 G needle and slid over the leading haptic so as to temporarily stabilize the haptic after being exteriorized. This avoids the surgeon's dependency on assisting nurse in holding the leading haptic while the trailing haptic is maneuvered.

X-NIT device[3] (**Fig. 7.5.4**) is a commercially available device (Aurolab, Madurai, India) which consists of a customized long (17 mm) 26 G needle prebent and preloaded with dual protection silicone stopper and attached to a handle which on the other end has sclerotomy markers to mark 1.5 mm distance from limbus for creating sclerotomies.

■ REFERENCES

1. Spandau U, Scharioth G. Complications during and after Cataract Surgery: A Guide to Surgical Management. Berlin, Germany: Springer; 2014.
2. Baskaran P, Ganne P, Bhandari S, Ramakrishnan S, Venkatesh R, Gireesh P. Extraocular needle-guided haptic insertion technique of scleral fixation intraocular lens surgeries (X-NIT). Indian J Ophthalmol. 2017;65(8):747-50.
3. Baskaran P, Venkatesh R, Ramakrishnan S, Sriram RD, Iyer G, Ramnath RK. A novel device for safe exteriorization of haptic in scleral fixation intraocular lens surgery. Indian J Ophthalmol. 2020;68(10):2205-7.

7.6 | Pediatric Retinal Imaging

Anand Vinekar
Department of Pediatric Retina, Narayana Nethralaya Eye Institute, Bengaluru
anandvinekar@yahoo.com

■ INTRODUCTION

Pediatric retinal imaging is more challenging than in adults due to several reasons. These include the fact that children, especially infants, are not the most cooperative patients, available devices are limited in its ability to image infants, adult devices are not always useable directly on children and finally the speed of image capture is not rapid enough. With advances in technology, imaging has gone beyond merely the retinal surface. For example, the faster spectral-domain optical coherence tomography (SD-OCT) which is now available as a handheld device is making imaging in infants more feasible.

Commonly used imaging devices are discussed in this chapter.

■ ULTRASONOGRAPHY

These include A scan for axial length measurement, B scan diagnostic ultrasonography (USG), and ultrasound biomicroscopy for anterior segment. The B scan is commonly used when the view of the retina is precluded by media opacities, corneal scars, cataracts, vitreous hemorrhage, and to ascertain the configuration of a retinal detachment and intraocular mass lesion or foreign body.

SECTION 7: Retina

■ FUNDUS PHOTOGRAPHY
Contact
The most common device used to image an infant retina has been the widefield retinal camera by the RetCam (Natus, California, USA). The portable version has been used in telemedicine programs in India and elsewhere. The RetCam 3 version has an additional ability to perform fundus angiography. The field is 130°. The camera has a resolution of 1,800 × 1,600 and saves the image in a proprietary format as well as Joint Photographic Experts Group (JPEG). An indigenous version developed since 2015-16, 3Nethra Neo or simply "Neo" has a resolution of 2,040 × 2,040, more portable and uses a liquid lens and a light-emission diode (LED) illumination system. Both devices are contact based and require a coupling agent as an interface between the camera tip and the eye of the infant.

The Icon (Phoenix, USA) is less portable and more expensive.

Noncontact
A more recent addition has been mobile phone-based devices which harness the coaxial light source and a handheld plus lens like the 20 D lens attached to a holder to create an indirect ophthalmoscopy like device. These are noncontact and therefore have the disadvantage of limited field of view, longer learning curve, less resolution, and nonintegration into health records or a telemedicine program.

Wide Field and Ultra-wide Field Retinal Imaging
These are based on scanning ophthalmoscope technology and utilize an ellipsoid mirror to capture a retinal image spanning a maximum of 200 internal degrees. The OPTOS Panoramic 200Tx (Optos PLC, Scotland, UK) is an example. These are useful for conditions like familial exudative vitreoretinopathy (FEVR).

■ FUNDUS FLUORESCEIN ANGIOGRAPHY
The most widely used device is the RetCam 3 (Natus, USA). It has been the only device which is capable of performing fundus fluorescein angiography (FFA) on supine infants. At the time of this publication, the Neo-HD unit from Forus Health, India has an angiography capable device as well. Sodium fluorescein 20% is injected intravenously as a bolus dose of 0.04 mL/kg (8 mg/kg). In older children who can be seated, the Optos angiography can also be used. FFA has been used to study retinopathy of prematurity (ROP), particularly the aggressive ROP (AROP) subtype, both before and after treatment with antivascular endothelial growth factor [antivascular endothelial growth factor (VEGF)] intravitreally. Other common conditions include FEVR, incontinentia pigmenti, and Coats disease.

■ OPTICAL COHERENCE TOMOGRAPHY (HH SD-OCT)
The availability of the handheld OCT (e.g., Envisu, Bioptigen, USA) has allowed imaging in awake infants in the outpatient without sedation. The most optimized OCT images in infants are possible when we consider:
- *Axial length:* It increases by 0.16 mm/week in the neonatal period, 1 mm/year in year 2, 0.4 mm/year from 2 to 5 years, and 0.1 mm/year from 5 to 15 years.
- *Refractive error changes with age:* Infants are more hyperopic by 40-52 weeks postmenstrual age (PMA). Astigmatism is also greater in infants and decreases by 6 months of age.
- The neonate's cornea is steeper than in adults. The power is between 48 and 58.5 D decreasing to adult values by 3 months.
- The OCT reference arm must be shortened (compared to adults) to allow the pivot point to return at the pupil.

SD-OCT in Normal Infants

The common layers and zones in the fovea of infants are summarized in **Table 7.6.1**. Compared to adult foveae, infants demonstrate **(Fig. 7.6.1)**:
- Shallow foveal depression
- Persisting inner retinal layers at the fovea [includes inner plexiform and inner nuclear layers (INLs)], this is called "retinal or foveal immaturity"
- Thinner retinal layers overall
- Attenuation of the photoreceptor layer (PRL) with absence of photoreceptor sublayers

Foveal Development on SD-OCT
- *Inner retinal development:* The persistence of the inner retinal layers in the foveal center is characterized by the presence of the ganglion cell layer (GCL),

TABLE 7.6.1: Definitions of the zones and layers.

	Layer(s) or zones	Definition
1.	Central foveal thickness (CFT)	The thickness of the entire retina from the inner aspect of the inner limiting membrane (ILM) to the inner aspect of the retinal pigment epithelium (RPE) at the foveal center
2.	Inner retinal layers (IRLs)	Retinal tissue from the inner aspect of the ILM to the outer border of the inner nuclear layer (INL)
3.	Outer retinal layers (ORLs)	Extends from the inner aspect of the outer plexiform layer (OPL) to the inner border of the RPE
4.	Photoreceptor layers (PRLs)	From the outer aspect of OPL to the inner border of RPE

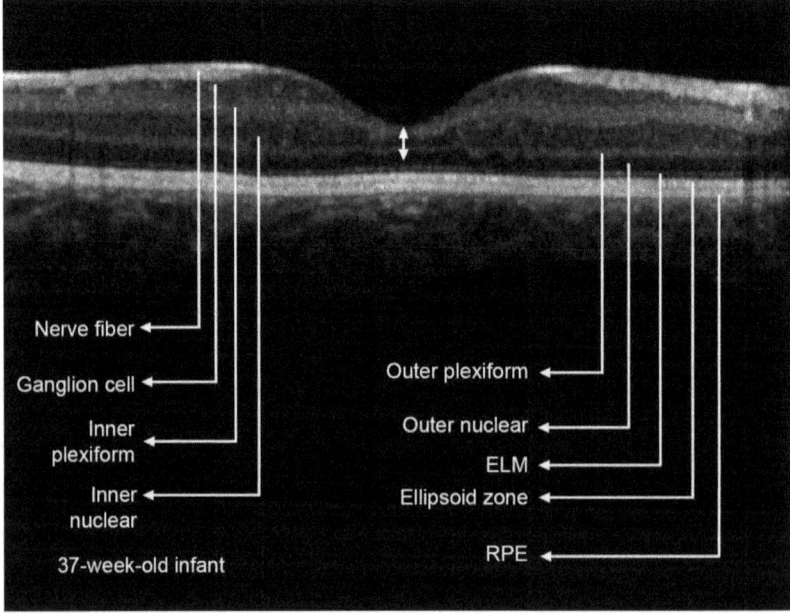

Fig. 7.6.1: SD-OCT of a 37-week-old preterm infant showing the layers and zones. The persistence of the inner retina (arrow) in the foveal center is suggestive of immaturity. These layers centrifugally migrate after a few weeks to form a single band. (ELM: external limiting membrane; RPE: retinal pigment epithelium; SD-OCT: spectral-domain optical coherence tomography)

inner plexiform layer (IPL), and the INL as distinct measurable layers at the foveal center. This "thins out" by centrifugal migration at the foveal center to condense into a single thin hyper-reflective band in older children.
- *PRL development:* The height of the PRL increases progressively from infancy to adulthood. This occurs rapidly after 38-week PMA in all the regions and especially in the cone-dense fovea.

SD-OCT in Retinopathy of Prematurity

The SD-OCT has been used to image clinically unseen or poorly detected retinal features in ROP:
- Preretinal neovascularization, especially in aggressive posterior ROP (APROP)
- Clinically undetected structures including retinoschisis, epiretinal membranes, retinal detachment, retinal pigment epithelium (RPE) changes, and atrophy
- Macular involvement in stage 4A, thereby changing the diagnosis to stage 4B
- Post lens-sparing vitrectomy to monitor the attachment of the fovea
- Macular edema detected in clinically normal looking fovea is a relatively new finding which was first reported in India in approximately 29% of cases with type 2 ROP. This foveal disruption is seen in two patterns (A and B) **(Figs. 7.6.2A and B)** and spontaneously resolves by 52 weeks PMA. This transient edema can influence long-term visual acuity changes in the first 1–2 years of life.

SD-OCT in non-ROP Retinal Conditions
- *Shaken baby syndrome (SBS):* Preretinal blood, localized vitreous detachment, premacular folds, and attachment of the vitreous to the inner limiting membrane (ILM) at the apices of the perimacular folds have been reported.

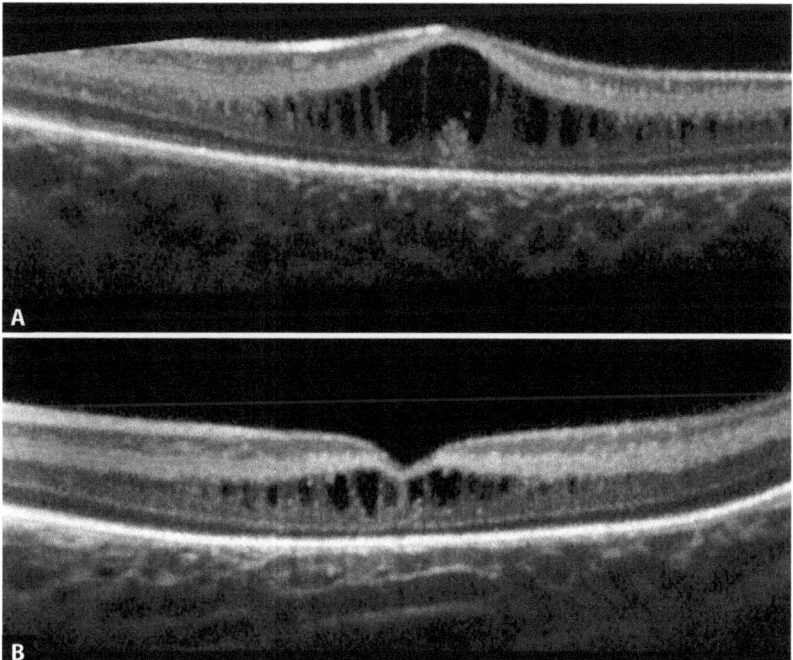

Figs. 7.6.2A and B: (A) Pattern A macular disruption was characterized by loss of foveal depression, increased central foveal thickness, and larger intraretinal cysts; (B) Pattern B macular edema showed less severe changes, better preservation of the foveal contour and smaller and shorter cysts.

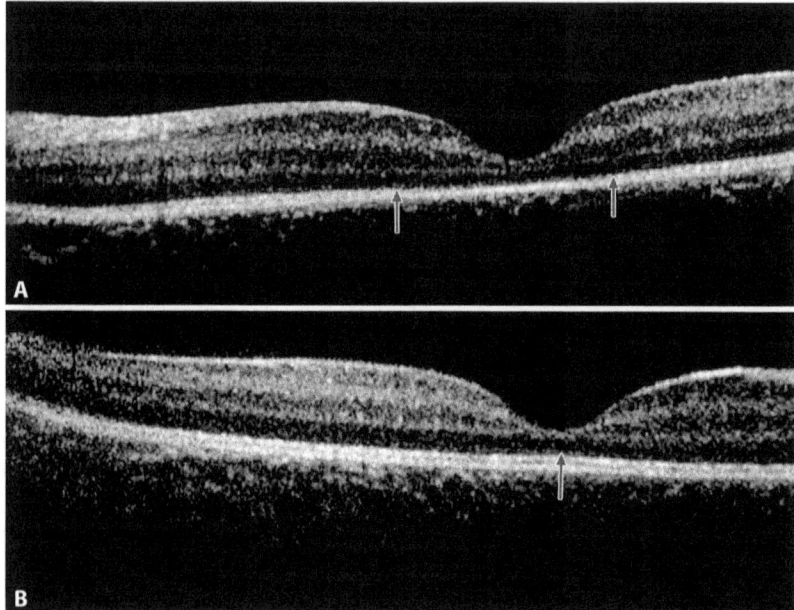

Figs. 7.6.3A and B: (A) The two vertical arrows indicate the position of the ellipsoid zone (IS-OS) at 46 weeks (PMA); (B) These centripetally grow toward the center of the fovea to converge at 48 weeks (PMA). (IS: inner segment; OS: outer segment; PMA: postmenstrual age)

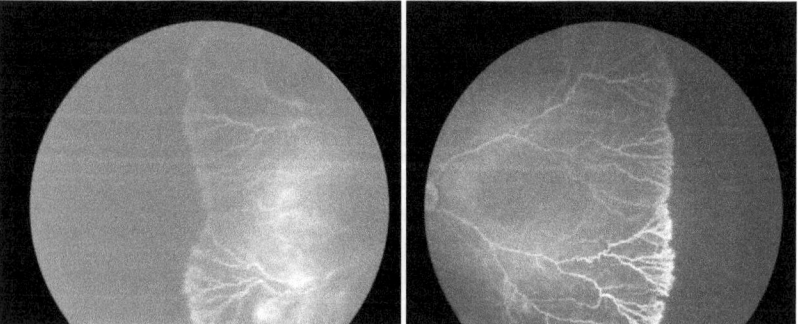

Fig. 7.6.4: Persistent avascular retinal (PAR) demonstrated on fluorescein angiography in an infant who had undergone intravitreal antivascular endothelial growth factor (VEGF) treatment 16 weeks prior in both eyes.

- Combined hamartoma of the retina and RPE, incontinentia pigmenti, retinal dystrophies and degenerations and retinoschisis are some of the other conditions.
- SD-OCT has been used to study the choroid in infants. Preterm infants had a thinner choroid when compared to term infants at the same age.

OCT-ANGIOGRAPHY IN INFANTS

A recent development has been the utilization of the "dyeless" angiography which has been adapted for imaging infants. The available systems can create automated cross-sections of retina at the superficial capillary plexus (SCP), deep capillary plexus (DCP), outer retina, and choriocapillaris (CC). OCT-angiography (OCT-A) allows separate analysis of these

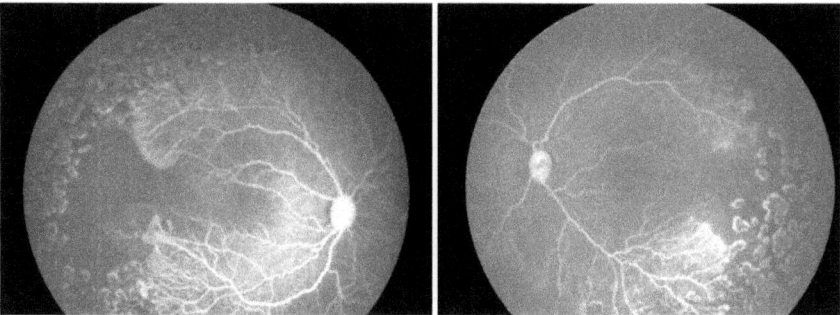

Fig. 7.6.5: Fluorescein angiography active neovascularization in both eyes and avascular retina in an undertreated case of aggressive posterior retinopathy of prematurity (ROP) and subsequent laser. The angiography reveals both flat and elevated neovascular tissue that is sometimes missed clinically.

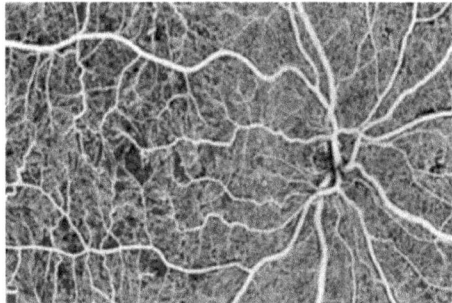

Fig. 7.6.6: Optical coherence tomography-angiography (OCT-A) image of the right eye showing an abnormal foveal avascular zone (FAZ) and superficial capillary plexus (SCP) in an 8-year-old child with a history of prematurity.

capillary plexuses and CC as compared to FFA where such detailed layer-wise image separation is not possible.

FUTURE TRENDS

Newer imaging tools such as the adaptive optics and oximetry are likely to be modified for the use in pediatric retina. Intraoperative use of microscope integrated OCT devices is likely to assist in pediatric retinal surgery. Low-cost wide field infant retinal cameras are now becoming available which may allow further expansion of tele-ROP programs. Integration of machine learning and artificial intelligence in retinal imaging of ROP has been shown to be useful in triaging, training, and telemedicine.

SUGGESTED READING

1. Agarwal K, Vinekar A, Chandra P, Padhi TR, Nayak S, Jayanna S, et al. Imaging the pediatric retina: An overview. Indian J Ophthalmol. 2021;69(4):812-23.
2. Azad R, Chandra P, Khan MA, Darswal A. Role of intravenous fluorescein angiography in early detection and regression of retinopathy of prematurity. J Pediatr Ophthalmol Strabismus. 2008;45:36-9.
3. Mallipatna A, Vinekar A, Jayadev C, Dabir S, Sivakumar M, Krishnan N, et al. The use of handheld spectral domain optical coherence tomography in pediatric ophthalmology practice: Our experience of 975 infants and children. Indian J Ophthalmol. 2015;63(7):586-93.

4. Temkar S, Azad SV, Chawla R, Damodaran S, Garg G, Regani H, et al. Ultra-widefield fundus fluorescein angiography in pediatric retinal vascular diseases. Indian J Ophthalmol. 2019;67:788-94.
5. Vijayalakshmi C, Sakthivel P, Vinekar A. Automated detection and classification of telemedical retinopathy of prematurity images. Telemed J E Health. 2020;26:354-8.
6. Vinekar A, Jayadev C, Mangalesh S, Shetty B. Role of tele-medicine in retinopathy of prematurity screening in rural outreach centers in India—a report of 20,214 imaging sessions in the KIDROP program. Semin Fetal Neonatal Med. 2015;20(5):335-45.
7. Vinekar A, Mangalesh S, Jayadev C, Maldonado RS, Bauer N, Toth CA. Retinal Imaging of Infants on Spectral Domain Optical Coherence Tomography. Biomed Res Int. 2015;2015:782420.
8. Vinekar A, Sinha S, Mangalesh S, Jayadev C, Shetty B. Optical coherence tomography angiography in preterm-born children with retinopathy of prematurity. Graefes Arch Clin Exp Ophthalmol. 2021;259(8):2131-7.

7.7 Branch Retinal Vein Occlusion

Aniruddha Agarwal
The Eye Institute, Cleveland Clinic Abu Dhabi, Abu Dhabi
Cleveland Clinic Lerner College of Medicine,
Case Western Reserve University, Cleveland, Ohio
Maastricht University, Medical Center+ (MUMC), Maastricht
aniruddha9@gmail.com

■ BRANCH RETINAL VASCULAR OCCLUSION

Branch retinal vascular occlusion (BRVO) is a common vascular disorder of the elderly. The visual loss in BRVO is due to the development of macular edema, hemorrhage, and nonperfusion of the perifoveal capillaries. In order to improve visual outcomes in patients with BRVO-associated macular edema, various randomized and nonrandomized trials have been performed to evaluate number of therapeutic agents employed for this condition.

■ PATHOGENESIS AND RISK FACTORS

The mean age of patients diagnosed with BRVO is 60–70 years. The location of BRVO could be variable. 62% BRVOs are superotemporal whereas 38% are inferotemporal. BRVO is usually mostly unilateral, 9% may be bilateral in occurrence. BRVO usually occurs at arteriovenous intersections as they share a common adventitious sheath. It is postulated that a rigid, arteriosclerotic artery compresses the retinal vein resulting in turbulent blood flow and endothelial damage, followed by thrombosis and obstruction of vein.

Systemic Factors

Hypertension is the most common risk factor for BRVO. Other systemic risk factors include history of cardiovascular disease, increased body mass index (BMI) at 20 years of age, and high serum levels of $\alpha 2$ globulin.

Local Factors

Local risk factors for BRVO include history of glaucoma, and other ocular diseases such as toxoplasmosis, Eales disease, Behçet's disease, and ocular sarcoidosis. In addition, the other risk factors include retinal macroaneurysms, Coats disease, retinal capillary hemangiomas, and optic disc drusen.

■ SIGNS AND SYMPTOMS

The visual symptoms of BRVO include diminution of vision, blurring, or central visual disturbance in patients with macular BRVO. Various signs of BRVO include segmental

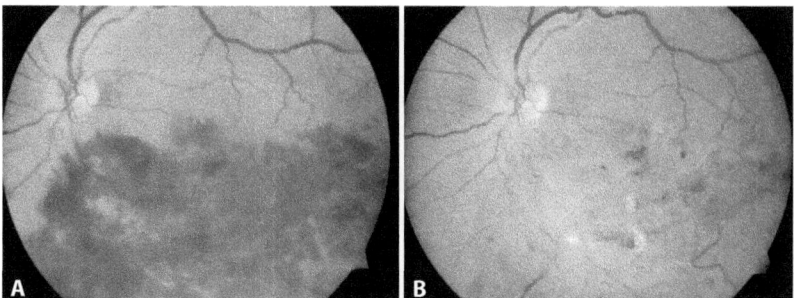

Figs. 7.7.1A and B: Inferotemporal branch retinal vein occlusion at presentation shows presence of multiple hemorrhages. At the subsequent follow-up, there is clearing of the hemorrhages.

distribution of retinal hemorrhages, flame-shaped and dot-and-blot hemorrhages, exudates, macular edema, and vascular tortuosity. Other features which are more common in old BRVOs include vascular sheathing and venous collaterals.

DIAGNOSIS AND ANCILLARY INVESTIGATIONS
The diagnosis of BRVO is mainly clinical. Various ancillary investigations used in the management of BRVO include:
- *Spectral-domain optical coherence tomography (SD-OCT):* On SD-OCT, one can quantify macular edema. Serial imaging using SD-OCT can help follow patients with macular edema and monitor the response to therapy.
- *Fluorescein angiography (FA):* FA in patients with BRVO shows venous filling delay, fluorescein column narrowed at the site of occlusion, blocked fluorescence, and areas of capillary nonperfusion.
- *Optical coherence tomography angiography (OCTA):* OCTA shows retinal vascular flow loss (hyporeflectivity) (termed as flow deficit) in eyes with BRVO. There can be accompanying retinal microvascular telangiectasia. The OCTA cannot differentiate between complications of BRVO such as collaterals and retinal neovascularization.

MANAGEMENT
Laser Photocoagulation
Macular Edema
Grid laser treatment was based on the outcomes of the branch vein occlusion study *[the Branch Vein Occlusion Study (BVOS)]*. The BVOS reported spontaneous improvement in about one-third of cases in the first 3 months. The laser spot size used is 100–200 µ, 0.1 second duration spaced one burn apart. Follow-up after 3 months, if edema persists, consider retreatment.

Retinal Neovascularization
Scatter laser photocoagulation (200–500 µ size, 0.05–0.1 second duration and spaced one burn apart) is performed with sufficient energy in patients with neovascularization to achieve a medium reaction covering the entire involved sector as defined by color photograph and FA. A quadrant usually requires 400–500 burns. Follow-up should be after 4–6 weeks. If neovascularization persists, retreatment is effective in inducing regression.

Intravitreal Steroids
Intravitreal triamcinolone acetonide (4 mg/0.1 mL) hastens the resolution of macular edema as per the results of *the SCORE trial*. Common side effects include increased

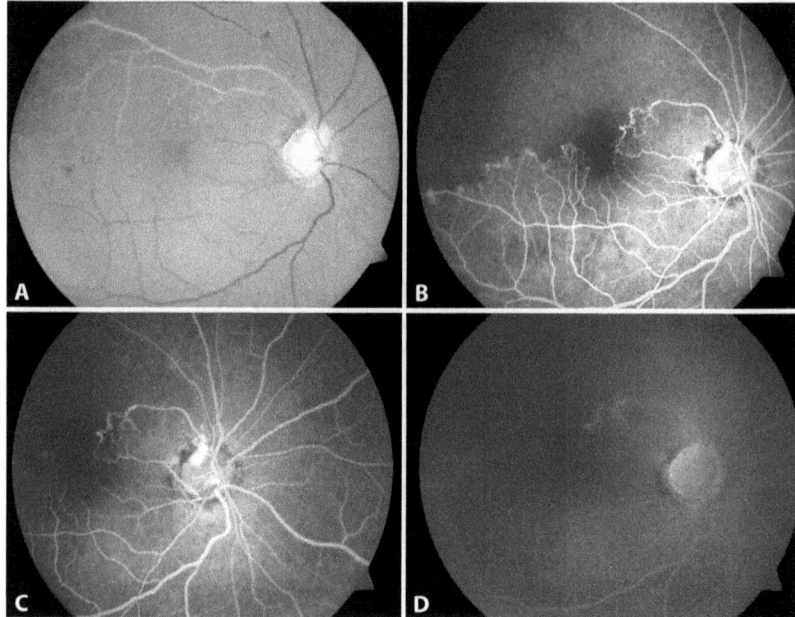

Figs. 7.7.2A to D: Superotemporal branch retinal vein occlusion at presentation shows presence of sheathed vessels. Fluorescein angiogram shows presence of nonperfusion in the area of the branch retinal vein occlusion.

intraocular pressure (IOP), cataract, and endophthalmitis. The use of intravitreal dexamethasone implant (Ozurdex®) has been evaluated by the *Ozurdex GENEVA study*. The results of this study indicated that Ozurdex® is very useful for the management of macular edema associated with BRVO.

Bevacizumab (1.25 mg/0.05 mL)

It is a humanized monoclonal antibody against vascular endothelial growth factor (VEGF) which increases capillary permeability. A comparison of the efficacy of bevacizumab to grid laser reported that bevacizumab treatment resulted in better and faster visual recovery. Bevacizumab was also efficacious with a treat and extend regime.

Ranibizumab

The efficacy of ranibizumab in these cases was investigated by Campochiaro et al. In a study comparing ranibizumab to sham, at the end of 6 months, there was a statistically significant improvement in visual acuity in the ranibizumab group (0.3 and 0.5 mg) compared to the sham group. Similarly, the reduction in central foveal thickness (CFT) was also significantly better in the ranibizumab group compared to the sham group. *The MARVEL study* evaluated the efficacy of bevacizumab compared to ranibizumab on a pro re nata (PRN) basis for the management of BRVO with macular edema. The study found that PRN administration of either bevacizumab or ranibizumab was effective in reducing macular edema with improvement in visual acuity (ranibizumab 18.08 letters; bevacizumab 15.55 letters).

Aflibercept

The VIBRANT study was a double-masked, multicenter trial to assess the efficacy of aflibercept compared to macular laser in eyes with macular edema secondary to BRVO.

At the end of 6 months, the eyes treated with aflibercept had more favorable outcomes in terms of reduced edema (aflibercept 280.5 μm/laser 128 μm) or visual improvement (aflibercept 17 letters/laser 6.9 letters).

Newer Agents
Brolucizumab and faricimab are not yet approved for the management of BRVO.

Arteriovenous Sheathotomy
In arteriovenous sheathotomy, the overlying artery is separated from the vein. However, this technique has a number of complications and is currently not preferred.

7.8 | Central Retinal Vein Occlusion

Aniruddha Agarwal
The Eye Institute, Cleveland Clinic Abu Dhabi, Abu Dhabi
Cleveland Clinic Lerner College of Medicine,
Case Western Reserve University, Cleveland, Ohio
Maastricht University Medical Center+ (MUMC), Maastricht
aniruddha9@gmail.com

■ INTRODUCTION

Central retinal vein occlusion (CRVO) is the occlusion of the central retinal vein at or just behind the level of the lamina cribrosa (**Fig. 7.8.1**). Typically seen in individuals above the age of 50 years, CRVO leads to a considerable loss of vision and is the second leading cause of visual loss due to a retinal vascular disease after diabetic retinopathy. Venous occlusion in CRVO induces an ischemic and hypoxic state that leads to visually significant sequelae including macular edema, and anterior segment and retinal neovascularization (NV).

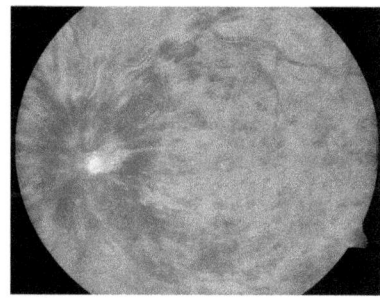

Fig. 7.8.1: Fundus photograph of the left eye of a patient showing presence of central retinal vein occlusion.

Central retinal vein occlusion consists of four distinct clinical entities:
1. Central retinal vein occlusion
2. Nonischemic CRVO
3. Ischemic CRVO
4. Hemicentral vein occlusion.

■ PATHOGENESIS AND RISK FACTORS
The risk factors of CRVO include:
- *Systemic factors:* Systemic hypertension, diabetes mellitus, and nocturnal arterial hypotension. Hematological factors such as protein C/protein S deficiency and procoagulable states are other risk factors for development of CRVO. In women, the risk of CRVO is decreased with the use of postmenopausal estrogen and increased with a higher erythrocyte sedimentation rate.
- *Local factors:* Various anatomical factors at the level of the lamina cribrosa predispose the eye to develop CRVO. The lumen of the central retinal artery and central retinal vein are narrower than they are in the orbital optic nerve, and the vessels are bound by a common adventitial sheath. The flow through the central retinal vein becomes increasingly turbulent as it progressively narrows at the lamina cribrosa, where it also

may be further impinged upon by arteriosclerosis of the adjacent central retinal artery. This turbulence damages the endothelium in the retrolaminar vein, which exposes collagen and initiates platelet aggregation and thrombosis. This triad (Virchow's triad) leads to the development of CRVO. Other local ocular risk factors include primary open angle glaucoma.

■ SIGNS AND SYMPTOMS

Patients with CRVO complain of sudden painless diminution of vision. Often, the visual loss is noticed on waking up in the morning.

Various signs of CRVO include flame-shaped or dot-and-blot hemorrhages, dilated tortuous veins in all four quadrants, cotton-wool spots, macular edema, disc edema, sheathing, collaterals (shunt vessels), and exudation. Differences between ischemic and nonischemic CRVO are given in **Table 7.8.1**.

■ DIAGNOSIS AND ANCILLARY INVESTIGATIONS

Various clinical and imaging modalities are available in order to diagnose and follow patients with CRVO. Spectral-domain optical coherence tomography (SD-OCT) and fluorescein angiography (FA) remain the most commonly used imaging modalities.
- *SD-OCT:* SD-OCT is useful to detect macular edema associated with CRVO.
- *FA:* On FA, patients with CRVO demonstrate delayed retinal vascular filling, increased retinal arteriovenous transit time, macular nonperfusion, macular edema, and retinal NV. In the acute phase of CRVO, FAs are poor due to the presence of overlying retinal hemorrhages.
- *OCT angiography (OCTA):* OCTA can provide distinct vascular network patterns that obscured by retinal hemorrhages on conventional FA. Using this technique macular ischemia in CRVO can be well documented. Recent studies have suggested that OCTA can be used to differentiate between ischemic and nonischemic CRVO. A flow deficit of >30% on OCTA wide field images is suggestive of an ischemic CRVO. OCTA, however, cannot be used to differentiate between collateral circulation and NV in eyes with CRVO.

■ COMPLICATIONS

The most serious complication of CRVO is development of retinal or optic disc NV. NV may also develop at the iris (NVI) or the angle (NVA). Almost 60% eyes with ischemic CRVO may develop NVI or NVA. Such eyes are predisposed to develop neovascular glaucoma (90-day glaucoma). In CRVO, vitreous hemorrhage may occur secondary to

TABLE 7.8.1: Differences between ischemic and nonischemic central retinal vein occlusion (CRVO).

Nonischemic CRVO	Ischemic CRVO
Presents with mild visual loss (≥20/120)	Presents with severe visual loss (≤20/200)
Relative afferent pupillary defect is rare	Relative afferent pupillary defect is common
<10 disc areas of nonperfusion on fluorescein angiography	>10 disc areas of nonperfusion on fluorescein angiography
Low risk of iris/angle neovascularization	High risk of iris/angle neovascularization
Less severe macular edema	Severe and often nonrefractory macular edema
Venous collaterals are less common	Venous collaterals are more common
B-wave amplitude on electroretinogram (ERG) is normal or slightly reduced	Markedly reduced B-wave amplitude on ERG

retinal or optic disc NV or due to rupture of the retinal blood through internal limiting membrane.

TREATMENT

Laser Photocoagulation

The Central Vein Occlusion group *(CVO Study)* (n = 728) investigated the efficacy of macular grid photocoagulation for the treatment of macular edema secondary to CRVO. In addition, the study aimed to determine whether photocoagulation therapy can prevent iris NV. There was no benefit of macular grid laser photocoagulation on comparing the treated and untreated eyes. Panretinal laser photocoagulation was shown to be beneficial for eyes with at least 2 hours of NVI or NVA.

Ranibizumab

Ranibizumab (RBZ) is an intravitreally injected, recombinant, humanized, and monoclonal antibody fragment that inhibits all isoforms of vascular endothelial growth factor (VEGF). The RBZ for the treatment of macular edema after CRVO *(the CRUISE Study)* trial evaluated the role of RBZ in CRVO. 392 patients with a visual acuity of 20/40–20/320 and macular edema for <12 months were included. At the 6-month follow-up, patients receiving RBZ gained a mean of >12.7 letters, compared with 0.8 letters in the sham group. The benefits of RBZ continued in the 12-month extension study with significant improvement in the central retinal thickness values.

Bevacizumab

Bevacizumab (BCZ) has been evaluated in various prospective randomized double-masked studies to assess its efficacy in the management of CRVO. At 6 months, there was a statistically significant greater proportion of patients in the treated versus sham group with 15 letter increase in visual acuity.

Aflibercept

Aflibercept (AFL) is a recombinant soluble VEGF receptor protein in which the binding domains of VEGF receptors 1 and 2 are combined with the Fc portion of immunoglobulin G.

- The Investigation of Efficacy and Safety in CRVO *(the COPERNICUS study)* (n = 189) investigated the efficacy and safety of intravitreal AFL in eyes with macular edema secondary to CRVO. At 24 weeks, treated eyes had a statistically significant higher percentage of patients reaching the primary endpoint versus the sham group.
- The General Assessment Limiting Infiltration of Exudates in CRVO with AFL *(the GALILEO study)* (n = 177) investigated the safety and efficacy of AFL in the treatment of macular edema associated with CRVO. At 6 months, both 15 letters gain in visual acuity compared to baseline and central foveal thickness reduction were significantly greater in the treated versus sham group.

Triamcinolone Acetonide

The Standard Care versus Corticosteroid for Retinal Vein Occlusion *(the SCORE study)* (n = 271) was a multicenter randomized clinical trial that studied the clinical benefits of intravitreal triamcinolone acetonide (IVTA) for treating macular edema associated with CRVO. The study compared 1 mg and 4 mg IVTA treatment versus standard care (i.e., observation). High rates of adverse events were observed in the 4 mg group compared to the 1 mg group and included cataract formation, elevated intraocular pressure (IOP), and glaucoma. Thus, the results of the study did not favor the use of IVTA in the management of CRVO.

Sustained-release Dexamethasone Implant

The safety and efficacy of implantable intravitreal dexamethasone implant (Ozurdex®) has been recently highlighted. This implant is composed of a biodegradable copolymer of lactic acid and glycolic acid-containing micronized dexamethasone. In the global evaluation of implantable dexamethasone in retinal vein occlusion with macular edema trial *(the Ozurdex GENEVA Study)* (n = 1,267; 437 patients with CRVO), patients were randomized to receive the implant with either 0.7 mg, or 0.3 mg or a sham implant. At 12 months, 32% of patients had a 15-letter gain in the 0.7 mg group. There was significant decrease in central foveal thickness in both the groups compared to the sham group. Cataract progression occurred in 90 of 302 phakic eyes that received two 0.7 mg implants versus 5 of 88 sham-treated phakic eyes. In the group receiving two 0.7 mg implants, there was a >10 IOP increase from baseline (12.6% after the first treatment and 15.4% after the second). The results of these studies indicate the therapeutic benefits of corticosteroids in the treatment of CRVO.

7.9 Management of Neovascular Age-related Macular Degeneration

Aniruddha Agarwal
The Eye Institute, Cleveland Clinic Abu Dhabi, Abu Dhabi
Cleveland Clinic Lerner College of Medicine,
Case Western Reserve University, Cleveland, Ohio
Maastricht University Medical Center+ (MUMC), Maastricht
aniruddha9@gmail.com

Deeksha Katoch
Advanced Eye Center, PGIMER, Chandigarh
drdeekshakatoch@yahoo.in

Mangat R Dogra
Grewal Eye Institute, Chandigarh
drmangatdogra@gmail.com

■ INTRODUCTION

Age-related macular degeneration (AMD) is the leading cause of central visual loss above the age of 65 years. Studies suggest that the prevalence of AMD is on the rise due to an increasing number of people living beyond 65 years of age. The exudative or neovascular form of AMD is characterized by choroidal neovascular membrane (CNV) growth **(Figs. 7.9.1A and B)** and/or serous retinal pigment epithelial (RPE) detachments. Various manifestations in patients with neovascular AMD such as subretinal hemorrhage, vitreous hemorrhage, fibrosis, and scarring are responsible for poor visual outcomes and legal blindness. The goal of therapy has been to salvage vision in this subset of patients with neovascular form of disease.

■ RISK FACTORS

- Various constitutional factors such as genetic composition, age, race, and family history demonstrate a consistently strong association with AMD in epidemiological studies.
- External factors such as smoking and cataract surgery are also major risk factors for AMD.

Recently, studies have suggested the role of various complement factor activation in the pathogenesis of AMD. Hypertension has also been linked in the pathogenesis of AMD.

SECTION 7: Retina

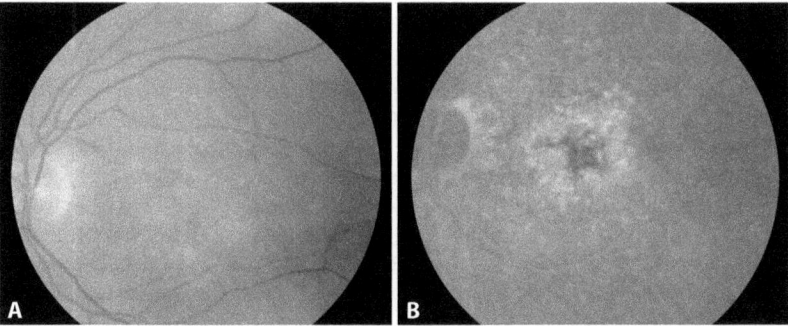

Figs. 7.9.1A and B: Fundus photograph of a patient with neovascular age-related macular degeneration (AMD). Fluorescein angiography shows presence of stippled hyperfluorescence. The patient was diagnosed with occult choroidal neovascular membrane (CNV) and started on monthly antivascular endothelial growth factor (VEGF) therapy.

SYMPTOMS

Neovascular AMD characteristically results in symptoms such as decreased vision and metamorphopsia. These signs may occur in very late stage of the disease. Unfortunately, by the time these symptoms occur, significant damage may have already occurred. More than one-third of patients may already have advanced fibrotic lesions before initial presentation.

DIAGNOSIS AND ANCILLARY INVESTIGATIONS

Various clinical and imaging modalities are available in order to diagnose choroidal neovascularization (CNV) associated with AMD. Spectral-domain optical coherence tomography (SD-OCT) and fluorescein angiography (FA) remain the best methods to detect CNV.

- *SD-OCT:* Once diagnosed, patients may be followed up on SD-OCT to assess response of therapy noninvasively.
- *FA:* On FA, the lesions of neovascular AMD can be classified as either (1) classic: discrete and early hyperfluorescence with late leakage of fluorescein dye or (2) occult: FA appearance of occult CNV is categorized into two basic forms:
  i. Late leakage of undetermined source or
  ii. Fibrovascular pigment epithelial detachment (PED)
  Both forms manifest as a region of ill-defined leakage in the early and late frames.
- *Indocyanine green angiography (ICGA):* ICGA helps in the detection of polypoidal choroidal vasculopathy (PCV) and retinal angiomatous proliferation (RAP).
- *OCT angiography (OCTA):* OCTA can provide distinct vascular network patterns that may be otherwise obscured by subretinal hemorrhage on conventional FA. OCTA may allow calculation of flow indices that may help in judging treatment response in neovascular AMD. The active CNV networks on OCTA appear as either medusa head or branching tree and inactive lesions can have a pruned tree appearance.

    Based on the OCTA appearance, the lesions of neovascular AMD can be classified as:
    - *Nonexudative neovascular AMD:* Evidence of CNV network on OCTA or the presence of a hot spot on ICGA, but no leakage on FA or presence of intraretinal/subretinal fluid on OCT. This term can be applied to lesions which are treatment naïve.
    - *Exudative neovascular AMD:* Evidence of network on OCTA or the presence of a hot spot on ICGA with leakage on FA and presence of intraretinal/subretinal fluid on OCT.

TREATMENT

Photodynamic Therapy

Verteporfin photodynamic therapy (PDT) selectively generates free oxygen radicals that cause cytotoxic damage and regression of CNV in patients with AMD. The Treatment of AMD with Photodynamic Therapy *(TAP study)* showed that percentage of patients losing <15 letters was significantly less in the PDT group compared to controls (classic CNV lesions). In the antivascular endothelial growth factor (VEGF) era, the use of PDT has declined due to its lower efficacy. However, current guidelines recommend the use of PDT in combination with anti-VEGF therapy for PCV *(EVEREST study*: Visual Outcome in Patients with Symptomatic Macular PCV Treated with Either Ranibizumab as Monotherapy or Combined with Verteporfin Photodynamic Therapy).

Ranibizumab

Ranibizumab (RBZ) is an intravitreally injected, recombinant, humanized, and monoclonal antibody fragment designed to actively bind and inhibit all isoforms of VEGF. It consists of two parts: a nonbinding human sequence (humanized), making it less antigenic in humans, and a high-affinity binding Fab fragment, which serves to bind the antigen.

- Historically, *ANCHOR and MARINA* proved the efficacy of RBZ using a monthly dosing regimen.
- More recently, the Prospective OCT Study with Lucentis® for Neovascular AMD *(PrONTO study)* (n = 40), a phase I/II prospective study, showed that with the OCT-based retreatment [*pro re nata (PRN)*], a mean improvement of 11.1 letters at 2 years was possible with a mean of 9.9 injections.
- *The SAILOR study* (n = 4307) (phase IIIb) used three initial monthly doses followed by PRN dosing at 3-month follow-up appointments.
- *The PIER study* (n = 184) was a phase IIIb multicenter, double-masked, sham-controlled trial of neovascular AMD patients. At 1 year, patients lost an average of only 0.2 letters from baseline compared to a loss of 16.3 letters in the sham cohort.
- *The SUSTAIN study* (n = 513) was a phase IIIb, multicenter, open-label, single-arm study analyzing results of PRN RBZ. At 1 year, mean best-corrected visual acuity (BCVA) increased 3.6 letters from baseline. This study encouraged the use of PRN dosing of RBZ in AMD.

Bevacizumab

Bevacizumab (BCZ) is a full-length humanized monoclonal antibody against human VEGF. Treatment with BCZ results in a much lower economic burden to the healthcare system as compared to RBZ. BCZ is still widely used off-label for the management of neovascular AMD.

- *The CATT study* (Comparison of Age-related Macular Degeneration Treatments Trial) (n = 1,208) was a multicenter, noninferiority trial comparing monthly and PRN BCZ and RBZ. At 2 years, the mean gains were 8.8 and 7.8 letters in the monthly RBZ and BCZ groups, respectively. The PRN groups gained 6.7 and 5.0 letters, respectively. These results showed noninferiority between RBZ and BCZ.
- *The LUCAS study* (Lucentis Compared to Avastin) trial (n = 441) is a recent, randomized, double-blind, multicenter, and noninferiority trial comparing BCZ and RBZ using a treat-and-extend strategy. Mean increase in visual acuity were 7.9 letters for the BCZ cohort and 8.2 letters for the RBZ cohort.

Aflibercept

Aflibercept (AFL) is a recombinant soluble VEGF receptor protein in which the binding domains of VEGF receptors 1 and 2 are combined with the Fc portion of immunoglobulin G.

- *The VIEW-1 and VIEW-2 trials* (n = 2,419) were two similarly designed, double-masked, multicenter, active-controlled, randomized, phase III studies comparing monthly and every 2-month dosing of intravitreal AFL and RBZ. Mean average BCVA gain was 8.1 and 9.4 letters in the RBZ groups, 10.9 and 7.6 letters in the monthly 2 mg AFL groups, and 7.9 and 8.9 letters in the bimonthly AFL groups. These results suggested better gains with AFL compared to RBZ.

Conbercept
Conbercept (CBP) (KH-902) is a novel, recombinant, and soluble VEGF receptor protein in which the binding domains of VEGF receptors 1 and 2 are combined with Fc portion of immunoglobulin G. In a phase I study, KH-902 was found to be safe with a dose of up to 3 mg. A recent phase III trial using KH-902 suggested beneficial effects on visual acuity.

Brolucizumab
Brolucizumab (BrL) is a newly approved anti-VEGF agent which is a single-chain antibody fragment against VEGF factor A (VEGF-A). The efficacy and safety of BrL in AMD has been studied in the two pivotal phase III HAWK and HARRIER studies. The HAWK and HARRIER were large, multicenter double-masked interventional clinical trials with over 1,817 patients.

Faricimab
Faricimab (FaB) is another recently approved agent which acts by inhibition of both angiopoetin-2 and VEGF-A in eyes with AMD. The TENAYA and LUCERNE were two large multicenter phase III clinical trials that led to the approval of FaB in the management of neovascular AMD. The highlights of FaB use are its long-lasting effect (over 16 weeks) in eyes with AMD.

Gene Therapy
Intraocular gene therapy for management of neovascular AMD has recently received attention. Various injectable genes incorporated into viral vectors include rAAV.sFLT1, AAV2.sFLT01, and RetinoStat.

Advances in Drug Delivery
Apart from development of newer drug formulations such as nanoparticles, there has been an emphasis on designing drug delivery devices. These include:
- Encapsulated cell technology
- Refillable reservoir devices
- Colloidal drug carriers
- Suprachoroidal drug delivery
- Transscleral delivery
- Pulsed high-intensity focused ultrasound (HIFU).

CONCLUSION
In the last decade, there have been numerous advances and breakthroughs in the management of neovascular AMD. With a comprehensive and rehabilitative approach, the management of AMD continues to advance.

7.10 Understanding Macular Holes

Atul Kumar
AK Institute of Ophthalmology, New Delhi
atul56kumar@yahoo.com

Divya Agarwal
Vikalp Eye Centre, Bareilly

Aman Kumar
AK Institute of Ophthalmology, New Delhi

■ INTRODUCTION

Macular hole is a vitreoretinal interface disorder where a partial (lamellar macular hole) or full thickness neural tissue defect occurs in macular region. It commonly occurs due to aging (idiopathic), trauma, and high myopia. It is mostly seen in sixth to seventh decade of life and seen twice more frequently in females, but maybe seen in younger patients, especially myopes. The disease may be seen bilaterally in 5-16% patients.

■ PATHOGENESIS

Vitreomacular traction leads to anteroposterior traction on the macula while the condensing posterior cortical vitreous provides a tangential traction over the macular area. Both these forces collectively cause a vitreomacular traction which leads to partial thickness retinal defect, or lamellar hole, or may directly lead to full thickness defect.

■ CLINICAL FEATURES AND INVESTIGATIONS

Patient complains of decreasing central vision, metamorphopsia, or central scotoma. It is clinically visible as loss of foveal reflex or full thickness retinal hole with round borders. It may have a surrounding cuff of fluid, drusen-like deposits, intraretinal edema, and cysts or associated posterior vitreous detachment (PVD) **(Fig. 7.10.1)**. Watzke-Allen test and laser aiming beam test maybe done to confirm diagnosis. An optical coherence tomography (OCT) is used to confirm and measure the retinal thickness and size of hole. Fundus autofluorescence indicates health of retinal pigment epithelium and has prognostic value. One can also do microperimetry which provides a topographic mapping of the retinal sensitivity and also aids in mapping of absolute and relative scotomas in macular holes both preoperatively and postoperatively.

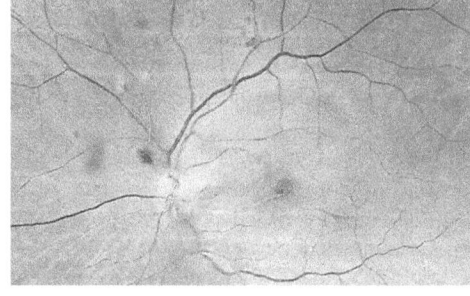

Fig. 7.10.1: Optos pseudocolor fundus imaging showing large full thickness macular hole associated with wrinkling of retinal surface suggesting an overlying epiretinal membrane.

Differential diagnosis includes lamellar macular holes and pseudoholes. In pseudohole, there is an absence of full thickness defect and has steep walls as opposed to a lamellar hole which has sloping edges and partial thickness defect. Watzke-Allen and laser aiming beam test will be negative in both of them differentiating them from true macular holes.

Macular hole stages are described in **Table 7.10.1**.

TABLE 7.10.1: Staging of macular holes.

Stage		Clinical (Gass)	OCT-based
Stage 0 (Chan et al.)		Perifoveal vitreous detachment	Elevation of cone outer segment tips (COST or Verhoeff's membrane)
Stage 1 **(Figs. 7.10.2 and 7.10.3)**	1A (impending macular hole)	Yellow spot, loss of foveal contour, 100–200 pm	Inner foveal pseudocyst, foveolar detachment of COST
	1B (occult hole)	Yellow ring, bridging vitreous cortex, 200–300 pm	Inner and outer retinal layer defect, intact foveal roof
Stage 2 **(Fig. 7.10.4)**		Full thickness defect <400 pm, associated operculum	Partial detachment of operculum at hole edge with attached posterior hyaloid
Stage 3		Full thickness defect > 400 pm, without PVD	Complete detachment of posterior hyaloid from fovea (irrespective of size of hole)
Stage 4 **(Fig. 7.10.5)**		Full thickness defect with complete PVD	Full thickness defect with complete PVD (not to be ascertained on OCT)

(COST: cone outer segment tips; OCT: optical coherence tomography; PVD: perifoveal vitreous detachment)

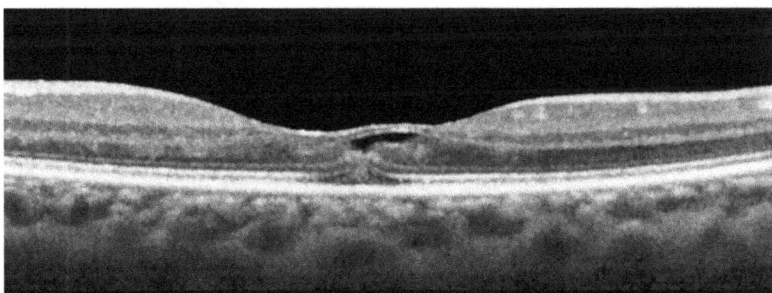

Fig. 7.10.2: Spectral-domain optical coherence tomography (SD-OCT) of stage 1a macular hole showing foveal cyst with disrupted cone outer segment tips (COST).

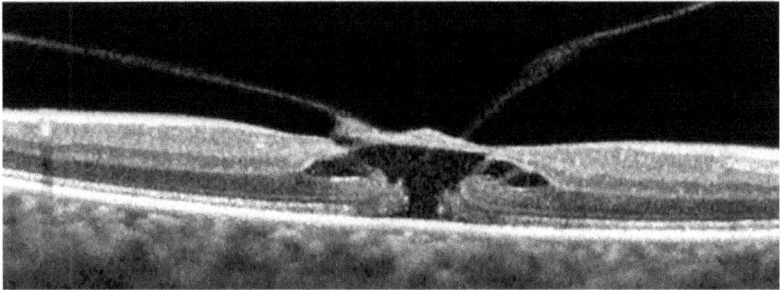

Fig. 7.10.3: Spectral-domain optical coherence tomography (SD-OCT) of macular hole stage 1B. Cystic space extends posteriorly with broken photoreceptor layer with surrounding cystic cavities. Posterior hyaloid attachment preserved to roof.

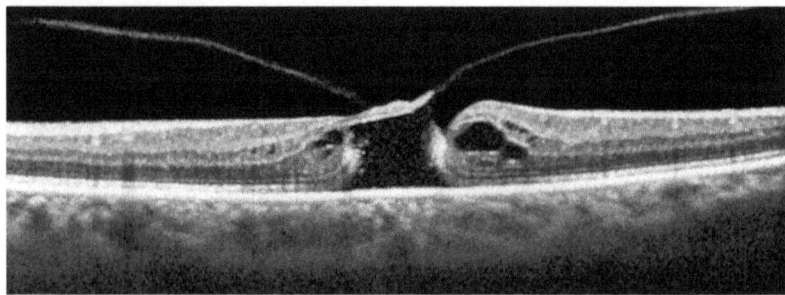

Fig. 7.10.4: Spectral-domain optical coherence tomography (SD-OCT) of macular hole stage 2. Attached posterior hyaloid to operculum with detached edge of foveal roof.

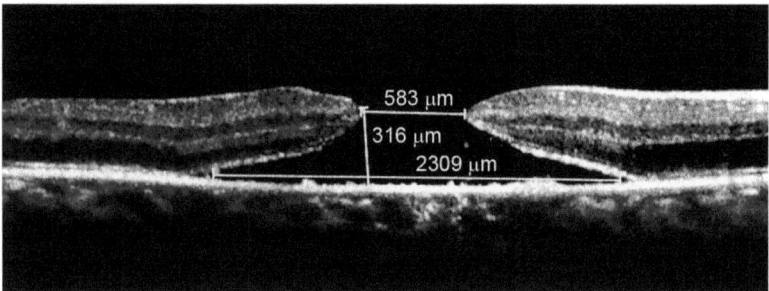

Fig. 7.10.5: Spectral-domain optical coherence tomography (SD-OCT) of macular hole stage 4. Full thickness macular hole with complete detachment of operculum. Macular hole index is calculated as height/base of macular hole.

■ VITAL STAINS IN MACULAR HOLE SURGERY

Vital stains have a promising role as they enhance and display internal limiting membrane (ILM), fine epiretinal membrane (ERM), posterior hyaloid, and vitreoschisis. Indocyanine green (ICG) stains the ILM, however, in vitro studies, have shown ICG exposure to lead to cytotoxicity of cultured retinal pigment epithelial (RPE) cells, while infracyanine green in 5% glucose did not demonstrate the same.

Trypan blue has an affinity for the cellular material composing ERMs, providing excellent visualization of same. Brilliant blue dye (ILM blue, DORC) (0.025%) is also effective for ILM staining. It may be combined with 4% polyethylene glycol (PEG) to increase relative molecular weight, better concentration at posterior pole, faster and better staining of ILM.

Membrane blue-dual combines trypan blue (0.15%), brilliant blue (0.025%), and 4% PEG for combined ERM and ILM staining.

Triamcinolone acetonide crystals with solvent removed provide excellent identification and help in peeling ERM/ILM in macular hole surgery. They have the added advantage of not possessing the toxic properties of dyes.

■ SURGERY FOR MACULAR HOLES

Careful patient selection is critical to a successful outcome. Observation is advisable for asymptomatic patients with early stage 2 macular hole. Post-traumatic macular holes can spontaneously close in 3–6 months, hence a wait and watch policy is mandatory for such patients. Surgical intervention can be done in stage 2, 3, or 4 macular holes with associated vision loss or significant metamorphopsia. Surgical repair of macular holes includes relief of all tangential, vertical traction, and retinal tamponade. Tangential traction is relieved by removal of the posterior hyaloid, fine ERM, and ILM around the hole. For large holes, inverted flap of peeled ILM attached to macular hole edge is placed over the hole, either tucked-in or in a multilayered fashion. An ILM tissue removed from distant site may be used as autograft to close the hole, especially in refractory or previously failed cases. Use of anterior or posterior lens capsule and amniotic membrane as autograft has also been described **(Figs. 7.10.6 and 7.10.7)**. At the end, tamponade is achieved by total gas-fluid exchange with air, 20–25% SF6, or 12–14% C3F8 gas mixture and face-down positioning is advised, generally for <1 week duration.

Microscope-integrated intraoperative OCT has shown promising role in macular hole surgery. It helps in identification of vitreoschisis and ensures proper placement of

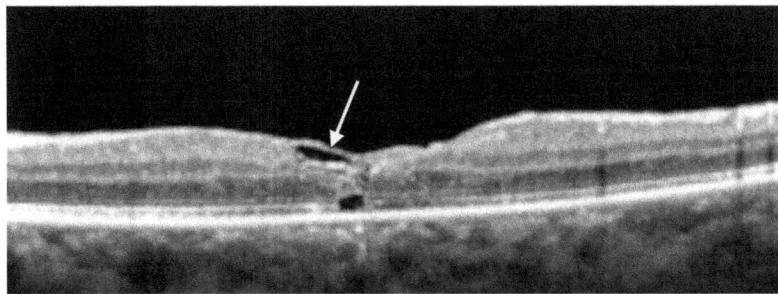

Fig. 7.10.6: Postoperative spectral-domain optical coherence tomography (SD-OCT) of patient with macular hole with type 1 closure. Note presence of internal limiting membrane (ILM) flap over healing edge of macular hole (arrow).

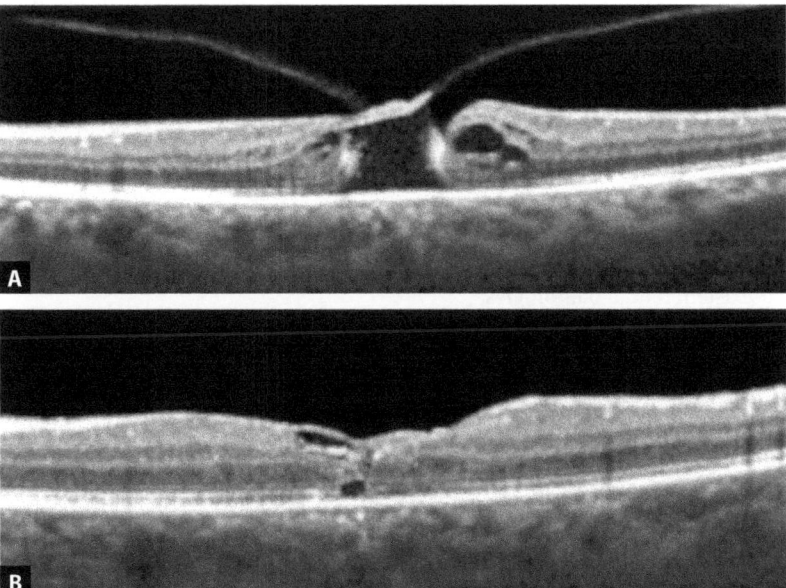

Figs. 7.10.7A and B: Preoperative and postoperative spectral-domain optical coherence tomography (SD-OCT) of patient with macular hole. (A) Stage 2 macular hole with attached posterior hyaloid; (B) Closed macular hole with remnants of inverted internal limiting membrane (ILM) flap at the healing edge.

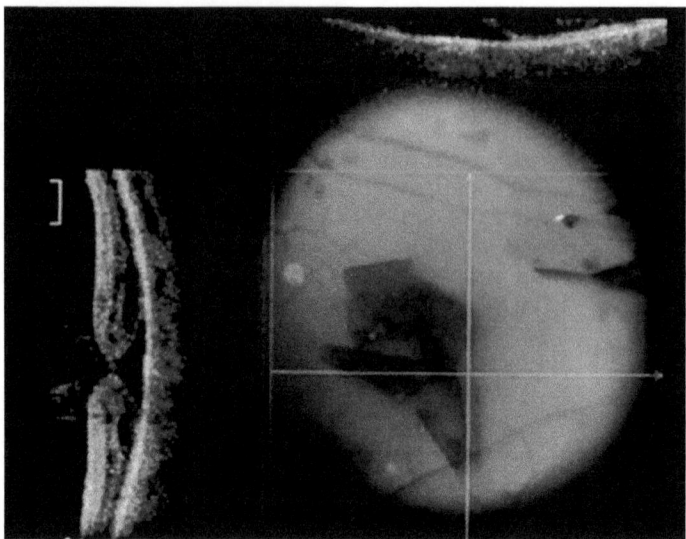

Fig. 7.10.8: Intraoperative optical coherence tomography (OCT) grab showing successful inverted internal limiting membrane (ILM) flap technique during digitally assisted vitreoretinal surgery using Ngenuity® (Alcon Inc.)

inverted ILM flap over macular hole which are difficult to visualize as in patients with pathological myopia with macular hole and retinal detachment, thereby increasing the anatomical and functional success. Nowadays, clinical outcomes of macular hole surgery using 3D viewing system are not inferior to that of conventional microscopes, and it has the added advantages of better ergonomics, reduced phototoxicity, peripheral visualization, magnification, and less asthenopia, and it serves as a good educational tool **(Fig. 7.10.8)**.

Autologous neurosensory retinal free flap is a new technique described by Grewal and Mahmoud for refractory myopic macular holes. It involves an endolaser applied to the area marked for graft harvesting, followed by diathermy to the blood vessels at the edge. A free retinal flap that is 0.5 disc diameter larger than the macular hole size is lifted and placed over the hole. This is done under perfluoro-n-octane heavy liquid followed by silicone oil exchange later.

Prognostic factors of visual recovery following macular hole surgery depends on presenting visual acuity, size, duration of macular hole, continuity of the outer retinal bands including the ellipsoid band (EZ) and the interdigitation zone (IZ) and presence of other co-existent retinal pathologies.

Postoperative anatomical appearance can be classified as type 1 closure, type 2 closure, and nonclosure. If the macular hole is observed to close without a foveal defect in the neurosensory retina, it is considered as type 1 closure **(Figs. 7.10.9A to C)**. If the foveal defect of neurosensory retina persists postoperatively with a reduction in hole diameter, it is considered to be a type 2 closure.

■ COMPLICATIONS

The most common complication of a vitrectomy for macular hole is the occurrence or progression of cataract. Other complications include retinal breaks, retinal detachment, late reopening of the hole, RPE loss under the hole, phototoxicity, and endophthalmitis. Dense wedge-shaped temporal and/or inferior visual field deficits have been noted upon gas resorption. Proposed origins include retinal ischemia of or direct trauma to the optic nerve head. Inner retinal dimpling and dissociation of outer nerve fiber layer (DONFL) have been observed postoperatively.

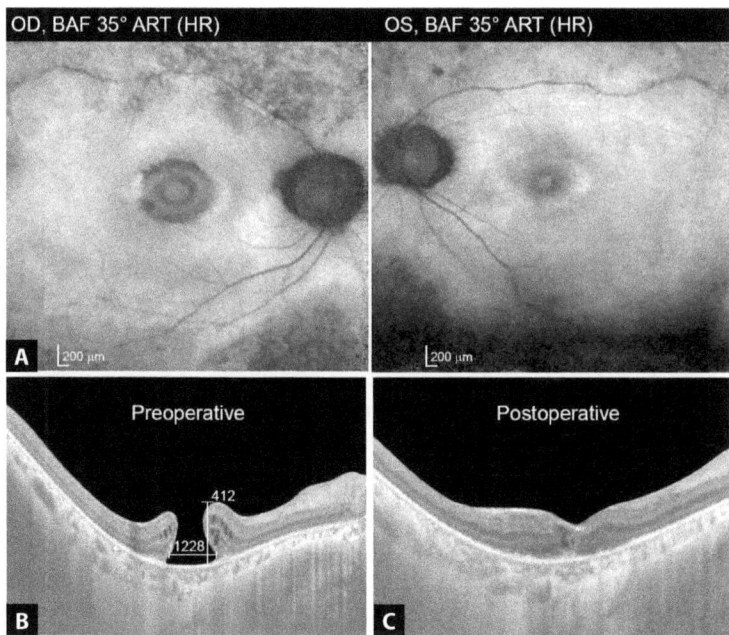

Figs. 7.10.9A to C: (A) Fundus autofluorescence imaging of a patient with inherited retinal dystrophy showing retinal pigment epithelial (RPE) hypo-autofluorescence in both eyes and macular hole defect in both eyes; (B) Large full thickness macular hole was also noted on OCT; (C) After macular hole surgery, type 1 macular hole closure was achieved.

SUGGESTED READING

1. Akiba J, Kakehashi A, Arzabe CW, Trempe CL. Fellow eyes in idiopathic macular hole cases. Ophthalmic Surg. 1992;23:594-7.
2. Kumar A, Agarwal D, Narde HK, Shaikh N, Kumar A, Sinha A, et al. Macular hole. In: Kumar A (Ed). Retina: Medical and Surgical Management, 2nd edition. New Delhi: Jaypee Brothers Medical Publishers; 2022.

7.11 | Retinitis Pigmentosa and Stem Cell Transplantation

Atul Kumar
AK Institute of Ophthalmology, New Delhi
atul56kumar@yahoo.com

Divya Agarwal
Vikalp Eye Centre, Bareilly

Aman Kumar
AK Institute of Ophthalmology, New Delhi

INTRODUCTION

Retinitis pigmentosa (RP) is a diffuse retinal degenerative disease, which initially predominately affects the rod photoreceptors with later degeneration of cone photoreceptors. It is the most common hereditary fundus dystrophy. As a result of photoreceptor degeneration, it presents initially with nyctalopia and dark adaptation difficulties and midperipheral scotoma, which later progresses to leave a tiny island of residual central vision.

CHARACTERISTIC TRIAD OF RETINITIS PIGMENTOSA

- Bone spicule retinal pigmentation (Fig. 7.11.1)
- Arteriolar attenuation
- Waxy disc pallor.

INHERITANCE

Age of onset, mode of progression, eventual visual loss, and associated ocular features are frequently related to the mode of inheritance. RP may occur as:

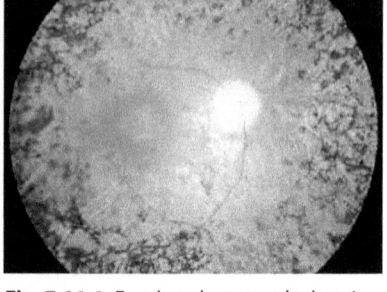

Fig. 7.11.1: Fundus photograph showing bone spicule retinal pigmentation.

- Isolated, without family history
- *Autosomal dominant (AD):* Common with good prognosis
- *Autosomal recessive (AR):* Less common with intermediate prognosis
- *X-linked recessive:* Least common with worst prognosis

CLINICAL FEATURES

Night blindness is the most common presenting feature in patients with RP. Gradual progressive contraction of the visual field (VF) is the second most common symptom of RP. Relatives often complain that the patients bump into objects frequently, especially at night. Superior field is affected first and VF loss tends to be symmetrical between the two eyes. Central vision is also involved later due to macular involvement.

Absence of pigment (RP sine pigmento) is just a stage in the development of typical RP. Virtually all RP would have bony spicule pigmentation sooner or later. Associated ocular findings are common in patients with RP.

These include:
- Posterior subcapsular cataract (PSC)
- High myopia and astigmatism
- Primary open angle glaucoma and keratoconus
- Vitreous cells are common and indicate ensuing rapid photoreceptor degeneration. Fine pigment-like dusting is also common.
- Optic disc drusen (seen in 10% of RP patients)
- Coats-like response and vasoproliferative tumor have also been reported.

VARIANTS OF RETINITIS PIGMENTOSA

- *Pericentral RP:* The pigmentary changes occur closer to the macula as compared to typical RP.
- *Sectoral RP:* Pigmentary changes are limited to a sector of retina, either a quadrant or two
- *Retinitis punctata albescens:* Fleck retinal degeneration with slowly progressive visual loss along with the macular atrophic degeneration
- Unilateral RP.

SYNDROMIC RETINITIS PIGMENTOSA

Several systemic disorders are known to occur in association with RP, most common being Usher syndrome. Others are Bardet–Biedl syndrome, Refsum disease, Bassen Kornzweig syndrome (abetalipoproteinemia), Kearns–Sayre syndrome, neuronal ceroid lipofuscinoses, Leber congenital amaurosis (LCA), and progressive cone dystrophy.

INVESTIGATIONS

- *Visual fields* are one of the most important modalities to note progression/worsening of RP. Initially, relative scotoma is seen in midperiphery which coalesces to form typical ring scotoma leaving behind tunnel vision in advanced stages.
- *Optical coherence tomography (OCT)* can detect macular abnormalities such as outer retinal layer abnormalities, macular edema, and epiretinal membrane.
- *Fundus autofluorescence* can monitor health of retinal pigment epithelium (RPE) on follow-up.
- In *electroretinography*, scotopic and combined responses are often severely diminished even when fundus may seem normal.
- *Prolonged dark adaptation* is seen in all types of RP irrespective of the stage of RP.

TREATMENT

Currently, no effective treatment exists for RP. Correction of refractive error, cataract extraction, treatment of macular edema whenever present, and low vision aids could be of great help in these patients. Supplementation of 15,000 IU of vitamin A has also been reported to slow down the progression of RP. Some researchers have also tried using oral valproate.

The US Food and Drug Administration has approved Luxturna (voretigene neparvovec-rzyl) in December 2017. Luxturna is the first directly administered gene therapy approved in the US that targets a disease caused by mutations in a specific gene, i.e., *RPE65* gene on chromosome no. 1. It works by delivering a normal copy of the *RPE65* gene directly to retinal cells. It is administered via subretinal injection and patients should be treated with a short course of oral prednisone to limit the potential immune reaction to Luxturna.

ROLE OF STEM CELL THERAPY

The use of autologous bone marrow derived stem cells for retinal degeneration offers neuroprotection and rescue from degeneration without immune rejection. The three distinct cell types which are conceivable targets for stem cell therapy in the retina are—neuroretina (photoreceptors, bipolar cells, and ganglion cells), retinal pigment epithelium, and vascular endothelial cells. Various stem cell types and their route of use are described in **Table 7.11.1**.

TABLE 7.11.1: Various stem cell types and their route of use.

	Replacement therapy	Rescue therapy
Cell type used	• Embryonic stem cells • Induced pluripotent stem cells • Retinal progenitor cells	Bone marrow-derived mononuclear stem cells
Route of injection	Subretinal	Intravitreal
Clinical trials	NCT 01344993[1]	• NCT 01518127[2] • NCT 01068561[3]

1. *NCT 01344993:* Safety and tolerability of subretinal transplantation of human embryonic stem cell (hESC)-derived retinal pigment epithelium (RPE) (MA09-h RPE) cells in patients with advanced dry age-related macular degeneration.
2. *NCT 01518127:* Intravitreal bone marrow-derived stem cells in patients with macular degeneration (safety/efficacy study).
3. *NCT 01068561:* Autologous bone marrow-derived stem cell transplantation for retinitis pigmentosa.

Studies Performed Thus Far
- Studied safety and feasibility of autologous bone marrow stem cell transplantation in various degenerative retinal disorders such as RP and dry AMD: Initial studies used a dose of 4 million cells/0.1 mL which was later increased to 8 million cells/0.1 mL.
- Studied efficacy of autologous bone marrow derived stem cells in various degenerative retinal disorders such as RP and dry AMD: Autologous stem cell injection improves and stabilizes central retinal visual function as shown by multifocal electroretinogram (mfERG).

SUGGESTED READING
1. Kumar A, Agarwal D, Narde HK, Shaikh N, Kumar A, Sinha A, et al. Retinitis pigmentosa and allied disorders. In: Kumar A (Ed). Retina: Medical and Surgical Management, 2nd edition. New Delhi: Jaypee Brothers Medical Publishers; 2022.
2. Minoru T, Yasushi A, Haruhiko Y, Takahashi K, Kiuchi K, Oyaizu H, et al. Bone marrow-derived stem cells can differentiate into retinal cells in injured rat retina. Stem Cells. 2002;20:279-83.

7.12 Vitrectomy for Diabetic Traction Retinal Detachment

Cyrus Shroff
cyrus_shroff@hotmail.com
Charu Gupta
Shroff Eye Centre, New Delhi

INTRODUCTION
Vitrectomy for diabetic traction retinal detachment (TRD) is indicated when there is TRD involving or threatening the macula, combined traction, and rhegmatogenous retinal detachment (RRD) or TRD with severe progressive fibrovascular proliferation threatening to progress to an irreparable stage **(Figs. 7.12.1A and B)**. Contraindications to surgery are old macular detachment with pale disc and grossly sclerosed blood vessels, poor prognosis with good vision in fellow eye, and ambulatory vision in an only eye which is stable.

VITREOSCHISIS
Vitreoschisis was first described in proliferative diabetic retinopathy (PDR) by Chu et al. and Schwartz et al. nearly 20 years back. An understanding of the process of posterior vitreous separation and vitreoschisis and identification of the appropriate surgical plane

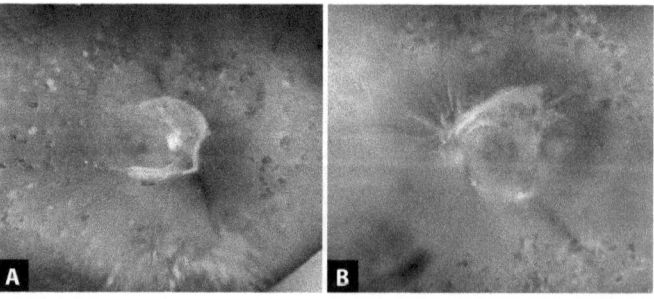

Figs. 7.12.1A and B: Fundus. (A) Extramacular tractional retinal detachment; (B) Advanced tractional retinal detachment involving macula.

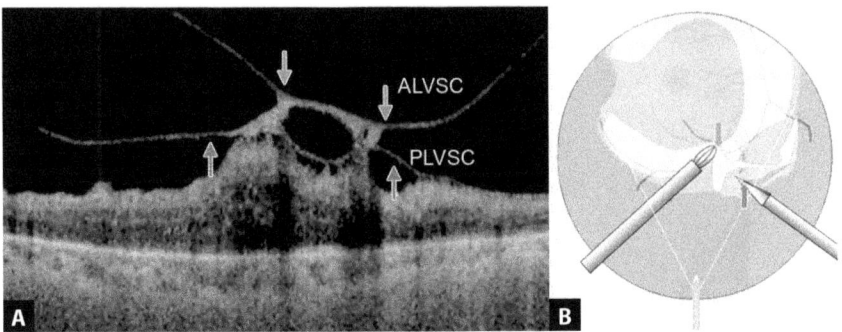

Figs. 7.12.2A and B: Vitreoschisis depicted on (A) Swept source optical coherence tomography and, (B) Diagrammatic representation. Anterior leaf of vitreoschisis cavity (ALVSC) (green arrow) is held with the forceps and the posterior leaf of vitreoschisis cavity (PLVSC), true plane (blue arrow) is teased out with the scissors.

during membrane surgery increases the ease of dissection and improves the surgical success. With newer swept source optical coherence imaging machines we are able to study the membrane attachments, their location and extent preoperatively **(Fig. 7.12.2A)**. We are also able to analyze the macular area in detail. This thorough preoperative assessment helps us to plan out the surgery and prognosticate the visual recovery.

The goals of surgery are twofold: Restoration of vision and stabilization of the neovascular process. This includes removal of vitreous blood and scaffold with fibrovascular proliferation, release of traction on macula, cataract removal if present, and photocoagulation of retinal breaks and ischemic retina. Eyes in which these surgical objectives are achieved and which have good outcome at 6 months tend to remain stable for many years.

Prognosis must be clearly explained. Surgery is generally performed under local anesthesia as most patients are high-risk cases.

■ PREOPERATIVE ANTIVASCULAR ENDOTHELIAL GROWTH FACTOR

In patients with florid neovascularization, intravitreal antivascular endothelial growth factor (VEGF) is given 3–5 days prior to vitrectomy. This decreases the chances of bleeding during dissection and makes the surgery cleaner and safe **(Figs. 7.12.3A and B)**. Cataract surgery when required is usually combined with vitrectomy. The cataract wound is sutured. A good visualization is critical to success of these challenging surgical procedures. Wide angle viewing is used. Xenon light source gives excellent illumination with self-retaining 25 G intraocular "chandelier" light enabling true *bimanual vitrectomy* to be performed safely.

Small incision microincision vitrectomy surgery (MIVS) is done. The gauge of instrumentation, 23 G, 25 G, or 27 G, can be the surgeon's choice. 25 G vitrectomy works well for these cases with better fluidics, less trauma to the vitreous base, and a cutter with its port close to the tip, which makes it a very versatile instrument. Core vitrectomy is performed and the membranes isolated from the periphery by the can opener technique. In cases with no or minimal hyaloidal separation the hyaloid is lifted at the disc with a forceps and the separation then extended with a cutter to isolate the membrane from the periphery. It is vital to differentiate the true posterior hyaloid from a large vitreoschisis cavity. Once the correct plane of dissection is identified, the edge of the fibrovascular membrane is lifted up with forceps and separated from the retina with scissors dissection, cutting the vascular connections very precisely and with minimal bleeding **(Fig. 7.12.2B)**. Iatrogenic breaks are also minimized this way. If an island of very adherent tissue remains, especially with broad attachment to a major vessel, it is segmented and diathermized.

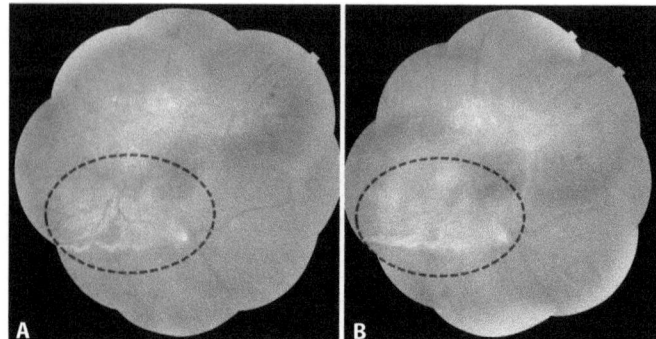

Figs. 7.12.3A and B: Fundus. (A) Tractional retinal detachment with florid vessels (dotted circle); (B) Postintravitreal bevacizumab with decreased vascularity.

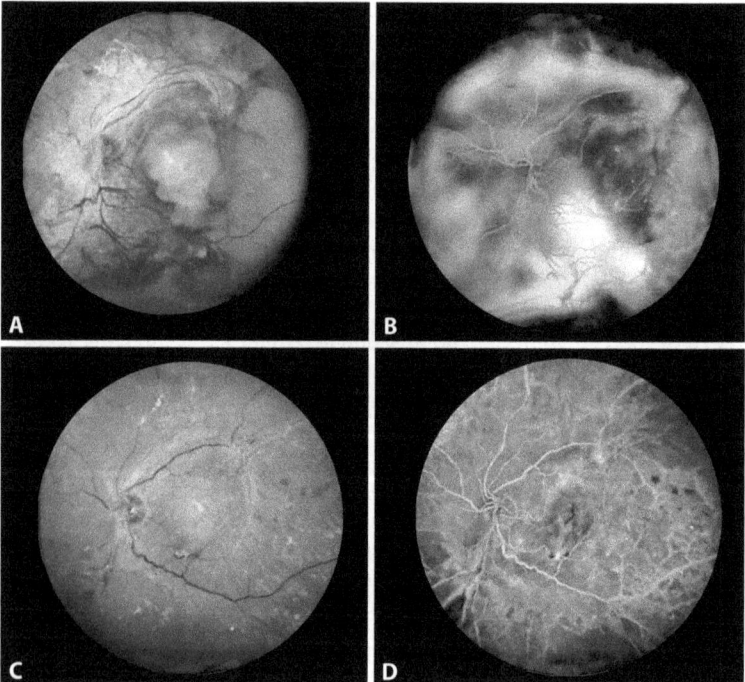

Figs. 7.12.4A to D: Preoperative (A) Fundus picture and (B) Fluorescein angiography showing tractional retinal detachment. Postoperative (C) Fundus picture and (D) Fluorescein angiography showing good anatomical result.

Hemostasis is important and should be achieved promptly to prevent formation of large adherent clots. Using bimanual technique we aspirate with one instrument and coagulate elevated or surface bleeders simultaneously with endodiathermy or endolaser. In some situations, manual pressure on the bleeder by a blunt instrument is helpful to achieve hemostasis.

Disc bleeds are usually controlled by raising the infusion bottle for up to 2 minutes at a time and then slowly lowering it. A good vitreous base excision with scleral depression is done irrespective of whether the vitreous is clear or hemorrhagic and even if the eye is phakic. This clears the sclerotomy area of vitreous and reduces risk of anterior hyaloidal fibrovascular proliferation, peripheral retinal breaks, and dialysis.

Laser photocoagulation is done to the breaks, if any, and panretinal photocoagulation is done as completely as possible up to the ora. Tamponade is required if there are preexisting or iatrogenic retinal breaks. If no tamponade is require an anti-VEGF agent is injected intravitreally at the end of the surgery.

Gas or oil tamponade are the options. Gas is preferred as there seems to be less postoperative bleeding and if it occurs, clears faster than with silicon oil. Eyes with silicon oil tamponade have a greater tendency to reproliferation and disc pallor.

Recurrent vitreous hemorrhage is the most common complication after this procedure. Intravitreal anti-VEGF injection helps in clearing the hemorrhage in most cases. An ultrasound is done prior to the intravitreal injection to rule out retinal detachment. In cases with persistent vitreous hemorrhage a vitreous lavage can be done. Cystoid macular edema (CME) is another complication faced postoperatively. Intravitreal dexamethasone implant and intravitreal anti-VEGF agents have been used successfully. Optic atrophy an irreversible cause of vision loss is seen in some cases despite a good anatomical result. With good case selection, appropriate instrumentation and correct technique this difficult surgery can be very rewarding **(Figs. 7.12.4A to D)**.

SUGGESTED READING

1. Shroff C, Gupta C, Shroff D. Bimanual surgery for diabetic retinopathy and vascular disorders. In: Narendran V, Kothari A (Eds). Principles and Practice of Vitreoretinal surgery, 1st edition. New Delhi. Jaypee Brothers Medical Publishers; 2014. pp. 399-412.

7.13 | Fundus Fluorescein Angiography

Deeksha Katoch
Advanced Eye Center, PGIMER, Chandigarh
drdeekshakatoch@yahoo.in

Ramanuj Samanta
AIIMS, Rishikesh
ramanuj.oph@aiimsrishikesh.edu.in

INTRODUCTION

Angiography comes from the Greek words *"Angeion"* meaning vessel and *"graphein"* meaning to "write or record". Fluorescein angiography (FA)[1,2] refers to photographing the retinal circulation following intravenous injection of fluorescein dye. It allows study of the retinal and to a certain extent choroidal circulation in normal and pathological states.

PRINCIPLE

Luminescence

Light energy is absorbed and then remitted by spontaneous decay of the electrons into their lower energy states. If this decay occurs in the visible spectrum, it is called luminescence.

Fluorescence

Fluorescence is luminescence that is maintained only by continuous excitation. In other words, excitation at one wavelength occurs and is emitted immediately through a longer wavelength.

Dye Used in Fluorescein Angiography

Sodium fluorescein is an orange-red crystalline hydrocarbon ($C_{20}H_{12}O_5Na_2$). It is effective at a pH of 7.37–7.45. 80% of the fluorescein is bound to protein and 20% remains free in the bloodstream, which is available for fluorescence. It is excreted by the kidneys and liver, usually within 24 hours. The most commonly used solution is a 3 mL vial of 20% fluorescein. Other concentrations available are 5 mL of 10% fluorescein and 10 mL of 5% fluorescein. If blue light (465–490 nm) is directed to unbound sodium fluorescein it will emit a light that appears green (520–530 nm). This is the fundamental principle of FA. For this the fundus camera has two types of filters: a blue excitation filter and a green barrier filter. These filters ensure that blue light enters the eye and only green light enters the camera. The blue flash of the fundus camera excites the unbound fluorescein within the blood vessels or the fluorescein that has leaked out of the blood vessels. The blue light then changes those structures in the eye containing fluorescein to green-yellow light at 520–530 nm. Blue light is reflected off the fundus structures that do not contain fluorescein. The blue reflected light and the green-yellow fluorescent light are directed back toward the film of the fundus camera. The barrier filter allows the green-yellow fluorescent light through but blocks the blue light. Therefore the only light that penetrates the filter is true fluorescent light.

■ PROCEDURE

Following pupillary dilatation, color fundus photograph and a red free photograph are taken first. This is followed by a control photograph with the filters in place to check for any pseudofluorescence. Then the fluorescein is injected rapidly into the antecubital vein over 4–6 seconds and photographs are taken at approximately 1–2 seconds interval between 5 and 25 seconds after injection. After transit phase has been photographed in the concerned eye, control photographs are taken of opposite eye. Late photographs can be taken 10 minutes and 20 minutes after injection.

■ PHASES OF A NORMAL ANGIOGRAM

Arm-retina time: Time taken for the first fluorescence to appear after the injection of dye. It is usually 10–12 seconds.

Choroidal flush: The early phase of choroidal fluorescence, which usually begins 1–2 seconds prior to appearance of dye in the central retinal artery, is called as choroidal flush. It appears patchy and irregularly scattered throughout the fundus due to the lobular architecture of the choroid. When present, a cilioretinal artery usually begins to fluoresce during this phase, prior to appearance of dye in the retinal arterioles **(Fig. 7.13.1)**.

Arterial phase: Appears at 10–15 seconds after the injection. After the central retinal artery begins to fill, the fluorescein flows into the retinal arteries.

Laminar flow: 14–15 seconds. When the fluorescein enters the veins the appearance of fluorescein in the veins is laminar. This occurs because the dye enters the veins along its walls. As the blood flow is faster in the center of a lumen than on the sides, the fluorescein seems to stick to the sides (hyperfluorescent) and the center remains dark (hypofluorescent) giving rise to the laminar flow.

Venous phase: 16–17 seconds. The fluorescence of the two laminae progressively thicken resulting in complete fluorescence of the veins.

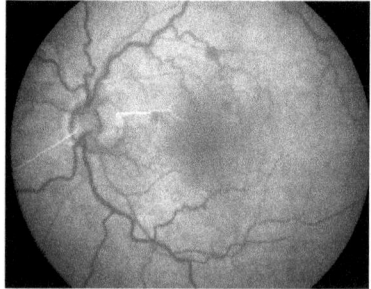

Fig. 7.13.1: Angiogram showing the choroidal flush with filling of two cilioretinal arteries. No dye is visible in the retinal arterioles as yet.

Peak phase: At around 20–25 seconds after the injection the fluorescence of the veins reaches its maximum.

Recirculation phase: The dye begins to slowly empty from the retinal and choroidal circulations. In majority of normal angiograms vessels are completely empty of fluorescein in approximately 10 minutes.

The large choroidal vessels and the retinal vessels do not leak fluorescein. However, the choriocapillaris do leak fluorescein. The extravasated fluorescein diffuses through the choroidal tissue, Bruch's membrane, and sclera. In the later phase of the angiogram, staining of Bruch's membrane, the choroid, and especially the sclera may be visible if the pigment epithelium is lightly pigmented.

■ PATTERNS OF ABNORMAL FLUORESCENCE

Hypofluorescence

Any abnormally dark area in the angiogram is termed as hypofluorescence. Hypofluorescence can be due to two possible causes:

1. *Blocked (masked) fluorescence:* Occurs due to a barrier (e.g., blood or pigment such as melanin or lipofuscin) anterior to either the retinal or choroidal fluorescence **(Figs. 7.13.2A to D)**.
2. *Vascular filling defect:* Results from obstruction to retinal and/or choroidal blood flow (e.g., capillary dropout in proliferative diabetic retinopathy) **(Figs. 7.13.2A to D)**.

The key to differentiate the two is to correlate the angiogram with the color fundus photograph. If there is a lesion that corresponds in size, shape, and location to the hypofluorescence on the angiogram, then it is blocked fluorescence. If there is no corresponding lesion on the color photograph, then the hypofluorescence is likely due to a vascular filling defect.

Hyperfluorescence

Abnormally bright area in the angiogram is called hyperfluorescence. There are three possible causes of abnormal hyperfluorescence:

1. *Preinjection fluorescence:* Hyperfluorescence seen before fluorescein dye in injected. It could result from structures that normally fluoresce (autofluorescence) or by

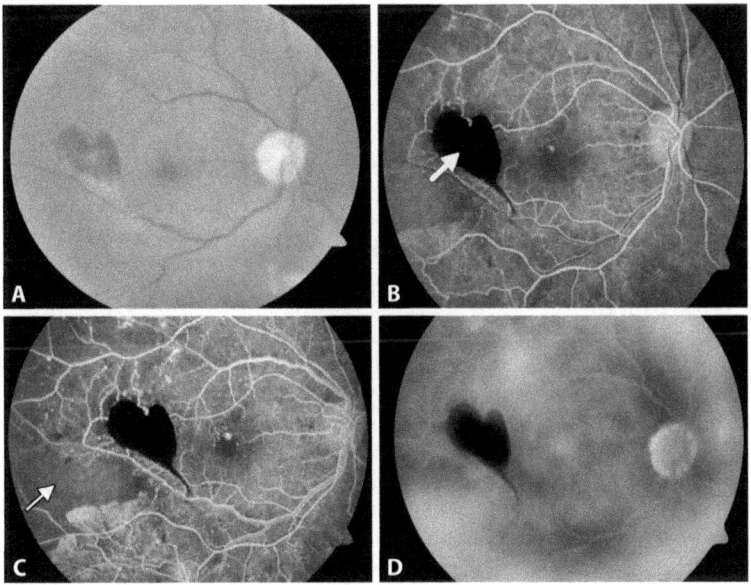

Figs. 7.13.2A to D: Fluorescein angiogram of a patient with proliferative diabetic retinopathy. Blocked fluorescence (B, yellow arrow) due to a preretinal hemorrhage corresponds exactly to the hemorrhage seen on the fundus photograph in size, shape, and location (A). In addition vascular filling defect due to capillary nonperfusion (white arrow, C) and leakage (D) in the late phase are seen.

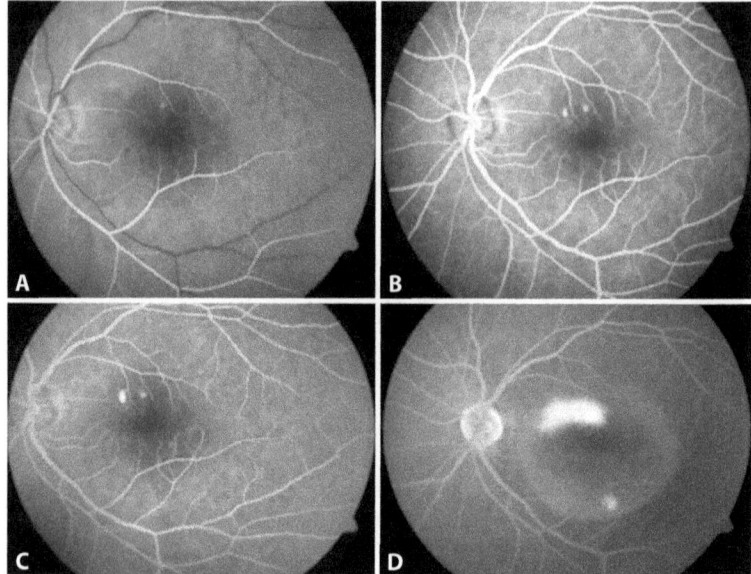

Figs. 7.13.3A to D: A patient of central serous chorioretinopathy showing appearance of early hyperfluorescence which assumes a smoke stack pattern in the late phases.

poorly matched filters (pseudofluorescence). Autofluorescence is seen in optic nerve head drusen and astrocytic hamartoma.

2. Early hyperfluorescence can occur with either retinal (e.g., neovascularization, aneurysms, and telangiectasia) or choroidal vessels [e.g., retinal pigment epithelial (RPE) window defect and choroidal neovascular membranes] **(Figs. 7.13.3A to D)**.

3. *Late hyperfluorescence:* Hyperfluorescence occurring in the late or extravascular phase of the angiogram could be normal (disc margins, crescent, or sclera) or due to leakage (e.g., cystoid macular edema), pooling, or staining **(Figs. 7.13.4)**.

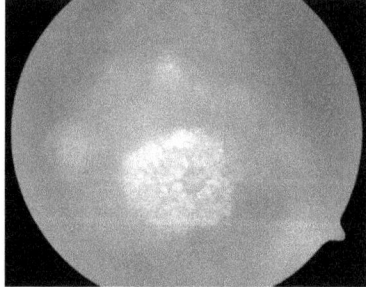

Fig. 7.13.4: Late phase angiogram showing leakage forming a classic petaloid appearance of cystoid macular edema.

When early hyperfluorescence increases in size and intensity with time, it is called leakage. This happens due to extravasation of dye from disruption of inner blood-retinal barrier (e.g., cystoid macular edema). If the intensity of hyperfluorescence increases with time but the size and boundary of the hyperfluorescence remains fairly same in subsequent phases of angiogram, it is denoted as pooling. It occurs due to disruption of outer blood-retinal barrier [e.g., subretinal pooling in central serous chorioretinopathy (CSCR) or sub-RPE pooling in pigment epithelial detachment]. If the hyperfluorescence appears early but its intensity, size, and boundary remains same in subsequent phases, it is called as transmission fluorescence or window defect (e.g., RPE atrophy).

CLINICAL USES

Some of the commonly used indications for fundus fluorescein angiography (FFA) include:
- *Diabetic retinopathy:* Detection of leaky microaneurysms, extent of capillary nonperfusion area, macular ischemia, and neovascularization

- *Age-related macular degeneration (AMD):* Differentiate dry from wet AMD by the presence of choroidal neovascular membranes
- *Vascular occlusions:* Detect degree of ischemia, reperfusion, and neovascularization
- *Intraocular tumors:* Melanoma, hemangioma, osteoma, etc.
- *Uveitis:* Retinal vasculitis, choroiditis, retinitis, cystoid macular edema, and ischemia
- CSCR (smoke stack, inkblot, or diffuse)
- *Optic nerve lesions:* Leakage and nonperfusion.

ADVERSE EFFECTS

- Mild yellowing of skin, conjunctiva for 6–12 hours and yellow-orange discoloration of urine may be noticed for the first day. Transient nausea and vomiting can occur in <5% cases.
- Injection site may have extravasation under the skin leading to sloughing, necrosis, and thrombophlebitis.
- Allergic reactions may range from mild itching to severe anaphylaxis. Vasovagal reaction, shock, and syncope may occur rarely.

CONTRAINDICATIONS

- It is absolutely contraindicated in patients with prior allergy to the dye.
- Severe hepatic or renal impairment, pregnancy (especially in the first trimester), and lactating mothers are relative contraindications.

NEW ADDITIONS TO STANDARD FLUORESCEIN ANGIOGRAPHY

Oral Angiography

As the conventional FFA is based upon intravenous fluorescein injection, it is difficult to perform in children and may need to be performed under anesthesia. Hence, oral FFA[3] has been proposed as an alternative to conventional intravenous FFA. Body weight adjusted oral fluorescein is mixed with fruit juice and the mixture is rapidly ingested in a quick gulp in oral FFA. While a standard intravenous fluorescein angiogram for an adult would use 20% fluorescein at 0.07 mL/kg, the same can be used in children at a dose of 0.0375 mL/kg for a 20% solution. Image acquisition is started immediately and continued till the late phase images are taken. Although the use of oral FFA has the limitation of poor information on the choroidal flush, arm to retina time, and unclear differentiation between various angiographic phases, it still provides reasonable information in some pediatric retinal diseases, such as familial exudative vitreoretinopathy (FEVR), Coats disease, and uveitis. Moreover, the rate and severity of adverse reaction with oral angiography is much less than in intravenous FFA.[4]

Ultra-widefield Angiography

These include the Optos® fundus camera (Optos Plc, Dunfermline, Scotland, UK) which can capture up to 200° of the fundus in a single photo, greater than the 30 or 50° images typically captured by standard fundus cameras. This allows better visualization retinal changes such as neovascularization and capillary nonperfusion as in diabetic retinopathy, retinal vasculitis, and familial exudative vitreoretinopathy (**Figs. 7.13.5A to C**). Another ultra-widefield angiography (UWFA) system is the Retcam (Clarity Medical Systems, Inc., Pleasanton, CA, USA), which can capture up to 130° and is especially useful for angiography of neonates in retinopathy of prematurity (**Fig. 7.13.6**). UWFA has the advantage of wider field of view, faster acquisition, high resolution images, and its ability to scan in nonmydriatic pupil also. UWFA has the disadvantage of high cost, peripheral distortion, and magnification of images (leading to error in peripheral measurements), pesudocolored fundus images, poor visibility of vertical peripheries as compared to horizontal peripheries, and artefacts from eyelashes or lid margins.

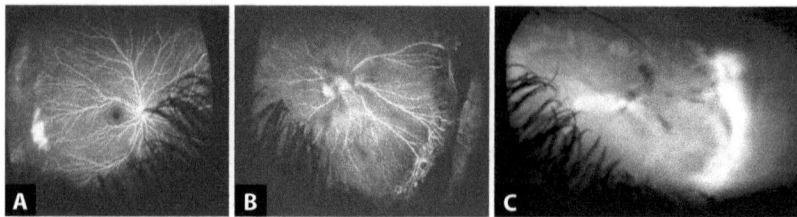

Figs. 7.13.5A to C: Ultra-widefield angiography of a patient with familial exudative vitreoretinopathy demonstrating peripheral avascular retina in the right (A) and left eye (B) with neovascularization causing leakage in the late phase (C).

Scanning Laser Ophthalmoscopy-based Angiography

Instead of a bright flash of white light as in traditional photography, scanning laser ophthalmoscopy (SLO) uses laser light to illuminate the retina. The advantages of using SLO over traditional fundus photography include improved image quality and resolution, suppression of scattered light, and improved patient comfort through less bright light. Examples of SLO-based imaging include Optos® camera (Optos PLC, Dunfermline, UK), and Spectralis® (Heidelberg Retina Angiograph, HRA 2, Heidelberg Engineering, Germany). HRA 2 allows multimodal imaging and simultaneous fluorescein and indocyanine green angiography is possible.

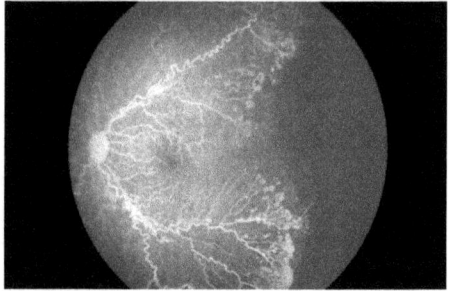

Fig. 7.13.6: Ultra-widefield fluorescein angiogram of the left eye of an infant with retinopathy of prematurity previously treated with antivascular endothelial growth factor (VEGF) therapy showing persistent vascularity of the peripheral retina with neovascular tufts at the vascular-avascular junction along with vascular tortuosity.

Optical Coherence Tomography Angiography

Optical coherence tomography angiography (OCTA) is a new noninvasive and motion contrast imaging modality. Based on two technologies, split-spectrum amplitude decorrelation angiography (SSADA) and motion correction technology (MCT), Angiovue® (Optovue Inc., Fremont, USA) is a dye-less depth resolved imaging system that allows imaging of the superficial as well as the deep capillary plexus not visible on the traditional angiograms. OCTA has the advantage of being quick, noninvasive, can acquire volumetric scans that can be segmented to specific depths, avoids dye-associated complications, can precisely determine size and location, visualize both retinal as well as choroidal vascularization, and provides structural and flow-based information in tandem. However, OCTA has the disadvantage of limited view, more artifacts (movement, blinks, and vessel ghosting) and it is unable to provide information about leakage.

■ REFERENCES

1. Ryan SJ, Schachat AP, Wilkinson CP. Fluorescein angiography: Basic principles and interpretation. In: Ryan SJ (Ed). Retina, 5th edition. Toronto: Elsevier; 2013. pp. 1-50.
2. Bennett TJ, Quillen DA, Coronica R. Fundamentals of Fluorescein Angiography. Insight. 2016;41(1):5-11.
3. Ali SMA, Khan I, Khurram D, Kozak I. Ultra-Widefield angiography with oral fluorescein in pediatric patients with retinal disease. JAMA Ophthalmol. 2018;136(5):593-4.
4. Sambhav K, Grover S, Chalam KV. The application of optical coherence tomography angiography in retinal diseases. Surv Ophthalmol. 2017;62(6):838-66.

7.14 Macular Telangiectasia

Dhananjay Shukla
Ratan Jyoti Netralaya, Gwalior
daksh66@gmail.com

Jay Kalliath
NMC Specialty Hospital, UAE

■ EVOLUTION OF THE NOMENCLATURE

The term "retinal telangiectasia" alludes to an irregular dilation and leakage of the retinal capillaries; this capillaropathy can occur anywhere in the fundus. Reese first used this term for a wide range of capillary anomalies from microaneurysms to Coat's disease. Gass and Oyakawa (1982) introduced a precise term *idiopathic juxtafoveolar retinal telangiectasis* to exclude the common and better-known telangiectasia secondary to retinal vascular diseases. Gass and Blodi later revised this classification (1993). Yannuzzi and colleagues simplified Gass' complex classification and called the condition *idiopathic macular telangiectasia*. The macular telangiectasia (MacTel) project, which started in 2005, has given a still simpler name to the condition: *macular telangiectasia* or just *MacTel*, which is the current, and hopefully the final nomenclature for this condition.

■ CLASSIFICATION AND STAGING OF MACULAR TELANGIECTASIA

Yannuzzi et al. (2006) recognized two distinct types of macular telangiectasia (MacTel): Type 1 or aneurysmal telangiectasia was a milder variant of Coat's disease, with similar demographics, clinical features, and response to treatment. Type 2 or perifoveal telangiectasia presented with subtle or occult telangiectasia and minimal exudation **(Table 7.14.1)**. Yannuzzi et al. described two stages of type 2 MacTel: a nonproliferative stage, and a later stage of intra- and subretinal neovascularization (SRNV), almost invariably associated with significant visual loss **(Fig. 7.14.1A)**. Type 2 MacTel typically appears as a gray opacification of macula, with or without intraretinal crystalline deposits, right-angled venules, and stellate plaques of inwardly migrating retinal pigment **(Fig. 7.14.1B)**.

TABLE 7.14.1: Two major types of macular telangiectasia.

	MacTel type 1	MacTel type 2
Mean age (years)	40	50–60
Sex	Male	No gender bias
Laterality	Unilateral	Bilateral; frequently asymmetrical
Clinical appearance	Clinically obvious telangiectasia and exudates	Telangiectasia subtle; graying of macula; fine crystalline deposits
Macular thickening	Significant and common	Thickening rare; atrophy common
Visual prognosis	Most lose vision if edema not treated	Most retain vision within 1–2 Snellen lines, unless neovascularization occurs
Angiographic leakage	Significant; extramacular leakage common	Subtle and wispy; only parafoveal
Treatability	Responds moderately to laser and antivascular endothelial growth factor (VEGF) injections	Treatment usually recommended only if neovascularization occurs

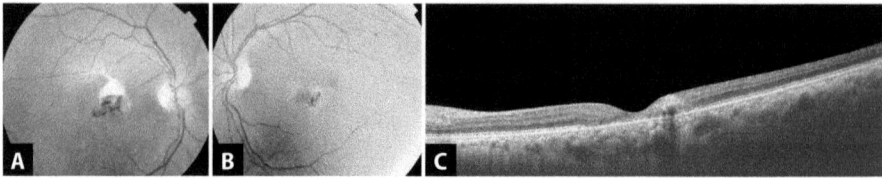

Figs. 7.14.1A to C: Proliferative and nonproliferative stages of type 2 macular telangiectasia (MacTel 2). (A) Right eye (RE) shows severe scarring and background pigment epithelial atrophy secondary to subretinal neovascularization. The stellate pigment plaques are the clue to MacTel; (B) Left eye (LE) of the same patient shows all the features of nonproliferative MacTel 2: doughnut-shaped gray opacification of the central macula resembling a bull's eye pattern, crystalline deposits, two parallel right-angled venules inferotemporal to center, and stellate pigmentary plaques at the tip of the superior venules of the pair. The faint microaneurysms and a dot hemorrhage are secondary to background diabetic retinopathy; (C) Spectral-domain optical coherence tomography (OCT) of LE shows foveal atrophy (central macular thickness: 94 µm), and perifoveolar collapse of the outer nuclear layer and outer retinal bands. Inner retinal hyper-reflectivity temporal to fovea corresponds to the stellate pigment plaques.

Telangiectasia, as mentioned before, is usually unnoticeable. Chew and colleagues from MacTel Study Group have recently proposed an optical coherence tomography (OCT)-based classification of MacTel 2, the MacTel type which predominates the current research and clinical experience (ARVO 2019). This review henceforth is focused on the most common type, MacTel 2; and refers to it by default, unless specified.

■ EPIDEMIOLOGY AND NATURAL HISTORY

MacTel has been frequently underdiagnosed and misdiagnosed, mainly due to low awareness about it. MacTel 2 is now known to be much more common than previously believed; Klein and colleagues estimated the prevalence of MacTel 2 to be 1 in 1,000 in subjects above 40 years of age in the Beaver Dam Study; and some authorities believe this figure might be an underestimation, as the fundus picture-based diagnosis was not aided by sensitive imaging tools such as fluorescein angiography (FA), OCT, and autofluorescence (AF) imaging. When we consider that a condition like central retinal vein occlusion, which most ophthalmologists are familiar with, has a similar prevalence, we begin to realize how frequently MacTel must be slipping under the radar.

MacTel is an enigma in natural history too: visual loss is invariable when SRNV (most commonly subfoveal) occurs; but the natural course of nonproliferative MacTel is not clear in the literature. Though Gass and Blodi suggested that gradual visual loss occurred due to foveal atrophy, its frequency, and diagnosis were not documented. Other authors disagree on the extent and frequency of visual loss. The MacTel study (report # 8) recently reported that the visual prognosis of MacTel 2 was not black-and-white: While a progressive neurodegeneration and corresponding visual decline does occur in most patients, the process is very gradual, so that >80% retain driving vision (6/12 or better) at least in one eye, irrespective of the development of SRNV. Severe visual loss (visual acuity of 6/60 or less) occurs in only a minority (<5%) of the eyes: the major cause is foveal atrophy; SRNV is less common. Visual acuity is therefore not a true reflection of the patient's symptoms. The measurements of visual scotoma, metamorphopsia, and near vision are more sensitive parameters of visual dysfunction than visual acuity.

■ CLINICAL FEATURES AND DIFFERENTIAL DIAGNOSIS

Impaired reading vision is the most common presenting complaint (≈80% patients). It is essential to suspect MacTel 2 clinically and differentiate it from the myriad similar conditions. In the earliest stage however, the macula looks normal, and the diagnosis is based on FA, AF, and OCT (discussed later). This elusive stage is sometimes picked up on imaging in the normal-looking fellow eye of an apparently unilateral MacTel 2, which is bilateral but frequently asymmetric in presentation. Later, the macula frequently develops a gray opacification, resembling *bull's eye* maculopathy; telangiectasia is still not visible. This is the earliest and the most frequent clinical appearance, and the cause of most confusion. Helpful clinical features include right-angled venules (which dip backward into retina), stellate pigment epithelial plaques, and crystalline deposits, which are much sparser, more superficial, and finer than hard exudates **(Fig. 7.14.2A)**.

The differential diagnosis includes many common retinal disorders, and includes not only vascular but also degenerative conditions. Diabetic maculopathy needs to be frequently differentiated from MacTel in a diabetic patient. In our experience, the most common mimics include heredomacular degenerations and drug toxicity (e.g., cone dystrophy, hydrochloroquine maculopathy) causing bull's eye maculopathy, chronic central serous chorioretinopathy, and (in the older patients), exudative age-related macular degeneration when MacTel is associated with SRNV. Less commonly, conditions causing crystal deposition in the posterior pole, including tamoxifen retinopathy and Bietti's crystalline dystrophy can also be mistaken for MacTel. In most of these scenarios, routine investigations such as FA and OCT, along with clinical evaluation, are sufficient to clinch the diagnosis.

DIAGNOSTIC INVESTIGATIONS

Gass and Blodi described FA as the key diagnostic investigation. It confirms the diagnosis in early and doubtful cases. In the earliest stage with no visible lesion in the macula, FA shows a characteristic faint, wispy late leakage from the telangiectasia, most prominently at the temporal aspect of foveal avascular zone **(Fig. 7.14.2B)**. When SRNV is present, its intense leakage is superimposed over the faint leakage of the telangiectasia.

Now spectral-domain OCT has become the most favored diagnostic tool for MacTel. The findings, though not pathognomonic, are very helpful in clinching the diagnosis. The most dramatic OCT feature of MacTel is foveal atrophy **(Fig. 7.14.1C)**, which is counterintuitive to the leakage seen on FA. Another common feature is foveal outer and inner lamellar cavitations. The earliest OCT sign is a temporal widening of the foveolar clivus. However, the key OCT correlate of visual deterioration is the loss of paracentral and then central ellipsoid zone, which occurs well before the foveal thinning. Outer retinal hyper-reflective lesions precede the clinical appearance of retinal pigment clumps, which in turn are a precursor of outer retinal and subretinal neovascular proliferation. Another interesting recent observation is that subretinal fluid on OCT may herald SRNV,

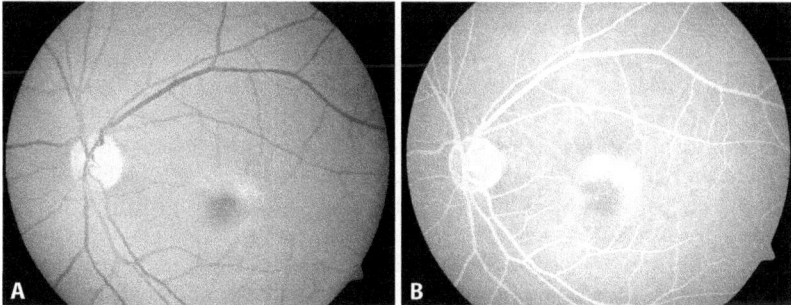

Figs. 7.14.2A and B: Nonproliferative MacTel 2: fluorescein angiography. (A) Fundus picture of left eye (LE): Besides the perifoveal gray discoloration, note the crystalline deposits, which are finer than hard exudates; (B) Late-phase fluorescein angiogram LE shows a wispy perifoveal capillary leakage, more prominent superiorly; this leakage is fainter and different in character (no honeycomb or flower petal pattern) from that seen in macular edema.

and in fact, represents a preproliferative stage of MacTel, amenable to pharmacotherapy. Rarely, full-thickness macular hole may occur in MacTel, but degenerative component makes surgery less rewarding.

Fundus AF imaging measures the accumulation of lipofuscin (a metabolic residue of phagocytosis and aging in the retinal pigment epithelium) in the fundus, a common sequel of several degenerative diseases of the outer retina and retinal pigment epithelium. Increased temporal parafoveal AF signal, due to the loss of luteal pigment, is considered one of the early and sensitive signs of MacTel. AF changes are almost universal in MacTel; and may serve not only as a diagnostic adjunct, but a standalone diagnostic tool for trained observers **(Fig. 7.14.3)**.

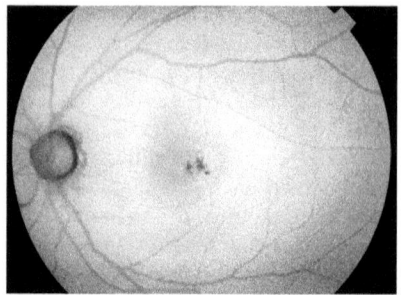

Fig. 7.14.3: Fundus autofluorescence imaging. Left eye (LE) of this patient clinically showed a nonproliferative MacTel 2 with pigment plaques. Autofluorescence imaging shows blocked signal from the plaques, as well as the characteristic increased autofluorescence of MacTel, especially temporally.

Optical coherence tomography angiography (OCTA) is useful in initially detecting bunching of deep perifoveal capillaries, indicating a preproliferative stage of MacTel (Venkatesh et al, 2020). Retinal subsidence due to vascular contracture and retinal thinning can masquerade SRNV on OCTA (projection artefact). Later, OCTA helps noninvasively in detecting outer retinal and SRNV and retinochoroidal anastomosis with disease progression. Intraretinal neovascularization is a characteristic feature of MacTel 2 and corresponds with the OCT feature of outer retinal hyper-reflectivity, both of which begin at the temporal edge of ellipsoid zone loss **(Figs. 7.14.4A and B)**.

Fundus microperimetry has already been used in MacTel to plot central scotomas; adaptive optics imaging was recently used to measure cone density in MacTel. As technology continues to improve, imaging for MacTel is likely to become progressively noninvasive, and yet more specific and sensitive for the pathology.

■ PATHOPHYSIOLOGY AND SYSTEMIC ASSOCIATIONS

Though MacTel was initially described by Gass and Blodi as a perifoveal capillary disease, the term now appears to be a misnomer; as more and more recent investigations point to a degenerative disease, primarily affecting the neural retina; vascular pathology merely adding to the disease manifestations. The foveal thinning and the absence of cystoid macular edema suggest that the primary pathology lies in perifoveal neural cells or Müller cells. Gass suggested that in this condition, the neovascularization originated from the outer retina rather than from choroid. This pattern of neovascularization was later called as type 3 neovascularization by Yannuzzi because the SRNV does not arise from choroid, it cannot be called either classic (type 2) or occult (type 1). Gass's suggestion of the role of Müller cell dysfunction in pathogenesis was endorsed by the subsequent immunohistochemical reports, which also confirmed the loss of macular pigment as a key pathological event, as also demonstrated in vivo by AF imaging.

Another pathogenetic aspect of MacTel was reported by Eliassi-Rad and Green, who demonstrated histopathological changes similar to diabetes in perifoveal capillaries: basement membrane thickening, loss of pericytes and capillary endothelial degeneration. Though systemic vascular/metabolic diseases such as diabetes, hypertension, obesity, and cardiovascular disease are not causally related to MacTel, several investigators including the MacTel study concur that these systemic associations are common compared to chronological peers in generally older communities and may share similar pathogenesis.

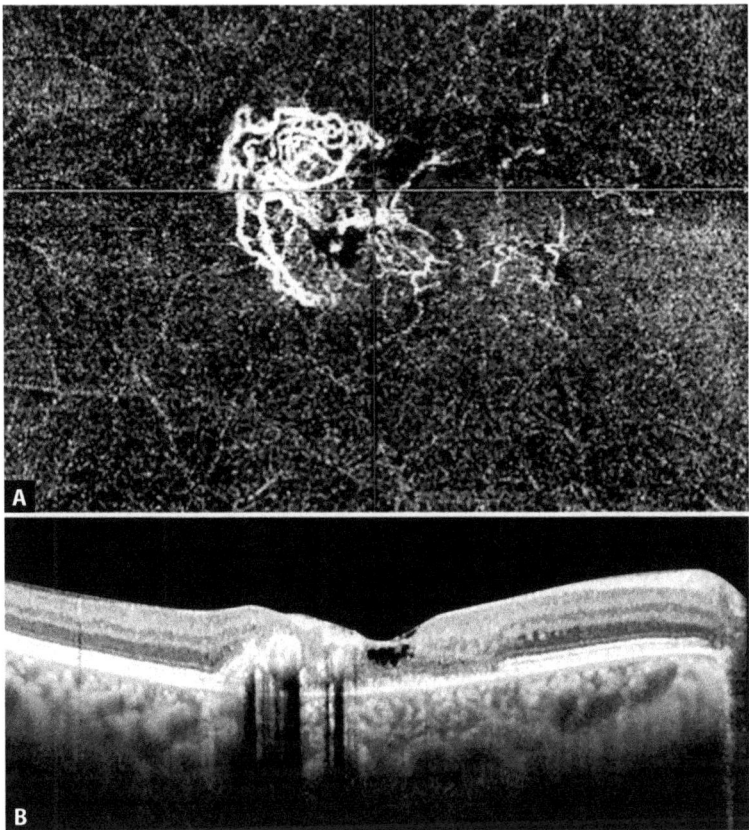

Figs. 7.14.4A and B: Optical coherence tomography (OCT) angiography and corresponding OCT. (A) Right eye (RE) of this patient with MacTel 2 reveals distinct outer retinal neovascularization temporal to fovea; (B) Horizontal OCT through shows central foveal cavitation with extensive loss of ellipsoid zone. Outer retinal hyper-reflectivity at the temporal edge of ellipsoid zone defect corresponds to intraretinal neovascularization, characteristic of MacTel 2.

TREATMENT

More than 80% of eyes which develop SRNV lose vision to 6/60 or less; proliferative stage of MacTel is therefore always treated. Treatment of nonproliferative MacTel has also been attempted by several authors, almost universally without success; and no treatment has been shown to prevent disease progression either. In fact, laser photocoagulation and anti-VEGF treatments may be harmful at the nonproliferative stage of MacTel. There is probably some rationale for anti-VEGF treatment at "preproliferative stage", specifically in presence of subfoveal fluid, when the degenerative element has been excluded by OCT (Mayanath et al, 2019). A role of antioxidant supplementation has been suggested in view of the neurodegenerative nature of MacTel. A phase 2 randomized multicenter trial of intravitreal injection of a neuroprotective agent [ciliary neurotrophic factor (CNTF)] has reported the safety and efficacy of CNTF, both in limiting ellipsoid zone loss (a surrogate for progressive neurodegeneration) and maintaining the reading speed. Two phase 3 trials are underway to evolve treatment recommendations.

Subretinal neovascularization in MacTel has historically been treated with trans-pupillary thermotherapy (TTT), photodynamic therapy (PDT), and anti-VEGF agents, standalone or in combination. Since the neovascularization starts intraretinally (type 3), surgical removal is contraindicated. Several studies have established the anti-VEGF drugs as the treatment of choice in proliferative stage of MacTel, with better safety and efficacy profile over subthreshold photocoagulation alternatives.

■ SUMMARY AND TAKE HOME MESSAGE

MacTel 2 is the most common, but ironically the most underdiagnosed and misdiagnosed type of primary retinal telangiectasia; and closely resembles several other common vascular and degenerative macular diseases. The complexity and urgency of diagnosis are increased by the coincidence of diabetes, and the subsequent confusion with diabetic macular edema. While photocoagulation helps in the treatment of diabetic macular edema, it can be harmful in nonproliferative MacTel. MacTel is usually not amenable to treatment at nonproliferative stage; but SRNV urgently requires treatment with anti-VEGF agents. Though a gradual, mild-moderate visual loss occurs over time due to progressive neurodegeneration in MacTel 2, most patients are likely to retain good vision in at least one eye. Neovascular complications develop only in a minority of the patients, severe vision loss is rare. Clinical suspicion and noninvasive tests such as AF, OCT, and OCTA can confirm diagnosis and avoid futile investigations and potentially harmful treatment for this enigmatic disease.

■ SUGGESTED READING

1. Chew EY, Spaide RF. Macular telangiectasia type 2. In: Sadda SR (Ed). Ryan's Retina, 7th edition. Amsterdam, Netherlands: Elsevier; 2022. pp. 1204-17.
2. Heeren TFC, Chew EY, Clemons T, Fruttiger M, Balaskas K, Schwartz R, et al. Macular Telangiectasia Type 2: Visual Acuity, Disease End Stage, and the MacTel Area: MacTel Project Report Number 8. Ophthalmology. 2020;127:1539-48.

7.15 | Polypoidal Choroidal Vasculopathy

Dinesh Talwar, Saurabh Arora
Centre for Sight, New Delhi
dineshtalwar@yahoo.co.uk

■ DEFINITION

Polypoidal choroidal vasculopathy (PCV) is a disorder characterized by abnormally branching choroidal vascular networks associated with polypoidal lesions that result in serosanguineous neurosensory and/or retinal pigment epithelial detachment (PED). The word "idiopathic" was later dropped from the nomenclature given initially to this disease. The definition of PCV as a clinical entity now considers it as prevalent either at the macula or in the peripapillary region in elderly people irrespective of race and gender **(Figs. 7.15.1A to C)**.

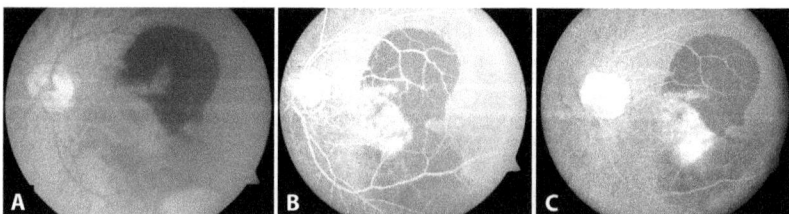

Figs. 7.15.1A to C: (A) Fundus photograph showing large subretinal hemorrhage; (B) Polyps in macular area on fundus fluorescein angiography (FFA); (C) Late phase of FFA shows increase in leakage in macular area.

HISTORY

The disease was initially described as peripapillary lesions in black women in the 7th and 8th decade by Yannuzzi in 1982 in a meeting of the Macula Society. Later, Kleiner et al. described a similar group of patients with the nomenclature "posterior uveal bleeding syndrome".

EPIDEMIOLOGY

Polypoidal choroidal vasculopathy shows a predilection for more heavily pigmented individuals, notably blacks, Asians and Hispanics. The disorder is most commonly seen in Asians, accounting for 23.0-54.7% of patients with neovascular age-related macular degeneration (ARMD) in people of Japanese descent, and 22.3-24.5% of patients of Chinese descent, with a male preponderance. However, it also accounts for 8-12% of exudative ARMD in Caucasians, with a female predominance. The disease has been described in African Americans and is also fairly common in other colored races including Indians. PCV occurs at a younger age than ARMD, and patients are usually between 50 and 65 years of age although the range in which the abnormality may first appear is wider and ranges from the third to the ninth decade of life.

CLINICAL FEATURES

Usual Presentation

Complaints of blurring of vision often of acute onset or relatively short duration but some time, the patient may present late, especially if the fellow eye vision is good.

Fundus Picture

Characteristic clinical features are one or more areas of moderate to large subretinal hemorrhage which is/are located subfoveally or in an extrafoveal location. The severity of the subretinal hemorrhage in PCV is significantly more than in cases of ARMD.

A characteristic feature, seen in many cases, is the presence of orange red polypoidal lesions due to dilated, choroidal vascular channels in peripapillary and macular area (single or multiple) **(Fig. 7.15.2)**. However, these are not always clearly visible due to the overlying retinal pigment epithelium (RPE) with pigmentation or could be obscured due to the subretinal hemorrhage.

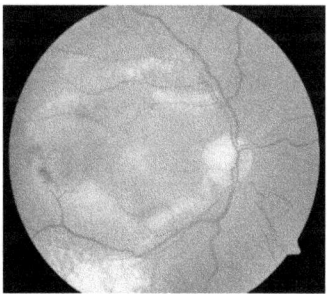

Fig. 7.15.2: Fundus picture demonstrating orange-red lesion with surrounding area of lipid exudation.

The subretinal hemorrhages and the polyps may or may not be associated with RPE detachment(s); sometimes there is a predominantly exudative response with extensive lipid deposition. Patients with extensive subretinal hemorrhage could occasionally develop vitreous hemorrhage also. The disease is often bilateral but asymmetrical.

Fluorescein Angiography

The fluorescein angiographic picture is that of an occult or minimally classic choroidal neovascularization (CNV). Early phase angiograms may show clusters of polyps and lead one to suspect the diagnosis based on the clinical picture and fluorescein angiogram alone. However, usually overlying intense fluorescence of the choriocapillaris masks the lesions of PCV which are in the inner choroid. Subretinal fibrinous material, if it exists, can be observed as an expanding fluorescent leakage that may simulate the classic lesion of exudative ARMD found by fluorescein angiography (FA).

Indocyanine Green Angiography

The diagnosis of PCV is confirmed only by indocyanine green angiography (ICGA). ICGA features of PCV are visible in the early phases of the angiogram and include polyps (which may appear pulsatile on video ICGA), and branching vascular networks (BVNs). Polyps are identified as typical focal areas of nodular hyperfluorescence within the first 5-6 minutes and are a sign of active disease **(Figs. 7.15.3A to D)**.

The definition of characteristic polyp lesion given in the EVEREST study includes early subretinal focal ICGA hyperfluorescence (appearing within the first 6 minutes of ICGA) and one of the following ICG angiographic criteria:
- Association with a BVN
- Presence of pulsation
- Nodular appearance when viewed stereoscopically
- Presence of hypofluorescent halo (in first 6 minutes)
- Orange subretinal nodule in stereoscopic color fundus photograph
- Associated with massive submacular hemorrhage (defined as size of hemorrhage of at least four disc areas)

Late phase of the ICGA may reveal staining of the area of the lesion. Polypoidal lesions most commonly appear in clusters, but could occur in isolation or in a string configuration

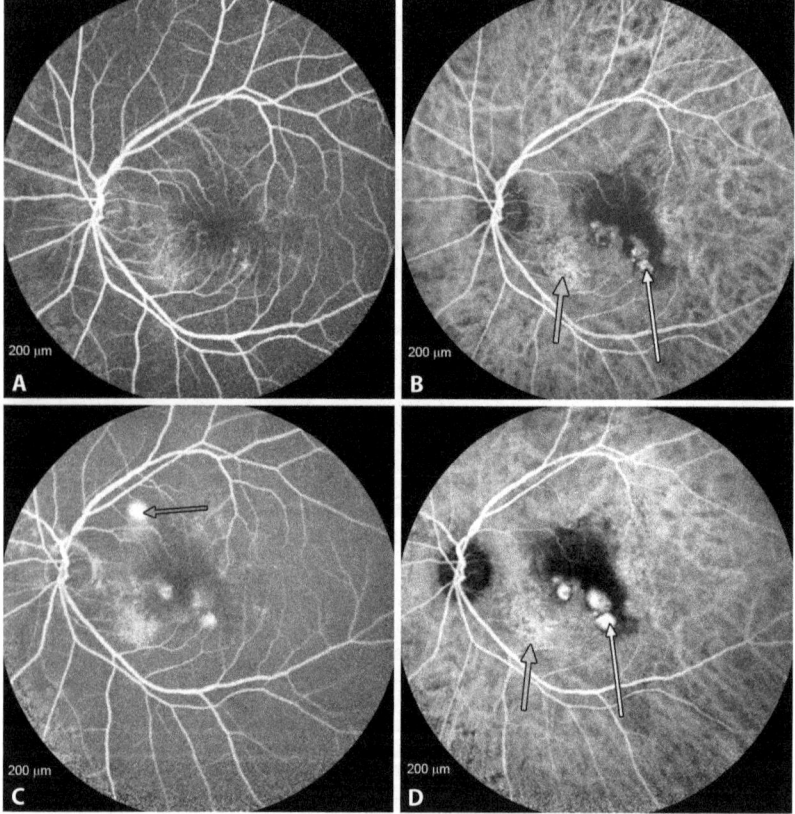

Figs. 7.15.3A to D: Indocyanine green angiography. (A) Revealing polyp in early phase which is staining in midphase; (B) Branching vascular network seen in peripapillary area (green arrow) with polyps in macula (yellow arrows); (C) Fundus fluorescein angiography (FFA) shows fibrinous material with increasing fluorescence (red arrow); (D) Late stage angiogram showing polyps (yellow arrow) and diffuse hyperfluorescence (green arrow).

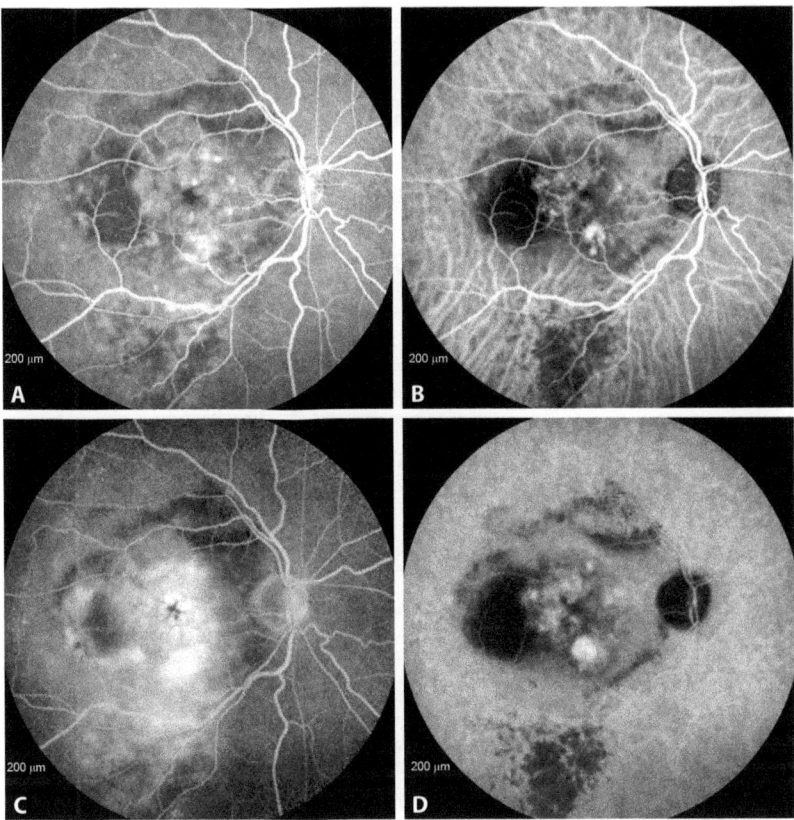

Figs. 7.15.4A to D: (A) Fundus fluorescein angiography (FFA)—midphase shows lesions suspected to be polypoidal in nature; (B) Indocyanine green angiography (ICGA) within first 6 minutes demonstrates presence of polyps; (C) Late phase FFA shows intense leakage with FFA suggestive of minimally classic choroidal neovascularization (CNV); (D) ICGA—late phase shows polyp with staining.

on ICGA **(Figs. 7.15.4A to D)**. ICGA is essential not only for the diagnosis but also for assessing response to treatment.

Optical Coherence Tomography

Optical coherence tomography (OCT) reveals the presence of subretinal fluid or blood, RPE detachments and polyps in areas delineated by FFA and ICGA. OCT is used as a guide to monitor the treatment response. Typical OCT changes seen in PCV are described here **(Figs. 7.15.5A to C)**. High-resolution OCT demonstrates the location of the polyps just beneath RPE and attached to the outer surface of the RPE. OCT features which are important include:

- *Tomographic notch sign* which is due to a sharply elevated "tall PED", which may overlie the polyp itself.
- *Double layer sign* which consists of two hyper-reflective lines, representing the RPE and Bruch's membrane, respectively, and corresponding to the extent of late geographic hyperfluorescence on ICGA. This sign represents the BVN invading into the space between the RPE and Bruch's membrane.
- Increased choroidal thickness.

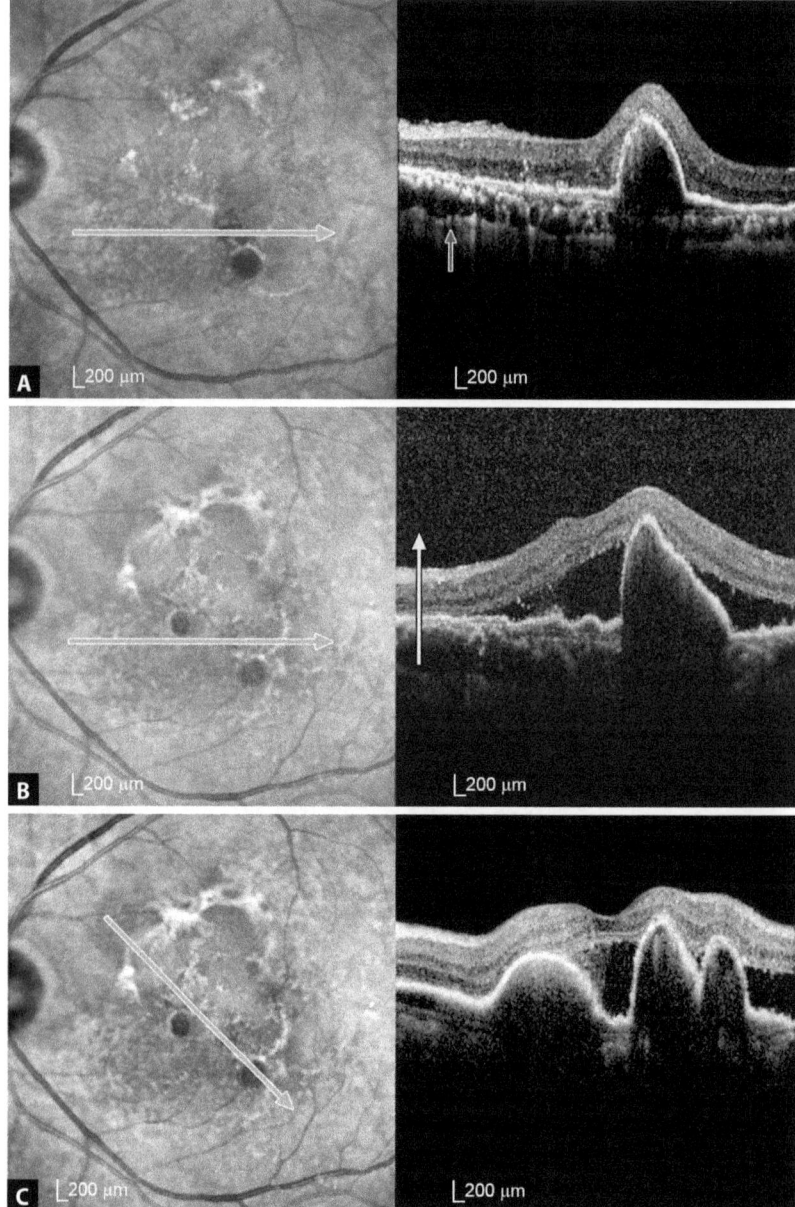

Figs. 7.15.5A to C: (A) Optical coherence tomography demonstrating retinal pigment epithelium (RPE) detachment with double layer sign adjacent it (blue arrow); (B) Tomographic notch due to sharply elevated "tall pigment epithelial detachment (PED)" (yellow arrow); (C) Multiple RPE detachments.

CLASSIFICATION

The Japanese Study Group proposed the classification of PCV into three categories:
1. *Quiescent:* Polyps in the absence of subretinal or intraretinal fluid or hemorrhage.
2. *Exudative:* Exudation without hemorrhage, which may include sensory retinal thickening, neurosensory detachment, PED, and subretinal lipid exudation.
3. *Hemorrhagic:* Any hemorrhage with or without other exudative characteristics.

The Japanese Study Group of PCV also differentiated definite cases of PCV from probable cases. Definite cases were defined as those with protruded orange-red elevated lesions on fundus examination and/or characteristic polypoidal lesions on ICGA as described earlier. Probable PCV was diagnosed if there was only an abnormal vascular network on ICGA or occurrence of recurrent hemorrhagic and/or serous detachments of the RPE was observed.

Further, subclassification of PCV into type 1 and 2 PCV has been done based on ICGA features since these two angiographic subtypes of PCV showed differences in their clinical course, genetic susceptibility, and response to therapy.

Polypoidal choroidal vasculopathy with apparent BVN is called "type 1 PCV" or "polypoidal CNV". Type 1 PCV usually has larger lesion sizes due to the larger and more distinct BVN, smaller polyp size on ICGA, smaller choroidal thickness, and lower response to photodynamic therapy (PDT) as compared to type 2 PCV. PCV with no or only faint BVN is called "type 2 PCV" or "typical PCV".

DIFFERENTIAL DIAGNOSIS

The diagnosis of PCV must be considered in all cases of occult or minimally classic choroidal neovascular membrane (CNVM) with large subretinal hemorrhages in the Asian populations.

Polypoidal choroidal vasculopathy forms a part of the emerging spectrum of what is known as pachychoroid disorders and can be sometimes difficult to differentiate from chronic central serous retinopathy (CSR) which in later stages may present a picture akin to PCV.

NATURAL COURSE

In general, the natural course of the disease is more favorable than in ARMD. Patients with PCV and acute serosanguineous complications may experience spontaneous resolution with little or no fibrous proliferation and complete or significant regression or even infarction of the membrane with consequent regression of the lesions. At the same time, bullous, even global detachments of the RPE and neurosensory retina have been seen with or without severe vitreous hemorrhage in some cases and some patients could even develop total retinal detachment with neovascular glaucoma and loss of the eye, a sequence of events that is very unlikely in ARMD. Half of study eyes had decreased vision due to massive hemorrhage or severe RPE atrophy after longer follow-up periods (24–54 months). Incidence of retinal hemorrhage or subretinal hemorrhage in PCV patients has varied from 30 to 64% in different studies and is often associated with vision loss.

MANAGEMENT

Treatment of progressive or vision threatening macular lesions is warranted. Management options for PCV include photocoagulation for extrafoveal lesions and PDT with verteporfin, antivascular endothelial growth factor (VEGF) drugs such as bevacizumab and ranibizumab and the newly available anti-VEGF drug such as aflibercept for subfoveal and juxtafoveal lesions.

Laser Photocoagulation

Treatment is done only for polyps which are extrafoveal in location and should be of mild to moderate intensity, as is done for laser treatment of a retinal arteriolar macroaneurysm. The objective is to induce a fibrotic response in the aneurysm wall. The entire vascular network or area of exudation does not need to be treated. Since many PCV lesions are extrafoveal, thermal laser photocoagulation has an important role to play in management of this condition.

Photodynamic Therapy

The role of PDT with verteporfin and anti-VEGF agents (ranibizumab) was investigated in the EVEREST trial, which studied the relative efficacy of PDT with or without ranibizumab and ranibizumab monotherapy in the treatment of PCV. PDT without or with ranibizumab was found to cause closure of polyps in 71 and 78% of patients at 6 months follow-up as compared to 28% in patients treated with intravitreal injection of ranibizumab. Occlusion of such leaky polyps is considered an important marker of treatment efficacy in clinical practice. Occlusion of polyps is also associated with improvement or stabilization of vision.

Photodynamic therapy with or without ranibizumab is therefore the treatment of choice for PCV with polyps. Anti-VEGF drugs such as bevacizumab and ranibizumab are not very effective in closure of polyps but can help to reduce the associated exudation consequent to the polyps and BVNs. Subsequently, the LAPTOP (Lucentis and Photodynamic Therapy On Polypoidal choroidal vasculopathy) study, conducted to assess the visual outcomes following PDT and anti-VEGF agents, demonstrated better visual outcomes following treatment with ranibizumab as compared to PDT, with a higher proportion of patients gaining >0.2 logMAR units in the ranibizumab arm (30.4% vs. 17.0%, $p = 0.039$) at 12 months. In addition, the mean gain in logMAR visual acuity was also greater in the ranibizumab arm at 12 months ($p = 0.011$) as well as at 24 months ($p = 0.025$). Therefore, in terms of efficacy in closing the polyps, PDT is more effective but it is associated with visual loss during long-term follow-up. Visual outcomes however seem to be better maintained by ranibizumab despite a lower closure rate for polyps. **Figures 7.15.6A and B** show the pretreatment (A) and post-treatment (B) fundus photograph and OCT of a patient treated with PDT.

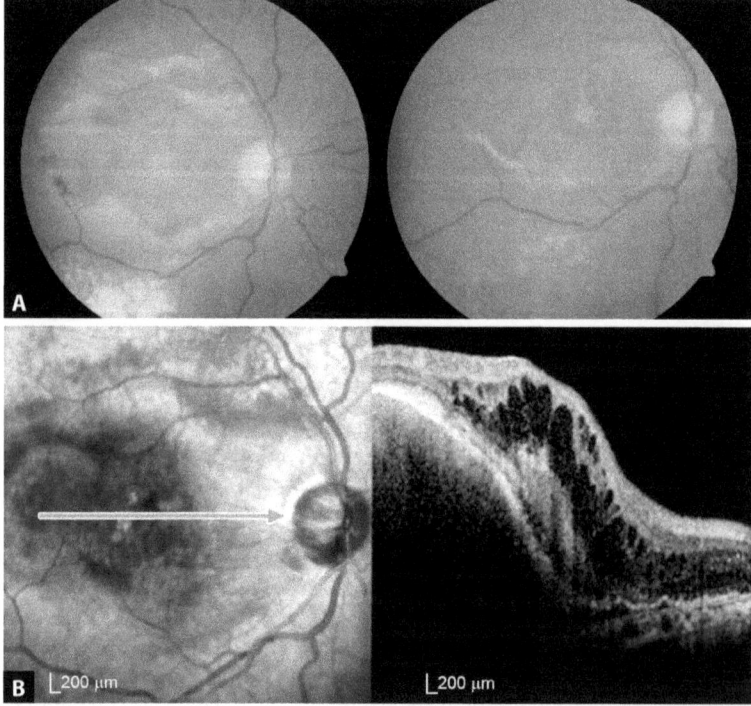

Figs. 7.15.6A and B: Pretreatment (A) and post-treatment (B) fundus photograph and optical coherence tomography (OCT) following photodynamic therapy.
Courtesy: Dr Lalit Verma, Centre for Sight.

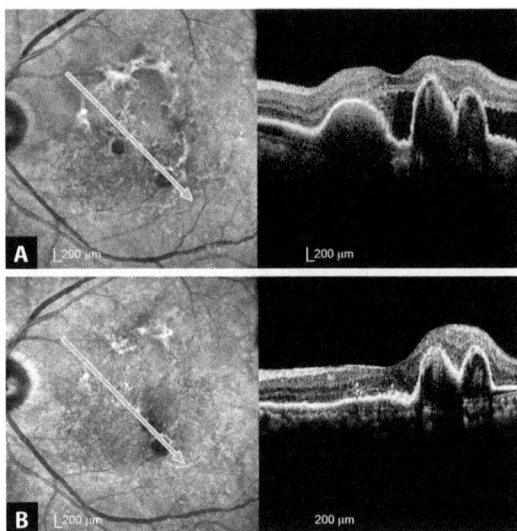

Figs. 7.15.7A and B: (A) Pretreatment; (B) Post-treatment with ranibizumab and then aflibercept showing resolution of subretinal fluid (SRF) and decrease in size of retinal pigment epithelium (RPE) detachment.

Aflibercept has demonstrated significant activity for closure of polyps in recent studies, with total closure being noted in over 50% of treatment naïve eyes treated with aflibercept at 12 months follow-up in one study and a similar closure rate in PCV patients refractory to treatment with ranibizumab in another study **(Figs. 7.15.7A and B)**. Treatment naïve patients with PCV treated with aflibercept; however, showed at least partial resolution of the RPE detachment in over 80% of the patients in the aflibercept injection (Eylea) for PCV with hemorrhage or exudation (EPIC) trial.

However, BVNs persisted with PDT as well as with anti-VEGF treatment and could be a source for recurrences later.

CONCLUSION

Among the currently available treatment modalities for PCV, PDT alone or PDT combined with VEGF inhibitors therapy seems to be the most promising. However, combined PDT with anti-VEGF therapy was superior to PDT monotherapy in terms of visual outcome and complications. PDT monotherapy causes regression of polyps and reduces fluid leakage, but polypoidal lesions have high recurrence rates over long periods.

Anti-VEGF drugs reduced exudative fluid and suppressed upregulation of VEGF, but the vascular lesions did not regress. Thus, the combination of PDT and an anti-VEGF agent seems to be a rational approach.

SUGGESTED READING

1. Honda S, Matsumiya W, Negi A. Polypoidal choroidal vasculopathy: clinical features and genetic predisposition. Ophthalmologica. 2014;231(2):59-74.

7.16 Wide-angle Viewing Systems

Hemanth Murthy
Retina Institute of Karnataka, Bengaluru
hemanthmurthy@yahoo.com

■ INTRODUCTION

Visualization of the fundus during posterior segment surgery has evolved over the years. Initially a hand-held contact lens was used later prismatic lenses helped surgery as it was independent of an assistant. These however have the drawback of limited field of view, i.e., 20–30°.

Wide-angle viewing systems work on the principle of indirect ophthalmoscope and have improved visualization of the fundus during retinal surgery. Wide-angle viewing systems are essential in improving outcomes of microincision vitrectomy surgery (MIVS).

■ TYPES OF WIDE-ANGLE SYSTEMS

Noncontact Systems

- Binocular indirect ophthalmomicroscope (BIOM) (field of view—60/90/120/130°)
- Erect indirect binocular ophthalmomicroscope system (EIBOS) (100/125°)
- RESIGHT system (60/120°) (**Fig. 7.16.1**)
- Optical fiber free intravitreal surgery system (OFFISS)

Contact System

- Volk (standard and self-stabilizing), 112–134°
- Ocular
- Advanced visual instruments (AVI).

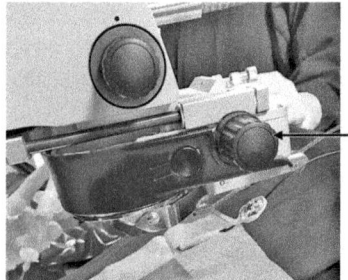

Fig. 7.16.1: RESIGHT system.

■ COMPONENTS OF WIDE-ANGLE

Like an indirect ophthalmoscope, the wide-angle systems consists of the condensing lens and objective lens, which are in a single piece or could be separated by an extension arm as in BIOM. The image thus formed, would be inverted like an indirect ophthalmoscope. Since the image formed is inverted, it needs to be reinverted to enable surgery. This requires the stereoscopic diagonal inverter (SDI).

The SDI is incorporated in the body of the microscope. It has a knob to change between normal and the reinverted image. However, in the EIBOS, the inverter is incorporated within it.

All wide-angle systems have a base plate, which is attached to the microscope. This is specific to the microscope. The other components are autoclavable and fix to this base plate in both BIOM and RESIGHT systems.

The RESIGHT system has the advantage of being in focus during surgery and the microscope zoom can be used independently. Once the objective lens swings in its place the fine focus is used to focus on to the area of interest. The condensing lens moves to get the fundus in focus and the objective lens remains stationary. The Lumera microscope with which it integrates has an Inverted-tube incorporated in the body, which reinverts the image.

The optics of the OFFISS system has a large objective lens and uses the specialized operating microscope light to visualize the fundus. This enables bimanual surgery and endoilluminator is not necessary. For effective use of OFFISS there is a need for the eye to be aphakic.

The BIOM system works similar to the RESIGHT system but once the objective is in place the microscope zoom needs to be adjusted and then the fine focus is adjusted to get a clear view of the fundus. Here the objective lens moves to bring the fundus into focus. Some modifications are available on BIOM 5 which has a microswitch which reinverts the image. A quartz lens which gives HD view of 130° is also available.

Peyman–Wessels–Landers (PWL) lens is a 132 D upright lens which initially was used with an attachment to the wrist support/OT table **(Fig. 7.16.2)**. However, nowadays a universal attachment to the microscope is available. It has a static view of 100° and dynamic 135°.

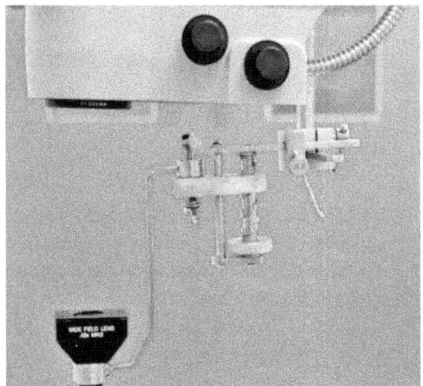

Fig. 7.16.2: Universal attachment to microscope for PWL lens.
Courtesy: Dr Raju Sampangi.

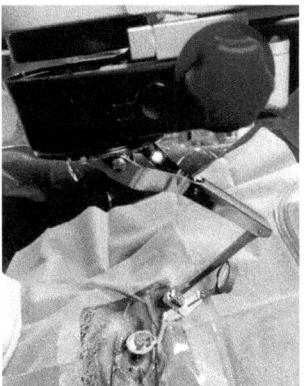

Fig. 7.16.3: Noncontact wide-angle viewing system—RESIGHT.

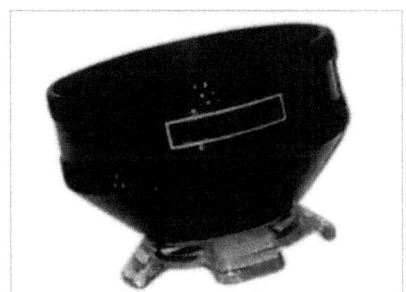

Fig. 7.16.4: Contact wide-angle—Volk MiniQuad XL self-stabilizing vitrectomy (SSV).

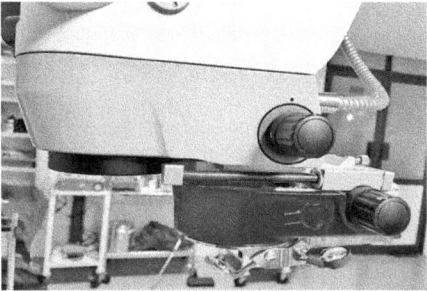

Fig. 7.16.5: The RESIGHT system slides back to allow anterior segment procedure.

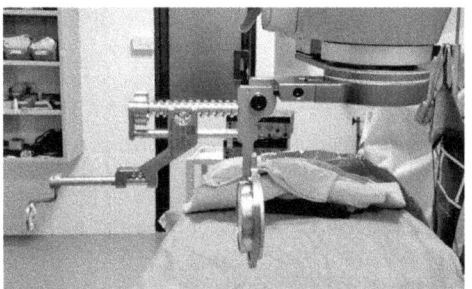

Fig. 7.16.6: Binocular indirect ophthalmomicroscope (BIOM 5) can be swung away to enable anterior segment work.

The contact wide-angle has the first lens on the corneal surface to neutralize the refractive power of the cornea and the second lens of 150 D is incorporated in the body of the lens. These lenses could either be self-stabilizing vitrectomy (SSV) which have flanges which support the lens on the eye during surgery or those without the flanges will require a ring to support the lens.

INDICATIONS FOR THE USE OF WIDE-ANGLE VIEWING SYSTEMS

Wide-angle viewing systems are essential for achieving good surgical outcome in all MIVS procedures. These are used for all vitrectomy procedures wherein peripheral retina needs to be visualized. They are particularly useful in:
- Retinal detachment with anterior proliferative vitreoretinopathy (PVR)
- Diabetic tractional retinal detachment
- Gas-fluid exchanges, perfluorocarbon liquid-silicone oil exchange

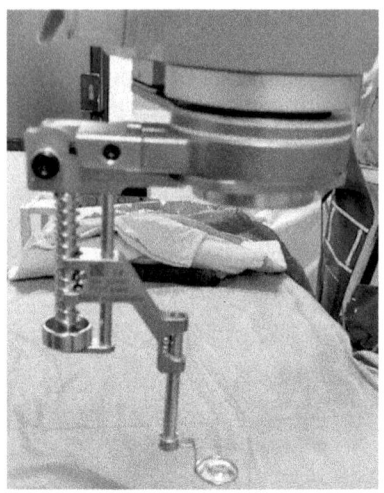

Fig. 7.16.7: Binocular indirect ophthalmo-microscope (BIOM 5) showing objective lens in position, fine focus is seen in the picture.

TABLE 7.16.1: Comparison between the regular landers lens system and wide-angle systems.

	Advantages	Disadvantages
Contact lenses	• Easily available • Inexpensive • Low maintenance • Adaptable to all microscopes • Stereopsis excellent, best for macula	• Corneal trauma • Blood can obscure image • Requires good pupil dilatation • Poor view and stereopsis of the periphery • Poor view in gas-filled eye
Wide-angle systems	• Good overall view • Ease of surgery, all areas of traction seen • Good view of periphery • Good view in gas-filled eye	• Higher initial cost • Learning curve • Not as good as contact lens for macular surgery

TABLE 7.16.2: Comparison between the contact and noncontact wide-angle systems.

	Advantages	Disadvantages
Noncontact system	• No assistant needed • No corneal trauma • Good in pediatric cases • Scleral depression is easier	• Adaptability to microscopes • Less optical resolution • Expensive • Reduces view on movement of eyeball • Fine focus to be done on the lens system
Contact system	• Better optical resolution • Wider field of view as movement of the eye is possible • Reduces haze due to surface irregularities • Can use microscope footswitch for fine focus	• Needs skilled assistant • Corneal trauma • Poor limbus access • Changes intraocular pressure (IOP) • Difficult to do scleral depression

- Cases requiring retinotomy in severe PVR
- Small pupil—pupil of at least 2.5–3 mm is required
- Subretinal fibrosis
- Retinopathy of prematurity—decreased scleral rigidity and small size of cornea
- Retained lens fragments and dislocated intraocular lens

PROBLEMS FACED WITH WIDE-ANGLE SYSTEMS

The SDI adds about 3 inches to the body of the microscope. While using the wide-angle systems the microscope needs to be raised. Since the microscope is raised, the scleral ports are not easily visualized. This is very irritating for the surgeons in the presbyopic age. The area visualized being very large, the usual illuminators with a small cone of light beam are very inadequate. Wide-angle endoilluminators and chandelier light source can overcome this problem.

PROCEDURE

Contact Wide-angle

After the ports are made the wide-angle lens is placed on the cornea with a viscoelastic coupling gel. The microscope zoom and focus is used to focus on the retina.

Noncontact Wide-angle Systems

There is a base plate, which is fixed to the microscope. The lens systems are fixed on to this base plate. Illuminate the disc with the endoilluminator and adjust the height of the microscope from the surface of the cornea (while using the objective lens) to focus on the retina. While using BIOM the objective lens is lowered or raised from the corneal surface using the fine focus ring to focus the retina. While using RESIGHT the system is positioned and the fine focus is used to focus the retina. The magnification can be changed on the microscope footswitch. Illumination with bullet light pipes, illuminating infusion line and chandelier illumination improve the visualization of the retina in wide-angle viewing.

Three-dimensional (3D) (heads-up) visualization systems have improved the visualization with higher magnification and lower illumination in addition to improved ergonomics.

SUGGESTED READING

1. Challam KV, Shah VA. Optics of wide-angle panoramic viewing system—assisted vitreous surgery. Surv Ophthalmol. 2004;49(4):437-45.
2. Paymen GA, Meffert SA, Chou F, Conway MD. Vitreoretinal Surgical Techniques, 1st edition. Florida, United States: CRC Press; 2000. pp. 99-106.
3. Raju Sampangi and Hemalatha BC Universal attachment- Proceedings.aios.org.2017

7.17 | Postoperative Cystoid Macular Edema

Jay Chhablani, Komal Agrawal
LV Prasad Eye Institute, Hyderabad
jay.chhablani@gmail.com

INTRODUCTION

With the change in trends of considering cataract surgery as a visually rehabilitative procedure to a refractive procedure, the expectations of outcomes after a cataract surgery have tremendously changed. Postoperative or pseudophakic cystoid macular edema (CME) is one of the most common causes for subnormal outcomes of cataract surgery (Fig. 7.17.1).

Cystoid macular edema after cataract surgery was first described by Irvine in 1953. Later, fluorescein angiography (FA) characteristics were described by Gass and Norton, hence, giving the name *Irvine-Gass syndrome* (Fig. 7.17.2).

RISK FACTORS

- *Type of cataract surgery:* Change in trend from intracapsular cataract extraction to extracapsular cataract extraction and small incision cataract surgery to now phacoemulsification techniques have shown a clear decrease in the incidence of CME.
- *Surgical complications:* Posterior capsular rupture and other causes of vitreous loss intraoperatively have been known to increase the incidence of CME. Retained lens fragments also increase inflammation and, hence, increase the incidence of CME.
- *Comorbidities:* Diabetic patients, especially, in preexisting diabetic retinopathy or diabetic macular edema show an increased propensity to develop CME postoperatively.
- *Ocular comorbidities:* Ocular inflammation or uveitis increases the chances of developing CME. Adequate control of inflammation is hence necessary before taking the patient for surgery.

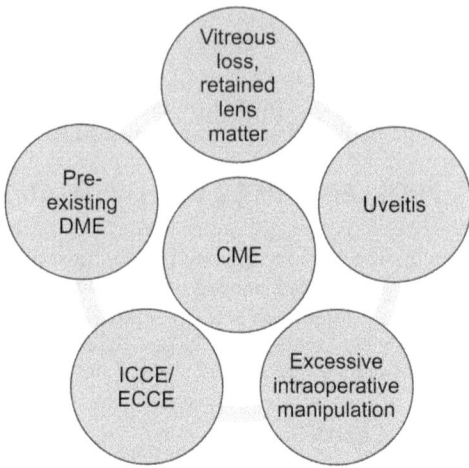

Fig. 7.17.1: Risk factors for pseudophakic CME. (CME: cystoid macular edema; DME: diabetic macular edema; ECCE: extracapsular cataract extraction; ICCE: intracapsular cataract extraction)

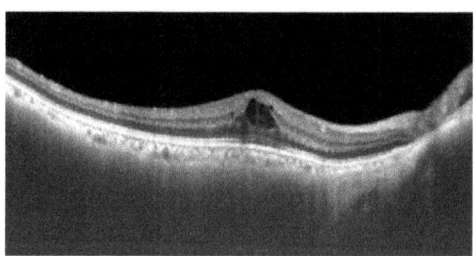

Fig. 7.17.2: Spectral-domain optical coherence tomography scan showing cystoid macular edema.

PATHOGENESIS

Multiple theories have been proposed for the pathogenesis of CME. However, role of inflammation in postoperative period in causation of CME postsurgery is the most widely accepted.

It has been hypothesized that surgical trauma to, especially, the more metabolically active tissues of the eye like iris and ciliary body leads to up regulation of cyclooxygenase (COX) enzyme pathway and, hence, causing overproduction of inflammatory mediators, prostaglandins, and leukotrienes. These are known to diffuse into the vitreous cavity and stimulate the breakdown of blood retinal barrier. Vascular permeability of the retinal vessels is, thus, increased causing accumulation of intraretinal fluid resulting in CME.

Apart from this, tractional forces on the foveal area due to vitreous disturbances caused during cataract surgery have also been implicated in development of CME. Minimal traction on vitreomacular interface in phacoemulsification might explain the less incidence of CME in such cases.

DIAGNOSIS

Patients usually complain of impaired vision after a period of improved vision after cataract surgery. It is usually seen to develop 4–6 weeks after surgery. The diagnosis is based upon:
- *Clinical examination:* It shows evidence of perifoveal cystic spaces.
- *Fundus fluorescein angiography:* It has been traditionally used to confirm the diagnosis of CME. Classic petaloid pattern of hyperfluorescence with or without late disc leakage (**Fig. 7.17.3**).
- *Optical coherence tomography:* Optical coherence tomography has now become indispensable in diagnosis of CME. It characteristically shows increase in macular thickness with cystic spaces in the outer plexiform layer. Occasionally subfoveal fluid can be seen.

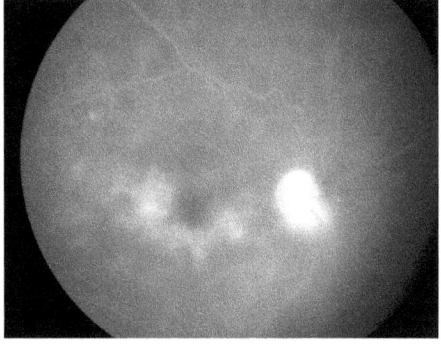

Fig. 7.17.3: Fundus fluorescein angiography showing typical petaloid pattern with disc hyperfluorescence.

Patients who are asymptomatic but show FA characteristics of CME are termed as having angiographic CME. Clinical CME is considered in patients having decreased visual acuity with angiographic and/or clinical evidence of CME.

> **CLINICAL PEARLS**
> - Preoperative risk factors
> - Intraoperative manipulation
> - Vitreous loss   Look for CME
> - Decrease vision postoperative
> - Yellow reflex at fovea

MANAGEMENT

- *Nonsteroidal anti-inflammatory drugs:* These drugs act by inhibiting by COX enzyme and, hence, reducing the load of inflammatory mediators.
    Topical nepafenac, diclofenac 0.1% and ketorolac tromethamine 0.5% are shown to have beneficial effect in both acute and chronic CME.
    Adverse effects include burning sensations, conjunctival hyperemia, and should be avoided in patients with preexisting ocular surface disorders.
- *Corticosteroids:* These act by inhibiting phospholipase A2 during arachidonic acid cascade and inhibit leukotriene and prostaglandin synthesis. They also play a role in reducing capillary permeability and inhibit macrophage and neutrophil migration:
  - *Topical corticosteroids:* Although these are routinely used after cataract surgery, their role as monotherapy in treatment for CME has not been well established. However, topical steroids in combination with nonsteroidal anti-inflammatory drugs have found to be beneficial for treatment of pseudophakic CME by various studies.
  - *Periocular and intravitreal steroids:* Both posterior subtenon injection and intravitreal injection of triamcinolone acetate are used, especially, for the treatment of refractory CME. They have the advantage of better bioavailability of drug as compared to topical administration. Side effects mainly include rise in intraocular pressure (IOP) in steroids responders, otherwise these are usually well tolerated.
  - *Intravitreal dexamethasone implant:* Significant improvement (>15 letter improvement) was seen in patients who received intravitreal dexamethasone implant (700 µg). This improvement persisted for 3 months in most patients.

It is a useful option in refractory CME. Although the implant is reported to be very well tolerated, IOP needs to be monitored in such patients.
- *Intravitreal antivascular endothelial growth factor (VEGF):* The role of VEGF as the mediator in development of postsurgical CME has not been well established. However, an interventional multicentric retrospective pilot study from Pan-American Collaborative Retina Study Group demonstrated improvement in best-corrected visual acuity (BCVA) more than two Early Treatment Diabetic Retinopathy Study lines in patients with refractory CME undergoing intravitreal bevacizumab injection (1.25 mg or 2.5 mg). However, the evidence regarding the use of anti-VEGF is not robust.
- *Surgical treatment (Pars plana vitrectomy):* Vitrectomy can be considered in chronic and refractory CME which involves vitreomacular traction as the etiological cause. However, no clear evidence is available regarding its use in pseudophakic CME in absence of vitreoretinal adhesions.

Another indication of this surgical intervention is presence of lens fragments in vitreous causing an increase in inflammation.

RECENT ADVANCES

Several other drugs have been tried in treatment of refractory pseudophakic CME in small pilot series. However, the use of these has not been supported by promising evidences.
- *Intravitreal diclofenac:* 500 µ/0.1 mL of intravitreal showed some improvement in BCVA, however, no significant change in central macular thickness (CMT) was observed in a small series by Soheillan et al.
- *Intravitreal Infliximab:* Seven eyes with refractory CME secondary to cataract surgery were studied for response to 1 mg of intravitreal infliximab by Wu et al. which showed significant improvement in BCVA and CMT.

SUGGESTED READING

1. Guo S, Patel S, Baumrind B, Johnson K, Levinsohn D, Marcus E, et al. Management of pseudophakic cystoid macular edema. Surv Ophthalmol. 2015;60(2):123-37.

7.18 Radiation Retinopathy

Karobi Lahiri Coutinho
Bombay Hospital Institute of Medical Sciences, Mumbai
doctorkarobi@gmail.com

Samyak V Mulkutkar
PD Hinduja Hospital and Medical Research Centre, Mumbai
Samyak.mulkutkar@gmail.com

INTRODUCTION

Radiation maculopathy (RM) is a sight-limiting consequence of radiotherapy. Radiation retinopathy (RR) and maculopathy are predictable complications resulting from exposure to any source of radiation, including external beam and plaque brachytherapy.

Radiation-induced damage to the eye can result in formation of cataracts, RM, or radiation-induced optic neuropathy.

Radiation retinopathy is a predictable complication following exposure to any source of radiation. It was first described in 1933 by Stallard following treatment of retinoblastoma. RR is a slowly progressive occlusive vasculopathy characterized by radiation induced damage to pericytes and endothelial cells causing an altered blood-retinal barrier.

The clinical spectrum is similar to that of diabetic retinopathy and presents as microaneurysms, areas of capillary drop-out, retinal hemorrhages, hard exudates, cotton-wool spots, macular edema in early stages and as intraretinal telangiectasias, neovascularization, and vitreous hemorrhage in late stages.

ETIOLOGY

Exposure to ionizing radiation including external beam and plaque brachytherapy can induce RR. External beam radiation is used as a treatment for nasopharyngeal, paranasal sinus, or orbital tumors, where there is limited protection to the eye and can often lead to clinically significant RR. Plaque brachytherapy used in the treatment of intraocular tumors can also cause severe damage to the immediate retina and the choroid.

Broadly speaking, RR is seen following radiation for ocular tumors such as retinoblastoma, choroid melanoma, angioma, head and neck cancers, optic nerve sheath meningioma, and Hodgkin's lymphoma.

RADIATION THERAPY

While radiation therapy is widely accepted as an appropriate vision-preserving therapy for the select tumors of the eye, the effects of radiation-related visual loss are also being increasingly recognized.

Effects of Radiation Treatment

Most side effects of mild radiation exposure to the human body are transient and self-limited. They include nausea, vomiting, focal alopecia, swelling, pain, and mild erythematous skin changes. Cranial nerve dysfunction, pituitary dysfunction, brain necrosis, hearing loss, and new tumor induction can also develop after decades.

RISK FACTORS

Radiation retinopathy is dose and dose-rate dependent. Parsons et al. have reported a 53% incidence of RR in patients who received 45–55 Gy to half or more of the retina during external beam radiation for extracranial tumors. Some authors have reported pretreatment tumor size as the single important factor for predicting maculopathy in a multivariate analysis. Shields et al. have found that tumor base >10 mm, thickness >8 mm, radiation of >33,000 cGy to tumor base and increasing dose to optic disc to be predictors of long-term poor visual acuity. The higher total radiation dose has been shown to increase the risk of RR. Larger tumors require larger dosage of radiation and increase the risk of RR. The incidence of retinopathy increases steadily at doses >45 Gy. RR has been reported in doses as low as 11 Gy but infrequent below 45 Gy dose. The proton beam irradiation is reported to be much more likely to induce RR changes.

Fractionation schedule, type of radiation, errors in treatment, and time elapsed in the course of treatment should also be accounted for. Hyperfractionation has been associated with a decreased incidence of RR. Patients who receive <25 Gy in fractions of 2 Gy or less are unlikely to develop significant retinopathy. An increased fraction size correlated with increase in retinal complications.

Ruthenium-106, for example, yields higher dosage versus iodine-125 or palladium-103 and is responsible for significant chorioretinal atrophy.

Proximity of the tumor to important ocular structures such as the fovea/macula and the optic disc would put these at an increased risk of damage causing RM and radiation optic neuropathy (RON), respectively.

A decreased distance to the fovea has also been associated with decreased time to maculopathy. Eyes considered at highest risk of RM are those with subfoveal or juxtafoveal locations and those eyes where the dose to the fovea has been created than or equal to 50–70 Gy irrespective of the radiation therapy source. Studies have shown that subfoveal melanomas carry the highest risk for RM and vision loss due to tumor location associated high radiation doses.

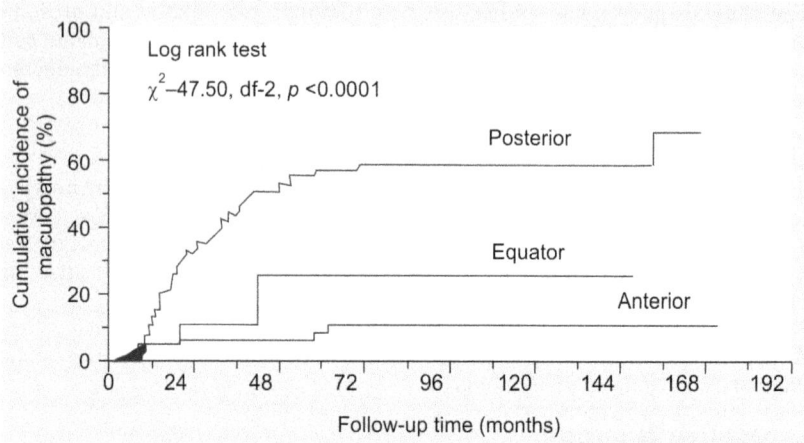

Fig. 7.18.1: Kaplan-Meier graph demonstrates the cumulative incidence of radiation maculopathy as a function of tumor location: Anterior, posterior, and equator.

With local or external beam irradiation patients may develop retinopathy from 6 months to 3 years after treatment.

With plaque brachytherapy, the risk of RR is related to total radiation dose. In the treatment of uveal melanoma, therapeutic apical doses range from 80 to100 Gy. Factors that affect total radiation dose such as tumor height and location also increase the risk of retinopathy. Tumor thickness >4 mm has been associated with a greater risk for RM (Fig. 7.18.1).

Concurrent chemotherapy also causes free-radical induced damage at cellular levels adding to the existing radiation damage.

COMORBIDITIES

The concurrent presence of diabetes is considered as one of the major patient associated risk factors for development of RR. The synergistic effect of diabetes and radiation on the capillaries is postulated to be the major reason for a highly increased risk of visual loss.

Comorbidities such as hypertension, autoimmune disorders, concurrent chemotherapy, younger age, and pregnancy are also associated with an increased risk of RR.

PATHOGENESIS

Radiation can cause both acute and chronic effects on retina. Acute changes occur within 6 hours of radiation and show nuclear pyknosis among rods, and edema in the outer retinal layers.

Ionizing radiation is responsible for the loss of retinal vascular pericytes and endothelial cells. However, there may be a preferential loss of vascular endothelial cells with relative sparing of the pericytes. It is hypothesized that the differential sensitivity between endothelial cells and pericytes is the result of direct exposure of the endothelial cells to high ambient oxygen and iron found in the blood which generates free radicals and leads to cell membrane damage.

The development of microaneurysms causing subsequent leakage and macular exudation is a direct effect of the pericyte loss. Loss of endothelial cells causes areas of capillary drop-out and cotton-wool spots. Exudation and capillary drop-out are both responsible for the vision loss in RR.

Recent imaging studies on optical coherence tomography-angiography (OCT-A) in the early stages have shown areas of capillary drop-outs both in the superficial and the deep capillary plexuses without clinical evidence of RM. In later stages, these may progress to widespread retinal ischemia, neovascularization, fibrovascular proliferation, and vitreous hemorrhage.

■ DIAGNOSIS
History
Patients will present with a history of radiation exposure, X-ray therapy, or radiotherapy few months to a few years duration. RR has been reported to develop anywhere from 1 month to 15 years but most commonly, it occurs between 6 months and 3 years. At times, patients may not be forthcoming with history of radiation exposure simply because they may not attribute their eye symptoms to radiation. This may happen in cases wherein, patients have not received the radiation or radiation therapy for ocular problems. In such cases, history of previous radiation exposure or history of past treatments in detail should be elicited by asking leading questions by the treating ophthalmologist to reach a complete diagnosis.

For example, a 45-year-old gentleman presented with solitary choroidal hemangioma **(Figs. 7.18.2 and 7.18.3)**. He had ruthenium-106 brachytherapy 3 years back, 4,500 cGy **(Figs. 7.18.4 to 7.18.6)**. He was diagnosed to have early RM but not requiring any treatment.

■ OCULAR EXAMINATION
Evaluation for RR includes a complete ophthalmologic examination including vision, intraocular pressures (IOPs), anterior segment, and dilated retinal examination to look for pathological features of retinopathy described here.

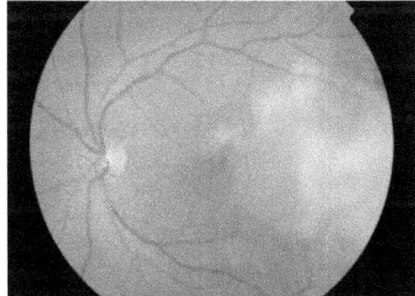

Fig. 7.18.2: Choroidal hemangioma encroaching fovea.

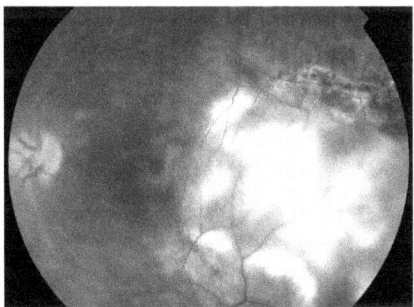

Fig. 7.18.3: Fluorescein angiography dye leakage with pooling.

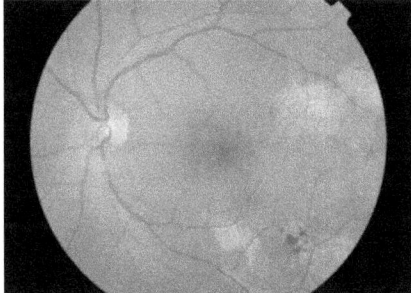

Fig. 7.18.4: Regression after ruthenium-106 brachytherapy early radiation retinopathy.

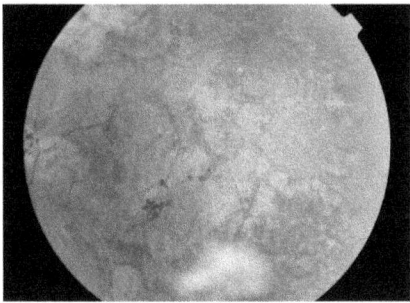

Fig. 7.18.5: Residual mass.

Symptoms

Those with subclinical or mild retinopathy may be asymptomatic but advanced disease can present with blurring of vision or floaters. Sudden loss of vision after radiation is not rare. Chronic blurring of vision, distorted vision, and defective color vision are also known to be occur.

Signs

Dilated funduscopic examination may reveal the following features that maybe unilateral or bilateral (**Fig. 7.18.7**):

- Retinal microaneurysms
- Retinal hemorrhages
- Retinal telangiectatic vessels
- Retinal hard exudates
- Macular edema
- Cotton-wool spots
- Retinal neovascularization
- Vitreous hemorrhage
- Tractional retinal detachment
- Capillary dilation
- Capillary closure
- Perivascular sheathing
- Retinal pigment epithelium (RPE) atrophy (a distinguishable feature from diabetic retinopathy)
- Central retinal artery or vein occlusion
- Optic disc edema, neovascularization of the iris, neovascularization of the angle, neovascular glaucoma, and cataract are associated features of the RR

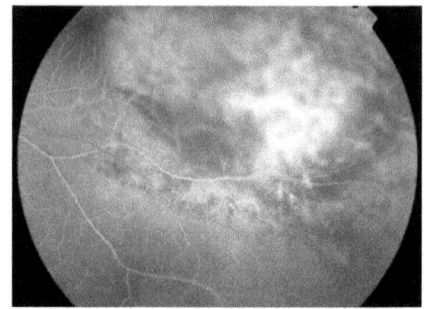

Fig. 7.18.6: Fundus fluorescein angiography.

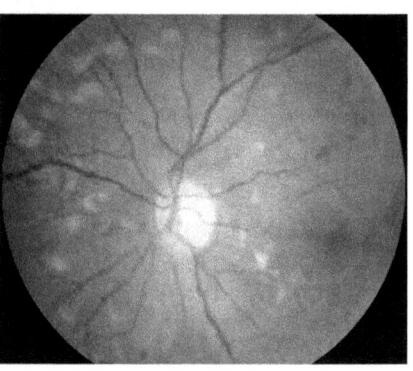

Fig. 7.18.7: Left radiation retinopathy with multiple cotton-wool spots and blot hemorrhages postradiation 1 year for left-sided brain tumor.

Visual impairment may range from mild to severe and is secondary to macular ischemia or edema. The most severe change is a progressive development of capillary nonperfusion (CPN) areas in periphery and posterior pole. These features are similar to changes in diabetic retinopathy with exception that microaneurysms are less frequent in RR. RPE atrophy due to vaso-obliteration is seen in RR.

In proliferative retinopathy, ischemia is seen in area that receives highest dose of radiation as compared to nasal location and diabetic retinopathy. Latency by radiation exposure and clinical manifestations of vascular changes may range either from 3 weeks to 7 years or 6 months to 3 years.

Radiation maculopathy includes hard exudates, cystoid and noncystoid edema, and serous detachment that can lead to significant visual loss.

Radiation optic neuropathy occurs in the acute phase which is marked by disc edema, intraretinal hemorrhages, hard exudates, and presence of subretinal fluid (SRF). The optic nerve appears progressively pale and atrophic with variable visual acuity during a few weeks or months.

■ BIOMICROSCOPY

Slit lamp biomicroscopic examination may show conjunctival hyperemia, conjunctival scars, signs of dry eye, symblepharon, corneal aberrations, corneal opacification, anterior uveitis, and cataract.

TABLE 7.18.1: The Finger Staging System for radiation associated vision loss.

Stage	Sign	Symptom	Location	Best viewed by	Risk of vision loss
1	Cotton-wool spots	None	Extramacular	Ophthalmoscopy	Mild
	Retinal hemorrhages	None	Extramacular	Ophthalmoscopy	Mild
	Retinal microaneurysms	None	Extramacular	Ophthalmoscopy	Mild
	Ghost vessels	None	Extramacular	Ophthalmoscopy	Mild
	Exudate	None	Extramacular	Ophthalmoscopy	Mild
	Uveal effusion	None	Extramacular	Ophthalmoscopy	Mild
	Chorioretinal atrophy	None	Extramacular	Ophthalmoscopy	Mild
	Choroidopathy	None	Extramacular	Angiography	Mild
	Retinal ischemia (<5 DA)	None	Extramacular	Angiography	Mild
2	Above findings	None	Macular	Both	Moderate
3	Any combination of the above plus retinal neovascularization	Vision loss	Extramacular	Angiography	Severe
	Macular edema—new onset	Vision loss	Macular	Angiography	Severe
4	Any combination of the above plus vitreous hemorrhage	Vision loss	Vitreous	Ophthalmoscopy	Severe
	Retinal ischemia (>5 DA)	Vision loss	Extramacular and macular	Angiography	Severe

Finger et al. have also devised *The Finger Staging System* **(Table 7.18.1)** for radiation associated vision loss. It assesses signs, symptoms, location, and best method for visualization and extrapolates it to the risk of vision loss with laser or antivascular endothelial growth factor (VEGF) treatment.

FINGER CLASSIFICATION
Radiation retinopathy is classified according to Finger into four stages:
1. *Stage 1:* It is located outside the macula and visual acuity is good.
2. *Stage 2:* It is located at the macula and has guarded prognosis.
3. *Stage 3:* It presents some vision loss and carries a severe risk of neovascularization, macular edema, and retinal ischemia.
4. *Stage 4:* Any above combination with vitreous hemorrhage and retinal ischemia affects vitreous, macula, and extramacular area (≥5 DA).

DIAGNOSTIC PROCEDURES
Clinical evaluation of above features usually gives an idea of retinopathy. *Fundus fluorescein angiogram* can be helpful in highlighting the microvascular features of RR, quantifying the extent of capillary nonperfusion as well as pick up early neovascular changes.

Indocyanine green angiography though is uncommonly performed for RR can reveal precapillary arteriolar occlusion and areas of choroidal hypoperfusion.

Amoaku classified the microvascular changes seen in RR based on fluorescein angiography.

AMOAKU CLASSIFICATION BASED ON MICROVASCULAR CHANGES DETECTED ON FLUORESCEIN ANGIOGRAPHY

- *Grade 1:* Small foci of dilated and irregular retinal capillaries along with isolated or small clusters of microaneurysms. Subtle evidence of capillary closure, without detectable microvascular incompetence or fluid accumulation, can be seen. Vision is usually very good.
- *Grade 2:* Multiple foci of dilated and telangiectatic capillaries and zones of capillary closure up to one optic disc area. Usually, numerous microaneurysms and focal leakage of dye from defective capillaries in later phase angiograms can be seen. It may be associated with clinically observable retinal edema. Visual acuity is relatively good.
- *Grade 3:* Characterized by widespread capillary dilatation, telangiectatic-like channels, microvascular incompetence, and significant areas of capillary closure (1–4 disc areas). These eyes can have significant macular edema with or without cystoid macular degenerative changes. Microaneurysms and intraretinal microvascular abnormalities commonly occur at the border of perfused and nonperfused retina. These eyes usually have poor visual acuity.
- *Grade 4:* Characterized by widespread disorganization of the retinal microvasculature with extensive inner retinal ischemia, nonperfused retina more than four disc areas, preretinal neovascularization, rubeosis iridis, and vitreous hemorrhage. Visual acuity is usually very poor.

Optical coherence tomography can be helpful in evaluating and quantifying the macular edema and response to treatment with anti-VEGF agents **(Figs. 7.18.8A to D)**. A study by Horgan et al. found that OCT was able to detect evidence of macular edema approximately 5 months earlier than clinically detectable RM. OCT can detect the

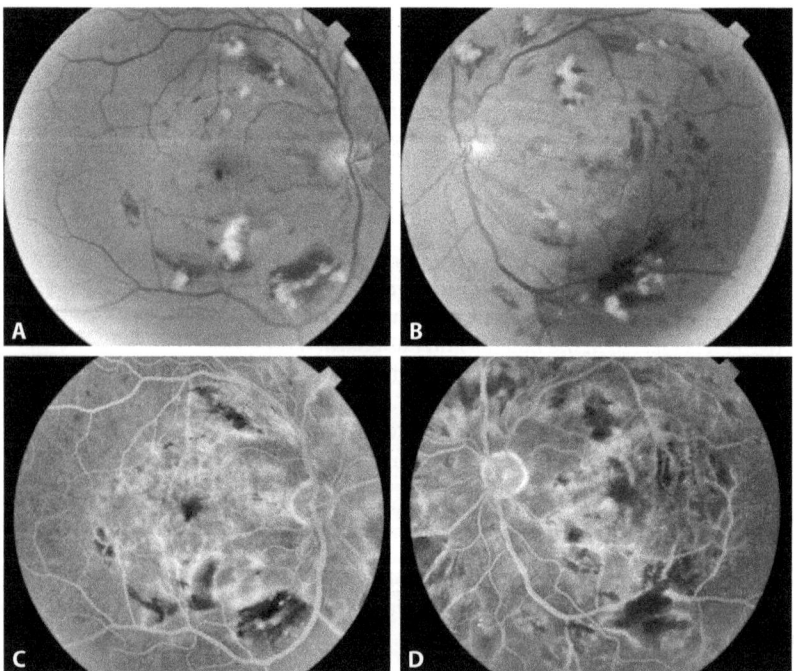

Figs. 7.18.8A to D: Fundus photograph reveals a macular hemorrhage, edema, cotton-wool spots as well as exudates, fundus fluorescein angiography showing blocked fluorescence, capillary nonperfusion (CNP) areas, and ischemic areas.

presence of subretinal fluid, hyper-reflective dots corresponding to intraretinal exudates, hyper-reflectivity of inner retinal layers suggesting retinal ischemia, disorganization of retinal layers, or outer retinal disruptions.

■ HORGAN CLASSIFICATION

Horgan et al. classified macular edema in five stages:
1. Grade 1—extrafoveal noncystoid macular edema
2. Grade 2—extrafoveal cystoid macular edema
3. Grade 3—foveal noncystoid macular edema
4. Grade 4—foveal cystoid macular edema—mild to moderate
5. Grade 5—foveal cystoid macular edema—severe

Optical coherence tomography angiography is a newer imaging tool that has shown to pick up capillary nonperfusion areas both in the superficial and deep capillary plexuses in very early stages before patients are symptomatic and significant clinical changes can be picked up on fundoscopy or on OCT. Broken or an enlarged foveal avascular zone (FAZ) can also be picked up on OCT-A and be a predictor of poor vision.

■ DIFFERENTIAL DIAGNOSIS

Following conditions should be considered in the differential diagnosis of RR:
- Diabetic retinopathy
- Branch retinal vein occlusion
- Central retinal vein occlusion
- Hypertensive retinopathy
- Coats' disease
- Perifoveal telangiectasia
- Hypercoagulation-associated retinopathy
- Anemia-associated retinopathy
- Ocular ischemic syndrome

■ MANAGEMENT

Medical

Antivascular Endothelial Growth Factor Therapy

Vascular endothelial growth factor has been shown to be elevated in vitreous and aqueous samples in eyes harboring melanoma and to have a positive association with larger tumors.

Treatment of radiation optic neuropathy: A prospective study by Finger and Chin evaluated bevacizumab for the treatment of RON in their prospective clinical case series on 14 patients with RON secondary to plaque radiotherapy for choroidal melanoma. Patients received a median of 13 injections every 6–8 weeks and showed reduction in the clinical evidence of RON in 100% of the patients.

However, Eckstein et al. have recently showed that RON patients treated with anti-VEGF injections and those followed up with the natural course of RON showed no statistically significant differences related to visual acuity or optic atrophy development.

Nevertheless, studies have shown that anti-VEGF drugs are safe and tolerated well in patients with anterior RON. However, anti-VEGF injections are not particularly helpful for treatment of posterior RON.

Treatment of RM: Finger et al. reported a 10-year data wherein, continuous treatment with anti-VEGF therapy every 4–12 weeks in patients with RM preserved vision: 80% of their 120 patients remained within two lines of their initial visual acuity or better with a mean treatment interval of 38 months. However, despite initial clinical improvement, this continuous treatment with anti-VEGFs, most patients did developed retinal manifestations. A few of them also required adjuvant retinal laser photocoagulation.

Radiation maculopathy continued to progress, albeit slowly despite continuous anti-VEGF therapy. Over a period of time, anti-VEGFs needed to be switched, intervals between injections required modifications and steroids were also required in some patients.

Subfoveal melanomas carry the highest risk for RM and vision loss due to inherent tumor location and associated high radiation doses. Additionally, they are not eligible for laser photocoagulation-induced VEGF suppression. Finger and Powell initiated periodic intravitreal anti-VEGF therapy, prior to the onset of RM at a mean of 24 days of plaque placement in case-matched groups. The last mean visual acuity in the anti-VEGF group was 20/32 as compared to 20/160 in the case-matched group. 64% cases in the anti-VEGF treated group showed improvement or no change in visual acuity, as compared to only 28% in the case-matched group. 70% in the case matched group lost more than three lines vision as compared with no patient in the anti-VEGF group ($p = <0.001$).

Studies have shown that intravitreal injection of the anti-VEGF drug Avastin (bevacizumab, Genentech), following early detection of RM with spectral-domain optical coherence tomography (SDOCT), may delay vision loss and maintain or possibly improve visual acuity. It appears to stabilize the vasculature and allow for visual improvement in a way similar to its benefits in diabetic macular edema (DME).

Effects—Decrease in macular edema, hemorrhages, exudates, microaneurysms, and improvement of visual acuity with decrease in macular edema.

Finger et al. reported on a larger series of 21 patients in which intravitreal bevacizumab (1.25 mg/0.05 mL) was injected every 6–12 weeks. At a mean follow-up of 7.8 months, 18 patients (86%) had improvement or stabilization of visual acuity, and three (14%) improved by two or more lines of vision. The authors also report improvement in vascular leakage as determined by fluorescein angiography. Another report by the same group investigated the use of ranibizumab for RR in five patients. A mean of 8.2 injections of ranibizumab (0.5 mg) was given over a mean follow-up of 8 months. Visual acuity improved by a mean of six letters, with four patients showing a modest improvement on average of 9.5 letters, and one patient losing seven letters. A decrease in vascular leakage and macular edema was seen, and central macular thickness (CMT) thickness decreased from 416 to 270 µm, a 35% reduction. Adverse effects were minimal, including subconjunctival hemorrhage at the injection site and transient postinjection IOP elevations. These studies show that periodic dosing, such as used in treatment of age-related macular degeneration (AMD), may be beneficial in sustaining a treatment effect.

At Bascom Palmer Eye Institute, a study was performed on a series of patients who were given 5,496 intravitreal bevacizumab injections for RR. Based on the observations, it was concluded that early identification of RR (using OCT), followed by early treatment, results in stability and often improvement.

It was also observed that combined therapy with triamcinolone and bevacizumab, in the radiation-induced macular edema, possibly has a synergistic effect. Contrary to earlier reports, a limited usefulness of anti-VEGF agents in RR was found on a longer follow-up. These preliminary reports and observations, therefore, warrant further studies to define the precise role of these agents in the management of RR.

Case

A 38-year-old male presented with complaints of watering and irritability of the eyes of 1 week duration. There was mild congestion of the conjunctiva bilaterally while the rest of the ocular evaluation including the fundus was unremarkable. He had underwent an uneventful brain surgery 1 year ago and the visual field evaluations pre- and postbrain surgery were normal. Lubricating eye drops were prescribed at this visit and 1 month later he was relieved of the ocular symptoms.

He presented 1 year later, with complaints of blurring of vision in the right eye. Dilated fundus examination showed presence of cotton-wool spots, hemorrhages, and microaneurysms in the right eye and microaneurysms in the left eye. Fluorescein angiography confirmed the fundus findings. There was leakage of the dye causing macular edema in the right eye. There was no neovascularization detected in either eye. OCT also showed macular edema in the right eye and normal fovea in the left eye **(Fig. 7.18.9)**.

Though he was not a known diabetic or a hypertensive, a detailed laboratory evaluation was performed to rule out any known causes. All tests were reported to be within normal limits. Detailed physician evaluation also was unremarkable.

Detailed evaluation of past medical records revealed that he had received chemotherapy for brain tumor along with tumor resection surgery 2 years ago. He had also received radiation therapy for the brain tumor which he had tolerated well. Hence, a definitive diagnosis of RR was made and 3 monthly intravitreal anti-VEGF injections were given for macular edema in the right eye. Macular edema responded well to the intravitreal injections **(Fig. 7.18.10)**. He was also advised close monitoring of retinopathy changes to look for progression of macular edema and development of neovascularization.

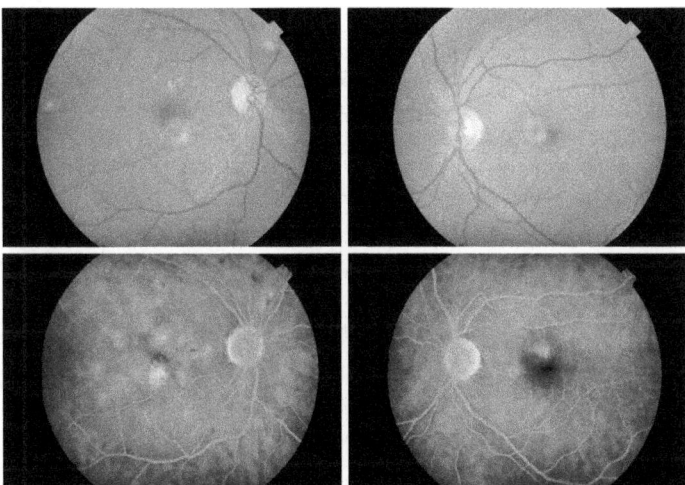

Fig. 7.18.9: Montage of fundus photograph and fluorescein angiography showing cotton-wool spots, hemorrhages, and microaneurysms in the right eye and microaneurysms in the left eye. Fluorescein angiography confirmed the fundus findings, presence of macular edema in the right eye.

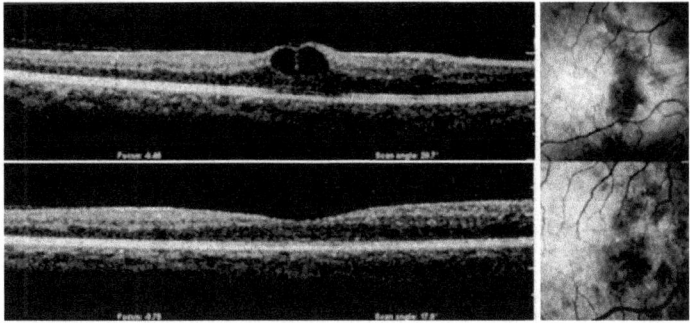

Fig. 7.18.10: Resolution of macular edema after intravitreal antivascular endothelial growth factor (VEGF) ranibizumab injection.

Practical Questions and Clinical Pearls

1. Which anti-VEGF agent is best?
There have been no published clinical trials comparing intravitreal bevacizumab (Avastin, Genentech, South San Francisco, CA), ranibizumab (Lucentis, Genentech) **(Figs. 7.18.11A to D)**, and aflibercept (Eylea, Regeneron, Tarrytown, NY). However, at the New York Eye Cancer Center, it was found that all three anti-VEGF therapies are able to suppress RM.

2. When to start anti-VEGF therapy?
Not all patients will develop RM, so select those who need close serial observation, early intervention, or prophylactic treatment. Therefore, balance the relative risks of intravitreal injection and ocular and systemic drug-induced side effects versus radiation-induced (typically monocular) vision loss.

Recent studies have shown that initiating early or even prophylactic treatments offer the best chance to prevent or (more likely) delay radiation vasculopathy-associated loss of vision. The calculated radiation dose to the fovea or the optic nerve head is the most important factor deciding the initiation of prophylactic treatment.

At the New York Eye Cancer Center, patients are divided into three risk groups depending upon the tumor size, location, and the preoperative calculation of radiation dose to the fovea:
- Patients at low risk (<25 Gy) for RM typically do not require treatment.
- Those at moderate risk (25–50 Gy) are offered close periodic observation until the first signs of RM occur (delayed strategy) and then prompt treatment.
- For eyes at high risk (>50 Gy) or those that are certain to develop RM (tumors within 2 mm, touching or beneath the fovea), the relative risks and potential benefits of delayed versus immediate treatment are discussed with the patient.

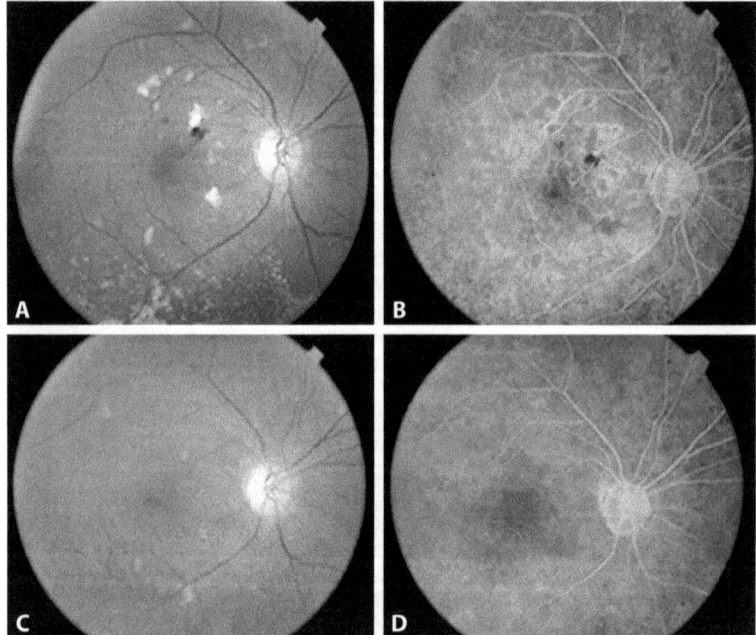

Figs. 7.18.11A to D: Clinical response to periodic intravitreal Lucentis (ranibizumab). A pretreatment fundus photograph (A) reveals a macular hemorrhage, edema, cotton-wool spots as well as exudates. Pretreatment angiogram (B) showed macular edema. Resolution is shown following Lucentis (C and D).
Source: JAMA.

3. **When should we stop anti-VEGF therapy?**
Anti-VEGF therapy suppresses and thus prolongs the evolution of RM. Almost all patients who significantly delay or stop anti-VEGF treatment develop "off-treatment" recurrent macular edema. Although these cases respond (a second time) after restarting anti-VEGF therapy, measurable damage has typically occurred in the interim. One has to remember that anti-VEGFs work, but they offer a time-limited suppressive effect, or they simply suppress radiation vasculopathy. The more consistent the treatment, the more likely it is that vision will be preserved. The bottom line is that do not stop therapy until there is no useful vision.

4. **What anti-VEGF dose is best?**
Anti-VEGF strength makes a difference. In Genentech-sponsored Investigator-Sponsored Trial (IST) testing 2.0 mg/0.05 mL ranibizumab RM trial, higher doses decreased radiation-associated macular edema in recalcitrant cases.

External beam radiation therapy (EBRT) treated patients often require higher doses to suppress their RM. This relationship is due to a more generalized radiation-induced retinal ischemia, with more resultant VEGF requiring more anti-VEGF therapy.

Finally, up to 3.0 mg/0.12 mL bevacizumab when lower doses have failed. The only current way to increase anti-VEGF dose is to shorten the time between intravitreal injections or to increase drug volume. Additionally, self-sealing "angled" injections allow for more drug (the prescribed amount) to be retained within the eye.

As a general rule, use the lowest dose and longest time interval that best restore the normal "OCT" anatomy of the macula and that preserve visual acuity.

Hence, the drug regimens, dosages, intervals, and drugs themselves need to be titrated to individual cases. One must consider the need to add steroids on a case to case basis in order to preserve vision.

Triamcinolone Acetonide Therapy

Triamcinolone acetonide is thought to downregulate various cytokines and regulate capillary permeability. It is used to treat macular edema secondary to various retinal pathologies and has similarly been used to treat RM.

While the data is limited, some studies suggest that intravitreal triamcinolone acetonide (4 mg/0.1 mL) does transiently reduce macular edema and improve visual acuity. Further studies are needed to determine whether these results are sustainable and whether the benefit of frequent injections outweighs the known risks of glaucoma, cataract, and endophthalmitis.

Laser

Grid Macular Laser Photocoagulation

Grid macular laser photocoagulation has been used to treat RM with variable success. Studies by Kinyoun et al. and Hykin et al. demonstrated a beneficial effect of photocoagulation in visual acuity. However, the effect was not sustained with longer follow-up in the study conducted by Hykin et al.

Sector scatter and pan-retinal laser photocoagulation: Sector scatter and pan-retinal laser photocoagulation has also been used to treat nonproliferative and proliferative RR. In a study by Finger et al. patients received sector scatter laser photocoagulation at the first sign of retinopathy, proliferative, or nonproliferative. Retinopathy regressed in 64% of their treated patients. Similarly, in a study by Bianciotto et al., pan-retinal photocoagulation was found to cause regression of neovascularization in 66% of eyes with proliferative RR. There are also case reports of successful treatment of RR using photodynamic therapy (PDT), hyperbaric oxygen, and oral pentoxifylline.

MicroPulse Laser Therapy

MicroPulse laser therapy (MPLT) is another option showing promise as a treatment for retinal vascular diseases. MicroPulse technology "chops" a continuous-wave laser beam into a series of short bursts, allowing the tissue to cool and thus preventing the buildup of thermal energy. Tissue damage is at least minimized and likely prevented, as there are no visible effects to the retinal tissue either during or after treatment.

MicroPulse laser therapy works by stimulating a biological response in cells that restores their integrity, rather than destroying it. The process is thought to improve RPE cell's tight junctions and pumping functions mediated by upregulation of metalloproteinase enzymes.

Monitoring on spectral-domain optical coherence tomography (SD-OCT) is the best means to observe the effect of MPLT. The focused subthermal delivery of laser energy is postulated to alter the microenvironment of the RPE that can be monitored with SD-OCT.

In conjunction with anti-VEGF treatments, MPLT has shown to restore foveal contours, resolved cystic edema and dramatically improved visual acuity in patients, without requiring retreatment.

Surgery

Advanced proliferative RR complicated by vitreous hemorrhage and/or tractional retinal detachment may require pars plana vitrectomy.

■ OTHER TREATMENTS

Various case reports describe other approaches for treating RR, including PDT, hyperbaric oxygen treatment, and oral pentoxifylline. PDT has been hypothesized to decrease hyperperfusion in affected areas of choriocapillaris in central serous chorioretinopathy, as well as to damage endothelial cells, causing occlusion of vessels.

A small study of four patients with radiation-induced macular edema demonstrated a decrease in hard exudates and improvement in visual acuity following PDT. Another case report described a patient with RR and subretinal neovascularization who had improvement in visual acuity following PDT for the subretinal neovascularization.

Hyperbaric oxygen treatment improves oxygenation and hypothetically counteracts the ischemia of RR and neuropathy. In one case report, a patient with both RR and optic neuropathy was treated with hyperbaric oxygen therapy. While retinal exudates and visual fields did improve, overall visual acuity was not significantly changed.

Finally, pentoxifylline, a drug commonly used to treat peripheral vascular disease, has also been used to treat RR. Pentoxifylline decreases the viscosity of blood, improves the flexibility of erythrocytes and leukocytes, and has a direct vasodilatory effect. It has also been shown to increase ocular blood flow. In one case report, a patient with RR was treated with oral pentoxifylline with improvement in visual acuity and improved capillary perfusion on fluorescein angiography.

■ PREVENTION

Two studies describe the use of periocular triamcinolone for prevention of RR. Periocular administration was chosen instead of intravitreal injection to avoid risks of endophthalmitis and tumor dissemination and possibly to decrease the risk of glaucoma following treatment.

In a comparative, nonrandomized, interventional study, 55 patients with newly diagnosed choroidal melanoma were treated with a periocular injection of triamcinolone at the time of iodine-125 plaque application and at 4 and 8 months postplaque. A comparison group of 32 patients was not treated with triamcinolone. At follow-up (median 24 months), the triamcinolone-treated group had a significantly lower rate of RM than the control group, but the difference in moderate and severe vision loss was not significant between the two groups.

A more recent randomized controlled study, published by the same group, randomized 163 patients with newly diagnosed choroidal melanoma to either a control group or a treatment group. Those in the treatment group received periocular injections of triamcinolone at the time of iodine-25 plaque application and at 4 and 8 months postplaque. At final follow-up (18 months), the treatment group had significantly less macular edema on OCT and significantly less moderate and severe vision loss compared to the control group.

Finally, one study described the use of laser photocoagulation in the prevention of RR and maculopathy. Plaque brachytherapy creates a predictable zone of ischemia in the tissue underlying and surrounding the plaque. In theory, treating this zone with scatter laser photocoagulation may prevent progression of RR. 16 eyes that were considered "high-risk" for developing RM given the posterior location of their melanomas were treated with laser photocoagulation in the region in and around the plaque. Photocoagulation was applied prior to the onset of clinically detectable RR. At final follow-up (mean 23.2 months), none of the eyes had lost more than three lines of vision.

RECOMMENDATIONS

Retinopathy with declining vision following brachytherapy remains a challenging adverse effect in the treatment of patients with choroidal melanoma. Although patients with larger, more posteriorly located tumors and those close to the fovea tend to have worse macular vision following radiation, it is difficult to identify which patients will develop RM and the time interval in which symptoms develop. It is important to inform patients from the outset that treatment of their tumors radiotherapy or brachytherapy will almost always result in some compromise of visual acuity. In patients who develop RM, one should discuss possible treatment options.

Following radiation therapy with external beam or brachytherapy:
- Periodic evaluation of the postradiation eye with evaluation of tumor response, treatment for neovascularization, and prescription of low vision aids when appropriate
- Careful monitoring of the fellow eye
- Regular evaluation for metastatic disease requires as much attention

CONCLUSION

No definitive treatments for RR and maculopathy have been established. The interventions discussed earlier may improve the clinical signs of RR along with transient improvement in visual acuity if predicted and treated in time. It is now a known fact that recurrent treatments are likely needed to sustain the effects.

SUMMARY

Ophthalmic radiation therapy continues to save the lives, vision, and eyes of cancer patients. All possible steps such as choosing the right source and modification of other technical parameters should be taken to reduce the radiation received by the eye. More importantly, one has to predict the development of RR or neuropathy and closely monitor even before symptoms occur. Despite best efforts, cases of RM are inevitable. Eyes with tumors posterior to the equator or in the macula and large tumors are at the greatest risk.

Newer evidence suggests predictive monitoring by OCT-A and prophylactic treatments with anti-VEGF therapy can suppress and delay the development of RM.

SUGGESTED READING

1. Al-Mefty O, Kersh JE, Routh A, Smith RR. The long-term side effects of radiation therapy for benign brain tumors in adults. J Neurosurg. 1990;73(4):502-12.
2. Horgan N, Shields CL, Mashayekhi A, Shields JA. Classification and treatment of radiation maculopathy. Curr Opin Ohthalmol. 2010;21(3):233-8.

3. Powell BE, Chin KJ, Finger PT. Early anti-VEGF treatment for radiation maculopathy and optic neuropathy: lessons learned. Eye (Lond). 2023;37(5):866-74.
4. Reichstein D. Current treatments and preventive strategies for radiation retinopathy. Curr Opin Ophthalmol. 2015;26(3):157-66.
5. Sahoo NK, Ranjan R, Tyagi M, Agrawal H, Reddy S. Radiation Retinopathy: Detection and Management Strategies. Clin Ophthalmol. 2021;15:3797-809.
6. Wen JC, McCannel TA. Treatment of radiation retinopathy following plaque brachytherapy for choroidal melanoma. Curr Opin Ophthalmol. 2009;20(3):200-4.
7. Yu HJ, Schefler AC. Radiation Retinopathy—A Review of Past and Current Treatment Strategies. US Ophthalmic Rev. 2020;13:34.

7.19 | Postoperative Endophthalmitis: An Update

Lalit Verma, Arindam Chakravarti, Anuja Patil
Centre for Sight, New Delhi
lalitretina@gmail.com

Postoperative endophthalmitis is the most devastating complication after intraocular surgery, which is commonly associated with a poor prognosis. Postoperative endophthalmitis can occur following any ocular surgery in which the globe is penetrated. However, 90% of postoperative endophthalmitis occurs following cataract surgery, because cataract surgery is one of the most frequently performed intraocular surgeries in the world. Fortunately, postoperative endophthalmitis after intraocular surgery is a rare clinical occurrence, but it often causes severe visual impairment or even the loss of an eye.

Worldwide, the reported incidence of postoperative endophthalmitis is 0.01-0.361%.[1] Postcataract surgery incidence is 0.265% (more with clear corneal incision), postkeratoplasty 0.382%, and postvitrectomy 0.05%. The incidence of bleb-associated infection is 0.2-9.6% **(Table 7.19.1)**. This range in the incidence of infection appears to be consistent across numerous patient populations from all over the world.[2] In a study of 10-year incidence of endophthalmitis rate at Bascom Palmer Eye Institute (1984-1994),[3] the incidence of postcataract surgery endophthalmitis was 0.09%. In a meta-analysis of Taban et al., the overall incidence rate of postoperative endophthalmitis was 0.128% from 1963 to 2003.[4] However, the incidence of postoperative endophthalmitis has changed over time and has increased to 0.265%/year over the last few decades, which coincides temporally with the development of self-sealing clear corneal incisions. Several retrospective, comparative, case-controlled studies found a significantly higher endophthalmitis rate associated with clear corneal incisions compared to sclera tunnel incisions. Recently, Nagaki et al. reported a statistically increased risk with clear corneal incisions (0.29%) compared to sclerocorneal incisions (0.05%).[5]

Though rare, it is potentially the most feared and devastating complication of intraocular procedures and can lead to a permanent, complete loss of vision. Endophthalmitis has been associated with severe visual loss in 20% of patients.[6] A series of endophthalmitis cases may force a temporary shutdown of the operation theater.

TABLE 7.19.1: Incidence of postoperative endophthalmitis after various surgical procedures.

Surgical procedure	Incidence
Postcataract surgery	0.265%
Postvitrectomy	0.05%
Postpenetrating keratoplasty	0.382%
Posttrabeculectomy	0.2–9.6%
Postintravitreal injection	0.028–0.056%

Infectious endophthalmitis is classified by the events leading to the infection and by the timing of the clinical diagnosis. The broad categories include postoperative endophthalmitis (acute-onset, chronic or delayed-onset, conjunctival filtering-bleb-associated), post-traumatic endophthalmitis, and endogenous endophthalmitis. Miscellaneous categories include cases associated with microbial keratitis, intravitreal injections, or suture removal. These categories are important in predicting the most frequent causative organisms and in guiding therapeutic decisions before microbiologic confirmation of the clinical diagnosis **(Box 7.19.1)**.

Results in the ESCRS (European Society of Cataract and Refractive Surgeons) postoperative endophthalmitis study, the Endophthalmitis Vitrectomy Study (EVS),[2] and other studies assessing the causative organism demonstrate that gram-positive organisms account for 90% or more of pathogens isolated in culture-positive cases of postoperative endophthalmitis following cataract surgery, with coagulase-negative staphylococci (i.e. *Staphylococcus epidermidis*) and *Staphylococcus aureus* representing the leading causes.[5,7]

Patient symptoms indicative of endophthalmitis include ocular pain, diminished vision, and headache. Although pain is an important symptom, it is not universal. It is important to differentiate infective endophthalmitis from sterile postoperative inflammation. Toxic anterior segment syndrome (TASS) is an acute postoperative inflammatory reaction in which a noninfectious substance enters the anterior segment and induces toxic damage to the intraocular tissues. Almost all cases occurred after uneventful cataract surgery. In TASS, most develop symptoms within 12–24 hours, there is decrease in visual acuity, corneal edema is from limbus to limbus, there is moderate to severe anterior chamber (AC) reaction with cells, flare, hypopyon and fibrin, pupil may be dilated and nonreactive and intraocular pressure (IOP) may be normal or raised. Differentiation is important as the management and prognosis of TASS is significantly different. Delay in diagnosis leads to delay in initiating appropriate treatment.

Postoperative endophthalmitis may be early or delayed. Most common causative agents are gram-positive coagulase negative organisms. However, in India, gram-negative organisms and fungi are important in etiopathogenesis.[8]

Endophthalmitis should be suspected when there is pain and increased in AC reaction on slit lamp examination on first postoperative day. However, pain may be absent in 25% cases. Decreased glow on distant direct ophthalmoscopy has high sensitivity but low specificity on first postoperative day.

On subsequent postoperative days, decrease in vision following initial improvement along with pain should immediately raise the index of suspicion. Presence of exudates

---

BOX 7.19.1: Classification of endophthalmitis (most frequent organisms in various clinical settings).

1. *Postoperative:*
   a. *Acute-onset postoperative endophthalmitis:* Coagulase-negative staphylococci, *Staphylococcus aureus, Streptococcus* species, gram-negative bacteria
   b. *Delayed-onset (chronic) pseudophakic endophthalmitis (>6 weeks postoperative):* *Propionibacterium acnes*, coagulase-negative staphylococci, fungi
   c. *Conjunctival filtering bleb-associated endophthalmitis: Streptococcus* species, *Haemophilus influenzae, Staphylococcus* species
2. *Post-traumatic (open globe): Bacillus* species, staphylococci.
3. *Endogenous: Candida* species, *S. aureus*, gram-negative bacteria
4. *Miscellaneous:*
   a. *Keratitis: Staphylococcus* and *Pseudomonas* species
   b. *Intravitreal injection (intravitreal triamcinolone, intravitreal ganciclovir, pneumatic retinopexy, etc.):* Coagulase negative staphylococci
   c. *Suture removal:* Both bacteria and fungi

in vitreous on indirect ophthalmoscopy is 100% specific. Presence of hypopyon and vitreous exudates is usually diagnostic of endophthalmitis. If there is no hypopyon, role of distant direct ophthalmoscopy, slit lamp examination, indirect ophthalmoscopy, and ultrasound B scan is very important in deciding surgical intervention, rule out other causes like masquerade. Slit lamp examination helps to see dilatability of pupil, wound margin (many cases related to suture removal). In cases with poorly dilating pupils and significant AC reaction (+++) and best corrected visual acuity better than 6/60, sterile reaction should be considered and treatment started with intravenous bolus steroids and topical steroids and antibiotics. However, if best-corrected visual acuity (BCVA) <6/60, endophthalmitis should be considered and patient should be administered intravitreal antibiotics. An USG B scan may aid in the diagnosis with nondilating pupils and severe AC reaction by demonstrating vitreous echoes. Presence of vitreous exudates clinches the diagnosis of endophthalmitis.

At present, best choice of intravitreal antibiotics is vancomycin (1 mg in 0.1 mL) combined with ceftazidime (2.25 mg in 0.1 mL) in separate syringes. Alternatively, vancomycin may be combined with amikacin (400 µg in 0.1 mL) **(Fig. 7.19.3)**. Topical treatment comprises ciprofloxacin/gatifloxacin/moxifloxacin 1 hourly or fortified cefazoline + tobramycin 1 hourly along with cycloplegics in the form of atropine every 6 hourly. The topical drug dosage is tailored according to response. Topical steroids are

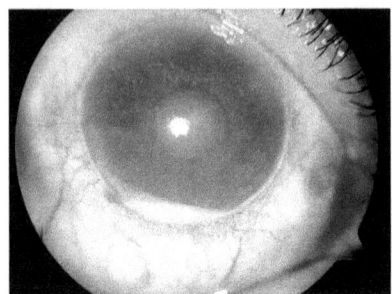

Fig. 7.19.1: Postoperative endophthalmitis: Before intravitreal injection HM+.

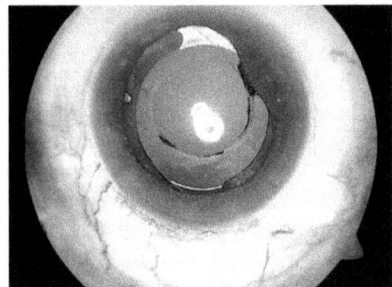

Fig. 7.19.2: Postoperative 3 weeks: Best-corrected visual acuity (BCVA) 6/6.

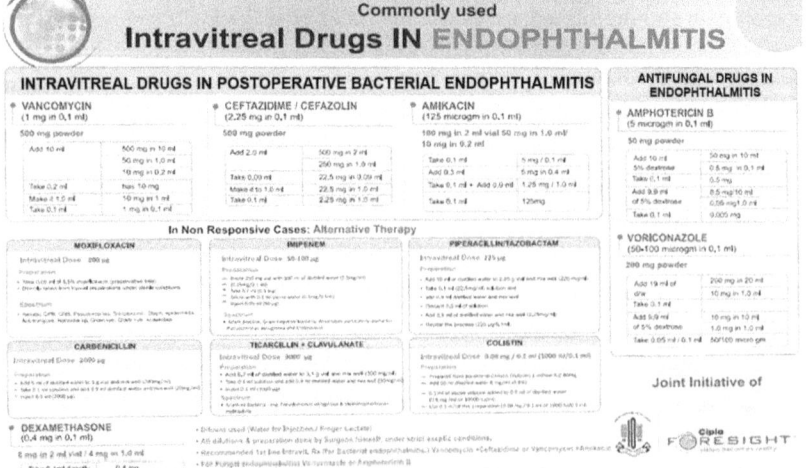

Fig. 7.19.3: Chart showing intravitreal dosage and preparation instruction of different intravitreal antibiotics and antifungal drugs and should be stuck on the OT wall.

added 1-2 days later. Intravenous ciprofloxacin 200 mg twice daily is required in very severe cases. Oral steroids administered as 1-1.5 mg/kg single dose along with oral antibiotics. Ciprofloxacin 750 mg twice daily for 7-10 days usually preferred although currently many clinicians prefer oral gatifloxacin or moxifloxacin. After intravitreal antibiotics, patient is monitored for 24-36 hours. If there is worsening, patient has to be taken up for surgical intervention in the form of pars plana vitrectomy (PPV). If there is no worsening, medical treatment can be continued for 48 hours following which decision regarding additional intravitreal antibiotics or surgical intervention is to be taken. Improvement in fundus glow with decrease in hypopyon is indicative of clinical improvement. Medical treatment should be continued.

However, in situations where there is a partial response to intravitreal antibiotics with resolution of hypopyon but persisting AC reaction (3-4+), further intravitreal antibiotics

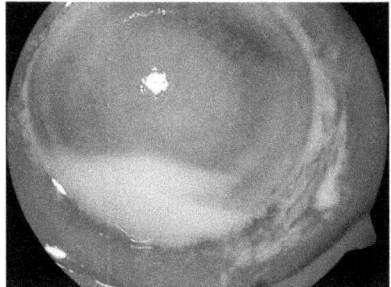

Fig. 7.19.4: Severe endophthalmitis: VA, PL+, no glow.

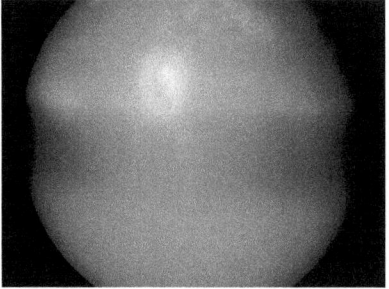

Fig. 7.19.5: Postradical PPV + IOL removal, day 9, VA: FCCF. (IOL: intraocular lens; PPV: pars plana vitrectomy)

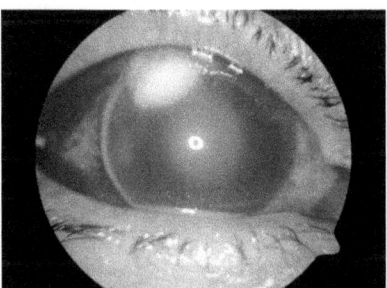

Fig. 7.19.6: Endophthalmitis with corneal abscess.

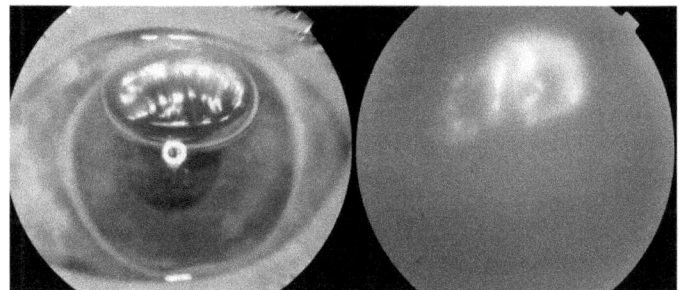

Fig. 7.19.7: Postcataract surgery endophthalmitis with retinal detachment with BCVA FCCF, PR accurate. (BCVA: Best-corrected visual acuity)

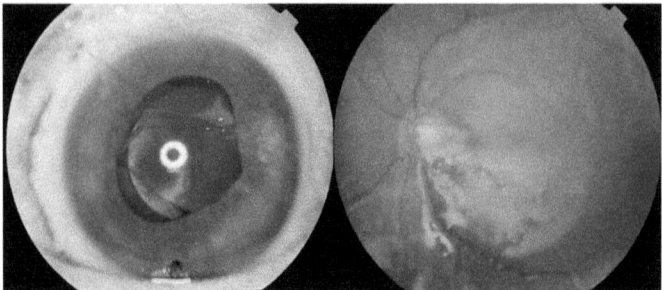

Fig. 7.19.8: Postvitrectomy VA improved to 6/9.

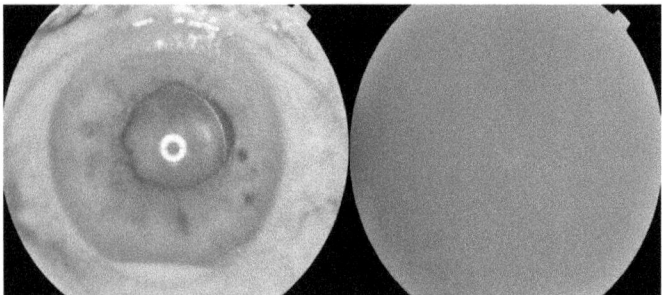

Fig. 7.19.9: A patient with CNVM due to ARMD developed postintravitreal anti-VEGF injection endophthalmitis, VA PL+, PR accurate. (ARMD: age-related macular degeneration; CNVM: choroidal neovascular membranes; VEGF: vascular endothelial growth factor)

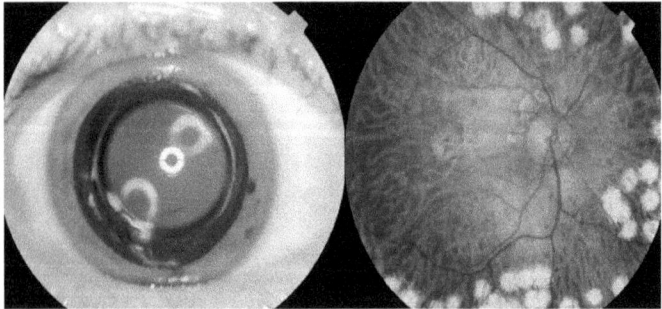

Fig. 7.19.10: Postvitrectomy VA improved to 6/9.

are not preferred, conservative medical management is continued and patient is readied for surgical intervention.

In situations where there is no response to intravitreal antibiotics or in very severe infection, radical PPV with peeling of hyaloid and base dissection is required. There is no role for core vitrectomy in this situation.

Intraocular lens (IOL) removal during vitrectomy for endophthalmitis may be indicated in severe endophthalmitis, *Propionibacterium acnes* (*P. acnes*) endophthalmitis, fungal endophthalmitis and recurrent endophthalmitis.

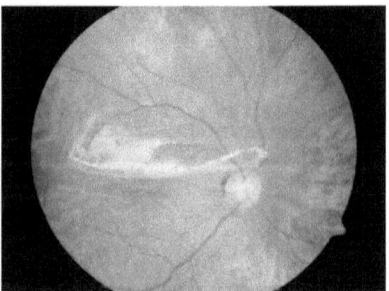

Fig. 7.19.11: Four weeks after radical vitrectomy with silicone oil, 6/24.

SECTION 7: Retina

■ FUNGAL ENDOPHTHALMITIS

Predisposing history may include diabetes mellitus, immunocompromised patient, injury with vegetable matter, and in patients on intravenous line. Usually a Quiter eye is encountered where signs are more prominent than symptoms. Vitreous balls, fungal granuloma may be seen. Smears, cultures may help. Treatment includes oral and intravitreal voriconazole (50–100 mg) or intravitreal amphotericin (5–10 mg). If on initial treatment, there is no/partial response or worsening, vitrectomy is the only hope. Often multiple vitrectomies are required; steroids should be stopped. Oral/intravenous antibiotics, cycloplegics, and topical antibiotics are usually continued.

■ CHRONIC ENDOPHTHALMITIS

Typical is *P. acnes*-related endophthalmitis. It runs a chronic course with multiple recurrences. Usual intravitreal antibiotic injections are not of much help.

Treatment Options

- "In the bag" vancomycin 1 mg/0.1 mL
- PPV + partial capsulectomy
- PPV + total capsulectomy + IOL explantation

Endophthalmitis after intravitreal Avastin: It is extremely severe due to direct inoculation of organism in vitreous. Prognosis is very poor and vitrectomy is the only answer. Lucentis scores over Avastin because of its efficacy and safety. Safety with regard to preparation of Avastin

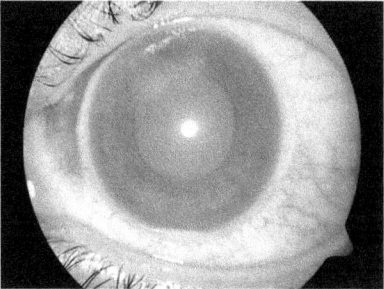

Fig. 7.19.12: Suspected fungal endophthalmitis with VA: HM.

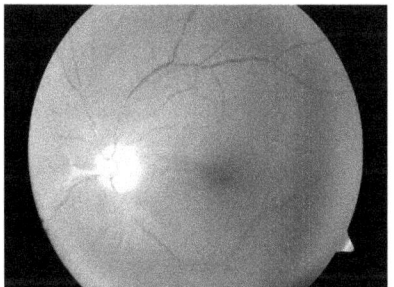

Fig. 7.19.13: After radical vitrectomy: BCVA: 6/9. (BCVA: best-corrected visual acuity)

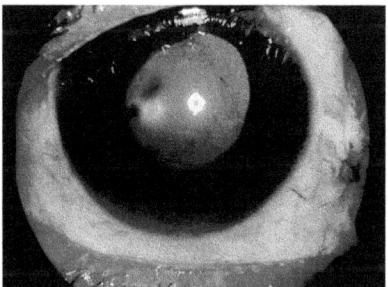

Fig. 7.19.14: Suspected *P. acnes* endophthalmitis.

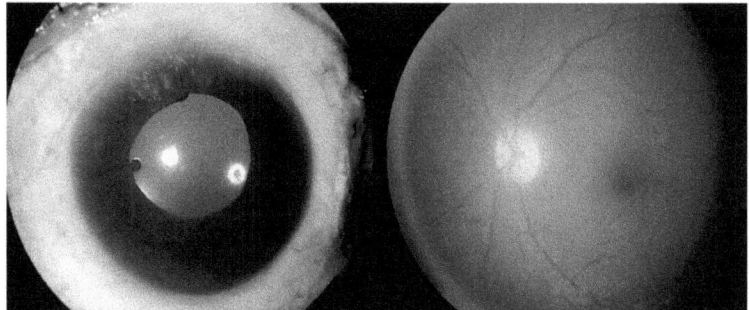

Fig. 7.19.15: Postoperative day 27: BCVA 6/18. (BCVA: best-corrected visual acuity)

is always a source of concern as there is no uniform method; multiple pricks are involved during alliquoting. There have been incidents of cluster endophthalmitis with Avastin.

In endophthalmitis with corneal involvement prognosis is generally poor. Management requires the help of a cornea specialist. Clinician has to depend upon intravitreal antibiotic injections + intensive topical treatment. Definitive vitreous surgery is difficult.

If no response: Can try core vitrectomy—if possible. Keratoprosthesis—Vitrectomy + penetrating keratoplasty (PK) or endoscopic vitrectomy.

■ NEWER INTRAVITREAL ANTIBIOTICS

Intravitreal injection of *piperacillin* and *tazobactam* could be effective in the management of multidrug-resistant endophthalmitis caused by gram-negative bacteria. *Enterobacter* species develop resistance rapidly to antibiotics due to their capacity to produce extended spectrum beta-lactamases. Piperacillin and tazobactam complement in their mechanism of action against beta-lactamase-producing organisms. Due to the production of high levels of beta-lactamase, combination therapy with piperacillin and tazobactam is a safe and effective alternative in the management of multidrug-resistant gram-negative infections. Combination of tazobactam and piperacillin is given in dosage of 225 µg/0.1 mL intravitreally based on available experimental data.

Intravitreal injection of *colistin* could be an option effective in the management of multidrug-resistant endophthalmitis caused by gram-negative bacteria. Colistin belongs to polymyxins, a group of polypeptide antibiotics which includes five different chemical compounds (polymyxins A, B, C, D, and E). Colistin binds to gram-negative bacterial cell membrane phospholipids, producing a disruptive physiochemical effect, which leads to the cell membrane permeability changes and ultimately cell death.[9] Most gram-negative microorganisms are susceptible to colistin, including multidrug-resistant *Acinetobacter baumannii* and *Pseudomonas aeruginosa* (*P. aeruginosa*) strains. Two forms of colistin are commercially available, colistin sulfate and colistimethate sodium (also called colistin methanesulfate, pentasodium colistimethanesulfate, and colistin sulfonylmethate). The target of antimicrobial activity of colistin is a bacterial cell membrane. The initial association of colistin with bacterial membrane occurs through electrostatic interactions between the cationic polypeptide (colistin) and anionic lipopolysaccharide (LPS) molecules in the outer membrane of the gram-negative bacteria, leading to derangement of the cell membrane. The endotoxin of gram-negative bacteria is the lipid a portion of LPS molecules and colistin binds and neutralizes LPS. Polymyxin E (colistin), only polymyxin B has been used in clinical practice in several countries. Polymyxin B has the same mechanism of action and resistance as does colistin. Colistin sulfate has greater activity than polymyxin B against *P. aeruginosa*. Intravitreal dose was 0.1 mg/0.1 mL (1,000 IU/0.1 mL) and IV dose was 2.5–5 mg/kg daily in 2–4 doses.

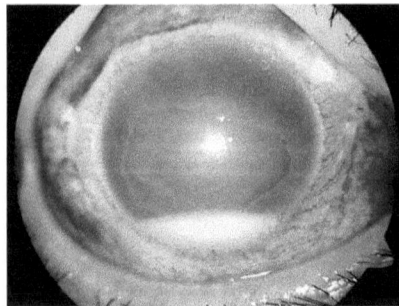

Fig. 7.19.16: Endophthalmitis after intravitreal Avastin.

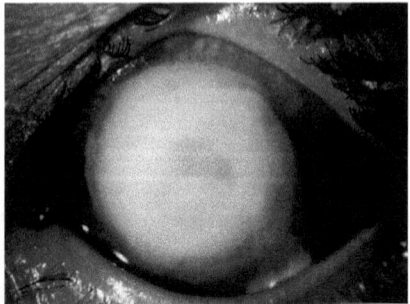

Fig. 7.19.17: Endophthalmitis with corneal involvement.

Imipenem has a broad spectrum of activity against both aerobic and anaerobic and gram-positive and gram-negative bacteria including *Pseudomonas* and *Enterococcus* species. It acts by inhibiting cell wall synthesis of various gram-positive and gram-negative bacteria. It is stable to hydrolysis by the common plasmid-mediated beta-lactamases produced by various bacteria and lacks cross-resistance with penicillins and third-generation cephalosporins. Intravitreal imipenem may limit intraocular inflammation and retinal tissue damage when given early in the course of *Pseudomonas* endophthalmitis. It is generally nontoxic in animal models at concentrations that are far higher than the minimum inhibitory concentration (MIC) 90 of 3.6–12.5 µg/mL against *Pseudomonas* infection and may offer promise in the treatment of endophthalmitis after intraocular surgery or perforating eye injuries.

WHEN TO REFER? (AFTER GIVING FIRST INTRAVITREAL ANTIBIOTIC INJECTION)

- Severe infection [very poor vision (PL +/-)]; posttrabeculectomy infection; after intravitreal injections; suspected fungal; endophthalmitis going on to panophthalmitis
- Nonresponse to first intravitreal injection
- Associated choroidal detachment or retinal detachment
- Associated corneal abscess
- Unsatisfied patient
- Cluster infection

WHAT TO DO IN CASE OF INFECTION?

Dialogue with patient and relatives; clearly explain the possible causes and pathophysiology of infection and further management. Need for cooperation and referral should be emphasized; all findings should be documented; review all sterility factors; have a peer review; referral to higher center; treat energetically with intravitreal antibiotics and supportive therapy; OT should be sealed and cultures for microbiological evaluation should be taken; batch numbers of all solutions used should be noted and samples sent for culture; all solutions used should be sealed and kept in safe custody; seek help from legal cell of All India Ophthalmological Society (AIOS).

WHAT TO DO IN CLUSTER INFECTIONS OR OUTBREAK?

Cluster endophthalmitis is defined as two or more endophthalmitis cases operated on the same day from the same operation room in one center and is a nightmare for the operating surgeon, hospital, and also patients. It usually results from a particular source of infection. Management of cluster endophthalmitis involves not only appropriate and timely treatment of infection but also identifying the source of infection and building confidence with the patient.[10]

Source of Infection (Table 7.19.2)

The causative organism in cluster endophthalmitis is usually gram-negative bacteria. *Pseudomonas* is the most common gram-negative bacteria reported to cause cluster

TABLE 7.19.2: Source of infection.

Patient-related	Healthcare worker-related	OT sterilization-related
Eye infection	Inappropriate hand wash technique	Improper OT sterilization
Poor eye hygiene	Not changing surgical gloves before each surgery	Contaminated surgical solutions, dyes, instruments
Immunocompromised state		

endophthalmitis in India.[11] Cataract surgery was the most common cause of cluster endophthalmitis around two decades ago. However, presently, cluster endophthalmitis is commoner in postintravitreal injection patients.

■ APPROACH TO CLUSTER ENDOPHTHALMITIS
What to do if Suspicion of Cluster Endophthalmitis?

An investigative team is formed which includes physicians, microbiologists, and operation room nurses. An investigation panel/team will not only find the reason for cluster endophthalmitis but also manage media, patients, and relatives effectively. The team must gather information about the recent treatment and clinical condition of the affected patients. Inform authorities—chief medical officer, medical superintendent, senior authority; Institute Infection Control Committees; inform AIOS and seek help of legal cell; engage and seek help of lawyer. Press has to be handled carefully to prevent pandemonium from spreading. It is desirable that medical superintendent/hospital committee does press briefing. Royal College of Ophthalmology, UK has given color-coded alerts based on number of cases in postoperative endophthalmitis:[12]

- Green—one case of endophthalmitis; 1 in >/= 100 cases; or 2 in >600 cases.
- Amber (0.4–0.7%)—one case in 75 cases, two cases in 300–500 cases, three cases in 700–800 cases.
- Red (0.8–4%)—two cases in ≤200 cases, three cases in ≤600 cases, four cases in ≤800 cases.

Green alert calls for reviewing the case with colleagues, alerting other consultants and reporting in the next audit. Amber alert requires the microbiology department to subtype any organism grown from second and subsequent cases. Red alert necessitates urgent immediate closure of the operation room until the cause of infection is identified along with the above-mentioned measures.

- *Treatment of endophthalmitis:*
  - Intravitreal antibiotics **(Fig. 7.19.14)**
  - Vitrectomy is usually needed

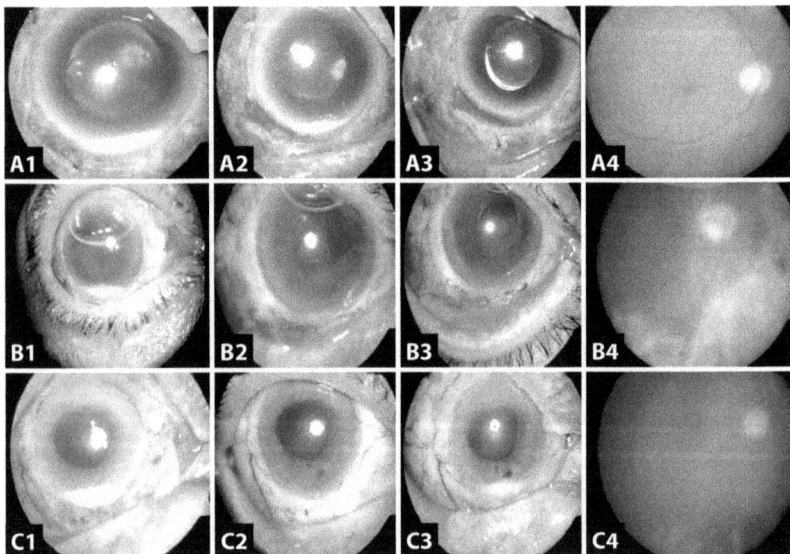

Figs. 7.19.18A to C: Three cases of operated silicone oil removal developed cluster endophthalmitis on postoperative day one (A1, B1, C1). All three cases responded well to intravitreal antibiotics (A2, 3, 4; B2, 3, 4; C2, 3, 4).

- Patients and their relatives should be properly counseled about their present condition, ongoing treatment, and future outcome
- *Identification of the cause of infection:*[13]
    - Patient-related factors—review patient's record for the presence of blepharitis, nasolacrimal duct obstruction (NLDO), immunocompromised condition, and poor eye hygiene
    - Surgeon-related factors—whether OT conduct guidelines were followed.
    - OT sterilization protocols followed in the center
    - Culture swabs from different areas of the OT, samples from irrigating solution, dyes, water, and hand scrub solution sent for culture.
- *Building confidence with the affected patients:*[10]
    - Counseling the patient and relatives is very essential.
    - They should be informed about the possible cause of the infection, ongoing treatment, and possible outcome.

TEN TIPS FOR MANAGING POSTOPERATIVE ENDOPHTHALMITIS

1. Suspect
2. Differentiate from TASS
3. Talk with relatives and patients
4. Peer review
5. Prompt intravitreal injection
6. Regular/daily review
7. Culture report
8. Early vitrectomy if required
9. Referral to higher center
10. Documentation

DECLARATION

This chapter is a modified version of the authors' prior publication in IJO 2017 with due citation of the same included in the references.

REFERENCES

1. West ES, Behrens A, McDonnell PJ, Tielsch JM, Schein OD. The incidence of endophthalmitis after cataract surgery among the U.S. Medicare population increased between 1994 and 2001. Ophthalmology. 2005;112(8):1388-94.
2. Results of the endophthalmitis vitrectomy study. A randomized trial of immediate vitrectomy and of intravenous antibiotics for the treatment of postoperative bacterial endophthalmitis. Endophthalmitis vitrectomy study group. Arch Ophthalmol. 1995;113(12):1479-96.
3. Aaberg TM, Flynn HW, Schiffman J, Newton J. Nosocomial acute-onset postoperative endophthalmitis survey: a 10-year review of incidence and outcomes. Ophthalmology. 1998;105(6):1004-10.
4. Taban M, Behrens A, Newcomb RL, Nobe MY, Saedi G, Sweet PM, et al. Acute endophthalmitis following cataract surgery: a systematic review of the literature. Arch Ophthalmol. 2005;123(5):613-20.
5. Nagaki Y, Hayasaka S, Kadoi C, Matsumoto M, Yanagisawa S, Watanabe K, et al Bacterial endophthalmitis after small-incision cataract surgery. Effect of incision placement and intraocular lens type. J Cataract Refract Surg. 2003;29:20-6.
6. Verma L, Chakravarti A. Prevention and management of postoperative endophthalmitis: A case-based approach. Indian J Ophthalmol. 2017;65(12):1396-1402.
7. Han DP, Wisniewski SR, Wilson LA, Barza M, Vine AK, Doft BH, et al Spectrum and susceptibilities of microbiologic isolates in the endophthalmitis vitrectomy study. Am J Ophthalmol. 1996;122:1-7.
8. Verma L, Venkatesh P, Tewari HK. (2000). Management of Endophthalmitis, AIOS CME Series-4. [online] Available from http://www.aios.org/cme/cmeseries4.pdf [Last accessed September, 2023].

9. Evans ME, Feola DJ, Rapp RP. Polymyxin B sulfate and colistin: Old antibiotics for emerging multiresistant gram-negative bacteria. Ann Pharmacother. 1999;33:960-7.
10. Das T. Management of cluster endophthalmitis does not stop at clinical care. Indian J Ophthalmol. 2020;68(7):1249-51.
11. Pinna A, Usai D, Sechi LA, Zanetti S, Jesudasan NC, Thomas PA, et al. An outbreak of postcataract surgery endophthalmitis caused by *Pseudomonas aeruginosa*. Ophthalmology. 2009;116:2321-6.
12. Ophthalmic service guidance, Royal College of Ophthalmology: Managing an outbreak of postoperative endophthalmitis 2016.
13. Desai SR, Bhagat PR, Parmar D. Recommendations for an expert team investigating a case of cluster endophthalmitis. Indian J. Ophthalmol. 2018;66(8):1074-8.

7.20 Retinal Detachment with Proliferative Vitreoretinopathy

Lingam Gopal
Sankara Nethralaya, Chennai
lingamgopal@gmail.com

■ INTRODUCTION

Proliferative vitreoretinopathy (PVR) is characterized by fibrosis in the vitreous cavity and along either of the surfaces of the retina resulting in failure in retinal reattachment. It is the most common cause of failure to reattach retina and of recurrent retinal detachment after initial success. Important predisposing factors are presence of choroidal detachment, giant retinal tear (and large tears), profuse hypotony, postperforating injury retinal detachments, failed surgery, long duration of retinal detachment, coexisting uveitis, etc.[1]

■ CLASSIFICATION

Retina Society Classification[1]
A—Vitreous haze and pigment clumps.
B—Surface retinal wrinkling, rolled edges of retinal tears, retinal stiffness, and vessel tortuosity.
C—Full-thickness retinal folds: C1—one quadrant; C2—two quadrants; and C3—three quadrants.
D—Fixed retinal folds in all quadrants: D1—wide funnel shape; D2—narrow funnel shape; and D3—closed funnel shape with no view of disc.

This classification had several lacunae including ignoring the anterior PVR, subretinal fibrosis, etc.

Updated Retina Society Classification (Partly Based on Silicone Oil Study Classification)[2]
Stage A and B are similar to the old classification.
A—Vitreous haze and pigment clumps.
B—Surface retinal wrinkling, rolled edges of retinal tears, retinal stiffness, and vessel tortuosity.

Stage C is divided into P and A.
CP—Posterior:
Description: Type "a"—focal star folds; type "b"—diffuse contraction in posterior retina; type "c"—subretinal membranes

Distribution: Number of clock hours of involvement is described.

CA—Anterior:
Type "a"—circumferential (retinal contraction inward at poster edge of vitreous base); type "b"—anterior contraction of the retina at vitreous base/CB detachment/epi ciliary membranes/iris retraction.

Distribution: Number of clock hours of involvement described.

RISK FACTORS[3]

These factors increase the dispersion of retinal pigment epithelium (RPE) cells and break down of blood ocular barrier.

Primary PVR: Large retinal tears, long duration of retinal detachment, vitreous hemorrhage, aphakia, and choroidal detachment.

Postoperative PVR: Large breaks, pre- and postoperative choroidal detachment, minor intra- or postoperative hemorrhages, signs of uveitis, extensive retinal detachment, cryopexy, and preoperative PVR.

MANAGEMENT

Preoperative Management

- *Preoperative steroids:*[4] Use of preoperative steroids has been found useful to resolve/reduce coexisting choroidal detachment and inflammation. However, the potential effect on incidence of postoperative PVR or recurrent PVR has not been conclusively demonstrated.
- *Early surgery:* In the presence of large retinal tears (especially giant retinal tears), early surgery is recommended to prevent the development of preoperative PVR.

Surgical Options

Scleral Buckle

Most cases of retinal detachment with PVR are not amenable for scleral buckle procedure alone.

Cases that can still be managed by scleral buckling alone include chronic retinal detachments secondary to lattice degeneration with atrophic holes, and a few cases of retinal dialysis with chronic retinal detachments. Even in the presence of a few subretinal bands, scleral buckling can succeed in some of the cases of lattice-related chronic retinal detachments.

Principles when scleral buckle is the chosen option:
1. One may have to produce a moderate buckle indentation in view of the relatively contracted retina. Encirclage is a must to maintain moderate and permanent buckle indentation (segmental buckle is likely to fail).
2. Drainage of subretinal fluid would be needed in most cases. Chronic retinal detachments have thick subretinal fluid that does not get absorbed fast enough to reattach the retina despite the buckle and there is a possibility the break may remain lifted off the buckle (nonclosure).

Vitreoretinal Surgery

In most other cases, a vitrectomy approach is chosen with or without additional encirclage.

Role of encirclage: Additional of a 360° silicone band helps in the overall goal of achieving attached retina due to:
- Further relieving traction in addition to what was achieved by vitrectomy and membrane peeling.
- *Supporting the vitreous base:* In phakic eyes, a thorough peripheral vitrectomy may not be possible and hence supporting the vitreous base can improve the success of surgery. Their role is also important in inferior breaks which have tendency to get lifted up asily.

Principles of vitreoretinal procedures:
- Thorough vitrectomy including vitreous base excision/debulking. Intravitreal triamcinolone can assist in identifying residual vitreous (especially in high myopic eyes)
- Preretinal membrane removal with instruments such as pic and forceps
- *Removal of subretinal membranes through:*
  - Isolated strategically placed retinotomies
  - Large peripheral circumferential retinotomies to access the subretinal space (for more extensive membranes)
- *Use of perfluorocarbon liquids (PFCLs):* Heavy liquids are useful at several steps of the surgery in PVR.
  1. To keep the posterior pole down and assist the dissection of membrane anteriorly
  2. To assist performance of relaxing retinotomies and retinectomies
  3. To drain subretinal fluid through an anteriorly located retinal break if one wants to avoid a posterior retinotomy
  4. To unfold the retina and reattach it as in cases of giant retinal tears/360 relaxing retinotomies
  5. *As short-term tamponading agents:* PFCLs are used mostly as intraoperative tools as mentioned earlier and replaced by other agents to provide postoperative tamponade. However, a few surgeons have used PFCLs as short-term postoperative tamponading agents and removed them by a second surgical procedure.
- *Lens management:* Predominantly posterior PVR can be managed by vitreoretinal (VR) procedures without sacrificing the lens. However, in the presence of severe PVR with extreme anterior loop traction caused by fibrosis bridging between ciliary processes and vitreous base, sacrifice of clear lens/intraocular lens may be required to facilitate complete dissection.
- *Fluid air exchange:* This step is performed after full mobilization of the retina and relief of all traction. It helps to reattach the detached retina. The fluid in subretinal space and vitreous cavity are removed and replaced by air. Entry of air into subretinal space indicates unrelieved traction. If it happens, one must replace the air with fluid, relieve the traction by looking for membranes and redo the fluid air exchange.
- *Drainage retinotomy:* This is a retinal hole deliberately made to facilitate drainage of subretinal fluid. In situations where the preexisting break is very anteriorly located and not easily reached or significant fluid is trapped posteriorly, one may have to perform this step. The location of the retinotomy is usually chosen superiorly and as far anteriorly as possible to have the least effect on visual field. (Refer for use of heavy liquids to avoid unnecessary posterior drainage retinotomy)
- *Relaxing retinotomies/retinectomies:* This refers to the performance of deliberate large cuts in the retina to achieve complete relaxation of the retina and facilitate its reattachment without any tension. The most common location is in the peripheral retina within the vitreous base where in total relief of traction may be sometimes impossible despite the membrane peeling.
- *Retinopexy:* Laser is preferred over cryopexy for performing retinopexy to surround all retinal tears including relaxing retinotomies.
- *Internal tamponade:* Supporting the retina from within is possible by use of gas or silicone oil once vitrectomy is performed and retina is reattached with fluid air exchange or use of perfluorocarbon liquids. For eyes with PVR, the gas most used is C3F8. Silicone oil is used when more long-term tamponade is desired. Both gas and routine silicone oil float in water and preferentially support superior retina better. Heavy silicone oil (Densiron, etc.) refers to a specific type of silicone oil that has specific gravity more than that of water and hence used when inferior retina needs to

be supported preferentially. Potentially, heavy silicone oils can be used like PFCLs to reattach the retina on the operation table as well as postoperative tamponade.
- *Ando iridectomy:* When using routine silicone oil in aphakic eyes, inferior iridectomy is performed to keep the oil in the pupillary plane by permitting the heavier aqueous to permeate into the anterior chamber from below.

Postoperative prone positioning is very often required to take help of the buoyancy of the gas or silicone oil in maintaining the pressure on the retina.

Second Surgeries

Retinal detachments with PVR often end up having multiple surgeries. The second intervention is needed for the following reasons:
- *Removal of silicone oil:* All cases that had oil injection are planned for an ultimate removal of oil to get an oil-free long-term success.
- *Revision surgeries for recurrent retinal detachment:* Recurrence of PVR is not uncommon and demands additional intervention.
- *Cataract surgery:* In phakic eyes, cataract development is 100% at some time or other following VR surgery with gas or oil tamponade.
- Management of band-shaped keratopathy
- Antiglaucoma surgery—usually in the form of tube implants

COMPLICATIONS OF SURGERY FOR PROLIFERATIVE VITREORETINOPATHY

- *Complications related to PVR:* These include failure to reattach the retina, limited recurrence of PVR leading to epiretinal membranes, gross recurrence of PVR leading recurrent retinal detachment.
- *Complications due to tamponading agents:*
  - *Gas-related:* Glaucoma and gas cataract
  - *Silicone oil-related:* Emulsification, hyperoleon (emulsified material collecting like inverse hypopyon in the anterior chamber), glaucoma, cataract, band-shaped keratopathy, etc.
- *Hypotony:* Hypotony is related more to the overall disease process (not surgery). Hypotony may not permit removal of silicone oil and perpetuate the complications.

PREVENTION OF PROLIFERATIVE VITREORETINOPATHY

Several approaches have been tried with conflicting results.
- Systemic steroids
- Intravitreal steroids[5]
- Intravitreal 2-fluorouracil with low-molecular-weight heparin[6]
- Decorin [a naturally occurring transforming growth factor (TGF)-β inhibitor][7]

Currently there is no proven method of prevention of PVR. Steroids continue to be used by most surgeons with a belief that control of inflammation can reduce the risk of PVR.

REFERENCES

1. Hilton G, Machemer R, Michels R, Okun E, Schepens C, Schwartz A. The classification of retinal detachment with proliferative vitreoretinopathy. Ophthalmology. 1983;90(2):121-5.
2. Heimann K, Wiedemann P. Cologne classification of proliferative vitreoretinopathy. In: Heimann K, Wiedemann P (Eds). Proliferative Vitreoretinopathy. Heidelberg, Germany: Kaden; 1989. pp. 148-9.
3. Nagasaki H, Shinagawa K, Mochizuki M. Risk factors for proliferative vitreoretinopathy. Prog Retin Eye Res. 1998;17(1):77-98.
4. Denwattana A, Prakhunhungsit S, Thoongsuwan S, Rodanant N, Phasukkijwatana N. Surgical outcomes of preoperative steroid for rhegmatogenous retinal detachment with associated choroidal detachment, Eye. 2018;32(3):602-7.

5. Gagliano C, Toro MD, Avitabile T, Stella S, Uva MG. Intravitreal Steroids for the Prevention of PVR After Surgery for Retinal Detachment. Curr Pharm Des. 2015;21(32):4698-702.
6. Sundaram V, Barsam A, Virgili G. Intravitreal low molecular weight heparin and 5-Fluorouracil for the prevention of proliferative vitreoretinopathy following retinal reattachment surgery. Cochrane Database Syst Rev. 2013;(1):CD006421.
7. Nassar K, Lüke J, Lüke M, Kamal M, Abd El-Nabi E, Soliman M, et al. The novel use of decorin in prevention of the development of proliferative vitreoretinopathy (PVR). Graefes Arch Clin Exp Ophthalmol. 2011;249(11):1649-60.

7.21 Retinopathy of Prematurity

Anand Vinekar
Narayana Nethralaya Eye Institute, Bengaluru
anandvinekar@yahoo.com

Gaurav Sanghi
Sangam Nethralya, Punjab
gaurav_pgi@yahoo.co.in

Mangat R Dogra
Grewal Eye Institute, Chandigarh
drmangatdogra@gmail.com

INTRODUCTION

Retinopathy of prematurity (ROP) is a vasoproliferative disorder affecting the retinae of infants, predominantly born premature, and/or with low birth weight.

Problem Statement

It is the leading cause of preventable infant blindness in the world. India has the highest number of premature infants worldwide, approximately 3.5 million annually. The incidence of ROP in India ranges from 20–50% of "at risk" babies. Of these, 150,000–200,000 infants are estimated to require treatment or risk blindness if not managed appropriately. There are few ROP specialists in India, and screening and treatment facilities are currently unavailable in most neonatal intensive care units.

FACTORS THAT INCREASE THE RISK OF RETINOPATHY OF PREMATURITY

The most important "risk" factors include preterm birth <34 weeks of gestational age, birth weight <2,000 g, and high exposure to unmonitored oxygen from birth. However, there are over 30 reported factors that include poor weight gain, sepsis, respiratory distress, transfusion of blood products, anemia among others, that also influence the disease.

RETINOPATHY OF PREMATURITY STAGING

The disease is classified according to the International Classification of Retinopathy of Prematurity (ICROP) classification. In 2021, the 3rd iteration (ICROP-3) was published and replaced the older classification of 2005. The new classification addresses the changing landscape of presentation of varying forms of disease, including aggressive retinopathy of prematurity (AROP), description of the notch, subclassification of stage 5 into A, B, and C, and defines regression and recurrence more clearly compared to its predecessors.

The International Classification of ROP (ICROP) is based on the location, extent, and stage of ROP.

Location

Three concentric retinal zones are centered on the disc and extend to the ora serrata. The location of the most posterior retinal vascularization or ROP lesion denotes the zone for the eye.

Zone I: It is defined by a circle with a radius twice the estimated distance from the optic disc center to the foveal center.

Zone II: It is a ring-shaped region extending nasally from the outer limit of zone I to the nasal ora serrata and with a similar distance temporally, superiorly, and inferiorly. A region of 2-disc diameters peripheral to the zone I border is defined as posterior zone II to indicate potentially "more worrisome" disease than ROP in the more peripheral zone II. A new term "notch" to describe an incursion by the ROP lesion of 1–2 clock hours along the horizontal meridian into a more posterior zone than the remainder of the retinopathy.

Zone III: It is the residual crescent of the peripheral retina that extends beyond zone II temporally.

Extent

Number of clock hours involved.

Stage

1. *Stage 1* is the demarcation line between the vascular and avascular retina.
2. *Stage 2* the line has acquired height and width and forms a ridge.
3. *Stage 3*, this ridge acquires extraretinal fibrovascular proliferation.
4. *Stage 4* is a subtotal retinal detachment (partial: 4A with fovea attached, 4B with fovea detached).
5. *Stage 5* is total retinal detachment (Stage 5A, in which the optic disc is visible by ophthalmoscopy (suggesting open-funnel detachment); Stage 5B, in which the optic disc is not visible because of retrolental fibrovascular tissue or closed-funnel detachment; and Stage 5C, in which Stage 5B is accompanied by anterior segment changes (e.g., marked anterior chamber shallowing, iridocorneolenticular adhesions, and corneal opacification), suggesting closed-funnel configuration.

■ PLUS AND PREPLUS DISEASE

Plus disease is defined by the appearance of dilation and tortuosity of retinal vessels, and preplus disease is defined by abnormal vascular dilation, tortuosity insufficient for plus disease, or both. These changes should be assessed by vessels within zone I.

■ AGGRESSIVE RETINOPATHY OF PREMATURITY

The term aggressive posterior ROP (APROP) was used previously to describe a severe, rapidly progressive form of ROP located in posterior zones I or II. This has been replaced in the 2021 classification by the term AROP because of increasing recognition that this may occur beyond the posterior retina and in larger preterm infants, particularly in regions of the world with limited resources like India. The hallmark of AROP is rapid development of pathologic neovascularization and severe plus disease without progression being observed through the typical stages of ROP.

■ OTHER NEW TERMS INTRODUCED IN ICROP-3 (2021)

Regression

Definition of ROP regression and its sequelae, whether spontaneous or after laser or anti-vascular endothelial growth factor (VEGF) treatment. Regression can be complete or incomplete. The location and extent of peripheral avascular retina (PAR) should be documented.

Reactivation
Definition and description of nomenclature representing ROP reactivation after treatment may include new ROP lesions and vascular changes. When reactivation of ROP stages occurs, the modifier reactivated (e.g., "reactivated stage 2") is recommended.

Long-term Sequelae
These include sequelae such as late retinal detachments, persistent avascular retina, macular anomalies, retinal vascular changes, and glaucoma.

■ RETINOPATHY OF PREMATURITY SCREENING
Retinopathy of prematurity screening in India is performed based on the National ROP screening guidelines. The current version was published by the Ministry of Health and Family Welfare and detailed in the operational guidelines in 2018.

Which Babies to Screen?
Babies born <2,000 g at birth and/or with a gestational age of <34 weeks are considered for screening. Those born between 34 and 36 weeks need of respiratory support, oxygen therapy for >6 hours, sepsis, episodes of apnea and need of blood transfusion, exchange transfusion, or unstable clinical course as determined by pediatrician.

When to Commence Screening?
Before 30 days of postnatal age. This is usually performed between 3 and 4 weeks of age. For infants born <28 weeks or <1,200 g, the first screening may be earlier and between 2 and 3 weeks of age.

How Often to Screen?
This would depend on the findings at the time of screening and are summarized in **Table 7.21.1**.

When to Terminate ROP Screening?
This is performed until complete vascularization of the retina is documented in cases without any ROP or if there was ROP, then the disease must show complete regression spontaneously. Those who are treated are followed up differently.

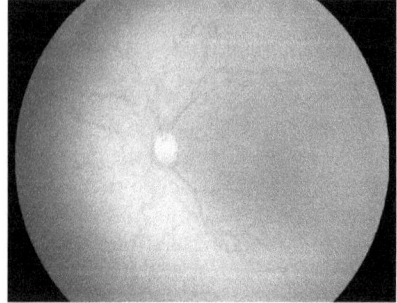

Fig. 7.21.1: Aggressive retinopathy of prematurity (AROP) in the left eye showing severe plus disease, closed loops, capillary nonperfusion, and poor vascular growth. No classical "ridge tissue" is noted in these cases leading to underdiagnosis.

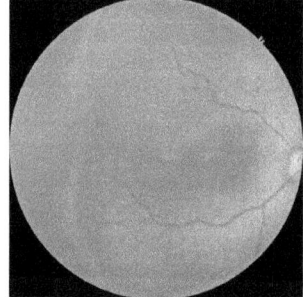

Fig. 7.21.2: Retinopathy of prematurity (ROP) stage 3 in zone 2 with plus disease. The fibrovascular proliferation with abnormal neovascularization is classical in classical stage 3. ROP requiring treatment with these "classical" (nonaggressive ROP) forms is called type 1 ROP.

TABLE 7.21.1: Follow-up schedule based on the clinical findings of the screening visit.

Zone	Stage	Follow-up interval
1	Immature	1–2 weeks
	Stage 1, 2, or regressing ROP	1 week or earlier
	Stage 3/AROP	Treat (**Table 7.21.2**)
2	Immature	2–3 weeks
	Stage 1	2 weeks
	Stage 2/regressing ROP	Treat if stage 2 has plus disease, follow-up 1–2 weeks if not present and regressing
	Stage 3	Treat if plus disease is present, 1 week or earlier if not present
3	Stage 1, 2/regressing ROP	2–3 weeks

(AROP: aggressive retinopathy of prematurity; ROP: retinopathy of prematurity)

How to Dilate the Pupil for Screening?

Pupillary dilation is achieved with 2.5% phenylephrine hydrochloride and 0.5% cyclopentolate or 1% tropicamide instilled twice after a gap of 15 minutes. Commercially available 5 or 10% phenylephrine should be diluted in distilled water to make it 2.5%.

Who Should Perform ROP Screening?

The National Operational Guidelines (2018) recommend that ROP screening can be performed by either a trained ophthalmologist using indirect ophthalmoscopy or a trained ophthalmologist using retinal imaging or a trained technician/district early intervention center optometrist/neonatal intensive care unit (NICU) nurse using retinal imaging.

■ LONG-TERM FOLLOW-UP SCHEDULE

It is recommended that preterm infants and those requiring ROP treatment must be followed up until 7 years of age (at least) for refractive errors, strabismus, cortical vision impairment, as well as other long-term sequelae mentioned earlier.

■ RETINOPATHY OF PREMATURITY TREATMENT

Laser Treatment

The gold standard for ROP treatment is laser photoablation. Traditionally the avascular retina anterior to the fibrovascular or neovascular ridge tissue is treated with near confluent laser spots. Historically 810 nm (infrared laser) was used. Currently, the 532 nm neodymium-doped yttrium aluminum garnet (Nd:YAG) green laser is preferred. The treatment is most often performed under topical anesthesia (paracain eye drops) with a supplement of oral "sugar pellets" used intraoperatively. Systemic monitoring is performed by a neonatologist or anesthetist during and following the procedure.

The current indications for laser are based on the Early Treatment for Retinopathy of Prematurity (ETROP) randomized trial and are summarized in **Table 7.21.2**. ROP laser is a relative ophthalmic emergency and must be ideally completed within 48–72 hours of diagnosis. Follow-up after laser treatment is usually after 1 week. Sometimes, a "laser add" is required based on the treatment strategy and the pretreatment diagnosis and is usually performed 2–4 weeks later. Following regression, long-term follow-up schedule (described earlier) must be followed.

TABLE 7.21.2: Treatment criteria based on the ETROP guidelines.

Zone I	No plus	Stage I	Close follow-up
		Stage II	Close follow-up
		Stage III	Treat
	Plus	Stage I	Treat
		Stage II	Treat
		Stage III	Treat
Zone II	No plus	Stage I	Follow-up
		Stage II	Follow-up
		Stage III	Follow-up
	Plus	Stage I	Follow-up
		Stage II	Treat
		Stage III	Treat

(ETROP: Early Treatment for Retinopathy of Prematurity)

Intravitreal Injections of Antivascular Endothelial Growth Factors

Intravitreal injections of anti-VEGF have more recently become popular for ROP treatment. There are currently no guidelines for its use and remains off label. Drugs used include, bevacizumab, ranibizumab, and aflibercept. The dose, timing, and indications for retreatment are currently not defined.

Anti-VEGF agents are most useful in posterior zone 1 or zone 1 ROP, especially AROP, before vitrectomy to reduce intraoperative bleeding, when laser treatment is difficult or the baby is systemically unstable to withstand laser, or where the traditional laser has poorer outcomes or requires more extensive laser treatment.

The procedure requires special consent and must be performed preferably in the operating room under prescribed protocols. Follow-up is imperative as persistent avascular retinae and late recurrences are common. A more common approach is a combination therapy where anti-VEGF injections are treated with laser a few weeks or months later. These guidelines are still evolving.

Retinal Surgery

Lens-sparing vitrectomy (LSV) and lensectomy-vitrectomy (LV) can be performed for retinal detachment cases in ROP. The former is used for stage 4A and selected cases of 4B and the latter for stage 5. LSV has a better anatomical outcome. The aim of surgery is the removal of as much of proliferation as possible. It is not possible to remove the hyaloid completely in an infant with ROP. Overall the outcome after stage 5 surgery is poor functionally or structurally.

■ RECENT ADVANCES

Some of the recent advances include low-cost, indigenous retinal cameras for ROP photo documentation and screening, tele-ROP programs that allow outreach screening in underserved areas, artificial intelligence that is able to diagnose ROP on wide-field retinal images, ultra-wide retinal imaging, fluorescein angiography to follow-up certain ROP cases, especially post-treatment with anti-VEGF agents, prediction of ROP using tear fluids, hand-held optical coherence tomography, and optical coherence tomography angiography (OCT-A) in ROP to evaluate preterm with and without ROP and online training modules. Medicolegal aspects in ROP management have become important and guidelines for screening and treatment must be carefully adhered to.

REFERENCES

1. Chiang MF, Quinn GE, Fielder AR, Ostmo SR, Chan RVP, Berrocal A, et al. International Classification of Retinopathy of Prematurity, 3rd Edition. Ophthalmology. 2021;128(10): e51-68.
2. Early Treatment for Retinopathy of Prematurity Cooperative Group. Revised indications for the treatment of retinopathy of prematurity: results of the early treatment for retinopathy of prematurity randomized trial. Arch Ophthalmol. 2003;121(12):1684-94.
3. Public Health Foundation of India. (2019). Project Operational Guidelines: Prevention of Blindness from Retinopathy of Prematurity in Neonatal Care Units. [online] Available from https://phfi.org/wp-content/uploads/2019/05/2018-ROP-operational-guidelines.pdf. [Last accessed July, 2023].

7.22 Choroidal Melanoma

P Mahesh Shanmugam
Sankara Eye Hospitals, Bengaluru
maheshshanmugam@gmail.com

INTRODUCTION

Uveal melanoma is the most common primary intraocular tumor with an incidence of 5.2–7/million Caucasians older than 60 years of age. It is rare in Asian Indians and occurs at a younger age (~45 years).

RISK FACTORS

- Choroidal nevi
- Congenital oculodermal melanocytosis
- Neurofibromatosis
- Light colored skin and eyes
- Occupational ultraviolet light exposure

CLASSIFICATION

Choroidal melanoma is classified based on cell type into:
- Spindle A
- Spindle B
- Epithelioid
- Mixed

The cell type has prognostic value for life with spindle cell tumors having the best prognosis and the epithelioid tumors the worst. Patients with choroidal melanoma can present with field loss or vision loss, pain due to secondary glaucoma or ciliary nerve involvement, and floaters due to pigment release or vitreous hemorrhage.

Fundus examination shows small melanomas to be nodular and large tumors to be dome or mushroom shaped (when growing through Bruch's membrane or retina) with gray or brown colored tumors (**Fig. 7.22.1**). Diffuse melanoma has a height that is <20% of the basal diameter.

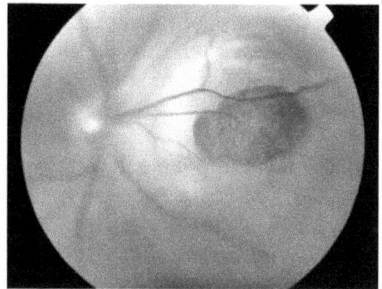

Fig. 7.22.1: Brown mushroom-shaped choroidal melanoma involving superotemporal quadrant.

SECONDARY EFFECTS

Secondary effects of the tumor on the following are as follows:
- *Retinal pigment epithelial:* Mottling, drusen, orange pigment, retinal pigment epithelium (RPE) detachments and choroidal neovascularization
- *Retina:* Secondary retinal detachment and cystoid changes
- *Vitreous:* Hemorrhage and seeds
- Extrascleral extension
- Secondary glaucoma
- Neovascular glaucoma

DIAGNOSTIC ANCILLARIES

Fundus fluorescein angiography shows tumor feeder vessels and pinpoint hyperfluorescence with late leakage. On ultrasonography, choroidal melanoma appear as dome or mushroom-shaped mass with high surface reflectivity, low internal reflectivity, choroidal excavation and orbital shadowing on magnetic resonance imaging (MRI), and the tumor appears as hyperintense to vitreous in T1-weighted image and hypointense in T2-weighted image. Extraocular or optic nerve invasion is better seen on MRI. Optical coherence tomography, particularly the ones with enhanced depth capability, can help differentiate between melanoma and nevi.
- *Differential diagnosis:* Choroidal nevus, choroidal metastasis, hemangioma, peripheral exudative hemorrhagic chorioretinopathy with subretinal hemorrhage, tubercular granuloma, melanocytoma of the optic nerve head, etc.

MANAGEMENT OF CHOROIDAL MELANOMA

Collaborative Ocular Melanoma Study (COMS), a multicentric study with patient accrual from 1987 to 1998, to determine:
- Efficacy of brachytherapy versus enucleation in treating medium melanoma (2.5–10 mm apical height; <16 mm in diameter)
- Effectiveness of enucleation with or without preenucleation radiation in treating large melanomas (>10 mm apical height; >16 mm in diameter)
- Observation of small melanomas (1.5–2.4 mm apical height: 5–16 mm in diameter).

Collaborative Ocular Melanoma Study results showed that there was no difference in 5-year and 12-year mortality in treating medium melanoma with brachytherapy or enucleation with approximately 50% of brachytherapy patients having severe visual loss. There was no benefit of preenucleation radiation when treating large melanomas. Older age, larger basal diameter, cell type, and extraocular extension were risk factors for mortality. Small melanoma with greater initial thickness and diameter, presence of orange pigment, absence of drusen, and absence of RPE alteration close to tumor were risk factors for growth.

Small melanomas are treated if they show diffuse orange pigment, subretinal fluid, proximity to disc or fovea and symptoms. Small tumors away from the disc and macula can be treated with transpupillary thermotherapy (TTT). COMS study showed intrascleral invasion of tumor which may account for recurrence after TTT. Hence, TTT alone is recommended to treat premalignant or small tumors in elderly. Medium melanomas are commonly treated with brachytherapy **(Fig. 7.22.2)**, charged particle radiation, and Gamma Knife being the other techniques of radiation.

Selected anteriorly placed tumors can be resected using partial lamellar sclerouvectomy following adjunct brachytherapy.

Large melanomas are enucleated. Melanoma metastasizes commonly to the liver, lungs, bone, and multiple sites. Localized hepatic metastasis can be treated with resection or hepatic arterial chemoembolization; generalized metastasis seldom responds to treatment.

Newer molecular insight shows that genetic defects within uveal melanoma, particularly monosomy of chromosome 3, loss of 3p, 1p, and 8q gain is associated with

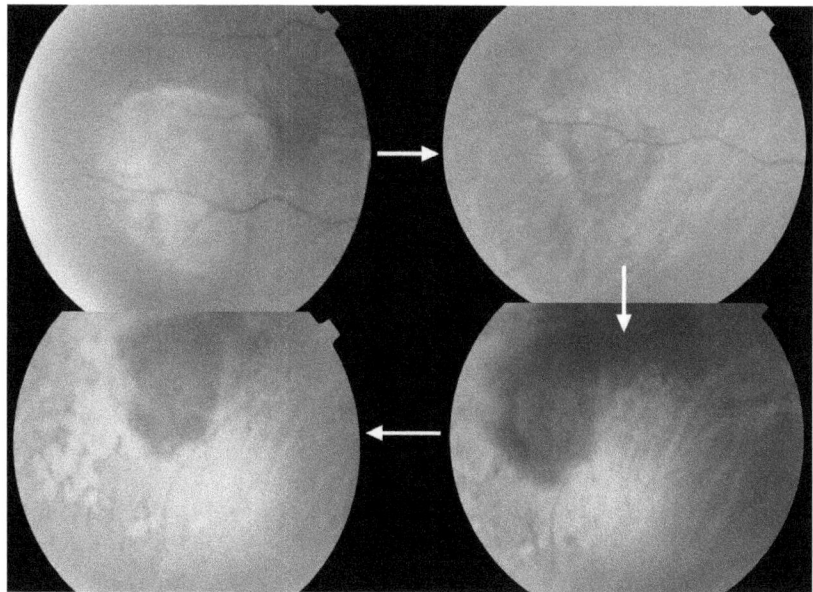

Fig. 7.22.2: Serial photographs showing regression of choroidal melanoma following ruthenium-125 brachytherapy.

increased risk of metastasis. Even with early diagnosis, 40–50% of patients may eventually die of melanoma metastasis.

■ SUGGESTED READING
1. Sallam A, Hungerford J. Choroidal melanoma. Br J Hosp Med. 2007;68(12):669-73.

7.23 | Transconjunctival 25-gauge Vitrectomy

P Mahesh Shanmugam
Sankara Eye Hospitals, Bengaluru
maheshshanmugam@gmail.com

■ INTRODUCTION

Transconjunctival 25-gauge instruments are 0.5 mm in diameter and scleral entry wound being 0.6–0.7 mm in diameter. This allows for self-sealing sclerotomies and transconjunctival surgery.

25-gauge vitrectomy is performed transconjunctivally, using self-retaining cannulas that are inserted through the conjunctiva and sclera using trocars. The conjunctiva is displaced from the proposed site of sclerotomy so that the conjunctival opening does not overlie the sclerotomy at the end of surgery. An angled entry resulting in a longer intrascleral track is used to create the sclerotomy thereby increasing chances of sutureless closure. Intraocular pressure presses on the inner lip of the sclerotomy, collapsing the track, aiding sutureless closure of the sclerotomy. Sclerotomy is placed by a two-step technique wherein the initial entry is tangential to the sclera for a longer scleral tract with the last part of the entry being completed by making the trocar perpendicular to the sclera.

Surgery is usually performed under peri- or parabulbar anesthesia though topical anesthesia has rarely been used. It is preferable to avoid chemosis of the conjunctiva, which makes sclerotomy placement difficult. The smaller bore of the 25-gauge vitreous cutter necessitates increased aspiration pressure (~500 mm Hg in contrast to 250 mm Hg for 23-gauge vitrectomy). Similarly, due to the smaller bore of the infusion cannula, infusion pressure is kept at 40–50 mm Hg.

At the conclusion of the surgery a cotton bud is rolled over the sclerotomy as the cannula is removed to allow for self-sealing of the sclerotomy.

ADVANTAGES

- Less postoperative discomfort from incisions in the absence of sutures
- Less intraocular inflammation
- Port optimization in the newer generation cutters has allowed the port to be placed closer to the tip of the vitreous cutter. This allows the cutter to be used close to the retina, within confined tissue planes to segment and delaminate tissue. Hence, the new generation cutters can be used in lieu of vitreous scissors in select diabetic vitrectomies.
- Relatively shorter operating time (as the sclerotomies need not be sutured)
- Topical medications can be used for a shorter duration (due to lesser intraocular inflammation and faster wound healing)
- Absence of conjunctival opening limits further limbal stem cell damage in predisposed eyes; does not compromise subsequent antiglaucoma surgery).

ADVANCES

Newer vitrectomy systems allow dual pneumatic cutting wherein both the to and fro movement of the cutter is driven pneumatically in contrast to the earlier spring loaded cutters. This allows increased cutting speed of up to 7,500 cuts/minute. Increased cutting rates make surgery safer. Some vitrectomy systems operate on a duty cycle which allows the used to dictate how long the port will remain open during a cutting cycle—longer port opening when removing thicker tissue and shorter opening when working close to the retina to avoid iatrogenic retinal damage.

DISADVANTAGES

- Smaller size of the instruments and decreased fluidics limit the use of 25-gauge vitrectomy in cases needing extensive intraocular manipulation or where significant membrane dissection is necessary. Recent modification of the tensile strength of the 25-gauge instruments have, however, made them less flexible and more durable, allowing them to be used to handle complicated vitreoretinal anatomy.
- Less intraoperative intraocular illumination with regular light sources.

COMPLICATIONS

In addition to all complications that may occur with conventional vitrectomy increased risk of hypotony (3.8–20%) is associated with 25-gauge vitrectomy. The increased risk of endophthalmitis earlier associated with 25-gauge vitrectomy has come down owing to better wound construction, instrumentation, and use of topical povidone iodine at the end of surgery.

Not Suitable

25-gauge vitrectomy is not well-suited for:
- Removal of dislocated nuclear fragments
- Though silicone oil injection and removal can be performed with 25-gauge systems, it is rather slow
- Management of severe proliferative vitreoretinopathy (PVR), particularly anterior PVR with thick membranes
- Intraocular foreign body

SUGGESTED READING

1. Khanduja S, Kakkar A, Majumdar S, Vohra R, Garg S, et al. Small gauge vitrectomy: Recent update. Oman J Ophthalmol. 2013;6(1):3-11.

7.24 | Suprachoroidal Hemorrhage

Mallika Goyal
Apollo Health City Campus, Hyderabad
drmallikagoyal1@gmail.com

INTRODUCTION

Massive suprachoroidal hemorrhage (MSCH) is an uncommon, potentially devastating event that may be perioperative, spontaneous, or traumatic.

It may be associated with severe pain, apposition of retinal surfaces, secondary glaucoma, and extrusion of intraocular contents.

PATHOGENESIS OF PERIOPERATIVE SUPRACHOROIDAL HEMORRHAGE

Suprachoroidal hemorrhage (SCH) occurs when the long or short ciliary arteries rupture, usually due to sudden or prolonged hypotony during or after surgery, and blood fills within the space between the choroid and the sclera. Vortex vein obstruction during scleral buckling is another mechanism. Preexisting damage to the posterior ciliary arteries, as with arteriosclerotic cardiovascular disease and hypertension, may increase their susceptibility to rupture.

SURGERIES ASSOCIATED WITH PERIOPERATIVE MASSIVE SUPRACHOROIDAL HEMORRHAGE

Any form of incisional intraocular surgery including minimally invasive vitrectomy, also with photodynamic therapy or cyclophotocoagulation.

Incidence

Cataract surgery (43.559%), glaucoma filtering surgery (10.26%), vitrectomy (10.26%), and scleral buckling (5.13%).

Spontaneous Massive Suprachoroidal Hemorrhage

Seen in age-related macular degeneration (up to 17.95% of all cases); following corneal perforation; following systemic thrombolysis for coronary or cerebral vascular events; on anticoagulants or antiplatelet therapy.

RISK FACTORS FOR PERIOPERATIVE MASSIVE SUPRACHOROIDAL HEMORRHAGE

- *Systemic factors:* Advanced age, use of anticoagulant or antiplatelet medication, uncontrolled hypertension, atherosclerosis, diabetes, and respiratory disease.
- *Ocular factors:* History of glaucoma, high myopia, elevated preoperative intraocular pressure (IOP), history of previous retinal detachment (RD) surgery, rhegmatogenous RD, excessive cryotherapy, scleral buckling, acutely made sclerotomy for external drainage of subretinal fluid, and associated ocular vascular anomalies (choroidal hemangiomas and Sturge-Weber syndrome).
- *Intraoperative factors:* General anesthesia, retrobulbar blocks, positive Valsalva maneuvers (coughing during local anesthesia and bucking on the endotracheal tube

during general anesthesia), prolonged hypotony, acute hypotony, injecting periocular anesthetics while there is air in vitreous cavity, intraoperative tachycardia, and arrhythmias.

■ MANAGEMENT AND COURSE

Role of B-Scan Ultrasonography

B-scan helps diagnose SCH, to differentiate SCH from serous choroidal detachment (heme shows higher reflectivity compared to clear fluid); to monitor response to therapy; to document extent, height and location of SCH; to assess fluidity of the blood for drainage; to identify appositional SCH; and to detect associated RD. The presence of last two factors is indication for intervention. The initial hyperechoic irregular clots are followed after 1-2 weeks by a hypoechoic and more homogeneous appearance indicating clot liquefaction which is an indication for drainage.

Medical Therapy

Systemic and topical steroids and cycloplegics stabilize choroidal vasculature, reduce inflammation, reduce adhesiveness of retinal surfaces, and build up IOP in cases with severe hypotony. Antiplatelet use to be avoided.

Surgical Management

During Primary Surgery

Immediate closure of all ocular incisions to prevent expulsion of contents and raise IOP.[1] Replace expelling ocular contents. If contents cannot be replaced, drainage of SCH to reduce IOP.[2] The latter can be done via transconjunctival 25-gauge trocar insertion.[3] Generally, it is best to avoid immediate SCH drainage during the primary surgery as that allows further continued bleeding.

Secondary Management

Indications for secondary management: Appositional SCH with central retinal apposition for more than a few days; associated RD.

Timing of secondary intervention: Surgery should not be delayed >7-14 days after the event. This interval allows inflammation to settle and maximal drainage of blood following clot lysis. B-scan aids monitoring heme liquefaction during this period.

Surgical steps: Include placing an anterior chamber (AC) maintainer, vitreous removal from AC, heme drainage through 1 or 2 radial sclerotomies (anterior or posterior, quadrant depending on maximal height of SCH identified by ophthalmoscopy or B-scan);[4] sclerotomes can be scleral cut down (**Fig. 7.24.1**) or trocar drainage (**Figs. 7.24.2 and 7.24.3**). If SCH is accompanied with RD, vitreoretinal traction, or vitreous hemorrhage then the drainage procedure may be combined with a vitrectomy or scleral buckle procedure.

■ POOR PROGNOSTIC FACTORS

Retinal detachment, vitreous in wound, afferent pupillary defect, central retinal apposition >14 days, delay in intervention >2 weeks, and increasing age.

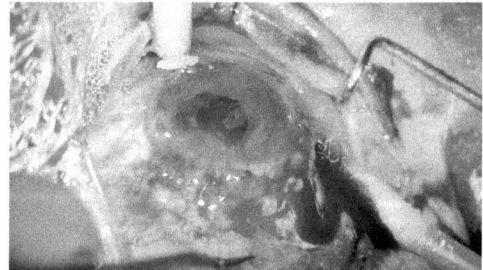

Fig. 7.24.1: Scleral entry and exit with a trocar at superotemporal pars plana leads to drainage of suprachoroidal hemorrhage (SCH) 2 weeks after the primary surgery.

SECTION 7: Retina

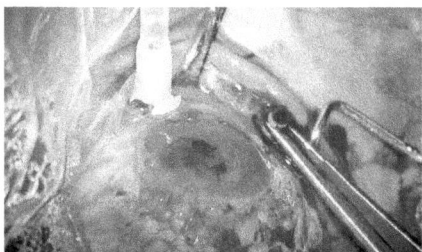

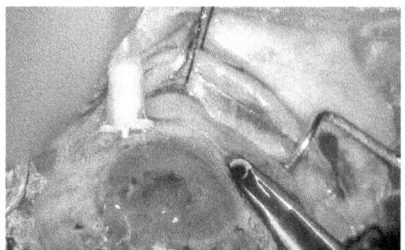

Fig. 7.24.2: Additional sclerotomy with 23-gauge trocar and cannula in the inferotemporal pars plana of same case as in Figure 7.24.1 leaving cannula in situ allows continued drainage of suprachoroidal hemorrhage (SCH) through the cannula.

Fig. 7.24.3: Tilting the cannula direction allows further drainage of suprachoroidal hemorrhage (SCH).

■ OUTCOME

Remains poor despite surgery. Phthisis bulbi, proliferative vitreoretinopathy, traction RD, and no light perception are common end results despite treatment.

■ PREVENTION

Per- and postoperative hypotony should be avoided when operating on patients with known risk factors.

■ REFERENCES

1. Mantopoulos D, Hariprasad SM, Fine HF. Suprachoroidal hemorrhage: Risk factors and diagnostic and treatment options. Ophthalmic Surg Lasers Imaging Retina. 2019;50(11):670-4.
2. Learned D, Eliott D. Management of delayed suprachoroidal hemorrhage after glaucoma surgery. Semin Ophthalmol. 2018;33(1):59-63.
3. Rezende FA, Kickinger MC, Li G, Prado RF, Regis LG. Transconjunctival drainage of serous and hemorrhagic choroidal detachment. Retina. 2012;32(2):242-9.
4. Roa TM, De La Rosa S, Netland PA. (2019). Five Pointers on Choroidal Effusion and Suprachoroidal Hemorrhage. [online] Available from https://glaucomatoday.com/articles/2019-july-aug/five-pointers-on-choroidal-effusion-and-suprachoroidal-hemorrhage. [Last accessed July, 2023].

7.25 | Submacular Hemorrhage

Manisha Agarwal
Dr Shroff's Charity Eye Hospital, New Delhi
agarwalmannii@yahoo.co.in

■ INTRODUCTION

Submacular hemorrhage (SMH) is defined as a collection of hemorrhage in the macular area in the potential space between the retinal pigment epithelium (RPE) and the neurosensory retina or sub-RPE in between the RPE and the choroid. There are several causes for a SMH the most common being macular neovascularization (MNV) secondary to neovascular age-related macular degeneration (AMD) and polypoidal choroidal vasculopathy (PCV).[1-4] An irreversible loss of vision may occur secondary to photoreceptor damage due to iron toxicity, fibrin meshwork contraction, and reduced nutrient flux, with subsequent macular scarring, especially if the hemorrhage is long standing. SMH is classified depending on the size of the hemorrhage.

Small submacular hemorrhage: Measures between 1 and 4 disc diameter (DD) in size.

Medium submacular hemorrhage: Measures minimum 4 DD in size but not extending beyond the temporal vascular arcades.

Large submacular hemorrhage: Extends beyond the temporal vascular arcades.

ETIOLOGY

Macular neovascular membrane (MNV) is the most common cause of SMH secondary to AMD and PCV. Patients with PCV often present with a large SMH with both subretinal and sub-RPE bleed. SMH has also been reported after treatment of MNV with photodynamic therapy and intravitreal injection of antivascular endothelial growth factor (VEGF) drugs. Anticoagulants and to a lesser extent antiplatelet drugs may increase the risk of SMH, particularly when combined with arterial hypertension.

Retinal arterial macroaneurysm (RAM) may cause bleed at any level including subretinal, intraretinal, and preretinal hemorrhage. The other causes of SMH are blunt or penetrating trauma from a choroidal rupture, coagulopathies, and systemic diseases.

Clinical Signs and Symptoms

The most common presenting symptom is diminution of vision and the other are central scotoma and metamorphopsia.

Prognostic Factors

The visual outcome after SMH depends on the following—amount of hemorrhage, size and thickness, and the duration of the hemorrhage.
- *Underlying disease process:* Visual prognosis is worse in eyes with subretinal hemorrhage from MNV than in eyes with hemorrhage secondary to other causes.[5,6]
- *Size and thickness of hemorrhage:* Increased size and thickness of the subretinal hemorrhage is inversely correlated with the visual acuity outcome as this causes increased distance between retinal photoreceptors and the RPE with the blood acting as a barrier for the diffusion of the nutrients to the photoreceptors.
- *Duration of the hemorrhage:* Duration of the subretinal hemorrhage correlates inversely with the final visual acuity due to iron toxicity. Recurrent subretinal hemorrhage also leads to poor visual prognosis.

MANAGEMENT

The main aim of management is to evacuate the hemorrhage as early as possible from the macular area. Early removal of hemorrhage also facilitates to detect the underlying disease process such as a choroidal neovascularization (CNV) through investigations such as:
- *Optical coherence tomography (OCT):* OCT which helps to localize the hemorrhage within the retinal layers and can objectively quantify the size and thickness of the SMH.
- *Fundus fluorescein angiography (FFA):* FFA helps to identify the underlying pathology when the SMH is thin, however, if the hemorrhage is thick and both subretinal and sub-RPE then there is significant blocked fluorescence and very limited information is provided regarding the underlying pathology.
- *Indocyanine green angiography (ICGA):* ICGA using infrared light which is able to penetrate the RPE and blood allowing in detecting an underlying CNV.
- *Optical coherence tomography angiography (OCTA):* It is a noninvasive test unlike FFA and ICGA which helps to identify the neovascular network without the injection of any dye.

A thin eccentric SMH is unlikely to cause a decrease of vision and requires observation only.

Treatment options aim at clearing the blood from the macular area at the earliest to minimize photoreceptor damage and they include the following:
- *Pneumatic displacement:* An undiluted volume of 0.3 mL of perfluoropropane (C3F8) or 0.5 mL sulfur hexafluoride (SF6) is injected into the vitreous cavity at 3-4 mm posterior to the limbus followed by an anterior chamber paracentesis to reduce the intraocular pressure (IOP). The patient is asked to maintain prone position for 12-14 hours for 2 weeks. It is said that pneumatic displacement has a better visual outcome than the natural history of SMH.[7]
- *Pneumatic displacement with tissue plasminogen activator (TPA):* An intravitreal injection of 25-100 µg per 0.1 mL TPA is given followed by 0.3-0.4 SF6 or C3F8 gas. The patient has to maintain a supine position followed by a face down position for 1-5 days so that the gas bubble through its buoyancy is able to displace the blood from the macula. TPA is a serine protease with fibrin-specific thrombolytic activity that forms a complex with fibrin to activate plasminogen to plasmin which then cleaves fibrin and dissolves the clot. This helps to reduce the fibrin-mediated damage to the photoreceptors. It is more effective in displacing subretinal hemorrhage in comparison to sub-RPE hemorrhage. This is followed by targeted treatment of the underlying cause. Complications include rise in IOP, retinal tear, retinal detachment, RPE rip, endophthalmitis and dose-dependent (TPA > 100 µg) exudative retinal detachment, retinal toxicity, and RPE mottling.[8]
- *Intravitreal anti-VEGF monotherapy:* Anti-VEGF monotherapy may be particularly helpful for patients with SMH secondary to MNV who are not suitable for pneumatic displacement, TPA, or surgery such as those who are unable to maintain a prone position. The other indications are patients having SMH superior to the fovea where an inferior displacement may lead to foveal involvement and patients with SMH older than 2-3 weeks as TPA and gas seem to be less effective in displacing the SMH.
- *Intravitreal anti-VEGF with pneumatic displacement:* Intravitreal anti-VEGF along with intravitreal 0.3-0.4 mL of SF6 or C3F8 is used to treat small size SMH secondary to MNV.[9]
- *Intravitreal anti-VEGF with TPA and pneumatic displacement:* Intravitreal anti-VEGF injection is given along with 25-100 µg per 0.1 mL of TPA is given followed by 0.3-0.4 SF6 or C3F8 gas.[10]

Surgical Management

Pars plana vitrectomy (PPV) in the management of SMH has the advantages of relieving any vitreomacular traction which may aggravate neovascular AMD, it may help in increasing the vitreous oxygenation and thereby reduce the VEGF levels and facilitate the diffusion of the VEGF away from the macula and lastly ensure a more complete removal of the SMH.
- *PPV, subretinal TPA, and gas:* PPV is done and a small retinotomy is made through which TPA (<50 µg/mL) is injected in the subretinal space using a flexible 41 gauge cannula and we wait for approximately 30-60 minutes followed by saline injection to evacuate liquefied hemorrhage. Fluid-air exchange and gas tamponade is subsequently done. Small retinotomy is said to close spontaneously without requiring a laser photocoagulation. Clot lysis with TPA avoids the need for to create the large retinotomies required to introduce forceps for removing the thrombus. This decreases the risk of retinal detachment and causes less damage to the photoreceptors during clot removal.[11,12]
- *Vitrectomy, anti-VEGF therapy, TPA and gas:* PPV combined with either subretinal or intravitreal TPA and subsequent intravitreal anti-VEGF injection is given to treat patients with AMD and SMH.
- *Vitrectomy and combined subretinal TPA and anti-VEGF therapy:* PPV and subretinal co-application of both anti-VEGF (0.05 mL) and TPA (0.05 mL) is done. The subretinal injection has to be done slowly using a 41 gauge subretinal flexible cannula with a total volume of 0.1 mL to avoid a macular hole formation.

- *Vitrectomy and subretinal TPA, anti-VEGF therapy, and filtered air (subretinal pneumatic displacement):* PPV is done followed by subretinal injection using a 41 gauge flexible cannula of 0.4 mL of TPA (50 µg) along with 0.1 mL of anti-VEGF and 0.2 mL of filtered air. The subretinal air aimed to reduce the hemorrhages' buoyancy relative to air and help displace it. This is followed by fluid-gas exchange. Postoperatively air remains in the macular region and the patient is asked to maintain an upright position which displaces the liquefied clot inferiorly.
- *Macular translocation:* This helps in relocating the functioning foveal neuroretina overlying a SMH from an area of compromised RPE to undamaged RPE. A PPV is performed followed by subretinal infusion to induce a retinal detachment followed by 360° retinectomy. The retina is then rotated and the fovea was relocated between 30 and 80° from the original site. This procedure should be performed for patients with very poor visual acuity as there is a risk of potential complications such as retinal detachment and choroidal hemorrhage. Patient may also suffer from torsional diplopia after the surgery.
- *Retinal pigment epithelium-choroid patch technique:* This is an alternative to macular translocation surgery, especially, in patients with good vision in the fellow eye where torsional diplopia maybe induced. A PPV is performed and the neovascular complex is extracted and an autologous peripheral full-thickness patch of the RPE-Bruch membrane—choriocapillaris is collected from the midperiphery and repositioned under the macula. This is presently not considered a standard treatment for SMH but future advancements in microsurgical techniques and instrumentation may lead to lesser traumatic removal of the neovascular complex and insertion of the RPE-choroid graft.

CASE 1

A 55-year-old male presented with drop of vision 2 days back in the right eye. The left eye had a history of poor vision secondary to amblyopia. On examination, the best-corrected visual acuity (BCVA) in the right eye was counting finger at 1 meter and left eye was 6/60, N36. Fundus examination showed a large submacular hemorrhage both subretinal and sub-RPE hemorrhage **(Fig. 7.25.1)**. He underwent intravitreal—C3F8 gas (100% 0.3 mL) + TPA (50 µg/0.05 mL) and bevacizumab (1.25 mg/0.05 mL) under topical anesthesia and strict aseptic precautions after an informed consent in the operation theater. Postoperatively was advised to maintain supine positioning for 6 hours followed by prone positioning.

There was displacement of the SMH seen at 1 week **(Fig. 7.25.2)** and at 2 weeks follow-up **(Fig. 7.25.3)**. Patient underwent FFA **(Figs. 7.25.4A to D)** confirming the presence of an extrafoveal MNV nasal to the fovea. Focal laser photocoagulation

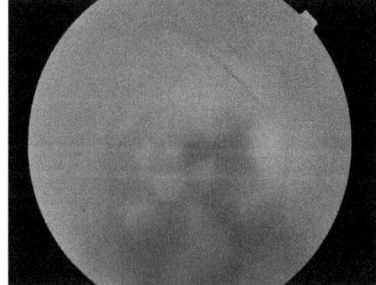

Fig. 7.25.1: Color fundus photo of the right eye showing large submacular hemorrhage (SMH).

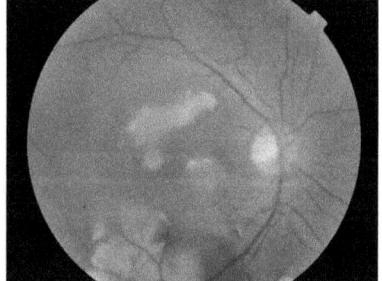

Fig. 7.25.2: Color fundus photo of the right eye at 1 week follow-up showing displacement of the submacular hemorrhage (SMH).

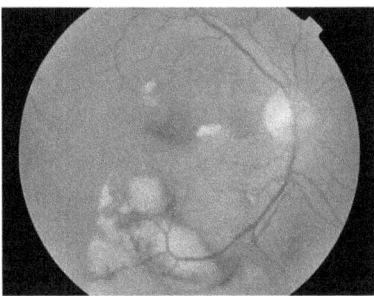

Fig. 7.25.3: Color fundus photograph of the right eye at 2 weeks follow-up showing displacement of the submacular hemorrhage (SMH).

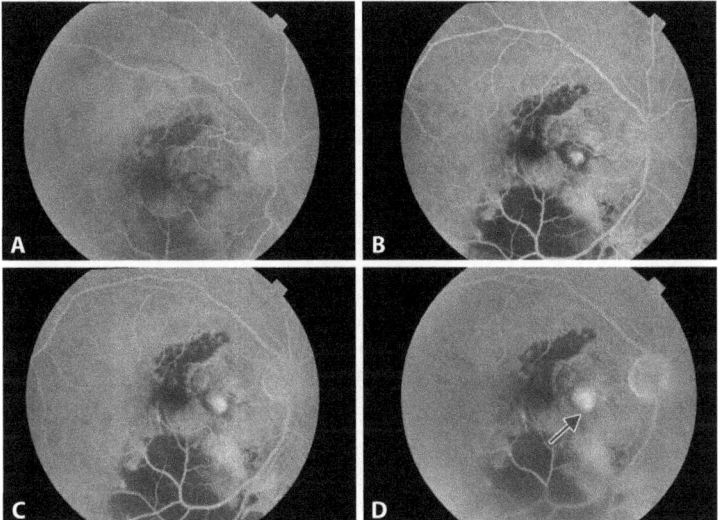

Figs. 7.25.4A to D: Fundus fluorescein angiography (FFA) of the right eye showing early hyperfluorescence with leakage nasal to the fovea suggestive of an active extrafoveal macular neovascularization (MNV).

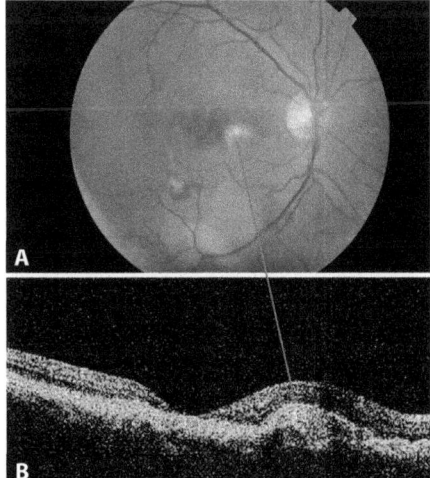

Figs. 7.25.5A and B: (A) Color fundus photo of the right eye at 3 months follow-up showing an extrafoveal scarred macular neovascularization (MNV); (B) Optical coherence tomography (OCT) of the right eye showing a scarred MNV with no evidence of subretinal or intraretinal fluid at 3 months follow-up.

was done to the extrafoveal MNV along with two more anti-VEGF injections given at monthly interval. At 3 months follow-up the BCVA in the right eye was 6/12, N9. Fundus examination showed a scarred MNV **(Fig. 7.25.5A)** which was also confirmed on OCT **(Fig. 7.25.5B)**. There was no recurrence of MNV at 1 year follow-up.

REFERENCES

1. Peyman GA, Nelson NC Jr, Alturki W, Blinder KJ, Paris CL, Desai UR, et al. Tissue plasminogen activating factor assisted removal of subretinal hemorrhage. Ophthalmic Surg. 1991;22:575-82.
2. Millsap CM, Peyman GA, Greve MD. Subretinal hemorrhage removal with multiple retinotomy sites in age-related macular degeneration. Ophthalmic Surg. 1994;25:723-5.
3. Ohji M, Saito Y, Hayashi A, Lewis JM, Tano Y. Pneumatic displacement of subretinal hemorrhage without tissue plasminogen activator. Arch Ophthalmol. 1998;116:1326-32.
4. Hochman MA, Seery CM, Zarbin MA. Pathophysiology and management of subretinal hemorrhage. Surv Ophthalmol. 1997;42:195-213.
5. Avery RL, Fekrat S, Hawkins BS, Bressler NM. Natural history of subfoveal subretinal hemorrhage in age-related macular degeneration. Retina. 1996;16:183-9.
6. Scupola A, Coscas G, Soubrane G, Balestrazzi E. Natural history of macular subretinal hemorrhage in age related macular degeneration. Ophthalmologica. 1999;213:97-102.
7. Gopalakrishan M, Giridhar A, Bhat S, Saikumar SJ, Elias A, Sandhya N. Pneumatic displacement of submacular hemorrhage: Safety, efficacy, and patient selection. Retina. 2007;27:329-34.
8. Krepler K, Kruger A, Tittl M, Stur M, Wedrich A. Intravitreal injection of tissue plasminogen activator and gas in subretinal hemorrhage caused by age-related macular degeneration. Retina. 2000;20:251-6.
9. Chawla S, Misra V, Khemchandani M. Pneumatic displacement and intravitreal bevacizumab: A new approach for management of submacular hemorrhage in choroidal neovascular membrane. Indian J Ophthalmol. 2009;57:155-7.
10. Hattenbach LO, Klais C, Koch FH, Gumbel HO. Intravitreous injection of tissue plasminogen activator and gas in the treatment of submacular hemorrhage under various conditions. Ophthalmology. 2001;108:1485-92.
11. Olivier S, Chow DR, Packo KH, MacCumber MW, Awh CC. Subretinal recombinant tissue plasminogen activator injection and pneumatic displacement of thick submacular hemorrhage in age-related macular degeneration. Ophthalmology. 2004;111(6):1201-8.
12. Fine HF, Iranmanesh R, Del Priore LV, Barile GR, Chang LK, Chang S, et al. Surgical outcomes after massive subretinal hemorrhage secondary to age-related macular degeneration. Retina. 2010;30(10):1588-94.

7.26 Antivascular Endothelial Growth Factor in Retinal Practice

Mohit Dogra, Simar Rajan Singh
Advanced Eye Center, PGIMER, Chandigarh
mohit_dogra_29@hotmail.com, simarrajansingh@gmail.com

INTRODUCTION AND RATIONALE

Angiogenesis is the process by which new blood vessels are created from preexisting vasculature. In the eye, angiogenesis occurs due to carefully balanced interplay of growth-promoting and growth-inhibiting factors. Vascular endothelial growth factor (VEGF) is one of the primary factors promoting abnormal angiogenesis within the eye. Elevated intraocular VEGF levels appear to be associated with neovascularization, a vascular abnormality that is common to many retinal conditions such as age-related macular degeneration (AMD), diabetic retinopathy (DR), and retinal vascular occlusion (RVO). This provides the rationale for pharmacological inhibition of abnormal angiogenesis to treat these retinal conditions.

INDICATIONS

- Choroidal neovascularization (CNV) secondary to:
  - AMD [including polypoidal choroidal vasculopathy (PCV)]
  - Myopia
  - Inflammation
  - *Others:* Idiopathic, choroidal osteoma, central serous chorioretinopathy (CSC), juxtafoveal telangiectasia (JFT), angioid streaks, and presumed ocular histoplasmosis
- DR:
  - Diabetic macular edema (DME)
  - Proliferative diabetic retinopathy (PDR)
- RVO:
  - Branch retinal vein occlusion (BRVO)
  - Central retinal vein occlusion (CRVO)
- Retinopathy of prematurity (ROP)
- *Others:*
  - Macular edema—pseudophakic, uveitic, and retinitis pigmentosa
  - Circumscribed choroidal hemangiomas
  - Radiation retinopathy
  - Retinal macroaneurysm
  - Vasoproliferative retinal tumors including capillary hemangiomas
  - Coat's disease
  - Vascularized choroidal granulomas
  - Intraocular metastasis
  - Retinal vasculitis.

ANTIVASCULAR ENDOTHELIAL GROWTH FACTOR AGENTS

- *Macugen (pegaptanib):* Pegylated anti-VEGF aptamer which specifically binds to 165 isomer of VEGF first agent to be the Food and Drug Administration (FDA) approved for intraocular use in 2005.
- *Avastin (bevacizumab):* Recombinant, humanized monoclonal antibody to VEGF. Not FDA approved for intraocular use, used off-label. Cost-effective with costs being about 30 times less than Lucentis.
- *Lucentis (ranibizumab):* Affinity-matured antigen-binding fragment derived from the parent mouse antibody to VEGF.
  Most widely used FDA approved agent for intraocular purposes. Most clinical trials are done using this agent.
- *Eylea (aflibercept):* Fully human fusion protein VEGF trap that inhibits VEGF-A and placental growth factor; FDA approved for intraocular use in 2011.
- *Razumab and RanizuRel (ranibizumab):* The Drugs Controller General of India (DCGI) approved biosimilar recently made available in India for intraocular use.
- *Pagenax/Beovu (brolucizumab):* FDA and DCGI approved anti-VEGF with longer duration of action, especially in cases with PCV.

ANTIVASCULAR ENDOTHELIAL GROWTH FACTOR IN DIABETIC RETINOPATHY AND RETINAL VASCULAR OCCLUSION

- First line for management of DME of nontractional variety. Monthly ranibizumab with or without prompt macular laser is the treatment of choice for center involving and center noninvolving DME. Aflibercept has been shown to be superior to ranibizumab and bevacizumab in patients with DME with visual acuity ≤20/50 at presentation.
- BRVO and CRVO with macular edema are managed with monthly anti-VEGF injections and grid laser (in BRVO). Repeated injections are needed in 40% of BRVO (3.2 injections) and 56% of CRVO (5.6 injections) patients even in the fourth year

after the initial event. Recently, ranibizumab has been shown to be superior to intravitreal steroids during the first 6 months after RVO.
- Anti-VEGFs have traditionally been used in PDR as rescue therapy before or with panretinal photocoagulation (PRP). Recent data from the DRCR.net has shown that treatment of PDR with ranibizumab injections alone was noninferior to PRP. Also, visual field loss, eyes developing DME and need for vitrectomy were lower in the anti-VEGF group.
- Use of anti-VEGFs for vitreous hemorrhage and prior to vitrectomy in PDR is also widely done. Clearing of vitreous hemorrhage (thus avoiding surgery), shrinkage of vascular component of fibrovascular proliferation (reducing intraoperative and early postoperative hemorrhage) and clearing of postvitrectomy re-bleeds are the main indications. Caution in patients of tractional retinal detachment (RD), as they should be taken up for surgery within 3–5 days of anti-VEGF injection, or they may end-up progressing to combined RD.
- Neovascular glaucoma (secondary to PDR or CRVO) is managed with intracameral or intravitreal anti-VEGFs, PRP and antiglaucoma medications. Anti-VEGF agents cause prompt regression of iris and angle neovascularization and are also helpful as adjuncts during glaucoma surgical procedures in these patients.

ANTIVASCULAR ENDOTHELIAL GROWTH FACTOR IN CHOROIDAL NEOVASCULARIZATION

- Anti-VEGF agents revolutionized the management of CNV in AMD. Ranibizumab has been shown to be superior to photodynamic therapy (PDT) and is now the treatment of choice. Aflibercept has also been shown to be equally efficacious in AMD, with the advantage of reduced number of injections.
- PCV is best managed with combination therapy—anti-VEGF and PDT, which has been shown to be superior to monotherapy with anti-VEGFs.
- Myopic CNV responds excellently to anti-VEGF treatment and aflibercept has been shown to be the best agent for the same.
- Other causes of CNV are also amenable to treatment with anti-VEGF agents, with variable response. While CNVs in JFT and CSC respond well and generally have a favorable outcome, those in patients of choroidal osteoma and angioid streaks tend to fare rather poorly.

ANTIVASCULAR ENDOTHELIAL GROWTH FACTOR IN RETINOPATHY OF PREMATURITY

- Systemic safety concerns in neonates regarding anti-VEGF use is the main issue. However, half dose ranibizumab has been shown to be superior to standard laser treatment for Zone 1 disease.
- Eyes with extensive tunica vasculosa lentis (TVL) with nondilating pupils, posterior Zone 1 aggressive posterior ROP, and eyes with multiple retinal hemorrhages with Zone 1 disease are common indications. However, laser ablation of avascular retina needs to be done to prevent late recurrence of disease and combination therapy (anti-VEGF + laser) should be employed in these cases.

SIDE EFFECTS

- *Ocular:*
  - Subconjunctival hemorrhage
  - Vitreous hemorrhage
  - Uveitis
  - Endophthalmitis
  - RD
  - Cataract

- Glaucoma
- Retinal pigment epithelial rip
- "Crunch phenomenon" tractional RD progressing to combined RD
■ *Systemic:*
- *Thromboembolic events:* Myocardial infarction, stroke, and peripheral vascular disease
- Elevated blood pressure
- Death

■ EMERGING THERAPIES (NOT YET AVAILABLE IN INDIA)

- *Conbercept:* Similar to aflibercept but having higher affinity for VEGF-B. Trials are underway in China to establish its superiority to ranibizumab.
- *Abicipar:* DARPin-based small protein against VEGF-A. Intrinsically more stable than immunoglobulin and, hence, having longer therapeutic effect and lower frequency of injections.
- The posterior MicroPump drug delivery system uses microelectromechanical system technology and can function reliably for >100 programmable injections of anti-VEGF corresponding to >8 years of therapy. It is implanted similar to glaucoma drainage device.
- The Port Delivery System (ForSight VISION 4, Menlo Park, CA, USA) is a refillable, nonbiodegradable drug delivery implant for the sustained release of ranibizumab. The implant is placed in the pars plana through a 3.2 mm sutureless scleral incision beneath the conjunctiva. The device can be refilled in the office using standard intravitreal injection technique.
- Vabysmo (faricimab) is combined VEGF and Ang2 receptor blocker with proposed longer duration and efficacy of action. It is FDA approved.
- High-dose aflibercept being tried to enhance the effect of the drug and prolong its action.

7.27 | Fungal Endophthalmitis

Janani Sreenivasan, Muna Bhende
Sankara Nethralaya, Chennai
drmuna@snmail.org

■ INTRODUCTION

Endophthalmitis is a serious ophthalmologic condition involving purulent inflammation of the vitreous and aqueous humor typically caused by a bacterial or fungal infection. Fungal endophthalmitis is less common than bacterial endophthalmitis but has a very poor prognosis. The mechanism of entry into the eye is either exogenous (postsurgery, trauma, contiguous spread from external ocular infection like keratitis and blebitis), or endogenous (via the bloodstream). Exogenous fungal endophthalmitis is more common than the endogenous type.

■ RISK FACTORS

Risk factors for endogenous fungal endophthalmitis are diabetes mellitus, systemic debilitating disease, malignancy, intravenous drug use, chemotherapy, systemic antibiotics and prolonged corticosteroid therapy, and alcoholism. Risk factors for the development of exogenous fungal endophthalmitis are not well studied but correspond to the exogenous cause. For example, in keratitis-associated exogenous fungal endophthalmitis, risk factors include contact lens use, trauma with organic matter, and laser-assisted in situ keratomileusis (LASIK).

Though high-powered studies have not been conducted, limited reports (Shroff et al. and Shah et al.) suggest that prolonged corticosteroid use and protracted hospital courses during the severe acute respiratory syndrome coronavirus 2 (SARS-CoV-2) or coronavirus disease-2019 (COVID-19) pandemic could result in an increase in rates of endogenous fungal endophthalmitis.

ORGANISMS

Normally, fungi are not residents of the human eye but are acquired from the surrounding. Fungi usually colonize on the lid margins and conjunctiva. *Aspergillus* species is the most common fungal isolate from the conjunctiva of healthy individuals reported from India.

The most commonly isolated species vary depending on the mode of infection (**Flowchart 7.27.1**).

CLINICAL FEATURES

The clinical features of fungal endophthalmitis vary widely from asymptomatic to fulminant infection. Ishibashi's classification of fungal endophthalmitis is depicted in **Table 7.27.1**. Risk factors for endogenous/exogenous endophthalmitis may be present (mentioned earlier) including a history of long-time topical and sometimes systemic corticosteroids. Ruling out systemic involvement is very important in fungal endophthalmitis, especially in endophthalmitis secondary to *Candida* species, *Aspergillus* species, *Cryptococcus* species, and *Coccidioides immitis*. In contrast to acute bacterial postoperative endophthalmitis which presents as a single episode of severe infection, fungal endophthalmitis has a slightly delayed presentation with an indolent and protracted course with a poor prognosis. The interval between the primary event and the occurrence of endophthalmitis is much longer than bacterial postoperative infection

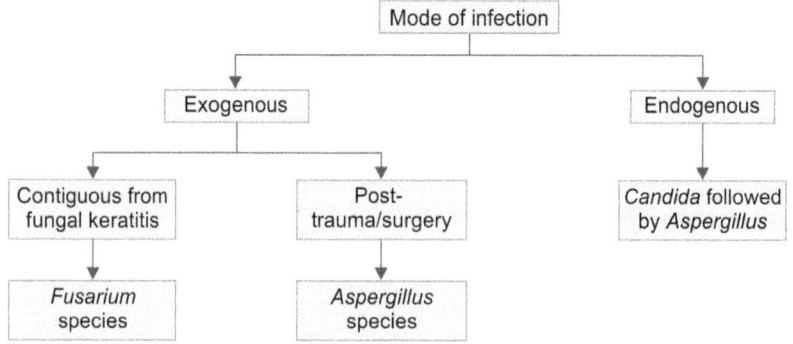

Flowchart 7.27.1: The mode of fungal infection and the common fungal species isolated.

TABLE 7.27.1: Ishibashi's classification of fungal endophthalmitis.

Stage	Follow-up interval
I	Inflammatory cells in the anterior chamber and vitreous
II	White round lesions in the posterior fundus
IIIA	Mild opacity of the vitreous
IIIB	Moderate-to-severe vitreous opacity
IV	Retinal detachment or opaque vitreous

and may range from 2 days to 7 months. A relatively quiet-looking eye with mild vitreous haze in a patient on prolonged topical and systemic steroids after intraocular surgery should raise the suspicion of fungal endophthalmitis.

The signs include a variable degree of lid edema, chronic conjunctival congestion, hypopyon, and intense vitritis. The more typical signs include yellow-white infiltrates at the corneoscleral wound (in cataract surgery), nodular exudates over the iris **(Figs. 7.27.1A and B)** and crystalline/intraocular lens surface, and vitreous exudates arranged like a string of pearls and creamy white circumscribed chorioretinal lesion. Vitritis is the most consistent presentation in endogenous endophthalmitis, sometimes with characteristic lesions in the vitreous and/or retina **(Figs. 7.27.2A and B)**. One also needs to look carefully for retroiridal fluffy exudates that may be seen only after dilatation **(Figs. 7.21.1A and B)**.

Fungal sclerokeratitis has been described as a rare postoperative complication of cataract surgery. It usually involves the scleral tunnel and extends to the cornea. A poorly constructed wound and loose or broken sutures have been identified as important predisposing factors. It can present with necrosis and can be confused with surgically-induced necrotizing scleritis (SINS). Rapid progression of scleritis and necrosis with corticosteroids may pinpoint an infective etiology.

The organism-specific features of the commonly isolated fungi are summarized in **Table 7.27.2**.

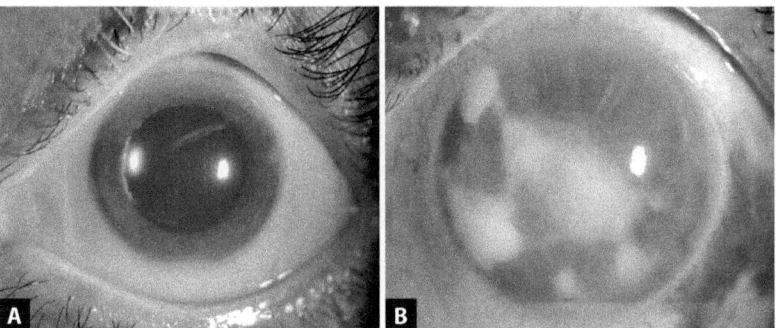

Figs. 7.27.1A and B: (A) A patient with fungal endophthalmitis having a fairly quiet eye with a streak of hypopyon and retroiridal exudate; (B) Anterior segment photograph of a patient with severe postoperative fungal endophthalmitis, showing exudates in the anterior chamber involving the pupillary area, iris, and wound entry site. Blood-tinged hypopyon is also seen.

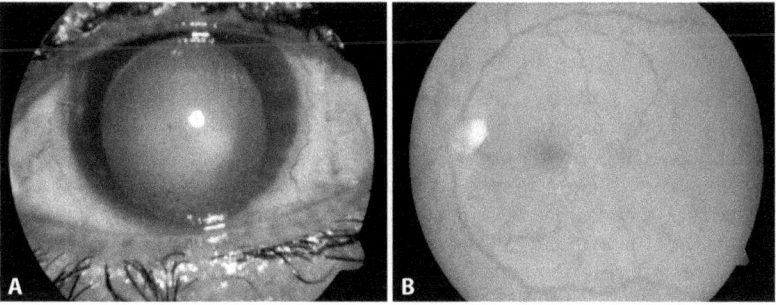

Figs. 7.27.2A and B: A case of *Candida* endogenous endophthalmitis. (A) An anterior segment photo depicting a yellow glow; (B) Fundus photo showing a creamy white lesion on the disc with exudates at the macula.

TABLE 7.27.2: Organism-specific features.

features/organism	Aspergillus	Candida	Fusarium
Specific clinical features	• Most common cause for exogenous type (due to its small spores) but can be endogenous with invasive aspergillosis • Histologically, it grows preferentially along the sub—RPE and subretinal space and has an affinity for macular area	• The earliest signs (respond well to antifungals) are peripheral creamy chorioretinal lesions with mild vitreous haze • Vitreous involvement—intravitreal puff ball-like lesions	Most frequent cause of exogenous endophthalmitis secondary to keratitis
Species commonly isolated	*Aspergillus fumigatus*, others—*A. niger, A. terreus*, and *A. flavus*	*C. albicans*; others—*C. krusei, C. glabrata, C. parapsilosis, C. tropicalis* and *C. guilliermondii*	*Fusarium solani*, others—*F. oxysporum, F. verticillioides, F. sacchari,* and *F. moniliforme*
Course and prognosis	Poor prognosis due to aggressive nature of the infection, macular involvement, and extensive chorioretinal necrosis	Better outcome than *Aspergillus* but in endogenous cases, mortality with candidemia is higher with coexisting endophthalmitis	Variable
Treatment	Early vitrectomy preferred amphotericin B, voriconazole	Amphotericin B, fluconazole, flucytosine, vitrectomy	Topical natamycin, intravitreal amphotericin B, voriconazole (topical, intravitreal and systemic), vitrectomy ± keratoplasty

■ INVESTIGATIONS

Direct Smear of Tissue/Fluid Specimens

The most common specimens collected are aqueous and vitreous. Direct isolation of fungi is the rapid and most used method. Available methods include KOH mount (most widely used), Grocott's methenamine silver stain, periodic acid-Schiff stain, Giemsa stain, Gömöri-methenamine silver, and Papanicolaou's stain. Special stains such as lactophenol cotton blue/calcofluor white improve the ease of identification due to the typical color-blue with the former, and fluorescence with the latter. *Cryptococcus* can be identified on India ink preparations.

Culture

An undiluted vitreous sample during vitrectomy is preferred. Vitrectomy samples are more sensitive for fungal cultures than vitreous needle biopsies. Retinal or choroidal biopsies can be performed when no organism is detected after multiple vitreous biopsies or in eyes with outer retinal or choroidal involvement. Culture must be retained for at least 4–6 weeks to ensure that slow-growing or fastidious fungal organisms are not missed. The commonly used media include selective media such as Sabouraud dextrose agar and potato dextrose agar and nonselective media like chocolate/blood agar/brain heart infusion broth. The selective media are incubated at 25°C for 2–4 weeks while others are incubated at 37°C for 1 week before reporting negative.

Molecular Techniques
Polymerase chain reaction (PCR) has a high degree of specificity and sensitivity. It reduces laboratory diagnosis time and is particularly useful in culture-negative cases. Pan-fungal primers ITS 1 and ITS 4 are used in PCR for the detection of fungal pathogens. Targeted high throughput sequencing (HTS) or next-generation sequencing (NGS) of the ocular fluid after deoxyribonucleic acid (DNA) extraction and amplification of internal transcribed spacer 2 (ITS2) region is an advanced method of identifying the fungal species.

Biomarkers in fungal endophthalmitis include galactomannan (cell-wall component of *Aspergillus*) and (1,3)-β-D glucan (a polysaccharide cell-wall component of *Aspergillus* and *Candida* species). Though evaluated in invasive *Aspergillosis*, the utility in fungal endophthalmitis is limited. These tests could be considered in conjunction with clinical and microbiological tests. The advantage is that the results of these tests are available within 2–3 hours compared to several days of conventional culture.

Systemic Investigations
Systemic investigations are essential in endogenous endophthalmitis. These investigations include full blood count, serum urea and electrolytes, liver function tests, culture of peripheral blood, sputum and urine, chest radiogram, liver ultrasonogram, and transthoracic echocardiogram. A thorough evaluation by a physician/infectious disease specialist to identify the systemic source of infection is important.

■ MANAGEMENT
The striking differences in managing fungal endophthalmitis from its bacterial counterpart are the low threshold for primary vitrectomy, multiple intravitreal injections, avoidance/judicious use of steroids (especially systemic), the important role of systemic antifungals, and need for prolonged treatment. Caution must be exercised in the use of corticosteroids in any form (topical, intravitreal, and systemic) in suspected fungal endophthalmitis. Achieving adequate concentrations of antifungal drugs in infected tissues is crucial to successful treatment.

Antifungal Agents
A standard treatment protocol for fungal endophthalmitis is not yet established. Initiation with a broad-spectrum systemic antifungal drug with or without an intravitreal antifungal drug is recommended. The injection may sometimes be performed into the capsular bag if sequestered infection is suspected. Systemic antifungal therapy has a more important role in endogenous infection. Important antifungal agents and their details are summarized in **Table 7.27.3**. All patients need weekly liver function tests when on systemic antifungal agents (especially azoles). Treatment needs to be continued for a minimum of 3 weeks and may go on for up to 6 months.

Surgical Management
Vitrectomy plays a crucial role in the management of fungal endophthalmitis, and early vitrectomy could be more beneficial. In view of the thickened choroid, it is prudent to use a longer infusion cannula (6 mm). An undiluted vitreous specimen is collected before the infusion begins. Amphotericin B may be used in the infusion fluid in certain cases. A complete vitrectomy is desired which includes the separation of the posterior hyaloid over

TABLE 7.27.3: Antifungal agents.

Properties	Polyenes	Azoles	Echinocandins	Flucytosine
Mechanism	Fungicidal (cell membrane damage)	Fungistatic (cell membrane damage)	D-glucan synthase inhibitor (cell wall synthesis)	Fungistatic inhibits nucleic acid synthesis
Drugs commonly used	Amphotericin B	Imidazoles and triazoles Most used—voriconazole and fluconazole	Caspofungin, micafungin, and anidulafungin	Flucytosine
Spectrum	Broad-spectrum *Candida*, *Cryptococcus*, and *Aspergillus* species	Fluconazole—*Candida*, *Cryptococcus*, and *Aspergillus* species Voriconazole—Broad-spectrum; *Aspergillus* species, fluconazole-resistant *Candida* species, *Paecilomyces lilacinus*, and *Cryptococcus neoformans*	*Candida* species and azole-resistant *Aspergillus* species	*Candida* and *Cryptococcus* species
Systemic use	Intravenous dose: 0.5–1 mg/kg	• Oral • Voriconazole and fluconazole—400 mg loading dose followed by 200 mg bd Itraconazole 100 mg bd	Limited data on utility in endophthalmitis	25 mg/kg four times daily
Intravitreal preparation	Available, 5–10 µg/0.1 mL	Available for voriconazole—50 µg/0.1 mL	Not available	Not available
Ocular penetration	Low	Good for voriconazole and fluconazole	Limited	Good
Side effects	Intravenous use—nephrotoxicity Intravitreal use—retinal toxicity	Hepatotoxicity and drug interactions	Need dose adjustments in renal and hepatic dysfunction	High-drug resistance, always used in combination

Flowcharts 7.27.2A and B: Algorithms for the management of fungal endophthalmitis.

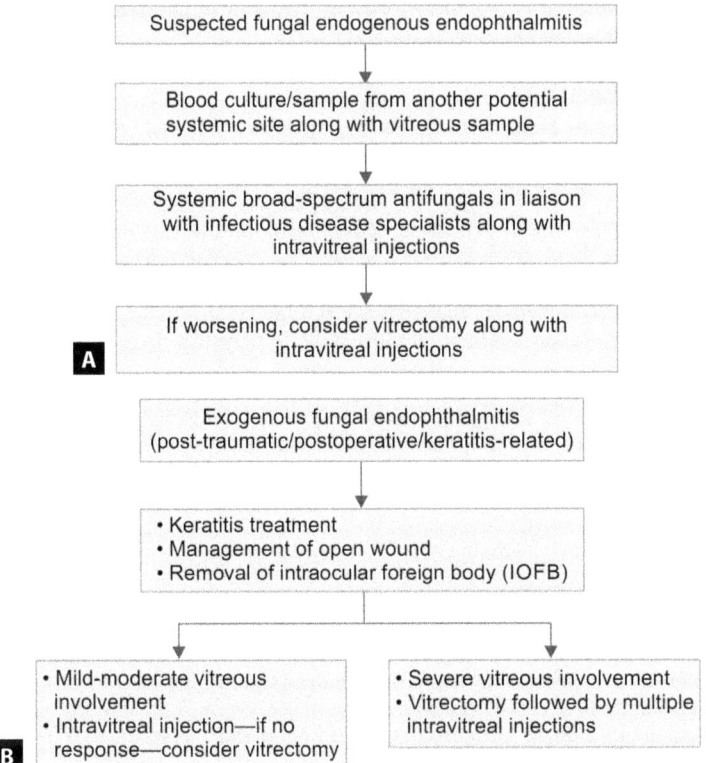

the posterior pole but staying short of the periphery. Adequate clearance of the anterior vitreous should be attempted in pseudophakic eyes as exudates tend to aggregate and harbor close to the ciliary sulcus. Inadequate clearance can lead to recurrent episodes of inflammation. Although removal of the entire capsule including the intraocular lens (IOL) may not be necessary in all cases, it must be considered in cases of recalcitrant infection, especially where the exudates are within the capsular bag. Complications of vitrectomy include retinal breaks/retinal detachment and hypotony. Silicone oil can occasionally be used as a tamponade in cases of retinal detachment as it is believed to act as a fungistatic agent. Suturing of sclerotomies is preferred to avoid hypotony even if self-sealing 23 g/23 g sclerotomies are made. The management of postoperative sclerokeratitis includes topical and systemic antifungal therapy with or without mechanical debridement and a scleral graft. Endoscopic vitrectomy (20/23 G endoscope) is an option when intraoperative visualization is poor due to corneal edema, inflammatory membranes, anterior/posterior segment hemorrhage (in traumatized eyes), and concurrent retinal detachment/large retained intraocular foreign body. In case the endoscopic vitrectomy facility is not available, there may be a need to combine penetrating keratoplasty with vitrectomy.

An algorithm for the management of exogenous and fungal endophthalmitis is shown in **Flowcharts 7.27.2A and B**.

CONCLUSION

Fungal endophthalmitis is rare but the prognosis is poorer (especially *Aspergillus* species) than its bacterial counterpart primarily due to delayed diagnosis. A high index of suspicion is necessary for diagnosing fungal endophthalmitis. Definitive diagnosis requires the isolation of the organism which can be aided by PCR. Systemic as well as intravitreal antifungal agents along with vitrectomy form the mainstay of the treatment. Prompt and prolonged treatment is needed to reduce significant visual loss.

■ SUGGESTED READING

1. Amphornphruet A, Silpa-Archa S, Preble JM, Foster CS. Endogenous Cryptococcal Endophthalmitis in Immunocompetent Host: Case Report and Review of Multimodal Imaging Findings and Treatment. Ocul Immunol Inflamm. 2018;26(4):518-22.
2. Bhattacharyya A, Sarma P, Sharma DJ, Das KK, Kaur H, Prajapat M, et al. Rhino-orbital-cerebral-mucormycosis in COVID-19: A systematic review. Indian J Pharmacol. 2021; 53(4):317-27.
3. Chhablani J. Fungal endophthalmitis. Expert Rev Anti Infect Ther. 2011;9(12):1191-201.
4. Das T, Agarwal M, Behera U, Bhattacharjee H, Bhende M, Das AV, et al. Diagnosis and management of fungal endophthalmitis: India perspective. Expert Rev Ophthalmol. 2020;15(6):355-65.
5. Das T, Joseph J, Jakati S, Sharma S, Velpandian T, Padhy SK, et al. Understanding the science of fungal endophthalmitis—AIOS 2021 Sengamedu Srinivas Badrinath Endowment Lecture. Indian J Ophthalmol. 2022;70(3):768-77.
6. Haider AA, Gallagher JR, Johnson JS, Benevento JD. Intravitreal Voriconazole for the Treatment of *Cryptococcus neoformans* Endogenous Endophthalmitis. Ochsner J. 2020;20(3):319-22.
7. Riddell J 4th, Comer GM, Kauffman CA. Treatment of endogenous fungal endophthalmitis: focus on new antifungal agents. Clin Infect Dis. 2011;52(5):648-53.
8. Sahu SK, Das S, Sahani D, Sharma S. Fungal scleritis masquerading as surgically induced necrotizing scleritis: a case report. J Med Case Rep. 2013;7:288.
9. Shah KK, Venkatramani D, Majumder PD. A case series of presumed fungal endogenous endophthalmitis in post COVID-19 patients. Indian J Ophthalmol. 2021;69(5):1322-5.
10. Shroff D, Narula R, Atri N, Chakravarti A, Gandhi A, Sapra N, et al. Endogenous fungal endophthalmitis following intensive corticosteroid therapy in severe COVID-19 disease. Indian J Ophthalmol. 2021;69(7):1909-14.

7.28 | Exudative Retinal Detachment

Neeraj Sandhuja, Anisha Seth
Delhi Retina Centre, New Delhi
neerajsanduja@yahoo.com, dranishasgupta@gmail.com

■ INTRODUCTION

Retinal detachment (RD) is the result of separation of the sensory retina from the retinal pigment epithelium (RPE). Exudative RD results from extravasation of fluid into the subretinal space from choroid or retinal blood vessels in absence of retinal hole.

■ PATHOPHYSIOLOGY

Under normal conditions, fluid flows from the vitreous cavity to the choroid. The direction of flow is influenced by the relative hyperosmolarity of the choroid with respect to the vitreous and the RPE that actively pumps ions and water from the vitreous into the choroid. When there is an increase in the inflow of fluid or a decrease in the outflow of fluid from the vitreous cavity that overwhelms the normal compensatory mechanisms, fluid accumulates in the subretinal space leading to an exudative RD.

- Any pathological process that affects choroidal vascular permeability can potentially cause an exudative RD.
- Damage to the RPE prevents the pumping action of fluid and can lead to fluid accumulation in the subretinal space.
- Several inflammatory, infectious, vascular, degenerative, malignant, or genetically determined pathological conditions have been recognized to cause exudative RDs.

- Abnormal retinal blood vessels which leak profusely or a broken blood-retinal barrier, increase the inflow of fluid into the subretinal space leading to exudative RD.
- Abnormally thick sclera, as seen in nanophthalmos, decreases the outflow of fluid.

SYMPTOMS

- *Decrease in vision or visual field defect:* Most common symptom
- Pain (e.g., uveitis or scleritis or any other inflammatory condition)
- Red eye (e.g., uveitic pathologies or inflammation)
- White pupil (leukocoria) due to RD.

SIGNS

- The anterior segment may show signs of inflammation—cells or flare in anterior chamber, keratic precipitates, and cataract.
- Bullous RD with convex configuration (like rhegmatogenous RD) but no retinal break.
- Smooth retinal surface without any retinal folds (unlike rhegmatogenous RD).
- Shifting subretinal fluid—the fluid gets collected in dependent position (most diagnostic) **(Figs. 7.28.1A and B)**.
- In chronic cases, deposition of hard exudates may be seen.
- Dilated telangiectatic vessels may be seen in Coats' disease.
- *Specific signs related to the underlying cause:* Retinal infiltrates or mass lesion.

CAUSES

- *Inflammatory:*
  - Vogt-Koyanagi-Harada syndrome
  - Scleritis
  - Sympathetic ophthalmia
  - Vasculitic entities (e.g., Wegener granulomatosis and rheumatoid arthritis)
  - Other uveitic conditions (e.g., toxoplasmosis and cytomegalovirus retinitis)
  - Dengue fever
  - Orbital pseudotumor
  - Tubercular granuloma
- *Idiopathic:*
  - Coats' disease
  - Central serous chorioretinopathy (CSCR)
  - Uveal effusion syndrome
- *Congenital:*
  - Nanophthalmos
  - Familial exudative vitreoretinopathy
  - Optic nerve head colobomas

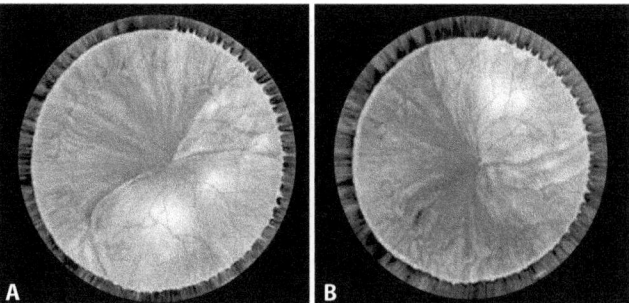

Figs. 7.28.1A and B: Exudative retinal detachment with shifting fluid: Fluid seen in inferior quadrant in sitting position; shifts to superior half in supine position.

- *Neoplastic:*
  - *Choroidal tumors:* Melanoma, hemangioma, nevus, and osteoma
  - Choroidal metastases
  - Retinoblastoma
  - Primary intraocular lymphoma
- *Iatrogenic:*
  - Excessive laser photocoagulation
  - *Scleral buckling:* Excessive cryopexy
- *Vascular factors:*
  - Malignant hypertension
  - Eclampsia
  - Exudative age-related macular degeneration (ARMD)

DIAGNOSIS

Investigations depend upon the suspected etiology. In the outpatient department settings, check blood pressure immediately. Ask for history of vitiligo or neurological auditory symptoms. Ask for history of trauma or other eye surgery, laser or cryopexy, recent pregnancy, and any ongoing systemic treatment.

- *Laboratory tests:* Mostly for inflammatory and infectious conditions:
  - Complete hemogram and erythrocyte sedimentation rate
  - TORCH
  - Kidney function tests
  - Venereal Disease Research Laboratory
  - Antineutrophil cytoplasmic antibodies
  - QuantiFERON gold for tuberculosis (TB)
  - Serum angiotensin-converting enzyme (ACE) level
  - Rheumatoid factor
- *USB scan:* Important investigative tool especially if media is hazy:
  - To detect choroidal thickness, choroidal detachment, and scleral thickness
  - To detect the presence or absence, the size, location, and internal character of choroidal masses.

  May be followed by magnetic resonance imaging with contrast for better diagnosis if choroidal tumors are suspected.
- *Fundus fluorescein angiography:* Extremely important for vascular causes—identifying areas of leakage in CSCR, Vogt–Koyanagi–Harada syndrome, Coats' disease, and exudative ARMD. Also helps in identifying choroidal vascular tumors and their feeder vessels.
- *Optical coherence tomography:* It can be done in cases with shallow detachments for monitoring treatment and resolution of fluid in follow-up.

MANAGEMENT

The management of exudative RDs is directed toward treating the underlying condition:
- Treat any causative systemic conditions such as hypertension and renal disease
- If suspecting steroid-induced CSCR, discontinue all forms of steroid use
- Infectious etiologies should be treated with antibiotics along with steroids or immunosuppressants
- Inflammatory conditions, such as scleritis, Vogt–Koyanagi–Harada syndrome, orbital pseudotumor, should be treated with anti-inflammatory agents
- Sick RPE/chronic CSCR may respond to systemic spironolactone and rifampicin
- Tumors need to be treated accordingly with radiation, chemotherapy, cryotherapy, or laser photocoagulation. In advanced cases, enucleation might be required.
- *Antivascular endothelial growth factor (VEGF) intravitreal injections:* Especially in Coats' disease and exudative ARMD.

- *Laser:*
  - *Focal laser:* In Coats' disease and familial exudative vitreoretinopathy—to ablate leaking vessels
  - *Photodynamic therapy or transpupillary thermotherapy:* For choroidal hemangiomas and other vascular tumors, exudative ARMD, and chronic central serous retinopathy
- *Vitrectomy:* Required in very rare cases—Coats' disease, optic disc pit, or coloboma.

SUGGESTED READING

1. Regillo CD, Mittra RA, Han DP. Exudative and traction retinal detachments: vitreoretinal disease. In: Regillo CD (Ed). Diseases of the Vitreous, Retina and Choroid. New Delhi, India: Thieme; 1999. pp. 491-503.

7.29 Familial Exudative Vitreoretinopathy

Parijat Chandra, Vinod Kumar
Dr RP Centre for Ophthalmic Sciences, AIIMS, New Delhi
parijatchandra@gmail.com

INTRODUCTION

Familial exudative vitreoretinopathy (FEVR) is a hereditary retinal vascular disorder initially described by Criswick and Schepens in 1969.[1] Though it is a bilateral disease, it tends to be asymmetric and usually presents in the first or the second decade of life. The primary cause of FEVR is a premature arrest of retinal vasculogenesis or retinal vascular differentiation, leading to incomplete vascularization of the peripheral retina.

Familial exudative vitreoretinopathy has a predominantly autosomal dominant inheritance, though autosomal recessive or X-linked cases have also been reported. Several identified genes are linked to FEVR such as *NDP, FZD4, LRP5, ZNF408,* and *TSPAN12*. Four out of these five genes have a role in Wnt signaling pathway, which is important for normal retinal vasculogenesis.

CLINICAL FEATURES

The hallmark feature of FEVR is avascular retinal periphery typically seen in the temporal retina. Retinal and preretinal neovascularization may occur at the junction of vascular and avascular retina which may result in fibrovascular proliferation. This results in temporal retinal traction causing vascular straightening, macular dragging and ectopia, and tractional and secondary rhegmatogenous retinal detachments (**Fig. 7.29.1**).

While mild presentations may remain asymptomatic till late, severe disease may present with blindness during the first decade of life. The other less common fundus features of FEVR include subretinal lipid exudation, supernumerary retinal vascular branching, falciform retinal folds, epiretinal membrane, and vitreous hemorrhage (**Fig. 7.29.2**). Also the apparently quiescent disease may develop neovascularization, vitreous hemorrhage, and retinal detachments and show chronic progression at any age.

CLASSIFICATION

Pendergast et al.[2] provided a detailed staging system and classified FEVR into five stages as given in **Table 7.29.1**.

DIFFERENTIAL DIAGNOSIS

The important differential diagnoses of FEVR are retinopathy of prematurity, Coats' disease, persistent fetal vasculature, Norrie disease, juvenile retinoschisis, and toxocariasis. The fundus picture in FEVR closely resembles retinopathy of prematurity, but these cases usually do not have history of prematurity or perinatal complications and are more asymmetrical. FEVR may be differentiated from Coats' disease which presents as unilateral involvement in young males, with typical retinal telangiectasias, intraretinal or subretinal exudation, and exudative retinal detachments. Norrie disease on the other hand is X-linked and seen in males and is associated with poor vision.

■ MANAGEMENT

Most mild (stage 1) and quiescent cases require no treatment. Peripheral scatter laser photocoagulation of avascular retina is recommended for active disease, angiographically leaking vessels and bleeding neovascularization (Stage 2). Wide field fluorescein angiography is especially useful to detect peripheral retinal changes such as peripheral retinal nonperfusion, neovascularization, and peripheral vascular anastomoses and helps to clearly delineate the junction between avascular and vascular retina, such that complete laser ablation can be performed **(Fig. 7.29.3)**. Advanced cases with vitreous hemorrhage and retinal detachments (Stages 3–5) require vitreoretinal surgery.

Diagnosing FEVR requires a high index of suspicion, careful family screening, and early detection to take prophylactic measures and prevent disease progression. Life-long regular retinal examinations and follow-up is essential.

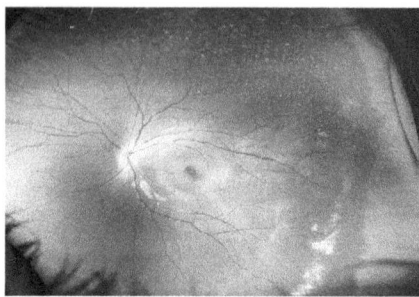

Fig. 7.29.1: Fundus photograph of left eye in familial exudative vitreoretinopathy showing temporal vascular straightening, exudation and peripheral avascular retina.

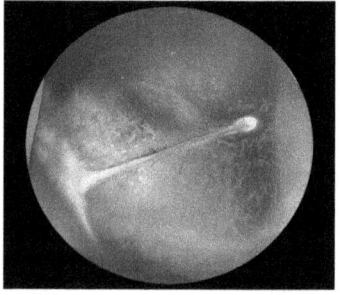

Fig. 7.29.2: Fundus photograph of right eye in familial exudative vitreoretinopathy showing temporal retinal traction with retinal falciform fold development, pigmentary changes and peripheral avascular retina.

Table 7.29.1: Five stages of familial exudative vitreoretinopathy.

Stage	Involvement
1	Avascular periphery
2	Retinal neovascularization A—without exudate B—with exudate
3	Extramacular retinal detachment A—without exudate B—with exudate
4	Subtotal macula-involving retinal detachment A—without exudate B—with exudates
5	Total retinal detachment

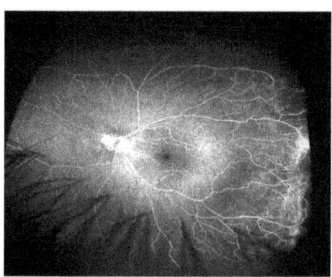

Fig. 7.29.3: Ultra-wide field fluorescein angiography of left eye with familial exudative vitreoretinopathy (FEVR) showing temporal drag of vessels, supernumerary vascular branching, periphery avascular retina, and vascular loop formation. There is leakage seen in relation to the neovascularization.

REFERENCES

1. Gilmour DF. Familial exudative vitreoretinopathy and related retinopathies. Eye (Lond). 2015;29(1):1-14.
2. Pendergast SD, Trese MT. Familial exudative vitreoretinopathy. Results of surgical management. Ophthalmology. 1998;105:1015-23.

7.30 Retained Lens Fragments in Vitreous

Pramod S Bhende
Medical Research Foundation, Chennai
pramod1999@yahoo.com

INTRODUCTION

Though posterior dislocation of lens material is an infrequent complication of cataract surgery, with increasing popularity of phacoemulsification the incidence of nucleus drop is on rise. It can occur during any phase of surgery but is more frequent during lens emulsification and cortical clean up. It can be either entire lens including capsule, only nucleus or part, only part of cortex, or fragments of both nucleus and cortex.

INCIDENCE

Overall incidence varies between 0.3 and 2.7% and the frequency decreases with increasing experience of surgeon.

RISK FACTORS

- Small nondilating pupil/deep-set eyes
- Traumatic cataract/hard nucleus/posterior polar cataract
- Uncooperative patient/inadequate anesthesia
- Pseudoexfoliation or zonular weakness due to any cause

MANAGEMENT

What the cataract surgeon should do?
Early recognition of the posterior capsule tear and prevention of anterior chamber (AC) collapse may help in preventing further extension of the tear, forward movement, and prolapse of the vitreous and posterior displacement of the lens matter. In case of any doubt, the surgeon should stop the surgery and do thorough assessment of the situation. The different situations are:

- *Only posterior capsule rupture but no vitreous disturbance:* Use adequate viscoelastics to prevent AC collapse. The surgeon can continue the surgery (depending on surgeon's competence). Please handle the tissues gently to avoid further damage.
- *Posterior chamber (PC) rupture and disturbance of anterior vitreous but no vitreous prolapse or loss:* Inject viscoelastics in AC to push the vitreous back. Depending on surgeon's experience, one can continue phacoemulsification or can convert to extra-capsular extraction.
- *Vitreous in the wound/lens vitreous admixture/lens fragments in anterior vitreous behind the iris plane:* It is important to perform thorough anterior vitrectomy. One can use second instrument through the limbus behind the fragment/s to push them in AC to deliver out through the limbal section.
- *Lens fragments in mid/posterior vitreous cavity:* Occasionally it may be possible to retrieve the lens matter from the vitreous using balanced salt solution (BSS)/Ringer lactate irrigation or lens loop. But it is important to understand that the other end of the vitreous fiber is adherent to the retina posteriorly. Any attempt of grasping or pulling of anterior vitreous can lead to unwanted posterior traction on the retina.

This risk is unacceptably high when a cryoprobe is used to retrieve the nucleus sinking in the vitreous. Apart from the risk of retinal detachment (RD) and giant retinal tear, it also increases the risk of corneal decompensation.

These eyes are best managed by pars plana approach by trained VR surgeon.

It is ideal to complete the surgery at the same sitting if instrumentation and VR surgeon is available or in case cataract surgeon himself is an experienced VR surgeon, to avoid the second surgery and psychological trauma to the patient.

If VR setting is not available, the cataract surgeon should clear the AC of vitreous/lens fragments. Ensure that the wound is water tight. One can implant intraocular lens (IOL) at this stage, if there is adequate capsular support and dislocated nuclear fragment/s is/are not very hard. During early postoperative period, the patient should be treated with topical steroids, cycloplegics, and antibiotics and should be referred to VR surgeon at the earliest. It is important to monitor the intraocular pressure closely.

How to get the nucleus back?
Observation is an option, if the nucleus piece is <10% size, or the dislocated material is only cortex (<25%). One needs to follow these patients closely till all the lens matter gets absorbed. Always look for any signs of chronic inflammation, high IOP, cystoid macular edema, or vitreoretinal traction.

INDICATIONS FOR VITRECTOMY

- Nuclear piece/large cortical fragments
- Persistent uveitis (incidence 56-100%)
- High IOP (incidence, 38.4-86.3%)
- Associated retinal break/s (11.0-21.5%), RD (3.0-7.0%), vitreous hemorrhage, or endophthalmitis

TIMING OF THE VITRECTOMY

Though controversial, generally, vitrectomy and removal of fragments is advisable within 2 weeks. Eyes with associated RD or infection need early surgery.

SURGICAL TECHNIQUE

Thorough fundus evaluation is important to rule out any associated posterior segment complication. If necessary, ultrasonography should be performed in eyes with media haze.

General/local anesthesia can be used. It is important to check cataract wound integrity and reinforce it, if needed. Standard 3 port pars plana approach should be preferred. Depending on availability and surgeons' experience and hardness of nucleus, 20 G, 23 G, or 25 G approach can be used. Please note that fragmatome is available only with 20 G and 23 G systems. Clear the vitreous from AC and cataract wound, if present. Complete vitrectomy before attempting retrieval of the lens fragments to avoid vitreous traction and associated iatrogenic retinal complications. Lens fragments can be lifted of the retinal surface using mild suction to perform phacofragmentation in mid vitreous cavity. Vitreous cutter can be used if the lens matter is soft; however, fragmatome is necessary to deal with hard nucleus. Very hard nucleus can be brought into AC to remove through the enlarged limbal section. Perfluorocarbon liquid (PFCL) can be used to float the lens matter, if needed. IOL can be implanted at this stage, if not implanted earlier. AC/PC or scleral fixated IOL can be used depending on the capsular integrity and surgeon's experience.

COMPLICATIONS

All the complications related to 3 port pars plana surgery such as retinal break/s, giant retinal tear, and dialysis should be reported. Retinal concussion injury can be due to dropped or flying lens pieces during ultrasound fragmentation within the vitreous cavity or can be due to instrument touch or direct impact of ultrasound energy on the retina.

VISUAL OUTCOME

If managed properly and at appropriate time, 20/40 or better vision is reported in 60–72% of eyes in the literature.

DON'TS FOR CATARACT SURGEON

- Do not follow fragments sinking in the vitreous.
- Avoid blind fishing or irrigation of vitreous cavity to retrieve the fragments.
- No phaco/active suction within the vitreous. Never use bare cryoprobe within formed vitreous
- Avoid excessive handling and damage to cornea and retina.
- Preferably avoid silicone IOL.

HOW TO AVOID THE DROP?

- Aim for larger rhexis
- Avoid touching edge of rhexis with metal instruments
- Avoid pushing movement during emulsification
- Do not advance phoco tip into the nucleus faster than the ultrasound energy can cut the path

To summarize—avoiding vigorous attempts to retrieve intravitreal lens fragment/s and timely referral to vitreoretinal surgeon for vitrectomy and complete removal of lens fragment/s can result in good visual recovery.

SUGGESTED READING

1. Baker PS, Spirn MJ, Chiang A, Regillo CD, Ho AC, Vander JF, et al. 23-Gauge transconjunctival pars plana vitrectomy for removal of retained lens fragments. Am J Ophthalmol. 2011;152:624-7.
2. Mathai A, Thomas R. Incidence and management of posteriorly dislocated nuclear fragments following phacoemulsification. Indian J Ophthalmol. 1999;47:173-76.
3. Merani R, Hunyor AP, Playfair J, Chang A, Gregory-Roberts J, Hunyor ABL, et al. Pars plana vitrectomy for the management of retained lens matter after cataract surgery. Am J Ophthalmol. 2007;144:364-70.
4. Monshizadeh R, Samiy N, Haimovici R. Management of retained intravitreal lens fragments after cataract surgery. Surv Ophthalmol. 1999;43:397-404.
5. Venkateswaran N, Medina-Mendez C, Amescua G. Perioperative management of dropped lenses: anterior and posterior segment considerations and treatment options. Int Ophthalmol Clin. 2020;60:61-9.
6. Watts P, Hunter J, Bunce C. Vitrectomy and lensectomy in the management of posterior dislocation of lens fragments. J Cataract Refract Surg. 2000;26:832-37.

7.31 Management of Myopic Maculopathy

Parveen Sen, Tarun Sharma
Sankara Nethralaya, Chennai
drps@snmail.org, drts@snmail.org

INTRODUCTION

- Myopic maculopathy (MM) is common in those eyes with myopia of >6.00 D sphere and axial length of >26 mm.
- The features of MM include—chorioretinal atrophy (CRA), lacquer cracks, Fuchs spots, posterior staphyloma, choroidal neovascular membrane (CNVM), retinoschisis or macular traction maculopathy (MTM), and dome-shaped maculopathy. These changes are usually present in various combinations.

CHORIORETINAL ATROPHY

- The CRA could be either diffuse or patchy. Diffuse CRA is characterized by marked and diffuse thinning of the choroidal layer. In patchy CRA, there is a complete loss of choriocapillaris, retinal pigment epithelium (RPE), and the outer retina; almost bare sclera is seen here.
- Matsui et al. in their META PM (META-analysis for Pathologic Myopia) study have classified myopic CRA into 0–4 categories:
    - *Category 0:* No macular lesion
    - *Category 1:* Tessellated fundus
    - *Category 2:* Diffuse CRA
    - *Category 3:* Patchy CRA
    - *Category 4:* Macular atrophy

The visual acuity remains unaffected in categories 0 and 1, while severe visual loss may be associated with other categories **(Figs. 7.31.1A to I)**.

LACQUER CRACKS

These cracks represent break or rupture in the Bruch's membrane. They are seen as yellowish linear lines either horizontal or vertical and may be associated with subretinal bleed without CNVM.

- *Fluorescein angiogram (FA):* Linear areas of hyperfluorescence radiating from the disc, due to the window defect caused by atrophy of overlying RPE. These eyes have an increased risk of CNVM.

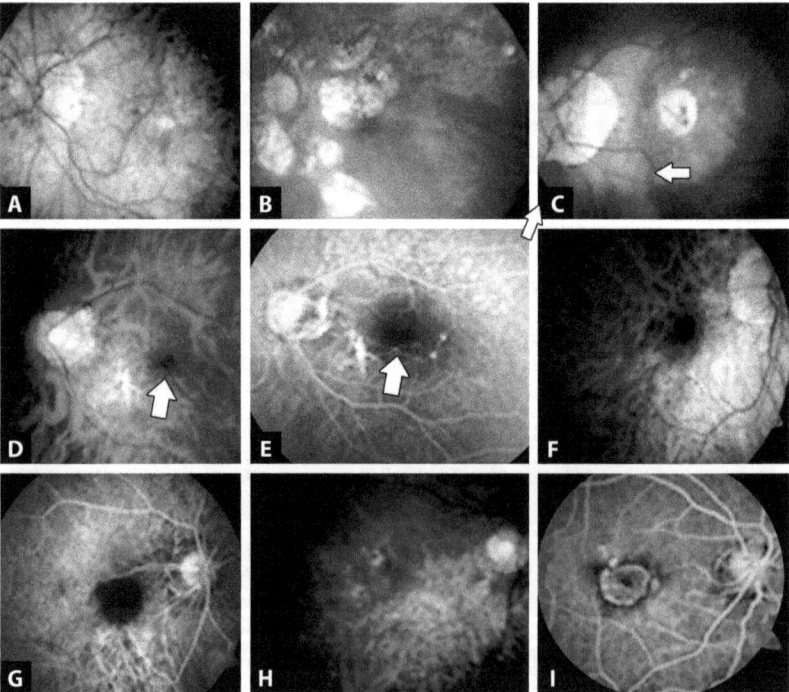

Figs. 7.31.1A to I: (A) Diffuse CRA; (B) Patchy CRA; (C) Macular atrophy with posterior staphyloma (white arrow); (D) Lacquer crack (white arrow); (E) FFA delineates the lacquer crack (arrow); (F) Focal hemorrhage which resorbs to give Fuchs spot; (G) FFA of same eye confirms the absence of CNVM; (H) Myopic subfoveal CNVM; (I) FFA shows the lacy network. (CNVM: choroidal neovascular membrane; CRA: chorioretinal atrophy; FFA: fundus fluorescein angiography)

FUCHS SPOT
- Spontaneous small areas of macular hemorrhages due to stretching of the retina and resorption of hemorrhages leads to a small circumscribed area of pigmentation, termed as Fuchs spot.
- These spots may cause metamorphosis and need FA to differentiate it from CNVM.

POSTERIOR STAPHYLOMA
- Usually associated with high myopia and increased stretching could result in macular hole or a retinal break close to the edge of the posterior staphyloma.
- Absence of a good contrast (due to atrophy of choroid and RPE) makes it difficult to identify these breaks and treat them.

CHOROIDAL NEOVASCULAR MEMBRANE
- *Epidemiology:* After age-related macular degeneration (AMD), myopic CNVM is the most common cause of CNVM, occurring in around 5–10% of eyes with myopia; lacquer cracks and patches of macular atrophy are important risk factors.
- *CNVM:* Usually type 2, classic, pre-RPE, well-defined, subfoveal, and less leaky.
- *Fundus:* Dark greenish-brown membrane with a surrounding thin layer of subretinal hemorrhage and some amount of retinal thickening.
- *FA:* Well-defined hyperfluorescence in the early phase and leakage in the late phase besides a rim of blocked hypofluorescence due to hemorrhage.
- *Optical coherence tomography (OCT):* Type 2 CNVM, hyper-reflective lesion with varying degrees of intraretinal fluid (usually less compared to AMD CNVM).
- *Treatment of thermal laser:* Usually avoided even in juxta- or extrafoveal ones as the laser burns could expand and run under the fovea.
- *Treatment of photodynamic therapy (PDT):* Not a favorable option in view of possible drop in vision due to choroidal ischemia and creeping laser scar.
- *Treatment of antivascular endothelial growth factor (VEGF):* Anti-VEGF injections are now the treatment of choice in managing myopic CNVM (mCNVM).
- *Radiance study, phase 3, randomized clinical trial (RCT):* It showed that eyes treated with ranibizumab had better visual gain (around 10 letters) than those treated with PDT. Over 12 months pro re nata (PRN) treatment regimens were able to improve and sustain visual gain, with nearly 65% of mCNVM showing resolution of leakage and a median of two to four injections were needed.
- *Ranibizumab versus bevacizumab:* RCT by Gharbiya et al. with 32 eyes with mCNVM treated with PRN intravitreal ranibizumab (0.5 mg) or bevacizumab (1.25 mg) revealed no significant difference in best-corrected visual acuity (BCVA) improvement (17 letters vs. 15 letters) as well as foveal central thickness on OCT.
- *Aflibercept:* MYRROR study (phase 3, sham-controlled RCT) reported a visual acuity gain of an average of 12 letters at 24 weeks in eyes treated with PRN intravitreal aflibercept 2 mg.
- *Follow-up:* Monthly with VA, OCT, and sometime FA (**Figs. 7.31.2A and B**).

MYOPIC RETINOSCHISIS
Myopic Traction Maculopathy
The term "MTM" was first used by Panozzo and Merchanti. Though asymptomatic in the early stages, this could cause visual loss in high myopia.

Pathophysiology
There are several factors that interplay and cause MTM.
- Progressive elongation of the globe results in posterior staphyloma and causes mismatch between the length of the sclera with that of the retina; so, stretching of

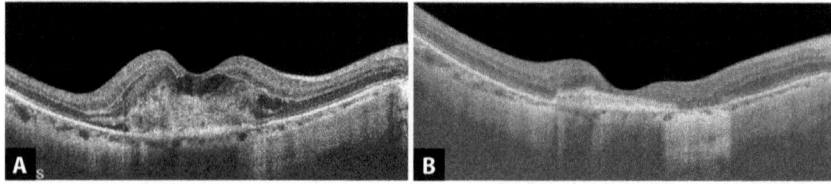

Figs. 7.31.2A and B: (A) Before and (B) after multiple antivascular endothelial growth factor injections. Good response is evident by decrease in subretinal fluid and central retinal thickness; choroidal neovascular membrane becomes more compact and well-defined with increased backscattering due to scarring.

the retina occurs with weakening of the adhesion between the neurosensory retina and the RPE.
- Incomplete posterior vitreous detachment (PVD) with vitreoschisis of the unhealthy vitreous gel in high myopia leads to anteroposterior traction.
- Increased tangential traction also occurs due to altered inner limiting membrane (ILM), epiretinal membrane, and stretched or rigid blood vessels.

Optical Coherence Tomography Features

It shows many pathognomonic signs:
- *Retinoschisis:* Splitting of the outer and inner retina with bridging columns; could also cause foveoschisis.
- Lamellar or full-thickness macular hole, with or without retinal detachment (RD).

Stages of Macular Traction Maculopathy

Shimida et al. described the development and progression of MTM.
- *Stage 1:* Focal irregularity of the thickness of the outer retina.
- *Stage 2:* Outer lamellar hole develops in the area of irregularity. Both stage 1 and stage 2 may be observed closely.
- *Stage 3:* Outer lamellar hole enlarges. Columns such as vertically elongated and horizontally separated structures overlying outer lamellar hole begins to appear.
- *Stage 4:* Increased retinoschisis and foveal detachment/RD. Stage 3 and stage 4 may need surgical intervention.

Indications for Surgery

- Troublesome metamorphopsia
- Progressive decrease in vision
- Foveal detachment
- Full-thickness macular hole **(Figs. 7.31.3A to C)**.

Surgery: Pars Plana Vitrectomy

- Pars plana vitrectomy (PPV) remains the mainstay of therapy. The aim of the surgery is to remove the anteroposterior traction caused by abnormal VR adhesion and remove tangential traction by removal of ILM.
- In view of the risk of development of full-thickness macular hole following surgery with ILM peeling, foveal sparing ILM peeling has been advocated.
- ILM peeling is somewhat more challenging in myopic eyes as compared to eyes with idiopathic macular hole due to several reasons: due to elongated globe, instrument tips may not reach to the end location for PVD induction/ILM peeling; difficulty in visualization due to lack of contrast/choroidal atrophy; and increased risk of iatrogenic retinal break due to thin retina **(Figs. 7.31.4A and B)**.

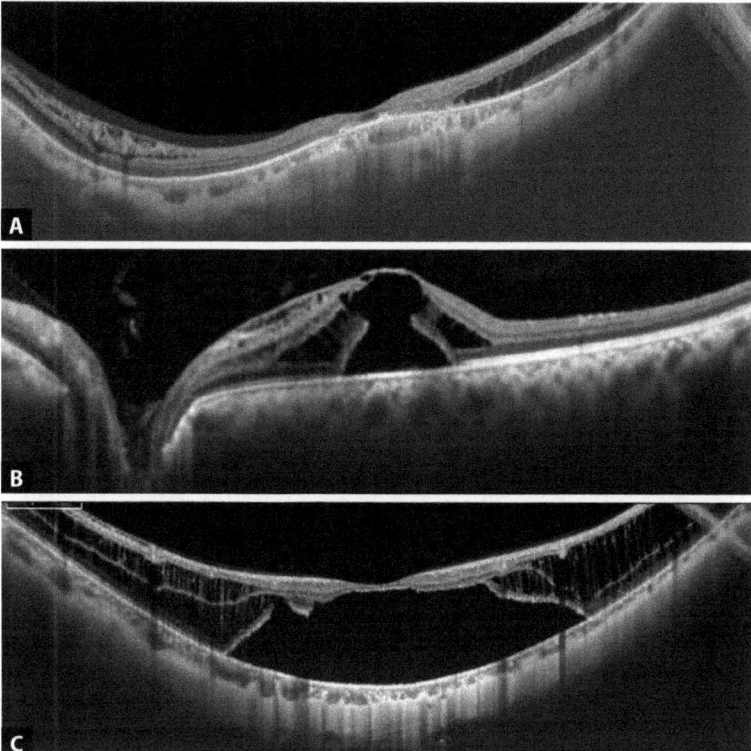

Figs. 7.31.3A to C: Swept source optical coherence tomography (OCT) showing various stages of macular traction maculopathy (MTM). (A) Extrafoveal thickening and irregularity of the outer retina; (B) Outer lamellar macular hole (LMH); (C) Advanced stage of retinoschisis.

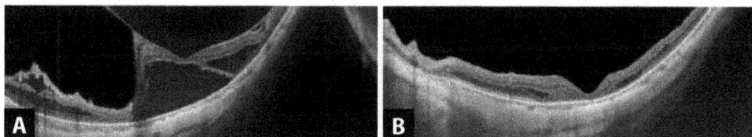

Figs. 7.31.4A and B: (A) Swept source optical coherence tomography (OCT) shows advanced macular traction maculopathy (MTM) along with foveoschisis; (B) Post-pars plana vitrectomy (PPV), 6 months follow-up, restoration of foveal contour, and vision improved from 3/60 to 6/18.

Factors Influencing Visual Outcome
- In some cases, despite surgical success, visual outcome may still be poor due to coexistent photoreceptor/choroidal atrophy.
- Preoperative ellipsoid zone disruption and reduced central foveal thickness on OCT.

Overall, macular hole closure rate after PPV is somewhat less in myopic eyes compared to idiopathic macular holes.

Macular Buckling
Rationale
It supports the globe posteriorly, reducing the anteroposterior traction on the neural retina caused by progressive staphyloma.

Indications

Myopic hole with posterior pole RD, in particular in eyes with posterior staphyloma having axial length of >30 mm or failure of closure of macular hole with persistent RD following PPV and ILM peeling.

Complications

Macular buckling is technically demanding and can be associated with various complications. Intraoperative or immediate postoperative complications include inadvertent globe perforation, damage to vortex veins or ciliary vessels/nerves, optic nerve abutting, and subretinal/choroidal/suprachoroidal hemorrhage. Late postoperative complications are buckle exposure/displacement, CNVM formation, limitation of eye movement causing diplopia, and focal RPE atrophy due to compression of the blood vessels.

◾ DOME-SHAPED MACULOPATHY

First described by Gaucher in 2008, dome-shaped maculopathy is defined as an inward bulge of the macula within the concavity of the posterior staphyloma, as evident on OCT. Serous macular detachment is a known complication of dome-shaped maculopathy; FA/indocyanine green (ICG) may show pinpoint leakage in the late phase and subretinal

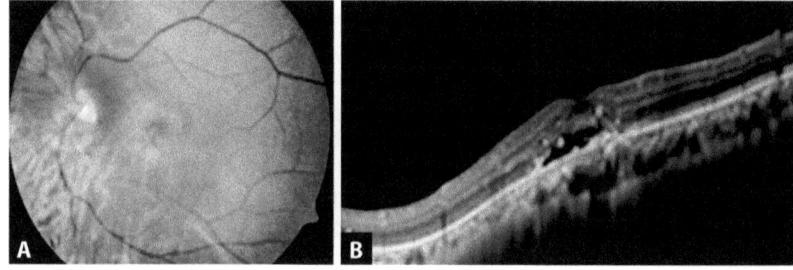

Figs. 7.31.5A and B: (A) Fundus photograph shows subretinal fluid at the macula with (B) serous macular detachment confirmed on optical coherence tomography (OCT) in the absence of choroidal neovascular membrane (CNVM); dome-shaped macula was seen on OCT in both eyes.

Flowchart 7.31.1: An algorithm for managing myopic maculopathy.

Myopic maculopathy
- Chorioretinal atrophy → Observe
- Lacquer cracks → FFA to rule out CNVM → No CNVM → Observe
- Fuchs spots → FFA to rule out CNVM → No CNVM → Observe
- Myopic CNV → FFA and OCT → Inactive → Observe; Active → Anti-VEGF (PRN)
- Myopic macular taction → Drop in vision, posterior pole RD, FTMH → PPV with ILM peeling → Mucular buckle

(CNVM: choroidal neovascular membrane; FFA: fundus fluorescein angiography; FTMH: full-thickness macular hole; ILM: inner limiting membrane; OCT: optical coherence tomography; PRN: pro re nata; RD: retinal detachment; VEGF: vascular endothelial growth factor)

fluid with increased choroidal thickness on OCT under the fovea. Treatment response to thermal laser, PDT or anti-VEGF drugs remain poor; use of spironolactone has shown some promise in few reported cases, and sometimes, spontaneous resolution of the fluid is also seen **(Figs. 7.31.5A and B)**.

CONCLUSION

Patients with high myopia need to be educated about the possibility of MM, and therefore, they must undergo periodical fundus evaluation **(Flowchart 7.31.1)**.

SUGGESTED READING

1. Gaucher D, Erginay A, Lecleire-Collet A, Haouchine B, Puech M, Cohen SY, et al. Dome-shaped macula in eyes with myopic posterior staphyloma. Am J Ophthalmol. 2008; 145(5):909-14.

7.32 Cataract Surgery in Diabetic Retinopathy

R Kim, V Muthukrishnan
Aravind Eye Hospitals and Postgraduate Institute of Ophthalmology, Madurai
kim@aravind.org

INTRODUCTION

The effect of cataract surgery on the progression of diabetic retinopathy (DR) remains an issue of debate.[1] Preoperative, intraoperative, and postoperative factors are of paramount importance in the management of diabetic patients undergoing cataract surgery. The Early Treatment Diabetic Retinopathy Study (ETDRS) suggested a trend toward increased retinopathy progression and worsening visual acuity (VA) in eyes undergoing cataract surgery compared to unoperated fellow eyes in diabetics.[2]

EFFECT OF PERIOPERATIVE GLYCEMIC CONTROL ON PROGRESSION OF DIABETIC RETINOPATHY AND MACULOPATHY

- Glycemic control does not influence the postoperative progression of retinopathy except in specific situations.[1]
- When there is a rapid preoperative glycemic correction (RPGC), the progression rate is significantly higher in moderate-to-severe nonproliferative diabetic retinopathy (NPDR) and in preexisting maculopathy.[1]
- RPGC should be avoided in patients with moderate to severe NPDR since it may increase the risk of postoperative progression of DR.[1]

RISK FACTORS FOR VISUAL OUTCOME

- Similar rate of progression has been observed in extracapsular cataract extraction and phacoemulsification.[1]
- Longer duration of surgery and complications like posterior capsular rupture may accelerate progression of DR.[1]
- The presence of diabetic macular edema (DME) and poor preoperative VA (reflecting diabetic maculopathy, ischemia, and traction) has been recognized as risk factors for poor postoperative VA.[2]

PRECAUTIONS DURING CATARACT SURGERY

- Diabetic eyes often have poor pupillary dilation, especially when active rubeosis iridis or even regressed neovascularization is present. Pupil stretching maneuvers should be avoided because these vessels can rupture and cause intraocular bleeding. Preoperative intravitreal antivascular endothelial growth factor (VEGF) agents may decrease the chances of bleeding from iris neovascularization.[1]

- Phacoemulsification may be combined with pars plana vitrectomy in the presence of coexistent cataract and nonclearing vitreous hemorrhage, macular traction retinal detachment (TRD), combined mechanism retinal detachment, and persistent DME not responding to intravitreal anti-VEGF agents and/or steroids.[2]

CHOICE OF INTRAOCULAR LENSES
- It is preferred to use hydrophobic acrylic intraocular lenses (IOLs) due to the lower incidence of posterior capsular opacification.[1]
- To avoid silicone IOLs in patients with preexisting proliferative diabetic retinopathy (PDR).[1]
- Multifocal IOLs should be avoided in eyes with vision threatening DR.[1,2]
- Preferable to use large optic IOLs.[1,2]

DIABETIC MACULAR EDEMA
- An uneventful phacoemulsification and IOL implantation results in a significant increase in VEGF, hepatocyte growth factor, interleukin-1 (IL-1), and pigment epithelium-derived factor concentrations culminating in worsening of DR and DME.[2]
- Macular edema (ME) arising after surgery (Irvine–Gass syndrome) resolves spontaneously over few months, and so early laser treatment of all diabetic postoperative ME is unnecessary and should be delayed for 6 months. Few studies have suggested that preoperative and postoperative use of nonsteroidal anti-inflammatory drugs such as diclofenac and nepafenac may reduce the chances of postoperative ME in patients with DR.[1,2]
- In patients with preexisting DME, cataract surgery can increase the risk of progression or recurrence to 20–50%. Thus, perioperative intravitreal steroids and anti-VEGF agents are a good option in these cases. In the current era of anti-VEGF therapy, the role of focal and grid laser photocoagulation has diminished generally for the treatment of DME and especially for DME following cataract surgery.[1,2]
- In a recent report by the DRCR.net, 11% of patients with DME not involving the foveal center on optical coherence tomography (OCT) developed center-involving DME in about 16 weeks after cataract surgery.[1]
- Patients with center-involving DME are treated until the level of edema is deemed stable, based upon OCT findings, clinical examination, and VA.[1]
- Given the data from the DRCR.net, patients without center-involving DME are to be evaluated 1 month after cataract extraction and no later than 16 weeks after cataract surgery to assess for DME occurrence.[1]

LASER AND CATARACT SURGERY
- In patients with severe cataract or posterior subcapsular cataract that obscures fundus observation, cataract surgery should be followed by treatment of macular edema or PDR,[1,2] if present.
- PRP should be considered for severe NPDR and early proliferative DR prior to cataract surgery.[1]
- When the cataract does not preclude laser treatment, effective control of retinopathy and maculopathy at least 3 months before surgery is advisable.[1]

RENAL FUNCTION
The presence of poor renal function increases the progression of retinopathy postoperatively.[1]

CONCLUSION
Diabetic patients with any type of retinopathy should be advised that cataract extraction may exacerbate preexisting DR. Prompt diagnosis and treatment of DR prior to cataract

surgery may enhance visual outcome.[1] Better understanding of various factors governing favorable outcome of cataract surgery in diabetic patients may guide us in optimizing results.[2]

REFERENCES

1. Squirrell D, Bhola R, Bush J, Winder S, Talbot JF. A prospective, case controlled study of the natural history of diabetic retinopathy and maculopathy after uncomplicated phacoemulsification cataract surgery in patients with type 2 diabetes. Br J Ophthalmol. 2002;86:565-71.
2. Kelkar A, Kelkar J, Mehta H, Amoaku W. Cataract surgery in diabetes mellitus: a systematic review. Indian J Ophthalmol. 2018;66(10):1401-10.

7.33 | Gene Therapy

Raja Narayanan, Taraprasad Das
LV Prasad Eye Institute, Hyderabad
dr_narayanan@hotmail.com, tpdbei@gmail.com

INTRODUCTION

Gene therapy is recognized as an important scientific achievement of the 20th century. The vector encapsulates therapeutic genes for delivery to cells. The vectors could be viral and nonviral in origin. The development of gene therapy in general has been limited by the host immune response to foreign antigens in the transgene and/or vector. Historically, the immune-privileged status of the eye has been demonstrated by clinical success in corneal transplantation and experimental delivery of tissue grafts to the eye. The first recombinant viral vectors were developed using the papilloma simian virus SV40, and it was demonstrated that retroviral vectors could correct the symptoms of hypoxanthine-guanine phosphoribosyltransferase deficiency and adenosine deaminase deficiency-severe combined immunodeficiency disease in vitro.

VECTORS

The development of gene therapy for retinal disease started >20 years ago with the first adenovirus-mediated gene transfer into the retina of adult mice.[1] In 2007, progressive refinement and innovation culminated in the first clinical trials for Leber congenital amaurosis (LCA).

Along the way, milestones were achieved to significantly reduce immunogenicity of adenoviral vectors, increase the payload capacity of adeno-associated viral (AAV) vectors, and optimize transduction efficiency and tropism of lentiviral vectors. Owing to their small size, lentiviruses easily cross biological barriers.

The limited packaging capacity of AAV remains the principal shortcoming of these vectors. Lentiviral vectors can partially overcome this challenge, accommodating coding sequences up to 10 kb in length.

Results from a trial involving subjects with LCA due to autosomal recessive mutations in *RPE65* demonstrated significant improvement of functional vision as measured by the primary end point, a multi-luminance mobility test, in those injected with SPK-*RPE65* (*voretigene neparvovec*) when compared with the untreated control group.

TROPISM AND MODES OF DELIVERY

Systemic delivery of gene therapy agents does not result in gene delivery to ocular structures. Intravitreal injection of vector leads to efficient gene delivery in retinal ganglion cells and Müller cells. Subretinal injection leads to efficient gene delivery in photoreceptors and retinal pigment epithelium (**Fig. 7.33.1**).

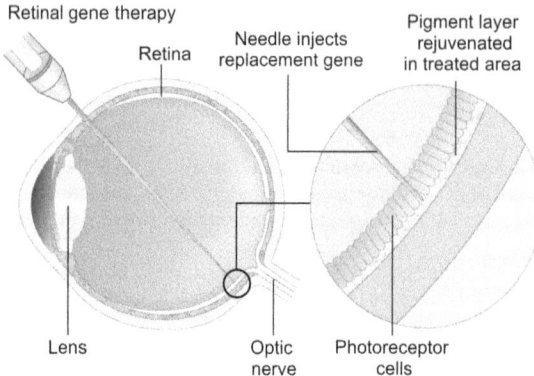

Fig. 7.33.1: Retinal gene therapy delivery.

■ RETINAL DISEASES

Clinical trials using AAV vectors are underway for the treatment of a variety of hereditary diseases. They include *X-linked retinoschisis* by the National Eye Institute (NCT02317887) and by AGTC (NCT02416622), and *achromatopsia* (NCT02599922). Lentiviral vectors are used by Sanofi to deliver lengthy genes, such as *ABCA4* and *MYO7A*, in the treatment of *Stargardt disease and Usher syndrome 1b*, respectively (NCT01367444 and NCT01505062). The AAV vectors coupled with targeting sequences are directing nuclear expression of a gene that encodes for a protein that will ultimately be transported into the mitochondria. Pioneering work in developing therapies for mitochondrial disease is currently carried out by three independent groups, each seeking to deliver a gene (*ND4*) encoding a subunit of mitochondrial complex 1, the defect in *Leber hereditary optic neuropathy* (NCT02161380, NCT02064569, and NCT01267422).

In the case of multifactorial retinal diseases like *age-related macular degeneration (AMD)*, gene transfer has been used in another strategy that differs from simple gene replacement. For patients with neovascular AMD, the goal of gene therapy is to provide a stable concentration of a naturally produced vascular endothelial growth factor (VEGF) receptor (sFLT-1) to reduce the complications and treatment burden of repeated intraocular injections. Phase 2 outcomes reported by Constable et al. showed safety and tolerability of sFLT-1 AAV2-mediated delivery. In recent years, the concept of gene editing as a new application of gene therapy has emerged. In this technique, viral vectors shuttle ribonucleic acid (RNA)-containing clustered regularly interspaced short palindromic repeats that complement the mutated gene sequence of interest and simultaneously introduce sequences encoding endonuclease Cas9.

Many angiostatic factors have been shown to counteract the effect of increasing local VEGF. The naturally occurring form of soluble Flt-1 has been shown to reverse neovascularization (NV) in rats, mice, and monkeys.

Pigment epithelium-derived factor (PEDF) also acts as an inhibitor of angiogenesis. The secretion of PEDF is noticeably decreased under hypoxic conditions allowing the endothelial mitogenic activity of VEGF to dominate, thus suggesting that the loss of PEDF plays a central role in the development of ischemia-driven NV. One interesting clinical finding shows that the levels of PEDF in aqueous humor of human are decreased with increasing age, indicating that the reduction may lead to the development of AMD.

■ KEY TO SUCCESSFUL THERAPY

Development of a successful strategy of gene therapy depends on several of the following factors:
- Clinically appropriate disease is identified.
- Molecular genetic basis of this disease is understood.

- Appropriate mechanism to deliver the desired gene to the therapeutic site is available.
- Strategy to ensure expression of therapeutic gene in appropriate cells and at appropriate level is in place.

CURRENT TRIALS

Gene therapy is currently explored in:
- Retinitis pigmentosa (RP)
- LCA
- Gyrate atrophy
- AMD
- X-linked retinoschisis
- Choroideremia

CONCLUSION

Notable progress has been made in understanding the genetic pathogenesis of ocular diseases and improving the safety and specificity of vector-based ocular gene transfer methods. These technical developments have been critical to the gene therapy successes achieved in experimental models of both retinal and nonretinal ocular diseases. The majority of experiments have been performed in mice, however, and more work is needed in animals with eyes that more closely resemble those of humans. Preliminary successes have been reported in clinical trials utilizing *RPE65* gene therapy for LCA and *PEDF* gene therapy for AMD. With the advancements in recent years and the establishment of proof-of-concept for gene therapy approaches targeting various retinal diseases, gene therapy may be an essential treatment strategy for ocular diseases in the near future.

REFERENCE

1. Bennett J, Wilson J, Sun D, Forbes B, Maguire A. Adenovirus vector-mediated in vivo gene transfer into adult murine retina. Invest Ophthalmol Vis Sci. 1994;35:2535-42.

7.34 Diabetic Macular Edema

Rajiv Raman, Chetan Rao, Vikas Khetan
Sankara Nethralaya, Chennai
rajivpgraman@gmail.com

INTRODUCTION

Diabetes is a systemic disorder affecting the small vessels of the body (microangiopathy) predominately affecting the three systems: the eye, the kidney, and the nerves.

Diabetic retinopathy (DR) results from the microangiopathy of the retinal vasculature leading to blindness in some individuals. A good understanding of the disease condition is important to treat and counsel patients.

EPIDEMIOLOGY

India is now regarded as the emerging diabetic capital of the world. According to the World Health Organization, in India in the year 2000 diabetics affected nearly 31.7 million people. It is expected to increase to 79.4 million by 2030, a matter of great concern for us.

According to a recent study on urban Chennai population they found 28.2% prevalence of diabetes and 3.5% prevalence of DR in general population. Among diabetics the prevalence of DR was 18%.[1]

The All India Ophthalmological Society Diabetic Retinopathy Eye Screening Study found the prevalence of DR to be 21%.

INITIAL ASSESSMENT OF DIABETIC MACULAR EDEMA

History
- Onset of ocular symptoms, duration, and progression to be taken in a chronological order. History of previous consultations, treatment underwent (eye drops, lasers, intraocular injections, and any surgeries), response to treatment, and compliance must be noted.
- Duration of diabetes, past glycemic control (hemoglobin A1C), systemic history (e.g., renal disease, cardiovascular events, systemic hypertension, serum lipid levels, pregnancy, smoking, anemia, and thyroid disorders).
- Ocular medications and other systemic drugs (insulin, oral hypoglycemic, antihypertensive, and lipid-lowering drugs)
- History related to drugs causing macular edema [thiazolidinediones, fingolimod (used in multiple sclerosis), tamoxifen, taxanes, niacin, interferons, and prostaglandin analogs]
- Any allergy, social and family history to be taken.

EXAMINATION

Systemic Examination
Evaluation of pulse, blood pressure, pallor, edema of face and extremities, weight, and height. A quick survey for wound infections in the foot, thyroid swelling, limb weakness, and peripheral sensations is required.

Ocular Examination
- Visual acuity [preferably by the Early Treatment Diabetic Retinopathy Study (ETDRS) or LogMAR chart] with and without correction.
- Anterior segment [to specifically look for neovascularization of the iris, cataract grading if any, gonioscopy to look for angle status and neovascularization of the angle, and intraocular pressure (IOP) estimation]
- Posterior segment [to grade DR status and presence of diabetic macular edema (DME), presence of peripheral artery disease, evidence of mixed or asymmetrical retinopathy, disc status for glaucomatous damage and any associated finding like myopic fundus, other associated macular pathology contributing to diminution of vision, and laser treatment evidence and its adequacy] **(Figs. 7.34.1A to D)**.

INVESTIGATIONS

Systemic Investigation
It must be done with consultation with a physician. It includes blood sugar profile, glycosylated hemoglobin, liver function test, kidney function test, thyroid screening, fasting lipid profile, hemoglobin estimation, ultrasound of whole abdomen, urine examination routine, and microscopy and electrocardiogram.

Ocular Investigation
Diabetic macular edema can be clinically significant or nonsignificant based on observation by slit lamp biomicroscopy, which is a subjective evaluation. However, further investigations will be needed to objectively assess the maculopathy. Objective assessment of macular vasculature or diabetic maculopathy is done by the following modalities:
- Invasive—fundus fluorescein angiography (FFA): Standard and ultra-wide field
- Noninvasive—optical coherence tomography (OCT) and OCT angiography **(Figs. 7.34.2A to C)**

The goal of investigations in management of DME is:
- To diagnose or distinguish the cause of macular edema
- As a baseline investigation to monitor disease progression and response to treatment

SECTION 7: Retina

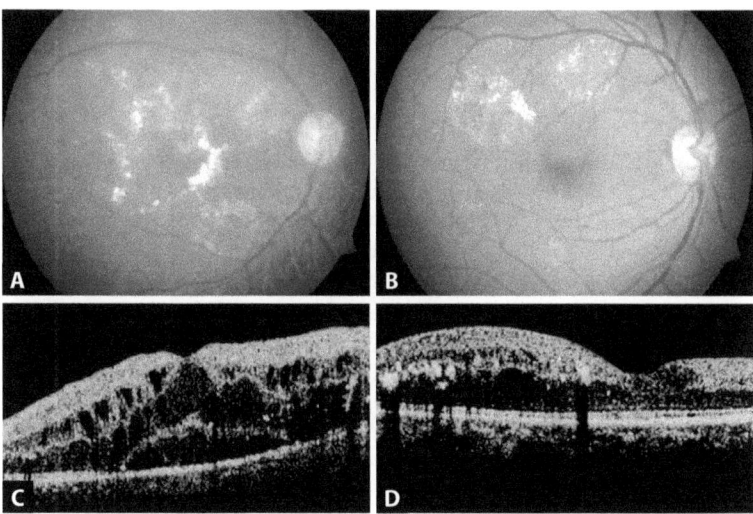

Figs. 7.34.1A to D: Center and noncentral involving diabetic macular edema.

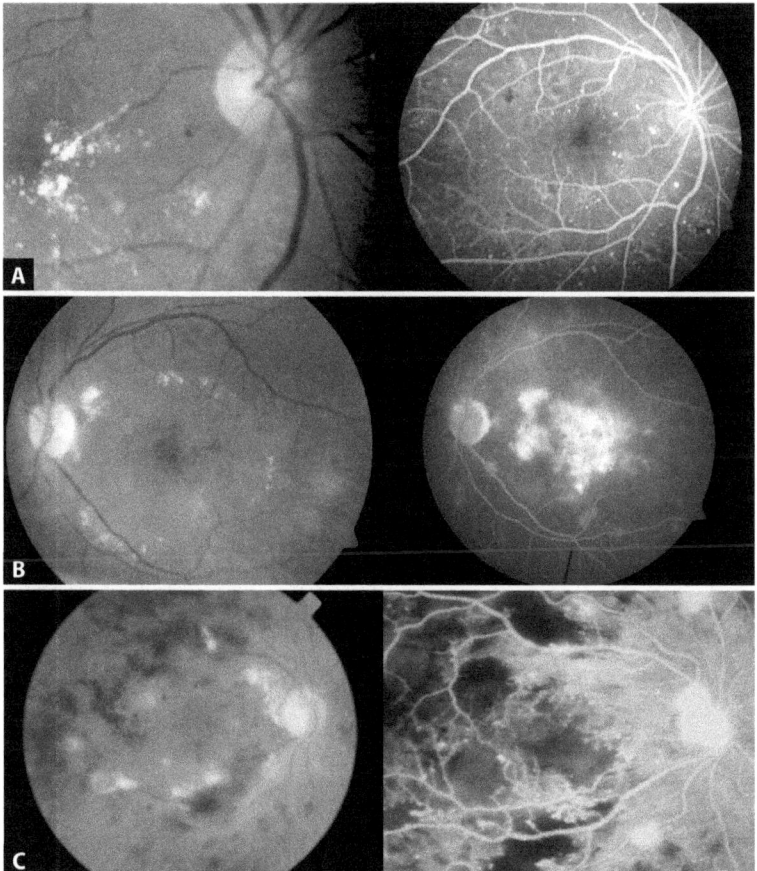

Figs. 7.34.2A to C: Fundus fluorescein findings in diabetic macular edema. (A) Focal leaks; (B) Diffuse leaks; (C) Ischemic maculopathy.

- To identify the pattern of leakage and the extent of disease
- To rule out macular ischemia
- To characterize the abnormal macular architecture

Fundus Fluorescein Angiography

Fluorescein angiography is the only modality that shows blood flow in the macular vessels and "leakage" functional assessment of retinal capillary health.

When the visual acuity is disproportionate to the amount of edema seen clinically. FFA can identify macular ischemia or damage to the foveal avascular zone (FAZ) as in these situations there is no leakage and there are well-defined areas of hypoperfusion or hypofluorescence.

To distinguish the cause of macular edema when it is disproportionate to the extent of retinopathy such as in mild central retinal vein occlusion or a small macular tributary retinal vein occlusion.

When the macula cannot be assessed clinically in case of decreased vision and dense asteroid hyalosis with DR.

To rule out the cause of nonresponse to treatment when the macular thickness on OCT persists.

Ultra-Wide Field Angiography

The ultra-wide field angiography images 200° of the retina up to the periphery in a single scan. It is available on the Optos 200Tx imaging system.

Recent studies show that peripheral ischemia may be one of the factors driving the development of DME. Targeted panretinal photocoagulation (PRP) to ischemic retina in the periphery may be a treatment modality as a first-line therapy or as an adjunct to antivascular endothelial growth factor (VEGF) therapy **(Flowchart 7.34.1)**.

Spectral-Domain Optical Coherence Tomography

Spectral-domain optical coherence tomography (SD-OCT) gives high resolution (around 3–6 μm transverse magnification) image of the retinal layers:
- It helps in characterizing the type of macular thickness in DME into cystoid, non-cystoid, or foveolar detachment.

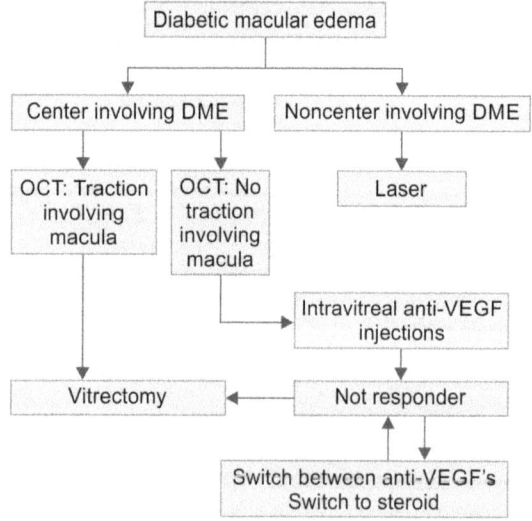

Flowchart 7.34.1: Management algorithm of diabetic macular edema (DME).

(OCT: optical coherence tomography; VEGF: vascular endothelial growth factor)

- It is used to monitor the progression of the disease and its response to various modalities (laser, anti-VEGF agents, and steroids).
- It can identify concomitant vitreoretinal interface disease such as thickening of the posterior hyaloid face or traction due to fibrous proliferative that may need surgical intervention for DME.

Optical Coherence Tomography Angiography

Optical coherence tomography angiography is a new imaging modality that uses the principle of Doppler to visualize the macular and choroidal vasculature. It has the advantage of clearly delineating the superficial and deep retinal capillary plexus and associated abnormalities by way of demonstrating FAZ abnormalities, areas of vascular tortuosity and remodeling, loss of capillary network, and the intercapillary distance, which signifies the progression of DR. However, its utility in managing DME is still being studied and needs further validation in clinical trials.

Center Involving Diabetic Macular Edema

Clinically: Definite retinal thickening involving the center of the macula.

On SD-OCT:
- Loss of foveal contour
- Cystic space or neurosensory detachment involving center of fovea
- *Retinal thickening:* Central subfield thickness on OCT ≥290 µm for women and ≥305 µm in men on spectral domain OCT (*Zeiss Cirrus*).

Noncenter Involving Diabetic Macular Edema

Clinically: Definite retinal thickening within 3,000 µm of the center of the macula but not involving the center.

On SD-OCT: Cystic spaces and/or retinal thickening in noncentral macular subfields.

We shall now see different clinical situations and the consensus statement on management in each of these.

Situation 1: Noncenter involving DME:
- *Treat:* Focal photocoagulation of individual microaneurysms that fill with fluorescein and/or leak on FFA within 500–3,000 µm from the center of macula.
- *Optional:* Treat microaneurysms <125 µm that did not fill with fluorescein; leaks within hemorrhages; microaneurysms or other focal points of leakage in the retina >2 DD from the center of the macula.
- *Avoid:* Nerve fiber layer retinal hemorrhage and blot hemorrhage >125 µm in size.
- Grid laser treatment of areas of thickened retina showing diffuse fluorescein leakage and/or capillary dropout.

Situation 2: Noncenter involving DME with few cystic spaces involving fovea (minimal center involvement):
- *If the vision is compromised:* Consider intravitreal anti-VEGF
- *If good vision (6/6), asymptomatic:* Laser according to the ETDRS guidelines
- *If symptomatic and vision is good (6/6):* Consider intravitreal anti-VEGF

Situation 3: Treatment naive center-involving DME:
Anti-VEGF therapy is the first line of treatment for all center involving DME patients without traction. On monthly follow-up, look for visual acuity and OCT for improvement:
- *OCT and vision shows improvement:* Continue anti-VEGF till vision improves to 6/6 and normal foveal contour obtained. Once injections are stopped, close monitoring with either pro re nata or a "treat and extend" treatment approach should be done.
- *OCT shows progressive improvement but vision not improving:* Continue anti-VEGF, but consider angiogram to look for ischemia at 3 months.

- *Vision improving but no OCT improvement:* Continue the treatment with anti-VEGF. Can consider adding laser. Also look for vitreomacular adhesion (VMA) on OCT.
- *Worsening or no improvement on OCT and visual acuity (defined as <10% decrease in central subfield thickness and less than five letters increase in visual acuity since the most recent injection):* At 3 months consider angiogram, look for other treatable lesions, ischemia, vitreomacular traction (VMT), systemic control, and then plan rescue treatment accordingly.

Situation 4: Previously treated center-involving DME with multiple anti-VEGF injections or steroid injections or laser:
- *Recurrent:* Evaluate with FFA and OCT. Treat with drug, which had shown good response previously. Evaluate the systemic factors for recurrence.
- *Resistant:* Evaluate with FFA and OCT.
  - Identify the ETDRS treatable lesions [microaneurysms located between 500 and 3,000 μm from the foveal center, microaneurysms located between 300 and 500 μm from the foveal center causing persistent clinically-significant macular edema despite first laser treatment, areas of diffuse retinal leakage that could arise from microaneurysms, dilated capillary bed or intraretinal microvascular abnormalities (IRMAs), and thickened ischemic zones] and treat if present.
  - Rule out VMT, macular ischemia.
  - Carefully evaluate the follow-up protocols and response of previous treatments.
  - Evaluate the systemic control of diabetes, lipids, and hypertension. Assess the renal status.
  - *Rescue plan:* Decide on switching over to other anti-VEGFs, steroids, addition of lasers, and combination of these in some patients.

Situation 5: Proliferative diabetic retinopathy with DME:
- *If no traction:* Complete PRP along with anti-VEGF or intravitreal triamcinolone acetonide (IVTA) (if not contraindicated) and then subsequent management of DME according to the protocol.
- *In the presence of extramacular traction:* PRP with burns 2 DD away from tractional retinal detachment, macular edema can be treated as usual protocol.
- *In the presence of traction threatening or involving fovea:* Vitrectomy is indicated.

Situation 6: Center involving macular edema with vitreoretinal surface abnormalities: Evaluate the vitreoretinal interface on OCT:
- *Focal VMT with DME:* Vitrectomy is the choice.
- *Extrafoveal traction site(s) without traction at the fovea:* Anti-VEGF treatment can be initiated, with a close watch at the extrafoveal traction site on follow-up. However, if the traction is significant, option of IVTA/Ozurdex can be considered.
- *Broad adherent epiretinal membrane (ERM) with retinal thickening attributed to DME:* Treat like center involving macular edema. However, these show a relatively poor response to pharmacological treatment.
- *Broad adherent ERM with retinal thickening with no associated DME and thickening attributable to ERM:* If asymptomatic; needs observation with OCT on follow-up visits. However, if symptomatic and shows worsening on follow-up visits can plan vitrectomy with ERM removal.

Situation 7: Center involving DME in pseudophakic eyes:
- *Differentiating Irvine–Gass from DME in presence of DR:* Diffuse petaloid type of leakage with disc leakage on FFA and with very few aneurysms and no hard exudates around the macula is suggestive of Irvine–Gass syndrome.
- *Presence of DME with no component of Irvine–Gass:* Treat as center-involving DME.
- *Presence of both DME and Irvine–Gass:* Can plan treatment of DME along with nonsteroidal anti-inflammatory drugs (NSAIDs). If no contraindications, intravitreal steroids are the first choice.

- *Time to start treatment of DME in fresh pseudophakia:* If macular edema is detected after cataract surgery, laser (macular) can be initiated after 1 month (after uncomplicated phacoemulsification); PRP if indicated can be done early (with IOL) and intravitreal anti-VEGF can also be planned after 1 month.

Situation 8: DME during pregnancy:
- Pregnancy may promote the onset or worsening of DR. Regular follow-up is must.
- The proliferative diabetic retinopathy (PDR) must always be treated; treatment should be earlier in pregnant women compared to nonpregnant women.
- Pregnancy can also cause macular edema; it spontaneously regresses during the postpartum and, therefore, does not require immediate treatment.
- However, if DME occurs early in the pregnancy and there is progressive deterioration of vision, laser or intravitreal steroids should be preferred and anti-VEGF avoided.

Situation 9: DME in young type I diabetes:
- Management of DME is similar to type 2, with optimal glycemic control.
- In cases of PDR with DME, there is an increased risk of thickened PHF contributing to edema. Clinical and OCT assessment of this is important.

Situation 10: Center involving DME in vitrectomized eyes:
- *Pseudophakic eyes with center involving DME:* Intravitreal steroids should be considered as first choice if not contraindicated. Consider choosing dexamethasone over IVTA to reduce IOP spikes.
- *In presence of recurrent vitreous hemorrhage with center involving DME:* Anti-VEGF is the better choice.
- *Selected cases where the risk of IOP spike and cataract is a concern:* Intravitreal anti-VEGF can be considered.

Situation 11: Ischemic macular edema:
- Access the ischemia with FFA and OCT: Normal FAA is defined as an FAZ <1,000 µ in the longest diameter, regular and round or horizontally oval in shape. Mild undulations of FAZ were also considered normal.
- *Grade ischemia on FFA:* Using ETDRS grading system, from 0 (normal), to 1 (questionable), 2 (less than half the original circumference destroyed), 3 (more than half the contour destroyed but some remnants remain), and 4 (capillary outline completely destroyed).
- *Accessing ischemia on OCT:* DME in presence of ischemia has retinal thickening in the total and outer retinal layers. Inner retinal layers, including the ganglion cell layer and retinal nerve fiber layer are thinned. There is also Haller's large vessel layer of the choroid thickened in presence of ischemia.
- *In FFA grade 1 and 2:* Treat as nonischemic (Center and noncenter involving).
- *FFA grade 3:* Avoid laser photocoagulation, can consider steroids in presence of center involving macular edema.
- *FFA grade 4:* Would not benefit from any treatment.

Situation 12: Center involving DME with history of cerebrovascular accident or myocardial infarction:
- If within last 3 months, do not initiate treatment with anti-VEGF. Treatment with laser or steroids can be considered in these patients.
- If the history is >3 months old, the treatment can be initiated with anti-VEGF. However, if systemic risks of thromboembolic phenomenon are significant, it is best to consult a physician first.

Situation 13: DME in glaucomatous eyes:
- *In eyes with established glaucoma or glaucoma suspect or ocular hypertension:* Avoid intravitreal steroids. Even if intravitreal anti-VEGFs are used, monitoring of IOP and if required medical augmentation of antiglaucoma medications is required.
- For rescue treatment in this group, laser photocoagulation is preferred.

Situation 14: Considering DME for vitrectomy:
- *Focal VMT:* Vitrectomy is the choice.
- *Broad vitreoretinal adhesion:* If treatment has failed and the ophthalmologist feels that there is a scope of improvement, vitrectomy can be considered.
- *Diffuse DME:* If treatment has failed, can be considered for vitrectomy with or without internal limiting membrane peeling. Patient's vision, optic disc status and macular perfusion and OCT structural integrity need to be evaluated first.

Situation 15: Cataract with DME:
- *DME with cataract:* If media is clear treat DME according to the protocol. Once macular edema is treated, one can plan cataract surgery.
- If the view is not good, cataract surgery can be done either along with intravitreal anti-VEGFs, or 2 weeks after surgery and subsequent protocol continued.
- *If during treatment of DME cataract has worsened:* Proceed as above.
- *If during treatment of DME, patient also develops posterior capsule opacification:* Neodymium-doped yttrium aluminum garnet (Nd:YAG) capsulotomy can be planned and treatment of DME can be continued as usual.

Situation 16: DME with optic nerve abnormalities: Differentiating nonarteritic anterior ischemic optic neuropathy (NA-AION), papillopathy and papillophlebitis:
- *NA-AION:* The optic disc edema may be diffuse or segmental, hyperemic or pale. ON perimetry shows generalized, altitudinal, and other pattern of field defect. FFA shows hypoperfusion with late leakage around affected segment.
- *Papillopathy:* Acute onset of unilateral or bilateral disc edema usually in young, type 1 diabetic, sometimes even type 2 diabetes, without the usual defects in visual field and pupillary function associated with NA-AION or optic neuritis. FFA shows very early leakage that increases through the late phases.
- *Papillophlebitis:* It typically shows more prominent retinal venous congestion and peripheral retinal hemorrhages. FFA to rule out vein occlusion.
- *NA-AION with macular edema:* Presence of DR lesions which cause edema (MA, diffuse leak, and IRMA) on FFA will help to clinch the diagnosis. If due to DME treat according to protocol. Otherwise treatment of NA-AION would resolve the edema. No intravitreal injections are required.
- *Papillopathy with DME:* Treat the DME according to protocol.
- *Papillophlebitis with macular edema:* If due to diabetes treat according to protocol.

Situation 17: DME with anemia:
- The anemia is related to renal dysfunction in most and may require subcutaneous erythropoietin injections for treatment. The macular edema improves with it; however, one should keep a close watch on proliferative component, as erythropoietin can worsen the same.
- Anti-VEGF can be the preferred agent in presence of anemia and center involving DME.

Situation 18 (miscellaneous) DME with mixed retinopathy:
- The management remains unchanged. History of cardiovascular risk factors should be sought and if required a physician consultation should be done.
- In cases of accelerated HT, anti-VEGF should be avoided.

Need for bilateral injection: Ideally a gap of a week/or at least 3 days should be kept between both the eyes.

Patient with Nonhealing Foot Ulcer

Surgeon or physician consultation must be taken and care provided. In presence of active infection, intravitreal injections should be avoided. The attendant and patient should be counseled to do foot dressing before doing ocular dressing or instilling the drops.

REFERENCE

1. Raman R, Rani PK, Rachepalle SR, Gnanamoorthy P, Uthra S, Kumaramanickavel G, et al. Prevalence of Diabetic Retinopathy in India Sankara Nethralaya Diabetic Retinopathy Epidemiology and Molecular Genetics Study Report 2. Ophthalmology. 2009;116(2):311-8.

7.35 Ultrasonography and Ultrasound Biomicroscopy Imaging for Vitreoretinal Diseases

Ramandeep Singh, Mohit Dogra, Simar Rajan Singh
Advanced Eye Center, PGIMER, Chandigarh
mankoo95@yahoo.com, mohit_dogra_29@hotmail.com, simarrajansingh@gmail.com

ULTRASONOGRAPHY

INTRODUCTION

Ultrasonography (USG) is a noninvasive diagnostic tool and is based on the piezoelectric principle. The conventional ultrasound for eye uses the lower frequencies of 8–12 MHz for imaging the posterior segment of the eye.

A thorough understanding of the ultrasound principles makes the diagnosis of variety of intraocular pathologies easy and quick. Ultrasound has A-scan and B-scan, which help us interpret the pathology in eyes with media opacity.

A-SCAN (AMPLITUDE SCAN)

The standard diagnostic A-scan is designed to display an echo intensity of 100% for retina when the sound waves are perpendicular to it. Choroid and sclera also produce 100% echo intensity. All other intraocular structures have <100% echo intensity.

B-SCAN (BRIGHTNESS SCAN)

It is a two-dimensional display, which uses the horizontal and vertical axis. An ultrasound probe will provide echo intensity of the structure, which is determined by the brightness of the dots on the screen.

The pointer of the probe marks the point that will appear superior on the screen. The probe by convention is kept nasal or superior. There are three types of scans, i.e., transverse, longitudinal, and axial. Interpretation of various scans is dependent on gain, time gain compensation (TGC), sector angle, display, probe position, and eye being scanned.

VARIOUS INDICATIONS

- *Vitreous hemorrhage:* On USG, multiple point-like echoes in the vitreous cavity on B-scan and low-to-moderate amplitude echo intensity on A-scan are seen. In long-standing vitreous hemorrhage, the point-like echoes may get settled inferiorly and the vitreous cavity is clear.
- *Endophthalmitis:* Multiple point-like echoes with low-to-moderate intensity, similar to vitreous hemorrhage. Clinical scenario helps to differentiate the two along with involvement of retinochoroid and subtenon space, seen on USG. Classical "T" sign is seen depicting progression to panophthalmitis and it can be picked up early with USG.
- *Posterior vitreous detachment (PVD):* Membrane-like structure seen on B-scan which may or may not be attached to the disc. Echo intensity of 50–60% on A-scan with after movements. The membrane disappears on reducing the gain. It is the most important differential diagnosis of retinal detachment (RD).

- *Intraocular foreign body (IOFB):* Metallic foreign bodies appear as hyperechoic dots with a back shadowing on B-scan and have 100% echo intensity on A-scan. Longitudinal scans at various clock hours are used to localize IOFBs.
- *Dislocated crystalline lens:* Posterior dislocation of the crystalline lens in the vitreous is seen as a cyst-like structure on B-scan with the anterior and posterior surfaces having high echo intensity on A-scan and the interior having moderate-to-high intensity, depending on the hardness of the lens.
- *Retinal detachment:* RDs appear as membrane-like structures attached to the optic disc with 100% echo intensity on A-scan **(Fig. 7.35.1)**. Old RDs loose mobility and appear to have no after movements and associated with retinal cysts.
- *Choroidal detachment:* Choroidal detachments appear as elevated membranes not reaching the disc. They may be touching each other, known as kissing choroidals. Hemorrhagic choroidals have bright dots on B-scan whereas serous choroidals have echo free interiors on B-scan. Serial ultrasounds are done in cases of hemorrhagic choroidals to look for clot liquefaction and appropriate time for surgery **(Fig. 7.35.1)**.
- *Intraocular tumors:* In retinoblastoma, high reflectivity with back shadowing is highly suggestive of calcification. Choroidal melanoma has collar stud appearance as one of the classic features on USG **(Figs. 7.35.2A and B)**. However, small melanomas can be seen as dome-shaped elevations. Choroidal hemangioma is seen as dome shaped on B-scan and shows high internal echogenicity on A-scan.
- *Parasitic cysts:* Cyst-like structure with high echo intensity in the center may be suggestive of a scolex. There may be surrounding low-to-moderate point-like echoes, suggestive of inflammatory reaction.

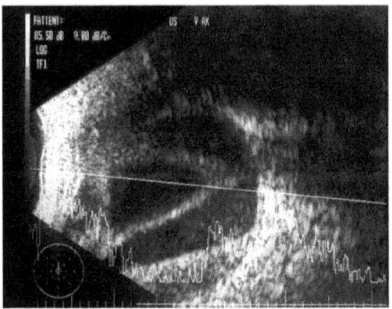

Fig. 7.35.1: Ultrasonography A- and B-scan showing highly reflective membranous structure attached to disc, i.e., retinal detachment and choroidal detachment in the periphery with echoes within suggestive of hemorrhagic choroidal detachment.

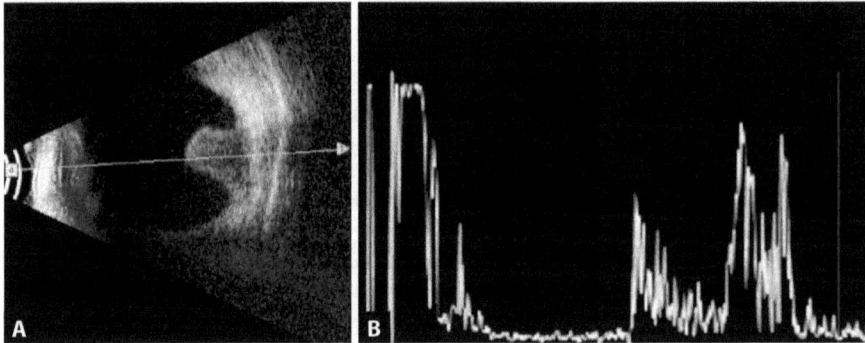

Figs. 7.35.2A and B: Ultrasonography A- and B-scan showing choroidal melanoma with acoustic hollowness and sound attenuation. Ultrasound is typically used to measure the melanoma size, evaluate internal reflectivity and its extrascleral extension.

ULTRASOUND BIOMICROSCOPY

INTRODUCTION

Ultrasound biomicroscopy (UBM) utilizes the same components as the conventional ultrasound except for the higher frequency of 35–100 MHz. This leads to higher resolution at the cost of depth of penetration, which provides better visualization of the anterior segment and ciliary body area. Scanning is performed with the patient in supine position through a plastic eye-cup filled with coupling solution or disposable silicon probe cover not requiring plastic cup in newer machines.

TYPES OF SCANS

The white line on the probe body indicates the direction of the linear movement of the transducer.
- *Radial/longitudinal:* UBM transducer is held over the area to be scanned and moved to and fro across the limbus, with the oscillations perpendicular to the limbus at the specific clock hour to be examined.
- *Transverse scan:* The probe is held at 90° to a radial line at the limbus. It takes the cross-section of the ciliary body when it is placed over it.
- *Sulcus to sulcus scan (axial):* It takes the scan of the anterior segment from front to back. The probe should be placed in the center of the cornea with the patient looking in the primary gaze.

VARIOUS INDICATIONS

- *Trauma:* Post-trauma UBM may be useful to examine anterior chamber details such as status of lens, angle recession, and suprachoroidal cleft. Accurate assessment of the structural damage and locating foreign bodies in the angle and ciliary body area are important uses of UBM in these cases **(Fig. 7.35.3)**.
- *Iris and ciliary body tumors:* UBM helps in diagnosis and management of iris and ciliary tumors by giving their anterior extent.
- *Retinal detachment:* UBM may help in localizing peripheral retinal breaks in the presence of media opacity and identifying presence of anterior proliferative vitreoretinopathy.
- *Uveitis-glaucoma-hyphema (UGH) syndrome:* UBM helps to find the cause of UGH syndrome, especially in postcataract surgery patients **(Fig. 7.35.4)**. Haptic rubbing on the iris or ciliary processes is the most common cause of UGH syndrome.

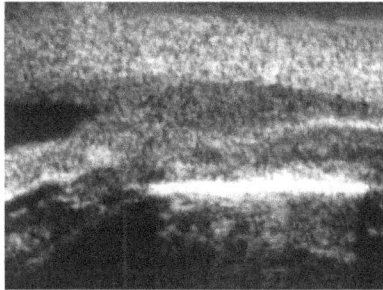

Fig. 7.35.3: Ultrasound biomicroscopy picture showing linear intraocular foreign bodies in ciliary body area with a back shadow.

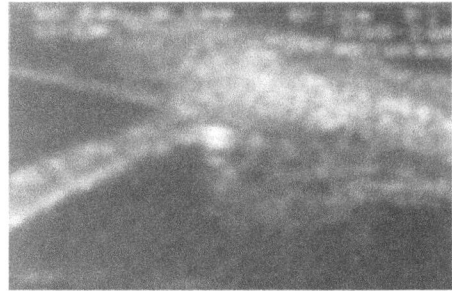

Fig. 7.35.4: Ultrasound biomicroscopy picture showing haptic of intraocular lens intruding the ciliary body area in a patient with pseudophakia with recurrent attacks of hyphema.

- *Scleritis:* Level of thickening on UBM helps in differentiating between episcleritis and scleritis. Different types of scleritis can also be differentiated based on UBM feature. Scleral necrosis presents as hyporeflective with loss of homogeneity.
- *Toxocara uveitis:* Toxocara granulomas are mostly peripheral and may not be visualized on routine ophthalmic examination. UBM may play a key role in documentation of these in the peripheral retina to aid in diagnosis.
- *Chronic hypotony:* Ciliary body and its processes can be visualized to narrow down the cause for the hypotony, i.e., ciliary body atrophy and cyclitic membrane.
- *Ciliochoroidal detachment:* Ciliochoroidal detachment due to various etiologies can be picked up with UBM.

7.36 | Intraocular Foreign Bodies

Ramanuj Samanta
All India Institute of Medical Sciences, Rishikesh
ramanuj.oph@aiimsrishikesh.edu.in

Shalaka Waghamare
Aravind Eye Hospital, Madurai
shalaka19293@gmail.com

■ INTRODUCTION

Intraocular foreign bodies (IOFBs) can be seen in up to 40% of traumatic ocular injury cases. Young males are generally most vulnerable due to occupational hazards such as hammering (one of the most common modes), using machine tools, automobile accidents, gun shot, and explosive injuries. Commonly encountered foreign bodies are iron, lead, copper, silver, gold, stone, glass, plastic, and wood. Foreign bodies can enter the eye through the cornea, sclera, or limbus, and can finally lodge into the anterior chamber (AC), lens, vitreous cavity, retina, or subretinal spaces and occasionally can perforate the globe to reach posterior sclera or orbit. The final visual prognosis depends upon multiple factors including time elapsed since injury, presenting visual acuity, location, extent, and severity of globe injury, composition of foreign body, presence or absence of concomitant endophthalmitis or retinal detachment or optic nerve injury, and various other factors.

■ SYMPTOMS

Patients may present early with decreased vision, pain, and redness in settings of open globe injury or may present at a later setting with symptoms of metallosis.

■ EVALUATION

A meticulous history should be elicited to know the mode of injury and likely nature of IOFB. Detailed ocular examination should be carried out including visual acuity, pupillary reaction, slit lamp examination (for conjunctival chemosis or hemorrhage/globe injury/iris holes/AC reaction/hypopyon/lens status), and fundus evaluation, if possible (without much pressure on the globe).

Metallic IOFB can produce specific signs of metallosis. Siderosis bulbi, caused by intraocular toxicity from iron, is characterized by a rust-colored corneal stroma, iris heterochromia, dilated and nonreactive pupil, and retinal degeneration. Intraocular toxicity of copper depends upon the amount of copper content in the IOFB. Acute chalcosis is seen with a copper content of 85% or more and is characterized by sterile endophthalmitis, corneal and scleral melt, hypopyon, and retinal detachment. Other clinical findings include a Kayser-Fleischer ring, iris heterochromia, a "sunflower" cataract, and retinal degeneration. Chronic chalcosis may be seen in IOFB with <85% copper content.

Organic IOFB (vegetable matter, thorn, and insect hairs) are more commonly contaminated and have a higher chance of endophthalmitis. Glass IOFBs are usually inert, but can cause mechanical injury to internal structures.

INVESTIGATIONS

X-ray is the most commonly performed primary imaging modality due to its easy availability and cost-effectiveness. However, very small and nonmetallic foreign bodies may not be picked up by X-ray.

Ultrasonography (USG) has a high sensitivity and can readily locate IOFBs, both radiolucent and radiodense. Metallic IOFB presents with a sharp hyperechoic lesion with an acoustic shadowing and high amplitude on the corresponding A-scan. Glass IOFB may have a reverberation artefact following the initial hyperechoic spike. Wooden and plastic IOFBs generally have lesser echogenicity as compared to metallic ones. USG also helps in planning surgery by providing details regarding the presence of any concomitant retinal or choroidal detachment, any vitreous incarceration, posterior perforation, etc. However, it is recommended to perform following repair of open globe injury.

Computed tomography (CT) has gained popularity because of its ability to precisely locate IOFB with minimum globe manipulation. Both axial and coronal cuts (ideally <1.5 mm) should be obtained. It is particularly helpful in the assessment of IOFB embedded in the scleral coats or gone beyond the ocular coats and helps in surgical planning or approach. However, CT can still miss small IOFBs <0.7 mm in size, wooden foreign bodies, IOFB embedded in the scleral wall, or glass IOFB near the lens.

Magnetic resonance imaging (MRI) is used in very selected cases with presumed plastic, wooden, or organic IOFB, which are likely to be missed by other imaging modalities. It should not be ordered in suspected metallic IOFBs.

Ultrasound biomicroscopy (UBM) may aid in detecting small IOFB lodged in the AC angle or in the sulcus.

Anterior segment optical coherence tomography (AS-OCT) helps in identifying IOFB located in the anterior segment in front of iris.

Electroretinogram (ERG) may be abnormal at subclinical stages of metallosis in metallic IOFB. It also helps to prognosticate visual recovery following surgical removal of IOFB in such patients.

MANAGEMENT

First and foremost, open globe injury should be repaired without delay to provide stability to the eye. Patient should be counseled regarding the nature of injury and explained about the possible surgical complications beforehand to avoid future unrealistic expectations.

Although the *precise role of systemic antibiotics* to decrease the incidence of endophthalmitis has not been proven conclusively, it is usually considered while awaiting definitive surgical therapy (if the surgery cannot be done within 24 hours). Owing to their broad spectrum of activity and bioavailability, third- and fourth-generation fluoroquinolones are generally recommended.

The *precise timing of surgery* for the removal of IOFB is controversial. It can be removed in conjunction with primary repair of globe injury; the advantages are reduced risk of endophthalmitis and retinal detachment, and avoidance of multiple surgeries. Such procedures are usually done if the wound is small and self-sealed, or in lacerations with optimum corneal clarity allowing posterior segment surgery, or in children under general anesthesia (to avoid hazards of repeated anesthesia). However, removal of IOFB may be planned at a later setting also (usually 2–7 days after primary repair). The advantages of second-setting IOFB removal are better wound stability and integrity, better corneal clarity, controlled intraocular inflammation, and ease of induction of posterior vitreous detachment (PVD) by the surgeon. Such a second intervention is preferred in hazy cornea, large unstable wounds, or where facilities for vitrectomy are not available. However, the choice also depends upon the personal experience of the individual surgeon and the availability of vitreoretinal surgical facility.

A few common principles of removal of any IOFB include minimum manipulation to avoid collateral damage, avoiding the entry wound for extraction (unless IOFB is partially visible/embedded at the entry wound), and extracting IOFB in the plane of the smallest cross-section, if possible.

Intraocular foreign body from AC may be removed with the help of intraocular forceps or magnets after placing AC maintainer or inflating the AC with viscoelastic substances. Pilocarpine drop may be used to prevent posterior migration of IOFB and prevent lens damage.

Intralenticular foreign body may need removal of IOFB with phacoemulsification or lensectomy. Anterior vitrectomy may be required following IOFB removal. Placement and type of intraocular lens (IOL) in the same setting primarily depend upon the status of residual capsular support, presence or absence of concomitant endophthalmitis or posterior segment injury, and other factors.

Intraocular foreign body in the posterior segment **(Figs. 7.36.1A and B)** requires vitrectomy and extraction can be done through limbus (after lensectomy/phacoemulsification) or through pars plana (sclerotomy incision). A limbal route is preferred in setting of large IOFB in the posterior segment, limited visibility, traumatic cataract with breached posterior capsule, very dense vitreous hemorrhage causing staining of posterior lens capsule, or in concomitant severe AC inflammation with fibrin/hypopyon (endophthalmitis). Peripheral capsular rim may be salvaged during lensectomy for future placement of IOL in the sulcus. Lens-sparing vitrectomy and extraction through scleral incision may be considered in presence of small foreign bodies, good media clarity, and clear lens status with an intact posterior lens capsule. If small pupil and posterior synechiae do not allow adequate dilatation, iris hooks may be applied for optimal posterior segment visualization.

Although the basic principles of pars plana vitrectomy (PPV) for the removal of IOFBs from the posterior segment remain the same, some points merit special mention:

- With the advent of modern instrumentation and sutureless vitrectomy system, 23-gauge and 25-gauge surgeries are being increasingly done. However many foreign body forceps and intraocular magnets require larger dimension ports; hence, one of the port sites can be extended for introducing such forceps/magnets or a new larger port (20-gauge) can be made in the vicinity of 23-gauge/25-gauge port (hybrid ports).
- Some surgeons prefer additional encirclage (240 band) as it reduces the chance of future retinal detachment. It is especially useful in phakic patients where peripheral shaving of the vitreous is compromised or in IOFB with retinal detachment or posterior perforation and/or peripheral vitreous incarceration.

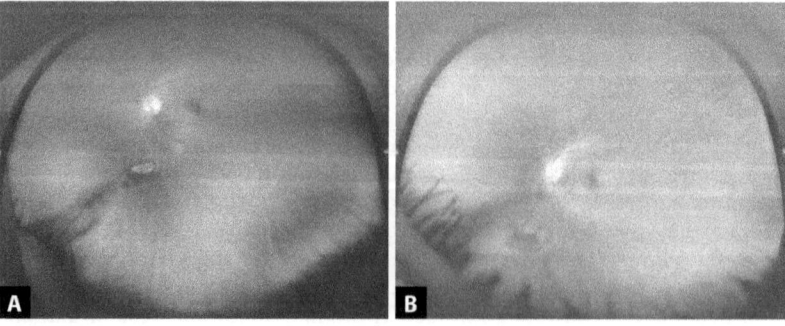

Figs. 7.36.1A and B: Ultra-wide field fundus photographs before and after removal of intraocular foreign body through sclerotomy incision.

- Triamcinolone-assisted PVD induction should be preferred. However, it should not be attempted vigorously in IOFB associated with endophthalmitis.
- Perfluorocarbon liquid may be injected to prevent iatrogenic trauma to the macula by repeated insult due to IOFB.
- Long-standing IOFB may be encapsulated with surrounding fibrotic adhesions. The capsule should be gently dissected out with a cutter to prolapse the IOFB instead of pulling it directly with forceps or magnet. Gentle cautery to the surrounding edge may be necessary to reduce bleeding.
- Before attempting removal of IOFB, all vitreous surrounding the IOFB and port sites should be cleared meticulously to avoid iatrogenic retinal break or giant retinal tear due to traction.
- Metallic foreign bodies can be removed with the help of intraocular magnets. Nonmagnetic foreign bodies require removal with forceps. Attempts should be made to align the IOFB in such a way so that the minimum dimension of the IOFB encounters the extraction incision. If successful alignment cannot be performed, a "handshake" technique may be employed by introducing a second forceps from the opposite port to grasp the IOFB in the anterior vitreous for removal.
- Following removal of IOFB, careful inspection of the entire periphery should be done to look for any retinal break. Foreign body impact site and any iatrogenic break should either be lasered or cryosed (excessive cryotherapy preferably be avoided to prevent proliferative vitreoretinopathy).
- A tamponading agent should be used if a retinal detachment is present or subretinal fluid is present around the IOFB impact site/iatrogenic break site. Endophthalmitis is a potentially devastating consequence of ocular trauma and develops in approximately 10% of IOFB cases.
- Delayed presentation and organic- or soil-contaminated IOFB pose a higher risk of endophthalmitis. If endophthalmitis is suspected, IOFB should be removed as earliest as possible. However, if vitreoretinal facilities are not available, primary repair should be done in conjunction with intravitreal antibiotics (most commonly vancomycin 1 mg/mL and ceftazidime 2.25 mg/mL) and should be referred to higher centers as early as possible.

CONCLUSION

Overall, IOFB if diagnosed and managed early can achieve a final visual acuity of ≥20/40 in approximately 70% of patients. Poor prognosis factors include poorer acuity at presentation, afferent pupillary defect, large blunt, and nonmetallic IOFB, posterior impact site, associated retinal detachment and endophthalmitis, and gunshot injury.

SUGGESTED READING

1. Yeha S, Colyerb HM, Weiche ED. Current trends in the management of intraocular foreign bodies. Curr Opin Ophthalmol. 2008;19:225-33.

7.37 | Optical Coherence Tomography Angiography

Reema Bansal, Simar Rajan Singh, Vinay Patil
Advanced Eye Center, PGIMER, Chandigarh
drreemab@rediffmail.com, simarrajansingh@gmail.com, vinaypatil4489@gmail.com

INTRODUCTION

Optical coherence tomography angiography (OCTA) is a novel noninvasive imaging technique that allows three-dimensional visualization of the retinal and choroidal vasculature. It employs motion-contrast imaging to generating high-resolution angiographic images in seconds without injection of a dye.

HOW DOES OPTICAL COHERENCE TOMOGRAPHY ANGIOGRAPHY WORK?

Optical coherence tomography angiography compares the difference between optical coherence tomography (OCT) signal intensity between sequential OCT B-scans taken at the same location to construct a map of blood flow. OCTA is based on the concept that in static tissue such as the neurosensory retina, the only dynamic structure is blood flow. Hence, visualizing flow-related changes reveals retinal and choroidal vasculature in high-resolution as well as a three-dimensional manner. Eye tracking eliminates bulk motion from patient movement, so the sites of motion between repeated OCT scans largely represent erythrocyte movement in retinal blood vessels (**Fig. 7.37.1**). By using en-face OCT technology, OCTA provides layer by layer details to identify areas of interest, such as the superficial and deep retinal vascular plexuses or the choriocapillaris. The deep retinal plexus is of special interest as it can neither be viewed by fluorescein angiogram (FA) or indocyanine green angiogram (ICGA). The potential differences of the OCTA over the conventional dye-based angiography are listed in **Table 7.37.1**.

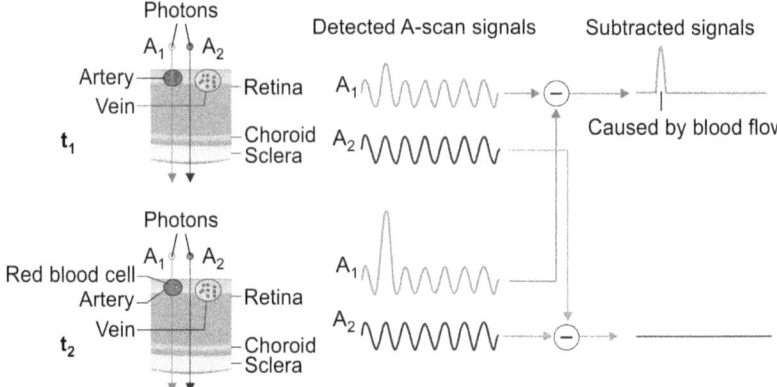

Fig. 7.37.1: As moving blood cells pass through vessels, they modify optical coherence tomography (OCT) signals. Based on this concept, a blood flow signal can be extracted by subtracting the OCT signals from the same location but at different time points (red path). The OCT signals will be different at these locations, while OCT signals from surrounding retinal tissues will remain steady (blue path).

Table 7.37.1: Fluorescein angiography versus optical coherence tomography angiography.

Fluorescein angiography	Optical coherence tomography angiography
Invasive	Noninvasive
Dye based	No dye used
Wider field of view	Field limited to 12 × 12 mm for now
Lower resolution	High resolution
Allows dynamic blood flow information such as leakage	Gives only static blood flow information, does not detect leakage
No segmentation possible, images superficial retina only	En-face imaging allows segmentation, can image superficial, deep, and outer retina and choriocapillaris at the same time
Less motion artifacts	More motion artifacts
5–30 minutes imaging time	<1 minute per eye

OCTA ALGORITHMS

Various algorithms have been developed to interpret the complex data from the sequential OCT B-scans to get the final angiographic images. Among them the most common ones are:
- *Speckle variance:* The variance of amplitude fluctuations between B-scans is calculated to visualize flow.
- *Amplitude decorrelation:* Uses correlation as metric to detect changes on OCT signal. A higher decorrelation value suggests areas of flow which implies the presence of vessels in the tissue.
- *Phase variance:* Uses the variance of the phase differences between various sequential OCT waveforms.
- *Optical microangiography (OMAG):* OMAG algorithm incorporates variations in both the intensity and phase information between sequential B-scans at the same position to generate the flow information

These algorithms are usually supplemented by different averaging methods to improve the signal-to-noise ratio and in consequence improving the visualization of vasculature. The most used ones are:
- *Split spectrum:* It relies on splitting the acquired interference spectrum into narrower overlapping bands which results in better vascular delineation at the cost of lower axial resolution.
- *Volume averaging:* These help in reducing the background noise and eye motion artifacts. This can be done by post image acquisition or by real-time eye tracking during the scan.

Different OCTA platform use various combinations of these algorithms and averaging methods to produce high-resolution images of the retinochoroidal vasculature. Our experience is based on the Avanti RTVue XR platform equipped with the AngioVue software (Optovue, Fremont, CA, USA) which uses the *split-spectrum amplitude-decorrelation angiography (SSADA)* algorithm with motion correction. While this technology is still in its infancy, here are some of the described applications in routine patient care.

OCTA PLATFORMS

- ZEISS AngioPlex™ OCTA imaging on CIRRUS HD-OCT platform with FastTrac software
- Optovue AngioVue® (Optovue, Inc., Freemont, CA), uses split-spectrum decorrelation amplitude angiography
- Topcon®, paired with SD-OCT, uses OCTA ratio analysis
- Heidelberg engineering® uses the active eye-tracking system (TruTrack™)

DIFFERENCES BETWEEN SPECTRAL-DOMAIN AND SWEPT-SOURCE OCTA

Differences between spectral-domain and swept-source OCTA are given in **Table 7.37.2**.

ARTIFACTS IN OCTA

- *Media opacities:* Media opacities such as corneal scarring, cataracts, posterior capsular opacification, and vitreous floaters may lead to signal attenuation and shadowing artifact. This results in poor image quality.
- *Projection artifact:* The light that traverses the blood vessels and the reflected by the deeper layers, produces projection artifact, which is seen in the final deep image, with similar vascularity as the superficial blood vessels.

TABLE 7.37.2: Differences between spectral-domain and swept-source OCTA.

Properties	SD-OCTA	SS-OCTA
OCTA	Spectral domain	Swept source
Wavelength	~840 nm	~1,050 nm
A-scans per second	70,000	400,000
B-scan repetition	2	4
Acquisition time	3s	6.7s
Axial resolution	5 μm	10 μm
OCTA volume	2 × 2 to 6 × 6 mm	Up to 12 × 12 mm
Penetration through RPE	Lower	Higher

(OCTA: optical coherence tomography angiography; RPE: retinal pigment epithelium; SD-OCTA: spectral-domain OCTA; SS-OCTA: swept-source OCTA)

- *Segmentation artifact:* Automated segmentation of the structurally abnormal retina produces segmentation artifacts, more commonly seen in myopic eyes due to increased curvature and optical aberration.
- *Motion artifact:* Excessive eye movements during the scanning causes motion artifact. Most platforms now have motion tracking to reduce motion artifact.
- *Masking and unmasking:* Due to light blockage and hypertransmission respectively.
- *Suspended scattering particles in motion (SSPiM):* Extravascular OCTA signals corresponding to hyperreflective intraretinal fluid.

CLINICAL APPLICATIONS

- *Diabetic retinopathy (DR):* OCTA is very useful in evaluating the foveal avascular zone (FAZ) and perifoveal intercapillary area, both of which show progressive enlargement as DR progresses. Microaneurysms and other microvascular abnormalities can also be visualized on OCTA but, as OCTA is dependent on flow of blood, some microaneurysms with flow below the OCTA threshold may not show up. En-face view of disruptions in the deep capillary plexus can explain many cases of previously unexplained visual loss. Proliferative disease [neovascularization at the disc/neovascularization elsewhere (NVD/NVE)] can also be picked up by taking en-face view in the vitreous plane over the suspected areas.
- *Age-related macular degeneration (ARMD):* Dry ARMD patients show decreased choroidal blood flow and increased drusen extent than that seen on clinical examination. An unparalleled visualization of choroidal neovascularization (CNV) is possible with OCTA. The morphology, presence of fibrovascular capsule, afferent feeders, and anastomosis can be clearly assessed. Owing to the noninvasive nature of OCTA, lesion monitoring is very convenient during treatment. Many cases of chronic central serous chorioretinopathy also have an underlying CNV which may go undiagnosed on routine fundus examination and even FA. OCTA can be invaluable in such cases.
- *Vascular occlusions:* OCTA can show focal areas of capillary dropout and nonperfusion, FAZ disruption, and collateral formation, in both superficial and deep vascular plexuses. However, as OCTA is like a snapshot in time, delayed arteriovenous transit time or progressive leakage of fluid from the capillaries cannot be demonstrated as in FA.
- *Posterior uveitis:* OCTA can provide high-resolution en-face imaging of inflammatory foci. In diseases such as Vogt–Koyanagi–Harada disease and multifocal choroiditis, OCTA shows areas of flow void in the choriocapillaris that correlate with ICGA

and decrease in number with treatment. This may also help in follow-up to detect recurrence early. Inflammatory CNVs, which may be missed on clinical examination due to extensive scarring in choroiditis, can also be picked up easily with OCTA.
- *Glaucoma:* OCTA can be useful to evaluate optic disc perfusion in glaucomatous eyes. Compared to conventional FA, which shows no microvascular network around the disc, OCTA shows a very dense peripapillary vascular network in both the superficial disc vasculature and the deeper lamina cribrosa. This network has been found to be greatly attenuated in glaucomatous eyes and may have a correlation with the severity/progression of glaucoma.
- *Quantitative OCTA:* Recently various quantitative parameters such as vessel area density, vessel skeleton density, nonperfusion area, and FAZ area have been developed by further analysis of the en-face OCTA images. These parameters can help in quantification of the vascularity and subsequent follow-up and decision making.

CONCLUSION

Optical coherence tomography angiography is a revolutionary imaging modality that is redefining our understanding of several retinal vascular disorders by giving us high-resolution depth resolved images of the retinal and choroidal vasculature. The technology, though promising, is still in its infancy and requires more research to validate its use and utility in everyday ophthalmic practice.

7.38 | Photodynamic Therapy

S Natarajan, Alay S Banker, Chinmay Nakhwa
Aditya Jyot Eye Hospital, Mumbai
prof.drsn@gmail.com, alay.bankar@gmail.com, drchinmay@adityajyoteyehospital.org

INTRODUCTION

Choroidal neovascularization (CNV) or wet age-related macular degeneration (AMD) is a leading cause of blindness in the world today. Generally, antivascular endothelial growth factor (VEGF) therapy is a first choice for wet AMD treatment. However, there is increasing evidence that a multipronged approach is essential for the best results in patients. CNV is stimulated and maintained by VEGF, but temporary inhibition of only VEGF is not enough to halt the disease development. Research has demonstrated that frequent intravitreal injections of anti-VEGF agents are necessary for satisfactory outcomes. In spite of these frequent injections, only few patients have complete inhibition of the CNV and improvement in vision.

Photodynamic therapy (PDT) was the first treatment to be approved by US Food and Drug Administration (US FDA) for CNV secondary to AMD. It brought about vision stabilization in CNV.[1]

MECHANISM OF ACTION

In PDT, a light-sensitive medicine called verteporfin is injected into the bloodstream. The dose of medicine is according to body surface area and given intravenously over a period of 10 minutes. The medicine collects in the abnormal blood vessels under the macula. The tissue to be treated is exposed to diode laser light for few seconds, which activates the medicine. This causes an excited oxygen molecule, producing thrombosis of the low flow vessels within the CNV lesion. This results in an inflammatory response, along with fibrosis and regression of the CNV.[1]

Generally, the effects of PDT monotherapy are temporary in most cases. Thus, the PDT therapy needs to be administered every 3 months during the first year. Since PDT inhibits CNV through a pathway which is different from anti-VEGF agents, PDT in combination with anti-VEGF therapy can reduce the frequency of treatments needed.[1]

■ BENEFITS

Photodynamic therapy seals the leaky blood vessels and by sealing the leaky blood vessels, PDT delays the buildup of fluid under the retina that distorts the shape and position of the macula. PDT also slows down the growth of scar tissue and the abnormal membrane under the retina, both of which can damage the cells in the macula. It can also slow down central vision loss.

■ LIMITATIONS

- Back pain during infusion
- Temporary vision loss after treatment
- After therapy, exposure to ultraviolet (UV) light needs to be reduced for at least 5 days
- The need for retreatments
- Induces stimulation and upregulation of VEGF after treatment which may stimulate CNV growth.[1]

■ COMBINATION THERAPY

Development of CNV involves many factors. A lot of growth factors and cytokines have an effect on different components of CNV growth. Similarly, many treatments have some side effects. Therefore, a combination therapy for CNV is advised. This is because negative side effects of one therapy can be alleviated by another therapy. For example, PDT causes thrombosis in small vessels but causes VEGF discharge and inflammation. Addition of anti-VEGF drugs can reduce the severity of VEGF release. Similarly, addition of steroids can decrease the inflammation and retinal edema. However, it should be noted that anti-VEGF drugs can be associated with rebound phenomenon of VEGF production 4–6 weeks after initial injection.

■ VARIATIONS OF COMBINATION THERAPY

Generally, PDT is combined with intravitreal injections of anti-VEGF agents with or without steroid. One treatment protocol suggestion is to combine PDT with an anti-VEGF agent at the same sitting. First the PDT and then anti-VEGF drug after few minutes. Combination therapy with steroids can be more complicated due to volume issues. Some studies indicate combination therapy may be associated with a reduced frequency of treatments with visual acuity similar to treatment with anti-VEGF alone. In some cases, where monotherapy alone is unsuccessful, combination therapy can be related to vision improvement and leakage reduction.

Usually, PDT is used in combination with anti-VEGF intravitreal injections with or without steroid. However, the amounts of injected medicine, the treatment sequence, and the PDT power employed may change. The reported results (FOCUS trial, uncontrolled series) suggest that combination therapy may be associated with following benefits: decrease in therapy frequency and visual acuity reduced frequency of treatments with visual acuity results similar to anti-VEGF monotherapy.

■ RECENT DEVELOPMENTS

In the 1980s, verteporfin a new photosensitizer was introduced by Dolphin, Levy, and colleagues. Verteporfin is a porphyrin derivative, which is activated at 690 nm. Its particular property of preferential uptake by neovasculature made it ideal candidate for use in PDT. In the year 2000, it received FDA approval for the treatment of wet AMD. It was the first medical therapy ever permitted for this disease, which is a major cause of vision loss.

In 1999, 1 year results of two randomized control trials (RCTs) [treatment of AMD with PDT (TAP) report 1] were reported. The study concluded that verteporfin therapy of subfoveal CNV from AMD can safely reduce the risk of vision loss and recommended verteporfin therapy for treatment of patients with predominantly classic CNV from AMD.

Another study done in University of Colorado Hospital Eye Center by Ammar and Kahook was reported in 2013. The study results suggested a potential use of PDT therapy for selective in vivo removal of targeted ocular cells beyond the use for destroying vascular endothelial cells.

Recently, a Japanese study reported that a modified PDT (ironing PDT) decreased subfoveal fluid and preserved visual acuity in some patients with AMD which cannot be treated effectively by standard treatment.

Another recent report came from an Italian study, which was aimed to demonstrate the efficacy of intravitreal ranibizumab (IVR) in combination with reduced-fluence photodynamic therapy (RF-PDT) in patients with pathologic myopia with secondary CNV. It was found that treatment with ranibizumab alone or along with RF-PDT enhanced best-corrected visual acuity (BCVA) and macular sensitivity in patients affected with myopic CNV, whereas mean central foveal thickness (CFT) results were reduced. SF-PDT combination regimen mostly stabilized vision at 48 weeks. When all patients groups were compared, the RF-PDT group has decreased frequency of retreatments with ranibizumab.

Recently, Chinese researchers performed a meta-analysis and systematic review of various treatments available for AMD. The study results reported in 2016 found that treatment with only anti-VEGF agent is more useful for improvement in visual acuity than combination therapy and more researches with larger sample size should be performed to study on the effect of the two therapy approaches on central retinal thickness (CRT) and number of injections.

The choroidal vascularity index (CVI) could be a useful index for early diagnosis of central serous chorioretinopathy (CSC) and to assess the treatment response of PDT.

■ SUMMARY

In the past, PDT had offered a new way to treat CNV, a major cause of blindness. PDT slows down the vision loss, but also requires multiple retreatments. Therefore, it should be considered in combination with other therapies to minimize negative effects and maximize positive outcomes.

■ REFERENCE

1. Visioncareprofessional. AMD Update. [online] Available from http://www.visioncare-professional.com/emails/amdupdate/index.asp?issue=1. [Last accessed July, 2023].

7.39 | Optic Nerve Head Pit with Serous Detachment (Kranenburg Syndrome)

Sangeet Mittal
Thind Eye Hospital, Jalandhar
sangeetmittal@rediffmail.com

■ PRESENTATION

Optic nerve pits are congenital abnormalities attributed to imperfect closure of upper end of embryonic fissure (**Fig. 7.39.1**). It is seen approximately in 1 out of 10,000 ophthalmology patients. The pits are usually unilateral (85–90%) with no significant racial or sex predilection. They may be slit like to oval and vary from yellow to black in color. 70% of the pits are located on the temporal side of the disc and about 20% are situated centrally. Optic pits are usually asymptomatic. 45–50% of affected individuals may present with serous detachment of macula.

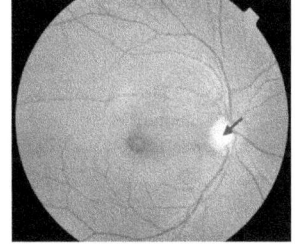

Fig. 7.39.1: Optic pit (blue arrow) with maculopathy.

Average age of presentation is 30 years. Though the exact pathology of serous detachment is disputed, the most recently accepted theory is that there is an abnormal communication between the intraocular and extraocular space. Vitreous traction over the pit is responsible for opening of this communication. This communication results in dynamic fluctuations in the gradient between intraocular and intracranial pressures that direct the movement of fluid (vitreous or cerebrospinal fluid) into the retina causing schisis like elevation of inner retinal layers. Detachment of outer layers of macula occurs as a secondary phenomenon and may present without any communication with the pit. Studies using optical coherence tomography (OCT) have confirmed the presence of schisis, bilaminar structure, and vitreous traction over the pit. If left untreated 80% of eyes lose vision to 20/200 or worse. Long-term macular changes include full thickness or lamellar holes, retinal pigment epithelium (RPE) mottling, or cystic changes in the macula. A gray fibroglial membrane appears to overlie the pit in many cases.

■ INVESTIGATIONS

Optic pits are associated with visual field defects ranging from arcuate scotomas to altitudinal hemianopia depending upon the size and location of the pit. Fluorescein angiography reveals initial hypofluorescence (filling defect) of the pit with staining in the later phases. The tract of the subretinal fluid extending from the disc also remains hypofluorescent. OCT of the optic disc reveals a gap in the area of the pit. Schisis of inner layer is seen extending from the optic disc margin to the fovea. A central serous separation of the fovea is seen in patients with maculopathy. Optic pits are not associated with brain malformations and thus no neuroimaging is required.

■ MANAGEMENT

Optic disc pit is a classic example of how the management has varied over a period of time depending upon the changing theories of pathogenesis. Various modalities of treatment had been attempted with variable results. Systemic steroids, optic nerve sheath compression, and scleral buckling have no role in the management. Both green and red lasers were used to produce photocoagulation burns in one or several rows between the area of serous retinal detachment and optic disc. Photocoagulation was effective for

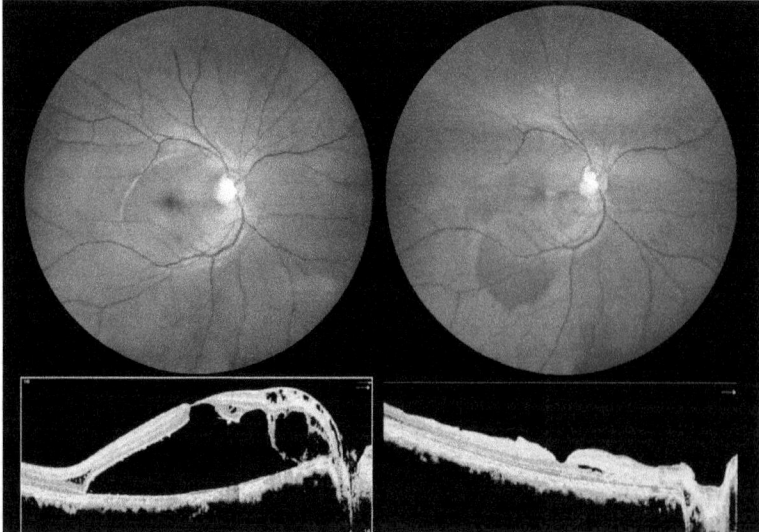

Fig. 7.39.2: A 23-year-old female with successful closure of optic pit after vitrectomy with fovea-sparing internal limiting membrane (ILM) peel and inverted ILM flap over pit.

flattening the retina but visual improvement was not significant and recurrences were common.

Permanent cure of maculopathy requires either elimination of translaminar pressure gradient or closure of pathway for fluid flow into the retina. This can be achieved by vitrectomy alone if vitreous traction can be demonstrated over the optic pit or by combining vitrectomy with gas tamponade and carefully titrated juxtapapillary laser to create a permanent barrier between intraretinal and subretinal fluid. Recently, covering the optic pit during vitrectomy with different materials such as inverted internal limiting membrane (ILM) flap, scleral plugs, and amniotic membrane have been tried with good postoperative results. Fovea-sparing ILM peeling is advocated in long-standing cases to avoid postoperative macular hole formation (**Fig. 7.39.2**).

SUGGESTED READING

1. Jain N, Johnson MW. Pathogenesis and treatment of maculopathy associated with cavitary optic disk anomalies. Am J Ophthalmol. 2014;158(3):423-35.
2. Ravani R, Kumar A, Karthikeya R, Kumar P, Gupta Y, Mutha V, et al. Comparison of inverted ILM-stuffing technique and ILM peeling alone for optic disc pit-associated maculopathy: long-term results. Ophthalmic Surg Lasers Imaging Retina. 2018;49(12):226-32.

7.40 | Photic Retinopathy

Saurabh Luthra, Shrutanjoy Mohan Das, Shweta Parakh
Drishti Eye Institute, Dehradun
drsaurabhluthra@gmail.com

INTRODUCTION

Photic retinopathy is also known as solar retinopathy, solar retinitis, solar eclipse retinopathy, foveomacular retinitis, laser-induced maculopathy, and Welder's retinopathy.

It refers to light-induced retinal damage, usually occurring at the fovea caused by direct or indirect solar viewing. Melanin granules facilitate light absorption in the retinal pigment epithelium (RPE) and choroid, and thermally enhance photochemical damage. Supranormal light exposure causes thermal denaturation of proteins, which overwhelms retinal defenses against toxic free radicals from light and oxygen. The damage manifests as a disorder of RPE and photoreceptor outer segments with relatively subtle clinical signs. Prognosis is usually favorable as visual recovery has been commonly described.

ETIOLOGY

Classically the disease entity is associated with solar eclipse viewing or sun-gazing. But it has also been reported following prolonged or high-intensity exposure to handheld laser pointers, ophthalmic operating microscopes, endoilluminators during vitreoretinal surgery, welding arcs, and photographical illumination.

RISK FACTORS

The risk factors include young age, clear lens, and photosensitizing drugs such as tetracycline and psoralens. High refractive errors, cataract [cataractous lens absorbs more of the shorter wavelength (300–400 nm) light], and darkly pigmented fundus (macular pigments zeaxanthin, lutein, and meso-zeaxanthin filter approximately 40% of relatively high-energy visible blue light) confer protection. Other determinants include direction of gaze, iris pigmentation, pupil diameter, and duration of transmission.

PATHOPHYSIOLOGY

Light or electromagnetic radiation can cause damage through photothermal, photochemical, and photomechanical means.

Photothermal damage to retina is irreversible when ambient temperature is raised by at least 10°C. At 2 days after exposure, there is RPE disruption with choroidal damage. Also, there are RPE pigmentary changes due to macrophages engulfing melanosomes. These changes resolve by day 10. Ultrastructurally, photoreceptors show vesiculation and fragmentation of lamellae, whirls within disc membranes, mitochondrial swelling, and nuclear pyknosis. RPE cells show plasma membrane changes, swelling of smooth endoplasmic reticulum, and lipofuscin granule structure alterations. The extent of damage can vary from apoptosis secondary to lower-level thermal damage (55–58°C), apoptosis and necrosis (60–68°C), and immediate cell death (72°C or greater).

Photochemical damage is the most common mechanism of damage. It is associated with both long-duration exposure times and lower wavelength (higher energy) light exposure. Photochemical damage is thought to occur due to exposure of retinal tissue to generated free radicals once the protective mechanisms of retina have been overwhelmed. This is mediated by chromophores in the retina and RPE, which include the photoreceptors, flavoproteins, heme proteins, melanosomes, and lipofuscin.

Photomechanical damage occurs due to sudden introduction of energy into the melanosomes of RPE resulting in thermoelastic expansion, which in turn forms microcavitation bubbles that are lethal.

■ CLINICAL FEATURES

Only 51% of subjects affected by solar retinopathy referred to a sun-gazing history or history of exposure to a strong source of illumination. These patients represent more of a diagnostic challenge.

Within 1–4 hours after exposure, patients complain of unilateral or bilateral decreased vision, metamorphopsia, central or paracentral scotomata, chromatopsia, photophobia, afterimages, and periorbital ache. Within the first few days there is outer retinal whitening. A small yellow spot with a gray margin may develop in the foveolar or parafoveolar area. The disciform lesion corresponds with the sun's image on the retina. Milder cases may not be detectable on ophthalmoscopy. Few days later, there are mild pigmentary changes, which evolve into coarse pigmentary changes over the next 1–2 weeks. The lesion evolves over the next few weeks to an outer lamellar hole. At about 4–5 weeks, epiretinal membranes may develop. After 3–6 months, yellowish plaque-like lesion may be the only residual change.

■ IMAGING

Fluorescein angiography may be normal, show window defects or mild foveal hyperfluorescence and leakage may be seen rarely in the acute stage. Ultrahigh-resolution optical coherence tomography (OCT) at presentation demonstrates a full-thickness isoreflective lesion traversing the fovea. Focal disruption at the level of the subfoveal RPE and outer retinal bands with an otherwise normal retinal architecture and contour are seen. There may be a small amount of subfoveal fluid. At 1-month follow-up, the external limiting membrane appears intact. There is a persistent wedge-shaped outer retinal defect involving the ellipsoid zone and the interdigitation zone (**Figs. 7.40.1A and B**). Pigment clumps reside in this potential space. The RPE appears restored in the later stages. There is persistent atrophy as evidenced by increased light transmission. Full-thickness macular holes have also been reported after laser exposure.

Parameters measured on OCT include central macular thickness (CMT), maximum defect thickness (vertical depth), and maximum horizontal dimension of the outer retinal defect at the scan through the fovea. Photic retinopathy index (PRI) is obtained by dividing the maximum defect thickness in the foveal scan with the CMT. Interestingly, subjective visual acuity improvement may be reported despite persistence of ellipsoid zone defect on OCT, even after 50 years of exposure, and visual acuity may not always correlate with structural findings. PRI and maximum defect thickness may be better

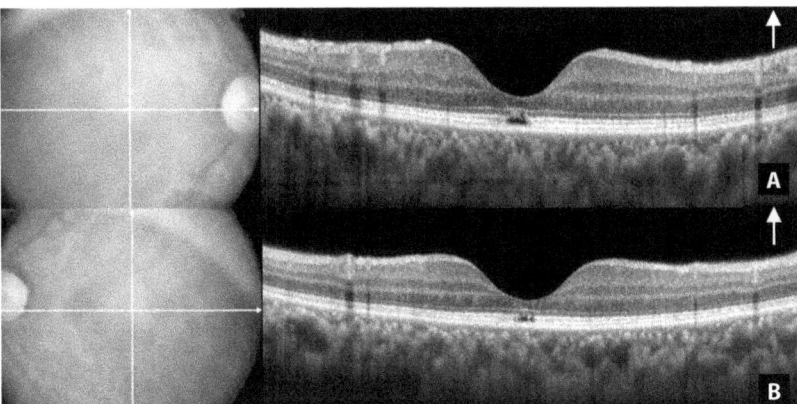

Figs. 7.40.1A and B: Spectral-domain optical coherence tomography in chronic solar maculopathy showing bilateral outer lamellar defect involving the ellipsoid zone and the interdigitation zone.

predictors of visual acuity. OCT-based ultrastructural features in photic retinopathy have poor correlation with presenting or final visual acuity.

Optical coherence tomography angiography of choriocapillaris layer was normal in acute solar retinopathy. OCT angiography captured 70 days later shows improved choriocapillaris flow with a higher signal than normal choriocapillaris in the affected area that could be caused by a window defect. Reperfusion of choriocapillaris can play a role in visual recovery and also can prevent the occurrence of complications like choroidal neovascularization.

Recent studies on macaque retinas, utilizing high-resolution autofluorescence imaging using an adaptive optics scanning laser ophthalmoscope, have shown an immediate decrease in autofluorescence of RPE cells following exposure of 568 nm light for 15 minutes. Follow-up autofluorescence showed long-term damage in RPE cells. Also, there was reciprocity between exposure duration and power. A hyperautofluorescent ring surrounding a well-demarcated area of hypoautofluorescence (that correlate to loss of the ellipsoid zone) is seen in the acute phase.

HISTOPATHOLOGY

Experimental studies in rhesus monkeys have shown the histological response to photochemical injury as occurring in three stages. Within 24 hours of the insult, the acute stage shows retinal edema, RPE pigment disorganization, photoreceptor irregularity, and abnormal pigmentary cells in the subretinal space. The reparative second stage occurs a week later and is marked by a macrophage response. The chronic degenerative third stage occurs weeks to months later and is characterized by RPE proliferation, with the RPE cells and macrophages forming a plaque between Bruch's membrane and retina.

DIFFERENTIAL DIAGNOSIS

Clinical and spectral-domain OCT (SD-OCT) features of acute solar retinopathy can sometimes mimic conditions such as ocular trauma, early stage idiopathic macular hole, persistent outer retinal defects in repaired macular hole, idiopathic juxtafoveal telangiectasis, and solitary macular cysts. Differential diagnosis is explored utilizing patient history combined with OCT findings.
- Macular telangiectasia (MacTel) type II
- Vitreomacular traction (VMT)
- Closed macular hole

- Alkyl nitrate abuse
- Tamoxifen
- Retinal pigment epithelitis
- Achromatopsia
- Early Stargardt disease

■ TREATMENT AND PROGNOSIS

No specific therapy exists. Role of oral corticosteroids is inconclusive. Within 6 months, almost complete recovery of vision to 20/20–20/40 range is seen but scotoma and metamorphopsia can remain.

■ WELDING ARC EXPOSURE

Retinal injury is rare. Photochemical effects from ultraviolet (UV) and short blue wavelength exposure produce it as retinal temperature elevation is below photocoagulation threshold. Clinical features are similar to solar retinopathy. There is no effective treatment.

■ LIGHTNING RETINOPATHY

Lightning maculopathy includes macular edema, macular hole, cyst, solar retinopathy-like picture, cataract, retinal detachment, retinal artery occlusions, and relative afferent pupillary defect. High-dose intravenous methylprednisolone therapy is beneficial.

■ RETINAL PHOTOTOXICITY FROM OPHTHALMIC INSTRUMENTS

Retinal injury has been reported following exposure to light from operating microscope and fiberoptic endoilluminators. It has been described following cataract surgery, epikeratophakia, combined anterior segment, and vitreous surgery. Photochemical damage from extended exposure of the retina by shorter wavelengths in the visible spectrum (450–550 nm) may be enhanced thermally. Intraocular lenses (IOLs) and microscopes with UV and infrared (IR) filters may lessen the risk of photic and thermal effects, respectively. A foveal lesion can produce severe, permanent visual loss. Within 24–48 hours of exposure, a yellow lesion at level of RPE develops. Retinal edema may also be seen. The shape of the lesion matches that of the illuminating source. Fundus fluorescein angiography (FFA) reveals leakage at level of RPE simulating a choroidal neovascular membrane (CNVM). The lesion evolves over weeks to result in areas of RPE clumping and atrophy. Long-term sequelae include postoperative erythropsia, epiretinal membranes, and CNVM adjacent to photic damage. Factors influencing microscope phototoxicity include brightness, wavelength, prolonged surgical duration, and surgical technique. Patient-related risk factors include higher body temperature, blood oxygenation, chorioretinal pigmentation, preexisting maculopathy, pupillary dilation, diabetes mellitus, retinal vascular disease, and vitamin A and C deficiency. No specific treatment is available, but spontaneous improvement is usually seen. Methods to reduce phototoxicity include reducing coaxial illumination and surgical time, use of IR and UV filters in microscope and IOL, use of air bubble in anterior chamber (AC), and use of eclipse filter or corneal cover.

■ SUGGESTED READING

1. Kumar K, Sen S, Anudeep K, Rajan RP, Kannan NB, Ramasamy K. Anatomical and functional features of photic retinopathy: a spectral domain optical coherence tomography-based longitudinal study. Graefes Arch Clin Exp Ophthalmol. 2022;260(2):415-23.
2. Ryan SJ. Medical retina. In: Ryan SJ (Ed). Retina, 4th edition. Philadelphia: Elsevier Mosby; 2006.

7.41 Hypertensive Retinopathy

Brijesh Thakkar, Soumyava Basu
Anant Bajaj Retina Institute
LV Prasad Eye Institute, Hyderabad
eyetalk@gmail.com

■ INTRODUCTION

Hypertension is a worldwide problem that affects up to one billion people worldwide and is the single most important modifiable risk factor for stroke. In India, 23.10% men and 22.60% women over 25 years suffer from hypertension, according to the WHO's global health statistics, 2012. The reason it has gained attention of physicians worldwide is that it acts as a silent killer many years before overt end organ damage is clinically apparent. Hence, improvised strategies to ensure reliable detection of hypertension-related end organ damage before it becomes symptomatic are making way into clinical practice.

■ RETINOPATHY

The retina provides a window to study the human circulation. Retinal arterioles can be visualized easily and noninvasively and share similar anatomical and physiological properties with cerebral and coronary microcirculation.

Hypertensive retinopathy, first described as "albuminuric retinitis", has traditionally been referred to as a spectrum of "retinal vascular signs" caused by elevated blood pressure. Marcus Gunn described it first at the end of the 19th century in a group of hypertensive patients with kidney disease. Previously, there has been little clinical or research interest in this field mainly because of subjectivity surrounding it together with uncertainty regarding the independent predictive value. New developments have paved way to the understanding of this common yet underdiagnosed condition.

■ ETIOPATHOGENESIS

The arteriosclerotic changes of hypertensive retinopathy are caused by chronically elevated blood pressure, defined as systolic >140 mm Hg and diastolic >90 mm Hg. **Table 7.41.1** summarizes the underlying mechanisms and corresponding fundus signs.

■ OCULAR SIGNS

The ocular fundus is an important target organ for detecting and, as well, monitoring hypertension. In detecting hypertension, arteriolar narrowing and focal constrictions seem to be the most sensitive indicators in the absence of hemorrhages and disc edema. Although many classification systems have been described (including the Keith-Wagener-Barker and Scheie systems), the Wong and Mitchell classification system has become widely accepted for systemic prognosis and management.

■ KEY POINTS IN EVALUATION

- First to be examined are the arterial vessels, including their size, regularity, color, course, light reflex, and visibility of the blood column. Unless the arterioles are narrowed dramatically, the most easily noted change in these vessels is irregularity of the caliber.
- Tortuosity of the arterioles may be seen on a congenital basis, where uniform tortuosity is present throughout the fundus. Segmental arterial tortuosity is always abnormal.
- The arteriovenous crossings should be evaluated for the degree of hiding of the venous blood column, as well as for changes in the course of the involved vein. These two changes, however, do not mean that there is impedance to the venous flow at this site.

TABLE 7.41.1: Pathophysiology of hypertensive retinopathy.

	Pathophysiological mechanism	Signs
Acute hypertension	• Vasospasm • Increased vascular tone	*Vasoconstrictive stage:* Generalized arteriolar narrowing
Chronic hypertension	• Intimal thickening, media wall hyperplasia, hyaline degeneration of arterioles • Compression of venules at their common adventitial crossings	• Diffuse and focal narrowing (copper wiring) and opacification (silver wiring) of arteriolar walls • *Arteriosclerotic stage:* Arteriovenous nicking
Severe hypertension	• Inner blood-retinal barrier breakdown • Necrosis of vascular smooth muscle and endothelial cells • Persistent damage to retinal microvasculature	• *Exudative stage:* Exudation of blood (retinal hemorrhages) and lipids (hard exudates) • Nerve fiber layer ischemia (cotton-wool spots)
Accelerated hypertension	• Intracranial pressure elevation • Optic nerve ischemia	• Hypertensive optic neuropathy/malignant retinopathy • Optic nerve ischemia • Optic disc swelling

- To determine if impedance to flow is present at an arteriovenous crossing, examination of the retina distal to the crossing is required. Impedance is evident when the distal vein is darker, larger, and more tortuous than the proximal segment. Additional signs of impedance are capillary changes, such as dilation of the capillaries, and retinal hemorrhage, edema, or cotton-wool spots. In frank obstruction, venous-venous collaterals may be noted.
- The disc must be carefully examined for edema.
- When each of the earlier mentioned parameters is evaluated, the examiner must compare them to the expected fundus picture in a similar age group of normal patients. Mild arteriolar light reflex changes and minimal arteriolar irregularity in a 70-year-old patient have a much lower chance of being associated with hypertension than do the same changes noted in a 20-year-old patient.
- In a young patient with recently diagnosed hypertension, irregular arteriolar caliber suggests long-standing or previous episodes of hypertension. Evidence of arteriolar necrosis (hemorrhage, cotton-wool spot, retinal edema, capillary nonperfusion, and/or disc edema, and venous obstruction) is a sign that the retinal vascular system is responding to elevated blood pressure and not to the process of aging.

HYPERTENSIVE CHOROIDOPATHY

Hypertensive choroidopathy is seen in association with acute hypertension. It occurs in relatively young individuals whose blood vessels are pliable and not sclerotic. Patients may show signs of malignant hypertension including encephalopathy. Hypertensive choroidopathy is primarily due to choroidal ischemia, which produces ischemic damage of the overlying retinal pigment epithelium (RPE), resulting in the development of the various ophthalmoscopically visible lesions.

Acute choroidal ischemia produces:
- Focal, whitish, and lobulated RPE lesions—Elschnig spots
- Serous retinal or RPE detachment, mostly bullous in nature

Chronic choroidal ischemia produces extensive RPE degeneration including hyper/hypopigmented patches. Normally, choroidal vessels are not seen on ophthalmoscopy.

In some of the eyes with extensive RPE degenerative lesions, the large choroidal vessels become unmasked and are seen as white lines due to choroidal sclerosis, and seen as Siegrist streaks.

Hypertensive retinopathy and choroidopathy are two independent and unrelated manifestations of renovascular malignant arterial hypertension. Until recently, the various manifestations of hypertensive choroidopathy have been considered to be part of retinopathy, and choroidopathy and retinopathy have been thought of as interrelated phenomena. But, the retinal and choroidal vascular beds have some fundamentally different properties, e.g., in the choroidal vascular bed:
- There is no autoregulatory mechanism for blood flow.
- There is sympathetic nerve supply. In response to systemic hypertension, the choroidal arterioles will initially undergo constriction. A further increase in blood pressure overcomes the compensatory tone of the sympathetic response, resulting in damage to the muscle layer and endothelium.
- The choriocapillaris has no blood-ocular-barrier (because of the presence of large fenestrations in its walls).

COMPLICATIONS

Patients with severe hypertensive retinopathy and arteriosclerotic changes are at increased risk for coronary disease, peripheral vascular disease, and stroke, as evident by the Wong and Mitchell classification systems prognostication. Since arteriosclerotic changes in the retina do not regress, these patients remain at increased risk for retinal artery occlusions, retinal vein occlusions, and retinal macroaneurysms. Most retinal changes secondary to malignant hypertension will improve once blood pressure is controlled. Damage to the optic nerve and macula, however, could cause long-term reductions in visual acuity.

ASSOCIATION WITH DIABETES

Diabetes and hypertension are both vascular risk factors and may share similar pathophysiological mechanisms. Both conditions are also linked by the metabolic syndrome. The prevalence of diabetes among patients with hypertension is high and type 2 diabetes may remain unrecognized for years before being diagnosed. Population-based studies detected hypertensive retinopathy in 2–14% of nondiabetic population aged 40 years and older. When diabetes is associated with hypertension, cardiovascular risk rises exponentially and retinopathy becomes more severe and rapidly progressive.

PREGNANCY-INDUCED HYPERTENSION

Hypertension is the most common medical disorder during pregnancy, affecting 6–8% of all pregnancies. According to the American college of Obstetrics and Gynecology Committee task force, hypertension is defined as either a systolic pressure of >140 mm Hg or an increase of >30 mm Hg (from a base line in the first half of the pregnancy) or as a diastolic pressure of >90 mm Hg or an increase of >15 mm Hg from the base line. Preeclampsia [pregnancy-induced hypertension (PIH)] is characterized by edema, proteinuria, and hypertension. Visual symptoms are reported in 25% of eclampsia and 50% of preeclampsia of PIH. In early studies of preeclampsia, the incidence of foveal retinal arteriolar abnormalities was reported to be 30–100%. The retinal vascular changes generally but not always correlate with severity of systemic hypertension. Vasospastic manifestations are reversible and the retinal vessels rapidly return to normal after delivery.

MAJOR OBSERVATIONS

Several major observations have emerged from recent research. First, studies have shown in the hypertensive population, patients with elevated blood pressure despite medical therapy had a higher frequency of retinopathy signs, compared with those whose blood pressure was controlled or those who were normotensive. This finding indicates that hypertensive retinopathy signs may be an indicator of blood pressure control.

Second, the patterns of specific retinal vascular changes vary with current and past blood pressure levels. Generalized retinal arteriolar narrowing and arteriovenous nicking usually appear in patients with long-term hypertension and are independently associated with past blood pressure levels measured up to 10 years before retinal assessment. In contrast, focal arteriolar narrowing and retinopathy lesions (retinal hemorrhages, microaneurysms, and cotton-wool spots) may indicate more transitory blood pressure changes and are related only to concurrently measured blood pressure.

Third, the association between blood pressure and retinal microvascular signs is weaker with age, possibly reflecting greater sclerosis of retinal arterioles in older persons.

Fourth, longitudinal data from recent population-based studies have demonstrated that smaller retinal arteriolar and larger venular calibers precede clinical stages of hypertension and predict the risk of hypertension in initially normotensive individuals.

DIFFERENTIAL DIAGNOSIS

The major conditions from which hypertensive retinopathy needs to be differentiated are:
- *Diabetic retinopathy:* The abnormal clinical findings are very similar to moderate hypertensive retinopathy (e.g., microaneurysms, hemorrhages, and cotton-wool spots). Microaneurysms arising from capillaries are seen in diabetic retinopathy. Proliferative diabetic retinopathy will show characteristic new vessels leaking on fundus fluorescein angiography (FFA). Choroidal filling and A-V transit time is usually normal.
- *Venous occlusions:* Central retinal vein occlusion (CRVO) and branch retinal vein occlusion (BRVO) can produce retinal hemorrhages similar in appearance; however, the onset of CRVO and BRVO are sudden versus hypertensive retinopathy's clinical signs which usually develop over time. Decreased visual acuity is a common finding in vein occlusions, but not hypertensive retinopathy. Moreover hypertensive retinopathy is bilateral. The venous dilatation and tortuosity will be prevalent as compared to arterial signs in hypertensive retinopathy. Sometimes a combined arterial and vein occlusion may show venous beading with arterial narrowing and nicking. Delayed A-V transit time on FFA clinches the diagnosis.
- *Arterial occlusions:* They will primarily present with attenuation/occlusion of arteries. The causative emboli can be visualized in the lumen of branching vessels. In CRAO, there is ischemia of the inner retina, the amplitude of the b-wave is decreased.

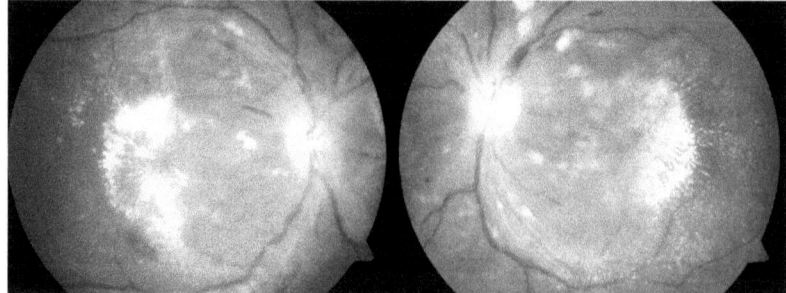

Fig. 7.41.1: A 37-year-old male, diagnosed as OU neuroretinitis elsewhere presented with complaints of sudden blurring of vision in both eyes since 3 weeks. Best-corrected visual acuity (BCVA) was 20/125 in OD and 20/200 in OS. Blood pressure (BP) recorded was 220/140 mm Hg. Fundus examination showed bilateral disc edema and hyperemia, retinal nerve fiber layer (RNFL) hemorrhages, soft exudates with macular star suggestive of grade 4 hypertensive retinopathy. The hemorrhages and disc edema resolved following BP control. Hard exudates however took weeks to resolve.

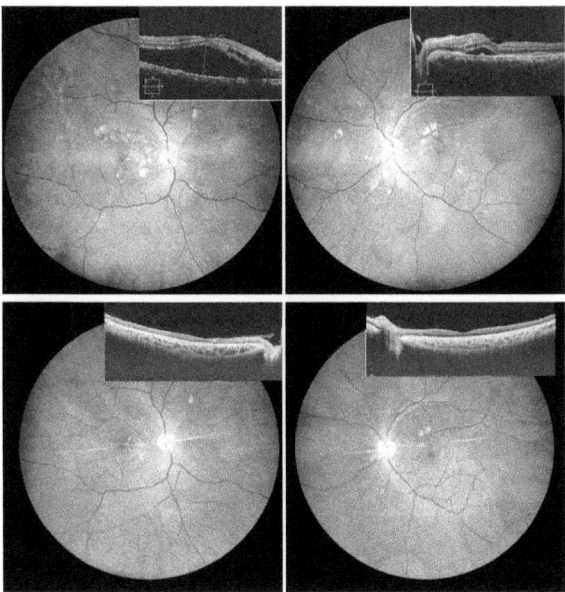

Fig. 7.41.2: A 35-year-old male with vision loss. The right-sided panel shows cotton-wool spots, early disc edema, and subretinal fluid with retinal pigment epithelium (RPE) changes and Elschnig spots. Optical coherence tomography (OCT) confirms presence of pigment epithelial detachments (PEDs) and subretinal fluid (SRF). This patient was suspected to have hypertension retinochoroidopathy. Evaluation initiated by ophthalmologist revealed low ejection fraction, malignant hypertension in a setting of chronic renal failure. Only blood pressure (BP) control led to restoration of vision and retinal-choroidal architecture as seen in the left-sided panel.
Courtesy: Dr Padmaja Rani, LVPEI, Hyderabad.

- *Ocular ischemic syndrome (OIS):* Characteristically unilateral, this will present with dilated and tortuous veins and neovascularization owing to long-standing ischemia. FFA will show delayed choroidal filling (most specific) as well as A-V transit time (most sensitive). Carotid Doppler studies are helpful in delineating the cause. Electroretinogram (ERG) studies have shown that in eyes with OIS where both the retinal and the choroidal circulation are compromised, there is ischemia of the inner and outer retina that results in decreased amplitude of both a- and b-waves.
- *Neuroretinitis:* This will closely resemble malignant hypertensive retinopathy however it has unilateral presentation, less of hemorrhages, and exudates. Usually there will be underlying systemic condition like syphilis. Other signs such as relative afferent pupillary defect (RAPD) and loss of color vision will be evident.
- *Hyperviscosity syndromes:* Fundus manifestations caused by serum or blood hyperviscosity include optic disc swelling, retinal capillary microaneurysms, cotton-wool spots, retinal hemorrhages, dilated retinal veins, and retinal venous occlusion. A basic workup should therefore include a complete blood cell count with differential, serum protein electrophoresis, and immunoelectrophoresis in patients presenting with bilateral CRVOs.
- *Radiation retinopathy:* The hallmark of radiation retinopathy on FFA is the presence of retinal capillary nonperfusion areas while macular edema or ischemia might also be seen in absence of other signs. It usually occurs within 3 years of initial radiotherapy although onset can vary from 1 month to 15 years after treatment. Visual loss in patients with radiation retinopathy is usually gradual and irreversible due to macular nonperfusion.

RECENT TRENDS

In the last decade, there has been a renewed interest in hypertensive retinopathy. New approaches have been developed that allow a more objective and precise assessment of hypertensive retinopathy characteristics from retinal photographs. Three major advances have occurred in research in hypertensive retinopathy over the past two decades.

The first advance has been the broad application of retinal photography (initial film and subsequently digital) to capture hypertensive retinopathy signs in clinical studies. As a result, elements of reproducibility in measuring early signs are no longer necessary.

The second advance is the application of computer-based techniques to measure early changes, such as generalized retinal arteriolar narrowing. The development of specific software packages have made it possible to objectively measure the arteriole-to-venule ratio (AVR) in selected standardized portions of the retina.

These techniques and their incorporation in artificial intelligence have allowed the third major advance, which is improved understanding of the relationship of these signs in large epidemiological studies with systemic conditions and target end organ damage, such as cerebrovascular, coronary, and renal diseases.

MANAGEMENT

The management of patients with hypertensive retinopathy should be based on the "simplified classification" shown in **Table 7.41.2**. This scheme allows clinicians to utilize retinal microvasculature as a model for assessing hypertensive patients for target organ damage risk stratification. Lifestyle modification in conjunct with antihypertensive drugs under the physician's care is essential. However, it is important to remember that medical treatment can only treat the acute changes of hypertension from vasospasm and vascular leakage. There is no treatment for arteriosclerotic changes of chronic hypertension. Retinal photocoagulation and antivascular endothelial growth factor (VEGF) therapies are mainly directed at preventing visual loss due to complications.

CONCLUSION

Hypertensive retinopathy remains a recognized manifestation of target organ damage in hypertensive patients. A thorough retinal examination along with digital imaging might

TABLE 7.41.2: Risk stratification and management guidelines of hypertensive retinopathy.

Retinopathy grade	Description	Systemic associations	Management
Mild	*One or more of the following signs:* Generalized arteriolar narrowing, focal arteriolar narrowing, arteriovenous nicking, and arteriolar wall opacity (silver wiring)	Weak associations with stroke, coronary heart disease, and cardiovascular mortality	• Routine care • Closer monitoring of vascular risk
Moderate	*Mild retinopathy with one or more of the following signs:* Retinal hemorrhage (blot, dot, or flame shaped), microaneurysms, cotton-wool spot, and hard exudates	Strong association with stroke, congestive heart failure, renal dysfunction, and cardiovascular mortality	• Exclude diabetes • Closer monitoring of vascular risk • Possible indication for hypertension treatment and other risk factors
Malignant	Moderate retinopathy signs plus optic disc swelling and macular edema	Associated with mortality	Urgent hypertension treatment

acquire a specific indication to predict [that is, consider cardiovascular disease (CVD) evaluation in presence of retinal microvascular lesions] and prevent (that is, role of retinal photography for CVD risk stratification) metabolic and/or cardiovascular events in the general population, even in the absence of overt hypertension or diabetes.

SUGGESTED READING
1. Couper DJ, Klein R, Hubbard LD, Wong TY, Sorlie PD, Cooper LS, et al. Reliability of retinal photography in the assessment of retinal microvascular characteristics: the atherosclerosis risk in communities study. Am J Ophthalmol. 2002;133:78-88.
2. Hayreh S, Servais G, Virdi P, Marcus M, Rojas P, Woolson R. Fundus lesions in malignant hypertension: III. Arterial blood pressure, biochemical and fundus changes. Ophthalmology. 1986;93:45-59.
3. Hayreh SS, Servais GE, Virdi PS. Fundus lesions in malignant hypertension. V. Hypertensive optic neuropathy. Ophthalmology. 1986;93:74-87.
4. Hayreh SS, Servais GE, Virdi PS. Fundus lesions in malignant hypertension. V. Hypertensive choroidopathy. Ophthalmology. 1986;93:1383-400.
5. JT Gillow, Gibson JM, Dodson PM. Hypertension and diabetic retinopathy: what's the story? Br J Ophthalmol. 1999;83:1083-7.
6. Kishi S, Tso MOM, Hayreh SS. Fundus lesions in malignant hypertension. II. A pathologic study of experimental hypertensive optic neuropathy. Arch Ophthalmol. 1985;103:1198-206.
7. Klein R, Klein B, Moss S, Wang Q. Hypertension and retinopathy, arteriolar narrowing and arteriovenous nicking in a population. Arch Ophthalmol. 1994;112:92-8.
8. The Sixth Report of the Joint National Committee on Prevention, Detection, Evaluation, and Treatment of High Blood Pressure. Arch Intern Med. 1997;157:2413-46.
9. Tso MO, Jampol LM. Pathophysiology of hypertensive retinopathy. Ophthalmology. 1982; 89:1132-45.

7.42 | Endogenous Endophthalmitis

Subina Narang, Varsha Jindal
Government Medical College and Hospital, Chandigarh
subina_navya@yahoo.com

INTRODUCTION
Metastatic endophthalmitis is a potentially blinding eye condition caused by the hematogenous spread of microorganisms to the eye. It is also known as endogenous endophthalmitis. It accounts for 2-8% of all cases of endophthalmitis. The risk of pediatric endogenous endophthalmitis is even lower and accounts for 0.1-4% of all endophthalmitis cases. Due to the rarity of the condition, there are no available guidelines in the literature for its management. The available data is in form of case reports or case series. It is misdiagnosed in >50% of cases. It is commonly misdiagnosed as granulomatous uveitis, fungal endophthalmitis, angle closure glaucoma, mucormycosis, cavernous sinus thrombosis, or orbital cellulitis.

Metastatic endophthalmitis can be classified as anterior (focal or diffuse), posterior (focal or diffuse), and panophthalmitis.

MICROBIAL SPECTRUM AND RISK FACTORS
The identification of preexisting predisposing conditions is possible in >90% of patients with proper history and examination. The most common systemic condition found is diabetes mellitus in 50% of endogenous endophthalmitis cases. The other predisposing conditions are immune-compromised patients with human immunodeficiency virus (HIV), malignancy, organ transplant, renal pathologies, liver failure, blood dyscrasias, or those on intravenous hyperalimentation, intravenous or indwelling catheter, hemodialysis, contaminated intravenous infusion, intravenous drug abuse (IVDA) etc. (**Fig. 7.42.1**).

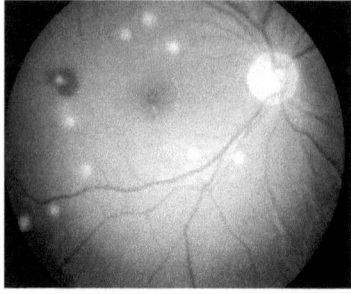

Fig. 7.42.1: Fundus photograph showing multiple retinal abscesses in IV drug abuser with *Candida* septicemia.

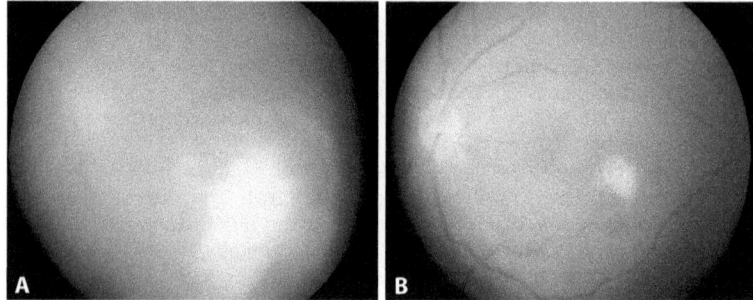

Figs. 7.42.2A and B: (A) Fundus photograph of a patient with history of intravenous dextrose 3 weeks prior to decreased vision showing fluff ball on retina; (B) Fundus photograph of the patient in (A) showing resolution after PPV and intravitreal amphoteric in (B).

The common sites of extraocular infection serving as a source of microorganisms in the eye are liver abscess, pneumonia, endocarditis, meningitis, soft tissue infection, gastrointestinal or urinary tract infection, renal abscess, pyonephrosis, brain abscess, etc.

The bacteria responsible for endogenous endophthalmitis include *Streptococcus pneumoniae, Staphylococcus aureus, Staphylococcus epidermis,* and *Listeria monocytogenes.* Methicillin-resistant *Staph. aureus* (MRSA) has been associated with a higher rate of retinal detachment in the presentation of endogenous endophthalmitis. The common fungal isolates include *Candida albicans, Candida tropicalis, Cryptococcus neoformans,* and *Aspergillus fumigatus.* Schiedler *et al.* demonstrated *Candida albicans* as a common cause of endogenous endophthalmitis in USA. Studies from Asia show *Klebsiella* liver abscess in a diabetic as the commonest cause of endogenous endophthalmitis. IVDA is an important cause of fungal infections. Gupta et al. reported *Aspergillus* endophthalmitis 4-6 weeks after a single intravenous fluid injection, in the rural Indian setting, as an important cause of endogenous endophthalmitis **(Figs. 7.42.2A and B)**. Atypical pathogens like *Mycobacterium tuberculosis,* nontuberculous mycobacteria, and *Nocardia.*

In coronavirus disease-2019 (COVID-19) pandemic, prolonged hospitalization, indwelling cannulas, use of antibiotics, and systemic steroids to manage the cytokine storm predisposed the patients to fungal endogenous endophthalmitis which typically presented 1–31 days after recovery. Severe acute respiratory syndrome coronavirus 2 (SARS-CoV-2) has also been detected in the vitreous samples of endogenous endophthalmitis vitreous sample. In addition to above, *Klebsiella* and MRSA have also been isolated from COVID patients with endophthalmitis.

■ CLINICAL FEATURES

The disease is uniocular to begin with and the other eye is subsequently affected in 15% cases. Binocularity is more common with *Meningococci, Klebsiella,* and *Escherichia coli.*

The male preponderance is seen and the peak age is in third decade in bacterial and <1 year and middle age in fungal. The right eye is twice as often prone for a focus of infection than the left, because of comparatively direct blood flow to the right carotid artery.

The patient typically presents with ocular pain, discharge, redness, blurred vision, lid edema and conjunctival chemosis, elevated intraocular pressure (IOP), corneal edema, anterior chamber and vitreous reaction including hypopyon, reduced red reflex, retinal cotton wool spots, Roth's spots, hemorrhages, choroidal abscess, or vitreous abscess. *Bacillus cereus* (*B. cereus*) is the common cause of metastatic endophthalmitis in drug abusers in whom the patients may exhibit a ring-shaped corneal ulcer with brownish anterior chamber exudates. If brownish hypopyon occurs without corneal involvement, then *listeria monocytogenes* should be considered as diagnosis. A red hypopyon may be seen in *Serratia*. Fungal endophthalmitis with *Candida* may have fluff balls in vitreous cavity. *Aspergillus* endogenous endophthalmitis usually presents with deep creamy white subretinal circumscribed lesions. A high index of suspicion is required to clinch the diagnosis.

■ DIAGNOSIS

Delayed diagnosis and initial misdiagnosis are common in cases of endogenous endophthalmitis. The disease could present unilaterally despite hematogenous spread. A high index of suspicion along with the ancillary tests could help us clinch the diagnosis. B-scan ocular ultrasonography is a useful adjunct to the clinical evaluation of infectious endophthalmitis especially in an eye with opaque media as it tells about vitritis and retinal detachment. Vitreous exudates are seen as low to moderate-intensity points like echoes in the vitreous cavity. The membranous structure seen on USG is thick posterior vitreous detachment (PVD) or retinal detachment (RD). Other investigations include blood cultures which give a higher positivity rate of up to 94% as compared to intraocular samples. It has a vitreous culture positivity rate of 59-65%% which is much higher than aqueous samples (32-47%). It is necessary to take cultures from multiple sites and also repeated samples if suspicion of endogenous endophthalmitis is strong. The vitreous specimen for cultures gives better yield with a vitreous cutter than by needle aspiration. The slide for microbiology assessment should be prepared from the centrifuged deposit of the vitreous sample for higher yield. The cultures are set up for aerobic bacteria, anaerobic bacteria, and fungi. The samples should be incubated for at least a week before giving a negative report.

The polymerase chain reaction is being increasingly used nowadays for the quick differentiation of bacteria from fungal endophthalmitis. Polymerase chain reaction (PCR) helps in a quicker assay in small quantity samples. It is highly specific (95-100%) and has 93% positive predictive value and 95% negative predictive value.

Optical coherence tomography (OCT) is a newer noninvasive tool that can be used in clear media. Intravitreal cells could be seen as preretinal hyperreflective aggregates. It helps us to localize the pathology which could be an intraretinal or chorioretinal pattern. *Candida* gives a classical "rain cloud sign", in which we have preretinal hyper-reflective aggregates with shadowing of retinal layers.

■ TREATMENT

Thorough history taking and examination is recommended to look for the primary focus of infection once the diagnosis of metastatic endophthalmitis is suspected. Systemic antimicrobials are the primary treatment in all cases of endogenous endophthalmitis which substantially decrease the chances of enucleation and evisceration. The primary focus of infection is the source of the ocular. Presuming the infection to be bacterial, empiric broad-spectrum antibiotic therapy is given. The commonly used antibiotic is ciprofloxacin 750 g twice a day. Alternatively, intravenous with vancomycin (1 g) and ceftazidime (1 g) twice a day can be given in sick patients. In case of fungal infection, intravenous fluconazole (loading dose of 12 mg/kg, then 400-800 mg od) or voriconazole

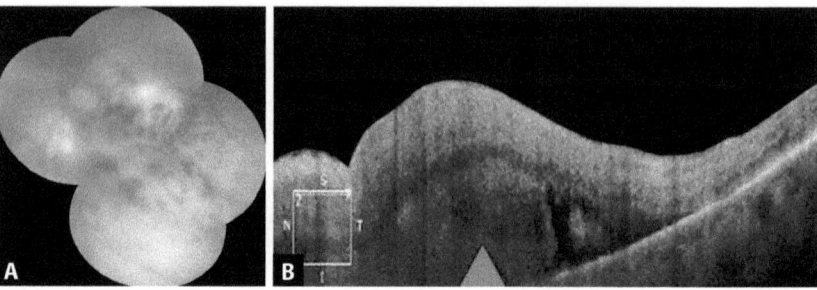

Figs. 7.42.3A and B: (A) Fundus photograph left eye showed subretinal exudates involving macular area with vessels overlying a few frosted branch vessels (suggesting retinitis involving both vein and artery) which was more obvious in the peripheral fundus and also associated with hemorrhagic spots (Roth spot); (B) Enhanced-depth imaging optical coherence tomography (EDI-OCT) suggesting subretinal abscess red arrow head shows hyper-reflective area suggesting abscess wall and area with purulent material.

(loading dose of 6 mg/kg, then 300 mg bd). The therapy can later be tailored depending on the culture reports if the patient does not respond. Systemic antifungals should be continued for at least 6 weeks. In patients with liver abscesses as the cause of endophthalmitis, our preference would be for cephalosporins or carbapenems.

Systemic therapy alone is sufficient when the infection is isolated to the retina and choroid. Prompt treatment with intravitreal antimicrobials and vitrectomy is an option in endophthalmitis with significant vitreous involvement. The broad spectrum antibacterials of choice are vancomycin (1 mg in 0.1 mL) for gram-positive organisms and ceftazidime (2.25 mg/0.1 mL) or amikacin 0.4 mg/0.1 mL for gram-negative organism coverage. In the case of fungal endophthalmitis antifungal of choice is amphotericin (5–10 µg/0.1 mL) or voriconazole (100–200 µg/0.1 mL) along with systemic azoles. Voriconazole in this dose achieves a final concentration of about 25–50 µg/mL in the vitreous and voriconazole has better coverage for *Aspergillus* species and some *Candida* species [such as *Candida glabrata* (*C. glabrata*) and *Candida krusei* (*C. Krusei*)] in which the other antifungals are ineffective.

Vitrectomy helps in decreasing the load of infection, toxins and ensures better accessibility of antimicrobials to intraocular structures. Surgery can result in improvement in ocular signs and visual acuity in a majority of patients. It has been seen that eyes that undergo pars plana vitrectomy are three times more likely to retain useful vision and more than three times less likely to require enucleation or evisceration. It has also been seen that intravitreal antibiotics lower the chances of evisceration and enucleation.

The definite indications for vitrectomy are:
- Worsening of signs and symptoms
- Rapid progression
- Retinal necrosis
- Extensive, subretinal abscess
- Retinal detachment

PROGNOSIS

The poor prognosticators for endogenous endophthalmitis include delayed diagnosis and treatment (>4 days), poor initial visual acuity <20/200, presence of hypopyon, and more virulent microorganisms. The visual outcomes are poor especially when it is *Klebsiella* species. Amongst fungal, *Aspergillus* has worse prognosis than *Candida*. Evisceration/enucleation is required in 25% cases. Only 5% of eyes with bacterial endogenous endophthalmitis can achieve visual acuity of 20/20 and 69% have vision worse than counting fingers.

SUGGESTED READING

1. Bariya S, Bhattacharya A, Narang S. Metastatic endophthalmitis presenting as sub-retinal abscess following a forearm furuncle. BMJ Case Rep. 2021;14(5):e241827.
2. Bilgic A, Sudhalkar A, Gonzalez-Cortes JH, March de Ribot F, Yogi R, Kodjikian L, et al. Endogenous endophthalmitis in the setting of COVID-19 infection: a case series. Retina. 2021;41(8):1709-14.
3. Gupta A, Gupta V, Dogra MR, Chakrabarti A, Ray P, Ram J, et al. See comment in PubMed Commons below Fungal endophthalmitis after a single intravenous administration of presumably contaminated dextrose infusion fluid. Retina. 2000;20:262-8.
4. Smith RS, Kroll AJ, Lou PL, Ryan EA. Endogenous bacterial and fungal endophthalmitis. Int Ophthalmol Clin. 2007;47(2):173-83.
5. Xie CA, Singh J, Tyagi M, Androudi S, Dave VP, Arora A, et al. Endogenous endophthalmitis—a major review. Ocul Immunol Inflamm. 2022;28:1-24.
6. Zhuang H, Ding X, Gao F, Zhang T, Ni Y, Chang Q, et al. Optical coherence tomography features of retinal lesions in Chinese patients with endogenous *Candida* endophthalmitis. BMC Ophthalmol. 2020;20:1-8.

7.43 Dry Age-related Macular Degeneration

Sunandan Sood, Meenakshi Chandel
Government Medical College and Hospital, Chandigarh
soods32@yahoo.co.in

INTRODUCTION

Age-related macular degeneration (AMD) accounts for 8.7% of blindness worldwide and is the most common cause of blindness in developed countries particularly in people of age ≥60 years. Demographic shift in the longevity will continue to increase the prevalence of the disease. According to recent National Eye Institute data, the estimated number of people with AMD will increase to more than double from 2.1 to 5.4 million between 2010 and 2050. Risk factors include age >50 years, Caucasian race, nutrition, smoking, atherosclerotic vascular disease, genetic factors, and sunlight exposure. The presence of drusen bodies and pigment abnormalities at the macula are the early signs of dry AMD.

TYPES OF DRUSEN BODIES

Small Hard Drusen

These are discrete, pale yellow seen better in red free light, fluorescing in the mid-venous phase; when few in number (<20) are not a risk factor for wet AMD.

Large Soft Drusen

These are yellow, confluent, and having sinuous shapes. On fundus fluorescein angiography (FFA), they fill more slowly, but remain fluorescent for a longer period. These have a risk of developing choroidal neovascular membranes (CNVM).

STAGES OF DRY AMD

Early AMD

Less than 20 medium-sized drusen (63–124 µm) with pigment abnormalities **(Fig. 7.43.1)**.

Intermediate AMD

At least one large drusen (>125 = width of retinal vein on the disc) and >20 medium-sized drusens or the presence of geographic atrophy not extending to the center of macula **(Fig. 7.43.2)**.

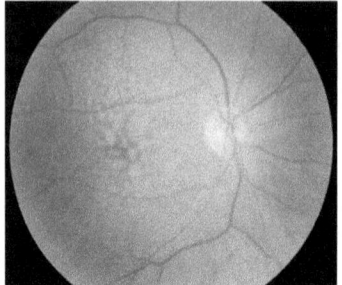

Fig. 7.43.1: Early AMD.

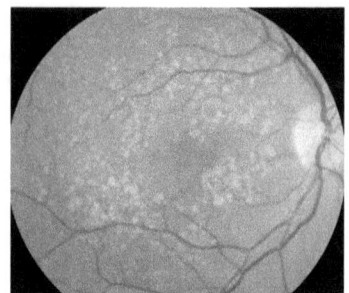

Fig. 7.43.2: Intermediate AMD.

Advance AMD

Results in geographic atrophy extending under the center of macula or signs of CNVM **(Fig. 7.43.3)**.

Geographic atrophy is the end result of the dry AMD. It is defined as any sharply delineated round or oval areas of hypopigmentation in which choroidal vessels are more visible than surrounding area which may or may not be involving fovea. The sparing of fovea for a longer time is attributed to the protective effect provided by lutein and zeaxanthin macular pigments [acting as antioxidants and ultraviolet (UV) light filters].

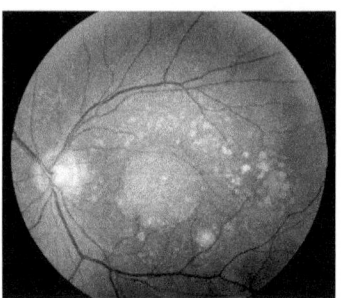

Fig. 7.43.3: Advanced AMD.

DIAGNOSIS

Dry AMD is mostly diagnosed clinically by 90D slit lamp examination. However, fundus autofluorescence (FAF) is the accepted modality of retinal imaging by which it can be diagnosed even when it is not apparent clinically. FAF is noninvasive in vivo method of retinal imaging by which the characteristics of lipofuscin in the fundus are ascertained. Lipofuscin, the metabolic byproduct found in retinal pigment epithelium (RPE), is responsible for FAF. Buildup of lipofuscin in RPE occurs in disease states including AMD, and increase FAF serves as a marker of RPE health and functionality. FAF patterns can predict progression from RPE atrophy leading to geographic atrophy and to vision loss (FAM study).[1] The FAF pattern in the junctional zone of geographical atrophy may predict the velocity of progression of disease **(Figs. 7.43.4A and B)**.

MANAGEMENT

Management depends on the stage of dry AMD. The recommendations of Age-Related Eye Disease Study-1 (AREDS-1) are as under:
- If there is no dry AMD or only early stage of AMD in the either eye, no management for AMD is indicated at that time. AREDS showed no benefit of taking dietary supplements (antioxidants) in reducing the risk of progression to advanced AMD.
- If the intermediate stage of AMD is noted in one eye but not in the fellow eye, the individual should consider taking dietary supplements such as that used in AREDS, the risk of progression to advanced AMD has been found to be decreased by 25% through at least 5 years.
  Vitamin C: 500 mg, vitamin E: 400 IU, β-carotene: 15 mg, zinc oxide: 80 mg, cupric oxide: 2 mg. However, vitamin E and β-carotene should be given with caution in cardiac patients and smokers.[1]
- If advance stage of AMD is noted in one eye and fellow eye has early or intermediate AMD, then dietary supplements should be considered.

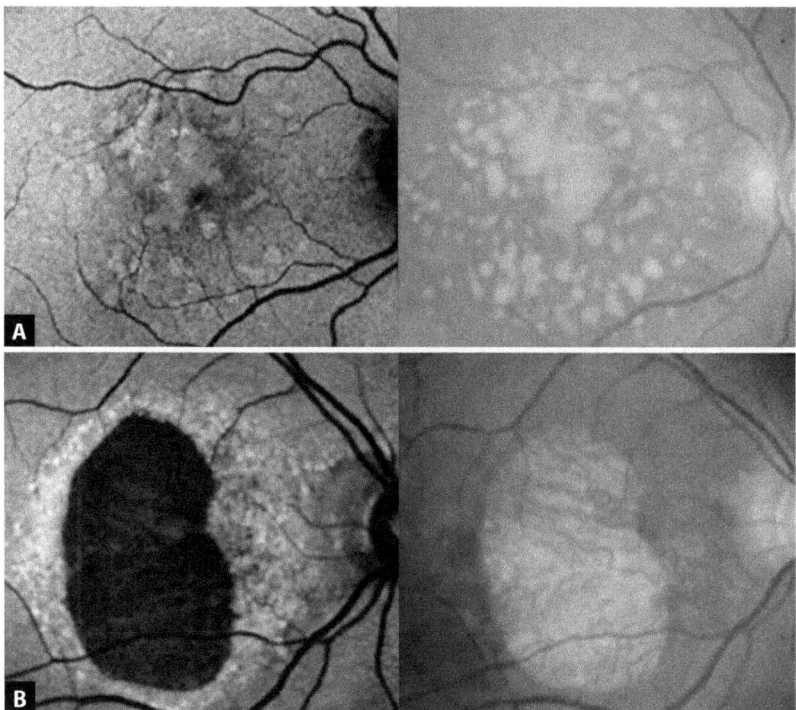

Figs. 7.43.4A and B: *Fundus photo with corresponding fundus autofluorescence images:* (A) Intermediate age-related macular degeneration; (B) Geographical atrophy.

- If both eyes have advanced AMD and one eye has relatively good vision (better than 6/24) consider dietary supplements.
- Advanced stage of dry AMD in both eyes and vision is 3/60–6/60; consider rehabilitation with low vision assessment (LVA).
- Individuals with intermediate stage of dry AMD should get follow-up every year in order to identify development of CNVM. Amsler grid can be given for early detection, and noninvasive optical coherence tomography (OCT) has been shown to identify early CNVM.

In 2004, the LAST (Lutein Antioxidant Supplementation Trial) showed that nutritional supplementation with lutein or lutein with antioxidants, minerals, and vitamins improved visual functions and symptoms in patients with atrophic AMD.

The TOZAL [taurine, omega 3 fatty acid (FA), zinc, antioxidant lutein] study used 18,640 IU natural β-carotene, 10,000 IU vitamin A, 200 IU vitamin E, 69.6 mg zinc, and 1.6 mg copper to decrease the potential side effects. 76.7% patients had stabilization or improvement of best corrected visual acuity (BCVA) at 6 months in this study without reporting any potential ocular or systemic side effects.

It has also been shown that oral supplementation of carotenoids can increase the measured level of macular pigment optical density (MPOD) to a variable degree, and thus MPOD measurements can be one of the ways to evaluate the treatment efficacy of oral supplementation of carotenoids.

MODIFICATION IN AGE-RELATED EYE DISEASE STUDY-2 FORMULATION

Recently there has been extension of AREDS-1 study titled as Age-Related Eye Disease Study-2 (AREDS-2) where the formulation of dietary supplements has been modified

SECTION 7: Retina

and the effect of removing β-carotene, reducing the level of zinc separately, and effect of removing β-carotene and reducing the level of zinc together has been examined and verified.

RESULTS
- Removing the β-carotene and lowering the zinc did not have an effect on the progression rate.
- Lung cancer rates were higher in the β-carotene group, mostly in former smokers.

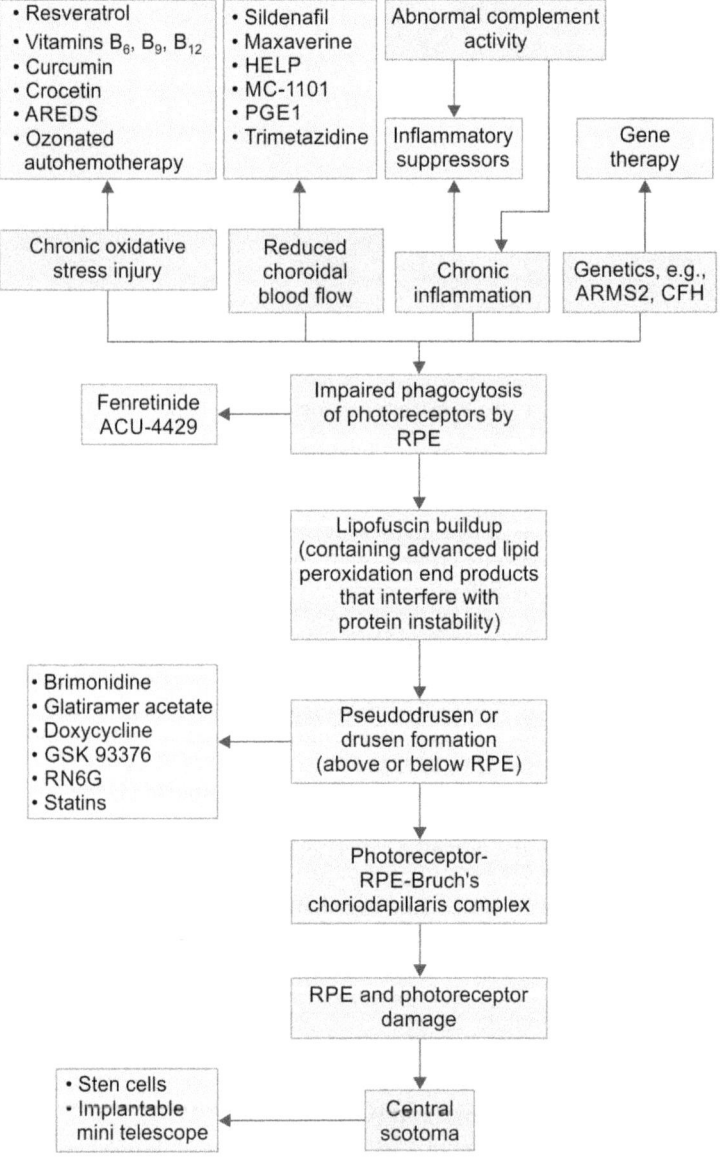

Flowchart 7.43.1: Molecular and physiological targets for treatment modality development in age-related macular degeneration (AMD).

(AREDS: age-related eye disease study; RPE: retinal pigment epithelium)

- Lutein and zeaxanthin are appropriate substitutes for β-carotene.
- Adding lutein and zeaxanthin provided about 20% reduction in the progression beyond the original AREDS with low dietary intake.
- The addition of omega-3 did not reduce the risk of progression.
- The development of cataract was not affected by any of the supplements.
- There was insufficient data to make recommendations about the level of zinc.
- *National Eye Institute recommend AREDS-2 formulation*: Vitamin C: 500 mg, vitamin E: 400 IU, lutein: 10 mg, zeaxanthin: 2 mg, zinc: 80 mg, copper: 2 mg.

There are number of other ongoing clinical trials to assess the role of lampalizumab, GSK933776, fluocinolone insert, MacuCLEAR eye drops, stem cells, sirolimus, and glatiramer in dry AMD but the results are awaited. Recently implantable miniature telescope (IMT) has been approved by US Food and Drug Administration for patients of 65 years and older with bilateral end-stage AMD. It was shown that significant preservation of improvement in best corrected distance visual acuity (BCDVA) is possible using IMT. Mean BCDVA improvement from baseline to 60 months was 2.41 ± 2.69 lines in all patients. Similarly studies to evaluate role of telescopic contact lenses is also underway for AMD management.

From the above it is obvious that there is no established treatment or cure for dry AMD else than prescription of dietary supplementation, change in lifestyle, and consumption of fresh fruits and vegetables on regular basis which may halt the progression of dry AMD **(Flowchart 7.43.1)**.

REFERENCE

1. Bindewald A, Schmitz-Valckenberg S, Jorzik JJ, Dolar-Szczasny J, Sieber H, Keilhauer C, et al. Classification of abnormal fundus autofluorescence patterns in the junctional zone of geographic atrophy in patients with age related macular degeneration. Br J Ophthalmol. 2005;89(7):874-8.

7.44 | Retinoblastoma: Current Update—2022

Usha Singh, Khushdeep Abhaypal
PGIMER, Chandigarh
drushasingh@gmail.com

INTRODUCTION

With the current advances in translational research of retinoblastoma gene (allele-specific assay) it is now possible to identify mutational mosaicism, in nearly 95% of bilaterally affected patients. These observations are likely to have a positive impact on treatment and reducing morbidity.

GENETICS

Current studies using microarray analysis have identified upregulated and downregulated genes localized to specific chromosomes. Even unilateral sporadic tumors may show loss of heterozygosity on chromosome 13 in addition to novel regions of amplification or loss on other chromosomes.[1-2] Sun J et al. have found significant copy number alteration (SCNAs) in enucleated specimens.[3] Recently developed organoids which are similar in all aspects with parental tumor, provide a specific and reliable model for therapeutic targets in retinoblastoma.[4-5]

LIQUID BIOPSY IN RETINOBLASTOMA

A liquid biopsy, or fluid biopsy from blood and aqueous provides noninvasive diagnostic and monitoring tool in retinoblastoma. Berry JL et al. in 2020 verified the presence of cell-free deoxyribonucleic acid (cfDNA) in aqueous humor of retinoblastoma patients which can be used to achieve genetic as well as epigenetic analysis of the tumor.[6] Liquid biopsy used to corroborate the efficacy of chemotherapeutic drugs in these children and prognosticate in cases with recurrence. Aqueous humor circulating tumor deoxyribonucleic acid (ctDNA) has been used to correlate lower tumor load in patients receiving intravitreal injections.[7] In further studies, gain of 6p chromosome was associated with aggressiveness of the tumor increasing the chances of enucleation by 10 times.[8] Tumor-derived cfDNA levels in the plasma of retinoblastoma patients too fell even after one cycle of chemotherapy proven by Kothari et al.[9]

ONCOLYTIC VIRUS VCN-01 TREATMENT IN RETINOBLASTOMA

Genetically modified oncolytic adenovirus (VCN-01) is a class of viruses used to selectively replicate in and terminate tumor cells. It was first demonstrated in 2016 to destroy tumor cells by exhibiting an altered RB1-E2F pathway, sparing the normal cells.[10] They provide exciting therapeutic avenues for retinoblastoma. VCN-01 administration in vitro kills retinoblastoma cultures and is proven to improve ocular survival.[11]

MICRORNAs

MicroRNAs regulate a variety of biological functions, gene expression at post-transcriptional level by inhibiting or destabilizing the transcripts. Various studies have reported the role microRNAs dysregulation in retinoblastoma being involved in its progression. This has prompted further studies to study its exact role.[12,13]

BIOMARKER p53 IN RETINOBLASTOMA

One recent study has shown that p53 and MDMX expression is strongly associated with age at diagnosis, laterality, and *RB* gene expression suggesting a hereditary factor.[14]

PRENATAL DIAGNOSIS OF RETINOBLASTOMA

Parents of familial retinoblastoma patients and families with germline mutations in retinoblastoma seek prenatal diagnosis for future planning. It is now possible to have a noninvasive prenatal diagnosis with the establishment of fetal cfDNA from peripheral maternal blood.[15]

ADVANCES IN IMAGING: SD-OCT IN RETINOBLASTOMA

Spectral-domain optical coherence tomography (SD-OCT) provides virtual biopsies of the retina due to its high resolution. In retinoblastoma it is useful in diagnosis of new lesions, monitoring treatment response, and detecting recurrences. Reports have established utility of SD-OCT in detecting subclinical recurrences.[16,17]

REFERENCES

1. Chakraborty S, Khare S, Dorairaj SK, Prabhakaran VC, Prakash DR, Kumar A. Identification of genes associated with tumorigenesis of retinoblastoma by microarray analysis. Genomics. 2007;90(3):344-53.
2. Ganguly A, Nichols KE, Grant G, Rappaport E, Shields C. Molecular karyotype of sporadic unilateral retinoblastoma tumors. Retina. 2009;29(7):1002-12.
3. Sun J, Xi HY, Shao Q, Liu QH. Biomarkers in retinoblastoma. Int J Ophthalmol. 2020;13(2):325-41.
4. Saengwimol D, Rojanaporn D, Chaitankar V, Chittavanich P, Aroonroch R, Boontawon T, et al. A three-dimensional organoid model recapitulates tumorigenic aspects and drug responses of advanced human retinoblastoma. Sci Rep. 2018;8(1):15664.
5. Lee C, Kim J. Chromatin regulators in retinoblastoma: Biological roles and therapeutic applications. J Cell Physiol. 2020;236(4):2318-32.

6. Jerry JL, Xu L, Polski A, Jubran R, Kuhn P, Kim JW, et al. Aqueous humor is superior to blood as a liquid biopsy for retinoblastoma. Ophthalmology. 2020;127:552-4.
7. Gerrish A, Stone E, Clokie S, Ainsworth JR, Jenkinson H, McCalla M, et al. Non-invasive diagnosis of retinoblastoma using cell-free DNA from aqueous humor. Br J Ophthalmol. 2019;103:721-4.
8. Berry JL, Xu L, Kooi I, Murphree AL, Prabakar RK, Reid M, et al. Genomic cfDNA analysis of aqueous humor in retinoblastoma predicts eye salvage: the surrogate tumor biopsy for retinoblastoma. Mol Cancer Res. 2018;16(11):1701-12.
9. Kothari P, Marass F, Yang JL, Stewart CM, Stephens D, Patel J, et al. Cell-free DNA profiling in retinoblastoma patients with advanced intraocular disease: An MSKCC experience. Cancer Med. 2020;9:6093-6101
10. Martínez-Vélez N, Xipell E, Vera B, Acanda de la Rocha C, Zalacain M, Marrodán L, et al. The oncolytic adenovirus VCN-01 as therapeutic approach against pediatric osteosarcoma. Clin Cancer Res. 2016;22:2217-25.
11. Pascual-Pasto G, Bazan-Peregrino M, Olaciregui NG, Restrepo-Perdomo CA, Mato-Berciano A. Therapeutic targeting of the RB1 pathway in retinoblastoma with the oncolytic adenovirus VCN-01. Sci Transl Med. 2019;11:9321.
12. Martin J, Bryar P, Mets M, Weinstein J, Jones A, Martin A, et al. Differentially expressed miRNAs in retinoblastoma. Gene. 2013;512(2):294-99.
13. Beta M, Khetan V, Chatterjee N, Suganeswari G, Rishi P, Biswas J, et al. EpCAM knockdown alters microRNA expression in retinoblastoma-functional implication of EpCAM regulated miRNA in tumor progression. PLoS One. 2014;9(12):e114800.
14. Martínez-Sánchez M, Moctezuma-Dávila M, Hernandez-Monge J, Rangel-Charqueño M, Olivares-Illana V. Analysis of the p53 pathway in peripheral blood of retinoblastoma patients; potential biomarkers. PLoS One. 2020;15(6):e0234337.
15. Gerrish A, Bowns B, Mashayamombe-Wolfgarten C, Young E, Court S, Bott J, et al. Non-Invasive Prenatal Diagnosis of Retinoblastoma Inheritance by Combined Targeted Sequencing Strategies. J. Clin. Med. 2020;9(11):3517.
16. Rootman DB, Gonzalez E, Mallipatna A, Vandenhoven C, Hampton L, Dimaras H, et al. Hand-held high-resolution spectral domain optical coherence tomography in retinoblastoma: clinical and morphologic considerations. Br J Ophthalmol. 2013;97(1):59-65.
17. Park K, Sioufi K, Shields CL. Clinically invisible retinoblastoma recurrence in an infant. Retina Cases Brief Rep. 2019;13(2):108-10.

7.45 Retinal Breaks and Vitreoretinal Precursors of Retinal Detachment: Diagnosis and Prophylaxis

Vasumathy Vedantham
Radhatri Nethralaya, Chennai
drvasumathy@gmail.com

Retinal breaks and other vitreoretinal precursors of retinal detachment (RD) are best diagnosed by a good indirect ophthalmoscopy and sometimes with a Goldmann three-mirror examination. Till date, there have been no prospective randomized clinical trials to evaluate the treatment of precursor lesions of RDs and interpretation of existing treatment results is not very useful due to the uncertainty of the natural course of the respective lesions. Of all the vitreoretinal lesions causing clinical RD, there is universal agreement that symptomatic horseshoe-shaped tears (HSTs) need prompt treatment, while the value of treating other lesions remains unclear **(Flowchart 7.45.1)**.

Preventive therapy is however desirable in the second eye (fellow eye) of patients with previous RD in the first eye and in patients with high-risk factors such as myopia, family history of RD, postcataract extraction, etc. **Flowcharts 7.45.2 and 7.45.3** are

Flowchart 7.45.1: Symptomatic eyes with acute posterior vitreous detachment.

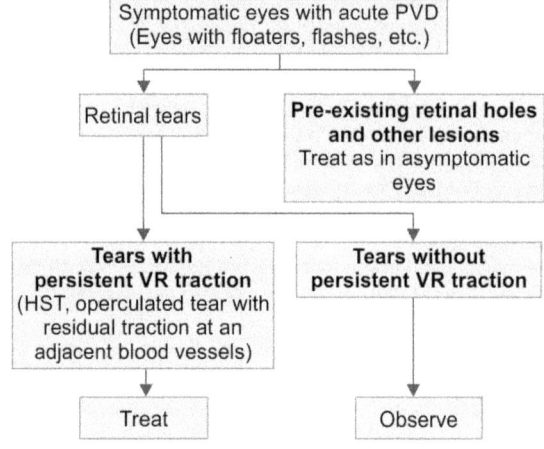

Flowchart 7.45.2: Asymptomatic fellow eyes.

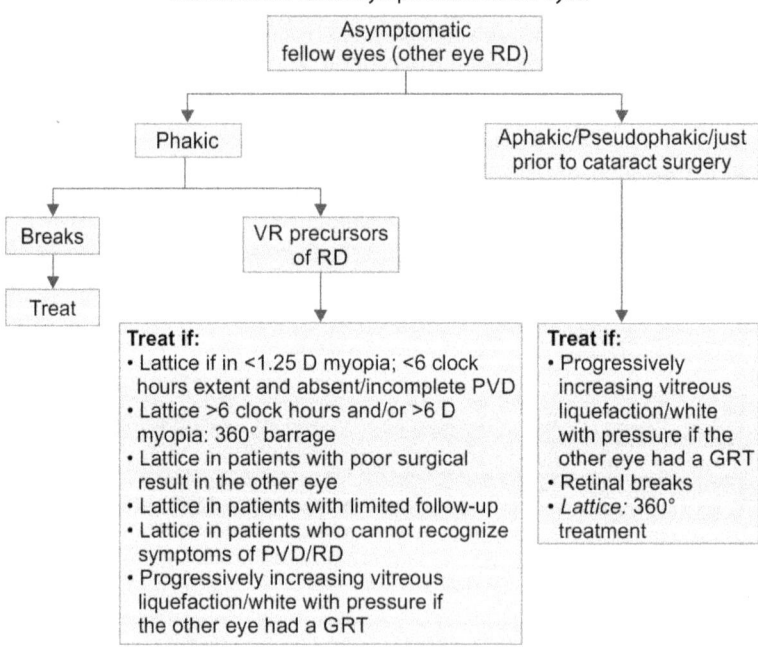

designed to provide basic guidelines in this regard. For simplification, the eyes can be categorized into those with symptoms due to acute posterior vitreous detachment (PVD) (symptomatic) and those without (asymptomatic). It is important to call back patients with acute PVD and no breaks for a second examination within 6 weeks as there is a 2% chance of the developing new breaks. Laser/cryoprophylaxis of the tear should be adequate and cover the anterior edge of the lesions and if not possible, treatment should extend to the ora serrata.

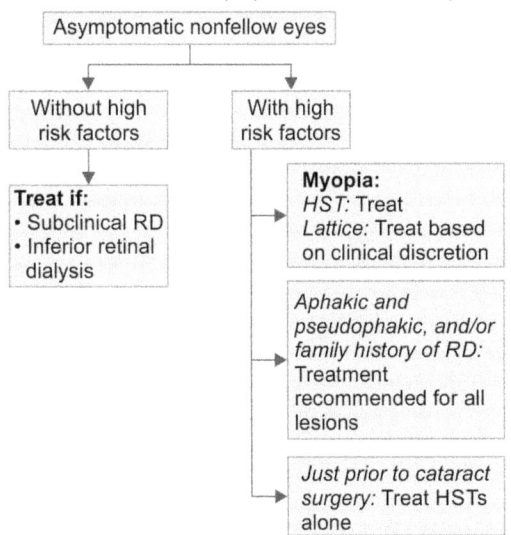

Flowchart 7.45.3: Asymptomatic nonfellow eyes.

SUGGESTED READING

1. American Academy of Ophthalmology. Posterior vitreous detachment, retinal breaks and lattice degeneration. Preferred practice pattern. San Francisco: American Academy of Ophthalmology; 2019.

7.46 Optical Coherence Tomography

Vishali Gupta, Mansi Sharma
Advanced Eye Center, PGIMER, Chandigarh
vishalisara@yahoo.co.in, dr.mansi.sharma@gmail.com

INTRODUCTION

Optical coherence tomography (OCT) enables noncontrast high resolution, cross-sectional, and in vivo imaging of tissue structure.

Optical coherence tomography can be used for both anterior and posterior segment imaging.

Optical coherence tomography in retina is particularly useful as it gives both quantitative and qualitative measurements.

PRINCIPLE

When light is directed into the eye, it is reflected from the tissue boundaries and backscattered with different intensities from tissues with different optical properties, distances and dimensions of different tissue structures can be determined by echo time delay of light back reflected or backscattered from structures at varying axial distances.

It is based on principle of interferometry wherein one optical beam is compared with another reference optical beam, to measure optical distances with tens of microns of resolution **(Fig. 7.46.1)**.

Retinal imaging is performed using infrared light at 800 nm.

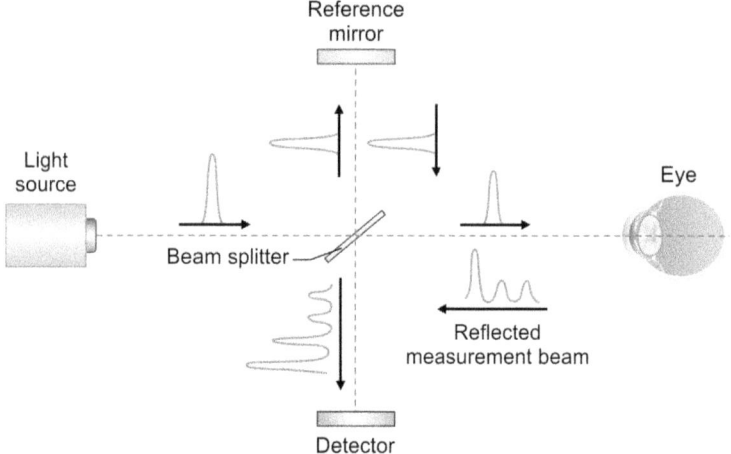

Fig. 7.46.1: Physics of optical coherence tomography devices.

■ TIME DOMAIN VERSUS SPECTRAL DOMAIN

In contrast to time domain which measures echoes as a function of delay, spectral domain (SD) measures all the echoes of light simultaneously owing to which it is highly sensitive, and imaging is much faster up to 50–100 times.

Better quality, highly accurate imaging, greater coverage, and reduced motion artifacts (due to higher speed of imaging and greater number of cross-sectional images) are its advantages.

■ OCT IN NORMAL RETINA

Retina is divided histologically into 10 distinct layers, including cell layers and neuronal interconnections **(Fig. 7.46.2)**.

Retinal nerve fiber layer, plexiform layers are highly backscattering appear bright on spectral-domain optical coherence tomography (SD-OCT), red on false color.

In contrast weak optically backscattering nuclear layers, i.e., ganglion cell layers, inner nuclear layers, outer nuclear layer, appear dark on SD-OCT, blue green on false color.

Boundary between photoreceptors IS and OS (inner segment and outer segment) is thin and highly backscattering band immediately anterior to retinal pigment epithelium (RPE) and choroid, reflection from this structure may be as a result of refractive index difference between photoreceptors IS and highly organized structure of OS containing stacks of membranous discs, rich in visual pigment rhodopsin.

Retinal pigment epithelium which contains melanin is also highly backscattering.

Choriocapillaris is vascular and strongly backscattering.

■ OCT SCANNING AND IMAGING PROTOCOLS

Scans of Macula

Three-dimensional Cube Scan

Three-dimensional structural information can be obtained using SD-OCT to acquire volumetric cubes of data **(Fig. 7.46.3)**.

Line Scan

The line scan gives an option of acquiring multiple line scans without returning to main window. The default angle is 0° and the nasal position is defined as 0°. The length of the

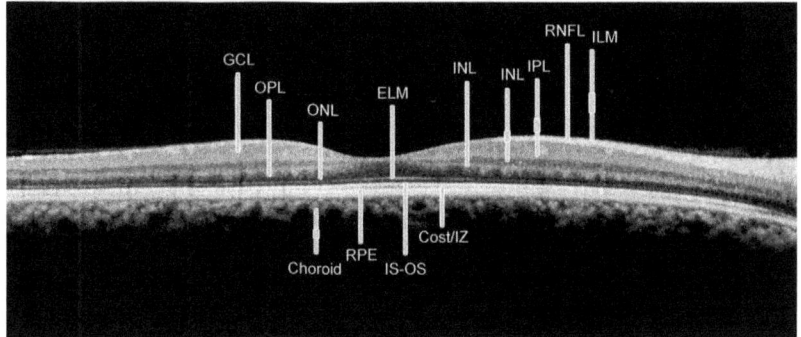

Fig. 7.46.2: OCT scan showing various retinal layers.

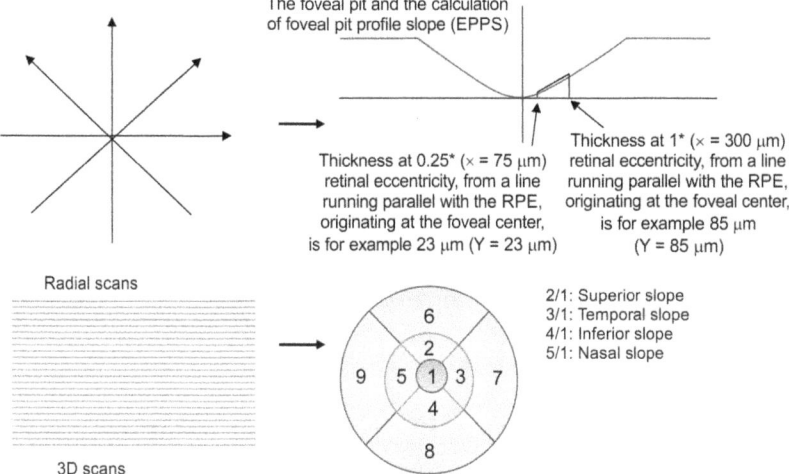

Fig. 7.46.3: Various scan protocols available for scanning the macula using OCT.

line scan can be altered, though one has to keep in mind that as the scan length increases, the resolution decreases.

By default, the length of line scan is 5 mm (A). Useful in acquiring images in high detail of retinal tissue because of high sampling density **(Figs. 7.46.4 and 7.46.5)**.

Raster

In this protocol we can acquire series of line scans that are parallel, equally spaced, and are 6–24 in number. Useful in obtaining scans at multiple levels.

Radial

This scan protocol consists of 6–24 equally spaced line scans that can be varied in size and parameters. All the lines pass through central common axis. The default setting has six lines of 6-mm length.

Repeat

This protocol enables us to repeat scan in consecutive visits using same set of parameters as used in previous protocol, especially helpful to monitor retinal changes.

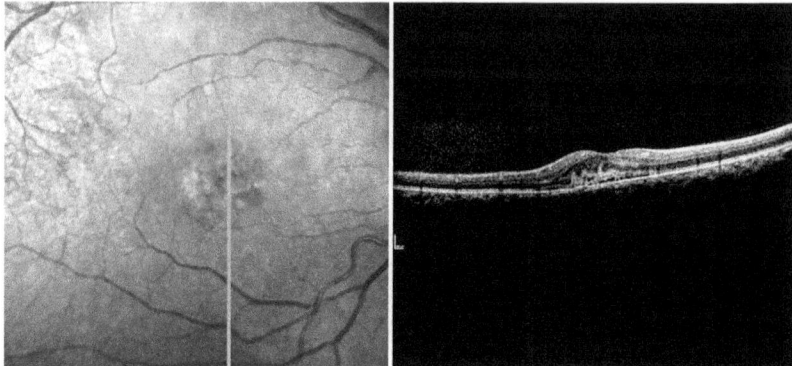

Fig. 7.46.4: Vertical line scan.

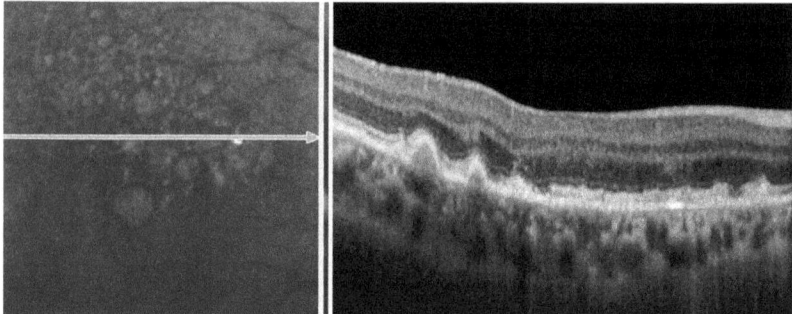

Fig. 7.46.5: Horizontal line scan.

■ QUANTITATIVE MEASUREMENTS OF RETINAL MORPHOLOGY

Retinal thickness measurement is done using computer image processing algorithms which automatically identify superficial and deep neurosensory retina boundaries to measure retinal thickness.

Quantification helps in tracking progression and monitoring response to intervention (**Fig. 7.46.6**).

■ OPTICAL COHERENCE TOMOGRAPHY IN RETINAL PATHOLOGY

General

Analysis of reflective pattern can help broadly classify lesions on OCT as:
- Hyperreflective—such as hard exudates, blood, scars, etc.
- Hyporeflective—serous fluid.

Diabetic Macular Edema

- Defining disease pattern (**Figs. 7.46.7 to 7.46.11**).
- Also useful in monitoring response to intervention at ultrastructural levels.
- Makes it relatively simpler to identify cases which will need surgical intervention, otherwise difficult to pick up on conventional modalities.

Macular Hole

Optical coherence tomography is useful in diagnosing and management of macular holes.

SECTION 7: Retina

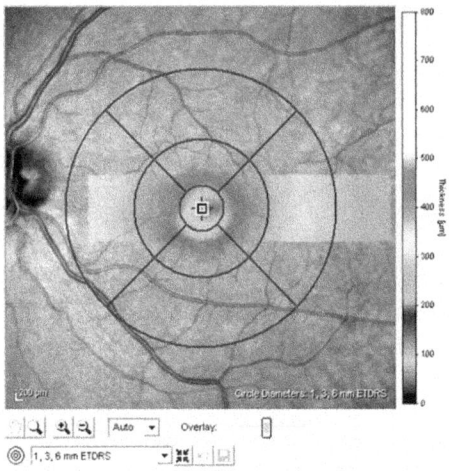
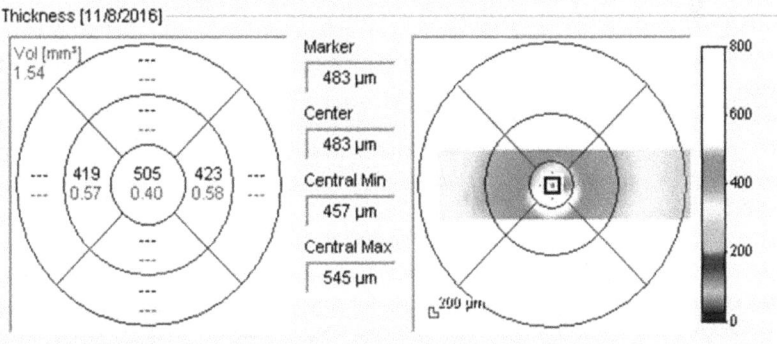

Fig. 7.46.6: Macular thickness measured using optical coherence tomography.

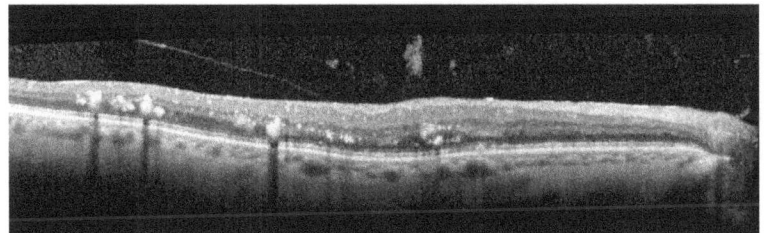

Fig. 7.46.7: Spongy retinal thickness.

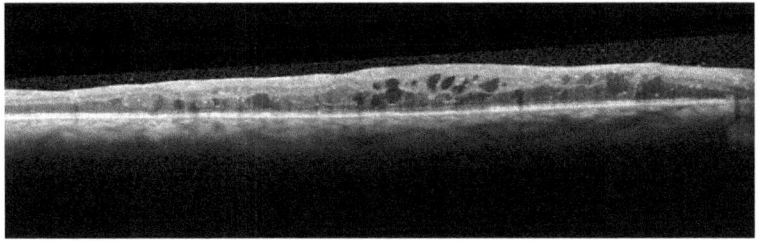

Fig. 7.46.8: Cystoid macular edema.

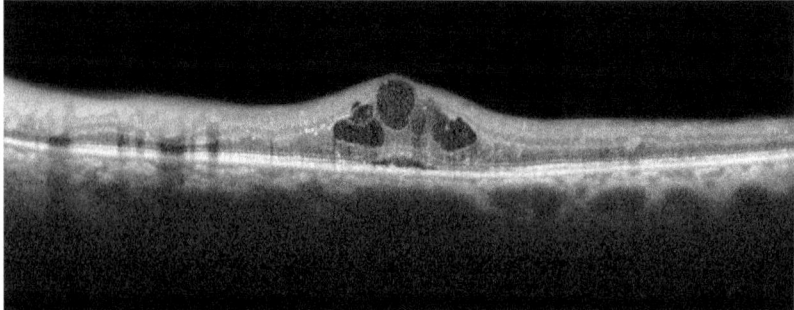

Fig. 7.46.9: Serous retinal detachment.

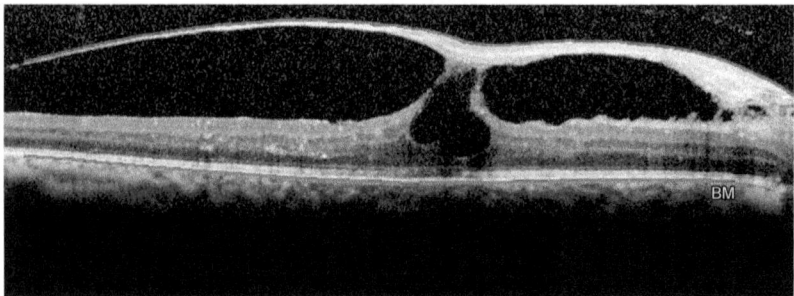

Fig. 7.46.10: Foveal tractional retinal detachment.

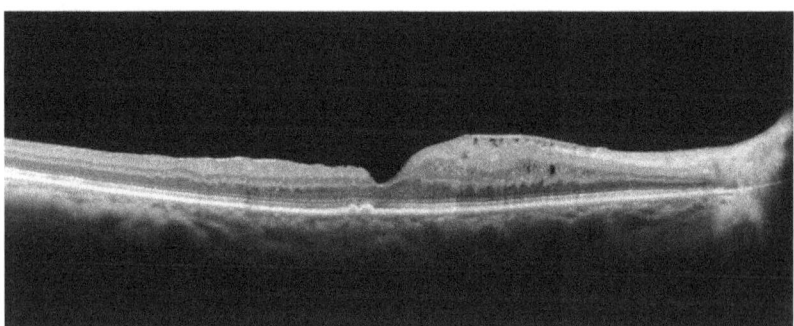

Fig. 7.46.11: Taut posterior hyaloid membrane.

CLASSIFICATION BASED ON OPTICAL COHERENCE TOMOGRAPHY

Stage 1A: Foveal pseudocyst.

Stage 1B: Impending macular hole and disruption of outer retina.

Stage 2: Lamellar macular hole.

Stage 3: Full thickness macular hole without PVD (posterior vitreous detachment).

Stage 4: Full thickness macular hole with PVD.

Based on macular hole size analyzed on OCT, it is also useful in prognosticating response to therapeutic intervention.

Also analysis of pattern of closure postsurgical intervention can be done **(Figs. 7.46.12 and 7.46.13)**.

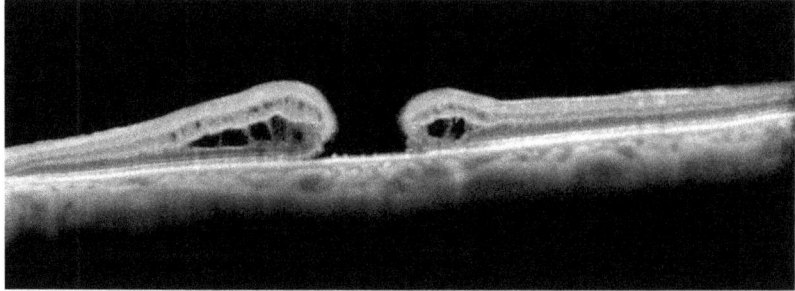

Fig. 7.46.12: Full thickness macular hole.

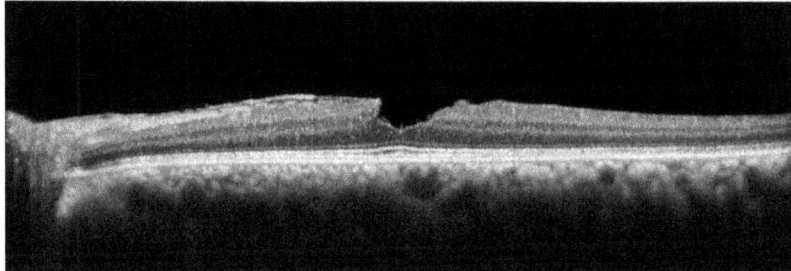

Fig. 7.46.13: Lamellar macular hole.

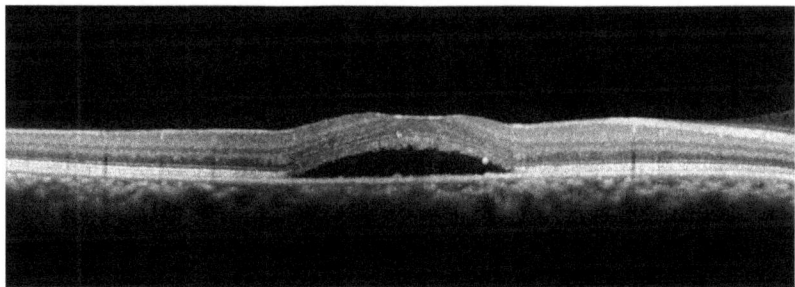

Fig. 7.46.14: Idiopathic central serous chorioretinopathy.

■ IDIOPATHIC CENTRAL SEROUS CHORIORETINOPATHY

Accumulation of fluid in between retinal pigment epithelium and neurosensory retina can be easily picked up; also differentiation between pigment epithelial detachment (PED) and neurosensory detachment can be made easily **(Fig. 7.46.14)**.

Retinal Vascular Occlusions

Optical coherence tomography is vital in management and diagnosis of retinal vein occlusions, wherein they show intraretinal fluid accumulation, serous retinal detachment, cystoids macular edema, and vitreoretinal traction including epiretinal membranes.

Quantification and tomography of macular edema help in monitoring response to therapeutic intervention with rapid noninvasive method **(Fig. 7.46.15)**.

Epiretinal Membranes

Optical coherence tomography helps in diagnosis and evaluating adhesiveness of the epiretinal membranes to the underlying retina, clearly marks its full extent, and also associated changes such as macular hole, vitreofoveal traction, and status of posterior hyaloids which are useful in planning and prognosticating surgery **(Fig. 7.46.16)**.

Age-related Macular Degeneration

Generally classified into: (a) neovascular and (b) non-neovascular.

Primarily and age-related pathology affecting choriocapillaris, Bruch's membrane, and RPE.

■ NON-NEOVASCULAR

- Drusenoid deposits can be pigment up as focal elevation of the RPE with shallow borders and no optical shadowing **(Fig. 7.46.17)**.
- Advanced cases with geographic atrophy show well demarcated retinal pigment epithelium and choriocapillaris atrophy.

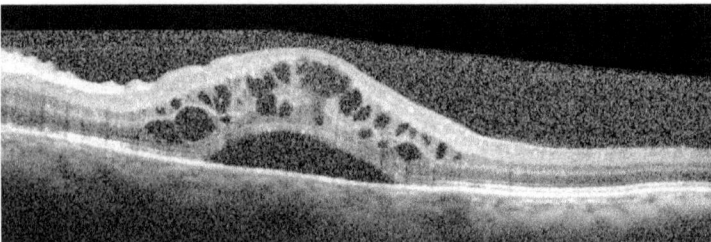

Fig. 7.46.15: Retinal vein occlusion.

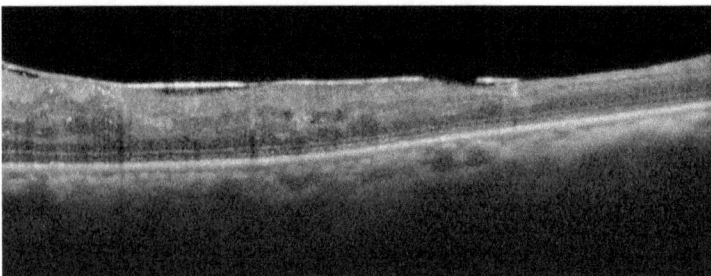

Fig. 7.46.16: Epiretinal membrane.

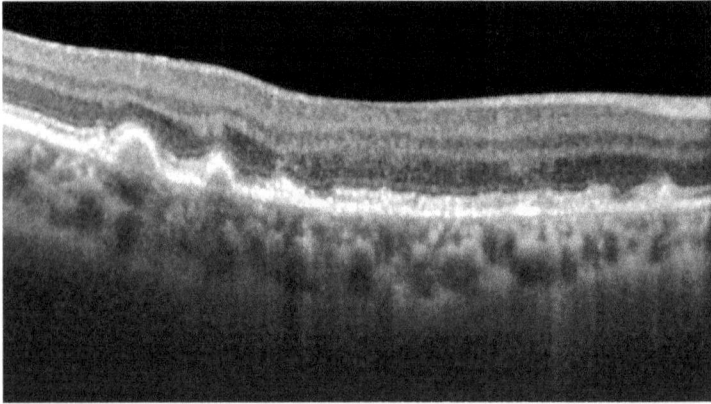

Fig. 7.46.17: Non-neovascular age-related macular degeneration.

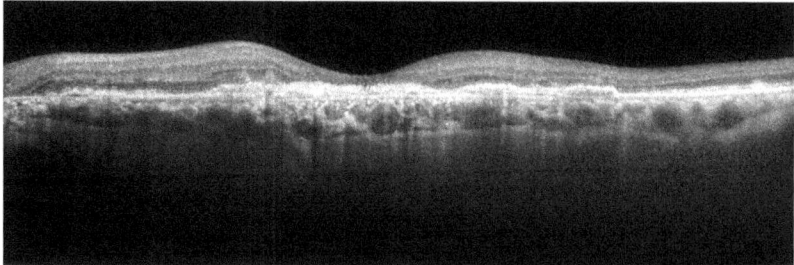

Fig. 7.46.18: Neovascular age-related macular degeneration.

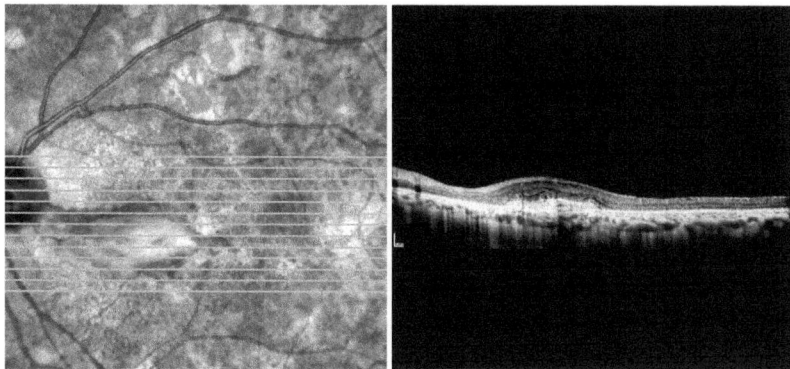

Fig. 7.46.19: Inflammatory diseases of retina and choroid.

■ NEOVASCULAR

Classic CNVM (choroidal neovascular membranes) is characterized by highly thickened reflective continuous band of RPE—choriocapillaris complex. It can additionally show cystoid spaces and subretinal fluid.

Occult CNVM is characterized by disruption of RPE-choriocapillaris complex where the boundaries are poorly defined.

Serous PED, hemorrhagic PEDs, and fibrovascular PED can also be seen **(Fig. 7.46.18)**.

Inflammatory Diseases of Retina—Choroid

Optical coherence tomography enables us to identify the extent, depth, and thickness of inflammatory lesions that helps in accurate localization of the retina choroid harboring the lesion which is extremely useful in diagnosis and monitoring progress as well as response to treatment.

Also associated secondary changes of cystoids macular edema, CNVM, epiretinal membrane, and subretinal fluid can be evaluated **(Fig. 7.46.19)**.

■ CONCLUSION

Optical coherence tomography as a diagnostic tool is immensely useful to perform cross-sectional imaging of biological tissues and easy accessibility of retinal tissues to light makes it ideal for management of retinal disorders.

Optical coherence tomography yields information about retinal tomography akin to conventional topographic techniques.

Especially with newer SD-OCT better visualization of retinal pathology with much higher resolution can be done making it an indispensable tool in current vitreoretinal disorder management.

7.47 Central Serous Chorioretinopathy

Manpreet Brar
Grewal Eye Institute, Chandigarh
dr.manpreetbrar@gmail.com

■ INTRODUCTION

Central serous chorioretinopathy (CSCR) is an idiopathic condition affecting young males in the age group of 30–50 years that causes visual impairment due to leakage of fluid in the macula. A dysfunction in the activity of the retinal pigment epithelium (RPE) and an increased vascular choroidal hyperpermeability seem to play a decisive role in the fluid collection.

■ TYPES OF CSCR

Depending on the duration the disease it is classified into acute and chronic CSCR.

Acute CSCR

The acute form presents with sudden onset painless blurred vision, usually unilateral. It is more commonly seen in people who are stressed, type A personalities, disturbed sleep pattern, or intake of steroids in any form (skin creams, inhalers, and oral steroids). On fundus examination, serous detachment of neurosensory retina is seen as a round well-defined transparent lesion at the central macula, yellowish subretinal material which is due to fibrin may also be seen (**Fig. 7.47.1A**). Optical coherence tomography scans are the most common noninvasive diagnostic modality to confirm the presence of subretinal fluid at the macula. Enhanced depth imaging optical coherence tomography (EDI-OCT) based studies have shown increased choroidal thickness in eyes with CSC as well as in the fellow eyes, compared to normal healthy subjects (**Fig. 7.47.1B**). Fundus fluorescein angiography helps to confirm the diagnosis by identifying the characteristic leakage pattern, i.e., either ink blot or smokestack pattern (**Figs. 7.47.1C and D**). On OCT angiography, no specific pattern has been observed, but it might be useful to differentiate CSCR from acute Vogt-Koyanagi-Harada (VKH). Optical coherence tomography angiography (OCTA) en-face images showed apparent areas of choriocapillaris *flow void* due to shadowing effect from overlying subretinal fluid and pigment epithelial detachment in CSC. However, eyes with VKH showed presence of *true* choriocapillaris flow void on OCTA that corresponded to choriocapillaris ischemia on indocyanine green angiography (ICGA) (**Fig. 7.47.2**). Acute CSCR usually resolves within 3 months in 90% of the patients without any treatment, sometimes leaving color vision and contrast discrimination difficulties in a few patients. Focal laser photocoagulation was the standard treatment option in nonresolving CSCR in the past that was effective in resolution of fluid in 80% of the cases (**Figs. 7.47.3A to F**). However, no consensus exists regarding the management. Subthreshold laser and half-fluence photodynamic therapy, diuretics are the other common treatment modalities.

Chronic CSCR

In many patients, it is a recurrent problem where the fluid builds up in the macula but does not resolve spontaneously. If the conditions persist beyond 6 months, it is then called chronic CSR. In recent times, chronic CSR is considered a disease entity under pachychoroid spectrum and history of organ transplantation; autoimmune diseases maintained on low dose oral corticosteroids for long duration are the common risk factors to develop chronic CSCR. The shallow subretinal fluid persists in the retina causes permanent RPE damage leading to irreversible visual loss. The pathophysiology of chronic CSC is complex and remains to be fully elucidated. However, it is thought

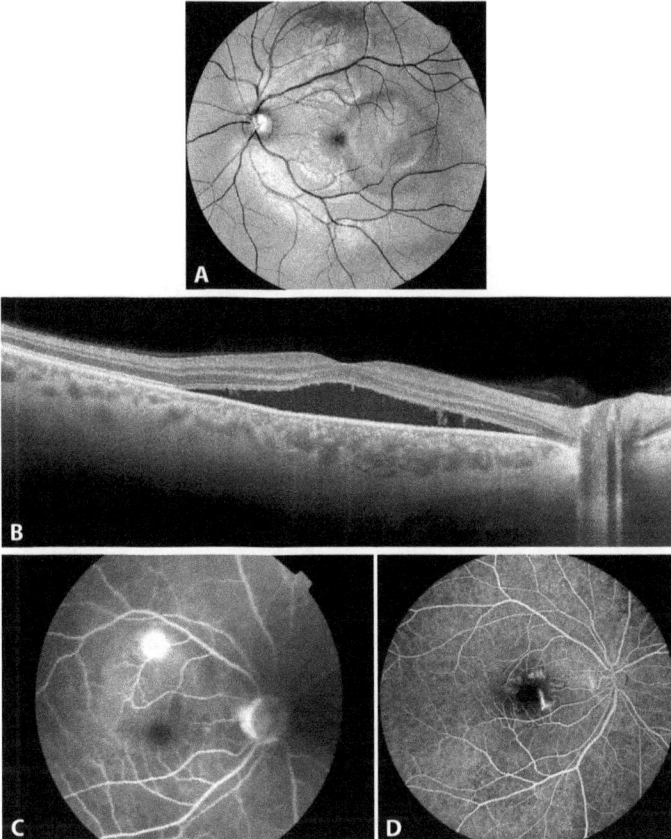

Figs. 7.47.1A to D: (A) The color fundus photograph shows a well-defined round elevated grayish lesion in the temporal macula suggestive of localized neurosensory detachment in patient with central serous chorioretinopathy. In the central part of neurosensory detachment, there is a ring like yellowish subretinal nodular deposits consistent with fibrin deposition; (B) Swept source optical coherence tomography photograph demonstrating sensory detachment of macula and increased choroidal thickness; (C) The fluorescein angiogram shows ink blot pattern of leakage in the extrafoveal region; (D) FFA identified a hyperfluorescent RPE point leakage in the early phase that rises in a smoke stack pattern.

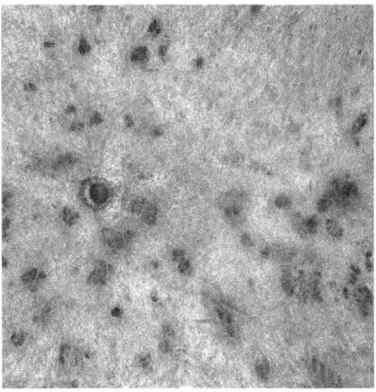

Fig. 7.47.2: ICG angiography.

that diffuse RPE decompensation impairs subretinal fluid absorption. Furthermore, indocyanine angiography studies have revealed alteration in choroidal permeability with changes in choroidal vascularity and a thickened choroid, perhaps leading to progressive fluid accumulation. Chronic CSCR is characterized by widespread RPE changes, pigment clumping, and RPE atrophy, develop gravitational descending tracts in inferior retina with RPE changes due to long standing accumulation of subretinal fluid. Chronic shallow subretinal fluid is best seen on OCT **(Figs. 7.47.4A to D)**. There is also

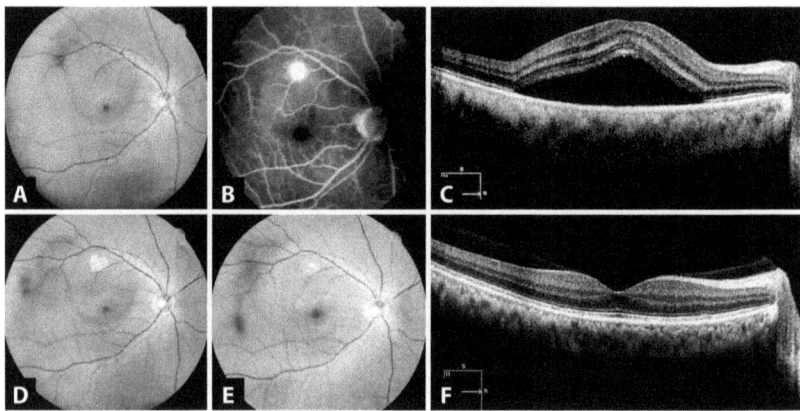

Figs. 7.47.3A to F: Typical case of acute CSCR (A) with extrafoveal leak on FFA (B) and subretinal fluid at the macula on OCT macula (C). Patient was treated with focal laser photocoagulation (D) and 6 week later laser scars are visible (E) with complete resolution of subretinal fluid on OCT (F).

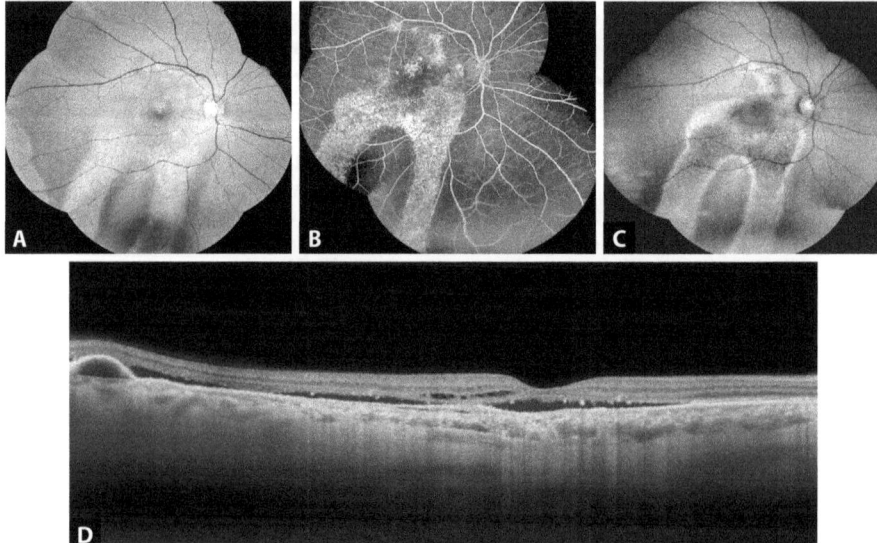

Figs. 7.47.4A to D: (A) Case of chronic central serous chorioretinopathy demonstrating inferior retinal tracts (diffuse retinal pigment epitheliopathy); (B) FFA shows multiple pinpoint leaks at the level of RPE suggestive of chronic CSCR along with an inferior tract of hyperfluorescent RPE staining; (C) Fundus autofluorescence of a descending tract in CSCR: Marked hypoautofluorescence suggests chronic disease and irreversible RPE damage surrounded by a hyperautofluorescent ring; (D) Swept source OCT scan demonstrating shallow subretinal fluid, few intraretinal cystic fluid pockets are also present due to chronicity of the disease condition.

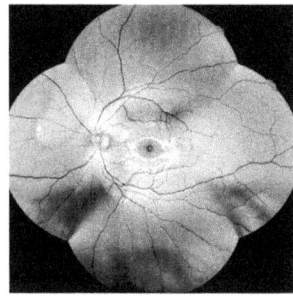

Fig. 7.47.5: Extramacular variant of central serous chorioretinopathy: Left fundus photograph of the same patient—macula was normal but nasal midperiphery shows round area of neurosensory detachment.

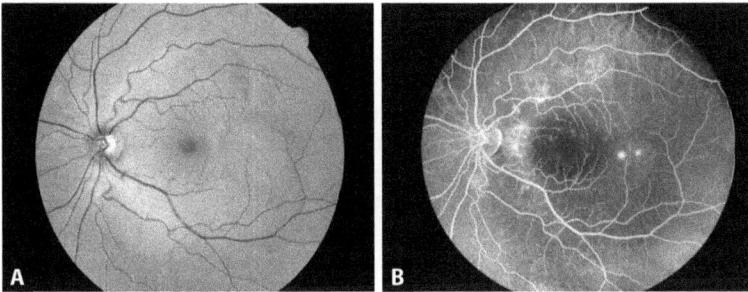

Figs. 7.47.6A and B: (A) Color fundus photograph of a case of multifocal central serous chorioretinopathy. Three scattered patches of retinal elevation were seen at the posterior pole; (B) FFA was suggestive of multiple RPE pinpoint leaks all along the posterior pole. Note the optic disc is normal unlike in VKH.

an increase in risk of choroidal neovascular membranes (CNVM) in cases of chronic CSR. Chronic CSCR are difficult to treat, photodynamic therapy, micropulse laser treatment, and anti-VEGF (antivascular endothelial growth factor) injections have been used with varying results.

OTHER TYPES OF CSCR

Extramacular CSCR
Even though the hallmark of CSCR is the presence of serous detachment of neurosensory retina in the posterior pole, but at times episodes may be limited to extramacular region that usually go undetected as they are asymptomatic.

Multifocal CSCR
Multifocal CSCR is a rare variant characterized by accumulation of subretinal fluid at the posterior pole of the fundus causing multiple areas of serous retinal detachment. Inflammatory disorder VKH is a common differential. Clinical history (absence of headaches/pain/tinnitus), absence of inflammatory cells on slit lamp examination, and fluorescein angiogram help to differentiate a CSCR from VKH.

Pregnancy-induced CSCR
Pregnancy, predisposed by endogenous hypercortisolism, probably represents a risk factor for central serous chorioretinopathy. Most CSCR heals spontaneously in 4–8 weeks postpartum, with recovery of visual acuity within 3–6 months.

SUGGESTED READING
1. Battaglia Parodi M, Arrigo A, Iacono P, Falcomatà B, Bandello F. Central Serous Chorioretinopathy: Treatment with Laser. Pharmaceuticals (Basel). 2020;13(11):359.

2. Chumbley LC, Frank RN. Central serous retinopathy, and pregnancy. Am J Ophthalmol. 1974;77(2):158-60.
3. Mudvari SS, Goff MJ, Fu AD, McDonald HR, Johnson RN, Ai E, et al. The natural history of pigment epithelial detachment associated with central serous chorioretinopathy. Retina. 2007; 27(9):1168-73.

7.48 Macular Function Tests for Patients Undergoing Cataract Surgery

Lingam Gopal
Sankara Nethralaya, Chennai
drlg@snmail.org

■ INTRODUCTION

Cataract surgery is the most common ophthalmic surgery performed by ophthalmologists. In view of the high expectation, there is need for proper prognostication. Macular diseases are also common in the age group when cataract surgery is needed. In the presence of medial opacity (cataract), the evaluation of the macula by clinical examination may be difficult and can potentially result in less-than-optimal postoperative outcomes. Tests are available to evaluate the macular integrity and function as well as to determine the potential recovery of vision after cataract surgery. It must be emphasized that none of them gives a foolproof prognosis for vision. The errors in estimates can go both ways—under and overestimation.

■ EYES WITH MILD-TO-MODERATE LENS OPACITIES

Structural Evaluation

1. *Direct macular evaluation:* Slit-lamp biomicroscopic evaluation is the best way of evaluating the anatomical integrity of the macula. Posterior polar opacities may however preclude proper evaluation of the same.
2. *Optical coherence tomography (OCT):* OCT scanning of the macula gives a very good structural evaluation. Features, such as macular hole, epiretinal membrane, foveal thickening, etc., can be detected. With increasing degree of cataract, the quality of the pictures deteriorates and may fail to give proper information. However, considering the infrared wavelength that is used, OCT can surprisingly give clear pictures even in the presence of significant cataracts.

Functional Evaluation

Pinhole Acuity

Principle: Pinhole eliminates optical aberrations and improves the vision.

Interpretation: In the presence of gross opacities, pinhole does not improve the vision. The test is less reliable in eyes with best corrected visual acuity less than 6/60. Pinhole potential acuity test was found more predictive than potential acuity meter (PAM) for eyes with best-corrected vision better than 6/60.[1]

Photo Stress Test

Principle: The macula is exposed to bright light for 10 seconds (using direct ophthalmoscope light) and the time taken for recovery original minus one line Snellen's vision is measured.

Interpretation: Normal recovery time is 20–30 seconds. Prolonged recovery time beyond 50 seconds indicates macular dysfunction.

Blue Field Entoptoscopy

Principle: When patients are made to look at a bright blue light, they notice flying corpuscles. This effect is produced by the WBC in the perifoveal capillaries and, hence, reflects indirectly the circulation in the macular area.

Interpretation: 99% of normal subjects visualize at least 15 or more corpuscles seen equally in different quadrants. Abnormal results are indicated by reduced number in one or more quadrants. Reasonable grasp and intelligence is needed to perform the test. Hence, a positive response is of more benefit in interpretation than negative one. This test was found to perform better than two-point discrimination test or Purkinje vascular entopic phenomenon test.[2]

Yellow Filter Test of Koch

If a transparent yellow filter is placed over reading material, it is noted to improve vision in eyes with macular degeneration but deteriorate the vision in eyes with only cataract.

Potential Acuity Meter

Principle: A miniature visual acuity chart is projected on the retina through areas of clarity in the lens and patient asked to read the letters. Focusing of the chart is done to permit patient to see clearly.

Interpretation: Best results are achieved in cataracts that have not progressed beyond 6/60 level. In general, if more than four-line improvement is predicted, the prognosis after cataract surgery is likely to be good. A predictive capability of 90% and above has been reported.[3] False-positives have been seen with some maculopathies. In general, it is supposed to underestimate rather than overestimate the recovery.

Laser Interferometry

Principle: Helium-neon laser provides a collimated beam that is optically split into two. The two beams are projected through clear spaces in the lens to meet behind the lens. This produces interference fringes. The size and orientation of the stripes so produced can be varied.

Interpretation: The patient is expected to identify correctly the orientation of the stripe as the test is repeated with finer stripes. Unlike the PAM test, focusing is not needed and so the refractive error does not affect the test. However, aphakic eyes are best tested with corrective lens. A conversion table indicates the maximal potential vision. The test tends to overpredict the visual potential in amblyopic eyes.

Lotmar Visometer

Principle: This test is similar to laser interferometer but uses white light instead of laser, and hence is less expensive. Moiré fringes are formed using two rotatable equal gratings. The fringes are split into two coherent beams and projected through pupil.

Interpretation: Interference stripes formed are similar to laser interferometry and interpretation is also similar. The predictions are in general more optimistic especially with macular diseases.

Illuminated Near Card Assessment

Principle: The device is a handheld instrument containing a brightly illuminated vision chart that is transported across a 7 mm by 38 mm viewing window. Visual angle subtended at 16 inches equals that subtended by a letter at 20 feet.

Interpretation: Illuminated near card (INC) was found to be more predictive in eyes with comorbid disease, in contrast to interferometers and PAM.

Vryghem Macular Function Test[4]

Principle: A simplified method of using near vision chart, the Vryghem test uses the Parinaud's near vision chart, a +8.00 diopter lens, and the Heine ophthalmoscope. The vision chart is placed 12 cm from the patient. +8.00 diopter lens is placed over the best distance vision correction in a trial frame. The chart is illuminated with the Heine ophthalmoscope light. Those reading the smallest numbers (Parinaud 1) are expected to be having good macular function.

Multifocal Electroretinogram

It can potentially indicate the macular function. However, dense cataracts do not permit multifocal electroretinogram (MFERG).

EYES WITH DENSE CATARACT

In eyes with dense cataract the approach to assess the potential for visual recovery would be different compared to those with mild-to-moderate cataracts. Here one must contend with the possibility of neither being able to see the macula clinically nor being able to image the same. Sometimes even the status of the retina (attached or detached) may not be possible to evaluate clinically and would need ultrasound examination.

Guidance from History

Perusal of old medical records can be of value to decipher previous notifications of macular diseases. History of poor vision since childhood can be due to amblyopia.

Clinical Evaluation

- *Perception of light and accurate projection:* Although accurate projection is encouraging, it excludes only large retinal detachments and absolute field defects and not macular diseases. Similarly, dense cataracts can so scatter light that inaccurate projection can still be compatible with good visual recovery.
- *Two-point discrimination:* Ability to distinguish two lights close together is a good sign but cannot exclude macular disease.
- *Color perception:* Although ability to identify colors is suggestive of potentially good macular function, macular degeneration is known to exist with good color perception.
- *Pupillary assessment:* This is perhaps the best objective evidence for presence or lack of gross posterior segment disease. Both extensive retinal disease and optic nerve disorders will produce afferent pupillary defect. Even total cataracts are known not to produce afferent pupillary defect if posterior segment is normal. However macular disorders are not excluded even if pupils are brisk.
- *Entopic visualization:* Eber and Friedman described a test wherein a light is gently rubbed on closed eye lids to-and-fro against the sclera. This can stimulate Purkinje vascular tree images. While some patients can detect the optic disc shadow and macula, others may not appreciate the detail despite having good macular function. It is most useful to compare between the two eyes.
- *Maddox rod test:* If light is shone behind a Maddox rod held in front of the eye, a continuous red streak will be made out. A break in the line indicates possible central scotoma.

A high index of suspicion is needed to suspect macular problems when there is mismatch between the vision and the degree of cataract. Information from more than one way of evaluation is needed for proper conclusions.

REFERENCES

1. Melki SA, Safar A, Martin J, Ivanova A, Adi M. Potential acuity pinhole: a simple method to measure potential visual acuity in patients with cataracts, comparison to potential acuity meter. Ophthalmology. 1999;106(7):1262-7.

2. Sinclair SH, Loebl M, Riva CE. Blue field entoptic phenomenon in cataract patients. Arch Ophthalmol. 1979;97(6):1092-5.
3. Ing MR. Potential acuity meter to predict postoperative visual acuity. J Cataract Refract Surg. 1986;12(1):34-5.
4. Vryghem JC, Van Cleynenbreugel H, Van Calster J, Leroux K. Predicting cataract surgery results using a macular function test. J Cataract Refract Surg. 2004;30(11):2349-53.

7.49 Other Causes of Choroidal Neovascularization

Rohan Chawla, Shakha Gupta
Dr RP Centre for Ophthalmic Sciences, AIIMS, New Delhi
dr.rohanrpc@gmail.com

INTRODUCTION

Choroidal neovascularization (CNV) is abnormal proliferation and extension of choriocapillaris through Bruch's membrane into the subretinal pigment epithelial or subretinal space.

On the basis of extension it can be classified into three types:
1. Type I—extends into subretinal pigment epithelial space.
2. Type II—extends into subretinal space.
3. Type III—extends into retina.

CAUSES

The cause of choroidal neovascular membrane (CNVM) could be any factor leading to break in integrity of Bruch's membrane and stimulating abnormal proliferation of the choriocapillaris. It can be broadly divided into:
- *Degenerative:*
  - Age-related macular degeneration
  - Parafoveal telangiectasia
  - Myopia
  - Angioid streaks
  - Postcentral serous chorioretinopathy or related to pachychoroid
  - *Hereditary causes:*
    - Vitelliform macular dystrophy
    - Fundus flavimaculatus
    - Optic nerve head drusen
- *Inflammatory:*
  - White dot syndromes:
    - Punctate inner choroiditis
    - Multifocal choroiditis and panuveitis
    - Serpiginous choroiditis
    - Birdshot chorioretinopathy
  - *Panuveitis:*
    - Vogt-Koyanagi-Harada syndrome
    - Sympathetic ophthalmia
    - Behçet's disease
- *Infectious:*
  - Ocular histoplasmosis syndrome
  - Toxoplasmosis
  - Toxocariasis
  - Rubella
- *Tumor:*
  - Choroidal nevus
  - Choroidal hemangioma

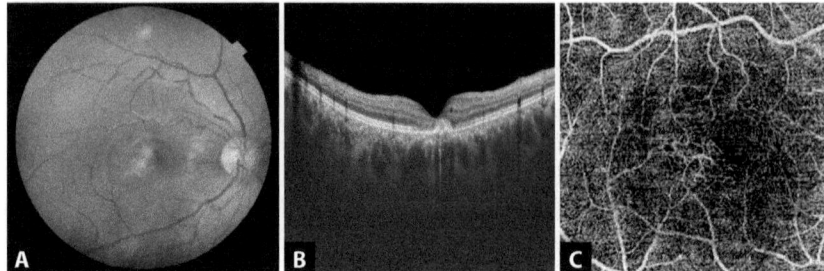

Figs. 7.49.1A to C: *Multimodal imaging of idiopathic CNVM.* (A) A yellowish lesion adjacent to fovea; (B) OCT shows a subretinal hyper-reflective membrane. Note there is no significant subretinal or intraretinal fluid; (C) OCTA shows the neovascular network in the parafoveal region.

- Metastatic choroidal tumors
- Hamartoma of retinal pigment epithelium
- *Trauma:*
    - Choroidal rupture
    - Intense photocoagulation
- Idiopathic CNVM **(Figs. 7.49.1A to C)**

PATHOPHYSIOLOGY

Prerequisites for CNVM formation generally are:
- Damage to Bruch's and pigment epithelium—the anatomical and physiological barrier.
- Presence of growth factors and inflammatory mediators.

Retinal pigment epithelium (RPE) secretes pigment epithelial derived factor (PEDF) which maintains the avascularity of subretinal space. PEDF is found in highest concentration at macula. Aged RPE cells produce less PEDF. The basal lamina on which RPE overlies separates epithelial cells from underlying stroma and provides an enzymatic substrate for antiangiogenesis, cell signaling, and inflammation. The elastic layer also provides an antiangiogenic barrier. It is more discontinuous at macula making macula more prone to CNVM. Endostatin derived by cleavage from collagen XVIII in Bruch's membrane can contributes to avascularity of the subretinal space. Laser-induced CNVM has reduced amount of endostatin. The elastic layer also provides an antiangiogenic barrier. It is more discontinuous at macula making macula more prone to CNVM.

Thus, damage to RPE-Bruch's complex breaches the physiological barrier and results in angiogenesis. Bruch's membrane may be disrupted by the balance between proteolytic enzymes such as matrix metalloproteinases and their inhibitors, tissue inhibitors of metalloproteinases.

Growth factors and inflammatory mediators involved in CNV formation:
- Vascular endothelial growth factor
- Fibroblast growth factor-2
- Integrins
- Ang1 and Tie2
- MMP2

CLINICAL FEATURES

Symptoms
- Blurring of vision
- Metamorphopsia
- Scotoma (positive)
- Can sometimes be asymptomatic

Signs
- Grayish or green elevation of tissue deep to retina
- Subretinal bleed
- Pigment epithelial detachment
- Subretinal scar

■ MYOPIC CHOROIDAL NEOVASCULAR MEMBRANE
Incidence
- Develops in 10% of eyes with high myopia.
- In 30% cases other eye is involved.
- Peak in fourth decade of life.
- More in eyes with shallow staphyloma—may be healthier resulting in stronger respond to injury and more neovascular growth.

Pathophysiology
Bruch's membranes (BM) show thinning, splitting, and rupturing. Lacquer cracks (BM rupture) are predisposing lesion; could be inflammatory in some eyes [punctate inner choroidopathy (PIC) and multifocal choroiditis].

Features
- Other features of myopia are also present.
- Small gray or pigmented discoloration at fovea with recent onset symptoms may suggest CNVM **(Fig. 7.49.2A)**.
- Easily visible due to thin retina.
- Bleeding usually absent due to thin stretched choroid. Coin-shaped hemorrhage may be present.
- Lacquer cracks may be seen which may also cause bleed.
- *Fluorescein angiography (FA):* Highly useful. Detects low activity CNVM. Mostly classic type **(Fig. 7.49.2B)**
- *Indocyanine green angiography (ICG):* No hotspot due to low activity of CNVM.
- *Optical coherence tomography (OCT):* Elevated lesion in subretinal space. Exudation and edema usually absent. Associated thin choroid and staphyloma **(Fig. 7.49.2C)**.
- *Optical coherence tomography angiography (OCTA):* Lacy wheel pattern with vascular network.

Management
Antivascular endothelial growth factor (anti-VEGF) first-line therapy:
- *REPAIR study:* Ranibizumab improves visual acuity in patients with active subfoveal and juxtafoveal CNVM.
- *RADIANCE study:* Ranibizumab is superior to verteporfin photodynamic therapy in patients with myopic CNVM.
- *MYRROR study:* Aflibercept is effective in patients with myopic CNVM.

■ ANGIOID STREAKS
Incidence
- Most common and significant complication of angioid streaks is CNVM.
- Usually bilateral but asymmetric.
- Occurs in 72–82% of eyes.
- Higher risk in patients with pseudoxanthoma elasticum.

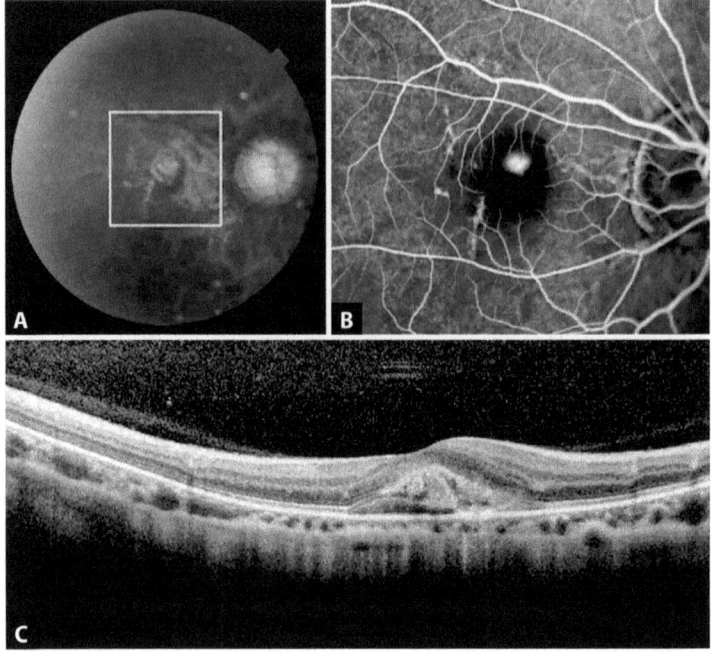

Figs. 7.49.2A to C: *Multimodal imaging of myopic CNVM:* (A) CNVM appears as grayish spot on macula with adjacent semilunar bleed. Associated features of myopic fundus such as tessellated appearance, lacquer cracks, and large disc with peripapillary atrophy also present; (B) FA shows classic CNVM with leak in early phase; (C) OCT shows type 2 CNVM (classic) in subretinal space with no exudation or edema and thin choroid.

Pathophysiology

Primary abnormality of Bruch's membrane fibers and increased deposition of metal salts resulting in brittle Bruch's membrane prone to rupture. Also, increased expression of MMP9 in BM resulting in BM degeneration and angiogenesis.

Features

- *Systemic associations present such as:* Pseudoxanthoma elasticum, Paget's disease, Ehlers–Danlos syndrome, Marfan syndrome, sickle cell anemia, thalassemia, abetalipoproteinemia, hypercalcinosis, and hyperphosphatemia.
- *OCT:*
  - Thinner choroid
  - BM undulations precede development of CNVM

Management

- Prevent trauma and development of breaks.
- Prophylactic treatment not recommended.
- *Anti-VEGF:* First-line treatment.

TRAUMA

Incidence

Approximately 10% develop CNVM within 1 month.

Pathophysiology

Choroidal rupture and the inflammatory response.

Features
- History of trauma present
- Concentric to optic disc

Management
- Anti-VEGF may produce response.
- *Other options:* Laser, photodynamic therapy (PDT), and surgical excision.

■ CHOROIDITIS
Incidence
- *Multifocal choroiditis:* 32–46%
- *PIC:* 17–40%
- *Serpiginous choroidopathy:* 10–25%

Pathophysiology
Chronic inflammation of choriocapillaris leads to nonperfusion, ischemia, and neovascularization.

Features
- Choroiditis may be active or healed. Ill-defined membrane may be seen adjacent to patch of choroiditis.
- Recent onset metamorphopsia suggestive of fresh development of macular pathology like CNV in such cases
- *Fundus fluorescein angiography (FFA):* Hyperfluorescence of CNV may be difficult to delineate separately from activity of choroiditis or macular edema.
- *OCTA:* Quite helpful in detecting an early network of vessels in inflammatory CNVM.

Management
- Control of active inflammation if any.
- Intravitreal anti-VEGF for the CNV.

■ PARAFOVEAL TELANGIECTASIA
Features
- Most commonly temporal to fovea (**Fig. 7.49.3A**).
- Preceded by right angle venule and intraretinal pigment hyperplasia (**Fig. 7.49.3A**).
- Pigment epithelial detachment (PED) absent.
- *OCT:* Inner retinal cysts (**Fig. 7.49.3B**).
- Mostly type 3 CNVM (**Fig. 7.49.3C**). It is of retinal origin (FA shows feeding arteriole and draining venule).

Management
- Intravitreal anti-VEGF for CNVM associated with parafoveal telangiectasia (PFT).
- Anti-VEGF, PDT, and laser ineffective for parafoveal telangiectasia.
- Ciliary neurotrophic factor (CNTF) under trial for PFT.

■ IDIOPATHIC CHOROIDAL NEOVASCULARIZATION
If no cause is found then the CNVM is said to be idiopathic. Such idiopathic CNVM can be seen in any age group. Patients typically present with recent metamorphopsia or drop in vision. A definite gray membrane or bleed may or may not be present. The only clinical

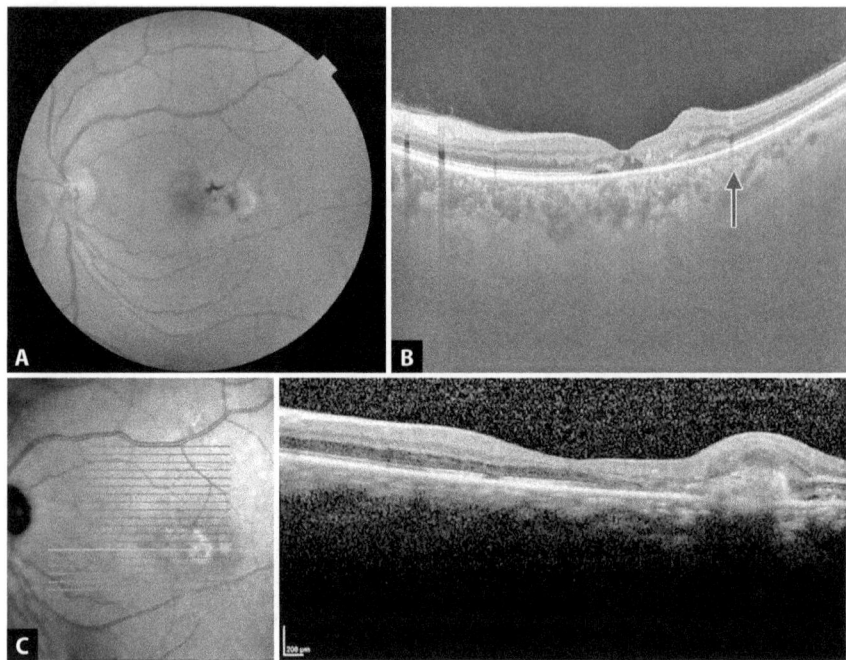

Figs. 7.49.3A to C: *Multimodal imaging of PFT-related CNVM:* (A) CNVM with bleed and pigmentary changes present temporal to macula. Associated right-angled venule and pigment migration into fundus also seen; (B) OCT shows inner retinal layers cavitation classic of PFT; (C) OCT scan passing through the CNVM shows intraretinal CNVM.

sign may be a yellowish lesion in the parafoveal area. OCTA is a very useful noninvasive investigation in such cases in picking up the neovascular network in the parafoveal lesion. Such CNVM generally respond well to intravitreal anti-VEGF therapy.

7.50 Posterior Segment Trauma: Clinical, Surgical Manifestations, and Management

Samendra Karkhur, Baldev Sastya, Sunil Verma, Richa Nyodu, Nikita Yadav

All India Institute of Medical Sciences, Bhopal

karkhurs@gmail.com

■ INTRODUCTION

Ocular trauma has always been a challenge for ophthalmic surgeons, especially when the injury has extended to posterior segment. From clinical and surgical perspective, any injury that either solely or in addition to anterior segment trauma involves vitreous, retina, choroid, optic nerve, etc., will constitute posterior segment trauma. With the advent of microincision vitrectomy surgery (MIVS) and other advanced vitreoretinal surgical paraphernalia; it has become progressively easier to achieve better surgical outcomes for the patients who present with posterior segment trauma. Another unique feature with such injuries is that, the visualization of posterior segment or its involved structures is often not possible and the surgeon must rely on ultrasound B-scan findings; thereby often requiring multiple surgical interventions to achieve desired visual and anatomical outcomes.

Depending on the kind of injury the following manifestations in the posterior segment are seen:
- Commotion retinae/Berlin's edema
- Dislocation of crystalline lens/intraocular lens (IOL)
- Retinal dialysis/tear/detachment
- Choroidal detachment/hemorrhage
- Subretinal hemorrhage
- Subhyaloid hemorrhage
- Vitreous hemorrhage
- Traumatic optic neuropathy
- Open globe injury/retained foreign body

COMMOTIO RETINAE

A concussive force to the globe results in whitening of the retina resulting in this clinical entity. Commotio retinae present in the posterior pole are called Berlin's edema. There is damage and edema of the photoreceptor layer of the retina. The visual prognosis is usually guarded when macula is involved. High dose corticosteroids have been tried with variable results to reduce the swelling and hasten recovery. In acute cases involving the macula the appearance of cherry-red spot may be misleading.

Important Considerations

All cases of commotio retinae should be subjected to peripheral fundus examination and gonioscopy to rule out any retinal tears and angle recession. This would help not only with discussion the prognosis and need for further follow-up but also further plan of management.

DISLOCATION OF CRYSTALLINE LENS/INTRAOCULAR LENS

Blunt trauma may leads to subluxation of clear crystalline or cataractous lens in the vitreous cavity. The IOL may also dislocate in a similar manner.

Ultrasonography (USG) B-scan is of immense help in this regard to formulate a management plan, especially in compromised media clarity especially with associated vitreous hemorrhage.

Management: The dislocated cataract or clear crystalline lens results in raised IOP per se, in addition to that due to trauma. Initial management entails antiglaucoma medications for control of IOP and achieves corneal clarity for better fundus visualization. This is followed by pars plana vitrectomy (PPV) and removal of crystalline lens with a vitrectomy cutter (usually 23G) since they are soft in younger individuals. Hard nucleus requires a phacofragmatome after PPV for phacoemulsification and removal of the dislocated cataract.

A dislocated IOL needs to be managed depending on the type of IOL. Rigid polymethylmethacrylate (PMMA) and single piece foldable IOLs usually need removal. However, multi-piece rigid or foldable lenses may be scleral fixated in the same sitting using various techniques available. Depending on various factors and the severity of trauma the secondary scleral-fixated or iris-fixated IOLs may be employed. It is to be kept in mind that secondary IOL fixation is associated with additional complications and may be avoided altogether in cases where visual prognosis in guarded due to posterior segment sequelae of trauma.

Important Considerations

- Thorough vitrectomy should be performed; especially at the port site; before introduction of the fragmatome. Since the latter is a wide-bore, high vacuum device; it may lead to active traction on the residual vitreous resulting in retinal tear.

- The 20G sclerotomy port should have preplaced mattress sutures before introducing the fragmatome; this is to ensure faster closure of a large sclerotomy wound after the fragmentation is completed and prevents fluctuation in infusion pressure.
- The port site needs constant irrigation to avoid charring (thermal damage) of the sclerotomy site by the heat generated during the process. The thermal damage could interfere with sclerotomy wound healing and predispose to leakage and therefore, hypotony and infection.
- After PPV and before initiating the phacofragmentation; a perfluorocarbon liquid cushion should be applied to prevent injury to the macula by the sharp fragments of the nucleus.
- Peripheral fundus examination should be performed before closing the ports.

■ RETINAL DIALYSIS/TEAR WITH RETINAL DETACHMENT

Blunt trauma may lead to formation of retinal breaks due to equatorial expansion of the globe, leading to retinal detachment. In younger individuals due to formed vitreous and strong vitreoretinal attachments, retinal dialysis may occur. The ensuing retinal detachment may be repaired using scleral buckling or pars plana vitreoretinal surgery and appropriate tamponading agent.

Important Considerations

- Patient presenting with blunt trauma should be thoroughly examined for peripheral fundus under dilatation. This may be deferred by a few weeks in cases with anterior chamber hyphema or superficial injuries and also keeping in mind the fact that patient would be more cooperative and comfortable for a peripheral fundus examination with indentation after some time has passed following injury.
- In younger individuals with clear crystalline lens, scleral buckling is preferred, since the vitreous is very strongly adherent to retina and induction of complete posterior vitreous detachment (PVD) is difficult. The removal of posterior cortical vitreous is also a challenge in younger individuals presenting with rhegmatogenous retinal detachment (RRD).

■ CHOROIDAL DETACHMENT/HEMORRHAGE

Choroidal detachment following trauma may be both serous or hemorrhagic in nature and shallow or "kissing" in extent. There may also be the present of ciliary body detachment along with choroidals. This usually presents with hypotony in the absence of any open globe injury. The management of each differs and requires ultrasound B-scan, not only in the diagnosis but also during follow-up to see clinical response to therapy.

Important Considerations

- Shallow serous choroidals may be observed and usually respond to topical atropine and systemic corticosteroids therapy.
- Kissing choroidal may require surgical draining in nonresponsive to medical management to prevent permanent retinal adhesion.
- Hemorrhagic choroidals often require drainage and the same is often carried out at 5-7 days following trauma to coincide with clot lysis. B-scan facilitates the same.
- Choroidals with ciliochoroidal detachment sometimes do not respond to therapy and require pars plana vitrectomy and internal tamponade using silicone oil.

■ SUBRETINAL/SUBMACULAR BLEED

This finding is usually associated with an underlying choroidal rupture. The heme is well defined and appears deep red to violaceous. If present in periphery it may be partially or fully dehemoglobinized and appears creamish or gray in color. No active intervention is required. If however it involves the posterior pole, the same may require intervention depending on the time of presentation following trauma.

Surgical management of subretinal bleed may be undertaken using following options:
- Pneumatic displacement by injection of an expansile gas bubble in the vitreous cavity and prone positioning of patient.
- Pars plana vitrectomy, subretinal injection of tissue plasminogen activator (tPA) to induce clot lysis and internal gas tamponade to facilitate displacement of heme away from macula, thus preventing iron-induced photoreceptor damage.
- The prognosis remains guarded in cases where the underlying choroidal rupture transects the papilla-macular bundle or foveal center.
- Also if the photoreceptor damage has been found to be irreversible only within first 24 hours of contact with heme.

SUBHYALOID HEMORRHAGE

Traumatic subhyaloid hemorrhages are a common occurrence either in isolation or associated with vitreous hemorrhage. A premacular subhyaloid bleed needs urgent intervention since the damage to photoreceptors may be irreversible.

The management is surgical and requires pars plana vitrectomy to induce a posterior vitreous detachment and internal limiting membrane peeling if necessary. The planning requires an optical coherence tomography (OCT) scan to delineate the level of blood before surgery. Pneumatic displacement with or without vitrectomy may also be employed.

VITREOUS HEMORRHAGE

Presence of blood in the vitreous cavity is a common occurrence after trauma especially in penetrating injury more than closed globe injuries. The origin of this bleed in blunt trauma is usually from ruptured retinal vessels. Apart from causing proportional visual loss, vitreous hemorrhage is important from a diagnostic perspective also, since it obscures any underlying posterior segment injury due to its presence. Therefore it becomes imperative to address vitreous hemorrhage (VH) in order to facilitate visualization of associated traumatic events such as retinal tears, optic nerve injury, etc. Management can be conservative or surgical depending on patient factors and associated posterior segment injuries.

Important Considerations
- All cases of blunt trauma with VH should undergo serial ultrasound B-scan on each follow-up to detect additional finding such as retinal detachment which may not be evident on first evaluation. This would change the line of management from conservative to surgical during the course of follow-up.
- Scant amount present inferiorly may be left alone and usually resolves spontaneously. However a detailed peripheral fundus examination is mandatory to rule out any retinal breaks, which mandate prophylactic barrage laser treatment.
- Very dense, nonresolving VH may require vitreous surgery, since it causes visual handicap and may predispose to ghost-cell glaucoma later on.
- Associated findings such as retinal detachment require a thorough USG B-scan study and should not be missed.
- Old nonresolving or gray vitreous hemorrhage may give the appearance of vitritis and needs to be differentiated from the latter.

TRAUMATIC OPTIC NEUROPATHY

This is a condition resulting in vision loss, arising from an acute injury to the optic nerve, due to direct or indirect trauma. Most common etiology is the forces transmitted to the optic canal from an orbital trauma. Other direct causes may be bony fragments and impact of projectile foreign bodies. The severity may range from a simple reversible contusion to complete avulsion of optic nerve from the globe.

The optic nerve head may appear normal initially on fundus examination, however optic atrophy sets in 4–6 weeks following traumatic event. Assessment of both direct and consensual pupillary reflexes is of paramount important in assessment of patients to rule out optic nerve injury; since visual assessment is often not possible.

Important Considerations
- Direct optic nerve injury requires multidisciplinary approach including neurosurgery, otolaryngology, and ophthalmology and needs urgent decompression of the affected portion.
- There is no clear guideline regarding the management of indirect optic nerve injury due to shearing forces, however most centers prefer pulse steroid therapy within 24 hours of trauma, if not contraindicated systemically.

■ OPEN GLOBE INJURY (RETAINED FOREIGN BODY)
Penetrating or perforating eye injuries constitutes an emergency situation and requires a well-planned approach to manage a patient successfully. This often requires multiple interventions with variable visual outcomes. Presence of retained intraocular foreign body further complicates the situation and requires specialized techniques for management depending on its nature and size.

Primary repair must be undertaken as soon as possible preferably under general anesthesia. This is followed by assessment of posterior segment using USG B-scan and radiopaque foreign bodies may further require CT-scan orbit to plan next management course.

All the above-mentioned aspects/findings of posterior segment trauma require thorough evaluation by a vitreoretinal surgeon and further management. Any to the above injuries should be suspected in a case of ocular trauma and must be timely referred to a specialist center for management.

7.51 Retinal Imaging in Adults

Manish Nagpal
Retina Foundation, Ahmedabad
drmanishnagpal@yahoo.com

■ INTRODUCTION
Retinal imaging techniques have evolved at a remarkable pace in the last two decades. Wide field imaging (WFI) and ultra-wide field imaging (UWFI) are now increasingly popular. WFI refers to imaging beyond 50° field area. UWFI systems can image up to 200°. They are well capable of imaging over 80% of the retinal surface area. The peripheral retina can be photographed with small pupils in instances where dilated peripheral fundus examination may be limited due to pupil size.[1,2] Also, availability of multimodal imaging enables the possibility of simultaneous acquisition of fundus fluorescein angiography (FA), indocyanine angiography (ICGA), fundus photography, fundus autofluorescence (FAF), including blue as well as green light fundus autofluorescence, infrared imaging (IR), optical coherence tomography (OCT), and optical coherence tomography angiography (OCT-A).

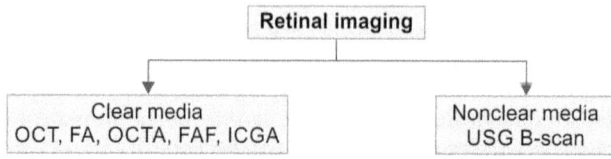

APPLICATIONS OF OCT IMAGING IN CLINICAL PRACTICE

Vitreomacular interface: Vitreomacular adhesion (VMA), vitreomacular traction (VMT), epiretinal membrane **(Figs. 7.51.1A and B)**, and macular hole **(Figs. 7.51.2A and B)**.

Intraretinal: Focal and diffuse retinal edema, pigmentary changes, scarring, and drusen.

Subretinal: Choroidal neovascular membrane (CNVM) and serous retinal detachment (RD)

Newer OCT biomarkers: Subretinal hyperreflective membrane, disorganization of retinal inner layer, outer retinal tubulations, leptochoroid, pachychoroid, and focal choroidal excavation.

APPLICATIONS OF FLUORESCEIN ANGIOGRAPHY IMAGING IN CLINICAL PRACTICE

Retinal vascular abnormalities such as diabetic retinopathy, branch retinal vein occlusion, and central retinal vein occlusion require proper evaluation peripheral avascular areas **(Fig. 7.51.3)**, neovascularization, macular ischemia, and vascular leakages. In cases of intermediate and posterior uveitis, it allows evaluation of activity, disease severity, progression, and treatment response. In cases of undiagnosed cases of familial exudative vitreoretinopathy (FEVR) in adults or regressed retinopathy of prematurity (ROP), peripheral areas of capillary nonperfusion can be identified. To identify and document activity of CNVM, to confirm the diagnosis of ocular ischemic syndrome, to identify the

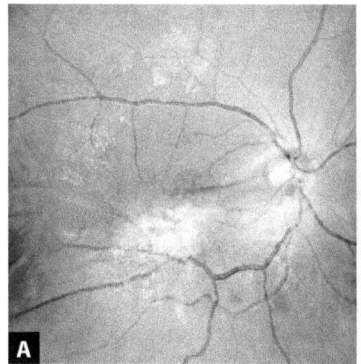
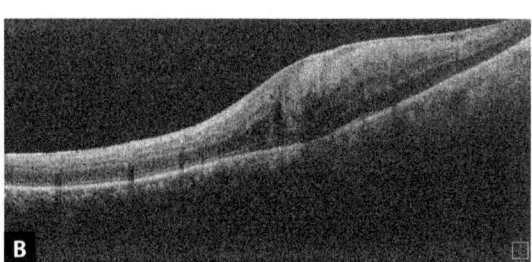

Figs. 7.51.1A and B: (A) Color fundus photograph of a patient with epiretinal membrane; (B) OCT demonstrating a primary epiretinal membrane with significant retinal thickening.

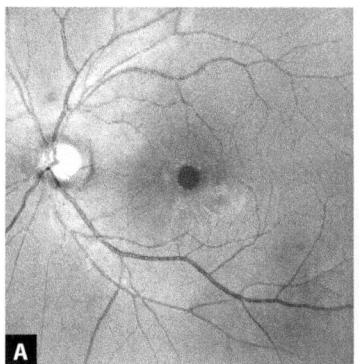
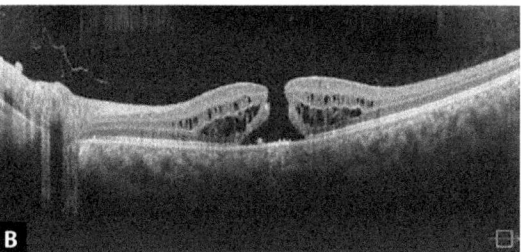

Figs. 7.51.2A and B: (A) Color fundus photograph of a patient with macular hole; (B) OCT demonstrating a full thickness macular hole.

type of leak in cases of central serous chorioretinopathy (CSCR) and to evaluate intraocular tumors, are a few other important indications.

APPLICATIONS OF OCTA IMAGING IN CLINICAL PRACTICE

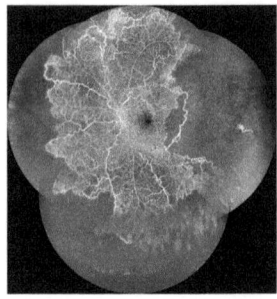

Fig. 7.51.3: Fluorescein angiography showing hypofluorescence due to filling defect suggestive of capillary nonperfusion.

Diabetic retinopathy where optical coherence tomography angiography (OCTA) offers the opportunity to evaluate the quantification of perfusion through vascular density maps, and the potential for feature identification such as identifying microaneurysms or specified regions of nonperfusion; vein occlusion where OCTA shows the areas of vascular nonperfusion, the dilated tortuous venous segments, the microvascular abnormalities, and the neovascularization; OCTA shows the prominent right-angle veins with the distortion of the foveal avascular zone with cavitations in macular telangiectasia and type 3 neovascularization can be visualized as a discrete high flow linear structure extending from the middle retinal layers into the deep retina, which sometimes extent throughout the retinal pigment epithelium on OCTA.

APPLICATIONS OF AUTOFLUORESCENCE IMAGING IN CLINICAL PRACTICE

In a normal fundus without retinal pathology, blood vessels will appear dark since blood is able to strongly absorb the blue or green light. The optic nerve will usually appear dark due to the absence of retinal pigment epithelium (RPE) or lipofuscin in this region. Fovea will usually be visualized as a spot of hypo-autofluorescence due to the high concentration of light-absorbing xanthophyll pigment in this area.

Abnormal regions of hyper-autofluorescence are a result of increased levels of lipofuscin/compounds with similar autofluorescent spectra, or increased transmission of fluorescence. Abnormal regions of hypo-autofluorescence are a result of decreased levels of lipofuscin, decreased RPE density, or blockage of fluorescence. Major indications include—geographic atrophy, retinitis pigmentosa, and rod-cone dystrophies, Stargardt disease, best disease and vitelliform maculopathies, hydroxychloroquine retinopathy, and other retinal drug toxicities (**Figs. 7.51.4 and 7.51.5**).

APPLICATIONS OF INDOCYANINE GREEN ANGIOGRAPHY IMAGING IN CLINICAL PRACTICE

Wet age-related macular degeneration (AMD) classifying it into focal spot or "hot spot", plaques, and mixed; idiopathic polypoidal choroidal vasculopathy revealed by the polypoidal lesions (**Figs. 7.51.6A to C**) and anomalous vascular network within the choroid on ICGA; choroidal tumors wherein melanoma varied from hypo-to-hypercyanscent in the late phase of the ICGA, hypocyanscence throughout the whole phase in choroidal metastatic tumor, more denser hypercyanscence in the early phase than in the late phase in choroidal melanomas; Vogt-Koyanagi-Harada disease shows early choroidal vessel hyperfluorescence. Intermediate to late phase fuzziness of choroidal stromal vessels, disc hyperfluorescence, and hypofluorescent dark dots and diagnosis of white dot syndromes are the major indications.

APPLICATIONS OF ULTRASONOGRAPHY B-SCAN IN CLINICAL PRACTICE

On B-scan of the normal eyeball, the optic nerve can be seen passing through the retrobulbar fat. The retrobulbar fat is echogenic, and the optic nerve is seen as a hypoechoic

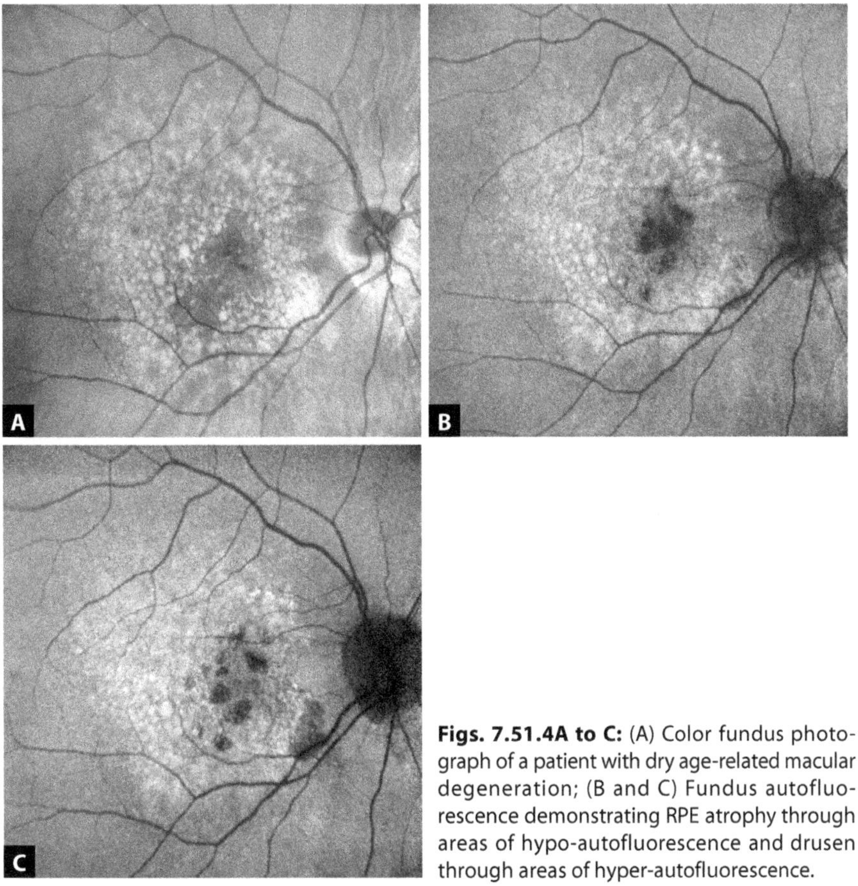

Figs. 7.51.4A to C: (A) Color fundus photograph of a patient with dry age-related macular degeneration; (B and C) Fundus autofluorescence demonstrating RPE atrophy through areas of hypo-autofluorescence and drusen through areas of hyper-autofluorescence.

tubular structure extending from the posterior pole of the eyeball toward the orbital apex. The axial length of the normal adult eye is 24 mm.

The detached retina is usually attached to the firm anchoring points of the ora serrata anteriorly and the optic nerve head posteriorly and, consequently, a total RD shows a funnel shape. In a choroidal detachment, B-scan shows fluid in the suprachoroidal space; the choroid is attached anteriorly to the ciliary body and posteriorly at the exit foramina of the vortex veins. It may be secondary to trauma or surgery or may even occur spontaneously. Choroidal melanoma **(Fig. 7.51.7)** is seen as a lenticular-shaped mass arising from the choroid where USG is used to assess scleral erosions and extraocular extension into orbital fat. B-scan revealing multiple

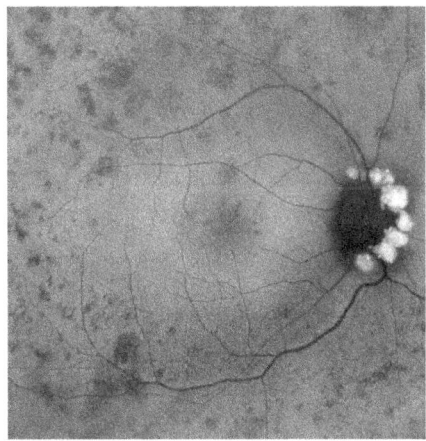

Fig. 7.51.5: Fundus autofluorescence demonstrating optic disc drusen through areas of hyper-autofluorescence and bony spicules in a case of retinitis pigmentosa through areas of hypoautofluorescence.

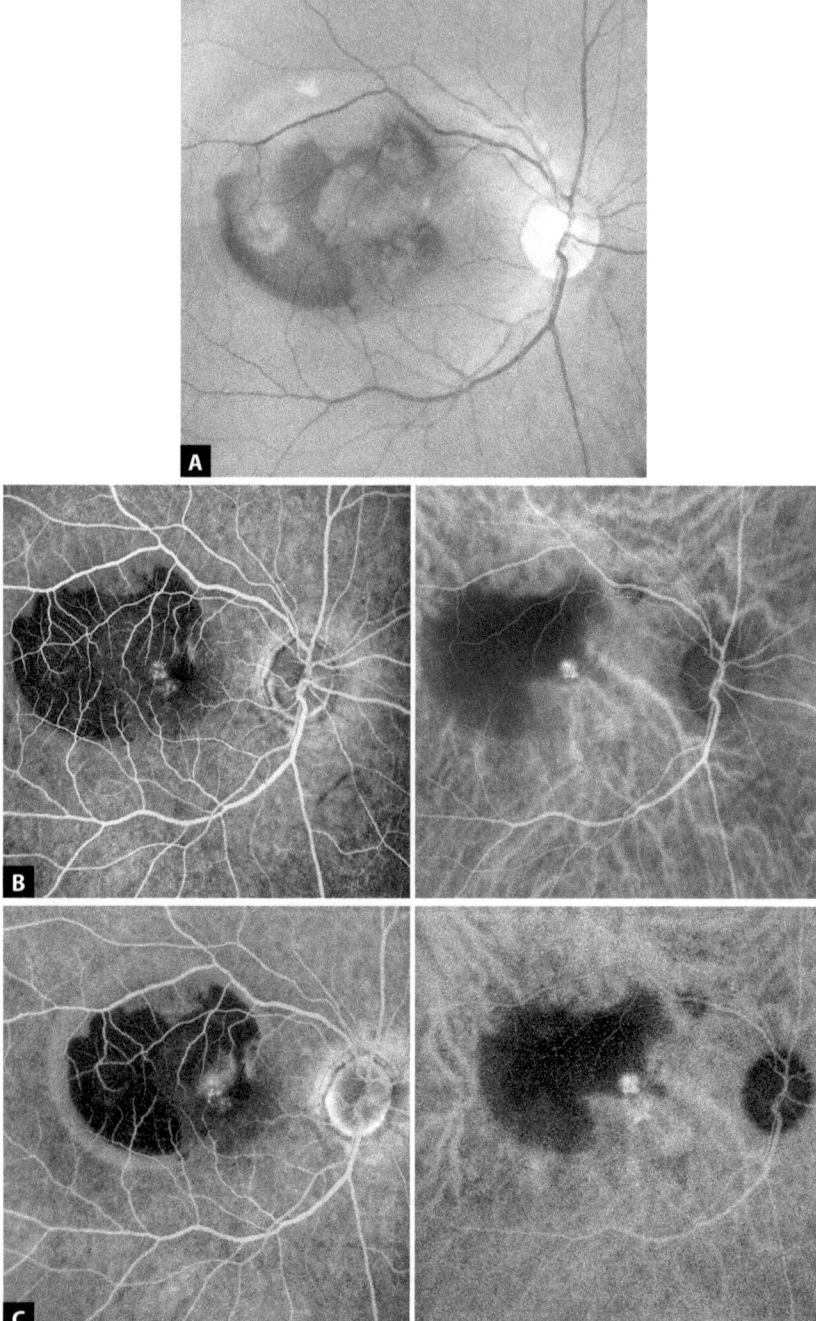

Figs. 7.51.6A to C: (A) Color fundus photograph of a subretinal bleed at posterior pole in a case of idiopathic polypoidal choroidal vasculopathy; (B) Early phase fluorescein angiography showing a patchy area of subretinal staining, along with hypofluorescence or blockage of the choroidal circulation by blood and early phase of indocyanine green angiography revealing presence of an inner choroidal vascular abnormality, ending in multiple small, hyperfluorescent polyps, and characteristic of polypoidal choroidal vasculopathy; (C) Late phases of fluorescein angiography and indocyanine green angiography.

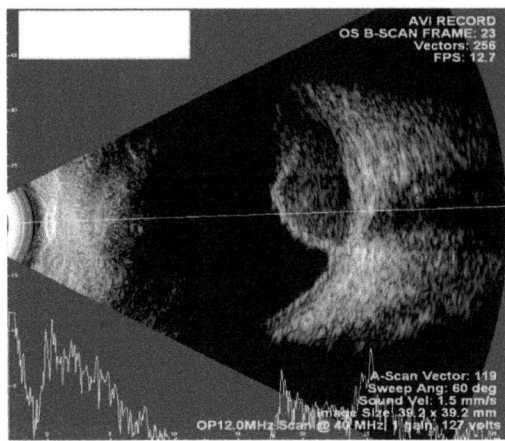

Fig. 7.51.7: USG B-scan showing a large mushroom-shaped mass lesion with an acoustically silent zone within suggestive of choroidal melanoma.

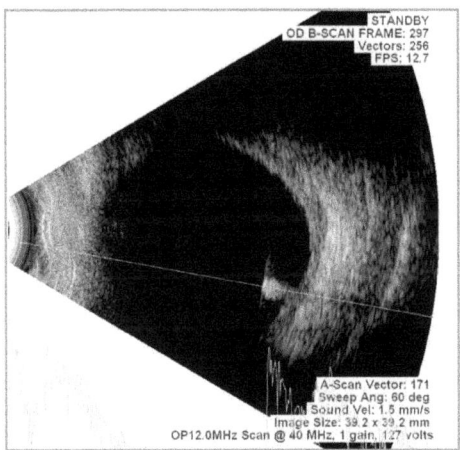

Fig. 7.51.8: USG B-scan of an IOL drop identified by high amplitude spike which is associated with acoustic reverberations.

hyperreflective mobile foci within the vitreous chamber that show after-movements on a dynamic scan without visual impairment is vitreous degeneration and with visual loss may be hemorrhage or exudation depending on the history **(Fig. 7.51.8)**.

CONCLUSION

A multimodal device combining conventional fundus photography, OCT, FA, FAF, ICGA, OCTA, and USG B-scan is a step forward in retinal diagnostic testing. As advancements continue to develop in the field of retinal imaging, our understanding of ocular disease processes continues to improve.

REFERENCES

1. Tripathy K, Chawla R, Venkatesh P, Sharma YR, Vohra R. Ultrawide field imaging in uveitic non-dilating pupils. J Ophthalmic Vis Res. 2017;12(2):232-3.
2. Tripathy K, Chawla R, Vohra R. Evaluation of the fundus in poorly dilating diabetic pupils using ultrawide field imaging. Clin Exp Optom. 2017;100(6):735-6.

SECTION 8

Neuro-ophthalmology

Editor: Rashmin Gandhi

8.1 **Optic Nerve Function Tests** 672
Rashmin Gandhi

8.2 **How do You Approach a Patient with Unilateral Disc Edema?** 673
Satya Karna

8.3 **Approach to a Patient with Bilateral Optic Disc Edema** 674
Peter J Savino

8.4 **Patient with Pale Discs** 676
Andrew G Lee, Ama Sadaka, Berry Shauna

8.5 **Optic Neuritis** 678
Rohit Saxena, Digvijay Singh, Rashmin Gandhi

8.6 **Approach to a Patient with Cranial Nerve Palsy** 679
Preeti Patil-Chablani

8.7 **Patient with Unequal Pupils** 684
Navin Jaykumar

8.8 **Patient with Ptosis** 686
Shubhra Goel, Akshay Nair

8.9 **Traumatic Optic Neuropathy** 687
S Ambika, Rashmin Gandhi

8.10 **Neuroimaging** 689
Olma Veena Noronha

8.11 **Different Magnetic Resonance Imaging Sequences** 691
Navin Jayakumar

8.12 **Electrophysiology in Neuro-ophthalmology** 693
Parveen Sen, Ramya Sachidanandam

8.13 **Role of Optical Coherence Tomography in Neuro-ophthalmology** 700
Devendra Venkatramani

8.14 **Radiation Tolerance of Ocular Structures** 702
Deepak Mishra, Ritusha Mishra, Himanshu Mishra

8.1 Optic Nerve Function Tests

Rashmin Gandhi
Foresight Worldwide, Hyderabad
rashmin.gandhi@gmail.com

■ INTRODUCTION

Optic nerve function tests help to determine the severity of optic nerve dysfunction and help in arriving at diagnosis.

■ VISUAL ACUITY

- In typical optic neuritis
  - There is acute loss of vision.
  - Typically will deteriorate for the next 2 weeks.
  - Improves in majority of cases by 2 months.
- In ischemic optic neuropathy, vision rarely improves.
- Compressive optic neuropathy, nutritional optic neuropathy, and hereditary optic neuropathy vision loss is progressive.

■ PUPILS

Check in dark room. Use a bright source of light. Ask patient to look at the distant target.
Irrespective of etiology, all unilateral optic neuropathy will produce relative afferent pupillary defect.

■ COLOR VISION

Optic neuropathy typically produces dyschromatopsia. Color vision loss is much more pronounced in inflammatory optic neuropathy, while in ischemic optic neuropathy color vision loss is proportional to visual acuity loss.

■ VISUAL FIELDS

In clinical settings, visual fields can be tested by:

Confrontation
- Tested monocularly
- Ask patient to fixate at your nose and project fingers in four quadrants and ask patient to count your fingers. Avoid projecting fingers bisecting horizontal or vertical meridians.
- Use red target to test the central visual field (eye drop top or a red pencil).

Amsler Grid
For the central visual fields.

■ BRIGHTNESS SENSITIVITY

Ask patient to look at a bright torch of light first with normal eye and then with eye with reduced vision. Most patients will be able to appreciate drop in brightness in diseased eye.

■ SUGGESTED READING

1. Walsh FB, Hoyt WF, Miller NR, Newman NJ, Biousse V, Kerrison JB. Walsh and Hoyt's Clinical Neuro-Ophthalmology. 6th edition. USA: Lippincott Williams and Wilkins; 2004.

8.2 How do You Approach a Patient with Unilateral Disc Edema?

Satya Karna
Jaypee Hospital, Noida
satyakarna@yahoo.com

ASSUMING NORMAL RETINA

Differential Diagnosis

- *Papillitis:* Painful, in young to middle aged female (20–40 years)
- *NAION (nonarteritic anterior ischemic optic neuropathy):* Hyperemic disc edema, segmental disc edema
- *AAION (arteritic anterior ischemic optic neuropathy):* Pale disc edema, elderly (above 55 years)
- *Neuroretinitis:* Disc edema with macular star of exudates.
- *Compressive:* Diffuse, elevated disc with blurred margins, without hemorrhages.

FEATURES

Papillitis
It is a painful, rapidly progressive visual loss over 5–7 days, followed by gradual recovery over 4–6 weeks. The vision may range from 6/6 to no perception of light. Chances of association with existing or later development of multiple sclerosis are around 10%.

Nonarteritic Anterior Ischemic Optic Neuropathy
Painless, usually sudden, static visual loss, may be gradually progressive over few weeks. Visual recovery may occur in less than half of the patients. Frequently the optic disc shows partial disc edema with the rest of the disc appearing normal. The other eye may show disc at risk.

Arteritic Anterior Ischemic Optic Neuropathy
Sudden visual loss along with headache, jaw claudication, fever, and other symptoms suggestive of temporal arteritis, with rapid involvement of the other eye within hours to days. Pale disc edema is the classical presentation.

Neuroretinitis
Sudden painful visual loss with disc edema and macular exudates in the form of a star with macular edema, usually associated with infective etiology, never associated with multiple sclerosis.

Compressive
Choked disc with no hemorrhages but associated with very gradual painless progressive loss of vision. It may be associated with proptosis or congestion of the globe. There may be associated disc pallor in chronic cases.

INVESTIGATIONS
Humphrey visual fields 30-2 both eyes. Almost all cases show central or centrocecal scotoma, arcuate defects, focal defects, or nonspecific defects. Altitudinal scotoma is suggestive of ischemic optic neuropathy. Virtually any visual field defect may occur with any optic neuropathy.

Flash and pattern visual evoked potentials are indicated in papillitis for documenting recovery. Magnetic resonance imaging (MRI) brain and orbits with contrast and fluid-attenuated inversion recovery (FLAIR) sequence in optic neuritis may show enhancement of the optic nerve sheath or demyelinating plaques in the periventricular areas or deep white matter.

Magnetic resonance imaging orbits with contrast are definitely indicated in suspected compressive pathology.

Fasting blood sugar, postprandial blood sugar, blood pressure, lipids, and carotid Doppler are indicated in suspected ischemic optic neuropathy.

Erythrocyte sedimentation rate (ESR), C-reactive protein (CRP), complete blood count (CBC), and temporal artery biopsy are needed to confirm AAION.

Serology for toxoplasmosis, toxocariasis, and syphilis is required in neuroretinitis.

■ TREATMENT

Papillitis
High dose intravenous methyl prednisolone 1 g/day for 3 days followed by tapering oral steroids at 1 mg/kg/day over 2 weeks.

Nonarteritic Anterior Ischemic Optic Neuropathy
No effective treatment.

Arteritic Anterior Ischemic Optic Neuropathy
High dose intravenous methyl prednisolone 1 g/day followed by slow tapering oral steroids at 2 mg/kg/day over few months until ESR and CRP are normal for few weeks.

Neuroretinitis
Treatment is aimed at the infection associated with pathology.

Compressive
Appropriate surgical biopsy and treatment is indicated in select cases.

■ SUGGESTED READING
1. Walsh FB, Hoyt WF, Miller NR, Newman NJ, Biousse V, Kerrison JB. Walsh and Hoyt's Clinical Neuro-Ophthalmology. 6th edition. USA: Lippincott Williams and Wilkins; 2004.

8.3 Approach to a Patient with Bilateral Optic Disc Edema

Peter J Savino
Shiley Eye Institute, San Diego
pjsavino@aol.com

■ INTRODUCTION
Rarely does the ophthalmologist encounter a medical condition that is life or sight-threatening to the patient and must be dealt with on an emergency basis. Bilateral optic disc edema may be a manifestation of such disorders.

When a patient presents with bilateral optic disc elevation, the primary differentiation must be made between *papilledema*, due to increase intracranial pressure and those more benign conditions that look like papilledema, so-called *pseudopapilledema*.

PSEUDOPAPILLEDEMA

This condition, often accused with acquired disc swelling due to increased intracranial pressure, is due to a congenital anomaly of the optic discs. In fact, another term for this is *congenitally anomalous optic discs*.

The congenitally anomalous disc can often be distinguished from papilledema on the basis of its ophthalmoscopic characteristics which are:
- There is no central optic cup.
- All of the large optic disc vessels appear to come from the center of the cup.
- There appear to be too many large blood vessels emanating from the optic disc.
- The color of the optic disc is yellow and not hyperemic.
- There is no edema of the retinal nerve fiber layer.
- Spontaneous and venous pulsations are present.
- A similar appearance of the optic disc may be seen in parents or siblings. The presence of such optic discs requires no investigation.

PAPILLEDEMA

Papilledema is a term that neuro-ophthalmologists reserved for bilateral (almost always), acquired optic disc elevation due to increased intracranial pressure. Initially the swelling is reflected in thickening and opacification of the retinal nerve fiber layer. In later stages, the optic disc itself becomes elevated and retinal nerve fiber layer hemorrhages may be seen. Spontaneous venous pulsations at the optic disc are lost.

The following symptoms may be experienced by a patient with increased intracranial pressure:
- Headache
- Pulsatile tinnitus
- Transient visual obscurations which are often posture early induced.
- Visual acuity is usually unaffected until chronic atrophic papilledema occurs.

The identification of previously unrecognized papilledema is a medical emergency. Cranial imaging must be done immediately to rule out one of the following causes:
- Intracranial tumor
- Hydrocephalus
- Cerebral venous sinus thrombosis
  Magnetic resonance imaging and magnetic resonance venography are the investigations of choice in patients with papilledema. If no structural lesion is identified, the next test should be a lumbar puncture to rule out a man meningitic process or *pseudotumor cerebri* also known as idiopathic intracranial hypertension (IIH).

ARTERITIC ANTERIOR ISCHEMIC OPTIC NEUROPATHY (AAION)

Anterior ischemic optic neuropathy is usually a unilateral process. However, when it is due to giant cell arteritis (GCA), bilateral simultaneous optic disc edema may occur.

This is a disorder that occurs in patients over 60 years of age and may be accompanied by any of the following signs or symptoms:
- Scalp tenderness
- Jaw claudication
- Neck stiffness
- Weight loss and loss of appetite
- Transient visual loss preceding fixed visual loss
- Pale swollen optic discs with possible concomitant retinal nerve fiber layer infarctions
- And elevated erythrocyte sedimentation rate (ESR), C-reactive protein (CRP), and platelets
- A positive temporal artery biopsy

When a patient is suspected of having GCA high-dose corticosteroids should be instituted immediately. Intravenous corticosteroid at a dose of 1 g/day is the usual therapy. This is instituted prior to performance of the temporal artery biopsy. If the biopsy is positive, the intravenous corticosteroids are switched to systemic oral corticosteroids at a dose of 100 mg/kg after 3 days of IV therapy.

The goal of the therapy is to prevent visual loss in a previously unaffected fellow eye or to prevent further visual loss in an affected eye. Return a vision with therapy is unusual.

LEBER'S HEREDITARY OPTIC NEUROPATHY

This condition is usually seen in young men at a ratio of 9:1 over women and presents as the sudden onset of visual loss in one eye followed by loss of vision in the fellow eye shortly thereafter. The optic disc is elevated with what has been described as pseudoedema. Often abnormal telangiectasia may be identified around the optic disc.

This is a genetic problem and specific blood tests are available to test for one of the several genetic defects that cause this disorder. No treatment is available.

SUGGESTED READING

1. Brude R, Savino P, Jonathan D, Trobe J. Clinical Diagnosis in Neuro-Ophthalmology. USA: Mosby; 2002.

8.4 Patient with Pale Discs

Andrew G Lee, Ama Sadaka, Berry Shauna
The Methodist Hospital, Houston
Aglee@houstonmethodist.org

INTRODUCTION

The evaluation of the patient with optic atrophy can be a difficult problem for the ophthalmologist. The most important first step is differentiating true optic atrophy from physiologic pallor of the disc.

The clinical signs of true optic atrophy due to an underlying optic neuropathy include the following:
- Symptoms or history of visual loss
- Decreased visual acuity or loss of visual field
- Poorly reactive pupils or a relative afferent pupillary defect in unilateral or bilateral but asymmetric cases
- Dyschromatopsia
- Visible or measurable loss of nerve fiber layer

In an asymptomatic patient, the normal structural eye examination (i.e., normal visual acuity, formal visual field testing, color vision, and pupillary examinations) suggests the diagnosis of physiologic rather than true pallor of the disc. A number of optical conditions (e.g., lens opacity, pseudophakia) can produce physiologic pallor especially if there is asymmetry of the disc appearance compared with a fellow eye that does not harbor the same optical or media findings.

Optical coherence tomography (OCT) or other quantitative assessment of the retinal nerve fiber layer might be helpful in establishing the diagnosis of physiologic pallor (i.e., normal retinal nerve fiber layer) and can be used to establish a new baseline. A normal retinal nerve fiber layer thickness on OCT or other quantitative nerve fiber layer assessment can be used as presumptive evidence in conjunction with a normal clinical exam for the diagnosis of physiologic pallor. If, however, there is clinical or OCT evidence for a true optic neuropathy as the cause of the disc atrophy then even in an asymptomatic patient, we would recommend that the clinician should search for an underlying etiology.

On the other hand, in a case of a suspected and symptomatic optic neuropathy, the clinician should perform a complete history and examination to establish an etiology. The two most common causes of an acute unilateral optic neuropathy in adults are optic neuritis and nonarteritic anterior ischemic optic neuropathy and a bilateral optic atrophy patient often has had bilateral sequential disease. Thus a prior history of optic neuritis in a young patient or a prior history of demyelinating disease (i.e., multiple sclerosis) might be sufficient to establish an explanation for optic atrophy. Conversely in an older patient with vasculopathic risk factors (e.g., hypertension, diabetes, hyperlipidemia, or smoking) a documented history of visual loss with examination evidence for sector or diffuse optic disc edema can establish a presumptive diagnosis of nonarteritic anterior ischemic optic neuropathy.

The bilateral central, cecocentral scotoma and optic atrophy narrow the differential diagnosis considerably and most commonly would be due to Leber hereditary optic neuropathy, ethambutol toxicity, or toxic-nutritional optic neuropathy. We still recommend neuroimaging for these cases however as an initial first step as compressive lesions might still present in this fashion. In addition, clinical or historical evidence for active or prior anterior or posterior uveitis should be sought that might suggest an inflammatory (e.g., sarcoid), infiltrative, or infectious (e.g., syphilis) etiology for the optic neuropathy.

Although there are many conditions that can produce optic atrophy typically these disorders do not present in isolation. The list includes systemic inflammatory conditions [e.g., sarcoidosis, or systemic lupus erythematosus (SLE)], infectious etiologies (e.g., Lyme disease in the United States, syphilis, or tuberculosis). In countries like India, which are not highly endemic for Lyme disease the history should focus on travel by the patient to Lyme endemic areas (e.g., the Northeastern United States). In addition, patients from different parts of the world (e.g., India, Asia, or Africa) might be more likely to harbor infectious etiologies that might be rare in the United States or Europe (e.g., tuberculosis, syphilis, Rift Valley fever, bejel). Although postinfectious optic atrophy in tuberculosis is usually the sequelae of prior meningitis, visual loss can also occur following the treatment of tuberculosis with ethambutol or rarely with isoniazid. Conversely, although demyelinating optic neuritis is a common cause of optic atrophy in Europe and in the United States the incidence and prevalence of multiple sclerosis in regions of India are probably lower and thus the emphasis of the evaluation should be directed at the etiologic diagnoses most prevalent in the geographic area of the patient.

■ SUMMARY RECOMMENDATIONS

The yield for an unfocused laboratory approach to testing in patients with optic atrophy is low. The first and most important step is to define "nonisolated" versus "isolated" cases of optic atrophy. Nonisolated optic atrophy includes patients with: (1) known ocular or systemic disorder producing the optic atrophy (e.g., retinal detachment, glaucoma, compressive lesion or other prior etiology for optic neuropathy); (2) other localizing neuro-ophthalmic findings (e.g., proptosis, other cranial neuropathies, other neurologic signs or symptoms) that should prompt neuroimaging and further evaluation directed at the topographical localization of the lesion; or (3) neuro-ophthalmic history suggestive of an etiology for optic atrophy (e.g., prior intracranial tumor, syphilis, giant cell arteritis, toxin exposure, nutritional deficiency, family history of optic neuropathy).

Second the clinician in India is urged to consider the endemic disorders in their patient cohort rather than simply using the European or American literature as the sole guide for diagnostic testing. For example, as stated previously certain conditions that might be common in the United States (e.g., sarcoidosis or Lyme disease) might be rare or nonexistent in India or present with different (e.g., less ocular involvement in sarcoidosis, less multiple sclerosis?) manifestations than reported in the European or United States experience and conversely some conditions that could cause optic atrophy may have a higher prevalence in India (e.g., tuberculosis) might be less common in the United States.

SUGGESTED READING

1. Lee AG, Chau F, Golnik KC, Kardon RH, Wall M. The evaluation of isolated optic atrophy. An update and review. Compr Ophthalmol. 2004;5:297-304.

8.5 | Optic Neuritis

Rohit Saxena
RP Centre for Ophthalmic Sciences, AIIMS, New Delhi
rohitsaxena80@gmail.com

Digvijay Singh
Noble Eye Care, Gurugram
drsingh.digvijay@gmail.com

Rashmin Gandhi
Foresight Worldwide, Hyderabad
rashmin.gandhi@gmail.com

■ WHEN DO I SUSPECT OPTIC NEURITIS?

Demography
Typically, optic neuritis occurs in young females (20–40 years); however, it may occur at any age and among males too.

Symptoms
- Acute or subacute blurred or reduced vision or altered quality of vision.
- Altered color perception/sensation.
- Pain behind the eyeballs particularly on eye movements.
- Vision loss shows spontaneous improvement over 2 weeks.

Signs
- Relative afferent pupillary defect in unilateral cases and sluggish pupils in bilateral cases.
- Hyperemic discs with mild edema (papillitis).

Associated Conditions
Multiple sclerosis.

■ HOW DO I INVESTIGATE A CASE OF OPTIC NEURITIS?

Ocular
- Visual acuity.
- Color vision (usually red-green color blindness).
- Contrast sensitivity (usually reduced).
- Visual fields (generally a central scotoma but any field defect can be present).
- Visual evoked potentials (a delayed P100 latency is seen in the affected eye).

Systemic
- Blood sugar (prior to giving steroids).
- Complete hemogram with erythrocyte sedimentation rate (in cases of atypical optic neuritis).
- Blood test for aquaporin-4 antibody and anti-MOG test.
- Autoimmune profile [rheumatoid factor (RF), antinuclear antibody (ANA), anti-neutrophil cytoplasm antibodies (ANCA), C-reactive protein (CRP), angiotensin-converting enzyme (ACE) (in cases of atypical optic neuritis)].

- Infectious diseases profile [venereal disease research laboratory (VDRL), Widal] (in cases of atypical optic neuritis).
- Cerebrospinal fluid analysis (in cases of atypical optic neuritis).
- Other tests (if a particular cause is suspected).

Radiological
- Chest X-ray (to rule out tuberculosis prior to giving steroids).
- Contrast-enhanced magnetic resonance imaging (CE MRI) head and orbits with fluid-attenuated inversion recovery (FLAIR) (to look for demyelination and prognosticate chances of multiple sclerosis).
- CE MRI spine (if suspicion of neuromyelitis optica).
- Ultrasound abdomen or CT chest (if a particular cause is suspected).

HOW DO I MANAGE A CASE OF OPTIC NEURITIS?
- The first decision is to ascertain whether the optic neuritis is typical or atypical.
- For typical optic neuritis, the standard treatment is in the form of pulse steroids followed by an oral taper. The decision to give steroids depends on the presenting visual acuity. Usually, I give therapy only if vision is worse than 6/12 in the affected eye (or at better vision if the patient is one eyed).
- For atypical optic neuritis (one which does not fit the symptoms and signs described above), directed investigations are done (mentioned above) to look for possible causes.
- Therapy for typical optic neuritis: Injection methylprednisolone 1 g IV pulse for 3 days followed by oral steroids in a rapid taper over 11 days. Methylprednisolone can be substituted by dexamethasone 200 mg.
- Therapy for atypical optic neuritis: Treatment of the cause with or without the addition of a pulse steroid therapy.
- Patients are followed up at 3 days, 2 weeks, 1 month, 3 months, and thereon 6 monthly after the initiation of treatment of optic neuritis.
- Patients with antibody-mediated optic neuritis may need a long-term steroid sparing immunosuppression.

8.6 Approach to a Patient with Cranial Nerve Palsy

Preeti Patil-Chablani
LV Prasad eye Institute, Hyderabad
drpreetipatil@gmail.com

PRESENTATION
How will this patient present? What history should you elicit?
- History of Double Vision:
  - *Monocular or binocular—most important question:* Ask the patient—does the diplopia go away on closing *either* eye?
  - *If truly binocular:* Is it vertical or horizontal or both? Is the image also tilted?
  - Does it vary with a change in gaze?
  - Does it vary depending upon the time of the day?
  - When did it start?
  - Is it getting worse or getting better?
  - Was there pain?
- History of Ptosis:
  - When did it start?
  - Is it getting worse or getting better?
  - Does it vary depending upon the time of the day?

- *General History:*
  - Always ask about pain, redness, swelling in or around the eye.
  - Trauma
  - *Systemic history:* Vascular risk factors such as diabetes, hypertension, previously diagnosed cancer, hyperthyroidism, etc.
  - Pain/tenderness
  - Headaches
  - Any other neurological signs/symptoms
- *Examination:*
  - Look for any obvious facial asymmetry.
  - Also look for proptosis, ptosis, enophthalmos or globe dystopia.
  - A complete ophthalmic evaluation is a must.
  - Visual acuity, refraction—distance and near.
  - Anterior segment evaluation—pay particular attention to lid edema, conjunctival congestion, chemosis, enlarged blood vessels (this may point toward a local orbital cause).
  - Corneal examination—any signs of exposure, edema
  - Anterior chamber
  - Fundus examination—look carefully for disc edema, choroidal folds, etc.

Pupils:
- A detailed examination of the pupils is a must—look for afferent/efferent defects
- Anisocoria—if present, is it worse in bright light or dim light?
- Relative afferent pupillary defect (RAPD)—if present, what is the grade?

Ocular Motility Examination:
- Note the presence of any abnormal head posture—a head tilt or a face turn.
- Corneal light reflex tests—these give a basic idea about the ocular deviation and are especially important in children where a detailed examination is not always possible, patients with poor vision where cover test may not be possible.
- Hirschberg light reflex test
- Krimsky/modified Krimsky tests—to measure the deviation with the help of a prism (which is used to center the corneal light reflex).
- Cover test—this remains the gold standard for measurement of strabismus and must be performed to measure the ocular deviations wherever possible.

Measurements must be carried out in all positions of gaze so that an incomitant strabismus will become evident.
- Motility examination—measurement of ductions and versions—in all gazes.
- Also carefully look for presence of any nystagmus or ocular oscillations.
- Saccades and pursuits
- Ancillary tests—Maddox rod test (to test a small tropia or unearth a phoria which may not be clearly evident on cover testing), double Maddox rod testing (to measure torsional deviations), diplopia charting and Hess charting will give idea about specific gazes which may worsen the diplopia and about underaction/overaction of specific muscles.

■ THIRD NERVE PALSY

The patient will present with exotropia and hypotropia, ptosis and may also have anisocoria. There may be incomplete involvement of the third nerve and all the features may not be present always.

The third nerve can be anatomically divided into the nuclear portion, fascicular part, subarachnoid space, cavernous sinus, and the orbital portion. The clinical signs differ depending upon the area of the nerve that it affected and can help in localizing the lesion.

Nuclear Third Nerve Palsy
- Rare
- Bilateral ptosis
- Weakness of the contralateral superior rectus
- Ptosis may be absent in extremely rostral lesions.
- May be associated with vertical gaze palsy.

Fascicular Portion
- Fascicles travel ventrally through midbrain tegmentum, the red nucleus and medial aspect of cerebral peduncles.
- Can cause partial palsy, involving only a few muscles—due to organized arrangement of the fibers in the fascicles.
- Syndromes associated with fascicular lesions include:
  - *Weber's syndrome:* Due to involvement of the superior cerebral peduncle—ipsilateral third nerve with contralateral hemiparesis.
  - *Benedikt's syndrome:* Due to involvement of the red nucleus—ipsilateral third nerve with contralateral extrapyramidal symptoms.
  - *Nothnagel's syndrome:* Due to involvement of the superior cerebellar peduncle—ipsilateral third nerve with ipsilateral ataxia.
  - *Claude's syndrome:* Features of Nothnagel's syndrome + Benedikt's syndrome.

Subarachnoid Portion
- The most common site of an isolated-acquired oculomotor paresis.
- The most important concern is the presence of an aneurysm of the PCA (posterior communicating artery).
- A subarachnoid oculomotor palsy may be complete, incomplete, or progressive.
- The pupillary fibers are superficial and dorsal in the nerve—pupillary involvement is variable and depends primarily on the nature and location of the lesion.
- Compressive lesions usually cause pupillary involvement and hence neuroimaging is mandatory in these cases (rule of the pupil).

Cavernous Sinus Lesions
- May produce isolated oculomotor nerve dysfunction but more often cause a unilateral cranial polyneuropathy.
- Characterized by paralysis or paresis of the 3rd, 4th, 6th nerves, usually with involvement of the ophthalmic division and the maxillary division of the trigeminal nerve.
- Horner's syndrome

Orbital Lesions
- May involve the superior division or the inferior division or both.
- Orbital apex involvement with visual loss.
- Other signs—chemosis, proptosis, inflammation are often present.
- Can cause polyneuropathy.

Work-up
Neuroimaging is a must in:
- Nonisolated third nerve palsy (multiple cranial nerve involvement)
- Acquired third nerve palsy in a young patient (<40 years)
- Pupil involving third nerve palsy (any age)
- Presence of severe pain
- Other neurological signs
- Aberrant innervation (except in traumatic and congenital cases)
- Progressive or nonresolving third nerve palsy (>3 months after onset)

Modality of Choice
- Magnetic resonance imaging (MRI) brain with contrast
- Magnetic resonance (MR) angiography—is an aneurysm, is suspected.
- *Computed tomography (CT) orbits and brain:* In cases post trauma to locate fractures, or where MRI is contraindicated.
- Catheter angiography: Gold standard can help pick up small aneurysms which may be missed by magnetic resonance angiogram.

In the absence of any other lesion, a complete systemic work-up for all vascular risk factors and a prothrombotic profile must be carried out.

■ SIXTH NERVE PALSY

The patient will present with esotropia, which is usually greater at distance when compared to near fixation, with abduction deficit.

Like the third nerve, the sixth nerve also can be anatomically divided into the nuclear, fascicular, subarachnoid, cavernous sinus, and orbital parts.

Nuclear Sixth Nerve Palsy
- Usually a gaze palsy—not isolated sixth nerve palsy [due to involvement of the parapontine reticular formation (PPRF)].
- May be associated with an ipsilateral seventh nerve palsy.
- Other signs of brainstem dysfunction—hemiparesis, hemisensory loss, a central Horner's syndrome—may be present.

Fascicular Sixth Nerve Palsy
- Fascicles of the sixth nerve are closely related to the cerebral peduncles, spinothalamic tract, cerebellar peduncle, seventh nerve nucleus, and fascicle.
- The various syndromes associated with sixth nerve palsy are:
  - *Millard–Gubler syndrome:* Ipsilateral sixth nerve and seventh nerve palsy with contralateral hemiparesis (due to involvement of the superior cerebral peduncle).
  - *Raymond's syndrome:* Ipsilateral sixth nerve with contralateral hemiparesis (due to involvement of the superior cerebral peduncle).
  - *Foville's syndrome:* Fifth, sixth, seventh, and eighth nerve involvement, with ipsilateral Horner's syndrome (due to involvement of the oculosympathetic central neuron) and horizontal gaze palsy (due to involvement of the PPRF).

Subarachnoid Portion
- Unilateral/bilateral sixth nerve palsy
- *Non-localizing sign:* Can occur due to raised intracranial pressure from any cause.
- *Involvement of the petrous apex:* Associated with other neurologic findings including involvement of other cranial nerves (e.g., fifth, seventh, and eighth) and facial pain.

Cavernous Sinus Lesions
- May produce isolated sixth nerve dysfunction: It is the earliest cranial nerve to get involved.
- Characterized by paralysis or paresis of the 3rd, 4th, 6th nerves, usually with involvement of the ophthalmic division and the maxillary division of the trigeminal nerve.
- Horner's syndrome

Orbital Lesions
- May cause isolated sixth nerve palsy—but usually causes a polyneuropathy.
- Orbital apex involvement—with visual loss.
- Other signs—chemosis, proptosis, inflammation are often present.

Work-up

Neuroimaging is a must in:
- Nonisolated sixth nerve palsy
- Presence of other neurological signs
- Fundus examinations showing papilledema
- Isolated sixth nerve palsy in a young patient (<40 years) with no known vascular risk factors.
- Progressive or nonresolving sixth nerve palsy (>3 months after onset)
- Presence of local orbital signs (chemosis, conjunctival congestion, proptosis)

Modality of Choice
- *CT scan:* Acute phase after trauma.
- *MRI brain with contrast:* For intracranial/cavernous sinus lesions.
- *Add MR venography (MRV):* In cases with papilledema—to rule out cavernous sinus thrombosis.

In the absence of any other lesion, a complete systemic work-up for all vascular risk factors and a prothrombotic profile must be carried out.

■ FOURTH NERVE PALSY

The patient usually presents with vertical diplopia and may have an anomalous head posture (head tilt).

The clinical features of a fourth nerve palsy are as follows:
- *Incomitant hypertropia:* Worse on contralateral gaze and ipsilateral head tilt—as diagnosed on Park's three-step test.
- *Variable excyclotorsion:* Subjective tilting of images and double Maddox rod testing/objectively by fundus examination.
- Underaction of superior oblique (SO) muscle.
- Overaction ipsilateral inferior oblique muscle (IOOA) (over-elevation in adduction).
- *Anomalous head posture:* Contralateral head tilt (most common), paradoxical ipsilateral head tilt (3%)
- One must always look for a bilateral palsy, which may be masked at times.

The features of bilateral fourth nerve palsy are as follows:
- Right hypertropia in left gaze and left hypertropia in right gaze—a reversing hypertropia.
- Positive Bielschowsky test on tilt to either shoulder—"double Bielschowsky test"
- Large excyclotropia (>10°)
- V-pattern esotropia
- Smaller hypertropia in primary position
- Bilateral SO underaction, IOOA
- The most common causes are congenital (which may manifest later in life) and traumatic.

Based on the anatomical localization, fourth nerve palsy may be classified into the following types:

Nuclear/Fascicular
- A nuclear lesion (in the midbrain) causes contralateral SO palsy (since the nerve decussates as it leaves the brainstem).
- Other brainstem signs—hemisensory loss, hemiparesis, and central Horner's syndrome are often present.
- Other brainstem cranial neuropathies—such as a third nerve palsy may be present
- Vertical gaze palsy may be present.

Subarachnoid Space
- Ipsilateral SOP
- Very rarely isolated IVth palsy
- Headache, neck stiffness, and multiple cranial neuropathies

Cavernous Sinus Lesions
- Characterized by paralysis or paresis of the 3rd, 4th, 6th nerves, usually with involvement of the ophthalmic division and the maxillary division of the trigeminal nerve.
- Horner's syndrome.

Orbital Lesions
- Usually causes a polyneuropathy.
- Orbital apex involvement—will be associated with visual loss.
- Other signs—chemosis, proptosis, and inflammation—are often present.

As in case of other cranial nerve palsies, neuroimaging is a must in acquired cases, those with progressive palsies, cranial polyneuropathies and in traumatic cases.

Always remember to consider investigating for *ocular myasthenia* in case the ocular deviation does not "fit" into a typical pattern or is very variable since myasthenia can mimic any cranial nerve palsy.

8.7 Patient with Unequal Pupils

Navin Jaykumar
Darshan Eye Clinic, Chennai
navinjay@yahoo.com

■ INTRODUCTION
Anisocoria implies a difference in pupil sizes.

It is considered physiological if the difference is <2 mm.

Pathological anisocoria is defined as any difference in pupil size >2 mm. This has to be evaluated in detail. Anisocoria always indicates a lesion involving the efferent pupillary pathway (either parasympathetic or sympathetic). It is *not* a sign of afferent pathway (optic nerve) disease.

■ KEY EVALUATION QUESTION: IS THERE REALLY AN ABNORMAL PUPIL?

Test 1: Perform Direct Light Reflex
Result

Any pupil that shows a brisk and sustained response to the direct reflex is a normal pupil irrespective of its size.

Test 2: Note Degree of Difference in Pupil Size in Bright and Dim Illumination
Result

No change in degree of anisocoria with any level of illumination—physiological. Anisocoria increases in bright illumination—parasympathetic palsy.

Anisocoria increases in dim illumination—sympathetic palsy (Horner's syndrome).

■ ANISOCORIA: PARASYMPATHETIC CAUSES
There are four important causes (**Table 8.7.1**) that can be differentiated by slit lamp examination of the pupil and pharmacologic testing with topical pilocarpine.

TABLE 8.7.1: Anisocoria: Parasympathetic causes.

Cause	Slit lamp	Contraction with pilocarpine	
		0.125%	2%
1. III nerve palsy	Normal	No	Yes
2. Tonic pupil	Segmental contraction	Yes	Yes
3. Sphincter trauma	Sphincter tears	No	+/−
4. Pharmacologic	Normal	No	No

Note: To prepare 0.125% pilocarpine from commercially available 2% solution:
Convert 2% pilocarpine into a 1% solution first as follows: Draw 0.25 mL of 2% pilocarpine eye drops into a 2 mL syringe. Dilute by drawing 0.25 mL (an equal amount) of water for injection (1:1 dilution). The syringe now contains 0.5 mL solution of 1% pilocarpine. Mix thoroughly and then discard 0.25 mL. What is left is 0.25 mL of 1% pilocarpine. Dilute further by drawing water up to the 2 mL mark (8 × dilution of 1% = 0.125%). Fit a cannula to the syringe for topical instillation.

ANISOCORIA: SYMPATHETIC PALSY (HORNER'S SYNDROME)
Test: With the Patient in Bright Ambient Illumination, Dim the Lights Rapidly

Result
Normally both pupils should dilate equally in 2–4 seconds when bright ambient light is suddenly dimmed (Note: The speed of the dilatation reflex is much slower than pupil constriction). A *dilatation lag* (anisocoria seen after 2–4 seconds of dark) implies a sympathetic palsy.

Horner's Syndrome
Localized as:
- Central
- Preganglionic
- Postganglionic

Evaluation
- Recognize Horner's syndrome clinically
- Look for associated signs for localization
- Pharmacologic localization if Horner's syndrome appears isolated.

Key Clinical Features of Horner's Syndrome
- Mild upper lid ptosis
- Apparent enophthalmos
- Small pupil
- Iris heterochromia (congenital Horner's only)
- Facial anhidrosis +/−

Associated Signs for Localization
Central: Look for hypothalamic, brainstem, and meningeal signs.

Preganglionic: Neck/arm pain, facial anhidrosis; examine neck and chest (cervicothoracic abnormalities).

Postganglionic: Cluster/migraine headache, cavernous sinus signs, no facial anhidrosis, internal carotid artery dissection (neck/face/orbit pain, amaurosis fugax/central retinal artery occlusion, neck bruit).

Pharmacologic Testing

Cocaine and hydroxyamphetamine are extremely difficult to come by. For practical reasons phenylephrine is useful.

Topical 1% phenylephrine dilates the postganglionic Horner's pupil, but not the non-postganglionic or normal pupil.

Phenylephrine 1% correlates well with the results of hydroxyamphetamine 1% in localizing the lesion to the post-ganglionic neuron.

■ SUGGESTED READING

1. Walsh FB, Hoyt WF, Miller NR, Newman NJ, Biousse V, Kerrison JB. Walsh and Hoyt's Clinical Neuro-Ophthalmology. 6th edition. USA: Lippincott Williams and Wilkins; 2004.

8.8 Patient with Ptosis

Shubhra Goel
Apollo Hospitals, Hyderabad
drshubhragoel@gmail.com

Akshay Nair
Advanced Eye Hospital and Institute, Navi Mumbai
akshaygn@gmail.com

■ CLASSIFICATION

Ptosis is classified in following categories:
- Aponeurotic, chronic progressive external ophthalmoplegia (CPEO), myotonic dystrophy
- 3rd nerve palsy, Horner's syndrome
- Neuromuscular junction related-myasthenia gravis

■ APPROACH

- Age of Presentation
  - Soon after birth—congenital
  - Young female—CPEO
  - Adult male—myotonic dystrophy
  - Middle-aged female—myasthenia gravis
  - Old age—aponeurotic
    - 3rd nerve palsy and ptosis due to trauma can occur at any age.
- Unilateral or bilateral
  - Unilateral   Congenital—70%
                      3rd nerve palsy
                      Horner's syndrome
                      Myasthenia gravis
                      Trauma
  - Bilateral   Congenital—30%
                      Aponeurotic
                      CPEO
                      Myotonic dystrophy Myasthenia gravis
- Progression
  - Stable   Congenital
                      Horner's syndrome
  - Worsening   Aponeurotic
                      CPEO
  - Fluctuating   Myasthenia gravis
  - Improving   Congenital
- Family history
  Myotonic dystrophy—autosomal dominant CPEO—mitochondrial inheritance.

MYASTHENIA GRAVIS
- Sudden onset
- Variable ptosis
- Diurnal variation
- Associated diplopia
- Associated intermittent phoria or tropia
- Good to poor levator action
- Fatigability
- Cogan's lid twitch
- Decrease speed of excursion of levator
- Decreased orbicularis oculi tone
- Asymmetrical extraocular movements limitation
- Positive ice test

CHRONIC PROGRESSIVE EXTERNAL OPHTHALMOPLEGIA
- Young female
- Congenital
- Progressive
- Bilateral and symmetrical
- Severe ptosis in later stages
- Chin elevation
- Poor levator action
- Limited ocular movements in all gazes

DYSTROPHIA MYOTONICA
- Old males
- Congenital
- Bilateral
- Weak facial muscles
- Progressive
- Poor levator action
- Limited ocular movements in all gazes
- Light near dissociation
- Pigmentary cataract

SUGGESTED READING
1. Walsh FB, Hoyt WF, Miller NR, Newman NJ, Biousse V, Kerrison JB. Walsh and Hoyt's Clinical Neuro-Ophthalmology. 6th edition. USA: Lippincott Williams and Wilkins; 2004.

8.9 Traumatic Optic Neuropathy

S Ambika
Sankara Nethralaya, Chennai
drsa@snmail.org

Rashmin Gandhi
Foresight Worldwide, Hyderabad
rashmin.gandhi@gmail.com

INTRODUCTION
Traumatic optic neuropathy (TON) is the chief cause of vision loss due to trauma in neuro-ophthalmology. It refers to acute injury of the optic nerve secondary to trauma.

The optic nerve axons may be damaged either directly or indirectly and the visual loss may be partial or complete.
- *Direct injury* that results from orbital or cerebral trauma that transgresses normal tissue planes to disrupt the anatomic and functional integrity of the optic nerve, e.g., bullet penetrating orbit. Vision loss is severe, immediate and recovery is unlikely.
- *Indirect injury* usually results from blunt trauma to the forehead that results in transmission of force through the cranium to the restrained intracanalicular portion of optic nerve. Vision loss may be delayed and recovery is poor.

They are classified into three types:
1. *Optic nerve avulsion:* Ophthalmoscopic appearance consists of a partial ring of hemorrhage or the avulsion can be seen as a dark crescentric area.
2. *Anterior optic neuropathy:* Injury within 10 mm of the globe. Central retinal artery occlusion or vein occlusion may occur.
3. *Posterior optic neuropathy:* Injury posterior to entrance of central retinal artery or vein.

CLINICAL FEATURES
- The condition may manifest immediately or within hours or days following the trauma. Occasionally, the vision loss may be insidious, and in some cases the patient may be not aware of any visual deficit until it is detected by routine examination.
- On examination patient can have variably reduced acuity with visual field defects. An afferent pupillary defect is characteristic, and dyschromatopsia may be noted in accordance with the severity of the vision loss.
- Initially a normal fundus may be seen. In other cases, a grossly edematous optic nerve head, vitreous hemorrhage, venous congestion or retinal edema may be seen. In the vast majority of cases, however, optic disc pallor ensues within few weeks of the injury.
- Multi-system trauma or serious brain damage with loss of consciousness may be present. Periorbital or ocular hemorrhage, ecchymosis or laceration may be present.

IMAGING
- In TON it is preferable to do a CT scan of orbit with 1–2 mm sections through the optic canal in the axial and coronal planes to rule out canal fracture compromising the canal. Routine sections of the brain should also be taken.
- Unenhanced CT scanning assists in delineating cases that have fractures of the optic canal, hemorrhage of the orbit or optic nerve sheath, orbital emphysema, or most penetrating orbital foreign bodies.
- MRI is superior to CT in imaging the soft tissue and discerning hemorrhages and hematomas.

MANAGEMENT
Recommendation
The CRASH trial, Spinal cord injury studies, and several animal studies have concluded a questionable or even harmful role of steroids-especially mega dose steroids in TON. Steroids in a dose usually administered in optic neuropathies may have a role in hyperacute optic nerve injuries without central nervous system involvement.

Role of steroids in TON is inconclusive. If started within first 48 hours of the injury it may help to reduce the damage because of axonal edema.

Optic Canal Decompression
Surgical intervention in form of optic canal decompression can be considered if there is a fracture of optic canal with bone fragment impinging on the optic nerve.

OPTIC NERVE AVULSION

Traumatic separation of optic nerve heads from the remaining portion of the nerve. Usually occurs following severe orbital trauma but can also occur in minor trauma. Fundus reveals hemorrhage over optic disc in classical avulsion. Ultrasonography may also demonstrate separation of the nerve head from the sclera.

Orbital CT scanning or MRI may reveal avulsion of the nerve but frequently shows the optic nerve sheath to be intact. There may be edema of the optic nerve head on imaging as an indirect sign of avulsion. Optic nerve transection and diffuse and localized orbital hemorrhage (hematoma) are the other causes of vision loss.

Traumatic optic neuropathy is true ophthalmic emergency. Early identification and prompt treatment can salvage vision.

SUGGESTED READING

1. Walsh FB, Hoyt WF, Miller NR, Newman NJ, Biousse V, Kerrison JB. Walsh and Hoyt's Clinical Neuro-Ophthalmology. 6th edition. USA: Lippincott Williams and Wilkins; 2004.

8.10 Neuroimaging

Olma Veena Noronha
Sankara Nethralaya, Chennai
olma_veena@hotmail.com

INTRODUCTION

Neuroimaging plays a very vital role in the diagnosis and management of patients with various visual pathway disorders. A neuro-ophthalmologist deals with various optic nerve disorders, ocular motility disorders, and visual disturbances which occur at different anatomical regions in the eye and brain. It is very important that a neuro-ophthalmologist after having clinically localized the lesion gives clinically relevant information to the radiologist, which would guide him in planning the study.

Magnetic resonance imaging (MRI) is the imaging modality of choice in most of the conditions pertaining to neuro-ophthalmology.

Computed tomography (CT) would be preferred in patients with disc drusen, trauma and in patients where MRI is contraindicated viz., metallic foreign bodies, pacemakers and cochlear implants.

OPTIC NERVE DISORDERS

Magnetic resonance imaging with contrast is the imaging modality of choice in patients suspected to have:
- Optic neuritis
- Optic neuropathy
- Optic nerve tumors

Optic Neuritis

- Coronal and axial T2 fat saturation images are most sensitive in identifying signal in the optic nerves.
- Post-contrast study should include axial, coronal and sagittal T1 fat saturation images parallel to the optic nerves.
- In patients suspected to have demyelination—brain and spine screening should always be performed.
- Brain contrast in patients with demyelinating plaques should be performed using magnetization transfer techniques.
- Magnetic resonance spectroscopy can be performed in patients with diagnostic dilemma.

Optic Nerve Tumors

One has to differentiate between meningioma and glioma, the two most common encountered tumors of the optic nerve **(Table 8.10.1)**.

TABLE 8.10.1: Differentiate between glioma and meningioma.

	Optic nerve glioma	Optic nerve meningioma
Age	Young	Relatively older
C/H	Visual loss is earlier	Vision loss is later
	Proptosis	Proptosis +/–
Imaging CT	• Intraconal heterogenous fusiform mass inseparable from the optic nerve • Optic canal widening • Calcification absent • Cystic changes +	• Intraconal homogenous mass inseparable from the optic nerve • Optic canal normal • Calcification +/– • No cystic changes
Imaging MRI	• Fusiform heterogenous intraconal mass inseparable from the optic nerve • Mixed signal in T2-weighted images • Intracranial extension better visualized	• Fusiform homogenous perioptic mass, encased optic nerve seen separately • Homogenous signal in T2-weighted images-mostly hypointense • Intracranial extension is better visualized

CHIASMAL COMPRESSIVE LESIONS

Magnetic resonance imaging should be done in patients suspected to have chiasmal lesions. CT would be a cost-effective modality in patients who cannot afford MRI.
- Magnetic resonance imaging is superior to CT
  - Identifying small lesions especially vascular
  - Characterization of the lesion
  - Extent and invasion of the surrounding structures
  - Helps in surgical planning
- CT is superior in identifying calcification and bony erosion.

CRANIAL NERVE PALSIES AND OCULAR MOTILITY DISORDERS
- Magnetic resonance imaging is the modality of choice.
- MRI with contrast is preferable in patients suspected to have cranial nerve palsies.
- MR angiogram should be done in patients with pupil involving third nerve, followed by digital subtraction angiography (DSA) if MRI is negative.
- Thin axial and coronal sections should be obtained to include the orbit, cavernous sinus and brainstem.

CAROTID CAVERNOUS FISTULAS
- Dynamic contrast-enhanced MRI should be done in patients suspected to have carotid cavernous fistulas (CCF) to confirm the diagnosis as it is noninvasive and helps to exclude other lesions. A negative MRI does not exclude CCF.
- MRI however cannot completely delineate the type of fistula.
- DSA is the confirmatory imaging modality.

TRAUMATIC OPTIC NEUROPATHY
- Computed tomography (CT) scan of the brain and orbit should be done to look for fracture of the optic canal.

- About 1-2 mm thick sections should be obtained in both axial and coronal planes if patient's general condition permits coronal imaging. The axial sections should be parallel to the optic nerves. Coronal sections are perpendicular to the axial sections.
- If CT scan does not show fracture, it should be followed by MRI to look for optic nerve contusion, avulsion or hematoma.
- MRI using surface coil is preferred in patients suspected to have optic nerve avulsion clinically.

The choice of the imaging modality should depend on the patient's clinical diagnosis, availability of the facility, and cost factor.

SUGGESTED READING

1. Radiology Clinics of North America. Vol.37. Jan 1999.

8.11 Different Magnetic Resonance Imaging Sequences

Navin Jayakumar
Darshan Eye Clinic, Chennai
navinjay@yahoo.com

Aim: "Not only to read the magnetic resonance imaging (MRI) report but also *try to interpret the images*!"

WHAT IS MAGNETIC RESONANCE IMAGING?

Magnetic resonance imaging is based on the principle of nuclear magnetic resonance (NMR).

How Does All This Work?

The MRI studies are images of the hydrogen nuclei (protons) present in our tissues (the *"Nuclear"* bit).

The subject is placed inside a giant superconducting magnet that causes randomly.

When these protons are stimulated by a radiofrequency (RF) pulse they absorb energy and spin in the direction of the pulse (the *"Resonance"* bit).

When the RF pulse is turned off, the protons relax back to their original alignment and give off the energy absorbed during the RF pulse. These energy signals are detected and converted the MRI image (the *"Imaging"* bit).

Discussion Plan

What are the commonly employed sequences and protocols?
What do the images look like?
When are they used?

Pulse Sequences

A pulse sequence is a preselected set of defined radiofrequency and gradient pulses, usually repeated many times during a scan.

The time interval between pulses and the amplitude and shape of the gradient waveforms will control the signal reception and affect the characteristics of the MR images.

Two Types

1. Spin Echo (SE) sequence
   - Most commonly used

2. *Gradient Echo (GRE) sequence*
   - Less commonly used
   - Especially useful in studying brain hemorrhage

T1 Image
- Shows anatomy well.
- Water (vitreous/CSF) appears dark.
- Fat (orbit) appears bright.

T2 Image
- Shows pathology well as bright signals.
- Water (vitreous/CSF) appears very bright.

Contrast Magnetic Resonance Imaging (Gadolinium) Image
- Looks like T1 image but blood vessels/extraocular muscles appear bright.
- Active lesions enhance (infections/MS plaques).
- Contraindicated in pregnancy/allergy to gadolinium.

Flair Image
- *Fl*uid *A*ttenuation *I*nversion *R*ecovery sequence.
- Water is suppressed and appears dark.
- Used in brain studies.
- Looks like a T2 image in that pathology appears bright but water (CSF) appears dark.
- Useful in studying deep white matter plaques adjacent to ventricles (the bright plaques are easily seen contrasted against the adjacent dark ventricles).

SPIR/STIR IMAGES
These are fat suppression images.
- STIR (short tau inversion recovery)
- SPIR (spatial presaturation inversion recovery)
  Fat suppression deletes orbital fat allowing visibility of small lesions in this location.
  Contrast studies in the orbit especially for optic nerve diseases require fat suppression to highlight bright signals from pathology.
  These improve detection of disease in the orbit, the pituitary gland, and around the skull base which has fat in the bone marrow.

Diffusion Weighted Image
- Usually an axial brain image
- Looks like a T1 image (water dark) but pathology may appear either as dark or bright patches.

Uses
- Diagnosis of early stroke (can differentiate between acute and chronic stroke)
- Multiple MS lesions—differentiate stages of lesion (acute/chronic)
- Tumors with high nuclear—cytoplasmic ratio appear brighter with diffusion weighted image (DWI).

MAGNETIC RESONANCE ANGIOGRAPHY
Two types: 2D or 3D time of flight magnetic resonance angiography (MRA) (common) and phase contrast MRA (less common).
  Images are not of the actual blood vessel itself as in a conventional arteriogram but blood flow characteristics within the vessel.

Uses
Clinical diagnosis/MR study suggests aneurysm or AV malformation.

MAGNETIC RESONANCE VENOGRAPHY (MRV)
Similar to MRA except it is commonly used to image dural venous sinuses.

Uses
Cavernous sinus thrombosis, idiopathic intracranial hypertension (hypoplasia or thrombosis of venous sinuses).

PROTON MAGNETIC RESONANCE SPECTROSCOPY (MRS)
Profiles biochemical alterations within brain lesions.

Common metabolites studied: Choline, creatine, N-acetyl-aspartate, lactate, lipids.

Image: Appears as a spectroscopic graph with various metabolite peaks, and a corresponding brain image with a box marking the area studied.

Uses
Brain tumor, stroke, focal cerebral lesions, MS, and intracranial hemorrhage. Not used for orbit lesions owing to smaller lesion size.

SUGGESTED READING
1. Radiology Clinics of North America. Vol.37. Jan 1999.

8.12 | Electrophysiology in Neuro-ophthalmology

Parveen Sen, Ramya Sachidanandam
Sankara Nethralaya, Chennai
drpka@snmail.org

INTRODUCTION
Optic nerve disorders may have varied clinical manifestations and neuro-ophthalmologists depend on electrophysiological investigations in addition to imaging modalities to reach at a correct diagnosis as well as to follow up of many of these neuropathies. The most commonly used electrophysiological test in neuro-ophthalmology is the visual evoked potential (VEP). The newer tests that are also being increasingly used include pattern electroretinogram (PERG), multifocal visual evoked potentials (mfVEP), multifocal ERG (mfERG), and photonegative response (PhNR).

Visual evoked potential evaluates the response of the visual system to light. The generator site of VEP is at the peristriate and the striate occipital cortex. This response can be in response to a bright flash of light (flash VEP) or in response to a pattern (pattern VEP).

Flash VEP is commonly used to assess the visual status in subjects with poor visual acuity, in opaque media or in infants and children. It may help to prognosticate the outcome by grossly picking up the optic nerve function. Pattern VEP is in response to pattern reversal or pattern onset and offset. Pattern reversal VEP is used more commonly in clinical evaluation because its results are more reproducible. Indications of pattern reversal VEP in neuro-ophthalmology include optic neuritis, multiple sclerosis, compressive optic nerve disease, unexplained visual loss, amblyopia, cortical blindness, traumatic optic neuropathy, and measuring visual acuity in non-cooperative individuals. Pattern onset/offset VEP is preferred over pattern reversal in malingering subjects and in patients with significant nystagmus.

INTERPRETATION OF VISUAL EVOKED POTENTIAL

Flash Visual Evoked Potential

The most important parameter in the analysis of flash VEP is the P2 latency and amplitude (**Figs. 8.12.1A to C**).

Since high degree of intersubject variability is seen in flash VEP parameters in the normal population, an interocular comparison is commonly used instead of comparison with the normative data.

Pattern Visual Evoked Potential

On pattern reversal VEP P100 is the most important parameter for analysis because of its narrow latency range in normal subjects. P100 is preceded by a negative waveform the N75 and followed by another negative wave form N 135 (**Fig. 8.12.2**).

Salient features on VEP in the commonly seen optic nerve disorders are given in **Table 8.12.1**.

Flash and Pattern VEP Responses in Optic Neuritis

Pattern VEP may be more sensitive in picking up an optic nerve disorder in certain situations and is especially useful in chronic optic neuritis when the magnetic resonance imaging (MRI) has become normal. Also, it is more economical for the patient especially when repeated investigations are required to know the progress of the disease (**Figs. 8.12.3A to D**).

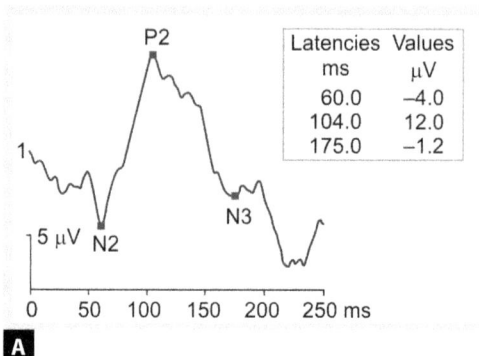
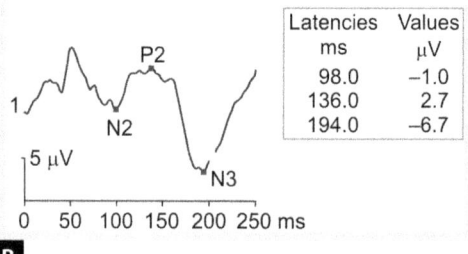
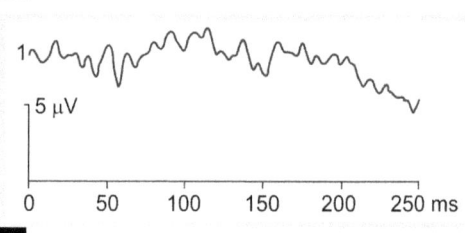

Figs. 8.12.1A to C: (A) Flash visual evoked potential with normal P2 latency; (B) Flash visual evoked potential with delayed P2 latency with reduced amplitude; (C) Non-recordable flash visual evoked potential.

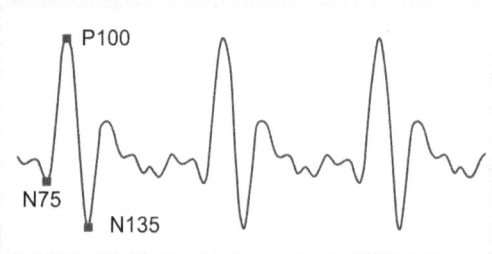

Fig. 8.12.2: Shows typical pattern visual evoked potential waveforms seen in normal subjects.

SECTION 8: Neuro-ophthalmology

TABLE 8.12.1: Features in visual evoked potential (VEP) in common optic nerve disorders.

Optic neuritis	Ischemic optic neuropathy	Compressive lesions
Marked latency delay	Latency delay not seen	Latency delay seen
Amplitude reduction seen which recovers	Predominant decrease in amplitude	Amplitude reduction seen
Waveform morphology maintained	Waveform morphology maintained	Distortion of the waveform seen
Changes in scalp distribution uncommon	Changes in scalp distribution uncommon	Abnormal scalp distribution seen
VEP changes seen during the course of the disease	Monophasic	VEP changes seen during the course of the disease

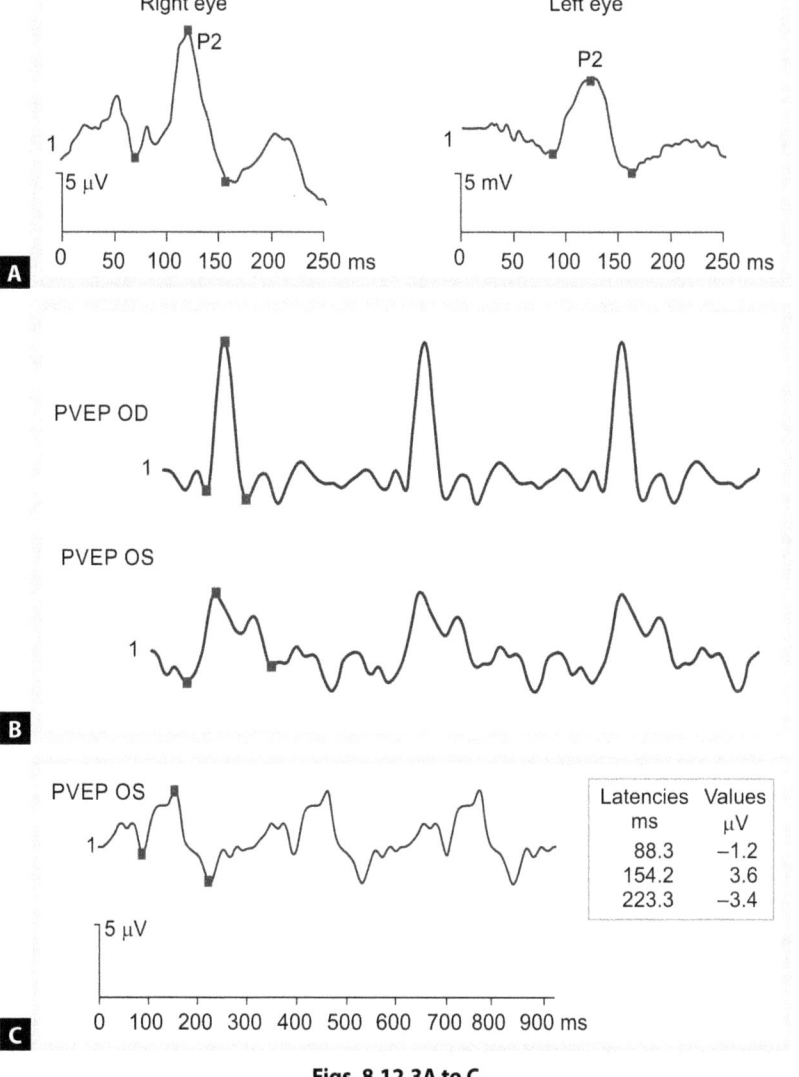

Figs. 8.12.3A to C

SECTION 8: Neuro-ophthalmology

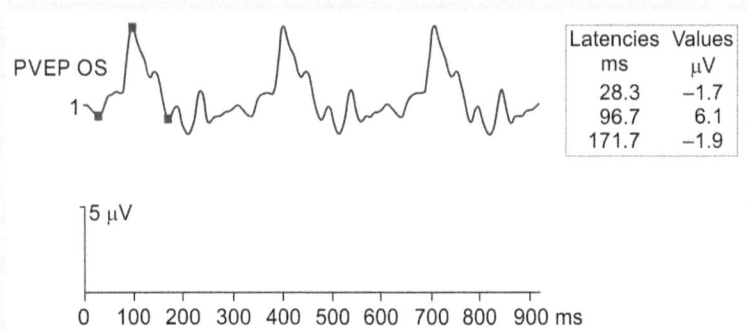

Fig. 8.12.3D

Figs. 8.12.3A to D: (A) Flash visual evoked potential showing delayed and reduced P2 component in the left eye; (B) Pattern visual evoked potential (PVEP) in optic neuritis: The right eye shows PVEP with normal latency and amplitudes whereas the left eye reveals delayed waveform with reduced amplitude; (C and D) Pattern visual evoked potential of left eye of a patient of optic neuritis, shows improvement in P100 latency and amplitude after treatment.

Flash and Pattern Visual Evoked Potential Responses in Ischemic Optic Neuropathy (Figs. 8.12.4A and B)

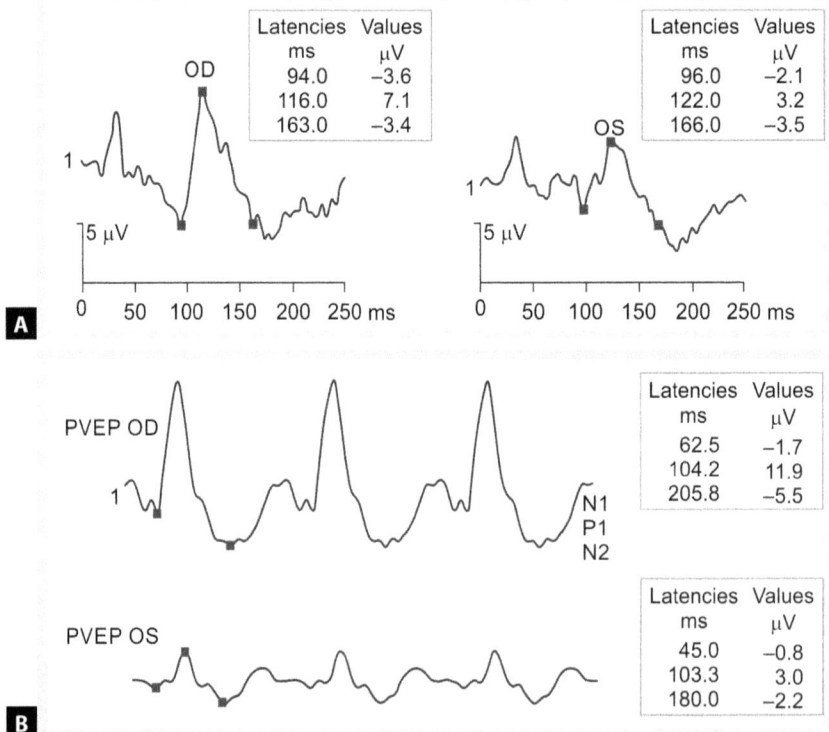

Figs. 8.12.4A and B: (A) Flash visual evoked potential (VEP) showing decrease in amplitudes in OS; (B) Pattern visual evoked potential (PVEP) showing a predominant decrease in amplitudes in a subject with ischemic optic neuropathy of the left eye. Note that the latency of the P100 remains largely same.

Flash and Pattern VEP Responses in Compressive Optic Neuropathy (Figs. 8.12.5 and 8.12.6)

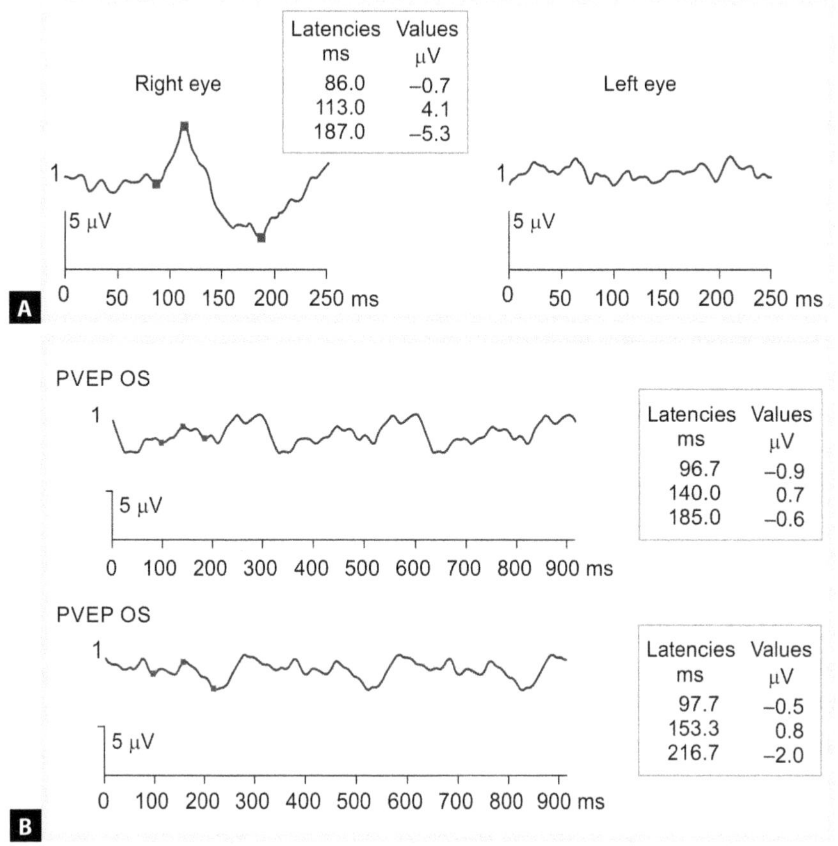

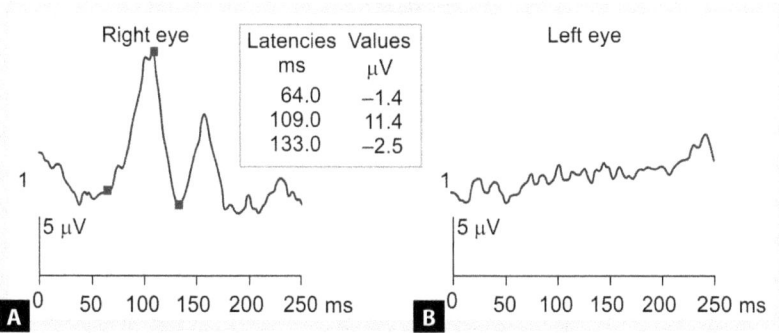

Figs. 8.12.5A and B: (A) Flash visual evoked potential in 8-year-old girl with compressive optic neuropathy due to optic canal narrowing. Right eye vision 2/60 and left eye no perception of light; (B) Pattern visual evoked potential of the same subject. OU reveals a distorted waveform reduced amplitude and delayed P100 latency OS >OD.

Figs. 8.12.6A and B: Flash visual evoked potential (VEP) in a 16-year-old boy who had injury to the left globe with no perception of light; shows normal waveform in the right eye while the left eye flash VEP is non-recordable.

Flash VEP Responses in Traumatic Optic Neuropathy

A normal VEP practically rules out an optic nerve disease anterior to the chiasma. However, chiasmal and retrochiasmal disorders may be missed until multichannel VEP recording is done.

Major limitation of use of VEP for nerve disorders is that it can be influenced by macular pathology as well since the majority of optic nerve fibers are from the macula. To differentiate between the reduced PVEP because of optic nerve disease or macular disorder *PERG* is used. *PERG* is a retinal biopotential that is produced when a stimulus pattern of constant mean luminance is viewed. *Transient PERG* has two components: P50 (positive component appearing at 50 ms) which shows macular function and N95 (larger negative component appearing at 95 ms) which shows ganglion cell function. In some patients an early small negative wave called the N35 is also seen **(Fig. 8.12.7A)**.

Pattern electroretinogram however has much lower amplitude (0.5–8 µV) than ERG and so special recording techniques need to be used to differentiate it from noise. Also, fixation is critical for a good PERG record; hence it cannot be used in patients with poor visual acuity **(Fig. 8.12.7B)**.

P50 component of PERG which reflects the macular function is complementary to full-field ERG. Normal ERG with a decrease in the P50 amplitude depicts macular dysfunction while an abnormal ERG with an abnormal PERG is a pointer toward a generalized retinal disorder. Extinct PERG may occur in macular dysfunction but is rarely seen in optic nerve dysfunction. Selective affection of the N95 component with a near normal P50 points toward optic nerve pathology; N95/P50 ratio could also be very useful in differentiating between the macular and optic nerve dysfunction. It remains unaltered in macular disease but decreases in optic nerve disorders.

Acute phase of optic neuritis shows a loss of visual acuity; hence PERG waveforms can be non-recordable. In chronic phase of optic neuritis P50 recovers while N95 abnormality persists with significant reduction in the N95:P50 ratio. This can be associated with the retrograde degeneration of the ganglion cells seen in the chronic stages of optic neuritis.

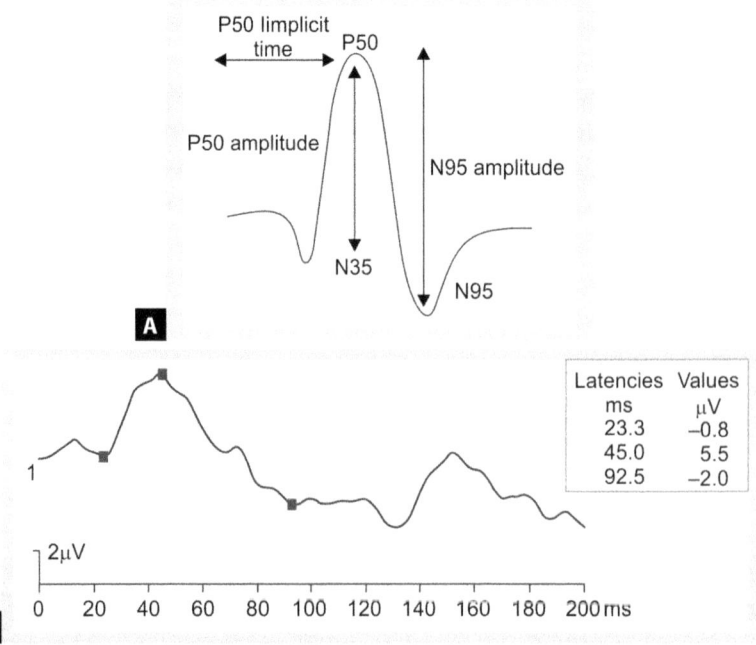

Figs. 8.12.7A and B: (A) The components of a typical pattern electroretinogram waveform; (B) A normal pattern electroretinogram waveform.

Subnormal N95 component is also seen in Leber hereditary optic neuropathy (LHON) and Kjer-type dominant optic atrophy (DOA) and in optic nerve compression. Though PERG can differentiate between a retinal and an optic nerve disorder it does not give us the topography of the disease process.

Photopic negative response which originates from retinal ganglion cells has also been used as an indicator for ganglion cell function especially in early glaucomatous neuropathy. The PhNR is a slow negative potential that is seen after the b-wave of a light adapted full field electroretinography (ffERG). It can be recorded as full-field PhNR, focal PhNR and multifocal PhNR **(Figs. 8.12.8A and B)**.

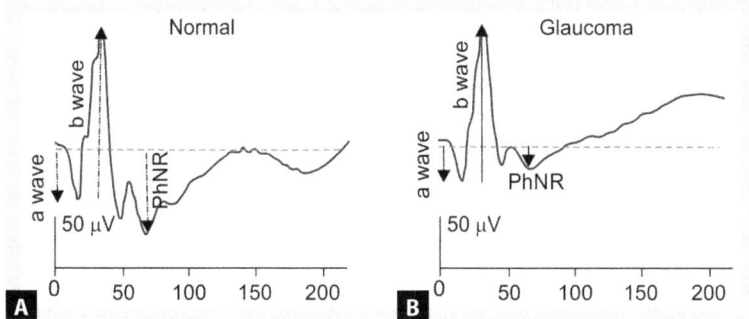

Figs. 8.12.8A and B: Showing photopic negative response (PhNR) in normal as well as glaucomatous eye. Note a significant decrease in the amplitude of PhNR in eye with glaucomatous neuropathy.

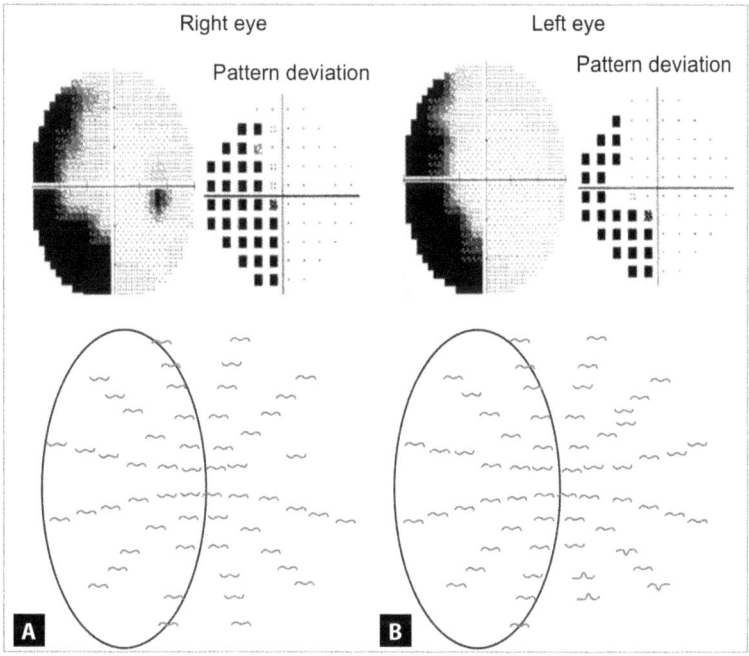

Figs. 8.12.9A and B: A 48-year-old male presented with field loss and best corrected visual acuity (BCVA) of 6/6 in both eyes. MRI revealed right occipital hemorrhagic infarct (A) Fields showed left homonymous hemianopia. (B) Multifocal visual evoked potential (MfVEP) trace array shows corresponding reduced amplitudes in nasal field. Optical coherence tomography (OCT) revealed normal retinal nerve fiber layer thickness in all quadrants.

Conventional VEP elicits global response and hence is unable to detect subtle or local pathology. For the topography of retinal and optic nerve disorders, multifocal techniques such as the multifocal VEP and the multifocal ERG are used. Most important application of *multifocal ERG* in neuro-ophthalmology is to rule out macular pathology as a cause of poor vision. A near normal fundus with a poor amplitude chart on mfERG and an abnormal VEP suggests macular pathology as the cause of poor vision.

Multifocal VEP can be particularly useful in picking up distribution of the optic nerve dysfunction and may be a pointer to the underlying pathology. For example, an altitudinal defect seen on mfVEP points toward an AION. MfVEP follows the visual fields but can also be effectively done in some subjects not cooperative for Humphrey visual field (HVF) 30-2 and in children. Just like macular pathology can affect the VEP, retinal disorders can also affect mfVEP **(Figs. 8.12.9A and B)**.

We have seen that no single test can give us the complete information and one has to rely on a combination of investigations to reach a diagnosis. Even though newer and better imaging techniques particularly MRI may have limited the use of electrophysiology in clinical setting, these tests still give useful information about the physiology of disease whereas the imaging modalities essentially give information on the structural damage. In most of the circumstances these could be complementary to patient care if intelligently used.

SUGGESTED READING

1. Acar G, Ozakbas S, Cakmakci H, Idiman F, Idiman E. Visual evoked potential is superior to triple dose magnetic resonance imaging in the diagnosis of optic nerve involvement. Int J Neurosci. 2004;114(8):1025-33.

8.13 Role of Optical Coherence Tomography in Neuro-ophthalmology

Devendra Venkatramani
Laxmi Eye Institute, Panvel
dev.venkatramani@gmail.com

INTRODUCTION

Optical coherence tomography (OCT) has revolutionized the diagnosis and management of patients with retinal diseases, and to a lesser extent, glaucoma. It is now also an invaluable tool in the assessment of patients with neurological and neuro-ophthalmic diseases.

Technological advances include vastly improved axial resolution, eye-tracking and reduction of motion artifact, increased penetration and choroidal imaging, and improvements in the analysis of data, including in the measurement of retinal nerve fiber layer (RNFL) thickness, ganglion cell complex (GCC), macular volume, and optic disc parameters. Its major advantages also include its noninvasive nature, and reproducibility and repeatability in longitudinal studies.

OPTIC NEURITIS

Whether isolated or associated with multiple sclerosis (MS), optic neuritis is characterized by axonal inflammation and degeneration.

Peripapillary RNFL Thickness

- Thickening can be demonstrated in eyes with optic disc edema due to papillitis, with subsequent thinning correlating with the severity of the episode.

- Optical coherence tomography can demonstrate subclinical damage even in the presence of normal acuity and field. In patients with MS thinning occurs even in the absence of optic neuritis.
- In general, thinning correlates with disease duration as well as visual and neurological function. Costello et al. detected a level of 75 microns to correlate with persistent visual dysfunction.

Ganglion Cell Complex Thickness
- Loss in the GCC occurs earlier and is a more sensitive marker than RNFL loss in relapsing-remitting MS (RRMS).
- Ganglion cell complex losses appear to correlate better with visual acuity and field than losses in RNFL.

Macular Edema in Multiple Sclerosis
Macular edema may occur in conjunction with intermediate uveitis in patients with MS. It may also be a side-effect of treatment with fingolimod. Microcystic macular edema (MME) is characterized by cysts in the parafoveal inner nuclear layer, and is thought to represent retrograde neuro-degeneration rather than exudation seen in typical cystoid macular edema.

PARACHIASMAL LESIONS
Danesh-Meyer and colleagues evaluated the pre- and postoperative RNFL thickness measurements in patients with parachiasmal compressive lesions. In this study, thinner preoperative RNFL thickness was associated with worse visual acuity and visual field changes. These patients were much less likely to experience improvement in visual acuity and visual fields than those individuals with normal OCTs. These findings enable neuro-ophthalmologists and neurosurgeons to advise patients more accurately in regard to the timing of surgery and the prospects for visual improvement.

DISC EDEMA

Papilledema
Peripapillary RNFL thickness values outside the normal range can readily demonstrate nerve fiber edema. This holds true even if the total retinal thickness in this region is measured, a parameter less easily affected by artifacts. Optic nerve head volume and height are other useful parameters.

Progressive thinning in the GCL-IPL (ganglion cell layer-inner plexiform layer) may reveal progressive optic nerve damage in papilledema and may warrant aggressive treatment, and a normal baseline thickness is prognostic for a better visual outcome.

Optic Nerve Head Drusen
Buried drusen may be hard to confirm clinically. On OCT, they may be differentiated from true disc edema, the latter showing an elevated ONH with smooth internal contour and subretinal hyporeflective space, as opposed to a lumpy-bumpy internal contour in drusen. SD-OCT shows the outer nuclear layer to smoothly cover the drusen. Quantitatively, there appears to be no difference in RNFL thickness in any quadrant in eyes with drusen or papilledema.

Ischemic Optic Neuropathy
Retinal nerve fiber layer thickening compared to the (presumed) normal fellow eye has been well documented in acute nonarteritic ischemic optic neuropathy (ION). By the second month there is significant RNFL thinning, with stability achieved by the 6th month. GCC measurements may be easier and more robust quantifiers.

While cupping of the optic disc has been more associated with arteritic ION, the nonarteritic form also shows cup:disc ratio asymmetry in the atrophic stages in many pairs of eyes.

Visual acuity has been found to correlate with RNFL thickness in the papillomacular bundle (PMB) and temporal quadrant. Visual field changes are also found to correlate well with sectoral (altitudinal) RNFL loss.

OTHER NEUROPATHIES

Toxic-Nutritional Optic Neuropathy
Retinal nerve fiber layer thickness may be normal or slightly increased in the acute stages, with subsequent thinning; thinning in the temporal quadrant and PMB correlate with visual acuity and field loss.

Traumatic Optic Neuropathy
Retinal nerve fiber layer thinning can occur as early as 2-4 weeks after trauma, prior to the clinical appearance of disc pallor.

Leber's Hereditary Optic Neuropathy
Retinal nerve fiber layer has been found to be thicker than normal in the presymptomatic and early disease state. RNFL thinning is seen in all quadrants in the late stages. A larger disc size appears to offer a prognostic benefit—a finding seen clinically as well as on OCT.

ALZHEIMER'S DISEASE
Retinal nerve fiber layer thickness in patients with Alzheimer's is significantly lower compared to age-matched normal. OCT biomarkers may play a valuable role in prognostication of patients with mild cognitive impairment (MCI) and their progression to Alzheimer's disease.

SUMMARY

Limitations of Optical Coherence Tomography
The normative database used in OCT is derived from adults over the age of 18 years. As such there is no normative data in use for children. Anatomic and pathological factors such as myopia, glaucoma, retinal disease, etc. affect measurements and act as confounders. Artifacts in OCT image segmentation can lead to errors in interpretation. Recent advances in image acquisition as well as interpretation seek to counter these.

SUGGESTED READING
1. Kardon R. The role of the macula OCT scan in neuro ophthalmology. J Neuroophthalmol. 2011;31(4):353-61.

8.14 Radiation Tolerance of Ocular Structures

Deepak Mishra, Ritusha Mishra, Himanshu Mishra
BHU, Varanasi
drdmishra12@yahoo.com

INTRODUCTION
Primary intraocular and orbital tumors are rare entities and pose a significant therapeutic challenge. Radiotherapy (RT) is one of the modalities used for treatment; both external beam RT (EBRT) and brachytherapy are used as per the clinical situation. Conformal techniques are now recommended to ensure maximal sparing of these sensitive structures

while achieving adequate tumor coverage. The incidence and severity of post RT injury are dose-dependent.

OCULAR STRUCTURES AND THEIR RADIATION TOLERANCE

Eyelids and Eyelashes
Eyelids have the thinnest skin of body capable of rapid flexible movements. Any inflammatory or fibrosing process is detrimental for this flexibility. Acute toxicity of eyelid skin is similar to skin at other sites and manifests as loss of eyelashes, erythema, and both dry and moist desquamation. Late effects can include telangiectasia and atrophy. It may subsequently lead to structural changes such as ectropion, entropion or corneal irritation due to trichiasis. Incidence of these permanent damages is very low up to doses of 45–50 Gy in conventional fractionated radiotherapy. Management includes proper local hygiene, dressings for moist desquamation, and instillation of artificial tears.

Lacrimal Apparatus
The function of lacrimal gland system is the secretion of tear film which consists of three layers—outer lipid, middle aqueous, and inner mucin. Deficiency of any of these components leads to the instability of tear film and may lead to the dry eye syndrome. Up to 30-40 Gy in fractionated doses, there are minimal complications, thereafter there is steep rise on increasing dose (around 50% for 50 Gy, nearly in all for doses >57 Gy). Lower incidence of these complications is observed when low dose (1.2 Gy twice daily) per fraction is used. Conformal techniques [intensity-modulated radiotherapy (IMRT)] can also minimize the risks of RT-induced xerophthalmia. Treatments available for RT-induced xerophthalmia are lubricants, punctal occlusion or tarsorrhaphy.

Cornea
There are five layers in cornea. Injury to epithelial and stromal layers is most critical for RT-induced damage. Punctate epithelial erosions can be seen after doses of 30–40 Gy. With further higher doses, corneal edema, ulceration or perforation can occur (at 60 Gy, the risk appears to be around 15–20%). Corneal toxicity can be reduced by using megavoltage beam thus minimizing the surface dose or by using commercially available eye shields without compromising tumor coverage.

Sclera
The sclera is relatively radioresistant as compared to other structures. RT-induced damage causes loss of episcleral vessels, scleral thinning or perforation rarely. Preservation of optimum scleral thickness is necessary to preserve the integrity of the globe.

Uvea
Similar to sclera, uvea is also relatively radioresistant. RT-induced damage is usually seen at the doses >70 Gy in conventional fractionation which manifests as neovascularization, rubeosis iridis and iridocyclitis leading to neovascular glaucoma. The primary treatments are topical steroids and cycloplegic drops. Laser photocoagulation may prevent or retard the progression of glaucoma if performed earlier. Trabeculectomy may be required in rapidly progressing cases.

Lens
The germinal layer is the most sensitive layer to radiation having actively proliferating cells and is responsible for most post-treatment cataracts. Older patients with other coexisting ocular problems may develop cataracts sooner. Total dose, fractionation schedule and age at the time of treatment are crucial to determine the probability of cataract formation. A dose of 1 Gy to the lens during childhood may cause significant damage

whereas in adults, higher doses (2.5–6.5 Gy) are associated with cataract; the latent period is around 8 years. With further increase in doses the latent period is decreased to around 4 years with a 66% risk. Customized lens shielding and fractionated RT helps to minimize the risk. The definitive management consists of surgery and the outcome is excellent.

Retina

Retinopathy is a late effect that usually presents 6 months to 3 years post RT. The threshold dose is usually considered to be 30–40 Gy; risk appears to increase drastically after doses of >50 Gy in conventional fractionation. Between 45 and 55 Gy, the incidence shows a strong correlation with the dose per fraction (>1.9 Gy) and with the use of chemotherapy. Incidence and severity are also increased by other coexistent ocular morbidities such as diabetic retinopathy, hypertension. Pan-retinal laser photocoagulation is used to treat severe ischemia, although the efficacy of this treatment is not conclusively proven.

Optic Nerve

Radiation-induced optic neuropathy (RION) is mainly a vascular ischemic phenomenon similar to diabetic retinopathy, manifests months or years after RT and the peak incidence is observed at 18 months. RION has a myriad of presentation mainly related to the nerve fibers most affected and usually seen as visual field defects. Risk of RION is almost nil with conventionally fractionated doses ≤50 Gy (maximum dose); thereafter the risk increases up to 7% at 55–60 Gy and is substantial increase at doses of >60 Gy. Fraction size is another most important parameter to be considered in RION. Since there is no known effective therapy for RION, efforts must be made to minimize the optic nerve dose within limits.

CONCLUSION

Ocular complications are common during and after radiation therapy, so proper precautions, dose limits, and early management of complications will minimize visual complications and maximize functional preservation.

SECTION 9

Oculoplasty

Editor: Kasturi Bhattacharjee

- 9.1 **Anatomy of the Eyelids** 707
  Nitin Trivedi
- 9.2 **Ptosis** 708
  Nitin Trivedi
- 9.3 **Lid Margin Anomalies** 714
  MV Vachhrajani
- 9.4 **Eyelid Infections** 718
  Ishan Acharya
- 9.5 **Cosmetic Eyelids Surgeries (Upper Lid and Lower Lid Blepharoplasty)** 723
  Kasturi Bhattacharjee, Divakant Misra, Komal Sawarkar
- 9.6 **Botulinum Toxin and Dermal Fillers** 730
  Kasturi Bhattacharjee, Obaidur Rehman
- 9.7 **Eyelid Tumors** 734
  M Subrahmanyam
- 9.8 **Eyelid Reconstruction: An Overview** 738
  Rajat D Maheshwari
- 9.9 **Benign and Vascular Eyelid Tumors** 744
  Usha Singh, Khushdeep Abhaypal
- 9.10 **Diagnosis and Management of Orbital Fractures** 752
  AK Grover, Rwituja Thomas
- 9.11 **Structural, Vascular, and Neoplastic Lesions of the Orbit** 758
  Ramesh Murthy, Santosh Honavar
- 9.12 **Vascular Lesions of the Orbit** 765
  Aditi Mehta, Kasturi Bhattacharjee
- 9.13 **Diagnosis and Surgical Management of a Case of Proptosis** 769
  Shaloo Bageja, Amrita Sawhney
- 9.14 **Infective and Inflammatory Disorders of Orbit** 778
  Amruthavalli KS, Tarjani Vivek Dave
- 9.15 **Adnexal Trauma** 795
  AK Grover, Shaloo Bageja, Rwituja Thomas
- 9.16 **Newer Techniques in the Management of Orbital and Ocular Tumors** 800
  Santosh G Honavar, Rolika Bansal
- 9.17 **Medical Management of Thyroid Eye Disease** 804
  Ashok Kumar Grover, Rwituja Thomas, Summy Bhatnagar
- 9.18 **Image-guided Orbital Surgery** 811
  Kasturi Bhattacharjee, Vatsalya Venkatraman
- 9.19 **Clinical Evaluation and Imaging of Lacrimal System** 815
  Prerna Sinha, Swati Singh
- 9.20 **Congenital Nasolacrimal Duct Obstruction** 823
  Usha Kim
- 9.21 **Chronic Dacryocystitis** 828
  Khushdeep Abhaypal, Manpreet Singh, Manpreet Kaur, Aditi Mehta
- 9.22 **Acute Dacryocystitis** 834
  Kamalpreet Likhari
- 9.23 **Canaliculitis** 839
  Ramesh Murthy
- 9.24 **Tumors of Lacrimal Drainage System** 841
  Lakshmi Mahesh, Smita Menon, Sonali Gaikwad
- 9.25 **Enucleation, Evisceration, and Exenteration** 846
  Kasturi Bhattacharjee, Deepika Kapoor

- 9.26 **Anophthalmic Socket** 852
  Bipasha Mukerjee, Ruhi Jange
- 9.27 **Orbital Implants** 856
  Kasturi Bhattacharjee, Deepak Soni
- 9.28 **Custom Fit Prosthesis** 861
  Usha Kim
- 9.29 **Orbital Imaging** 868
  Akshay Gopinathan Nair
- 9.30 **Surgical Approaches to the Orbit** 873
  Obaidur Rehman
- 9.31 **Pathologies and Surgeries Related to Punctum and Canaliculus** 875
  Nandini Bothra, Mohammad Javed Ali
- 9.32 **Peripheral Nerve Sheath Tumors** 879
  Maya Hada, Nikita Jain

9.1 Anatomy of the Eyelids

Nitin Trivedi
CH Nagri Eye Hospital, Ahmedabad
trivedinitinv54@gmail.com

INTRODUCTION

Two movable eye lids have prime function of protection and to give rest to eye balls. Upper lid is very mobile but lower one has very minimal mobility. Upper lid has average height of 10-12 mm and average width of 25-30 mm. In straight gaze, upper lid covers about 2 mm of upper part of cornea cutting corneal border from 11 to 1 o'clock. Each eye lid has two laminae, i.e., anterior containing skin and orbicularis muscle and posterior containing tarsal plate and conjunctiva. Anterior to posterior layers are:
- Skin
- Subcutaneous tissue
- Protractive muscles (orbicularis oculi)
- Orbital septum
- Orbital fat
- Retractor muscles [levator palpebrae superioris (LPS) and Müller's muscle]
- Tarsal plate
- Conjunctiva

SKIN

Lid skin is one of the thinnest in body. It is very elastic and has sparse hairs.

SUBCUTANEOUS TISSUE

It lies in the space between skin and tarsal plate. It works as bonding agent between the two layers but allows separation in old age.

ORBICULARIS OCULI

This muscle is mainly responsible for closure of palpebral fissure.

ORBITAL SEPTUM

It is a thin layer of fibrous tissue separating orbit into pre- and postseptal compartments. In upper lid, it extends from upper orbital rim periosteum. Lower part fuses with LPS anastomosis in non-Asian races. In Asian races, it extends down up to the lower border of the upper lid.

In the lower lid, it extends from lower border of lower level of lower tarsal plate to lower orbital rim.

ORBITAL FAT

Pad of fat in lower lid overlying maxillary and zygomatic periosteum is called suborbicularis oculi fat (SOOF). It is equivalent to upper lid fat pad present behind eyebrow called superiorly located retro-orbicularis oculi fat (ROOF). It fills the space between orbital septum in front and LPS muscle on back in upper lid. In lower lid, it is bounded by orbital septum in front and lower lid retractor (capsulopalpebral ligament) on back. Two pads of fat, medial yellow and central gray, are present in upper lid. Three pockets i.e., medial, central, and lateral are present in lower lid. All pockets are separated by thin fibrous tissue.

RETRACTORS

Upper Lid Retractors

Levator Palpebrae Superioris

It originates from apex of orbit above upper part of annulus of Zinn. It is about 40 mm long running horizontally forward close to roof of orbit. There are two parts of LPS muscle. Anterior is aponeurotic part and posterior tendinous part. Aponeurotic part spreads out like wings called two horns and attaches to lower third of front of tarsal plate. Medial horn is attached to medial palpebral ligament. Temporal part is stronger, attached to lateral orbital rim. It divides lacrimal gland into two parts; orbital above and palpebral bellow. Posterior tendinous part of LPS muscle continues at a horizontal fibrous tissue band called Whitnall's ligament which is about 14–20 mm from upper border of tarsal plate and works as an internal sling.

Lower Lid Retractor

Capsulopalpebral ligament is equivalent to Müller's muscle in upper lid. It pulls lower lid down by one-fourth of eye ball movement making lower vision possible. It also keeps lower lid margin apposed to globe. In old age, laxity of ligament allows lower lid to separate from globe giving rise to lower lid entropion. Consequently lower lid lashes rub globe irritating cornea and leads to watering.

CONJUNCTIVA

Palpebral conjunctiva is a nonkeratinized squamous epithelium. It contains mucin-secreting goblet cells. It also contains glands of Wolfring along nonmarginal tarsal border and glands of Krause along fornices. They help in secretion of basic lacrimal fluid.

LID MARGIN

It is divided into two parts by a gray line. Anterior is lined by keratinized squamous epithelium with special strip of orbicularis oculi called muscle of Riolan. Posterior is nonkeratinized conjunctival epithelium with tarsal plate. Lines of lid lashes are on the anterior line.

BLOOD SUPPLY

Lids are highly vascular structures promoting and helping in prevention of infection. Branches of internal and external carotid arteries anastomose vertically in front of tarsal plate. There are two venous plexuses in lid. Post-tarsal drains into ophthalmic vein and pretarsal into subcutaneous vessels.

Lymphatics from medial part of lids drain into submandibular lymph glands. Tissues from temporal side drain first to preauricular glands and then to deeper cervical lymph nodes.

9.2 Ptosis

Nitin Trivedi
CH Nagri Eye Hospital, Ahmedabad
trivedinitinv54@gmail.com

INTRODUCTION

Blepharoptosis is a condition in which the upper eyelid comes down lower than its normal position, i.e., covering about 2 mm of upper part of cornea. It mostly leads to a cosmetic blemish but may cover the pupillary area obstructing the vision and sometimes resulting into amblyopia.

ETIOLOGICAL CLASSIFICATION
- *Myogenic ptosis:*
  - Levator maldevelopment
    - Simple
    - With superior rectus weakness
  - Blepharophimosis syndrome
  - Chronic progressive external ophthalmoplegia
  - Oculopharyngeal syndrome
  - Progressive muscular dystrophy
  - Myasthenia gravis
  - Congenital fibrosis of the extraocular muscles
- *Aponeurotic ptosis:*
  - Senile ptosis
  - Late developing hereditary ptosis
  - Stress or trauma to levator aponeurosis such as cataract surgery, local trauma, pregnancy, Graves' disease, and long-term use of corticosteroids
- *Neurogenic ptosis:*
  - Lesions of third nerve
    - Post-traumatic ophthalmoplegia
    - Misdirected third nerve ptosis
  - Marcus Gunn jaw-winking ptosis
  - Horner's syndrome
  - Ophthalmoplegic migraine
  - Multiple sclerosis
- Mechanical ptosis
- *Apparent ptosis:*
  - Due to lack of posterior eyelid support
  - Due to hypotropia
  - Due to dermatochalasis

Myogenic Ptosis
This is a major cause of ptosis comprising >60% of all cases. Levator maldevelopment is due to deficiency of striated fibers in the muscle which leads to inelasticity of the structure causing defective elevation. This result into ptosis and also lid lag on down gaze, as the muscle fails to relax. It is mostly sporadic, but some familial cases have been reported. In 15–20% of cases, it may be associated with superior rectus weakness.

Myasthenia Gravis
The condition is due to deficiency of acetylcholine at myoneural junction. Thought to be autoimmune in nature, it may be associated with thymus hyperplasia, dysthyroidism, collagen diseases, or Lambert–Eton syndrome. In most of the cases, ptosis, unilateral or bilateral, is the presenting feature. Later on the extraocular muscles may be involved followed by muscles of all over body. The symptoms are classically more in the evening and after exercise. Difficulty in deglutition and respiration are present in advance case which may terminate in death. The condition is highly under diagnosed. Cogan's lid twitch sign is useful in which the patient is asked to look up and down repeatedly or to stare in upgaze. Due to fatigue, the lid shows flicking and gradually droops down. Diagnosis is usually done by injecting neostigmine or edrophonium (Tensilon). Ice pack test is a reliable and simple, noninvasive test which can be easily done in outpatient department (OPD). Ice packed in gauze piece or rubber glove is kept on the affected lid for 1 minute. Average 3–4 mm of correction is noted. Electromyography (EMG) is conclusive. Treatment is almost always medical. Minimal ptosis surgery can be performed in longstanding cases with caution.

Different forms of myopathies are rare conditions mostly associated with affections of extraocular muscles. As the Bell's phenomenon is absent in almost all cases, surgery is contraindicated and elevation of the lids by mechanical means like crutches or contact lenses is the only way of management. Frontalis sling surgery may be done with elastic synthetic materials like silicone.

Aponeurotic Ptosis

Levator aponeurosis is either disinserted from the tarsal plate or there are areas of dehiscence in it. Lid crease recedes up and so the margin-crease distance is increased (**Fig. 9.2.1**). Treatment is always surgical reattachment or repair.

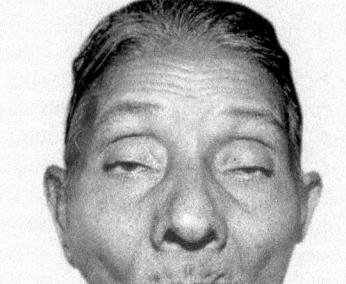

Fig. 9.2.1: Aponeurotic ptosis.

Neurogenic Ptosis

Third nerve palsy may be congenital or due to trauma, vascular lesions, tumors, demyelination, and inflammation or systemic diseases like diabetes mellitus. Ocular movements are mostly affected; therefore, management of the case should be done after proper assessment of the squint. Spontaneous recovery is possible up to 6 months; so any surgical intervention should be done after that time interval except in children in whom chances of amblyopia is there.

Horner's syndrome is due to paralysis of the Müller's muscle supplied by the sympathetic nerve. Ptosis produced is 2–3 mm. The other features include ipsilateral miosis, enophthalmos, and anhidrosis of the face.

Synkinetic ptosis is due to aberrant connections within the central nervous system. The most common variety is the Marcus Gunn or jaw-winking phenomenon in which trigeminal nerve supplying the muscles of mastication aberrantly involves the levator. Clinically, the ptotic lid shoots up on opening the mouth or shifting the jaw to same side.

Mechanical Ptosis

Excessive weight of the upper lid due to any cause like edema or mass lesion, or scarring of the conjunctiva with tethering of the levator muscle.

■ EVALUATION OF PTOSIS

- *History:* To ascertain whether the ptosis is congenital or acquired as the amount of levator resection required for the former group is more than that for the latter. Examination of the eye visual acuity is assessed to detect the presence of amblyopia.
- *Examination of the lid:* Lid crease is a good guide to determine the function of the levator. Absence of lid fold indicates very poor levator action. Higher lid crease indicates disinsertion of the levator in aponeurotic ptosis. Lid lag is a sure sign of congenital ptosis due to muscle maldevelopment (**Fig. 9.2.2**).
- *Assessment of lid position and amount of ptosis:* It is determined by measuring the distance of the lid margin from different structures such as limbus, pupil, or orbital margin, and then comparing it with the other eye or the standard. The most commonly practiced method is to assess the vertical height of the normal size. Care is taken to neutralize the function of the frontalis muscle by pressing with a thumb. As the vertical diameter of the cornea is 11 mm and the upper lid and the size of the palpebral fissure is on an average 9 mm. The ptosis can be graded according to the amount of ptosis (**Fig. 9.2.3**).
  - Mild ptosis means 2 mm or less
  - Moderate ptosis means 3 mm
  - Severe ptosis means 4 mm or more

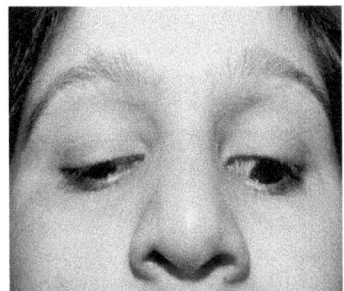

Fig. 9.2.2: Left eye lid lag.

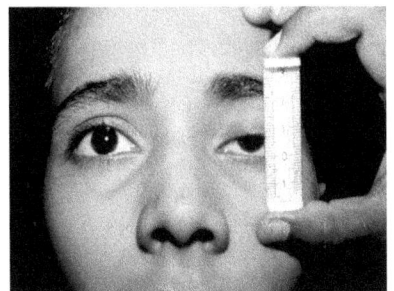

Fig. 9.2.3: Lid level assessment.

- *Assessment of levator function:* It is done by measuring the amount of eyelid excursion, i.e., movement from down to up. Normal function is 15 mm.
  Good   8 mm or more
  Fair   5-7 mm
  Poor   4 mm or less
- *Ocular movements and cover test:* This helps in detecting presence of pseudoptosis in cases of hypotropia.
- *Abnormal synkinetic movements:* Asking the patient to open the mouth and turn the jaw from side to side to demonstrate the Marcus Gunn phenomenon. Size of the palpebral fissure is assessed, while the patient is asked to look from side to side, to detect the presence of Duane's retraction syndrome.
- *Bell's phenomenon:* Absence or weak Bell's phenomenon should be an absolute contraindication for any type of ptosis surgery as it can lead to exposure keratitis.
- Tear film and corneal sensations are tested to prevent postoperative dryness.
- *Phenylephrine test:* Elevation of lid by instillation of phenylephrine usually indicates good result after Fasanella-Servat surgery.

SURGICAL TREATMENTS

Points to be considered before surgery:
- *Age:* Formative surgery is done at or after 5 years of age, because it is not possible to assess the child thoroughly before this age. Further, the structures of the lid are very tiny and friable and hence it is difficult to identify and handle them while operating. In severe ptosis, temporary frontalis sling surgery can be done to prevent amblyopia and deformity of the spine. According to the recent studies, it has been observed that amblyopia in ptosis patients is more commonly due to astigmatism or anisometropia rather than prolonged occlusion.
- *Laterality:* If unilateral, surgery is done early as there are more chances of amblyopia.
- *Amount of ptosis and levator function:* Both these interrelated effects decide the nature of the surgery to be undertaken.
  Commonly done surgeries with general guidelines:
  - Mild ptosis → Excellent levator function → Fasanella-Servat operation
  - Moderate ptosis → Good levator function → Levator resection surgery
  - Severe ptosis → Poor levator function → Frontalis sling surgery

Fasanella-Servat Operation (Transconjunctival Müllerectomy)

Its indications are minimum congenital ptosis, Horner's syndrome, and minimal residual ptosis. Vertical shorting posterior lamina of the lid is achieved by resecting a strip of upper part of tarsus along with some part of conjunctiva and underlying Müller's muscle.

Surgery is mainly done under local anesthesia. Lid is everted and three traction sutures are taken at the tarsoconjunctival junction. Line of resection is marked at about 3 mm from the tarsal border so that to give a total tarsoconjunctival resection to be 6 mm.

A heavy scissors is used to cut all the three layers of conjunctiva, tarsus, and Müller's muscle in one go. The two cut ends are brought together with 6/0 plain catgut continuous suturing to have minimum exposure on the conjunctival side to reduce chances of suture rubbing the cornea hence minimizing chances of corneal irritation and abrasion. Advantage of this surgery is minimum invasion and so faster recovery without disturbing the lid fold. The main objection to the surgery is a possibility of development of dry eye.

Levator Resection

It is indicated in moderate ptosis with good levator palpebrae superioris (LPS) function. The muscle can be exposed from the skin side: Eversbusch surgery, conjunctival side: Blascovich surgery.

Frontal approach is easier and maximum LPS resection can be done with good lid crease formation. Posterior approach produces less inflammation and so recovery is faster.

Surgery is preferably done under local anesthesia so that lid level can be adjusted with precision. Skin incision is marked at the level of existing lid crease or at the site where it is present on the opposite side. Skin and orbicularis muscle are separated to expose the orbital septum which is cut and orbital fat prolapse is ensured. LPS aponeurosis is seen easily under the fat as glistening white fanned out structure. Aponeurosis is detached from the front of the tarsal plate and from the underlying conjunctiva. Dissection is carried out upward up to the Whitnall ligament. It is advisable to preserve the two horns to get better lift of the lid. Levator resection is done according to the preoperative evaluation and the new lower end of LPS is sutured back to the front of the tarsal plate with nonabsorbable material like 6/0 prolene. Lid level is gauged with patient lying down or preferably in sitting position. Skin incision is closed with five to six interrupted sutures taking the bites from the LPS stump to form the lid crease. Frost suture is taken from the lower lid up to prevent exposure keratitis in the immediate postoperative period.

In congenital ptosis, preoperative assessment of LPS function and lid level is done meticulously to determine the amount of resection. Formula for resection of LPS in congenital ptosis is up to 8 mm there is no correction, and then each 3 mm resection gives rise to 1 mm of correction. But in acquired cases, no formula of preoperative assessment is perfect and on table adjustment is preferred. In severe cases, the lid is adjusted 1 mm above the upper limbus; in moderate cases, it is kept at limbus; and with good action, it is adjusted to remain 1 mm below the limbus.

Frontalis Sling Surgery

Indications

- Poor LPS function
- Marcus Gunn jaw-winking phenomenon
- Myopathic ptosis

Frontalis sling or suspension surgery aims at attaching tarsal plate to the frontalis muscle as the LPS function is poor **(Fig. 9.2.4)**. Ideally, it should be done bilaterally to give symmetry. Different techniques are employed for the suspension.

In Crowford's technique, two triangles are made with apices at the forehead and then the two ends are tied in the center. In pentagonal technique, material is passed in a single running fashion with knot tied in the center of forehead.

Different materials are used as the sling, but autogenous fascia lata is most commonly used as it is well-tolerated and maintains strength. The other materials employed are strips of sclera,

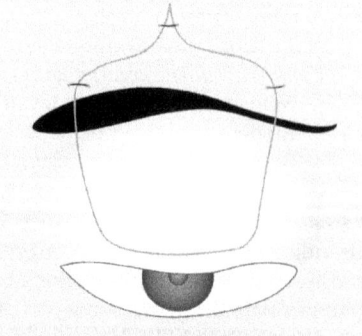

Fig. 9.2.4: Frontalis sling pentagon technique.

silicon roads or bands, and synthetic sutures. Silicone is the best of the synthetic materials fulfilling all the criteria to be an ideal sling material. Lid lag can is a constant feature of the surgery and so an attempt should be made to minimize it without compromising with the height. Main complications are lid lag, extrusion of sling material, recurrence of ptosis, and suture granuloma.

Other Surgeries

- *Anderson's Whitnall advancement surgery:* Whitnall ligament is brought forward and sutured to the front of the tarsal plate without disturbing LPS aponeurosis—Müller's muscle complex.
- *Supramaximal LPS resection:* In cases of severe congenital ptosis, >20 mm resection is done to get desired result. The disadvantage is the lid lag.
- *Putterman surgery:* It is a modification of posterior laminar shortening in which graduated excision of conjunctiva and Müller's muscle is carried out keeping tarsal plate intact.

PTOSIS IN SPECIAL SITUATIONS

- *Marcus Gunn jaw-winking phenomenon:* Levator muscle is excised on both sides and bilateral frontalis sling surgery is performed to remove the element of lid retraction and to attain bilateral lid symmetry.
- *Blepharophimosis syndrome* **(Fig. 9.2.5)**: Blepharophimosis and ptosis are traditionally in two stages but they can be combined to save time and exposure to anesthesia. Telecanthus is traditionally corrected by transnasal wiring. Instead, screw and plate can be fixed to the bone or thick nonabsorbable suture can be used to plicate medial canthal tendon. Epicanthal fold is corrected preferably by Mustarde's operation of double Z plasty or by elliptical skin excision. Temporal widening of palpebral fissure can be done by lateral canthoplasty.
- Squint, especially the vertical one, is diagnosed, assessed, and corrected first before ptosis correction.

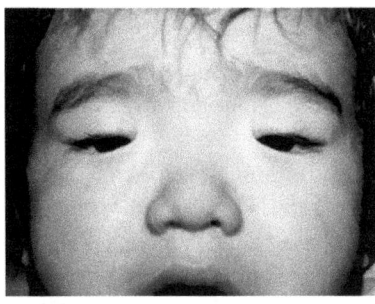

Fig. 9.2.5: Blepharophimosis syndrome.

COMPLICATIONS OF PTOSIS SURGERY

- Under correction
- Over correction
- Lid-lag lagophthalmos—keratitis
- Entropion, lash ptosis, and ectropion
- Conjunctival (fornix) prolapse
- Loss of lashes
- Asymmetrical lid contour—lid fold
- Hemorrhage and edema
- Infection and granuloma **(Fig. 9.2.6)**

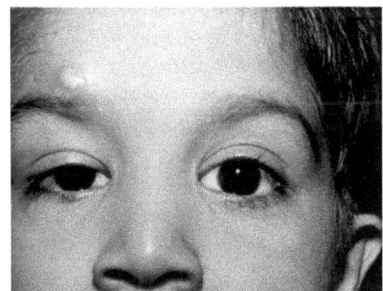

Fig. 9.2.6: Suture granuloma.

SUGGESTED READING

1. American Academy of Ophthalmology. Orbit, Eyelids, and Lacrimal System. San Francisco, United States: American Academy of Ophthalmology; 2012.

9.3 Lid Margin Anomalies

MV Vachhrajani
Tolat Eye Hospital and Oculoplasty Clinic, Ahmedabad
dr.vacchrajani@gmail.com

■ INTRODUCTION

Entropion and *ectropion* (i.e., in-turning or out-turning) are the common lid marginal malpositions encountered in day-to-day practice. This disrupts the normal tear film and causes symptoms such as epiphora and foreign body sensation which are detrimental to the corneal health.

■ APPLIED ANATOMY: RELEVANT TO MANAGEMENT OF ECTROPION AND ENTROPION

The normal position of the lids is a delicate interplay between:
- Anatomical and functional integrity of the canthal tendons
- Anatomic and functional integrity of the pretarsal and preseptal parts of the orbicularis
- Normalcy of the two lamellae of the lid
- Normal tone and insertion of the lower lid retractors
- Gravity (in cases of ectropion of the lower lid especially)

Skin: It is thinnest in the body. Lid crease and lid fold are of significance and to be repaired at the time of surgical correction.

Superficial musculoaponeurotic system (SMAS): In the lower lid, attachments between the SMAS and the dermis are present. The SMAS has attachments to the deeper bone (especially significant in deep injuries and their repair).

Protractors: The orbicularis is of special importance in the lower lid where the interplay between its two parts the preseptal and pretarsal determines whether the lid turns in or out.

Preseptal part is of significance in causing spastic entropion.

Paralysis of the Horner's muscle (a part of orbicularis responsible for the pump mechanism of the lacrimal sac) plays a role in aggravating the paralytic ectropion because of frequent rubbing in response to epiphora.

The preseptal orbicularis also forms the lateral tarsal raphe whose integrity and lack thereof has a role to play in the genesis of involutional entropion. Surgeries directed at tightening or reinserting the raphe have been most successful in the management of both involutional *ectropion* and *entropion*.

The muscle of *Riolan*, the gray line is also sometimes implicated in the paralysis which straightens the lashes thus contributing to the trichiasis worsening the entropion.

Lower eyelid retractor, a muscle analogous to levator palpebra superioris (LPS) (but not as well differentiated), is responsible for maintaining the lower tarsal plate in position.

Disinsertion or weakening of its insertion onto the tarsal plate results in in-turning of the margin and many surgeries directed at reinserting to the tarsal plate produce excellent results. Sometimes done in conjunction with lateral tarsal strip (LTS).

Marginal anomalies can be:
- Congenital
- Traumatic
- Senile

SECTION 9: Oculoplasty

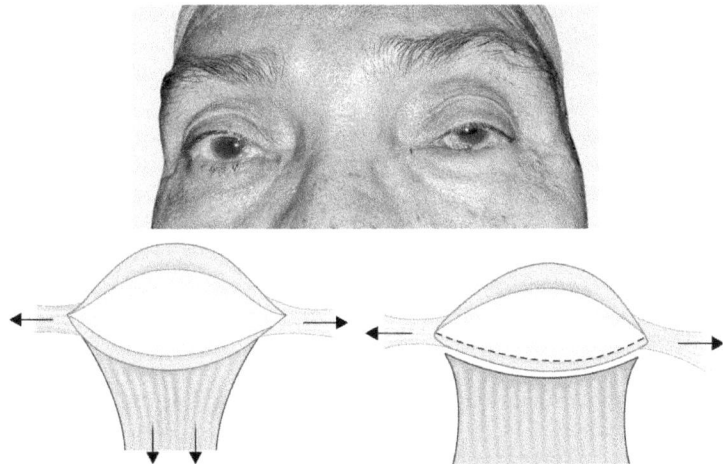

Fig. 9.3.1: Disattachment of LPS from tarsal plate.

CONGENITAL MALPOSITIONS

Congenital eyelid anomalies result from a fetal insult during second month of gestation.

Congenital malpositions are seen in:
- Blepharophimosis eyelid syndrome (BPES)
- Downs
- Ichthyosis
- Nonsyndromic entropion

In *blepharophimosis* syndrome, there can be medial *entropion* because of epicanthus inversus, and lateral part of the lower lid may show *ectropion* secondary to vertical insufficiency of the anterior lamella in the lateral half of the lower lid.

In *euryblepharon*, here we see ectropion of the lower lid because of increased length and vertical shortening of the lateral part of lower lid. The lateral canthus is also inferiorly displaced. This is also seen in *centurion* syndrome.

For total correction of these defects, LTS with augmentation of the internal lamella with tarsoconjunctiva, palatal mucoperichondrium, and correction of vertical shortening of the external lamella with skin graft is required.

In *epiblepharon*, pretarsal orbicularis rides above the lid margin and lashes assume vertical position, and irritate the cornea in down gaze.

In ichthyosis/collodion babies anterior lamellar shortening results in ectropion of both the lids.

True congenital entropion is rare and is a result of either retractor dysgenesis or tarsal defects or relative shortening of posterior lamellae.

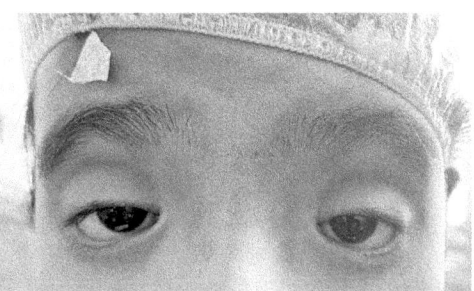

Fig. 9.3.2: Euryblepharon.

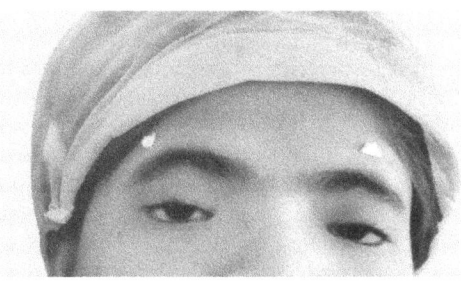

Fig. 9.3.3: Blepharophimosis eyelid syndrome.

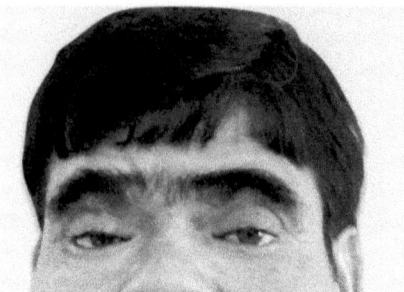

Fig. 9.3.4: Epiblepharon.

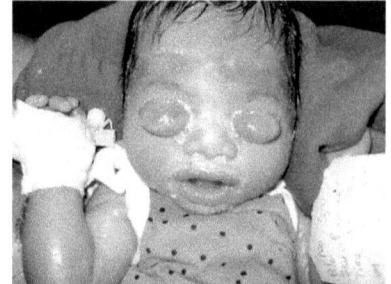

Fig. 9.3.5: Ectropion in ichthyosis.

This always requires surgical intervention in the form of anterior lamellar shortening or retractor advancement.

Marginal rotating sutures are often beneficial.

Congenital distichiasis though not true entropion causes similar symptoms.

■ ACQUIRED MALPOSITIONS

Floppy Eyelid Syndrome

It is not a true ectropion but eversion of the upper lid due to flaccidity of the upper lid occurs due to tarsal dysgenesis on the slightest trigger. Often this is associated with obesity, keratoconus, rubbing of eyes, and sleeping in a prone position. Often these patients also suffer from sleep apnea.

Management is surgical and by horizontal lid shortening.

Ectropion of the acquired variety can be classified based on etiology as:
- Involutional
- Paralytic
- Cicatricial
- Mechanical

Involutional

It occurs mainly in the lower lid. The main pathology is age-related laxity of medial and lateral canthal tendon.

The ectropion can range from mild punctual eversion to eversion of the entire lower lid.

Most procedures for correction are surgical and involve some form of lateral or medial canthopexies. In addition, shortening of the lid may also be required, if the ectropion is complete and long standing. The stretched out lower lid retractors also must be reinserted surgically.

Paralytic

In 7th nerve palsy, either temporary or permanent, the orbicularis becomes inactive and there by resulting in flaccid ectropion of the lower lid.

Management again depends on degree of flaccidity, superimposed senile, and atrophic changes in older individuals and in long-standing palsies.

Canthopexies may suffice in younger individuals with resent onset palsy.

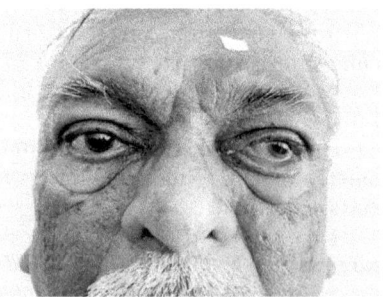

Fig. 9.3.6: Floppy eyelid syndrome.

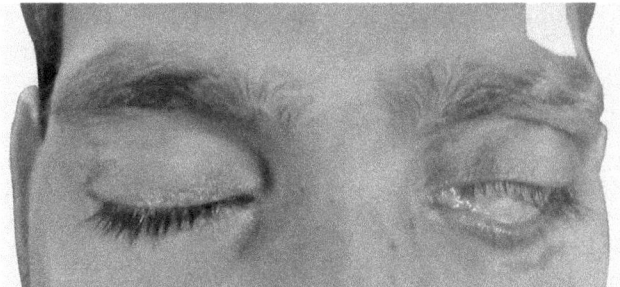

Fig. 9.3.7: Lower lid ectropion with exposure.

Suspension procedures and vertical augmentation grafts are also required in more severe case along with canthopexy.

Cicatricial
In this, there is anterior lamellar shortening, secondary to thermal or chemical burn.

It can involve both lids to varying degrees.

Management is by release of cicatrix and skin grafting. Sometimes, if the lid has been stretched, lateral canthopexy may also be required.

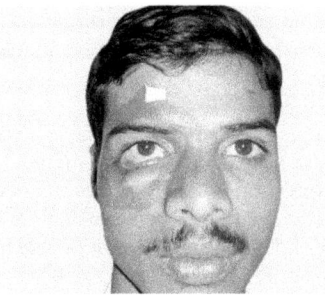

Fig. 9.3.8: Cicatricial ectropion of lower lid.

Mechanical
Tumors of the lower lid, ill-fitting spectacles can pull the lid down by their weight thus also causing stretching and laxity of the canthal tendons.

Management is by excision of the tumors and tightening medial and lateral canthal tendon.

Entropion
Entropion or in-turning can be classified as:
- Acute spastic
- Involutional
- Cicatricial

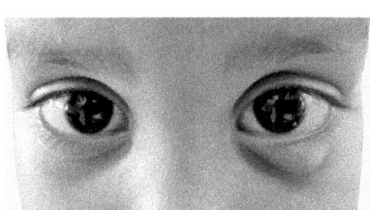

Fig. 9.3.9: Mechanical ectropion of lower lid.

Acute Spastic
This is a temporary type of entropion occurring mainly due to acute spasm of the orbicularis due to corneal ocular surface disease.

It can be relieved by treating the corneal conditions and taping the in-turned lid.

In more severe spasm, botulinum toxin can be used to temporarily paralyze the preseptal orbicularis.

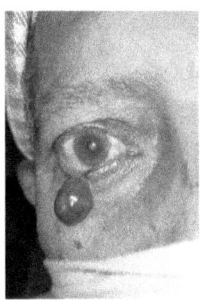

Fig. 9.3.10: Lower lid entropion.

Involutional
Generally, occurs in the lower lid.

Here, in addition to involutional laxity of the canthal tendon, there is also disinsertion of the retractors which allow in-turning of the lid margin.

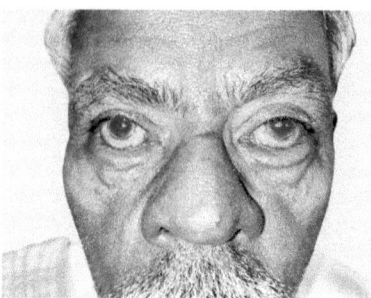

Fig. 9.3.11: Bilateral lower lid entropion with lower lid laxity.

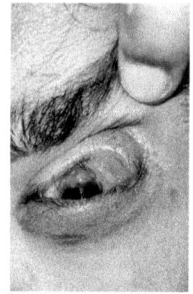

Fig. 9.3.12: Keratopathy due to entropion.

Management is again surgical, requires canthopexy and reinsertion of the retractors. Any excess skin and prolapsed fat may also be excised.

Cicatricial

It occurs because of the cicatrix involving the inner lamellae, secondary to autoimmune disease like cicatricial pemphigoid, inflammation as in Stevens-Johnson syndrome (SJS), and infections such as herpes zoster ophthalmicus (HZO) and trachoma.

Management is by releasing the cicatrix and mucous membrane grafting either from upper lid of the other eye or buccal mucous membrane. In very mild cases, advancement of posterior lamellae can be tried.

Tarsal fraction and wedge resection are also useful in some cases.

All patients must in addition be put on intense lubrication. Treatment of the coexistent or resultant corneal condition is mandatory.

Prognosis is poor in autoimmune disorders.

9.4 | Eyelid Infections

Ishan Acharya
Orbit Eye Hospital, Vadodara
ishan_ach@rediffmail.com

■ INTRODUCTION

The eyelids are subject to a variety of infectious diseases. Essentially any organism that infects the skin can also infect the eyelids. The eyelids may be the primary site of infection, or they may be part of a larger, multisystem infectious disease.

■ ETIOLOGICAL CLASSIFICATION

- Bacterial
- Viral
- Fungal
- Mycobacterial
- Parasitic

■ BACTERIAL

Blepharitis

Blepharitis refers to a group of disorders characterized by inflammation of the eyelids and associated adnexal structures including skin, lashes, and meibomian glands. It typically occurs bilaterally. Disease is usually chronic with intermittent exacerbations **(Figs. 9.4.1A to D)**.

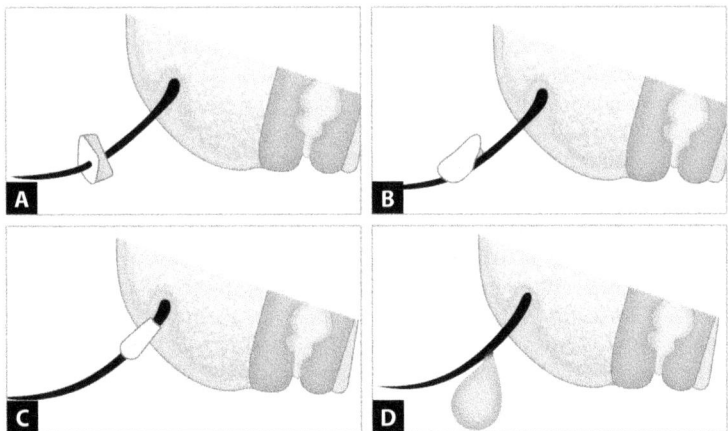

Figs. 9.4.1A to D: Lash appendages in blepharitis. (A) Collarette: Crenelated fibrin coagulum impaled on eyelash in staphylococcal blepharitis; (B) Scurf: Greasy skin squame stuck on eyelash in seborrheic blepharitis; (C) Sleeve: Translucent keratin collar encasing base of eyelash in demodectic infestation; (D) Nit: Egg case of *Pthirus pubis* mite attached to lash in crab louse infestation.

Classification

- *Anterior blepharitis:* It primarily involves the eyelid skin, base of the eyelashes, and the eyelash follicles.
  - Staphylococcal
  - Seborrheic
  - Angular
- *Posterior blepharitis (meibomian gland dysfunction):* It primarily affects the meibomian glands located on the posterior lid.
  - *Anterior blepharitis:*
    - *Staphylococcal:* It is the most common cause of anterior blepharitis. It is also the most common cause of bacterial eyelid infections. Symptoms include redness, itching, burning, and crusting of the eyelid. The diagnosis involves physical examination and a swab test. With chronic blepharitis, the patient may have madarosis, ulceration of eyelid margin, distichiasis, and trichiasis. There may be signs of ocular surface inflammation also.
    - *Seborrheic:* Seborrheic blepharitis is a nonulcerative form of blepharitis in which waxy scales form on the eyelids. It is usually associated with *seborrheic dermatitis* of the surrounding skin. Seborrheic marginal blepharitis is commonly associated with acne rosacea, keratitis sicca, and dermatitis.
    - *Angular:* It is characterized by maceration, fissuring, scaling, and erythema at the lateral or the medial canthus or both. Frequently, there is an associated papillary conjunctivitis, moderate mucopurulent discharge, and adherent exudate. Classically, the causative organism is *Moraxella lacunata*, a gram-negative diplobacillus. *Staphylococcus aureus* and herpes simplex may also be found. Localization of the infection to the canthi is thought to result from the predilection of *Moraxella* to accumulate at the canthal angles.
  - *Posterior blepharitis (meibomian gland dysfunction):* In posterior blepharitis, both quantitative and qualitative changes of the meibomian glands and their secretions have been described. The etiology of these alterations is unknown. One hypothesis involves the action of microbial lipases. *Propionibacterium acnes, S. aureus,* and *S. epidermidis,* all of which have been found on the blepharitic lid, produce lipases that act on esters secreted from the meibomian glands, producing toxic-free fatty

acids that ultimately disrupt gland integrity and function. The pathophysiology of posterior blepharitis involves structural alterations and secretory dysfunction of the meibomian glands.

Patients complain of burning, irritation, photophobia, and redness. Signs include frothy tear film, rounding of posterior margin, anterior migration of conjunctiva, inspissated mucus in meibomian gland orifices, and loss of orifices.

Diagnosis

Diagnosis is usually clinical. Lid biopsy is indicated in atypical cases to exclude malignant conditions. Lid margin culture may be indicated in cases of recurrent anterior blepharitis with severe inflammation or cases not responding to therapy and to know antibiotic susceptibility. This includes cases of unilateral lid changes, significant lid architecture alteration, lash changes or loss, recurrent chalazion, and cases not responsive to treatment for blepharitis.

Management

Patients must be counseled chronic nature and partial response to the therapy. It is partial symptomatic relief rather than cure of the disease.

Eyelid hygiene measures
- Warm compresses for 5–10 minutes twice daily are aimed at raising the temperature above the melting point of meibomian gland secretions and aiding in expression.
- Eyelid scrubs will clear away the scales on the lashes. Gently scrub the eyelids with a moist washcloth with diluted baby shampoo or other commercially available eyelid-cleansing agents twice daily. Patients should receive specific instructions on how to properly perform lid margin (not eyelid skin) hygiene using cotton-tipped applicators that are wet with tap water or a dilute solution of baby shampoo, or proprietary formulations of mildly detergent chemicals. The applicators should be used to scrub back and forth across the lid margins once or twice each day. Failure is most commonly due to improper technique. Eyelid massage is thought to help express meibomian gland secretions and may be performed by the ophthalmologist at the slit lamp examination.

Treat underlying disease
Omega-3 fatty acids: It improves tear film break-up time, dry eye symptoms, and meibum score. 2,000 mg orally in divided doses daily.

Artificial tears or topical ophthalmic ciclosporin: Because of the frequent association of dry eye syndrome with all forms of blepharitis, its presence needs to be assessed and treated accordingly with artificial tears on an "as-required" basis. Topical ophthalmic ciclosporin has been shown to improve ocular symptoms, lid margin vascular injection, tarsal telangiectasias, and fluorescein staining and to decrease meibomian gland inclusions compared with artificial tears.

Topical antibiotic therapy: In cases where symptoms do not respond to eyelid hygiene measures, topical antibiotics effective for gram-positive microorganisms should be used. Erythromycin or bacitracin ointment is an option.

Topical corticosteroid therapy: In the acute phase of inflammation, especially if there is marginal keratitis or corneal phlyctenules, patients may benefit from a short course of a topical ophthalmic corticosteroid, which is tapered after symptoms improve. A minimum effective dose should be used, and dose should be tapered (usually decreasing by one drop daily per week) once acute episode resolves.

Antibiotic lid scrubs: Tea tree oil (*Melaleuca alternifolia*) or metronidazole lid scrubs can be used to treat *Demodex* blepharitis.

Oral antibiotic therapy: Chronic suppressive oral antibiotics are indicated in cases of visual impairment. Tetracyclines are the preferred antibiotics. Patients with posterior blepharitis more frequently require oral antibiotics than those with anterior blepharitis. Doxycycline: 40-100 mg orally once or twice daily for usually 1 month, then discontinue or taper to maintenance dose of 40-50 mg per day or tetracycline: 250 mg orally four times daily for usually 1 month, then discontinue or taper to maintenance dose of 250 mg per day.

Acute Infection of Sebaceous Glands and Chalazion

Zeis glands and meibomian glands are sebaceous glands in the eyelid. Infection of the either can produce a localized abscess of that gland. Infection of a Zeis gland results in an external hordeolum, where the abscess is centered around an eyelash and usually points anteriorly onto the eyelid skin. Infection of a meibomian gland results in an internal hordeolum. Acute infection of a meibomian gland may lead to chronic granulomatous inflammation known as a chalazion. This may be a sterile inflammatory reaction to lipoidal material.

The patient should be advised hot moist compress four to six times a day. Topical antibiotic eye drops and ointment should be given. Systemic antibiotic is advised if clinical features are severe.

Localized Skin Abscess and Preseptal Cellulitis

Infection of Zeis gland is called external hordeolum or commonly stye. Pus points externally at the root of a lash. Infection of meibomian gland is known as internal hordeolum. Usually, the causative organism is staphylococci. Treatment includes hot compresses and topical antibiotic eye drops and ointment. In severe cases systemic antibiotic can be given.

Preseptal cellulitis is a deep infection of the eyelid tissues. It does not breach orbital septum. All try should be done to prevent the spread to orbit by treating the condition aggressively with systemic antibiotic. The presence of any constitutional symptoms such as fever, chills, or significant leukocytosis should be looked for closely. The patient should be advised for timely hospital admission to prevent further complications.

Streptococcal Infections

Impetigo

Impetigo is a superficial skin infection. The organisms responsible are staphylococci, group A streptococci, or both. The face is often affected. In impetigo, the infection begins as small red macules that quickly become vesicles. In classic staphylococcal bullous impetigo, the vesicles progress to large bullae that rupture and form thin crusts often accompanied by local lymphadenopathy. Oral erythromycin or azithromycin is usually effective.

Erysipelas

Erysipelas is superficial cellulitis usually caused by group a streptococci and it is common on face and eyelid. Clinical features are painful, elevated, red, sharply demarcated, and shiny induration of the skin. It is accompanied by systemic signs.

Necrotizing Fasciitis

It is the infection of all layers of skin. The patient presents with swelling, pain, blackening of lid skin, and constitutional symptoms. The patient is often diabetic or immunocompromised. The organisms responsible are anaerobes, facultative anaerobes, or group A β-hemolytic *Streptococcus* with or without *S. aureus*. Treatment must be very aggressive and consists of intravenous (IV) penicillin G with appropriate coverage for anaerobes in an intensive care unit. Frequent surgical debridement is often necessary.

MYCOBACTERIAL

Tuberculosis

Tuberculosis of the eyelid is rare. It may results from contiguous spread from other facial skin involvement or there may be a fistulous tract due to infection of any of the sinuses or orbit. They are chronic. Clinical presentation may be a brownish plaque with pus discharge. Scarring is common. The combination of tarsoconjunctival granuloma and local lymphadenopathy is known as Parinaud's syndrome. High degree of suspicion is required for the diagnosis.

VIRAL

Herpes Simplex

The clinical manifestations of herpes simplex infection can be the result of primary infection or recurrence. Primary infection of the eyelids typically presents as single or multiple pinhead-sized vesicles containing a clear fluid that later becomes seropurulent. The rupture of these vesicles leads to crusting, which heal without scarring in approximately 7 days. Nothing other than supportive treatment for the skin is necessary. Topical antivirals are recommended for concurrent corneal disease and consideration of oral acyclovir in recurrent disease (**Fig. 9.4.2**).

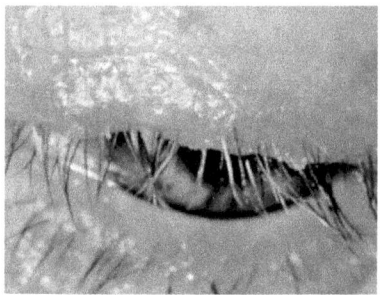

Fig. 9.4.2: Crusting, lash loss, and ulceration of the lid margin caused by staphylococcal lid disease.

Herpes Zoster

Zoster ophthalmicus occurs as a result of reactivation along the ophthalmic division of Vth cranial nerve. Lesions present as grouped vesicles on an erythematous base. Ulceration and scarring of the vesicles can lead to eyelid abnormalities. Therapy consists of topical or oral antibiotics to prevent superinfection. Oral acyclovir is most effective when started within 3 days of onset.

Varicella

Causative agent is *herpes zoster*. Eyelid involvement characterized by nongrouped vesicles on an erythematous base can be associated with conjunctival or corneal involvement. Lesions heal without scarring. Treatment consists of topical antibiotics to prevent superinfection.

Molluscum Contagiosum

Molluscum contagiosum is a double-stranded deoxyribonucleic acid (DNA) poxvirus transmission in children occurs by direct contact or via fomites. Autoinoculation is common. Transmission from sexual contact is more common in adults. Eyelid lesions appear as multiple, round, and waxy umbilicated skin papules. Incision and expression of the viral bead with a curette is usually curative. Topical and IV cidofovir may be indicated in recalcitrant or disseminated cases in immunosuppressed individuals.

PARASITIC

Phthiriasis

Pthirus pubis, the crab louse, is usually found in the hairs of the genital region. Transmission occurs by direct contact or contact with infested articles. Presents as blepharoconjunctivitis with tiny, pearly white nits attached to the lashes. Lice are almost transparent unless they contain blood, and are easily missed on examination. Though many treatment options exist, 1% yellow mercuric oxide ointment qid for 14 days is considered the treatment of choice. Adjunctive measures to treat all contacts and delouse personal effects are needed.

Demodex

Demodex folliculorum is a type of Demodex mite that lives mostly within the hair follicles on the face and the eyes and is usually found on the eyelids and lashes. The Demodex mite can cause blepharitis, resulting in inflammation of the eyelids and severe dry eye.

Symptoms of demodicosis include itching, redness, scaling, and thickening of the skin. In severe cases, it can lead to hair loss and secondary bacterial infections. It is treated by trimming the lashes from the base, eyelid scrub, and application of an eye ointment.

FUNGAL

Rarely, *Pityrosporum orbiculare* and *ovale* may be found in patients with seborrheic blepharitis. *Candida albicans* may uncommonly cause a marginal blepharitis in immunosuppressed patients.

9.5 Cosmetic Eyelids Surgeries (Upper Lid and Lower Lid Blepharoplasty)

Kasturi Bhattacharjee, Divakant Misra, Komal Sawarkar

kasturibhattacharjee44@hotmail.com

UPPER LID BLEPHAROPLASTY

Introduction

The natural process of aging can cause the eyes to appear tired, but there are ways to rejuvenate the face and achieve a more youthful look. Eyelid rejuvenation plays a vital role in this process. Blepharoplasty is the preferred surgical procedure for revitalizing the eyelids, resulting in eyes that look younger and more vibrant. This procedure involves carefully removing excess eyelid skin, reshaping the orbicularis oculi muscle, and sculpting the orbital fat to achieve improved cosmetic and functional outcomes. It is important to approach the surgery with caution and discretion to avoid complications such as postoperative lagophthalmos and exposure keratopathy.

Elderly patients often present with various concerns related to their eyes, including restricted visual field, excess eyelid skin, deteriorated vision quality, increased skin wrinkles and folds, and strain, and headaches caused by prolonged lifting of the upper eyelids. Additionally, these changes contribute to a tired appearance. Some patients may also experience irritation and excessive tearing. While younger patients primarily seek upper eyelid blepharoplasty for cosmetic reasons, older and middle-aged individuals often have both cosmetic and functional issues. Specifically, younger individuals, particularly those of Asian and North-East Indian descent with typical Asian eyelid features, may request the creation or modification of an eyelid crease, achieving higher or symmetrical creases, or forming a double lid fold in eyes with a single lid fold.

When evaluating patients for blepharoplasty, the surgeon must consider various factors. In addition to conducting a comprehensive ophthalmologic examination, it is important to obtain a thorough medical and ocular history. This should include any history of trauma or previous surgeries. The patient should also be evaluated for thyroid disease and dry eye disease. The function of the seventh cranial nerve should be assessed as well. Any history of bleeding disorders or the use of anticoagulants such as aspirin should be documented and appropriate precautions taken. Preoperative photographs should be taken with the eyes in the primary position and from a lateral view. It is crucial to carefully examine the patient's best corrected visual acuity, palpebral fissure height and contour, upper eyelid position, eyelid crease and fold distance, eyebrow position, frontalis muscle action, and tear film health. Elaborate written and informed consent of the patient should be obtained before the surgery day to avoid any kind of preoperative dilemmas and anxiety.

Surgical Technique

The upper lid blepharoplasty includes the following main steps:
- Skin marking
- Anesthesia
- Skin incision
- Skin and muscle excision
- Fat excision
- Closure

Marking Incision

The upper limit of skin excision and the skin crease are critical components of blepharoplasty marking. The marking can be done using any dye that will not be completely washed out when the patient is prepared.

Classical lid marking techniques are:
- Classic Rees incision
- Scalpel-shaped incision
- Bellinvia's incision

Authors prefer their own technique of skin marking. The marking process is performed with sufficient lighting while the patient is comfortably seated and looking straight ahead. Point A is marked 10 mm above the central margin of the eyelid. Point B is marked 6 mm above the inner corner of the eye (medial canthus). Point C is marked at the lowest point of the excess skin or hooding on the outer corner of the eye. Then, a pinch test is conducted to determine point D. Point E is marked 8 mm above and

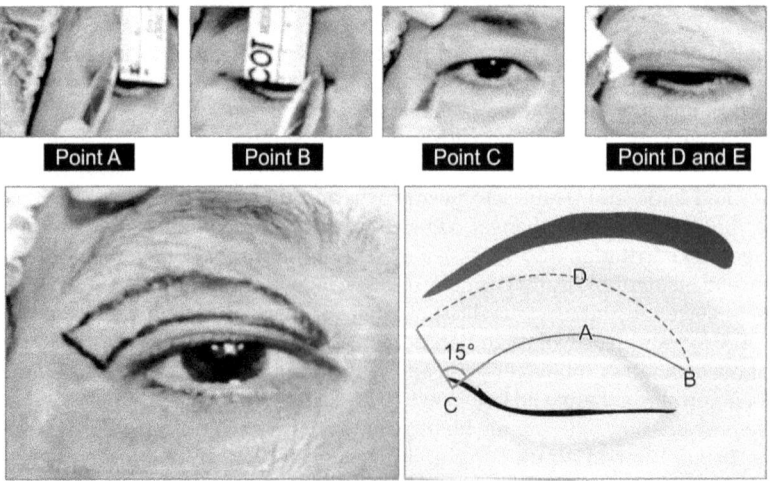

Fig. 9.5.1: Marking technique.

at a 15° angle from point C. All of these points are connected in an ellipsoid manner to complete the marking of the eyelid **(Fig. 9.5.1)**.

Anesthesia

Upper lid blepharoplasty is frequently conducted using local anesthesia. A disposable needle with a gauge size of 27 or 30 is used to inject 2–3 mL of 2% lidocaine containing 1:100,000 epinephrine subcutaneously. This injection is administered over the previously marked areas of the upper eyelid and lateral canthus to provide anesthesia and control bleeding.

Skin Incision, Muscle, Fat Excision, and Closure

Once the skin incisions have been made, one edge of the wound is lifted, and the excess skin is carefully removed using a fine angled empire tip on a radiofrequency cautery device. A section of the preseptal orbicularis muscle is excised, and small incisions are made over the septum to gain direct access to the preaponeurotic fat pads. The medial (whitish) and central (yellow) fat pads, which can be distinguished by their color and embryonic origin (medial-neural crest derived), are gently teased out through the small openings in the orbital septum. Before excision, it is important to secure the fat pads with a hemostatic clamp and use radiofrequency cautery for their removal. The remaining stump in the hemostatic clamp is cauterized and then retracted **(Fig. 9.5.2)**.

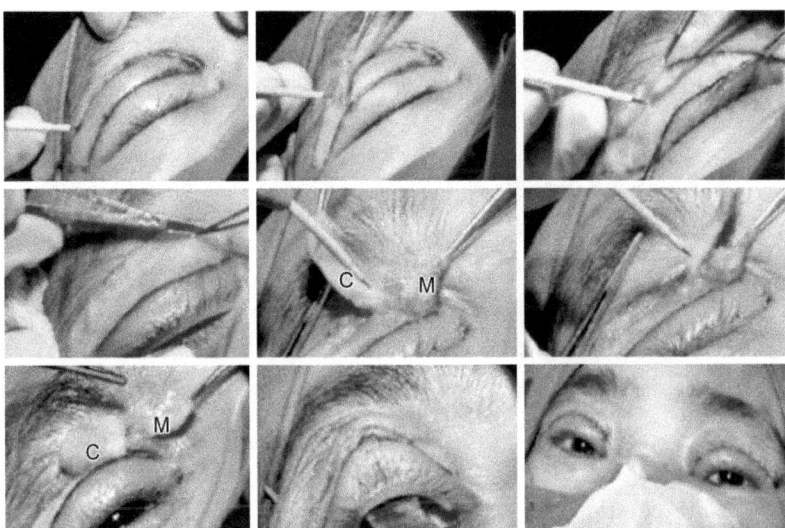

Fig. 9.5.2: Surgical steps of upper lid blepharoplasty.

The retro-orbicularis oculi fat is carefully repositioned to restore eyebrow volume and is internally fixed in the desired position, typically 2–3 mm above the supraorbital rim, using two nonabsorbable sutures. The orbicularis muscle is then closed with interrupted sutures using an absorbable material of size 6-0. To create a well-defined and desired eyelid crease, an interrupted, horizontal mattress suture is applied, involving the pretarsal skin, orbicularis oculi muscle, levator fibers, and skin. Finally, the skin is meticulously approximated using continuous or interrupted sutures, preferably nonabsorbable and of size 8-0 prolene.

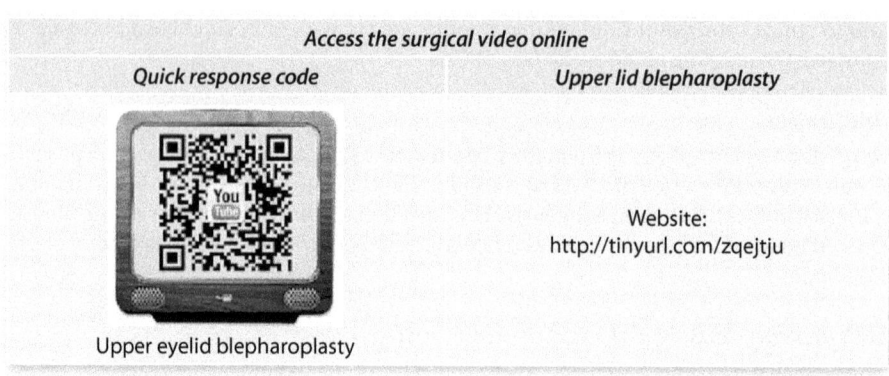

Postoperative Advice

- Avoid lifting heavy weights.
- To avoid anticoagulants for 1 week.
- To avoid direct sunlight exposure and use of sunscreens to avoid scar pigmentation and scar irregularities.
- Intermittent use of ice packs (3-4 times/day) along with head end elevation while sleeping (to reduce/minimize the edema).
- Generous use of lubricating drops for preventing exposure-related corneal dryness.
- Avoid eye make-up for minimum of 10-14 days.

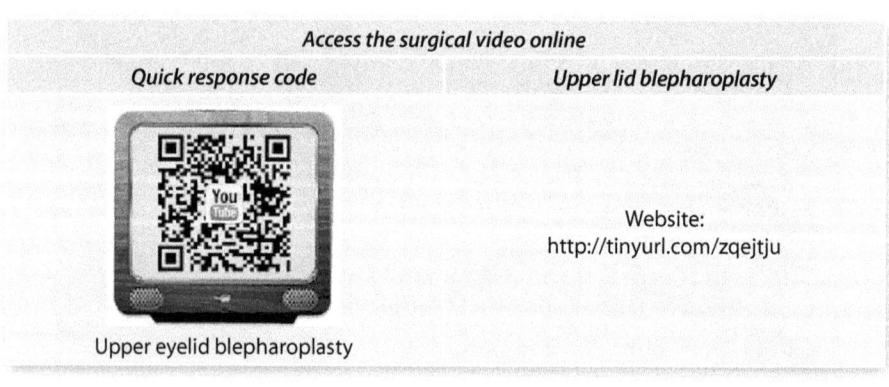

Complications

- *Superficial ecchymosis:* Superficial ecchymosis, characterized by intramuscular or subcutaneous hematoma, can be a common complication. Preoperatively, it may occur during the administration of local anesthesia. Intraoperatively, bleeding from the orbicularis oculi muscle may contribute to ecchymosis. Fragile blood vessels in the early postoperative period can also lead to this condition. To prevent or minimize superficial ecchymosis, proper injection techniques, optimal control of blood pressure, and discontinuation of blood thinners before surgery are essential. The use of radiofrequency cautery has reduced the incidence of intraoperative muscular or fat bleeding. Applying ice packs to the eyelid can help reduce pain, hematoma, edema, and erythema.
- *Asymmetry:* Asymmetry is a significant complication to address. Achieving symmetry between the two eyelids is one of the goals of upper eyelid blepharoplasty.

Since the lid crease serves as a surgical and cosmetic landmark, any asymmetry becomes readily noticeable. When correcting asymmetry, surgery is performed on the lid with a higher crease. Lowering a lid crease is easier than elevating it, as there is typically enough residual upper lid skin available. Residual upper lid fat or excessive fat resection can lead to superior sulcus asymmetries. Dog-ears can result in fine asymmetric scars. Therefore, it is crucial to maintain appropriate symmetry from the creation of skin incisions to wound closure. While lateral scar asymmetry can be prevented, medial webbing of scars can be managed with V-Y plasty. Digital massage and creams with vitamin supplements can aid in the early postoperative period.

- *Lagophthalmos:* Lagophthalmos may occur due to upper lid retraction resulting from postoperative fibrosis of the levator aponeurosis caused by excessive cautery or significant postoperative inflammation. Longer anesthetic effects, hematoma, or trauma can contribute to lagophthalmos in the early postoperative period. In later stages, excessive excision of skin and muscle can shorten the anterior lamella, leading to a cicatricial type of lagophthalmos.
- *Ptosis:* Ptosis can arise due to inadequate preoperative eyelid examination, leading to an overlooked existing blepharoptosis. The blepharoptosis becomes more apparent once the dermatochalasis resolves after surgery. Direct intraoperative injury to the levator palpebral superioris (LPS) or inadvertent damage during intraocular surgeries like cataract surgery can also cause ptosis. In such cases, levator surgery is required and can be performed via the same incision site. Transient mechanical ptosis may occur due to lid edema postoperatively or levator paresis following aggressive fat resection or cautery. It typically resolves without treatment within several weeks.
- *Scar-related issues:* Wound infections and scars are rare due to the rich vascularity of the eyelids. Applying generous amounts of ointment to the wound during the first postoperative week can help avoid suture cysts. Certain problems related to wound healing and modulation, such as pigmentation, scar hypertrophy, and persistent scar erythema, can occur. Local vitamin E cream, directional digital massage, subcutaneous injections of antifibrotic agents, and steroid creams can be helpful in such situations. Silicone-based gels are effective and safe options for scar management. Epithelial inclusion cysts may require excision or marsupialization. Wearing larger sunglasses and using sunscreens is advised to protect the surgical area from direct sunlight exposure.
- *Orbital hematoma/compartment syndrome:* Orbital hematoma/compartment syndrome is considered a postoperative emergency in patients undergoing upper lid blepharoplasty. It mainly occurs in the immediate postoperative period. Patients may experience severe, sudden-onset pain along with profound vision loss. Active hemorrhage may not be recognized during the procedure due to the retraction of bleeding vessels back into the orbit, leading to routine wound closure. Postoperatively, the hematoma enlarges and can cause ischemic damage to the optic nerve due to increased intraorbital pressure. Patients present with a proptosed and congested globe, limited ocular movements, and a dilated pupil. In such cases, the wound is reopened, bleeders are located, and hemostasis is achieved. Immediate lateral canthotomy and cantholysis are performed if the pupil is dilated. Systemic steroids and osmotic agents may be used.
- *Lymphedema:* Postoperatively, a chronic type of eyelid edema may occur due to the severing of lymphatics during the eyelid incision. This edema gradually resolves as the lymphatics regain their function.

- *Ocular motility disorders:* Although rare, ocular motility disturbances resulting from extraocular muscle injuries have been described in upper eyelid blepharoplasty. Transient ocular motility issues can occur due to deeper diffusion or extravasation of the anesthetic agent. During fat resection, injury to the trochlea and superior oblique muscle can also lead to postoperative diplopia.

LOWER EYELID BLEPHAROPLASTY

Introduction

Baggy lower eyelids result from hypertrophic or lax orbicularis, excess skin, and herniated orbital fat. Lower lid blepharoplasty incorporates a set of complicated maneuvers to rejuvenate the lower lid.

Preoperative Evaluation

A full medical and ocular history should be collected, along with a complete ophthalmologic examination. A thorough preoperative evaluation of the eyelid is important for successful surgery and to minimize the risks of complications. Evaluation of the tone of the lower lid is crucial which can be done by doing a snap test. It is crucial to evaluate the tone of the lower lid as ectropion and retraction can occur in lax lids. "Snap test" is done by pulling the lid downwards and then releasing it. Brisk and spontaneous return to normal position denotes normal tension in the lid. Preoperative photographs should be taken with the eyes in primary position. A well elaborated written and informed consent of the patient should be taken before the surgery to avoid any kind of preoperative dilemmas and anxiety.

Surgical Technique

Approaches

Previously, lower lid blepharoplasty was all about removal of skin and fat which led to lower eyelid retraction, rounding of lateral canthal angle and canthal dystopia. Then came the transconjunctival approach of fat excision but was found to be associated with sulcus deformity and sunken eyes. However, lower blepharoplasty is now performed by fat repositioning. This can be done either by anterior transcutaneous approach or by transconjunctival approach. The anterior transcutaneous approach is associated with postoperative complications such as lower eyelid retraction due to middle lamellar cicatrix and hence not preferred nowadays.

Transconjunctival approach: In transconjunctival approach an incision through conjunctiva beneath the tarsus is given, which avoids disruption of skin, orbicularis or orbital septum and allows rapid and direct entry into the orbital fat.

Conjunctival incision of approximately 4 mm below the tarsus is given which allows safe entry into fat compartments. From the edge of the caruncle to the lateral canthus an "open sky" like exposure is necessary for good exposure. Once the fat pads are visualized the connective tissue septa can be further dissected, this can also be performed with blunt dissection with Stevens scissors. For a wide exposure of the central and lateral fat pockets fascial band can be cut. The lateral fat pad, as it is deeply seated and covered with more septa, so may not come forward easily. Blunt dissection down to the arcus marginalis at the inferolateral orbital rim should be done as identification of the internal orbital surface is very useful for identification of lateral fat pad. Care should be taken to visualize central fat pad. Belly of the inferior oblique separates the central and medial fat compartments. Careful fat isolation should be done beginning with the central fat pad and prominent vessels should be coagulated. The surgeon should check external eyelid contour intermittently during the procedure. Endpoint of fat excision is reached when the fat is flushed with orbital rim while applying light pressure on the globe. Over resection may cause sunken or deskeletonized appearance of the orbit. It has been observed that only orbital fat removal leads to prominence of tear trough groove. So repositioning of the fat over the inferior orbital rim onto the superior face of the maxilla helps to overcome the deformity and is cosmetically more acceptable. Debulking of the lateral fat pad is done conservatively and central and medial fat pads should be repositioned into the tear trough deformity. Laser resurfacing and botulinum toxin injection are the best treatment for fine wrinkling and orbicularis creases, respectively. In some cases conservative skin pinch along with transconjunctival approach may be tried.

Complications

- *Corneal abrasion:* Corneal injury is a common postoperative complication but can easily be avoided by careful instrumentation and by the use of protective corneal shields.
- *Infection:* Postoperative wound infections are rare occurrences as the result of the rich vascular supply of the orbit and eyelid.
- *Orbital hematoma:* Hematomas develop either under a skin or skin-muscle flap. Small hematomas can be managed conservatively. Large or progressive hematomas need exploration and control of the hemorrhage.
- *Acquired diplopia:* It is due to inadvertent iatrogenic injury to the inferior oblique muscle while excising the medial fat. An indication for inferior oblique injury is excessive bleeding which is caused when the belly of the muscle is cut. The diplopia usually resolves on its own and a surgery should be considered only if it lasts for >6 months.
- *Lower lid malpositions:* These are caused due to imbalances in the dynamic forces acting on the lid. A malposition may present as lateral scleral show, rounding of the lateral palpebral fissure and lower lid laxity leading to ectropion. It should be initially conservatively managed with gentle massage and observation. If unresolved in 2–3 months' time, a lid tightening procedure can be performed.

BROW LIFT/BROWPEXY

Introduction

Pathophysiological changes in the anatomy of the upper lid lead to varying degree of dermatochalasis and ptosis. The eyebrows play an important role in accentuating these changes. Failure of recognition and correction of brow abnormalities lead to comprised results of upper eyelid surgeries. Browpexy is a procedure which involves the fixation of brow structures of the supraorbital rim area.

Surgical Approaches

Several surgical approaches to brow lift surgery have been described. These approaches include:

- *Direct brow lift:* This technique involves the excision of supraorbital skin and subcutaneous tissue above the eyebrow. The subcutaneous tissue and skin are then closed.
- *Temporal brow lift:* In this approach, the incision is made behind the temporal hairline. The dissection plane is over the fascia temporalis proper, extending toward the lateral orbital rim. Soft tissue fixation is performed during the procedure.
- *Transpalpebral browpexy:* This technique involves fixing the lateral brow to the frontal periosteum through an upper lid crease. The fixation is done at a more cephalad (higher) position.

- *Pretrichial brow lift:* An incision is made just in front of the hairline for this approach. The purpose is to lift the brow using this incision.
- *Mid forehead lift:* This technique utilizes deep forehead creases to place the incision. Skin and subcutaneous tissue are excised, and direct closure is performed without tension.
- *Coronal brow lift:* This technique is known as an "open sky" technique. It involves the excision of skin and subcutaneous tissue several centimeters behind the hairline.
- These various approaches offer different options for brow lift surgery, allowing surgeons to choose the most suitable technique for each patient.

9.6 Botulinum Toxin and Dermal Fillers

Kasturi Bhattacharjee, Obaidur Rehman
Sri Sankaradeva Nethralaya, Guwahati
kasturibhattcharjee44@hotmail.com, obaid.rehmann@gmail.com

BOTULINUM TOXIN

What is Botulinum Toxin?

Botulinum toxin, popularly known as "Botox" in routine clinical practice is in fact the most potent of all known toxins. This neurotoxin is produced by *Clostridium botulinum*, an anaerobic gram-positive spore forming bacteria. Based on antigen specificity, eight different serotypes have been identified, namely type A, B, C1, C2, D, E, F, and G. Botulinum toxin type A, the most widely used for therapeutic purpose, is the most powerful and longest acting of all. It is composed of a heavy and light polypeptide chains linked together by a disulfide bond. It is synthesized as an inactive single peptide chain with a molecular mass of 150 kD. Although clinical experience is emerging with botulinum toxins B, C, and F, toxin type A has been used in clinical practice for almost two decades, with a great efficiency and safety profile.

Mechanism of Action

Botulinum toxin acts by inhibiting the release of the cholinergic neurotransmitter acetylcholine (Ach), the primary site of action being the neuromuscular junction. Normally, at the junction, when action potential depolarizes the axon terminal, Ach is released from the synaptic cleft. This process is facilitated by a transport protein, named SNARE (soluble N-ethylmaleimide-sensitive factor attachment protein receptor) complex. The SNARE proteins are responsible for fusion of vesicle of Ach with nerve cell membrane. The toxin inhibits this aggregation and complex formation.

After injection of the toxin into a target tissue, it is proteolytically cleaved into 100 kD of the heavy chain and 50 kD of the light chain. The heavy chain is responsible for binding of the molecule with the nerve terminals, which is followed by internalization of the molecule. Light chain, then acts by inactivating the SNARE proteins, which leads to inhibition of release of the Ach from the junction and resulting in paralysis of the muscle. The inhibitory effect lasts for around 3 months, after which restoration of the SNARE protein complex occurs. Axonal sprouting and endplate elongation are also responsible for the reversal of the muscle action.

Indications

Botulinum toxin was first approved by the Food and Drug Administration (FDA) in 1989 for the treatment of strabismus and blepharospasm as well as spastic lid disorders involving the facial nerve such as hemifacial spasm and Meige syndrome.

Botulinum toxin comes as a sterile 100 units or 200 units vacuum-dried powder which is reconstituted with sterile, preservative-free 0.9% sodium chloride injection. It can be used in a concentration of 1.25–5 IU/0.1 mL.

Functional Indications

- *Benign essential blepharospasm:* The initial dose is 1.25–2.5 units injected into the medial and lateral pretarsal orbicularis oculi of the upper lid and into the lateral pretarsal orbicularis oculi of the lower lid. Each site is injected with 0.1 mL of botulinum. The effect of the injection is seen after 3 days and reaches the peak by 1st to 2nd week. It usually lasts for 3 months following which injection can be repeated with titration of the dose.
- *Hemifacial spasm and Meige syndrome:* Treatment with botulinum toxin should be considered to reduce the involuntary facial muscle contractions only after ruling out organic causes for hemifacial spasms. 5–10 units are injected into the muscles of the mid face while platysma muscle may require up to 10–20 units. For the first time, it is rational to start with 2.5 units per injection site and increase up to 5 units to avoid any facial asymmetry.
- Cervical dystonia
- *Various types of strabismus*
- *Chronic migraine:* 15 or more days each month with a headache lasting for 4 or more hours each day. Botulinum is injected at multiple head and neck muscle specific areas.
- *Hyperhidrosis:* Sweating in excess of what is required for physiological regulation of body temperature can be cumbersome. Botulinum toxin by inhibiting acetyl choline releases and prevents the hyperstimulation of eccrine sweat glands.

Cosmetic Indications

When evaluating the patient for cosmetic purposes, it is essential to provide the patient with a hand mirror to allow identification of an area that the patient would like to discuss and get treated for. After identification and appropriate marking of the areas, 2.5–5 units of botulinum toxin are usually injected into the facial musculature.

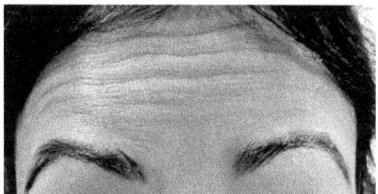

Fig. 9.6.1: Transverse forehead lines pre-Botox.

Indications are as follows:
- Frown lines between the eyebrows (glabellar lines) in adults
- Transverse forehead lines **(Figs. 9.6.1 and 9.6.2)**
- Orbicularis rhytides or crow's feet
- Nonsurgical brow lift
- *Bunny lines:* Transverse lines over nasal bridge **(Figs. 9.6.3 and 9.6.4)**
- *Marionette lines:* Downward turning of the lateral corners of the mouth
- Perioral lines
- Platysmal bands

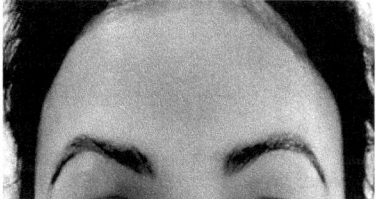

Fig. 9.6.2: Transverse forehead lines post-Botox.

Off-label uses:
- Chronic daily headache and tension headache
- Reflex brow elevation after ptosis repair
- *Thyroid orbitopathy:* To reduce upper lid retraction and glabellar furrows
- Chemical tarsorrhaphy in corneal ulceration following 5th or 7th nerve palsy
- *Crocodile tears:* Hyperlacrimation following 7th nerve injury or Bell's palsy

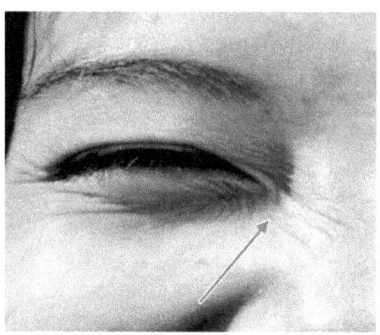

Fig. 9.6.3: Bunny's line pre-Botox.

- *Dry eye:* Injection into the medial upper and lower lids to evert puncta and decrease tear drainage
- Spastic lower lid entropion
- Apraxia of eyelid opening

Complications

Patient can develop following complications hours to weeks after injection:
- Extraocular muscle weakness
- Diplopia
- Ptosis
- Swelling of eyelid
- Corneal exposure and ulceration
- Blurred vision
- Dysphonia, dysarthria, dyspnea, and dysphagia
- Allergic reaction or anaphylaxis
- Exacerbation of the pre-existing neuromuscular disorder
- Death

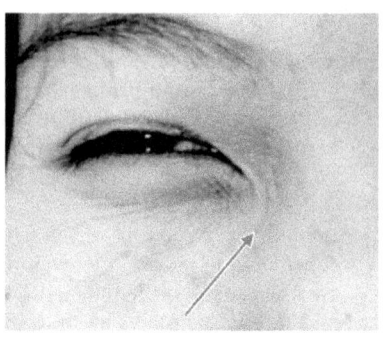

Fig. 9.6.4: Bunny's line post-Botox.

Precautions

Cosmetic use of botulinum toxin is not recommended for use in individuals younger than 18 years of age, while therapeutic use is limited to >12 years of the age.

It is contraindicated in following situations:
- Previous allergic reaction
- Infection at the injection site
- Lactating mother or pregnancy
- Neuromuscular disorder such as myasthenia gravis or Lambert–Eaton syndrome
- Urinary tract infection or urinary retention

▌DERMAL FILLERS

Dermal fillers are used for facial rejuvenation in patients seeking nonsurgical means for correcting age-related changes to their facial skin. Over many years, different substances such as mineral oil, paraffin, and liquid silicone have been used as soft tissue fillers.

Basically, there are two types of wrinkles: dynamic and static. Repeated contraction of the muscle of facial expressions leads to the development of dynamic wrinkles. Regardless of facial dynamics, static wrinkles or static rhytides appear as a result of intrinsic changes in the dermal ground substances. Also, external factors such as gravity, smoking, and sun exposure are responsible for the development of static wrinkles. Development of these dynamic and static rhytides depends on the natural collagen support of the dermis.

The recent introduction of the newer agents has increased interest in dermal fillers as they have better outcomes and lesser side effect profile. Fillers are effective mean to correct facial aging changes along with botulinum toxin injections, especially in the lower face.

Based on the bioavailability and longevity of the effect, they are divided into temporary agents, semipermanent agents and permanent agents.
- *Temporary biodegradable agents (<1 year):*
  - *Collagen compounds:*
    - Bovine collagen (Zyderm 1 and Zyderm 2)
    - Human collagen (Cosmoderm)
  - *Hyaluronic acid (HA) compounds:*
    - Restylane and Perlane
    - Hylaform/Hylaform Plus

- Puragen/Puragen Plus
- Juvéderm Ultra and Juvéderm Ultra Plus
- Juvéderm Voluma
- *Semipermanent biodegradable compounds (1–2 years):*
  - Calcium hydroxyapatite (Radiesse)
  - Poly-L-lactic acid (PLLA) (Sculptra)
  - Cadaveric fascia lata (Fascian)
- *Permanent Nonbiodegradable (>2 years):*
  - Silicone (Silikon 1000)
  - PMMA (polymethylmethacrylate) spheres (ArteFill)

Hyaluronic Acid Derivatives

Hyaluronic acid is a glycosaminoglycan, a major component of the connective tissue and a building block of the dermis. HA is a monomer which is a combination of sodium glucuronate and N-acetyl glucosamine. For filler injection, it comes in a polymerized form. In its noncross-linked form, it is in a liquid form. To increase its hardness, cross-linked polymer is added which forms a gel-like consistency. The hardness of the commercially available HA gel depends on the amount of cross-linked polymers that is present in the preparation.

It has the following properties:
- Immunologically inactive
- No species or tissue specificity
- Bind to water molecules
- Expands in volume

Use of HA-based fillers:
- Fine superficial wrinkles
- Glabellar furrows
- Tear trough deformities **(Figs. 9.6.5 and 9.6.6)**
- Nasolabial lines
- Lip augmentation
- Marionette lines
- Nonsurgical facelift
- Chin augmentation

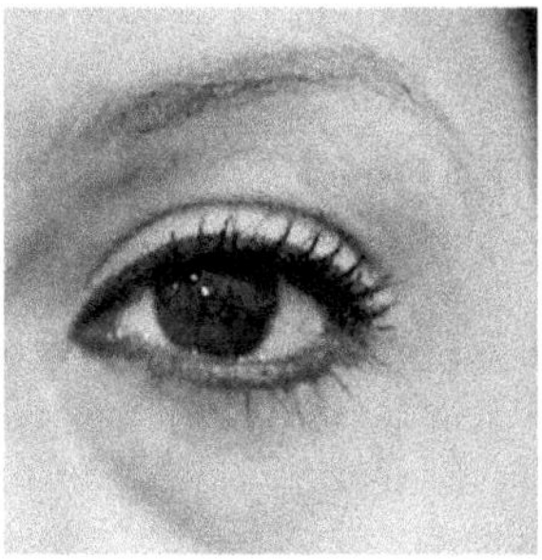

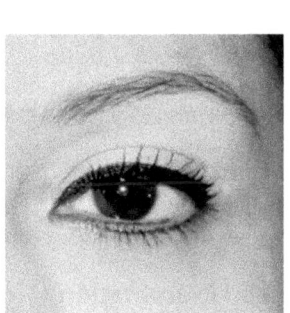

Fig. 9.6.5: Tear trough deformity prehyaluronic acid filler.

Fig. 9.6.6: Tear trough deformity posthyaluronic acid filler.

Adverse Reaction

Common side effects following injection of HA are pain, erythema, swellings, itching, bruising, and tenderness. These are transient and resolve within few days of the injection.

Other adverse reactions can be:
- Hypersensitivity-related:
  - Urticaria
  - Granuloma formation
  - Tissue necrosis leading to scar formation
- Nonhypersensitivity:
  - Bruising, infection at injection site, and reactivation of the herpes
  - Bluish discoloration of the skin, known as the Tyndall effect
  - Serious complications such as tissue necrosis and intravascular injection have also been documented
  - Central retinal artery occlusion leading to blindness can occur in 1 in 10,000 cases.

Newer Developments

The US-FDA has recently approved resilient hyaluronic acid, known as RHA dermal filler. It is supposed to be a modern dermal filler that can adapt to the dynamic facial lines and gives a more natural look.

SUGGESTED READING

1. Czyz CN, Burns JA, Petrie TP, Watkins JR, Cahill KV, Foster JA. Long-term botulinum toxin treatment of benign essential blepharospasm, hemifacial spasm, and Meige syndrome. Am J Ophthalmol. 2013;156(1):173-7.e2.
2. Doft MA, Hardy KL, Ascherman JA. Treatment of hyperhidrosis with botulinum toxin. Aesthet Surg J. 2012;32(2):238-44.

9.7 Eyelid Tumors

M Subrahmanyam
Hyderabad

INTRODUCTION

Neoplasia of various types arises from any of the eyelid structures. It is beyond the scope of this chapter to discuss all of them. Hence, only the common and important tumors will be discussed.

BASIC EXAMINATION

Certain basic examination techniques are described when looking for eyelid tumors.

Present History

Most often the lid tumors present with structural symptoms such as abnormal appearance and asymmetry compared to the fellow eyelid. Rate of onset and progression are also indicative of malignancy as for any other tumor in the body. Most are of a long duration, painless, and slowly progressive.

Past History

Look into the risk factors such as past history of irradiation, sun exposure, tobacco use, and similar growths elsewhere. Most important risk factors include elderly age, immunosuppression [receivers of organ transplants, human immunodeficiency virus (HIV)], exposure to ionizing radiation, and psoralen ultraviolet light A (PUVA) treatment.

Face Examination

First the entire face should be looked at to know the Fitzpatrick type of skin. Fair skin carries a higher risk for cutaneous malignancy, especially basal cell carcinoma.

Eyelid Examination

Measure the dimensions of the tumor with a scale in order to document the progress on later visits. Examine the lids for elevation of the mass, ulcerations, edges, pearly translucency and loss of lashes, rounding of the posterior lid margins, associated telangiectasia, and diffuse conjunctival thickening. Eyelid functions should be documented such as levator action, corneal sensations, and lagophthalmos.

Adnexal Examination

Palpate for the preauricular nodes, submandibular nodes, and anterior cervical lymph nodes.

CLASSIFICATION

These have been variously classified but the current classification that is followed internationally divides the eyelid tumors into six broad categories:
1. Epidermal tumors
2. Adnexal tumors
3. Stromal tumors
4. Secondary tumors
5. Metastatic tumors
6. Inflammatory and infectious lesions simulating neoplasms

From the point of simplification and to discuss the common ones, the three most common tumors namely, basal cell carcinoma, sebaceous gland carcinoma (SGC), and squamous cell carcinomas will be briefly described.

Basal Cell Carcinoma

Basal cell carcinomas are considered to be the most common tumors of the eyelid contributing 80–90% of the cases in western literature.

Risk factors known for this malignancy are:
- Fair skin type with inability to tan
- Ultraviolet (UV) radiation exposure
- Systemic immune dysfunction
- Arsenic compounds
- Genetic diseases such as xeroderma pigmentosa, Gorlin–Goltz syndrome, and albinism

Basal cell carcinoma is thought to arise from the basal cells of the epidermis. It usually presents in the sixth decade and above, but can also be seen in young adults in cases of genetic predispositions as mentioned earlier. Most of them arise from the lower eyelid, followed by medial canthus, upper lid, and lateral canthus in order of frequency. It can present as nodular mass or a noduloulcerative mass. It begins as a small papule, enlarges to a pearly nodule and may ulcerate. Ulcer has been described as having raised everted edges with telangiectasias. They are usually firm on palpation, painless, and associated with loss of lashes in that region. Another important clinical presentation is the morpheaform which extends both in superficial plane and in depth and is often associated with pigmentation. Orbital extension can occur in neglected cases. Metastasis is extremely rare.

Management commonly includes excision biopsy with frozen section or Mohs micrographic surgery. Cryotherapy is used for localized small tumors with well-defined borders, but not popular in Indians because the depigmentation that occurs due to cryotherapy leaves a patch resembling vitiligo. Chemotherapy is usually reserved for nonresectable tumors. Imiquimod has been tried, but it produces very severe local inflammatory response. Intralesional interferon can also be tried. Vismodegib causes tumor shrinkage in 46–58%. Orbital extension may require exenteration. Alternately radiation/vismodegib can be tried for chemoreduction to reduce the size of the tumor and then excise it to save the eye.

Squamous Cell Carcinoma

It is an invasive epithelial malignancy arising from squamous cell layer of the epidermis. It is not so common tumor of the eyelid.

Risk factors described are:
- Sunlight exposure
- UV radiations
- Immunosuppressive states such as acquired immunodeficiency syndrome (AIDS) and postrenal transplants
- Arsenic exposure
- Xeroderma pigmentosa and albinism

It usually presents in the sixth decade but can also be seen in young adults in cases of genetic predispositions and HIV.

Most of them arise from the lower eyelid followed by medial canthus, upper lid, and lateral canthus in order of frequency. It can present as nodular mass or a noduloulcerative mass. It presents as painless, elevated nodular, or plaque-like lesions with chronic fissuring and scaling. Some may ulcerate with irregular rolled out edges. Look for systemic associations like Bowen's disease elsewhere. Orbital extension can occur either due to direct extension or due to perineural invasion.

Management commonly includes excision biopsy with frozen section or Mohs micrographic surgery. Cryotherapy is used for localized small tumors with well-defined borders. Radiotherapy can be used as adjunctive or as palliative for advanced/metastatic tumors/in those not willing for surgery. Chemotherapy is usually reserved for nonresectable tumors. Drugs used include cisplatin, doxorubicin, bleomycin, methotrexate, 5-fluorouracil, and cetuximab.

Follow-up after management should be for 5 years as most of the recurrences are noted during this period.

Sebaceous Gland Carcinoma

This is the most lethal of the eyelid tumors described. Though it accounts for only 5% in Western literature, the incidence is very high among the Indian population, varying from 55 to 70% and common in South East Asian countries. This marked difference is because we are protected from basal cell carcinoma by the melanin in our skin **(Fig. 9.7.1)**. It arises from meibomian glands, glands of Zeiss, and sebaceous glands in caruncle and brow.

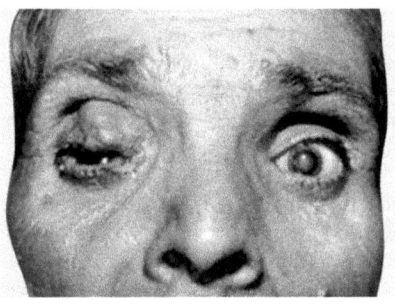

Risk factors known include:
- Ocular or facial irradiation
- Immune dysfunctional states
- Elderly
- Females
- Possible relation with human papillomavirus (HPV)

Fig. 9.7.1: Sebaceous gland carcinoma.

It usually affects the elderly but children may also develop it following radiotherapy for tumors. Majority of SGC arise from the meibomian glands but may also arise from glands of Zeis and caruncle. Upper lids are more commonly involved than the lower lid since upper lid has more meibomian glands.

This usually presents as a solitary nodule fixed to the tarsus, just like a chalazion, may assume yellow color. It is mandatory to have histopathology evaluation for any recurrent chalazion or on the table the "supposed chalazion" looks atypical. In my experience more than half of the cases of meibomian carcinomas were subjected to surgery for chalazion, a few as many as five times. Associated loss of lashes, conjunctival ulceration, or diffuse thickening of the tarsus point toward malignant lesion. Another subtle way of SGC presenting is the pagetoid variety which can be commonly misdiagnosed as chronic blepharoconjunctivitis. The catch points are diffuse thickening of the conjunctiva and tarsus, posterior rounding of the lid margin, loss of lashes, blocked meibomian orifices and telangiectasia and not responding to treatment for blepharitis.

Clinical diagnosis can be confirmed by biopsy. In cases where pagetoid variety is suspected a conjunctival map biopsy is done to establish the diagnosis and extent of spread histopathologically.

Management commonly includes excision biopsy with wide margins of 5 mm under frozen section or Mohs micrographic surgery and reconstruction. Cryotherapy is used when resection of the wide margins is not possible. Chemotherapy is usually reserved for nonresectable tumors or ones with regional extension or for chemoreduction before exenteration. Radiotherapy is usually not used as it is quite radioresistant. Of late topical mitomycin C drops are found to be effective in certain pagetoid varieties.

Malignant melanoma and lymphoma are the other malignant neoplasia of the lids which are very rare.

Melanoma is extremely rare. The risk factors include intense, intermittent exposure to UV radiation, changing nevus, >50 nevi that are >2 mm in size, family history of melanoma, and immunosuppression. The clinical presentation includes asymmetry, border irregularity, change in the color, diameter >6 mm, and enlarging lesion with elevated surface. Treatment comprises of excision with 10 mm clear margin and reconstruction. Radiotherapy and chemotherapy can be tried in extensive lesions to avoid exenteration.

WHEN TO SUSPECT MALIGNANCY?
- Chronic and painless progression of a tumor
- Ulceration
- Loss of cilia
- Telangiectasia
- Rounding of posterior lid margin
- Recurrent chalazion
- Chronic blepharitis not responding to treatment

Among the benign tumors the more common types include hemangioma, neurofibroma, nevus, and papilloma.

Capillary Hemangioma
Capillary hemangioma is typically diagnosed by its port-wine stain or by the color of the raised tumor. It can involve the upper or lower lid, usually grows for a few months and then starts to regress. Hence, treatment is indicated only when the mass is big enough to occlude the pupil or induce significant astigmatism to cause amblyopia. Till that time periodic examination is needed **(Fig. 9.7.2)**.

However, remember that it can be associated with Sturge–Weber syndrome and look for choroidal and intracranial hemangiomas.

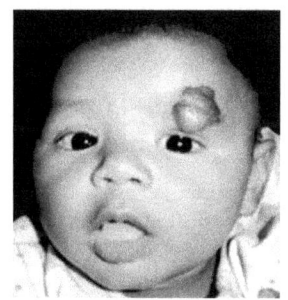

Fig. 9.7.2: Capillary hemangioma.

Neurofibroma
Neurofibroma presents as plexiform type or nodular, in association with von Recklinghausen's disease or can be a solitary tumor. The presence of Lisch nodules on the iris, café-au-lait spots, and family history point out the diagnosis. Surgery is indicated when there is a possibility of amblyopia or for cosmetic reasons. But the results are often not satisfactory and recurrence is almost always **(Fig. 9.7.3)**.

Nevus is commonly nonpigmented and occurs at three margins. Rarely pigmented kissing nevus is seen from birth, involving both the lids symmetrically. While evaluating a lid tumor, look for the changes that suggest malignancy. When in doubt, histopathological evaluation is important for early diagnosis and management of the tumor.

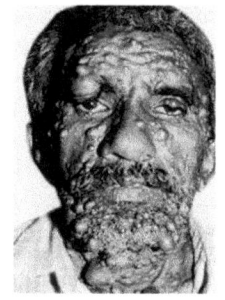

Fig. 9.7.3: Neurofibroma.

9.8 Eyelid Reconstruction: An Overview

Rajat D Maheshwari
Netraseva, Jalna, Maharashtra

■ INTRODUCTION

Eyelid reconstruction is the most fascinating ophthalmic plastic procedure, it is like a zigzag puzzle and we have so many alternatives/combinations to work with. I usually plan it beforehand considering the site involved, age of the patient and extent of defect.

It is always best to be prepared with an alternative plan in case intraoperative the original one does not work well. I have just given a frame work which I have found worked well for almost all types of eyelid defects in my career of more than two decades.

Most of the procedures are the gold standards well described in literature and I deliberately have kept this simple as a flowchart to have a bird's eye view of the reconstruction methods.

The goals of eyelid reconstruction are:
- Adequate globe coverage
- Dynamicity of eyelids function
- Preservation the tear film
- Restoring the aesthetic appearance of the eye

■ GENERAL PRINCIPLES

- When both anterior and posterior lamella has to be reconstructed one of the lamella must be a vascularized flap
- The inner side of the lid need to have a mucus membrane lining
- Proper canthus fixation
- Avoid vertical tension on the lower eyelid
- Provide good closure of the eyelids
- Preserve the lacrimal drainage system

■ DONOR TISSUES FOR RECONSTRUCTION

Skin
- Preauricular
- Retroauricular
- Supraclavicular
- Medial side of the arm
- Sliding flaps from adjacent areas

Mucosal Grafts
- Conjunctival graft
- Tarsoconjunctival flap
- Tarsal graft
- Lip mucosa
- Cheek mucosa
- Nasal mucosa with septal cartilage

■ EYELID DEFECTS INVOLVING ANTERIOR LAMELLA ONLY

- Primary closure (if defect is small)
- Primary closure may be assisted with cantholysis if direct closure not possible

Flaps
Various types of flaps can be fashioned to close the anterior lamellar defects, which are as follows:
- Transposition flap
- Advancement flap
- Rotation flap
- Bilobed flap
- Rhomboid flap
- Z-plasty
- V-Y/Y-V plasty

Grafts
- Full thickness grafts
- Split thickness grafts

FULL THICKNESS EYELID DEFECTS
Upper Eyelid
- *<25%:* Direct closure
- *25–50%:* Direct closure assisted with cantholysis
- *50–75%:*
  - Tenzel flap
  - Cutler–Beard flap
- *>75%:*
  - Cutler–Beard flap
  - Mustards lid rotation
  - Bucket handle flap

Lower Eyelid
- *<25%:* Direct closure
- *25–50%:* Direct closure assisted with cantholysis
- *50–75%:*
  - Tenzel flap
  - Hughes flap with full-thickness skin graft (FTSG)
  - Reverse Cutler–Beard flap
- *>75%:*
  - Hughes flap with FTSG
  - Reverse Cutler–Beard flap

SPECIAL SITUATIONS
- *Medial canthal defects:*
  - Glabellar flap
  - Median forehead flap
- *Lateral canthal defects:*
  - Lateral tarsal strip
  - Lateral periosteal strip

Figures 9.8.1 to 9.8.11 are animated pictures of some common procedures which I believe are sufficient to manage majority of eyelid repairs. Readers are requested to refer texts in detail as it is not possible to cover in detail the procedures here.

I also believe a thorough knowledge of the facial anatomy is must for good results.

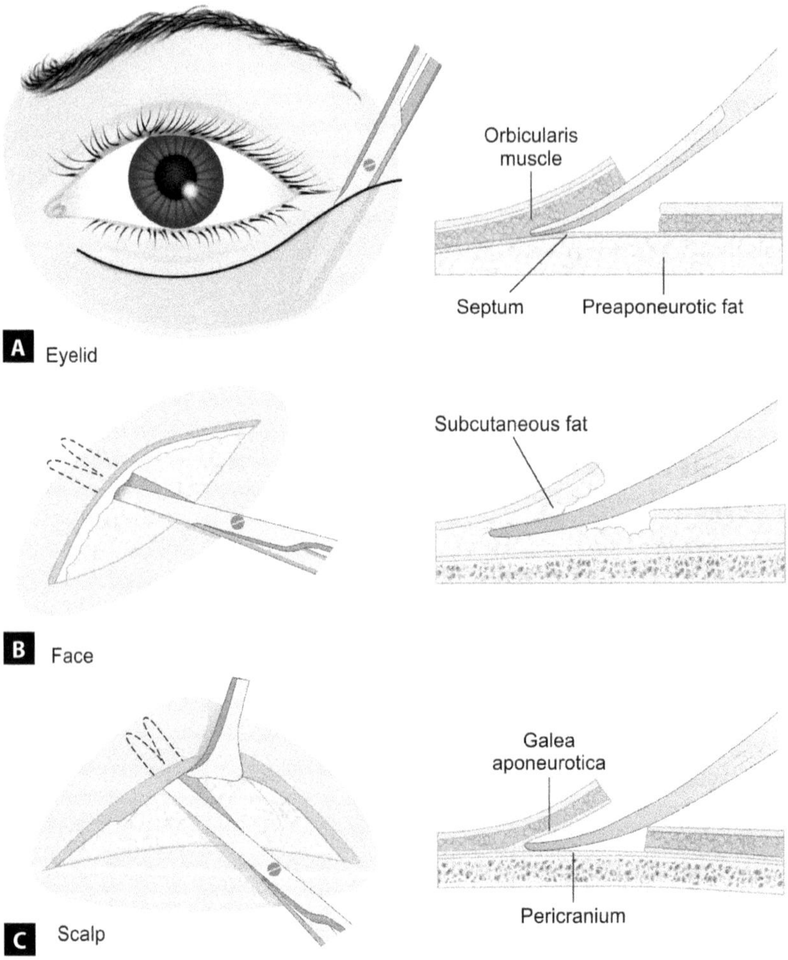

Figs. 9.8.1A to C: Dissection planes for making flaps in facial area. (A) Eyelids: Dissection plane is under the orbicularis muscle (preseptal plane); (B) Cheek: Within the subcutaneous plane; (C) Scalp: Loose areolar tissue plane anterior to the periosteum and posterior to the galea or frontalis.
Source: Nerad JA. Techniques in Ophthalmic Plastic surgery: A Personal Tutorial, 1st edition. Philadelphia: Saunders Elsevier; 2010.

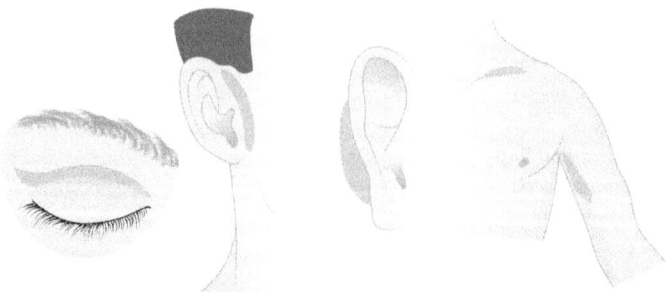

Fig. 9.8.2: Donor site for full-thickness skin graft. Upper eyelid, preauricular, retroauricular, supraclavicular, and medial side of the upper arm.
Source: Nerad JA. Techniques in Ophthalmic Plastic surgery: A Personal Tutorial, 1st edition. Philadelphia: Saunders Elsevier; 2010.

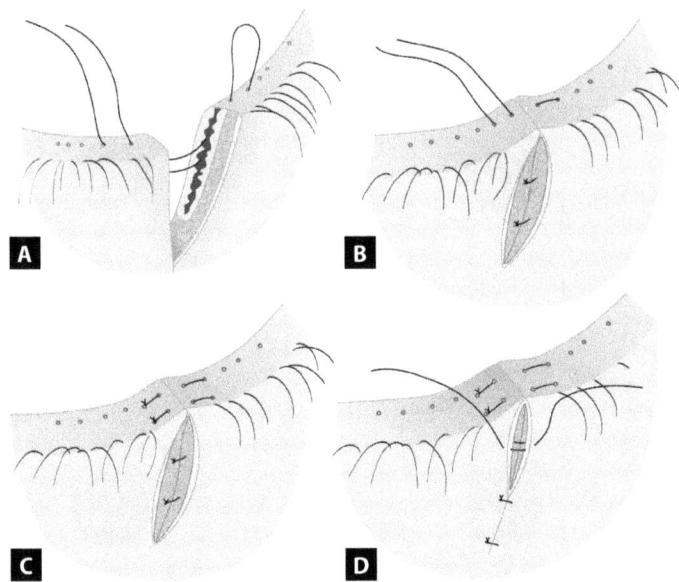

Figs. 9.8.3A to D: Direct closure of eyelid margin. (A and B) Align the eyelid margin by a horizontal mattress suture passing through the meibomian gland orifice creating an eversion; (C) Suture the tarsal plate; (D) Skin closure.
Source: Nerad JA. Techniques in Ophthalmic Plastic surgery: A Personal Tutorial, 1st edition. Philadelphia: Saunders Elsevier; 2010.

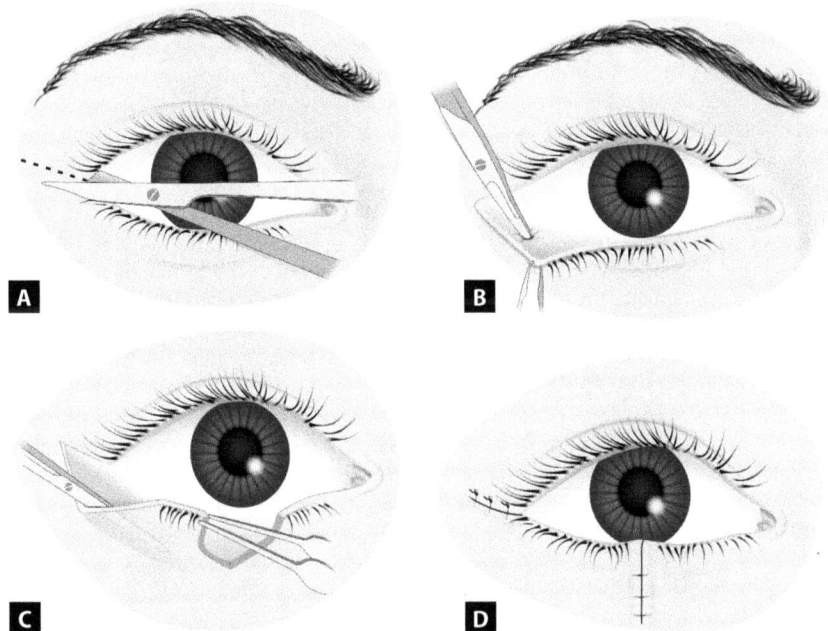

Figs. 9.8.4A to D: Canthotomy and cantholysis for full thickness eyelid defects. (A) Canthotomy angled superiorly for lower eyelid; (B) Cantholysis; (C) Free the orbital septum and lower lid retractors; (D) Repair the lower lid margin and closure of the canthotomy.
Source: Nerad JA. Techniques in Ophthalmic Plastic surgery: A Personal Tutorial, 1st edition. Philadelphia: Saunders Elsevier; 2010.

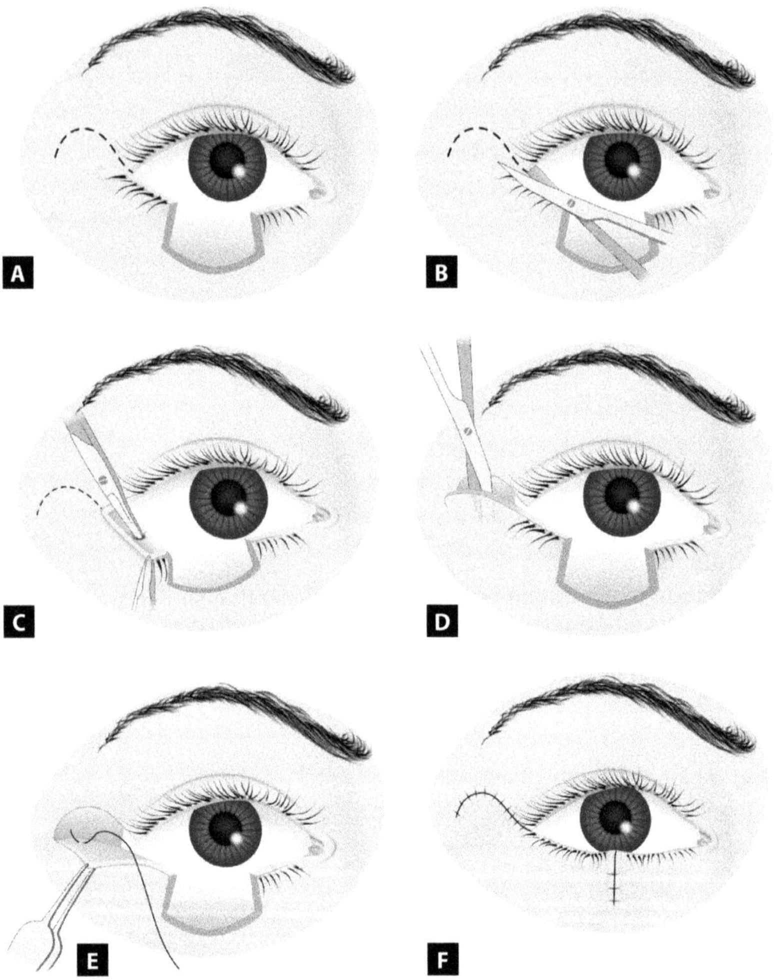

Figs. 9.8.5A to F: Tenzel flap for full-thickness lower eyelid defect. (A) Marking the Tenzel flap (remember frontal nerve passes from the trigs to the tail of the brow); (B) Canthotomy; (C) Cantholysis; (D) Mobilize the tense flap (dissection in the suborbicularis plane); (E) Anchor the flap to the lateral at the periosteum of the lateral orbital rim; (F) Close the lid defect and the flap.
Source: Nerad JA. Techniques in Ophthalmic Plastic surgery: A Personal Tutorial, 1st edition. Philadelphia: Saunders Elsevier; 2010.

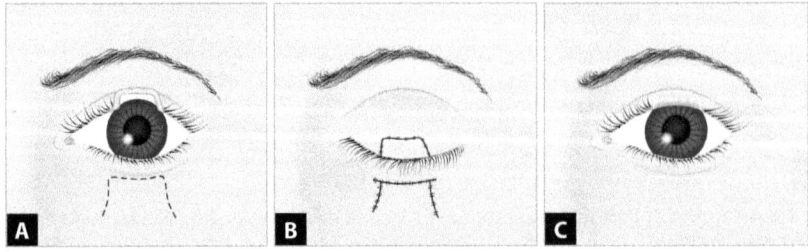

Figs. 9.8.6A to C: Cutler–Beard flap. It is a two-staged lid sharing procedure. Full-thickness lower eyelid flap below the tarsal plate is used to form full-thickness upper eyelid defect. The flap is separated after 4–6 weeks.

SECTION 9: Oculoplasty

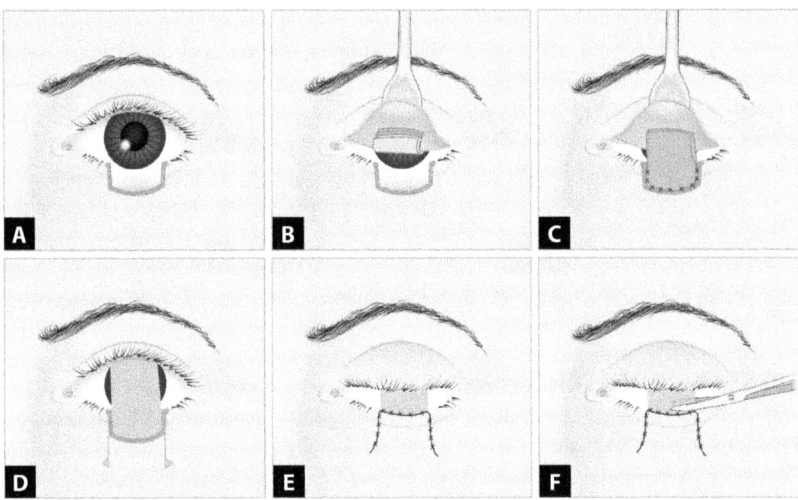

Figs. 9.8.7A to F: Hughes flap. (A) Appropriate size defect for a Hughes flap; (B) Conjunctiva and tarsus incised. Horizontal border of flap is at least 4 mm superior to lid margin; (C) Composite flap advanced into the lower lid defect; (D) Anterior lamella reconstructed with advancement flap; (E) Superior border or advancement flap suture 1–2 mm above upper border of tarsus; (F) Pedicle divided 4–6 weeks after initial reconstructive stage.

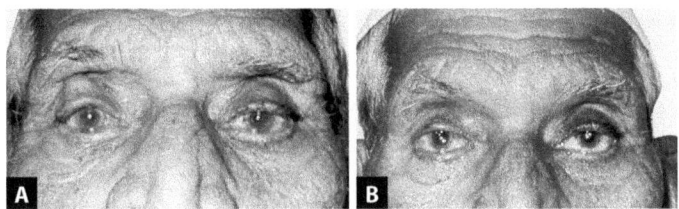

Figs. 9.8.8A and B: (A) Right upper eyelid sebaceous carcinoma; (B) Excision with direct closure after canthotomy and cantholysis.

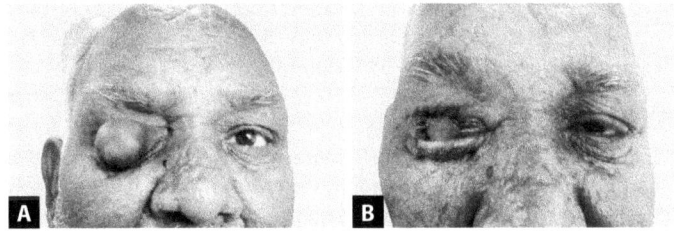

Figs. 9.8.9A and B: (A) Right upper eyelid sebaceous carcinoma; (B) Excision with Cutler–Beard flap for repair.

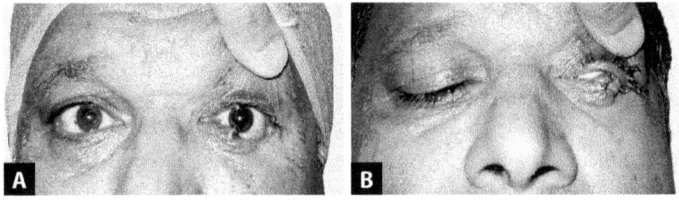

Figs. 9.8.10A and B: (A) Left lower lid defect; (B) Hughes flap forming the posterior lamella and anterior lamella formed by full-thickness skin graft from preauricular area.

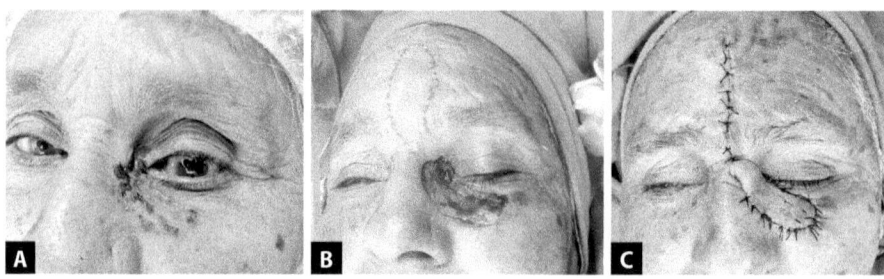

Figs. 9.8.11A to C: (A) Left lower lid BCC; (B) Excised tumor; (C) Repaired with medial forehead flap.

■ SUGGESTED READING

1. Alghoul MS, Kearney AM, Pacella SJ, Purnell CA. Eyelid Reconstruction. Plast Reconstr Surg Glob Open. 2019;7(11):e2520.
2. Bernardini F, Skippen B. Principles and techniques of eyelid reconstruction. In: Chaugule S, Honavar S, Finger P (Eds). Surgical Ophthalmic Oncology. New York: Springer, Cham; 2019.
3. Nerad JA. Techniques in Ophthalmic Plastic Surgery: A Personal Tutorial. Philadelphia: Saunders Elsevier; 2010.
4. Somenek M. Eyelid defect reconstruction. Plast Aesthet Res. 2022;9:16.
5. Subramanian N. Reconstructions of eyelid defects. Indian J Plast Surg. 2011;44(1):5-13.

9.9 Benign and Vascular Eyelid Tumors

Usha Singh, Khushdeep Abhaypal

Advance Eye Centre, Post Graduate Institute of Medical Education and Research, Chandigarh

drushasingh@gmail.com

■ INTRODUCTION

Benign eyelid lesions are commonly encountered by ophthalmologists during their daily practice having a heterogeneous clinical spectrum. It is prudent to differentiate all benign lesions from premalignant and malignant lesions. The management will be guided by a careful history including questions on duration and rate of growth of the lesion and associated symptoms of tenderness, discharge or bleeding. It has been established in various studies that about 80–85% of eyelid lesions are benign.[1,2]

■ APPLIED ANATOMY OF EYELID

Eyelid consists of numerous histological elements which give rise to various benign and malignant eyelid tumors. The eyelids are composed of four layers: skin and subcutaneous tissue, striated muscle (orbicularis oculi), tarsus, and conjunctiva. The skin epithelium is keratinized stratified squamous epithelium. Melanocytes are spread in the basal layer of the epithelium. The eyelids are rich in glandular tissue: The eccrine glands—the sweat glands of the eyelid skin and the accessory lacrimal gland of Krause and Wolfring; the apocrine gland of Moll; and the sebaceous glands—the meibomian glands and the glands of Zeis.

Majority of benign lesions including premalignant arise from epidermal cells (46%). Rest of benign lesions arise from miscellaneous tissues, commonly being melanocytic nevus, seborrheic keratosis (13.7%), squamous cell papilloma (13.0%), and epidermal cysts (11.5%).[3]

■ EPIDEMIOLOGY

Incidence of benign tumors has a wide regional geographical variation **(Table 9.9.1)**.

TABLE 9.9.1: Frequency of benign lid tumors in large studies from various geographical regions.

Author/Year/country	Total number of lid tumors	Most common	Second most common	Third most common	Others
Sha-Sha Yu et al., 2018, China[3]	1,910	Seborrheic keratosis 24.6%	Squamous cell papilloma	Epidermal cysts	Dermoid cysts, inverted follicular keratosis, and keratoacanthoma
Huang YY, 2015, Taiwan[4]	4,294	Intradermal nevus (905; 21.1%)	Seborrheic keratosis (540, 12.6%)	Xanthelasma (483; 11.2%)	• Epidermal cyst (8.2%) • Chronic inflammation (7.5%) • Verruca vulgaris (5.9%)
Wang L, 2021 China[5]	2,413	Papilloma (658, 27.9%)	Pigmented nevi (578, 24.4%)	Cysts (427, 18.1%)	• Angioma (222, 9.4%) • Verrucae (212, 9%)
Rathod A, 2015, India[6]	61	Intradermal nevus (17, 27.9%)	Squamous papilloma (11, 18%)	Compound nevus (8, 13.1%)	• Capillary hemangioma (6, 9.8%) • Papilloma (3, 4.9%)
Deprez M, 2009, Switzerland[7]	4,087	Squamous cell papilloma (1,063, 26%)	Seborrheic keratosis (876, 21%)	Melanocytic nevus (816, 20%)	• Hidrocystoma (326, 8%) • Xanthelasma (246, 6%)
Bagheri A[8]	880	Squamous papilloma (237, 27%)	Seborrheic keratosis (120, 14%)	Melanocytic nevus (161, 18%)	• Hidrocystoma (128, 15%) • Actinic keratosis (31, 4%) • Keratoacanthoma (20, 2%) • Inverted follicular keratosis (18, 2%) • Syringoma (16, 2%)
Gundogan FC, 2015, Turkey[9]	1,424	Squamous papilloma (336, 23.6%)	Nevus (279, 19.6%)	Seborrheic keratosis (266, 18.67%)	• Hidrocystomas (164, 11.52%) • Xanthelasma (116, 8.1%) • Epidermal cysts (111, 7.8%)

■ CLASSIFICATION

Benign eyelid lesions can arise from epidermis, dermis, hair follicles, adnexal structures, and of vascular origin as depicted in **Flowcharts 9.9.1 and 9.9.2 and Box 9.9.1**.

■ BENIGN EPITHELIAL EYELID TUMORS

- *Squamous papilloma (acrochordon or skin tag):*[10] They are most common benign eyelid lesion of epithelial origin occurring with higher frequency in middle age to older patients. They have polypoidal lesion with a stalk and keratinized surface.

Flowchart 9.9.1: Eyelid tumors arising from epidermis, hair follicles and adnexa.

```
                        Benign eyelid tumors
         ┌──────────────────────┼──────────────────────┐
     Epidermis              Hair follicles      Adnexal and cystic lesions
```

Epidermis

Nonmelanocytic
- Squamous cell papilloma
- Seborrheic keratosis
- Inverted follicular keratosis
- Reactive hyperplasia

Melanocytic
- Ephelis or freckles
- Lentigo simplex
- Solar lentigo
- Congenital nevus
- Acquired nevus

Hair follicles
- Trichoepithelioma
- Trichofolliculoma
- Trichilemmoma
- Pilomatrixoma

Adnexal and cystic lesions

Sebaceous gland
- Sebaceous gland hyperplasia
- Sebaceous gland adenoma

Sweat and lacrimal gland
- Syringoma
- Papillary syringadenoma
- Eccrine spiradenoma
- Eccrine acrospiroma

Other cystic lesions
- Epidermal inclusion cyst
- Sebaceous cyst
- Retention cyst
- Eccrine hidrocystoma
- Apocrine hidrocystoma
- Trichilemmal cyst
- Other benign cystic lesion

Flowchart 9.9.2: Eyelid tumors having stromal origin.

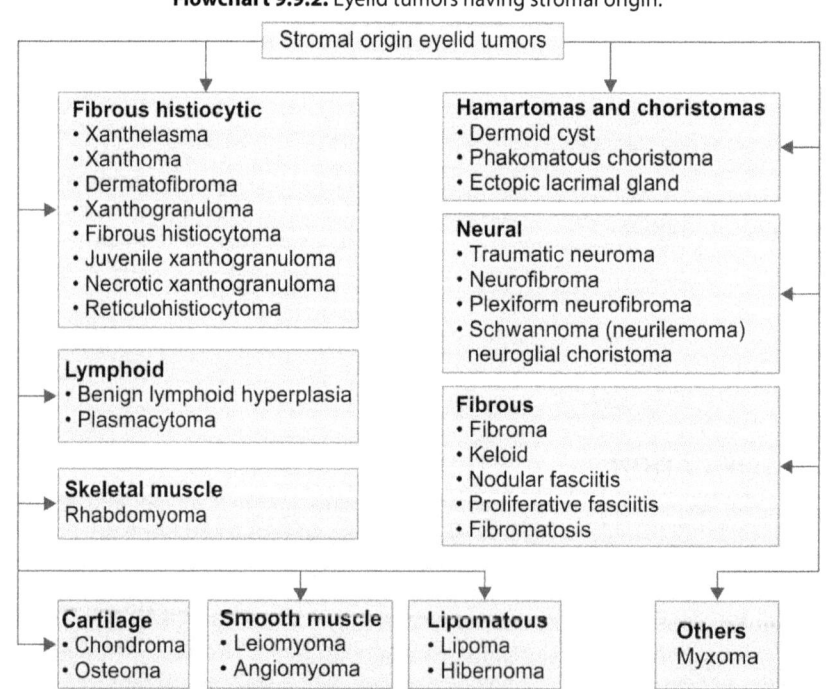

Stromal origin eyelid tumors

Fibrous histiocytic
- Xanthelasma
- Xanthoma
- Dermatofibroma
- Xanthogranuloma
- Fibrous histiocytoma
- Juvenile xanthogranuloma
- Necrotic xanthogranuloma
- Reticulohistiocytoma

Lymphoid
- Benign lymphoid hyperplasia
- Plasmacytoma

Skeletal muscle
Rhabdomyoma

Hamartomas and choristomas
- Dermoid cyst
- Phakomatous choristoma
- Ectopic lacrimal gland

Neural
- Traumatic neuroma
- Neurofibroma
- Plexiform neurofibroma
- Schwannoma (neurilemoma) neuroglial choristoma

Fibrous
- Fibroma
- Keloid
- Nodular fasciitis
- Proliferative fasciitis
- Fibromatosis

Cartilage
- Chondroma
- Osteoma

Smooth muscle
- Leiomyoma
- Angiomyoma

Lipomatous
- Lipoma
- Hibernoma

Others
Myxoma

> **BOX 9.9.1:** Benign vascular tumors of the eyelid.
>
> *Vascular:*
> - Nevus flammeus (port wine stain)
> - Papillary endothelial hyperplasia
> - Capillary hemangioma
> - Cavernous hemangioma
> - Venous hemangioma
> - Arteriovenous malformation
> - Lymphangioma
> - Epithelioid hemangioma (angiolymphoid hyperplasia)
>
> *Perivascular:*
> - Hemangiopericytoma
> - Glomus tumor

On histopathology, the papillomatous structure has a fibrovascular center. They are managed with surgical excision or shave biopsy.
- *Seborrheic keratosis:*[11] They present as well-demarcated warty plaques of various size, shape, degree of pigmentation and greasy surface in people >50 years old. Increased prevalence is seen with sun exposure and positive family history. Histopathological examination reveals proliferation of basaloid cells with keratin-filled cystic inclusions and variable hyperkeratosis. Shave excision is done at the junction of the dermis and epidermis. Leser–Trélat sign is characterized by multiple seborrheic eruptions and is associated with gastrointestinal adenocarcinoma.
- *Inverted follicular keratosis:*[12] A solitary nodular or papillary keratotic mass occurring at the eyelid margin in patients >60 years of age with increased sun exposure. It may be confused with squamous cell carcinoma. Prominent squamous eddies with papillomatosis and acanthosis are seen on histopathology. Biopsy with complete excision is the treatment of choice.
- *Keratoacanthoma:*[13] It is most commonly seen in lightly pigmented females between 50 and 69 years of age as a dome-shaped nodule with a central keratin-filled crater and elevated, rolled margins. The lesion is excised with 4 mm margins due to the association with squamous cell carcinoma. Histopathology reveals thickened epidermis in the shape of a cup surrounding a central plug of keratin.

BENIGN MELANOCYTIC EYELID TUMORS

May arise from nevus cells, melanocytes of the epidermis, and melanocytes of the dermis; all derive embryologically from the neural crest.
- *Freckles (ephelis):*[14] They appear as small, flat brown skin spots scattered over sun-exposed areas, including the eyelids in light skin individuals with blond or red hair and characteristically become darker when exposed to sunlight. These lesions are usually observed.
- *Lentigo simplex:*[15] They are small, flat brown to black lesions present at birth and not affected by sunlight. They are clinically indistinguishable from junctional nevi. On histopathology there is increase in the number of nevus cells (melanocytes) as well elongation of the rete ridges and the presence of melanophages in the upper dermis. They can be observed or removed with chemical peels, surgical excision, skin laser, or cryotherapy.
- *Solar lentigo (sun spots, liver spots, and age spots):*[15] They are light to dark brown lesions developing in chronically sun-exposed areas of the skin. Histopathological examination reveals increase in the number of nevus cells with club-shaped rete ridges. They are usually observed or treated with skin lightening agents such as cysteamine 5% cream as well as skin laser or cryotherapy.

CONGENITAL NEVI

- *Split nevus:*[16] It is a rare compound nevus located on the upper and lower eyelid with only around 30 cases reported worldwide.
- *Oculodermal melanocytosis:*[17,18] It has a prevalence of 0.038% in Whites and 0.014% prevalence in Blacks. It presents as unilateral bluish discoloration of the eyelid and periorbital skin, in addition to blue scleral discoloration. Histopathology displays dendritic and plump polyhedral nevus cells in the deeper dermis layer. Oculodermal melanocytosis may be associated with glaucoma thus warranting semiannual monitoring for glaucoma as well as melanoma of the skin, iris, and choroid.
- *Giant hairy pigmented nevi:*[19,20] It is an uncommon congenital nevus presenting as flat dark nevus, often covered with hair growing till 40 cm.
- *Blue nevi:*[21] It is dark blue, smooth, dome-shaped, and round nevi seen more commonly in females with a prevalence of 3-5% in Asians, compared to 1-2% in Whites. It is of two types: the common blue nevus which is smaller and the cellular blue nevus is larger than 1 cm. Dendritic nevus cells are seen deeper in the dermis on histopathology.

ACQUIRED NEVI

- *Spitz and reed nevi:*[22] It is an uncommon nevus occurring in <0.01% of the population. Spitz nevus appears as pink and dome-shaped lesion during the first two decades. Reed is a variant of a Spitz nevus that is black with feathered edges. On histopathology, it presents as compound nevus with mitotic figures while reed nevus has more spindle-shaped nevus cells.
- *Melanocytic nevi (junctional, intradermal, and compound):* They occur in about 60% of the population.
  - *Junctional:* 1-10 mm flat or slightly elevated, round or oval macule with a uniform medium to dark brown pigmentation. Nevus cells are located in the dermoepithelial junction of the skin on histopathology.
  - *Intradermal:* 5-10 mm, elevated, and nonpigmented lesion that may have hair with nevus cells are located in the dermis.
  - *Compound:* 1-10 mm lesion, displaying a symmetrical central raised area surrounded by a flat area, with variable pigmentation that is symmetrically distributed. The nevus cells are located in both the dermis and the dermoepithelial junction.
- *Dysplastic nevi:* They are often >6 mm, with a darker pigmentation pattern in the center ("fried egg" appearance) seen in 2-18% of the population. On histopathology there are four characteristic features: intraepidermal lentiginous hyperplasia, cytological atypia of nevus cells, lamellar and concentric fibroplasia, and architectural atypia, and they are present in dysplastic nevi.

BENIGN TUMORS OF SWEAT GLANDS

- *Syringomas:*[23] They are 3 mm or smaller yellow to skin-colored papules seen on lower lid seen in 1% of the population. They occur with increased frequency in females during puberty. There are multiple treatment options including: removal with a CO_2 laser, excision, dermabrasion, trichloroacetic acid, electrocautery, electrodesiccation, or cryotherapy. Histopathology shows small ductal elements lined with two layers of epithelial cells (no myoepithelial cells) inside dense fibrous tissue.
- *Pleomorphic adenoma:*[24] It accounts for 0.01% of all benign adnexal tumors seen in middle-aged men presenting as a slow-growing subdermal mass of 2-6 cm in size. The tumor is completely excised with a few millimeters of margin to avoid recurrence with histopathology revealing epithelial cells arranged in nests and bands that may contain apocrine, eccrine, or mixed glandular components. In the eyelids, the epithelial cells rest in a myxoid matrix.

- *Eccrine spiradenoma:*[25] It is a rare flesh-colored, gray, pink, purple, red, or blue nodule about 10 mm in size that is soft and tender to palpation. Single lesions are surgically excised while multiple lesions can be removed with a CO_2 laser.

BENIGN HAIR FOLLICLE TUMORS
- *Trichoepithelioma:*[26] It is a very rare lesion originating from hair follicles in sun-exposed areas on the face and scalp. It presents as two subtypes:
    1. *Multiple familial and desmoplastic trichoepithelioma:* Inherited in an autosomal dominant fashion with increased penetrance in females and presents as multiple skin-colored lesions 2–8 mm in size.
    2. *Solitary trichoepithelioma:* Sporadic form presenting as a single lesion.
    On histopathology, these hamartomatous lesions may have overlap with basal cell carcinoma (BCC) consisting of abortive hair papillae, branching nests of basaloid cells, and horn cysts.
    They can be managed with laser treatment, skin transplantation, electrodesiccation, imiquimod, and retinoic acid application.
- *Trichofolliculoma:*[27] It is a rare tumor resembling a sebaceous cyst with a central umbilication containing white hair. It is removed using simple surgical excision with histopathology revealing central dilated cystic hair follicle lined with stratified squamous epithelial strands and buds showing different stages of pilar formation protruding from the wall of the lesion.
- *Trichilemmoma:*[28] It is a relatively common hair follicle tumor with an estimated prevalence of 1 in 2,500 consisting of solitary or multiple smooth and well-defined papules or verrucous growths which may resemble verruca or BCC. It is removed using a shave biopsy with histopathology showing lobules of squamous epithelial cells along with palisading cells in the periphery.
- *Pilomatrixoma:*[29] It is a solitary, subcutaneous, pink to purple, painless, and firm nodule with a calcified center found in the upper eyelid or eyebrow and can resemble a chalazion seen in the first two decades of life. It is surgically excised with wide surgical margins to avoid recurrence.

BENIGN SEBACEOUS GLAND TUMORS
- *Sebaceous gland hyperplasia:*[30] It is a yellow, elevated, and soft nodule with umbilication seen in >60-year-old. The nodule is excised and sent for histopathological analysis displaying umbilicated lesion containing sebaceous glands that are larger than normal.
- *Sebaceous gland adenoma:* Clinically it is similar to sebaceous gland hyperplasia and histopathology shows dense layers of blue basaloid cells surrounding the glands. Multiple adenomas in young patients should raise suspicion of Muir-Torre syndrome.

NEUROGENIC TUMORS
- *Plexiform neurofibroma:*[31] It is a rubbery lesion presenting clinically with ptosis or a classic "S-shape" of the eyelid margin in about 10% of patients with neurofibromatosis type I (NF1). It is prudent to have 6 monthly ophthalmic examinations. On histopathology lesion is surrounded by a thickened perineurium and contains axons, Schwann cells, and endoneurial fibroblasts.
- *Solitary neurofibroma:*[32] It is the most common peripheral nerve sheath tumor presenting as chalazion or ptosis or fullness of the eyelid without pain in 20–40 years age group. It is essential to test for neurofibromatosis and can be managed with observation or surgical excision if medically indicated. The lesion contains collagen in the stroma and bundles of peripheral nerve sheath cells enclosed in a pseudocapsule without a clear perineurium on histopathology.

- *Schwannoma:*[33] It is a painless, gradual growth with an incidence of five cases per 100,000 adults/year adults and about 0.4 cases per 100,000/year in children. It is managed with complete excision with a clear margin to allow histopathological analysis revealing encapsulated lesion containing compact spindle cells and/or larger, round, clear cells with Antoni A and Antoni B patterns, respectively.

BENIGN VASCULAR TUMORS

- *Pyogenic granuloma:*[34] It is a fleshy, pink to red, vascularized, and lobulated lesion found on the tarsal conjunctiva most commonly in second and third decades of life usually associated with a preceding history of tissue disruption from surgery or injury to the tarsal plate from a chalazion. Histopathology shows thin-walled capillaries are embedded in a fibrous stroma that contains fibroblasts and inflammatory cells organized into lobules, each with a central feeder vessel. The lesion responds to topical corticosteroids.
- *Capillary hemangiomas:*[35] It is the most common benign childhood orbital lesions affecting 1–5% of infants with a female predilection. It may present with a cutaneous, subcutaneous, or orbital lesion with lesions becoming deeper red and lobulated during the first year of life. They are hamartomas or abnormal proliferation of normal tissue in a normal location, namely endothelial cells. First-line treatment includes systemic beta-blockers or oral and intralesional corticosteroids. Surgical treatment can include CO_2 and other laser photocoagulation treatments for more superficial lesions. Radiation and surgical excision are other options.
- *Angiofibromas:*[36] These are dome-shaped, skin-colored to red papules with small apical telangiectatic vessels that are densest in the maxillary area, over the bridge of the nose, around the nasolabial folds, and the chin and extending onto the lower eyelid associated with tuberous sclerosis and multiple endocrine neoplasia type 1 and Birt–Hogg–Dubé syndrome. Histopathology presents proliferation of stellate and spindled cells around blood vessels within the dermis with the overlying epidermis pushed up and atrophic. They are managed by ablation with lasers as well as shave excision and electrodesiccation. Sirolimus ointment has been used successfully in reducing the severity of facial angiofibromas.
- *Nevus flammeus (port-wine stain):*[37] It affects 0.3–0.5% of newborns with no gender predilection and strongly associated with Sturge–Weber syndrome. It presents as flat, pink, or red homogenous skin lesion with geographic borders at birth. Histopathology reveals high density of telangiectatic capillaries containing a single cell layer of endothelial cells located in the dermis and subcutaneously. Pulsed dye laser photocoagulation can be used for cosmesis.

ADVANCEMENTS

Li Z et al. demonstrated the potential of using artificial intelligence on 1,417 photographic images from 851 patients. Its utility is in early differentiation between benign and malignant lesions and early treatment.[38]

Laser Therapy of Eyelid Tumors

Recently, studies have reported the use of modified argon laser in the treatment of benign lesions such as nevi, and papillomas.[39] It acts by photoablating the tumor surface. The tumor surface had been stained which increased the amount of thermal laser energy absorbed by the target tissue. Filipe Sousa-Neves et al. reported excellent outcome and cosmesis on treating benign lesions with neodymium-doped yttrium orthovanadate (Nd:YVO) laser-assisted photocoagulation.[40]

Other lasers used to treat benign lesions are super pulse carbon dioxide laser and dual-wavelengths copper vapor to treat benign lesions.[41] Zhang et al. used carbon dioxide laser in large series of 99 benign eyelid tumors, some of which involved the eyelid margin, causing thermal necrosis. He also used it treating nevi (30%), viral warts (18.8%), squamous papillomas (17.5%), cystic lesions (13.8%), seborrheic keratosis (8.8%), granulomas (3.8%), vascular lesions (angiomas or telangiectasia) (3.8%), xanthelasma palpebrarum (1.3%), trichofolliculomas (1.3%), and fibroepithelial polyps/skin tags (1.3%).[42]

REFERENCES

1. Herwig-Carl MC, Löffler KU. Eyelid Tumors: Clinical Aspects of Ophthalmic Pathology. Klin Monbl Augenheilkd. 2018;235(7):776-81.
2. Kersten RC, Ewing-Chow D, Kulwin DR, Gallon M. Accuracy of clinical diagnosis of cutaneous eyelid lesions. Ophthalmology. 1997;104(3):479-84.
3. Yu SS, Zhao Y, Zhao H, Lin JY, Tang X. A retrospective study of 2228 cases with eyelid tumors. Int J Ophthalmol. 2018;11(11):1835-41.
4. Huang YY, Liang WY, Tsai CC, Kao SC, Yu WK, Kau HC, et al. Comparison of the Clinical Characteristics and Outcome of Benign and Malignant Eyelid Tumors: An Analysis of 4521 Eyelid Tumors in a Tertiary Medical Center. Biomed Res Int. 2015;2015:453091.
5. Wang L, Shan Y, Dai X, You N, Shao J, Pan X, et al. Clinicopathological analysis of 5146 eyelid tumours and tumour-like lesions in an eye centre in South China, 2000–2018: a retrospective cohort study. BMJ Open. 2021;11(1):e041854.
6. Rathod A, Pandharpurkar M, Toopalli K, Bele S. A clinicopathological study of eyelid tumours and its management at a tertiary eye care centre of Southern India. MRIMS J Health Sci. 2015;3(1):54.
7. Deprez M, Uffer S. Clinicopathological features of eyelid skin tumors. A retrospective study of 5504 cases and review of literature. Am J Dermatopathol. 2009;31(3):256-62.
8. Bagheri A, Tavakoli M, Kanaani A, Zavareh RB, Esfandiari H, Aletaha M, et al. Eyelid Masses: A 10-year Survey from a Tertiary Eye Hospital in Tehran. Middle East Afr J Ophthalmol. 2013;20(3):187-92.
9. Gundogan FC, Yolcu U, Tas A, Sahin OF, Uzun S, Cermik H, et al. Eyelid tumors: clinical data from an eye center in Ankara, Turkey. Asian Pac J Cancer Prev. 2015;16(10):4265-9.
10. Ramberg I, Heegaard S. Human Papillomavirus Related Neoplasia of the Ocular Adnexa. Viruses. 2021;13(8):1522.
11. Eren S, Fritz K, Salavastru CM, Tiplica GS. The most common benign cutaneous neoplasms of the epidermis and appendages and their treatment. Hautarzt. 2022;73(2):94-103.
12. Boniuk M, Zimmerman LE. Eyelid tumors with reference to lesions confused with squamous cell carcinoma. II. Inverted follicular keratosis. Arch Ophthalmol. 1963;69:698-707.
13. Krema H, Gursel Ozkurt Z, Lando L, Altomare F. Complete cure of a large resistant keratoacanthoma of the eyelid with intralesional methotrexate. Can J Ophthalmol. 2021;56(5):e162-4.
14. Sawant O, Khan T. Management of periorbital hyperpigmentation: An overview of nature-based agents and alternative approaches. Dermatol Ther. 2020;33(4):e13717.
15. Yates B, Que SK, D'Souza L, Suchecki J, Finch JJ. Laser treatment of periocular skin conditions. Clin Dermatol. 2015;33(2):197-206.
16. Rajput GC, Mahajan D, Chaudhary KP, Deewana V. Kissing naevus arising from neural crest cells presenting as upper and the lower lid mass. J Neurosci Rural Pract. 2015;6(3):417-9.
17. Mittal K, Azad SV. Oculodermal melanocytosis. Indian J Med Res. 2020;151(6):613-4.
18. Williams NM, Gurnani P, Labib A, Nuesi R, Nouri K. Melanoma in the setting of nevus of Ota: a review for dermatologists. Int J Dermatol. 2021;60(5):523-32.
19. Bhatnagar V, Mukherjee MK, Bhargava P. A Case of Giant Hairy Pigmented Nevus of Face. Med J Armed Forces India. 2005;61(2):200-2.
20. Hashmi GS, Ahmed SS, Khan S. Congenital giant melanocytic nevi. Rare Tumors. 2009;1(1):e9.
21. Sayed-Ahmed I, Murillo JC, Monsalve P, Ulloa JP, Fernandez MP, Wong J, et al. Blue Nevi of the Ocular Surface: Clinical Characteristics, Pathologic Features, and Clinical Course. Ophthalmology. 2018;125(8):1189-98.
22. Yeh I, Busam KJ. Spitz melanocytic tumours—a review. Histopathology. 2022;80(1):122-34.
23. Walvekar PV, Jakati S, Bothra N, Kaliki S. Isolated eyelid chondroid syringoma: a study of two cases. BMJ Case Rep. 2021;14(12):e245354.

24. O'Rourke MA, Cannon PS, Shaw JF, Irion LC, McKelvie PA, McNab AA. Cutaneous pleomorphic adenoma of the periocular region—a case series. Orbit. 2022;41(3):361-4.
25. Hartford JB, Sweeney AR, Allen RC, Yen MT. Rapidly Enlarging Hidradenoma of the Eyelid. Ophthalmic Plast Reconstr Surg. 2021;37(3S):S149-51.
26. Gupta A, Ali MJ, Mishra DK, Naik MN. Solitary Trichoepithelioma of the Eyelid: A Clinico-Pathological Correlation. Int J Trichology. 2015;7(2):80-1.
27. Kapoor AG, Vijith VS, Mittal R. Trichofolliculoma of the Eyelid Margin: A Case Report and Review of Literature. Ophthalmic Plast Reconstr Surg. 2019;35(3):e74-6.
28. Pihlblad M, Chelnis J, Schaefer D. Eyelid desmoplastic trichilemmoma: 2 case reports and review. Ophthalmic Plast Reconstr Surg. 2014;30(5):e136-8.
29. Siadati S, Campbell AA, McCulley T, Eberhart CG. Clinicopathological Features of 19 Eyelid Pilomatrixomas. Ocul Oncol Pathol. 2022;8(1):30-4.
30. Jakobiec FA, Cortes Barrantes P, Milman T, Yoon M. Sebaceoma of a Meibomian Gland of the Upper Eyelid. Ocul Oncol Pathol. 2020;6(4):297-304.
31. Alkhairy S, Baig MM. Ocular Neurofibromatosis. Cureus. 2021;13(9):e17765.
32. Poonam NS, Alam MS, Das D, Biswas J. Solitary eyelid neurofibroma presenting as tarsal cyst: Report of a case and review of literature. Am J Ophthalmol Case Rep. 2018;10:71-3.
33. Shapira Y, Juniat V, Dave T, Hussain A, McNeely D, Watanabe A, et al. Orbito-cranial schwannoma-a multicentre experience. Eye (Lond). 2023;37(1):48-53.
34. Tan IJ, Turner AW. Pyogenic Granuloma of the Conjunctiva. N Engl J Med. 2017;376(17):1667.
35. Achibane A, Taouti H, Belghamaidi S, Hajji I, Moutaouakil A. Management of an infantile eyelid hemangioma. J Fr Ophtalmol. 2021;44(9):1474-5.
36. Nguyen QD, DarConte MD, Hebert AA. The cutaneous manifestations of tuberous sclerosis complex. Am J Med Genet C Semin Med Genet. 2018;178(3):321-5.
37. Guedes Neto HJ, Kuramoto DAB, Correia RM, Santos BC, Borges ADC, Pereda MR, et al. What do Cochrane systematic reviews say about congenital vascular anomalies and hemangiomas? A narrative review. Sao Paulo Med J. 2022;140(2):320-7.
38. Li Z, Qiang W, Chen H, Pei M, Yu X, Wang L, et al. Artificial intelligence to detect malignant eyelid tumors from photographic images. NPJ Digit Med. 2022:2;5(1):23.
39. Han J, Lee SH, Choi CY, Khoramnia R, Kim J, Shin HJ. Modified argon laser therapy for benign tumor of the eyelid dermal nevi and papilloma. BMC Ophthalmol. 2022;22(1):383.
40. Sousa-Neves F, Cardoso da Costa J, Braga J, Prazeres S. Treatment of benign eyelid lesions with Nd:YVO laser: a prospective study (Neodymium-doped yttrium orthovanadate). J Cosmet Laser Ther. 2020;22(3):146-9.
41. Ponomarev IV, Topchiy SB, Andrusenko YN, Shakina LD. The successful treatment of eyelid intradermal melanocytic nevi (Nevus of Miescher) with the dual-wavelengths copper vapor laser. J Lasers Med Sci. 2021;12:e23.
42. Zhang J, Duan J, Gong L. Super pulse CO_2 laser therapy for benign eyelid tumors. J Cosmet Dermatol. 2018;17(2):171-5.

9.10 Diagnosis and Management of Orbital Fractures

AK Grover, Rwituja Thomas
Vision Eye Centres, New Delhi
akgrover55@yahoo.com

■ INTRODUCTION

Fractures of the orbit are common and pose several management challenges. They require special attention because both surgical and nonsurgical approaches can potentially affect vision or alter the position of the eyeball. Orbital fractures typically occur more frequently in males during the second decade of life. Road traffic accidents and assault are the most common causes, while falls and sports-related injuries are more common in pediatric patients. Orbital fractures are often referred to as "blowout" fractures, although not all orbital fractures are confined to the orbit alone. They can occur in isolation or in combination with other fractures, such as those involving the head, neck, spine, or the maxillofacial region, including Le Fort II and III fractures, zygomatico-maxillary complex (ZMC) fractures, and naso-orbito-ethmoid (NOE) fractures.

Surgeons typically classify orbital fractures based on their location within the orbit, involving the floor, medial wall, lateral wall, or roof. Various classification systems have been proposed to differentiate between isolated, multiwalled, and comminuted orbital fractures, taking into account the involvement of soft tissues.

Evaluation of an orbital fracture begins with a thorough history to understand the cause and extent of the injuries. Patients who have experienced blunt orbital trauma should undergo a comprehensive ophthalmic examination to rule out associated eye injuries, as ocular injuries are reported to occur in up to 29% of cases. The eye examination includes assessments of vision, intraocular pressure (IOP), ocular motility, pupillary reflexes, slit-lamp examination, fundus examination, and a general external examination. If possible, a complete eye examination should be performed in conscious and cooperative patients.

Typical signs of an orbital fracture include swelling around the eyes (periocular edema), bruising (ecchymosis), protrusion of the eyeball (proptosis) in the acute stages, sunken appearance of the eyeball (enophthalmos) in larger fractures, redness and swelling of the conjunctiva (chemosis), reduced sensation in the area below the eye (infraorbital hypoesthesia), and bleeding beneath the conjunctiva (subconjunctival hemorrhage). It is important to rule out any obvious or hidden perforation of the eyeball. Signs of a ruptured globe may include extensive subconjunctival hemorrhage, an irregularly shaped pupil, and a flattened anterior chamber. The eyelids and tissues surrounding the eye should be examined for the presence of air trapped beneath the skin (subcutaneous emphysema).

Any proptosis (eyeball protrusion) or enophthalmos (eyeball sinking) should be measured. Drooping of the upper eyelid (ptosis), which is usually caused by nerve or muscle injury, should be noted. In cases of midface injuries involving the inner corner of the eye (medial canthus), the lacrimal system should be carefully evaluated.

The patient should be asked to open and close their mouth to check for any associated difficulty or limitation in jaw movement (trismus), which may suggest fractures involving the zygomatic complex. A forced duction test is performed to assess the presence of muscle entrapment at the fracture site.

Elevated IOP can occur due to orbital compartment syndrome resulting from bleeding behind the eyeball, which can lead to optic nerve damage. Traumatic optic neuropathy has been reported in 3% of cases with isolated orbital fractures. If the IOP exceeds 40 mm Hg, immediate lateral canthotomy (incision of the outer corner of the eye) and cantholysis (separation of the eyelid) should be performed. IOP below 40 mm Hg can be managed with antiglaucoma medications.

Other associated injuries can include corneal abrasions, subluxated or dislocated lens, hyphema, commotio retinae, and retinal detachment. Ocular motility assessment is imperative in children as they can have a variant called white-eyed fracture, in which there are no obvious ocular findings other that motility restriction. Children more commonly have trapdoor fractures which can lead to muscle entrapment and result in pain with eye movement, nausea, vomiting, and bradycardia which can require urgent surgical intervention.

RADIOLOGIC EXAMINATION

X-ray

- *Water's view:* Demonstrates the orbital floor, roof, zygomatic bone, and the temporal arch **(Fig. 9.10.1)**.
- *Caldwell's view:* It is useful in evaluating margins and walls, superior orbital fissures, sphenoid ridges and temporal, ethmoid, frontal, and nasal fossae.
- *Lateral view:* It is used to interpret anterior-posterior relationships.
- *Optic canal view (Rhese):* Demonstrates optic canal contours and fractures.

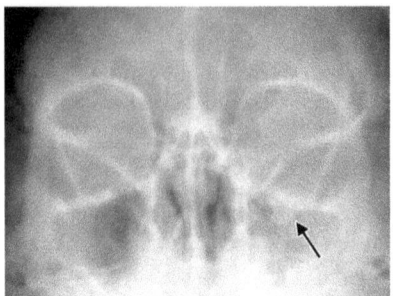

Fig. 9.10.1: Water's view showing the orbital floor fracture.

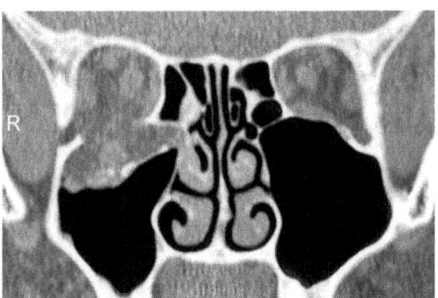

Fig. 9.10.2: Coronal cut in computed tomography scan showing right-sided orbital large floor fracture with incarceration of orbital contents.

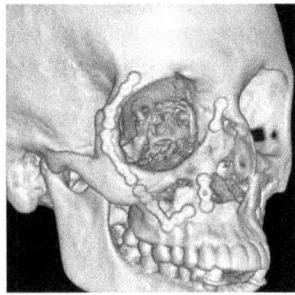

Fig. 9.10.3: Three-dimensional scan showing previously repaired facial bony defects.

Computed Tomography Scan

In the context of trauma, computed tomography (CT) is the most effective method for evaluating orbital injuries and assessing potential cranial or facial injuries. To obtain detailed information, a CT scan of the orbits and face with approximately 2 mm cuts is ideal. Coronal and sagittal views provide the best visualization of orbital floor fractures, while coronal sections also allow for the detection of soft tissue and extraocular muscle entrapment. In cases of inferior entrapment, the normal round shape of the inferior rectus muscle on coronal cuts may appear elongated in a vertical oval shape **(Fig. 9.10.2)**. Axial views are useful for tracking the course of extraocular muscles within the orbit. Three-dimensional (3D) reconstruction images are best for understanding the spatial orientation of more extensive fractures, but they have limited utility in isolated orbital fractures **(Fig. 9.10.3)**. The CT bone window is effective in visualizing bone displacement, while the soft tissue window is better for assessing soft tissue herniation and muscle entrapment. The degree of bone displacement observed on imaging helps determine the need for surgical repair, as larger orbital floor fractures with greater tissue displacement are more likely to result in enophthalmos (recession of the eyeball) and require surgical intervention. It is important to thoroughly examine the CT images for associated fractures involving the frontal bone, maxilla, zygoma, nasal bone, and mandible. Other potential findings include opacification of the maxillary sinuses and displacement of the eyeball.

ORBITAL FRACTURES

These fractures can be categorized as pure or blowout fractures (involving the orbital floor, medial orbital wall, or both with an intact bony margin) or impure fractures (combined with orbital rim fractures).

Clinical Signs
- Eyelid bruising/hematoma
- Reduced sensation in the area below the eye (infraorbital hypoesthesia)
- Limitation of upward eye movements and double vision (diplopia)
- Protrusion/recession of the eyeball and lower eyelid (enophthalmos/hypophthalmos)
- Deformity of the upper eyelid sulcus/pseudoptosis

Management: Conservative Management
- Applicable when there is minimal diplopia and normal eye motility
- Absence of muscle entrapment
- No significant enophthalmos
- Small fractures unlikely to cause late enophthalmos

Conservative management involves cold compression to reduce orbital swelling and bleeding. Patients should be advised to avoid blowing their nose or performing Valsalva maneuvers to prevent orbital emphysema and proptosis (protrusion of the eyeball). Oral steroids may be prescribed to expedite the resolution of periorbital swelling and facilitate decision-making regarding surgical intervention. Prophylactic antibiotics are recommended if the wound is contaminated or if there is a cerebrospinal fluid (CSF) leak.

Indications for Surgery

Emergent Treatment
- Early onset of enophthalmos/hypophthalmos
- White-eyed fractures in children
- Trapdoor fractures that may appear well-aligned with minimal swelling or bleeding but exhibit severe motion restriction and oculocardiac reflex (a reflex slowing of the heart rate upon eye movement). These fractures require immediate management to prevent ischemic damage and necrosis of the muscles.

Within 2 Weeks
- Persistent limitation of upward eye motility causing clinically significant diplopia after 10–14 days.
- Large fractures at risk of enophthalmos.

Timing of Surgery
Surgeons have varying opinions when it comes to the timing of surgery. It is generally recommended to wait for a period of 1–2 weeks as there is a decrease in bleeding and swelling, which often leads to natural improvement. The main objective of surgical repair is to address the bony defect and prevent the displacement of orbital tissues into the sinuses.

Surgical Technique

Approaches
- Orbital
- Caldwell's approach—rarely used
- Bicoronal scalp approach

Advantage of Orbital Approach
Ophthalmologists are familiar with the anatomy. It permits direct visualization of fracture and release of entrapment is possible. The implant can be placed under direct visualization.

Choice of Materials

The perfect implant should be simple to insert and handle, biologically inert, resistant to infection and displacement, capable of secure attachment to surrounding structures, cost-effective, and should not stimulate the formation of fibrous tissue.

Implants Used (Box 9.10.1)

- Autologous materials like bone or cartilage.
- Alloplastic implant such as porous polyethylene (Medpor), silastic, Teflon, titanium mesh, and extended polytetrafluoroethylene (ePTFE). Preformed titanium mesh is available especially for floor and medial wall fractures. These are designed to restore the orbital contour at these sites.
- Dissolvable alloplastic materials such as Gelfilm and Lactosorb are used in small fractures.
- Allogenic material such as banked bone or lyophilized cartilage.

BOX 9.10.1: Options for orbital implants.

- Alloplastic implants
- Nonporous implants
  - Nylon implant
  - Silicone
  - Polytetrafluoroethylene (Teflon)
  - Titanium (premade and moldable or patient-specific implant (PSI))
  - Polyetheretherketone (PSI)
- Porous implants
  - Porous polyethylene (Medpor)
  - Porous polyethylene with embedded titanium
- Autogenous tissues
  - Bone grafts–cranial bone, iliac crest, and rib

Autogenous Bone Grafts

They are usually preferred in large and multiple fractures. Cancelous bone grafts are preferred over cortical because cancellous bone grafts revascularized rapidly and completely.

Material of Choice—ePTFE, Porous Polyethylene, and Titanium Mesh

- Nonimmunogenic
- Biologically and chemically nonreactive
- Highly resistant to infection
- Readily integrated into the host tissue

Surgical Procedures

Surgery is performed under general anesthesia. A forced duction test (FDT) should be performed before, during, and at the conclusion of the surgery.

Incision

- Transcutaneous
- Transconjunctival (preferred)

Transcutaneous approach: Incision can be subciliary, lower lid crease or over inferior orbital margin, through previous scar. Author's choice is subciliary incision as it prevents prolonged postoperative lymphedema.

The medial orbital wall may be approached via a lynch incision or a transcaruncular approach.

Transconjunctival approach: This approach utilizes an incision through the conjunctiva of the inferior fornix combined with lateral canthotomy and cantholysis (swinging eyelid approach). The eyelid is detached from the lateral orbital rim, improving the exposure **(Figs. 9.10.4A to F)**.

Patient-specific implants made of polyetheretherketone (PEEK) are the latest in the repair of complex orbital and facial fractures. They consist of 3D printed implants

SECTION 9: Oculoplasty

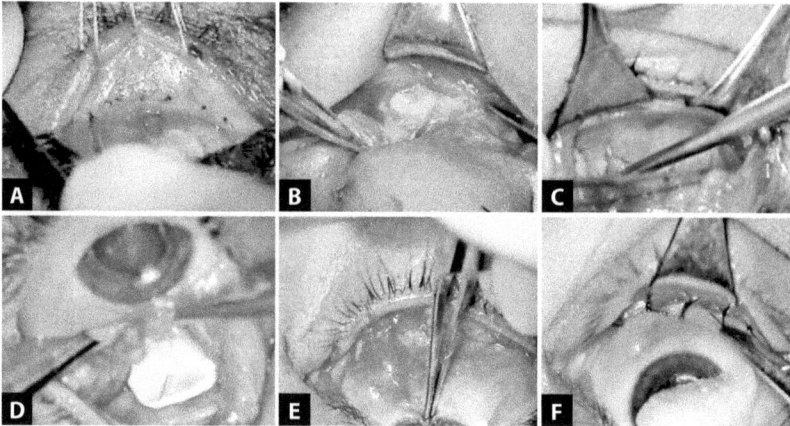

Figs. 9.10.4A to F: Steps of surgery. (A) Stay suture are placed through the gray line to provide traction. Transconjunctival incision is given about 4 mm below the lower border of tarsus; (B) The dissection is carried out between the orbicularis muscle and septum till the orbital rim and the periosteum is incised 2 mm below the inferior orbital margin. This is then elevated with periosteum elevator along with periorbital rim; (C) Prolapsing contents should be repositioned using two instruments in hand-over-hand fashion. All the margins of fracture should be exposed. Aggressive posterior dissection should be avoided as it risks damage to optic nerve; (D) Once the prolapsing contents are lifted up, the extended polytetrafluoroethylene (ePTFE) implant is bridged across the fracture. The implant of adequate size is placed. One should avoid large implant to avoid compression to apical structures; (E) Forced duction test is repeated after placement of implant to ensure motility; (F) Subcutaneous closure is done with polyglactin suture. It is not necessary to suture periosteum. The conjunctiva edges are closed using 6-0 Vicryl.

whose measurements are based on the orbital architecture of the normal side and can be modified by the surgeon. They are modeled on a 3D printed bone that mimics that of the patient, prior to inserting into the defect on table **(Fig. 9.10.5)**.

Postoperative Management

Prophylactic broad-spectrum antibiotics along with anti-inflammatory for a week postoperatively.

Complications

These are:
- Loss of vision
- Prolonged postoperative lymphedema
- Extrusion of implant
- Lower lid retraction
- Lower lid entropion
- Ectropion
- Symblepharon formation
- Undercorrection of enophthalmos

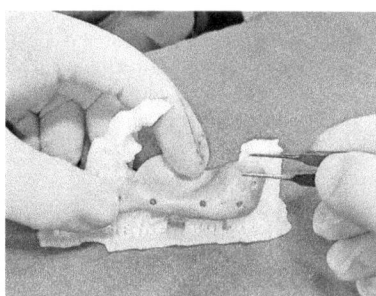

Fig. 9.10.5: Applying patient-specific implant (PSI) made of polyetheretherketone (PEEK) to 3D printed skull bone model.

■ ZYGOMATIC COMPLEX FRACTURES

These fractures involve displacement of the zygoma and may constitute tripod fracture. The fracture involves the frontozygomatic suture, zygomaticomaxillary suture and the zygomatic arch, orbital floor, and the back wall of the maxillary sinus.

Surgical Management

Small, undisplaced fractures are managed conservatively. The treatment of choice is open reduction with internal fixation of the displaced zygoma.

■ NASO-ORBITO-ETHMOID FRACTURE

These are the most common fractures affecting the facial skeleton. It results in flattening of the nasal bridge, displacement of the medial canthus leading to telecanthus, and may be associated with lacrimal injuries.

Medial canthal tendon injuries are classified into three types:

1. *Type I:* Single-piece bone segment with intact canthal tendon insertions (**Fig. 9.10.6**)
2. *Type II:* Fragmented central bone segment with fractures located outside the medial canthal tendon insertion (**Fig. 9.10.7**)
3. *Type III:* Fragmented single piece with fractures extending into the bone that supports the canthal insertion.

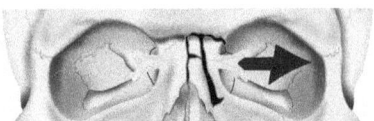

Fig. 9.10.6: Type I medial canthal injury.

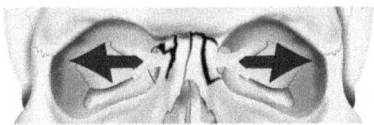

Fig. 9.10.7: Type II medial canthal injury.

Management

Open reduction and internal fixation of the fractures with transnasal wiring or miniplates along with medial canthus anchorage provides best cosmetic results.

■ SUGGESTED READING

1. Boyette JR, Pemberton JD, Bonilla-Velez J. Management of orbital fractures: challenges and solutions. Clin Ophthalmol. 2015;9:2127-37.
2. Chepurnyi Y, Chernogorskyi D, Kopchak A, Petrenko O. Clinical efficacy of peek patient-specific implants in orbital reconstruction. J Oral Biol Craniofac Res. 2020;10(2):49-53.
3. Donald PJ, Holt GR. Upper facial trauma. In: Resident Manual of Trauma to the Face, Head and Neck, 1st edition. Alexandria, Virginia: American Academy of Otolaryngology-Head and Neck Surgery; 2012. pp. 41-73.
4. Grob S, Yonkers M, Tao J. Orbital Fracture Repair. Semin Plast Surg. 2017;31(1):31-9.

9.11 Structural, Vascular, and Neoplastic Lesions of the Orbit

Ramesh Murthy
Axis Eye Clinic, Pune
drrameshmurthy@gmail.com

Santosh Honavar
Centre for Sight, Hyderabad
santosh.honavar@gmail.com

■ STRUCTURAL LESIONS

These comprise approximately 15% of all orbital lesions and can be congenital or acquired.

Dermoid Cyst

- Arises from ectodermal rests pinched off at suture lines
- Most commonly located in the upper outer quadrant of the orbit, they are slow growing and cause bony excavation

- Dermoids are lined by keratinized epithelium and contain adnexal structures, while epidermoids are lined by squamous epithelium alone
- Dermoid can be superficial or deep
- Superficial dermoid cysts present in infancy as round periorbital masses
- Deep dermoids have rounded anterior margins with deeper extension. Imaging may reveal dumbbell components into the temporalis fossa, intracranial cavity and the sinuses. Complete excision of the cyst and its lining should be performed. Care must be taken not to rupture the lesion, since leaking of keratin into the surrounding tissues leads to severe granulomatous inflammation.

Congenital Cystic Eye
- Results due to arrested development of the optic vesicle
- Can be associated with profound malformations of the brain.

Microphthalmos with Cyst
- Results due to failure of closure of the optic fissure
- Usually unilateral, this may be associated with systemic abnormalities
- Generally located in the inferior orbit, in contrast to the cystic eye where the lesions are present in the upper lid.

Orbital Cephaloceles
- Result from failure of separation of the surface ectoderm and the neuroectoderm, which leads to a dehiscence of bone and protrusion of dura (meningocele) or brain (encephalocele)
- Midline facial anomalies could be associated
- Usually present superomedially, they may show pulsation and change in size with the Valsalva maneuver
- Management consists of excision, closure, and ligation of the base with patching of the bony defect from the orbital aspect. When large, a transfrontal craniotomy is necessary.

Dermolipomas
- These are ectopic lesions and are seen as a pinkish mass with the presence of hair on the superolateral epibulbar surface.
- Excision is performed for cosmesis as an ellipse avoiding aggressive orbital dissection.

Teratomas
- Arise from pluripotent embryonic tissues and are composed of tissues derived from all three germ layers
- Presentation is as a rapidly growing tumor of the infant orbit with extreme unilateral proptosis usually as a primary lesion
- Usually benign, on imaging they are seen as heterogeneous masses with cystic and solid components, foci of fat and heterotopic bone and teeth.

Craniofacial Dysostosis
Most commonly presents with extreme orbital shallowing due to arrested cranial bone growth. Crouzon's and Apert's syndrome present with marked proptosis and large exodeviations. Narrowing of the optic canal can lead to optic atrophy.

Orbital Implantation Cysts
Occur due to prior trauma or surgery most commonly muscle surgery. Management is by excision of the cyst.

Mucoceles

- Frontoethmoidal mucoceles present with fullness in the superomedial and medial canthal regions and cause outward and downward displacement of the globe.
- Mucoceles originating in the sphenoid and posterior ethmoid sinus present with visual symptoms, retrobulbar pain or nasal symptoms. Enophthalmos may occur due to orbital floor erosion due to a maxillary sinus mucocele (silent sinus syndrome).
- On imaging, mucoceles expand the sinus with thinning of the sinus walls and destroying the normal internal septae. Surgical excision of the entire cyst lining, reestablishment of normal drainage, or obliteration of the sinus is performed.

■ VASCULAR LESIONS

Presentation is usually in the first few weeks of life.

Signs

- Superficial tumors are bright red
- Preseptal tumors are dark blue.

A large tumor may enlarge and change the color to a deep blue during crying or straining, but there is no pulsation. 30% of the lesions resolve by 3 years and 70% by the age of 7 years.

Treatment

Indications

- Amblyopia due to induced astigmatism, anisometropia, and occlusion
- Optic nerve compression
- Exposure keratopathy
- Severe cosmetic blemish, necrosis, or infection

Oral propranolol is very effective in a dose of 1–2 mg/kg body weight as a daily dose under the supervision of a pediatrician.

Intralesional steroids in the form of triamcinolone acetonide 40 mg/mL or betamethasone 4 mg/mL are effective during the early active stage. A maximum of 1–2 mL is injected in multiple sites. Complications include occlusion of the central retinal artery, skin depigmentation and necrosis, bleeding, and fat atrophy.

Systemic steroids can also be given for orbital lesions.

Capillary Hemangioma

- Most common vascular tumor of the orbit in children
- Usually seen as a fluctuant bluish mass deep to the eyelid
- Gradual enlargement occurs in the first year, followed by gradual regression
- Main complications are amblyopia and refractive error. If obstructing the visual axis treatment is essential with oral or intralesional corticosteroids.

Cavernous Hemangioma

- Most common vascular tumor of the orbit in adults
- Benign lesion presents with slowly progressive axial proptosis
- Imaging reveals a well-circumscribed mass in the intraconal space
- More common in females with a preponderance of 70%
- Management is by observation for small asymptomatic lesions and surgical excision for larger tumors. Complete excision is essential to avoid recurrence.

Hemangiopericytomas

- These are an abnormal proliferation of pericytes surrounding blood vessels usually seen in adults.

- Usually benign, they may become locally aggressive and rarely undergo malignant transformation.
- Complete excision of the tumor with the capsule should be performed. If recurrent it may need orbital exenteration or irradiation.

Lymphangiomas
- Are slowly progressive tumors with onset in childhood
- Presentation may be with sudden onset hemorrhage. In addition there may be lesions on the palate and cheek.
- Imaging reveals a diffuse multiloculated mass with cystic spaces filled with blood "chocolate cysts".
- Observation is advocated if there is no threat to vision. Aspiration of hemorrhagic cysts can be performed. Complete surgical excision is not possible; however, debulking can be performed if the tumor is massive or cosmetically disfiguring.

Orbital Varix
- It is a venous malformation which usually presents in young adults with positional proptosis with worsening on Valsalva maneuver.
- Imaging may not reveal a mass unless Valsalva maneuver is performed especially with contrast.
- Minimally symptomatic lesions can be observed. If large or symptomatic, surgical excision using glue embolization can be performed.

Malignant Hemangioendothelioma
It arises from the endothelial cells of blood vessels. This is seen in young adults and is locally aggressive but rarely metastasizes.

NEOPLASTIC LESIONS

Peripheral Nerve Sheath Tumors

Neurilemmoma (Schwannoma)
- This usually occurs in young adults with progressive proptosis.
- Imaging reveals a solid mass usually outside the muscle cone along the supratrochlear or supraorbital nerve.
- Management is by surgical excision.

Neurofibroma
- Most common is the plexiform variety which presents with S-shaped ptosis.
- Management is often by debulking when complete surgical removal is not possible.

Alveolar Soft Part Sarcoma
It is a highly malignant tumor in children with frequent metastasis to the lungs and needs aggressive chemotherapy and irradiation.

Optic Nerve Tumors

Optic Nerve Glioma
- Most common optic nerve tumor in childhood
- Presentation is usually in the first or second decade with slowly progressive proptosis and visual loss with a strong association with neurofibromatosis
- Imaging reveals an ovoid tumor with a mid-portion kink
- Management is by radiotherapy in older children, especially when the tumor involves the chiasm and brain, chemotherapy is considered in children <4 years of age. In cases with total vision loss and unacceptable proptosis, removal of the mass by lateral orbitotomy is advocated sparing the eyeball.

Meningioma
- Benign tumor arising from the meninges; can be a primary optic nerve sheath type or a sphenoid wing meningioma, both of which are common in middle-aged women
- Presentation is with visual loss and gradual proptosis with the presence of retinochoroidal shunt vessels on the optic disk
- Conservative management is advocated with recourse to radiotherapy and rarely surgery for progressive disease with visual loss.

Myogenic Tumors
Rhabdomyosarcoma
- Presentation is in the first two decades of life with rapidly progressive proptosis, conjunctival chemosis, and globe displacement
- Embryonal type is the most common, while the alveolar variety is the most malignant
- Prompt biopsy for confirmation of diagnosis followed by radiotherapy and chemotherapy is needed.

Fibrous Connective Tissue Tumors
Includes nodular fasciitis, fibroma, fibrosarcoma, and fibrous histiocytoma.

Fibrous Histiocytoma
- Usually presents in adults as a circumscribed orbital mass with proptosis and globe displacement and occurs in the superior and nasal extraconal areas
- Management is by complete surgical resection, incomplete excision leads to recurrence.

Osseous Tumors, Fibro-osseous, and Cartilaginous Tumors
Osteomas
Originate from the orbital bones and protrude mainly into the orbit. Management is needed only if symptomatic.

Osteosarcoma
- Highly malignant tumor with poor prognosis and can be primary or secondary to orbital irradiation for retinoblastoma
- Management is by wide surgical resection combined with irradiation and chemotherapy.

Fibrous Dysplasia
Onset in the first or second decade, involves the frontal bone commonly. The polyostotic variety is associated with Albright's syndrome. Surgical intervention is considered when there is optic canal encroachment or cosmetic disfigurement.

Ossifying Fibroma
It is seen in the second decade of life and on imaging is seen to have localized bone expansion. Management is by surgical removal.

Lipomatous and Myxomatous Tumors
Dermolipoma
It is a benign lesion with the presence of visible hairs and can be a part of Goldenhar's syndrome.

Histiocytic Lesions
Juvenile Xanthogranuloma
- Which presents as a solitary orbital mass with typical Touton giant cells on histopathology
- Management is by complete excision and corticosteroids

Eosinophilic Granuloma
Most common subtype of Langerhans cell histiocytosis occurring in the first decade of life as a superotemporal mass. Following biopsy intralesional steroids is recommended.

Lacrimal Gland Tumors
Dacryops
Benign epithelial tumor of the lacrimal gland arising from the palpebral lobe, presenting as a cystic mass and does not need excision unless symptomatic.

Pleomorphic Adenoma
- Usually arises from the orbital lobe, commonly in adults and on imaging is seen as a circumscribed round mass with fossa formation
- Complete excision without prior biopsy is essential to prevent recurrence and malignant transformation.

Pleomorphic Adenocarcinoma
Arises due to incomplete excision and subsequent malignant transformation of a pleomorphic adenoma.

Adenoid Cystic Carcinoma
- Presents with down globe displacement and pain due to invasion of the nerves
- This aggressive tumor needs biopsy for confirmation of diagnosis. Complete surgical excision along with adjuvant radiotherapy and chemotherapy is needed.

Metastatic Tumors
- *Adults:* Commonly occurs from the breast, prostate, lungs, and gastrointestinal tract
- *Children:* Commonly occurs from neuroblastoma, Wilms' tumor, and Ewing's tumor.

Lymphoid Tumors and Leukemia (Figs. 9.11.1 to 9.11.3)
Orbital Lymphoma
- Presents as a unilateral or bilateral anterior orbital mass with a salmon patch appearance and on imaging is seen to mold to the adjacent structures
- Most are B cell type and are managed by chemotherapy and radiotherapy.

Granulocytic Sarcoma (Leukemia)
It presents as a rapidly growing mass in children. Peripheral blood smear may identify the presence of systemic leukemia. Most being myeloblastic in nature, prognosis is poor.

Secondary Orbital Tumors
These can arise from the eyelid—sebaceous gland carcinoma, basal cell carcinoma, squamous cell carcinoma and cutaneous melanoma, intraocular tumors like melanoma, and retinoblastoma or invasion from paranasal sinus tumors like carcinomas.

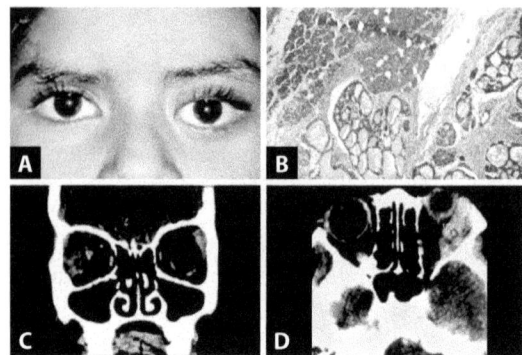

Figs. 9.11.1A to D: (A) An 8-year-old child presented with a superolateral orbital mass in the left eye; (B) Following biopsy, histopathology [hematoxylin and eosin (H&E) stain; 100X] showed the presence of acini arranged in a cribriform pattern suggestive of adenoid cystic carcinoma of the lacrimal gland; (C) Computed tomography scan orbits coronal; (D) Axial showed the presence of a diffuse mass in the superolateral part of the left orbit involving the lacrimal gland, lateral and superior rectus.

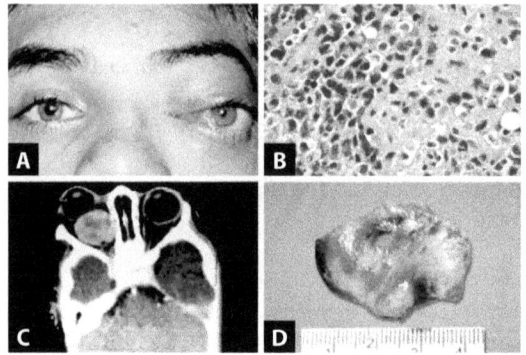

Figs. 9.11.2A to D: (A) This 12-year-old boy presented with rapidly progressive proptosis of the left eye with congestion and inflammation of 10 days duration; (B) Histopathology revealed the presence of a round cell tumor, which was confirmed to be rhabdomyosarcoma on immunohistochemistry; (C) Computed tomography scan axial sections showed a well-defined mass behind the globe; (D) Biopsy yielded a white and friable mass.

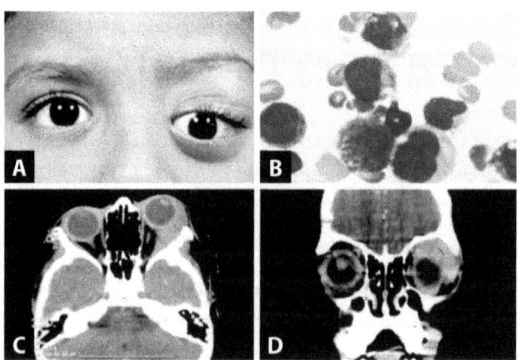

Figs. 9.11.3A to D: (A) A 5-year-old child presented with a left superolateral orbital mass; (B) Peripheral blood smear revealed the presence of cells of myeloblastic lineage with large nuclear cytoplasmic ratio and the presence of Auer rods suggestive of acute myeloid leukemia; (C and D) Computed tomography scan axial and coronal cuts revealed the presence of a diffuse soft tissue mass involving the superolateral orbit of the left eye.

9.12 Vascular Lesions of the Orbit

Aditi Mehta
Grewal Eye Institute, Chandigarh
aditimehta7@gmail.com

Kasturi Bhattacharjee
Sri Sankaradeva Nethralaya, Guwahati, Assam
kasturibhattachajee44@hotmail.com

■ INTRODUCTION

Pediatric ocular-adnexal vascular lesions include two types—malformations and neoplastic lesions.[1] Neoplastic lesions are commonly benign. They originate from proliferation of transformed vascular endothelial cells. Amongst these, most common is infantile hemangioma (IH), formerly known as capillary hemangioma. It presents in first year of life. Others include rapidly involuting, partially involuting, and noninvoluting type of congenital hemangioma, spindle cell hemangioma, epithelioid hemangioma, and pyogenic granuloma. Locally infiltrative lesions include tufted angioma, reticular or composite Kaposiform hemangioendotheliomas, Kaposi sarcoma—these are quite rare. Large hemangioendotheliomas may cause sequestration of circulating platelets and lead to coagulopathy—Kasabach-Merritt phenomenon. Malignant lesions are angiosarcomas as well as epithelioid hemangioendothelioma. Occurrence is extremely rare and they are highly metastatic.

Vascular neoplasms must be differentiated from the malformations which are usually noninvoluting in nature, grow commensurately with patient's age, usually do not show endothelial proliferation and can also expand hemodynamically.[2] These lesions histologically have small or large vascular channels lined by flat endothelial cells with a unilamellar basement membrane. The International Society for the Study of Vascular Anomalies (ISSVA) Classification (year 2018) serves as clinical standard to categorize the lesions based on patient demographics, presenting features, imaging and/or histopathology findings. This helps avoid misdiagnosis and wrong nomenclature.[3,4]

Capillary hemangioma, which is now known as infantile hemangioma, is the commonest vascular tumor, affects the pediatric age group and shows rapid growth followed by spontaneous regression. Watchful observation may be useful in small lesions.[5] Rarely, when a diagnostic dilemma arises, imaging with histopathology confirmation is required. IH shows endothelial positivity for GLUT-1 on IHC (immunohistochemistry). Intervention is needed if the lesion causes visual axis obstruction leading to induced astigmatism and amblyopia, compression of the optic nerve, exposure keratopathy, necrosis, infection or significant cosmetic blemish.[6-8] Systemic involvement or presence of large lesions (>5 cm) warrants assessment for likely associated high output cardiac failure. Mass effect from extensive facial hemangiomas with perioral, nasal or subglottic lesions can compromise airway. Since 2017, oral beta blocker (propranolol) has received FDA approval as the recommended first line therapy for IH in a dose of 1.7 mg/kg/day in two to three divided doses for about 6 months duration **(Figs. 9.12.1A and B)**. Institution and end treatment discontinuation should be gradual with a step up and step down dosing over 2 weeks to avoid systemic symptoms such as bradycardia, poor feeding, and lethargy.[9,10] Topical beta blockers (timolol maleate gel) have shown promising results in localized skin surface lesions and minimize systemic complications. A third route is direct intralesional beta blocker (propranolol or labetalol) which has shown high efficacy in small localized hemangiomas.[11] Other drugs used to treat include systemic and local glucocorticoids. Pulsed-dyed laser is useful for treating superficial lesions.

Pyogenic granuloma usually has a history of minor trauma preceding its onset. Morphologically, it consists of a lobular dilation of capillaries, similar to hemangioma and

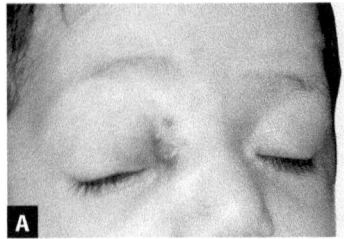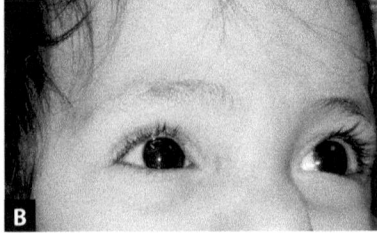

Figs. 9.12.1A and B: Infantile hemangioma; (A) At presentation; (B) After 6 months of oral propranolol with near total resolution.

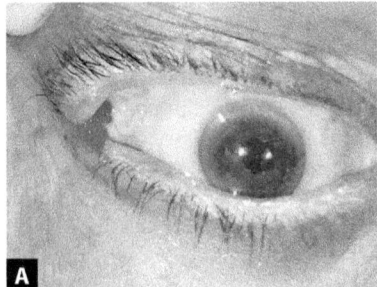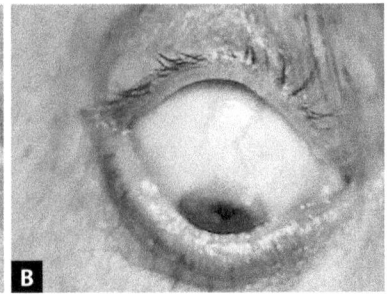

Figs. 9.12.2A and B: Pyogenic granuloma at lateral canthus before (A) and after (B) surgical excision.

has a tendency to bleed on touch. Surgical curettage and excision is definitive treatment **(Figs. 9.12.2A and B)**.[12]

Kaposi sarcoma is rare in the pediatric age. It has a malignant potential, and is associated with human herpes virus (HHV)-8 infection of the endothelial cells causing lymphatic reprogramming.[13] In eyelid lesions, a metastatic work up should be followed by debulking with cryotherapy or intralesional bleomycin.

Hemangiopericytomas arise from vascular pericytes, and fall in the spectrum of solitary fibrous tumors. Histologically, they are characterized by staghorn shaped dilated vessels and surrounding spindle cells.[14] In children, these lesions are usually self-limiting with low malignant potential, unlike adults. Treatment involves preoperative embolization followed by surgery and radiotherapy in combination with systemic therapy.

On the basis of angiographic imaging, malformations may be divided into: (a) no/minimal flow—lymphatic malformation (LM) which are microcystic or macrocystic and capillary malformations; (b) slow flow distensible—varices; slow flow nondistensible—cavernous venous malformation (VM); and (c) high flow—arteriovenous malformation.

Lymphangiomas commonly involving the facial region usually present at birth (in about 60%) or by 2 years of age (>90%).[1] Lesions may be confined to skin or ocular surface or may involve deeper tissues. In patients with periocular lymphangiomas, evaluation of buccal mucosa can show associated lesions. Clinical presentation can be diverse as these lesions may produce facial asymmetry and hypertrophy, neurovascular dysfunction or airway obstruction **(Fig. 9.12.3)**. Enlargement and painful proptosis occurs when there are associated respiratory tract infections causing intralesional hemorrhage. In this situation, urgent aspiration is required to avoid orbital compartment syndrome and avert vision decline. Treatment is largely symptomatic rather than being curative as the lesions are significantly infiltrative. Percutaneous drainage with ablation is the first line of management. Oral doxycycline and sirolimus (an inhibitor of mammalian target of rapamycin (mTOR)) have shown good results in microcystic LM.[15] Intralesional bleomycin is preferred in macrocystic lesions.[16]

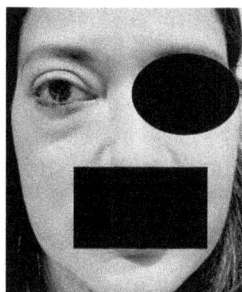 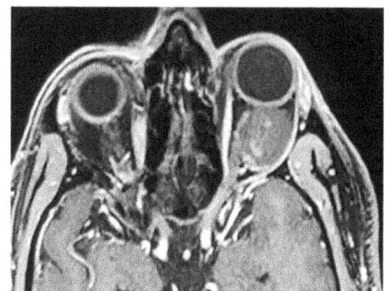

Fig. 9.12.3: Lymphangioma of right orbit and maxillary region with proptosis and facial asymmetry.

Fig. 9.12.4: Magnetic resonance imaging of left sided intraconal well-defined cavernous venous malformation leading to proptosis.

Capillary malformations are sporadic and congenital venule malformations and produce a classic port-wine stain. They may be associated with the Sturge-Weber syndrome. Ophthalmic evaluation for ipsilateral congenital glaucoma and intracranial pial angiomas is necessary.[1]

Venous malformations of distensible type include *varices*. These may affect the conjunctiva, eyelids, and the orbit. Enophthalmos may be noted in long standing lesions due to resultant fat atrophy. Evaluation includes tests for compressibility, postural variation of size, and enlargement of lesion on Valsalva maneuver—which is diagnostic.[17] Small asymptomatic lesions may be observed. The conjunctival lesions have a bunch of grapes appearance which may bleed on trivial trauma causing subconjunctival hemorrhage. Intralesional sclerotherapy with bleomycin has shown effective results.

Non-distensible malformations (*cavernous venous malformation*) present in middle age and have a female preponderance. Occasionally, they present early with puberty or enlarge during pregnancy, due to hormone-associated growth because of estrogen and progesterone. These lesions are located intraconally. Radiological imaging is diagnostic **(Fig. 9.12.4)**. Complete surgical excision with cryoprobe-assisted extraction is the preferred treatment.

Arteriovenous malformations (AVM) cause functional morbidity, cosmetic disfigurement, and have a risk of associated high output cardiac failure.[1] When these lesions are suspected, retinal evaluation for Wyburn-Mason syndrome is needed. Widespread cutaneous telangiectasias may be seen in hereditary hemorrhagic telangiectasia (HHT), also known as the Osler-Weber-Rendu syndrome. This has multiple AVMs which affect the brain, liver, lungs, and orbit. Treatment involves obliteration of the nidus via percutaneous, endovascular, and/or surgical routes.[3]

Once the diagnosis is established, proper counseling should be done to explain regarding the chronic nature of disease especially in malformations with syndromic associations. The ophthalmologists must always keep in mind the psychological impact when parents and caregivers are anxious about the associated cosmesis and long-term prognosis.[1]

■ SECONDARY ORBITAL INVOLVEMENT

Sometimes intracranial vascular lesions may at first present with ophthalmic symptoms. Timely neuroimaging is paramount in such cases. Acquired (traumatic) carotid cavernous fistulas post blunt head trauma may cause axial proptosis, secondary orbital congestion, chemosis, tortuous corkscrew scleral vessels as well as persistent headaches and diplopia. Due to an extensive communication between the two cavernous sinuses, presentation can be bilateral, involving both orbits.[18] Though not life threatening, they may cause vision loss. Neuroimaging reveals dilated and tortuous superior ophthalmic vein with increased bulk of extraocular muscles due to passive congestion and dilated cavernous venous sinus. Surgical or endovascular ligation of external and/or internal carotid arteries and fistula embolization is therapeutic.[19]

■ SUMMARY

Vascular anomalies of the head and neck are not limited to hemangiomas. Early clinical assessment, keeping in mind the presenting age, growth pattern and proliferation can help classify the lesions into tumors or malformations. The International Society for the Study of Vascular Anomalies (ISSVA) Classification provides standardized nomenclature. Periocular presentation can often be dramatic and potentially disfiguring. In addition they may cause stimulus deprivation amblyopia and thus affect vision potential. Clinical diagnosis is complemented by radiological imaging for assessment of extent of orbital involvement, characterization of intralesional vasculature (capillary/arterial/venous/mixed), and for diagnosing rare infiltrative/malignant tumors. Management is often multidisciplinary, especially in presence of systemic involvement or syndromic associations. Molecular targeted therapy is under evolutionary research and may soon help pave the way for enhanced management of such complex lesions.

■ REFERENCES

1. Mahady K, Thust S, Berkeley R, Stuart S, Barnacle A, Robertson F, et al. Vascular anomalies of the head and neck in children. Quant Imaging Med Surg. 2015;5(6):886-97.
2. Adams DM, Brandão LR, Peterman CM, Gupta A, Patel M, Fishman S, et al. Vascular anomaly cases for the pediatric hematologist oncologists-an interdisciplinary review. Pediatr Blood Cancer. 2018;65(1):10.
3. ISSVA.ORG. (2018). ISSVA classification for vascular anomalies. [online] Available from http://www.issva.org/UserFiles/file/ISSVA-Classification-2018.pdf. [Last accessed August, 2023].
4. Wildgruber M, Sadick M, Müller-Wille R, Wohlgemuth WA. Vascular tumors in infants and adolescents. Insights Imaging. 2019;10(1):30.
5. Kanski JJ, Bowling B, Nischal KK, Pearson A. Clinical Ophthalmology: A Systematic Approach. 7th edition. Edinburgh, New York: Elsevier/Saunders; 2014. pp. ix, 909.
6. Tambe K, Munshi V, Dewsbery C, Ainsworth JR, Willshaw H, Parulekar MV. Relationship of infantile periocular hemangioma depth to growth and regression pattern. J AAPOS. 2009;13(6):567-70.
7. Stigmar G, Crawford JS, Ward CM, Thomson HG. Ophthalmic sequelae of infantile hemangiomas of the eyelids and orbit. Am J Ophthalmol. 1978;85(6):806-13.
8. Cuttone JM, Durso F, Miller M, Evans LS. The relationship between soft tissue anomalies around the orbit and globe and astigmatic refractive errors: a preliminary report. J Pediatr Ophthalmol Strabismus. 1980;17(1):29-36.
9. Bang GM, Setabutr P. Periocular capillary hemangiomas: indications and options for treatment. Middle East Afr J Ophthalmol. 2010;17(2):121-8.
10. Pierre Fabre Pharmaceuticals, Inc. (2014). HIGHLIGHTS OF PRESCRIBING INFORMATION for Hemangeol. [online] Available from https://www.accessdata.fda.gov/drugsatfda_docs/label/2014/205410s000lbl.pdf. [Last accessed August, 2023].
11. Mehta A, Bajaj MS, Pushker N, Chawla B, Pujari A, Grewal SS, et al. To compare intralesional and oral propranolol for treating periorbital and eyelid capillary hemangiomas. Indian J Ophthalmol. 2019;67(12):1974-80.
12. Patrice SJ, Wiss K, Mulliken JB. Pyogenic granuloma (lobular capillary hemangioma): a clinicopathologic study of 178 cases. Pediatr Dermatol. 1991;8(4):267-76.
13. Abalo-Lojo JM, Abdulkader-Nallib I, Pérez LM, Gonzalez F. Eyelid Kaposi Sarcoma in an HIV-negative Patient. Indian J Ophthalmol. 2018;66(6):854-5.
14. Gengler C, Guillou L. Solitary fibrous tumour and haemangiopericytoma: evolution of a concept. Histopathology. 2006;48(1):63-74.
15. Adams DM, Trenor CC 3rd, Hammill AM, Vinks AA, Patel MN, Chaudry G, et al. Efficacy and Safety of Sirolimus in the Treatment of Complicated Vascular Anomalies. Pediatrics. 2016;137(2):e20153257.
16. Balakrishnan K, Edwards TC, Perkins JA. Functional and symptom impacts of pediatric head and neck lymphatic malformations: developing a patient-derived instrument. Otolaryngol Head Neck Surg. 2012;147:925-31.

17. Smoker WR, Gentry LR, Yee NK, Reede DL, Nerad JA. Vascular lesions of the orbit: more than meets the eye. Radiographics. 2008;28(1):185-325.
18. Jain C, Mehta A, Bhatia V, Gupta P. Isolated contralateral abducens palsy in direct carotid-cavernous fistula. BMJ Case Rep. 2020;13(12):e238746.
19. Sundar G. Vascular lesions of the orbit: conceptual approach and recent advances. Indian J Ophthalmol. 2018;66(1):3-6.

9.13 Diagnosis and Surgical Management of a Case of Proptosis

Shaloo Bageja, Amrita Sawhney

Sir Ganga Ram Hospital, New Delhi

bagejashaloo@yahoo.co.in, amrita.sawhney3@gmail.com

INTRODUCTION

Proptosis is defined as forward protrusion of the globe in relation to the skull. It can be caused by an isolated orbital pathology or could be a manifestation of a systemic disorder.

Orbital disorders are relatively uncommon and challenging to manage. It is difficult to diagnose every orbital disorder clinically and imaging may be required to identify the nature of the pathology. The disease process may have originated in the orbit or extended from adjacent sinuses or cranial cavity. A systematic and comprehensive evaluation is necessary in every case of proptosis to achieve an appropriate diagnosis and plan further management.

ETIOLOGY

The surgeon should approach the patient of proptosis, keeping in mind five basic processes which may occur independently or in combination: (1) inflammation (cellulitis, Graves' disease and pseudotumor), (2) neoplasia (lymphoma, secondary metastasis, and lacrimal gland tumor), (3) vascular disorders (hemangioma and lymphangioma), (4) structural disorders (dermoids and mucocele), and (5) degenerations/depositions (amyloidosis and scleroderma).

Age of onset is one of the important factors that one must consider while listing the differentials in cases presenting with proptosis.

The most common orbital lesions encountered in adults are idiopathic orbital inflammatory disorder, myocysticercosis, thyroid disorders, lacrimal gland tumors, cavernous hemangioma, meningioma, lymphoid lesions, and occasionally metastatic disease.

Children or younger adults with proptosis are more likely to have the following underlying pathologies—dermoids, capillary hemangiomas, orbital cellulitis, optic nerve glioma, orbital extension of retinoblastoma, lymphangioma, and rhabdomyosarcoma.

Pseudoproptosis, defined as abnormal prominence of the globe not associated with anterior displacement of the globe, must be ruled out while assessing a patient with bulgy eyes.

Causes of Pseudoproptosis

- Buphthalmos
- Unilateral high myopia
- Contralateral enophthalmos
- Asymmetric orbital size (shallow orbits)
- Asymmetric palpebral fissures (contralateral ptosis and ipsilateral eyelid retraction)
- Paralysis of extraocular muscles

HISTORY

A detailed history is essential to achieve a provisional diagnosis.
- Age of onset
- The course and duration of the disease
- Progression
- Any association with pain, swelling, redness, diplopia, or visual disturbance
- Any associated neurosensory loss
- Any increase in proptosis with coughing, straining, Valsalva maneuver, or bending forward
- Any history of trauma or relevant systemic disease
- Any positive family history
- Any significant previous episodes/history

EXAMINATION

A detailed systemic and ophthalmic examination is necessary. A careful examination of the type of proptosis, ocular motility, pupillary reaction, ophthalmoscopy, and any associated periorbital changes may provide important clues to the underlying disorder.

Systemic Examination

Systemic diseases such as thyroid disorders, other autoimmune diseases, and malignancies require thorough systemic workup. Cutaneous examination is simple but essential and can be carried out in an ophthalmology setup. Certain cutaneous vascular lesions suggest orbital lymphangioma and café-au-lait spots are one of the major criteria to diagnose neurofibromatosis. It is imperative to palpate the lymph nodes. Detailed cranial nerve examination should be performed including the corneal sensations.

Ocular Examination

Visual Acuity

The best corrected visual acuity should be documented.

Color Vision and Red Color Desaturation

Deterioration in color vision (Ishihara chart) or red color desaturation suggests optic nerve involvement.

Pupillary Reaction

Both direct and consensual reflex must be checked. Swinging flashlight test should be carried out to assess any afferent pupillary defect. Anisocoria, if present, should be further assessed both in dark and light conditions.

Intraocular Pressure

A rise in intraocular pressure, more prominent in up-gaze, is seen in restrictive orbitopathy like thyroid eye disease.

Orbital Examination

General Face Appearance
- Facial asymmetry must be looked for to rule out any congenital deformities.
- The extent of periorbital fullness, edema, and erythema must be noted as conditions such as preseptal cellulitis can have edema extending to the forehead and cheeks whereas well demarcated swelling, that abruptly ends at the orbital rim at the arcus marginalis (respecting the attachments of the orbital septum) is a postseptal swelling seen in orbital cellulitis.

Evaluation of Proptosis

Measurement of proptosis: Hertel's exophthalmometer is used to quantify proptosis, measured by protrusion of corneal apex in front of the lateral orbital rim. The normal range is being 14–21 mm with an average of 16 mm. A value of >21 mm as an absolute reading or >2 mm difference between the two eyes is usually considered as abnormal.

Types of proptosis: It can be unilateral (tumors, cysts, vascular anomalies) or bilateral (thyroid eye disease, lymphoproliferative diseases, cavernous sinus thrombosis, leukemia) and sometimes bilateral but presenting as unilateral disease due to marked asymmetry like in thyroid eye disease. Proptosis can be axial or abaxial. Axial displacement is caused by an intraconal lesion such as cavernous hemangioma, glioma and meningioma. Inferomedial displacement can result from mass in the superolateral quadrant such as lacrimal gland tumor and dermoid cyst. Inferolateral displacement is usually due to frontoethmoidal mucocele, abscesses or sinus lesion. Proptosis can also be classified as pulsatile versus nonpulsatile, common causes of pulsatile proptosis being caroticocavernous fistula, neurofibromatosis associated with sphenoid wing aplasia and meningocele.

Palpation and retropulsion: Palpation around the globe may reveal any mass in the anterior orbit, check for the extent of the mass, its fixity to the underlying structures and overlying skin, transillumination, fluctuation, reducibility, compressibility, associated bony defects, and lymph node enlargement. Increased resistance to retropulsion is either due to orbital mass or diffuse inflammation as in thyroid eye disease.

Thrills and bruit: The orbit should be palpated for thrills and auscultated for bruits. These result due to abnormal vascular flow as in arteriovenous communications such as caroticocavernous fistula or defect in bony orbital walls as in meningocele, neurofibromatosis, and sinus mucocele.

Variability of proptosis: Increase in proptosis with Valsalva maneuver, bending forward, straining, or crying may point toward venous orbital lesions such as orbital varices.

Ocular motility: Restriction in ocular motility may be due to restrictive inflammation (thyroid eye disease), infiltration (leukemia) or neuromuscular junction deficit (myasthenia gravis).

Periorbital Changes

Along with orbital examination one should also review lid, conjunctiva, iris, and fundus. Signs such as eyelid retraction and lid lag suggest thyroid eye disease, S-shaped eyelid deformity is seen in neurofibromatosis, optociliary shunt vessels may suggest optic nerve meningioma, salmon patch lesion may indicate lymphoma.

Photographic Documentation

It is necessary in all cases. It helps in comparison and evaluation postoperatively.

DIAGNOSIS

Laboratory Diagnosis

Various orbital disorders are a manifestation of systemic disease. A number of investigations that are helpful in establishing the diagnosis: (1) thyroid function tests and antibodies—thyroid eye disease, (2) angiotensin converting enzyme—sarcoidosis, (3) antinuclear cytoplasmic antibody (c-ANCA)—Wegner's granulomatosis, (4) immunology screening—systemic lupus erythematosus, and (5) serum immunoglobulin G4 (IgG4) levels – IgG4 disease.

Orbital Imaging

With advancement, the imaging modalities have become an important tool in orbital lesion diagnosis and surgical planning. The imaging modalities available are:

(1) radiographs, (2) ultrasonography (USG), (3) computed tomography (CT scan), (4) magnetic resonance imaging (MRI), (5) magnetic resonance angiography (MRA), (6) orbital venography, and (7) orbital arteriography.

Radiographs

Plain film radiographs are nowadays rarely used. They were used to identify any orbital wall fractures, bony optic canal fractures and foreign bodies. Chest X-rays are used to diagnose systemic conditions such as tuberculosis (TB), sarcoidosis, Wegner's granulomatosis, and bronchogenic carcinoma.

Ultrasonography

It is a suitable and inexpensive tool, providing significant dynamic information about orbital disorders. Brightness amplitude scan (B scan) provides two-dimensional images of the orbital tissue. A scan exhibits spikes of different heights suggesting the internal characteristics of the lesion.

It is especially useful in identification and localization of the disease process in the anterior orbit and extraocular muscles, and to assess the optic nerve. Color Doppler demonstrates the vascular flow in the mass.

Computed Tomography Scan

It is an important tool in delineating the shape, location, extent, and character of the lesion. A density value is assigned to each tissue proportional to their coefficient of absorption of X-rays. A two-dimensional image is constructed from these density measurements.

Orbital images can be obtained in axial, coronal, and sagittal plane (**Fig. 9.13.1**). Simultaneous evaluation of axial and coronal views permits three-dimensional assessment of orbital tumors. Thin cuts of 2–3 mm are essential. Intravenous contrast may be useful in vascular and inflammatory tumors. Bone windows should be ordered where bony lesions are suspected.

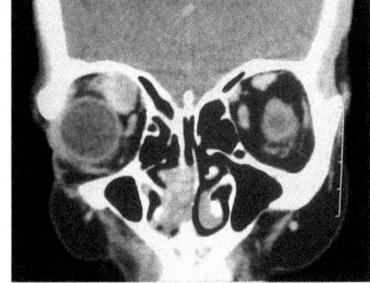

Fig. 9.13.1: Computed tomography scan—coronal view showing well-defined mass in superonasal quadrant.

Spiral CT, with the use of the newer hardware, provides continuous data set. It can later be reconstructed into thin sections in any required plane thus reducing the radiation exposure and is especially useful in uncooperative patients and children.

Magnetic Resonance Imaging

Patient is placed in a magnetic field leading to movement of protons in the tissues based on which the images are created. The aligned protons in the magnetic field are excited by a radiofrequency pulse emitted from a coil. These radio waves are modified to produce T1-weighted (dark appearance of vitreous) and T2-weighted (bright appearance of vitreous) images (**Fig. 9.13.2**).

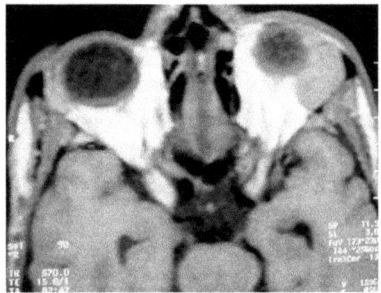

Fig. 9.13.2: T1-weighted (axial view) magnetic resonance imaging showing lacrimal gland mass in the left orbit.

It has the advantage that ionizing radiations are not required, and it provides excellent soft tissue delineation. It is the preferred method for imaging the optic nerve especially the intracanalicular and intracranial tract. Intravenous gadolinium is used as a contrast medium which helps in better identification of various pathologies such as vascular lesions. Fat suppression technique further improves the imaging of these lesions.

Contraindications of the Use of Magnetic Resonance Imaging
- Pacemakers
- Cochlear implants
- Metallic foreign body
- Clips/staplers
- Claustrophobia

Magnetic Resonance Angiography
It is a noninvasive investigative modality in certain orbital vascular disorders. It does not utilize any contrast medium and is without any exposure to ionizing radiation. When using the arterial phase, vascular lesions and aneurysms of ophthalmic artery and cavernous sinus lesions >4 mm can be diagnosed. When the venous phase is utilized, arteriovenous malformation, superior ophthalmic vein enlargement, or venous thrombosis can be visualized.

Orbital Venography
The procedure is not in much use nowadays. It was used earlier before the advent of CT or MRI scan to assess the extent and location of orbital masses and to diagnose orbital varices or to study the cavernous sinus.

Orbital Arteriography
The technique is used in patients with high suspicion of arterial disease like aneurysm or arteriovenous malformations. Some of these lesions can be treated by interventional radiologists by placing intralesional coils via the transarterial or transvenous routes.

Orbital Biopsy
Although imaging studies provide quite a bit of information, biopsy is required in some conditions to obtain a definitive diagnosis. Orbital biopsy can be incisional or excisional or may be attained by fine needle aspiration.

Incisional biopsy is carried out in cases of diffuse or infiltrative orbital diseases such as suspected malignancy or inflammation. Benign well circumscribed lesions, such as cavernous hemangioma and suspected pleomorphic adenomas, undergo excisional biopsy. Fine needle aspiration biopsy is mainly indicated to diagnose anterior orbital lesions or nonresectable lesions in the deep orbit.

ORBITAL SURGERY
Management of orbital disorders is quite challenging, and a thorough knowledge of eyelid and orbit anatomy is imperative.

Imaging is a must, wherever feasible, to identify the location, size, and nature of the orbital lesion along with its relationship to the surrounding structures, prior to surgery. A meticulous planning with other departments (in case multidisciplinary approach is required) and the patient is important. The risks and benefits associated with the surgery must be outlined in detail to the patients and their relatives, and get an informed consent signed.

Improved instrumentation and advancement in the techniques have greatly reduced the risks associated with orbital surgery.

The choice of surgical approach depends upon the:
- Surgical space occupied by the lesion
- Size and extent of the lesion
- Suspected pathology

- Relationship to the surrounding structures
- Goal of surgery—incisional or excisional

Advancement in Orbital Surgery

- *Endoscopic-guided orbital surgery:* Use of endoscope improves visualization and assessment of deeper orbit and has been used in medial wall decompression for thyroid eye disease and orbital abscess drainage.
- *Navigation system:* It is computer-assisted technology. This system enables real-time surgical navigation using preoperative computed tomographic images. The system includes a monitor, a computer, an optical camera, a reference head frame, and specialized optical probes. The reference frame and each optical probe contain infrared emitting diodes which transmit infrared light to the optical camera. The camera identifies the location of each source of light and relays this information into the computer. The computer then determines the exact location in space of the tip of the probe. Allows the intraoperative location and mapping of the extent of the tumor. It is useful in identification of risk zones especially blood vessels.
- *Stereotactic navigation guidance* also improves anatomic localization and precision during orbital decompression surgery in cases of thyroid eye disease as it helps the surgeon to maximally decompress the lateral wall to achieve significant reduction in proptosis with relatively lower risk of inducing new onset postoperative diplopia.
- *Piezoelectric bone surgery:* The device produces ultrasonic micro-vibration at frequency ranging from 20 to 30 kHz. It causes cutting with cavitation phenomenon. Used for precise bone cutting sparing surrounding soft tissues. It also improves visibility in the surgical field, decrease blood loss and provides good aesthetic results.

Surgical Approaches

The most common approaches used for orbitotomies are:
- Anterior orbitotomy
- *Medial orbitotomy:* It can be approached transcutaneous, transconjunctival, endoscopically and through retrocaruncular incision.
- Lateral orbitotomy
- Transcranial
- Combined approach
- *Anterior orbitotomy:* Anterior orbital lesions for incisional or excisional biopsy are approached via transcutaneous or transconjunctival approach.
  - *Transcutaneous:* A skin crease incision or sub-brow incision in the upper lid allows access to superior extraconal or subperiosteal space **(Fig. 9.13.3)**. Subciliary or skin crease incision in the lower eyelid allows access to anterior inferior orbit. One should avoid incision over the inferior orbital margin as it leads to persistent postoperative lymphedema.
  - *Transconjunctival:* Conjunctival incision is made in the inferior fornix. It may be combined with lateral canthotomy and cantholysis (swinging eyelid incision) providing excellent exposure to deep inferior and lateral orbit especially in cases of orbital floor fracture repair or orbital mass removal. Inferior forniceal incision can also be extended medially to approach medial orbit via retrocaruncular approach. Orbital septum or periosteum is breached depending upon the site of the lesion in the extraconal or subperiosteal space.

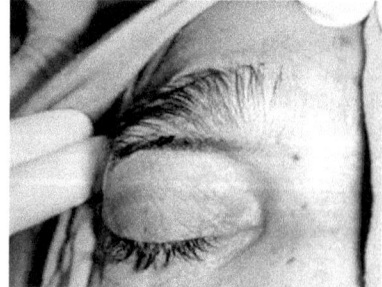

Fig. 9.13.3: Marking for sub-brow incision to approach superior extraconal space.

Eyelid Split Technique

It is used to approach large superomedial orbital mass. The upper eyelid is split vertically just lateral to the periosteum.

The lesion is exposed with the help of retractors and dissected out (**Fig. 9.13.4**). Meticulous hemostasis is obtained. Orbital septum is not closed. Closure is done in two layers subcutaneous with 5'0 polyglactin (vicryl) and skin with 6'0 silk. Conjunctiva is closed with 5'0 vicryl suture. Lateral canthotomy if performed needs to be repaired with 6'0 silk vertical mattress sutures.

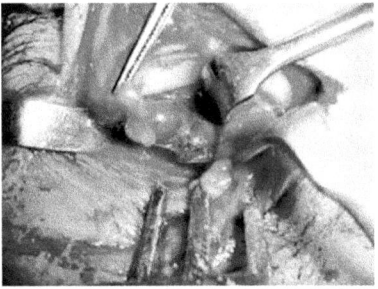

Fig. 9.13.4: The lesion being exposed with help of retractors and being removed.

Medial Orbitotomy

Transcutaneous (Lynch) Incision

It is used to approach the medial extraconal or subperiosteal space. A curvilinear skin incision is placed midway between a line joining medial canthal angle to the bridge of the nose by Bard parker No. 11 blade or radiofrequency needle. Subcutaneous tissue is incised and orbicularis separated apart to expose periosteum. Periosteum is incised along the full length of the wound and reflected. Anterior and posterior ethmoidal vessels can be cauterized.

This approach is useful for drainage of a subperiosteal abscess or repair of the medial wall fracture.

Transconjunctival

It is used to access Tenon's or intraconal space or to perform optic nerve decompression. A medial 180° peritomy is performed. Radial relieving incisions can be made to improve exposure. Tenon's capsule is bluntly separated from the sclera. Medial rectus muscle is hooked and disinserted from its insertion at the globe if deep intraconal dissection is anticipated. The lesion is exposed with the help of retractors. It is biopsied or removed depending upon the nature of the lesion. The medial rectus muscle is reattached to its insertion and conjunctiva is closed with 5'0 vicryl.

Retrocaruncular

The approach is used to repair medial wall fracture, to perform ethmoidectomy as a part of orbital decompression or for the drainage of a hematoma. An incision is made between the caruncle and the plica. Blunt dissection is carried out by Stevens scissors. Medial orbital wall posterior to posterior lacrimal crest is exposed. Good retraction is required to improve the exposure. Periorbita may not be closed. Conjunctival closure is achieved with 5'0 vicryl.

Lateral Orbitotomy

The lateral orbitotomy provides excellent access to extraconal and intraconal space lateral to optic nerve. This approach is commonly used for removal of lacrimal gland tumors, intraconal tumors and as a part of an orbital decompression procedure.

Surgical incisions used are:
- An extended upper eyelid crease incision—our preference for deeper orbitotomies
- Lateral canthotomy approach—our preference for lesions occupying lateral orbit
- Berke-Reese incision
- Stallard-Wright incision—obsolete

Extended Upper Eyelid Crease Incision

The procedure is performed under general anesthesia. An upper eyelid skin crease incision extending to the lateral canthus is marked. Infiltration of 2% xylocaine with adrenaline and bupivacaine is given along the lateral orbital margin and deep into the periosteum. 4'0 silk suture is passed through the lateral rectus muscle for traction. A tarsorrhaphy is done to protect the cornea. Skin incision is made with a No. 11 blade or radiofrequency needle. The upper eyelid orbicularis muscle is cut down to the orbital septum. At the lateral canthus subcutaneous tissue is dissected up to the periosteum (**Fig. 9.13.5**). The periosteum is incised 2 mm lateral to the orbital rim extending superiorly above the frontozygomatic suture and inferiorly beyond the superior aspect of zygomatic arch. Posterior relieving incisions are made in the periosteum. It is reflected carefully posteriorly toward the temporalis fascia to allow access to temporalis muscle (**Fig. 9.13.6**). Periosteum is reflected from the inner aspect of lateral orbital wall using the periosteal elevator (**Fig. 9.13.7**).

Bone cuts are marked. The groove can be made with the help of hammer and chisel before cutting the bone with the Stryker saw (**Fig. 9.13.8**). The temporalis muscle is cut with the help of radiofrequency or cutting cautery. The lateral orbital wall is held with a large bone rongeur, and bone is removed. It is placed in a bowl of a saline mixed with antibiotic. Periorbita is opened in a T-shaped fashion and is gently dissected from the orbital contents. The lateral rectus muscle is identified after opening the periorbita. The mass is gently palpated in the orbit with the finger. The orbital fat is retracted with the help of retractors. The lesion is bluntly dissected from the surrounding orbital tissue, keeping the dissection close to the mass. The mass may be delivered using a cryoprobe (**Fig. 9.13.9**). Surgeon should assess the pupils at regular intervals intraoperatively.

Once the mass is removed, adequate hemostasis is achieved before closure. Periorbita is closed with 5'0 vicryl. Bone is placed in position. Mostly it fits snugly into its position and does not require any fixation. A suction drain is placed into the temporal fossa. Periosteum is closed over the bone with 5'0 vicryl suture. After the subcutaneous closure with 5'0 vicryl, skin is closed by interrupted or continuous sutures.

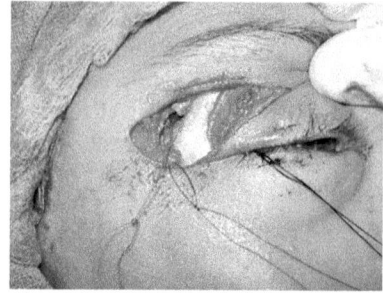

Fig. 9.13.5: An eyelid crease given. Subcutaneous dissection done to expose periosteum.

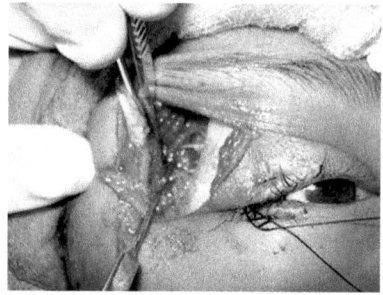

Fig. 9.13.6: Periosteum is reflected back and temporalis muscle is exposed.

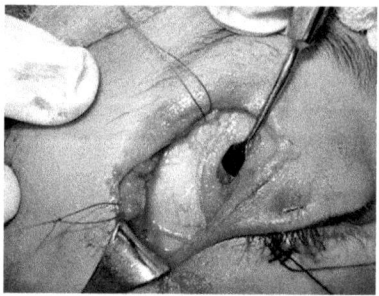

Fig. 9.13.7: Periosteum is reflected from the inner aspect of the lateral orbital wall using periosteal elevator.

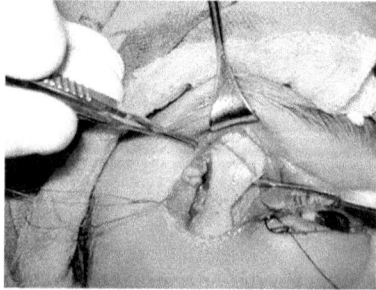

Fig. 9.13.8: Bone is cut and removed with Stryker saw.

Lateral Canthotomy Orbitotomy

In this approach, lateral canthal tendon is split along the horizontal raphe without detachment of either of the limbs from Whitnall's tubercle, no bone is removed. Traction sutures are placed along the upper and lower canthal tissues thereby creating a rhomboid entry into the lateral orbit. The closure is carried out by aligning the lid margins.

This is an excellent approach to access lesions in the optic nerve and lateral two-thirds of the orbit, both extraconal and intraconal, with the flexibility to increase the exposure peroperatively by performing inferior cantholysis (swinging the lower lid) if required.

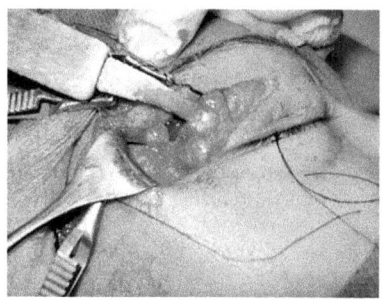

Fig. 9.13.9: Periorbita is cut—mass is delivered by the use of a cryoprobe.

Transcranial Orbitotomy

A lesion at orbital apex or with intracranial extension such as optic nerve glioma or meningioma requires a frontal craniotomy via a bicoronal flap technique. This is undertaken in collaboration with neurosurgeon.

Combined Orbitotomies

The orbitotomies may be used in combination if required as in cases of multiloculated lymph-angioma, neurofibroma, or benign apical lesions.

Postoperative Management

Visual acuity and pupillary reaction should be assessed few hours after the surgery.

The patient is prescribed systemic antibiotic, anti-inflammatory, and corticosteroids (1 mg/kg/day) for 7 days.

Exenteration

The surgical procedure involves the removal of globe and surrounding orbital and periocular soft tissues.

Indications

- *Benign lesions:*
  - Benign orbital tumors such as aggressive meningioma
  - Life-threatening infection—rhino-orbital mucormycosis
  - Severe orbital deformity as in neurofibromatosis.
- *Malignant lesions:*
  - Malignant eyelid tumors with orbital extension, e.g., basal cell carcinoma and squamous cell carcinoma
  - Malignant conjunctival lesions, e.g., melanoma
  - Malignant lacrimal gland carcinoma—most commonly adenoid cystic carcinoma
  - Extensive malignant eyelid tumors which are unrepairable such as sebaceous cell carcinoma.

Types

- *Total exenteration:* Globe and associated soft tissue of the orbit and adnexa are removed. This could be *lid sparing*, where eyelid skin is preserved like in cases of mucormycosis or *nonlid sparing* such as in cases of eyelid malignancy with Orbital extension.
- *Subtotal exenteration:* In this technique, globe is preserved but the surrounding adnexal tissues are excised. This technique has been used in medial orbital spread of basal cell carcinoma of the eyelid.

- *Extended exenteration:* Involves resection of adjoining structures such as paranasal sinuses. The socket may be reconstructed by spontaneous granulation, full thickness skin grafts, local, or free flaps. The prosthesis is applied to improve the cosmesis of the patient.

SUGGESTED READING
1. Hamed-Azzam S, Verity D, Rose G. Lateral canthotomy orbitotomy: a rapid approach to the orbit. Eye. 2018;32:333-7.
2. Leatherbarrow B. Orbital disorders. In: Oculoplastic Surgery. St. Louis: CV, Mosby; 2002.
3. Millar M, Maloof A. The application of stereotactic navigation surgery to orbital decompression for thyroid-associated orbitopathy. Eye. 2009;23(7):1565-71.

9.14 Infective and Inflammatory Disorders of Orbit

Amruthavalli KS
dramruthaoph@gmail.com
Tarjani Vivek Dave
LV Prasad Eye Institute
tvdeye@gmail.com, tarjani@lvpei.org

INFECTIOUS DISORDERS OF THE ORBIT

Most cases of orbital cellulitis are bacterial in etiology that can originate following direct inoculation after trauma, or spread from surrounding sinuses or rarely have hematologic spread from distant infections such as endocarditis or pneumonia.

Orbital infections can be bacterial, fungal, or parasitic in etiology.

Bacterial Orbital Infections

Chandler's classification[1] based on the location and severity has been used that has implications on the management.
- *Group 1:* Preseptal cellulitis
- *Group 2:* Orbital cellulitis
- *Group 3:* Subperiosteal abscess (SPA)
- *Group 4:* Intraorbital abscess
- *Group 5:* Cavernous sinus thrombosis (CST)

Preseptal Cellulitis[2]

Key diagnostic features:
- Infection of soft tissues anterior to the orbital septum
- Acute onset of lid edema, tenderness, and erythema
- Quiet eye with normal vision, ocular motility, pupillary reaction, and position of the globe

Treatment guidelines:
- *Mild preseptal cellulitis:* Topical antibiotics and topical warm compresses
- *Severe preseptal cellulitis:* Oral antibiotics can be added
- *Severe preseptal cellulitis with eyelid abscess:* Incision and drainage may be needed
- If the patient does not respond to antibiotics within 48 hours, or if there is evidence of orbital involvement, imaging studies along with prompt culture and sensitivity and revising antibiotic therapy help.

Orbital Cellulitis

Key diagnostic features:
- Potentially life-threatening
- Infection of soft tissues posterior to the orbital septum

- *Systemic signs:* Fever, leukocytosis, malaise, and loss of appetite
- *Ocular signs:* Signs of preseptal cellulitis along with proptosis, ptosis, chemosis, and restriction of ocular movements **(Figs. 9.14.1A to D)**
- Associated diminution of vision, color vision defect, and relative afferent pupillary defect indicate optic neuropathy due to compression on the nerve and need aggressive management.
- Complications such as meningoencephalitis, intracranial abscess, CST, and sepsis may occur in patients with a suppressed immune system.

Treatment guidelines:
- Admit for intensive medical care
- *Laboratory investigations:* Complete blood count, culture, and sensitivity
- *Imaging:* To rule out abscess formation, cavernous, and intracranial spread; to assess compression on nerve; and to look for presence of gas suggestive of infection with a gas forming organism **(Figs. 9.14.2A and B)**
- *Medical management:* Prompt empirical intravenous (IV) antibiotic with broad-spectrum gram-positive and gram-negative coverage is instituted

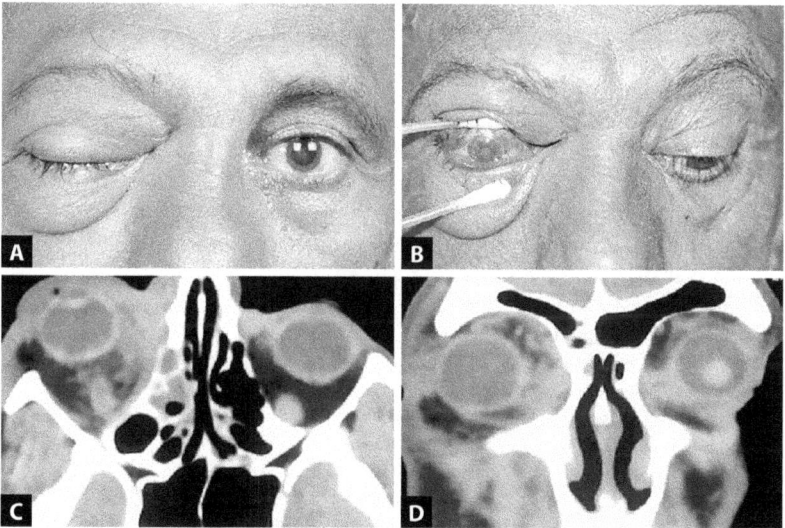

Figs. 9.14.1A to D: (A) Standard clinical photograph showing right periorbital edema and ptosis; (B) Retracted eyelids in downgaze, shows chemosis and restricted ocular motility; (C) Axial CT scan image demonstrating ill-defined and isodense lesion in the medial extra- and intraconal space with right proptosis; (D) Coronal CT scan image demonstrating the ill-defined isodensity centered inferomedially.

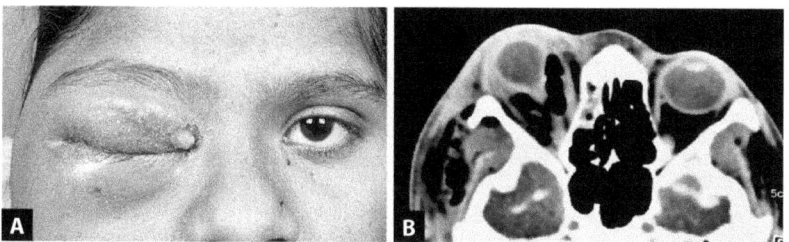

Figs. 9.14.2A and B: (A) Standard clinical photograph showing right periorbital edema, ecchymosis with excoriation of the skin, and superior discharging sinus; (B) CT scan, axial cut demonstrating proptosed right eye with globe tenting and gas in the intraconal space.

- In adults, the infection is usually polymicrobial.
- In children, orbital cellulitis is most often caused by a single organism, streptococci group being commonly implicated.
- Amoxicillin-clavulanate for broad-spectrum gram-positive and gram-negative coverage along with metronidazole (if anaerobic infection is suspected) should be administered.[3]
- Treatment is tailored once culture and sensitivity results are available.
- Treatment with IV corticosteroids after 48 hours of initiation of systemic antibiotics in bacterial infections leads to faster resolution of inflammation, although the timing and dose remain controversial.[4]
- Sinusitis causing orbital cellulitis should be identified which may require treatment by otolaryngologist.

Subperiosteal Abscess[2]

Key diagnostic features:
- Accumulation of purulent material between periorbita and orbital bone
- Located adjacent to opacified paranasal sinuses
- *Common locations:* Medial and the roof
- Progressive proptosis, globe displacement, and lack of response to appropriate antibiotic therapy suggest abscess formation.
- *Imaging:* Subperiosteal, well-defined collection with homogenous hypodensity, internal appearance, and smooth convex surface with contrast-enhancing capsule adjacent to an infected sinus **(Figs. 9.14.3A to C)**

Treatment guidelines:
- Admission and institution of appropriate IV antibiotics
- Surgical drainage either via needle aspiration on via incision and drainage during an orbitotomy if any of the following criteria is present:
  - Patient aged ≥9 years
  - Presence of frontal sinusitis
  - Nonmedial SPA location
  - Large SPA (volume >3.8 mL)
  - Suspicion of anaerobic infection

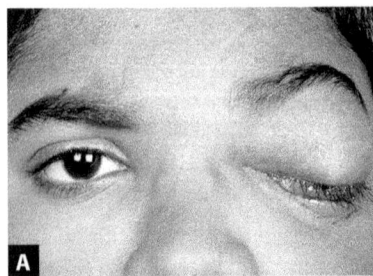
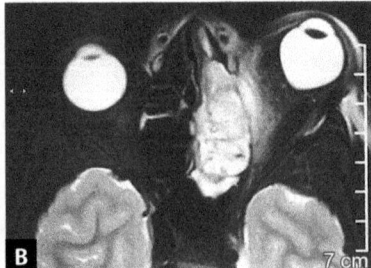
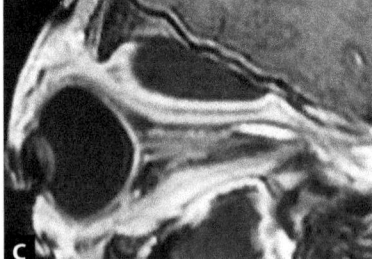

Figs. 9.14.3A to C: (A) Standard clinical photograph showing left complete ptosis, periorbital edema, and chemosis; (B) Axial T2-weighted images of MRI orbit demonstrating fullness of the left ethmoid sinus with adjacent hyperintense area in the medial extraconal space. Left globe tenting and proptosis can also be seen; (C) T1-weighted image demonstrating the subperiosteal abscess superiorly.

- Recurrence of SPA after prior drainage
- Evidence of chronic sinusitis
- Acute optic nerve or retinal compromise
- Infection of dental origin (anaerobic infection more likely)
■ To start IV steroids after 48 hours of antibiotics

Intraorbital Abscess[1]

Key diagnostic features:
■ Discrete collection of pus within the orbital tissues
■ Secondary to progressive and localizing orbital cellulitis
■ Pus may exit anteriorly through the eyelid
■ Difficult to differentiate intraorbital abscess from orbital cellulitis clinically
■ Contrast imaging is imperative to distinguish an abscess from cellulitis which reveals peripheral enhancement with nonenhancing areas in the center

Treatment guidelines: Treatment is similar to that of SPA.

Cavernous Sinus Thrombosis[2]

Key diagnostic features:
■ The most severe complication of orbital cellulitis which is fatal if not treated promptly
■ Rapidly worsening proptosis with severe pain
■ Loss of sensation in the distribution of maxillary division of the trigeminal nerve
■ Limitation of ocular motility in the contralateral eye of a previously unilateral orbital cellulitis is an early sign of CST
■ Imaging:
  • Enlarged extraocular muscles and superior ophthalmic vein (**Figs. 9.14.4A to C**)
  • Loss of concavity of the lateral border of the cavernous sinus (**Figs. 9.14.5A and B**)

Treatment guidelines:
■ IV antibiotics with broad-spectrum coverage are the main stay of treatment.
■ Role of anticoagulants is controversial.

Necrotizing Fasciitis[2,5]

Key diagnostic features:
■ Severe and potentially a sight-threatening and life-threatening infection involving the skin and the subcutaneous soft tissues with rapid progression.

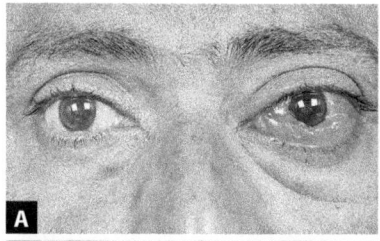
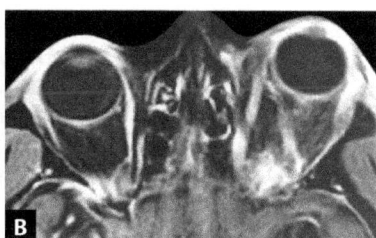
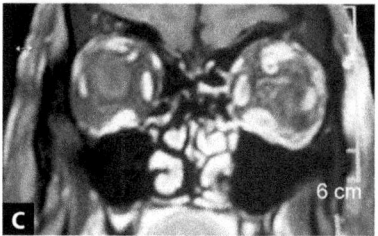

Figs. 9.14.4A to C: (A): Standard clinical photograph showing left eye chemosis; (B) T1-weighted image in axial cut demonstrating contrast enhancement at the left orbital apex and thrombosis of superior ophthalmic vein (SOV); (C) Coronal cut demonstrating thrombus within the SOV.

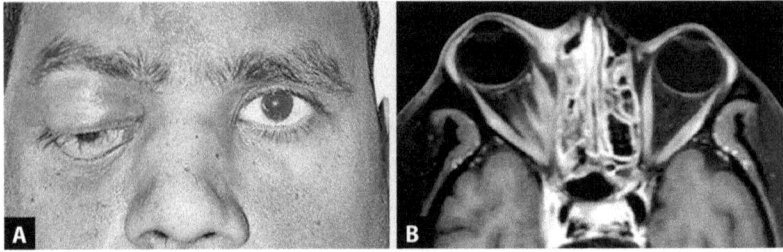

Figs. 9.14.5A and B: (A) Standard photograph with right ptosis, chemosis with restricted ocular motility; (B) T1-weighted MRI showing bilateral ethmoid sinus thickening with thickened right medial rectus and involvement of cavernous sinus. Perineural involvement can also be appreciated.

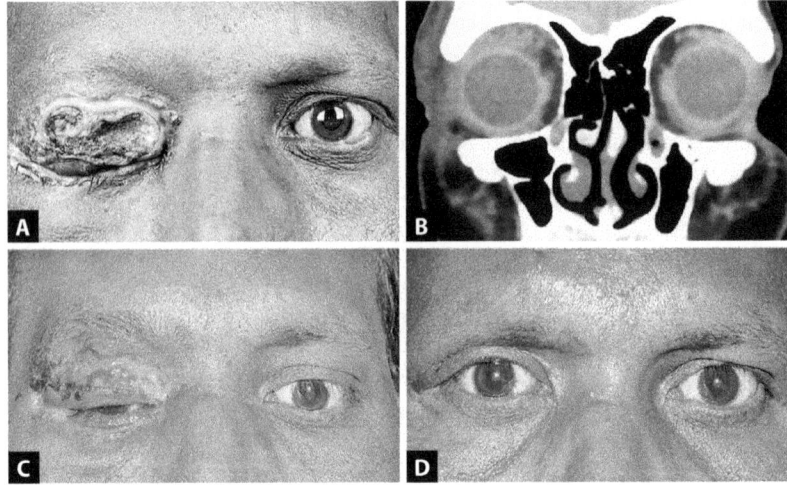

Figs. 9.14.6A to D: (A) External photograph showing necrosis of the skin and the periocular tissues on the right side; (B) CT coronal cut demonstrating ill-defined isodense area in the superior extraconal space corresponding to the areas of the necrosed tissues; (C) The same patient with necrotizing fasciitis immediate postdebridement with healthy granulation tissue; (D) At 1 month postdebridement.

- Most common organism involved is group A β-hemolytic *Streptococcus* but can be caused by aerobic or anaerobic, gram-positive or gram-negative bacteria.
- There may be disproportionate pain along with other signs such as skin color changes with bullae formation and frank cutaneous necrosis along with features of orbital or preseptal cellulitis **(Figs. 9.14.6A to D)**.
- An early sign may be anesthesia over the involved area, as necrotizing fasciitis tends to track along the avascular planes and involves the deep cutaneous nerves.

Treatment guidelines:
- Early surgical debridement till healthy granulation tissue bleed is seen along with IV antibiotics.
- Clindamycin is effective in treating infection caused by group A β-hemolytic *Streptococcus*.
- Adjunctive treatment with corticosteroids under broad-spectrum antibiotic coverage has been advised to limit the inflammatory damage caused by the toxins.
- Severe cases may experience rapid deterioration, culminating in hypotension, renal failure, and adult respiratory distress syndrome.

Fungal Orbital Infections

Rhino-orbital-cerebral Mucormycosis[6,7]

Key diagnostic features:
- Organisms that belong to the class zygomycetes can lead to rhino-orbital-cerebral mucormycosis (ROCM) which is an opportunistic infection.
- Predisposing factors include systemic disease with associated diabetes mellitus, iron overload, hematologic malignancy, bone marrow/solid-organ transplant and treatment with immunomodulators, steroids, and now infection with the delta strain of severe acute respiratory syndrome coronavirus 2 (SARS-CoV-2).
- Most common organism leading to ROCM is *Rhizopus oryzae* (90%).
- Found in soil, decaying fruit and vegetables, and animal feces.
- The most common mode of infection is by invasion from adjacent paranasal sinuses or pterygopalatine fissure.
- These fungi invade the blood vessels producing thrombosing vasculitis, and produces tissue necrosis, termed as angioinvasion.
- Early symptoms and signs include fever, sinusitis, nasal discharge, and orbital pain.
- Black eschar over the skin, nasal mucosa or palate is characteristic.
- Eyelid edema, chemosis, proptosis, and features of orbital apex syndrome like ptosis, decreased vision, decreased corneal sensations, and internal and external ophthalmoplegia are common ophthalmic features **(Figs. 9.14.7A to D)**.
- KOH mount of the suspected cases show nonseptate branching fungal filaments arranged at right angles. Histopathology shows thrombosing arteritis with vessel walls invaded with fungal hyphae and areas of necrosis.
- MRI with contrast is the imaging modality of choice.
- T1 and T2 postcontrast fat suppressed images give the most information in orbital involvement.
- Extent of sinus involvement and the presence or absence of contrast enhancement in the orbit guide the treatment.
- Optic perineuritis and globe tenting or the guitar-pick sign are seen in severe cases.

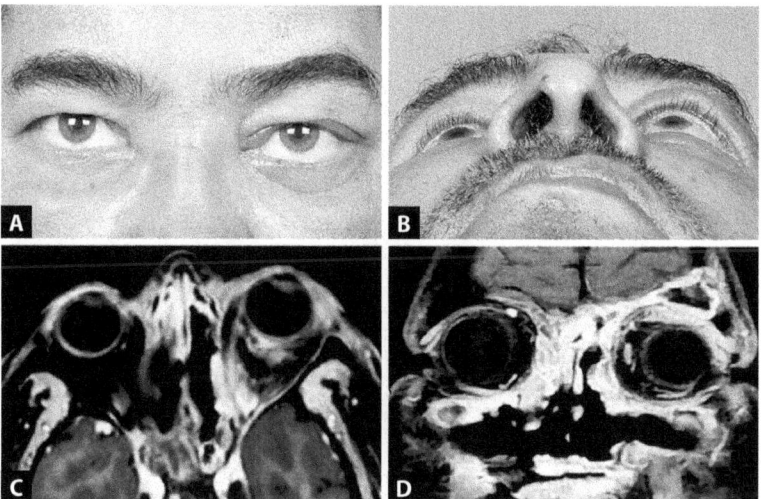

Figs. 9.14.7A to D: (A) Standard clinical photograph of mucormycosis patient presenting with left eye lid edema; (B) Worm's eye view demonstrating left eye proptosis; (C) T1-weighted images in axial cut postcontrast, showing enhancing lesion in the posteromedial orbit extending up to the apex; (D) Anterior coronal cut showing bilateral involvement of the ethmoid sinus, and left frontal sinus, loss of contrast is seen superiorly, extending in to the basifrontal region.

Treatment guidelines:
- Treatment includes multidisciplinary approach to address the sinus disease along with the orbital and intracranial component.
- Prompt correction of the diabetic ketoacidosis, or the underlying immunodeficiency and reducing the free serum iron is imperative.
- Antifungal therapy consists of a loading dose of IV liposomal amphotericin B (LAMB) for 2 weeks followed by a short bridge therapy with IV and oral antifungal for 1–2 days and a step-down to oral antifungals such as isavuconazole or posaconazole for 3–6 months.
- Dose of LAMB is based on rhino-orbital or rhino-orbital-cerebral presentation.
- Transcutaneous retrobulbar amphotericin B (TRAMB) may be considered in addition to the systemic therapy for cases with orbital involvement that demonstrates contrast enhancement.
- Surgery and local debridement of the necrotic areas (areas of loss of contrast enhancement) should be promptly performed.
- Diffuse involvement of the orbit with large areas of loss of contrast enhancement warrant orbital exenteration to prevent intracranial extension.

Aspergillosis[7]

Key diagnostic features:
- Aspergillosis is a fungal disease caused commonly by *Aspergillus fumigatus, Aspergillus flavus,* and *Aspergillus niger.*
- It can affect the immunocompromised and immunocompetent hosts.
- The infection occurs in two forms, noninvasive and invasive aspergillosis.
- In noninvasive (allergic) aspergillosis, orbital involvement is rare and proptosis occurs secondary to expansion of the sinus cavities.
- Invasive orbital aspergillosis can present with orbital pain, decreased vision, proptosis, ptosis, and limitation of extraocular movements. However, the eye may be quiet with no signs of inflammation.
- CT scan will detect localized sino-orbital with bony erosion and infiltrating the orbit. MRI shows contrast enhancing masses that are hypointense on both T1 and T2 **(Figs. 9.14.8A to D)**.

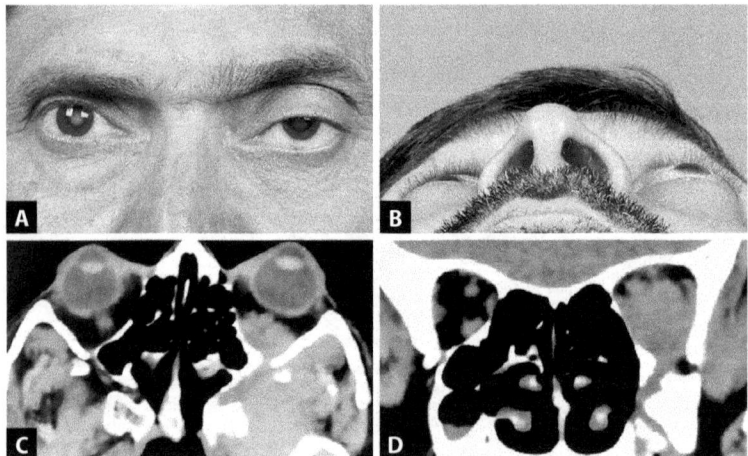

Figs. 9.14.8: (A) Standard photograph showing left side ptosis; (B) Worm's eye view showing left eye proptosis; (C) Ill-defined isodense lesion seen at the left orbital apex in CT scan axial cuts; (D) Coronal cuts demonstrating the lesion in the posterior orbit extending in to the pterygopalatine fossa.

- Diagnosis is confirmed by orbital biopsy from the epicenter of the lesion. Grocott-Gömöri's methenamine silver nitrate stain show septate hyphae with dichotomous branching at 45° angle.
- Newer serological techniques such as serum galactomannan (GM) and beta-D-glucan (BG) have found a new place in the diagnosis of aspergillosis.

Treatment guidelines:
- Strict glycemic control
- Systemic voriconazole has better efficacy and fewer side effects compared to LAMB in invasive orbital aspergillosis.
- Retro-orbital, intralesional injections of TRAMB, or voriconazole can be attempted.

Parasitic Diseases

Parasitic diseases of the orbit include cysticercosis and echinococcosis.

Orbital Cysticercosis[8]

Key diagnostic features:
- Cysticercosis is a parasitic infestation caused by cysticercosis cellulosae, which is a larval form of *Taenia solium* (pork tapeworm).
- Tissues involved include the extraocular muscle, conjunctiva, eyelid, vitreous, optic nerve lacrimal gland, and orbit.
- Patient presents with pain, eyelid edema, conjunctival congestion, limitation of ocular motility worst in the direction opposite to the involved muscle, axial or nonaxial proptosis, and diminution of vision (due to rare involvement of the optic nerve or by compression)
- Cyst in the levator muscle will present with ptosis.
- Cyst, which has migrated anteriorly, will be present at the insertion of the muscles.
- Rarely cyst may be palpable and may extrude spontaneously. If cyst ruptures in the orbit it causes intense inflammation.
- Orbital ultrasonography (USG) demonstrates well-defined lesion having clear contents, and a high reflective echo dense nodule within, suggestive of a scolex.
- CT may show well-circumscribed lesion in the thickened muscle, as hypodense lesion with central hyperdensity and surrounding soft tissue shadows **(Figs. 9.14.9A to D)**.
- Neurocysticercosis is the infection of central nervous system (CNS) and its meninges by the larva and should be ruled out.
- Presents with seizures, hydrocephalus, and focal neurological deficits.

Treatment guidelines:
- Oral albendazole 15 mg/kg/day for 1 month.
- Systemic corticosteroids 1-2 mg/kg/day is started concurrently and tapered over 6 weeks to reduce inflammatory effects.
- Serial B-scan is used to monitor the disease.
- Surgical excision, if required, the cyst should be excised in toto.

Orbital Hydatid Cyst[9]

Key diagnostic features:
- Caused by *Echinococcus granulosus* (dog tapeworm), manifests as hydatid cyst, within the orbit.
- Hydatid cysts involve multiple areas in the body. Common sites are liver, lung, and brain.
- Presenting clinical features are similar to orbital cellulitis.
- Imaging reveals single or multiple hypodense cystic with an iso to hyperdense cyst wall.
- B-scan reveals a single cyst or multilobulated cysts with echo-lucent centers.

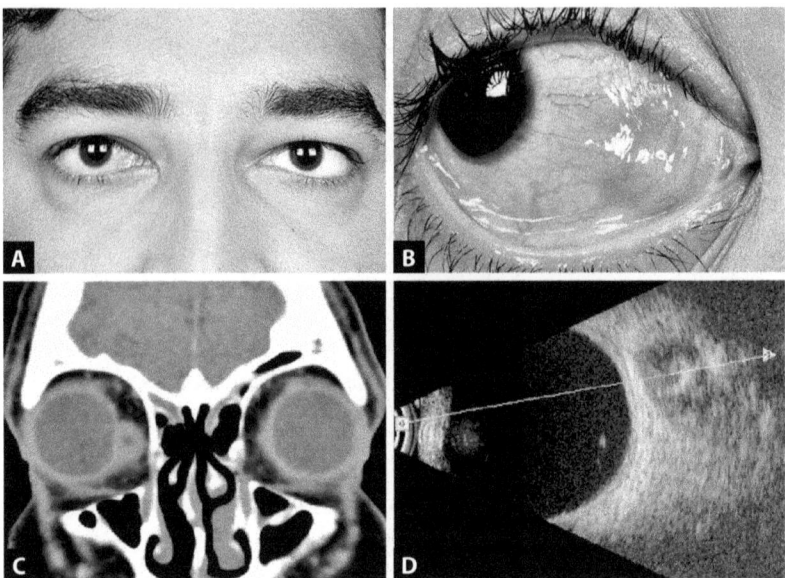

Figs. 9.14.9A to D: (A) External photograph showing conjunctival congestion of right eye; (B) Chemosis and conjunctival congestion on the medial aspect of the right eye; (C) Hypodense area is seen involving the thickened right medial rectus on CT scan, coronal cut; (D) Ultrasound B-scan showing hypoechoic lesion with central hyperechoic area suggestive of scolex.

Treatment guidelines:
- Orbitotomy and excision biopsy of the cysts
- Rupture of the cyst leads to severe inflammation
- Systemic albendazole (15 mg/kg/day for 1 month) can be prescribed for recurrent cysts.

INFLAMMATORY DISORDERS OF THE ORBIT

Autoimmune Inflammations

Thyroid Eye Disease[2,10]

Key presenting features:
- Thyroid eye disease (TED) is an autoimmune disorder that affects the orbital adipocytes and the extraocular muscles leading to proptosis, diplopia, and at times diminished vision.
- Females are more commonly and males are more severely affected.
- TED commonly occurs in individuals with Graves' hyperthyroidism.
- Cigarette smoking has been considered the strongest risk factor in the development of TED
- Eyelid retraction is the most common feature and results from the fibrosis of tissues and due to increased sympathetic activity. Lateral flare of the upper eyelid is an early sign.
- A patient with TED can also develop ptosis where myasthenia gravis, aponeurotic ptosis due to constant stretch on the levator, and compression at the apex should be ruled out.
- Dysthyroid optic neuropathy (DON) occurs in 5–7% of patients with TED.
  - Early detection is possible by testing color vision and relative afferent pupillary defect. Vision may diminish in more severe cases.

- Arcuate or altitudinal defects, paracentral scotomas, and generalized constriction represent the most common visual field defects in TED.
- Visual evoked potential (VEP) provides a useful diagnostic and monitoring tool in DON
■ On CT scan, TED is usually bilateral, the eye appears proptosed and optic nerve appears straightened. There will be bilateral fusiform enlargement of extraocular muscles sparing the tendons (cola bottle sign) with smooth borders.
■ The disease can be classified into adipogenic or myogenic based on the radiology **(Figs. 9.14.10 and 9.14.11)**.
■ *Clinical course:* TED is a self-limiting disease, with the active phase lasting for 1–3 years. Rundle and Wilson described the orbital changes in three phases:
  1. *Inflammation (initial phase):* Associated with orbital and periorbital signs including proptosis and eyelid retraction
  2. *Static phase:* Heralds little clinical improvement despite reduced inflammation
  3. *Quiescent phase:* Gradual improvement in lid retraction and ocular motility
■ Several clinical scoring systems such as Clinical Activity Score (CAS) and vision, inflammation, strabismus, and appearance (VISA) exist to guide TED evaluation and management.

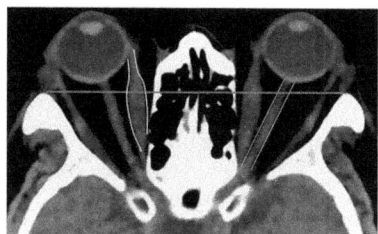

Fig. 9.14.10: CT scan orbit axial cut demonstrating bilateral proptosis (shown with blue horizontal line), fusiform enlargement of medial rectus, sparing the tendons, known as cola bottle sign (highlighted in yellow), and straightening of optic nerve (highlighted in orange).

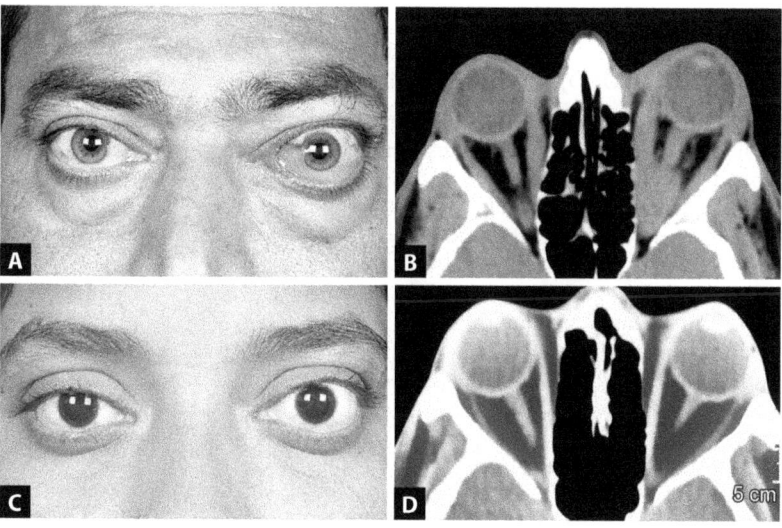

Figs. 9.14.11A to D: (A) Standard clinical photograph showing bilateral eyelid retraction with lateral flare of left eyelid, congestion, and chemosis of left eye; (B) CT scan axial cut of the same patient demonstrating bilateral proptosis and enlarged medial rectus; (C) Standard photograph of a different patient demonstrating left eyelid retraction with lateral flare; (D) CT scan axial cut of the same patient demonstrating predominantly enlarged fat spaces with normal extraocular muscles.

TABLE 9.14.1: Clinical Activity Score (CAS) (amended by EUGOGO after Mourits et al.).

For initial CAS, only score items 1–7

1. Spontaneous orbital pain
2. Gaze evoked orbital pain
3. Eyelid swelling that is considered to be due to active GO
4. Eyelid erythema
5. Conjunctival redness that is considered to be due to active GO
6. Chemosis
7. Inflammation of caruncle or plica

Patients assessed after follow-up (1–3 months) can be scored out of 10 by including items 8–10

8. Increase of >2 mm in proptosis
9. Decrease in uniocular ocular excursion in any one direction of >8°
10. Decrease of acuity equivalent to 1 Snellen line

(EUGOGO: European Group on Graves' orbitopathy; GO: Graves' orbitopathy)
Source: Barrio-Barrio J, Sabater AL, Bonet-Farriol E, Velázquez-Villoria A, Galofré JC. Graves' Ophthalmopathy: VISA versus EUGOGO Classification, Assessment, and Management. J Ophthalmol. 2015;2015:249125.

- The CAS and VISA systems, each assign points for various findings, CAS adds parameters for follow-up visits. CAS is composed of seven items. TED is defined as active if the score is ≥3/7 on first visit or ≥4/10 on follow-up **(Table 9.14.1)**.
- VISA uses same scale for initial and follow-up visits. While CAS is binary (absent/present, 0/1) for each item VISA inflammatory score assigns a higher score for more severe forms of eyelid and conjunctival inflammation (0 to 2) **(Table 9.14.2)**. Also on CAS equal weightage is provided to the "soft tissue signs" and the "impaired function items". Therefore a patient with low CAS score may still have DON and need high dose steroids.[11]
- Severity of the disease can be classified based on the European Group on Graves' orbitopathy (EUGOGO) severity score **(Table 9.14.3)**.[12]

Treatment guidelines: Treatment for TED needs to be individualized based on the severity and activity of TED. Supportive measures include:
- Smoking cessation
- Establishment of euthyroid state
- Topical lubricants and topical cyclosporine for dry eye and ocular surface symptoms
- Salt restriction
- Elevation of head end of bed
- Oral selenium supplementation
- Temporary prism glasses to relieve diplopia
- Botulinum toxin injection to reduce upper eyelid retraction

CAS ≤3 or VISA inflammatory score ≤4

- Lubricants
- Selenium supplementation for 6 months
- If the quality of life is impaired, low-dose immunomodulator therapy is given for the active disease and rehabilitative surgery is done in inactive cases

CAS ≥3 or VISA ≥4

- *First-line treatment:*
  - Intravenous methylprednisolone (IVMP) with or without mycophenolate mofetil is the first-line treatment

TABLE 9.14.2: VISA inflammatory index (I) (Dolman and Rootman 2006,[10] ITEDS modified).

Sign or symptom	Score
Caruncular edema	0: Absent 1: Present
Chemosis	0: Absent 1: Conjunctiva lies behind the gray line of the lid 2: Conjunctiva extends anterior to the gray line of the lid
Conjunctival redness	0: Absent 1: Present
Lid redness	0: Absent 1: Present
Lid edema	0: Absent 1: Present but without redundant tissues 2: Present and causing bulging in the palpebral skin, including lower lid festoon
Retrobulbar ache At rest With gaze	0: Absent; 1: Present 0: Absent; 1: Present
Diurnal variation	0: Absent; 1: Present

(VISA: vision, inflammation, strabismus, and appearance)
Source: Barrio-Barrio J, Sabater AL, Bonet-Farriol E, Velázquez-Villoria A, Galofré JC. Graves' Ophthalmopathy: VISA versus EUGOGO Classification, Assessment, and Management. J Ophthalmol. 2015;2015:249125.

TABLE 9.14.3: The European Group on Graves' orbitopathy (EUGOGO) classification.

Mild GO (one or more of the following signs)	Moderate-to-severe GO (two or more of the following signs)	Sight threatening GO (very severe)
Lid retraction <2 mm	Lid retraction >2 mm	Dysthyroid optic neuropathy
Mild soft tissue involvement	Moderate or severe soft tissue involvement	Corneal melt
Exophthalmos <3 mm	Exophthalmos >3 mm	
No or intermittent diplopia Corneal exposure	Inconstant or constant diplopia	

(GO: Graves' orbitopathy)
Source: Bartalena L, Kahaly GJ, Baldeschi L, Dayan CM, Eckstein A, Marcocci C, et al. The 2021 European Group on Graves' orbitopathy (EUGOGO) clinical practice guidelines for the medical management of Graves' orbitopathy. Eur J Endocrinol. 2021;185:G43-67.

- 12 weekly infusions of methyl prednisolone (500 mg weekly for 6 weeks and 250 mg weekly for 6 weeks) with a cumulative dose of 4.5 g
- Write steroid protocols (weekly, daily)
- *Second-line treatment:* If response to primary treatment is poor, a second course of IVMP, starting with high single doses (750 mg)
- Oral prednisolone combined with cyclosporine or azathioprine
- Orbital radiotherapy combined with oral or IV glucocorticoids
- Biologic agents used in the treatment of TED are teprotumumab, rituximab, and tocilizumab

- *Teprotumumab:* A human monoclonal antibody inhibitor of insulin-like growth factor type I receptor (IGF-IR), reduced proptosis and CAS in patients with active TED[13]
- *Rituximab:* Affects clinical course of the disease by blocking CD20 receptor on B lymphocytes
- *Tocilizumab:* A monoclonal interleukin-6 (IL-6) antibody may reduce inflammatory signs via an upstream effect on inflammatory cycle.

Sight-threatening (very severe) TED:
- High-single dose of IVMP (1 g/day) for 3 consecutive or alternate days is given and assessed after 1 week.
- If there is response, continue IVMP (500 mg/week) for five additional pulses.
- If there is poor or no response within 1–2 weeks, consider urgent orbital decompression surgery.
- Recent globe subluxation may need orbital decompression.
- Severe corneal exposure should be urgently treated medically or with tarsorrhaphy.

Inactive TED: When the disease is stable for 6–9 months, rehabilitative surgery (orbital decompression/squint/lid surgery) as needed or required by the patient.
- Surgical decompression creates more space for the swollen tissues by expanding the walls of the bony orbit (bone decompression) or by removing the orbital fat (fat decompression).
- Decompression should precede strabismus surgery as it may produce or worsen diplopia.
- Surgery to recess the rectus muscles can change eyelid position, so strabismus surgery should precede eyelid repositioning surgery.

Idiopathic Orbital Inflammatory Disease[14,15]

Key diagnostic features:
- Idiopathic orbital inflammatory disease (IOID) is an inflammatory condition of the orbit without identifiable local or systemic causes.
- The etiology of IOID remains unknown. It may be caused by subclinical infection or immune process secondary to infection.
- The peak incidence is in sixth decade and there is no sex predilection except in myositis (common in females).
- The most commonly used classifications are as follows:
  - Dacryoadenitis
  - Myositis
  - Anterior (sclera, uvea, and Tenon's capsule)
  - Apical
  - Diffuse (two or more of the mentioned structures are involved)
- Optic perineuritis, where optic nerve sheath is the target tissue is considered a form of apical subset.
- *Dacryoadenitis:*
  - Clinical features include pain, periorbital edema, enlargement of lacrimal gland, and palpable in the superotemporal orbit. Eyelid shows S-shaped deformity, due to localized edema.
  - On CT there is diffuse enlargement with homogenous enhancement. Preservation of gland shape and involvement of both orbital and palpebral lobes is characteristic **(Figs. 9.14.12A to D)**.
- *Myositis:*
  - Diplopia is the predominant feature of myositis along with pain on ocular movements and proptosis.
  - CT scan usually shows unilateral asymmetric enlargement of the muscles with strong enhancement. Surrounding infiltration making ragged and fluffy margins

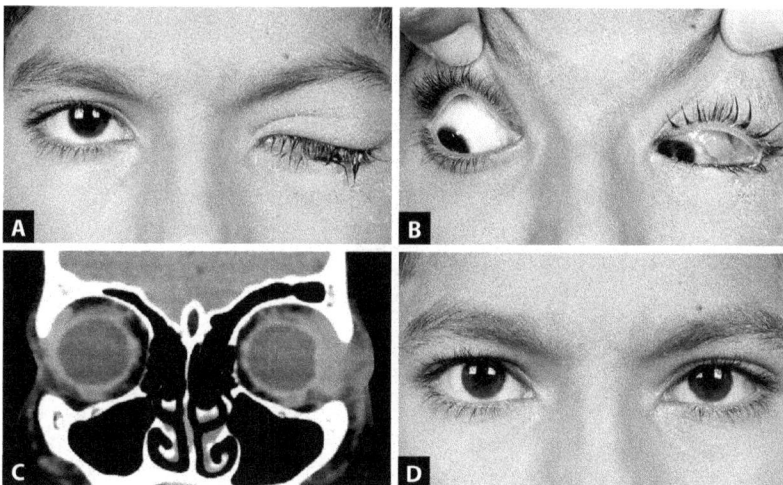

Figs. 9.14.12A to D: (A) Standard clinical photograph showing left side periorbital edema and S-shaped deformity of upper eyelid; (B) Enlarged lacrimal gland visible in dextrodepression; (C) CT scan coronal cut demonstrating enlarged lacrimal gland; (D) Standard photograph postresolution.

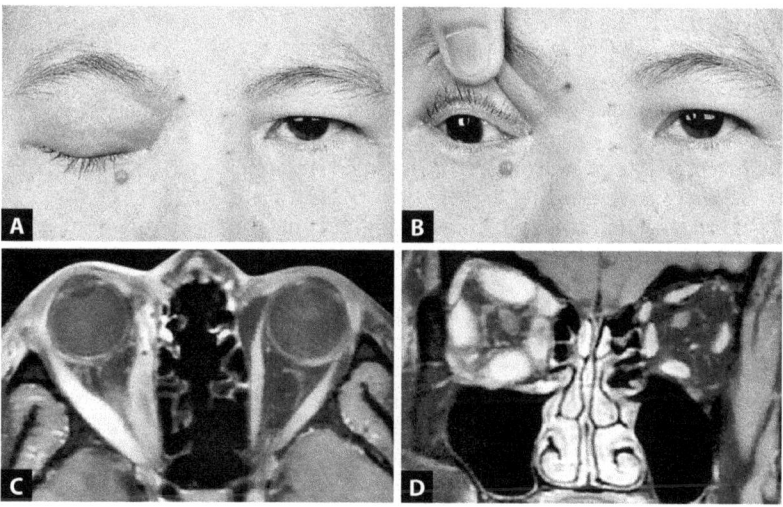

Figs. 9.14.13A to D: (A) External photograph showing right complete ptosis and periorbital edema; (B) Retracted upper eyelid showing limited ocular motility; (C) T1-weighted MRI axial cut postcontrast demonstrating bulky medial rectus (MR) and lateral rectus (LR) involving the tendons on the right side; (D) Coronal cut with bulky extraocular muscles on right side.

are characteristic. Tendon thickening along with belly differentiates it from TED (**Figs. 9.14.13A to D**).
- *Anterior IOID:*
    - *Clinical features:* Acute onset of pain, edema, and erythema. Chemosis is the most common feature, followed by proptosis.
    - On imaging there is localized soft tissue shadows involving the anterior part of the orbit.

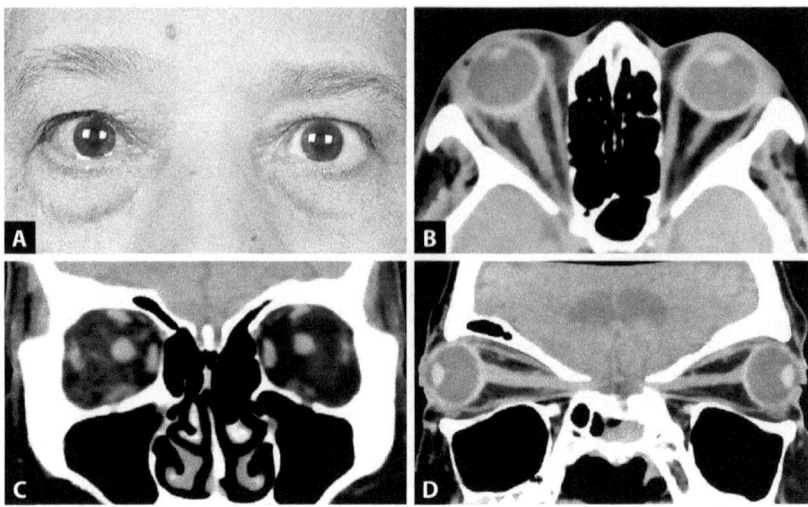

Figs. 9.14.14A to D: (A) External photograph showing right eye conjunctival congestion; (B) CT scan axial cut showing right thickened optic nerve with perineural involvement; (C) Thickened optic nerve appreciated on coronal cut; (D) Sagittal reconstruction image demonstrating perineuritis.

- *Apical IOID:*
  - *Clinical features:* Pain, proptosis, diplopia, ptosis, and evidence of optic nerve dysfunction **(Figs. 9.14.14A to D)**
  - CT scan demonstrates inflammatory soft tissue at the orbital apex
- *Diffuse IOID:*
  - *Clinical features:* Acute onset of pain, eyelid edema, chemosis, proptosis, diplopia, and rarely visual loss
  - On imaging, there will be diffuse soft tissue involvement with irregular outline, shadowing the entire orbit
- It is a diagnosis of exclusion.
- Laboratory tests such as complete blood count, basic metabolic panel, erythrocyte sedimentation rate (ESR), C-reactive protein (CRP), rheumatoid arthritis (RA) factor, serum angiotensin-converting enzyme (ACE) cytoplasmic antineutrophil cytoplasmic antibody (c-ANCA), perinuclear ANCA (p-ANCA), Antinuclear antibody (ANA), and total serum immunoglobulin G4 (IgG4) are done to exclude other possible diseases.
- In 2016, the orbital society established consensus that tissue biopsy is recommended for nonmyositic IOID, while corticosteroids can be tried for myositic nonspecific orbital inflammatory disease (NSOID).

Treatment guidelines:
- Mild cases may resolve spontaneously.
- However early and adequate treatment is required to reduce inflammation effectively, to prevent recurrence and to protect the orbital tissue from scarring.
- Therapeutic options include: (1) Corticosteroids, (2) immunomodulating agents, (3) biological agents, (4) radiation therapy, and (5) surgical debulking.
  - *Oral corticosteroids:* Primary choice except for severe cases with optic nerve dysfunction. Initial dose is 1 mg/kg/day prednisolone. Dramatic improvement of signs and symptoms within 24–48 hours is typical.
  - *Immunosuppressive:* Methotrexate is most commonly used steroid sparing agent. Azathioprine, cyclosporine A, and mycophenolate mofetil are used in recurrent cases.

- *Rituximab:* For treating refractory cases of IOID. Infliximab is promising as a steroid sparing therapy for recalcitrant IOID. Adalimumab, tocilizumab, and daclizumab were reported to be effective in some cases.
- *Radiation therapy:* Effective in recalcitrant cases or in patients with contraindication to steroids. Low-dose radiation 15–20 Gy delivered in 10 fractions over 2–3 weeks is used.

Immunoglobulin G4-related Disease[16]
Key diagnostic features:
- Immunoglobulin G4-related Disease (IgG4-RD) comprises a significant proportion of what was previously labeled IOID.
- IgG4-RD is a fibroinflammatory disorder that may affect one or more organs.
- Within the orbit, it commonly affects the lacrimal gland.
- Patient presents with eyelid edema, ptosis, proptosis, and limitation of extraocular movements **(Figs. 9.14.15A to D)**.
- Histologic examination shows lymphoplasmacytic infiltrates with large number of IgG4 positive plasma cells, storiform fibrosis, obliterative phlebitis, and eosinophil infiltration.
- Serologic testing shows elevated IgG4 and peripheral eosinophilia.

Treatment guidelines: Corticosteroids, immunosuppressants, and biologic agents including rituximab.

Specific Orbital Inflammations[17]
Key diagnostic features:
- Noninfective specific causes of orbital inflammation include granulomatosis with polyangiitis (GPA), previously known as Wegener's granulomatosis, sarcoidosis **(Figs. 9.14.16A and B)**, xanthogranulomatous inflammation, Sjögren's syndrome, and Rosai-Dorfman disease

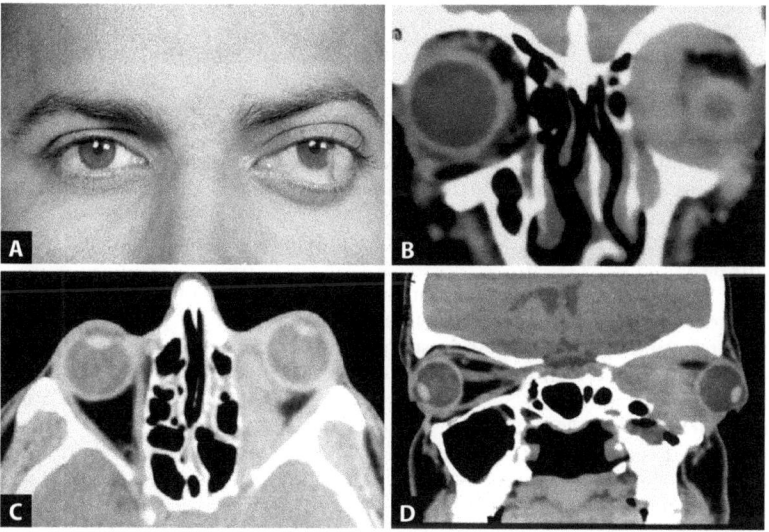

Figs. 9.14.15A to D: (A) Standard clinical photograph showing left proptosis and lower eyelid retraction; (B) CT scan coronal cut demonstrating ill-defined isodense lesion occupying the medial, superior, and inferior orbit; (C) CT scan axial cut demonstrating lesion occupying the extraconal and intraconal space extending till the apex; (D) Sagittal reconstruction image demonstrating the same.

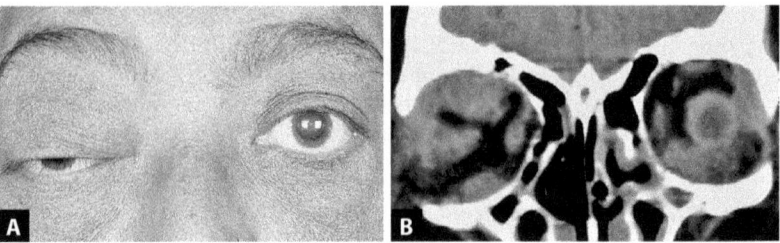

Figs. 9.14.16A and B: (A) Standard clinical photograph showing right side ptosis; (B) CT scan coronal cut demonstrating isodense lesion occupying the superior extraconal space of the right orbit, superior rectus-levator palpebrae superioris (SR-LPS) cannot be seen separately, and inferomedial quadrant on the left side.

- Present with subacute disease with features of mass in the orbit
- Associated with other ocular and systemic features

Treatment guidelines:
- Management approach involves biopsy, tailored systemic and serologic investigations such as c-ANCA (for GPA), p-ANCA (polyarteritis nodosa), ACE levels, lysozyme and calcium (sarcoidosis), ESR, CRP, and RA factor.
- Treatment involves a combination of corticosteroids, immunosuppressants, and biologic agents.

REFERENCES

1. Chandler JR, Langenbrunner DJ, Stevens ER. The pathogenesis of orbital complications in acute sinusitis. Laryngoscope. 1970;80:1414-28.
2. Korn BS, Burkat CN, Carter KD, Perry JD, Setabutr P, Steele EA, et al. Orbital inflammatory and infectious disorders. In: Korn BS (Ed). Oculofacial Plastic and Orbital Surgery. San Francisco: American Academy of Ophthalmology; 2022. pp. 43-70.
3. Wong SJ, Levi J. Management of pediatric orbital cellulitis: A systematic review. Int J Pediatr Otorhinolaryngol. 2018;110:123-9.
4. Pushker N, Tejwani LK, Bajaj MS, Khurana S, Velpandian T, Chandra M. Role of oral corticosteroids in orbital cellulitis. Am J Ophthalmol. 2013;156:178-83.
5. Elwood ET, Sommerville DN, Murray JD. Periorbital necrotizing fasciitis. Plast Reconstr Surg. 2007;120:107.
6. Nair AG, Adulkar NG, D'Cunha L, Rao PR, Bradoo RA, Bapaye MM, et al. Rhino-orbital mucormycosis following COVID-19 in previously non-diabetic, immunocompetent patients. Orbit. 2021;40:499-504.
7. Mukherjee B, Raichura ND, Alam MS. Fungal infections of the orbit. Indian J Ophthalmol. 2016;64:337-45.
8. Salim S, Alam MS, Backiavathy V, Raichura ND, Mukherjee B. Orbital cysticercosis: Clinical features and management outcomes. Orbit. 2021;40:400-6.
9. Kumar A, Parihar V, Yadav YR, Shrivastava V, Patel NK. A rare case of giant primary orbital hydatid cyst. World Neurosurg. 2019:S1878-8750/30087-7.
10. Dolman PJ, Rootman J. VISA classification for Graves orbitopathy. Ophthalmic Plast Reconstr Surg. 2006;22:319-24.
11. Barrio-Barrio J, Sabater AL, Bonet-Farriol E, Velázquez-Villoria A, Galofré JC. Graves' Ophthalmopathy: VISA versus EUGOGO Classification, Assessment, and Management. J Ophthalmol. 2015;2015:249125.
12. Bartalena L, Kahaly GJ, Baldeschi L, Dayan CM, Eckstein A, Marcocci C, et al. The 2021 European Group on Graves' orbitopathy (EUGOGO) clinical practice guidelines for the medical management of Graves' orbitopathy. Eur J Endocrinol. 2021;185: G43-67.
13. Smith TJ, Kahaly GJ, Ezra DG, Fleming JC, Dailey RA, Tang RA, et al. Teprotumumab for thyroid-associated ophthalmopathy. N Engl J Med. 2017;376:1748-61.

14. Mombaerts I, Bilyk JR, Rose GE, McNab AA, Fay A, Dolman PJ, et al. Consensus on diagnostic criteria of idiopathic orbital inflammation using a modified Delphi approach. JAMA Ophthalmol. 2017;135:769-76.
15. Lee MJ, Planck SR, Choi D, Harrington CA, Wilson DJ, Dailey RA, et al. Non-specific orbital inflammation: Current understanding and unmet needs. Prog Retin Eye Res. 2021;81: 100885.
16. McNab AA, McKelvie P. IgG4-related ophthalmic disease. Part II: clinical aspects. Ophthalmic Plast Reconstr Surg. 2015;31:167-78.
17. Chaudhuri Z, Vanathi M, infections of the orbit and orbital inflammations—pathological lesions of the orbit, postgraduate ophthalmology, 2012;1316-1317.

9.15 Adnexal Trauma

AK Grover, Shaloo Bageja, Rwituja Thomas
Sir Ganga Ram Hospital, New Delhi
akgrover55@gmail.com, bagejashaloo@gmail.com, thomas.rwituja@gmail.com

■ INTRODUCTION

The incidence of adnexal injuries is increasing due to factors such as road traffic accidents, industrial mishaps, and intentional assaults. These injuries can involve the eyelids, lacrimal system, or orbital wall, either in isolation or in conjunction with midfacial injuries. Before addressing the localized injury, it is crucial to evaluate the basic airway, breathing, and circulation (ABC). The decision of whether to repair the wound immediately or delay the repair depends on factors such as tissue edema, presence of hematoma, or infection.

In cases of eyelid injury, a thorough examination of the globe is necessary. Assessing visual acuity is important, and if it is difficult to evaluate the visual system, optic nerve and retinal functions can be assessed by observing pupillary reactions. Confrontation visual field examination should be performed to detect any field loss. It is important to observe the ocular adnexa before manipulating the injured eye. In the absence of signs of penetrating ocular injury, a comprehensive examination of the anterior segment, intraocular pressure (IOP) measurement, and fundus evaluation should be conducted. The presence of exophthalmos may indicate a retrobulbar foreign body or hemorrhage. Subcutaneous emphysema, anesthesia of the infraorbital skin, or bony step-offs of the orbital rim are indicative of orbital bone damage. If there is significant lid edema, a Desmarres Lid Retractor may be used. Classification of adnexal trauma is presented in **Flowchart 9.15.1**.

Flowchart 9.15.1: Classification of adnexal trauma.

Eyelid	Lacrimal system	Orbit
Soft tissue edema	Canalicular tears	Foreign bodies
Ecchymosis	• Nasolacrimal duct obstruction	Fractures
Laceration/avulsion	• (Naso-orbital fractures)	Extraocular muscle damage
Malpositions		
Tissue loss		
Burns, scars		

■ EVALUATION OF THE LID INJURY

- *Duration:* The time that has passed since the injury occurred plays a crucial role in determining the approach to wound repair.
- *Mode of injury:* Differentiate between injuries caused by sharp or blunt objects. Contaminated wounds from dog bites require preventive measures. Chemical and thermal injuries often require delayed secondary wound repair.
- *Site of injury:* Assess whether the lid margin is intact or lacerated. Injuries in the medial canthus region may be associated with lacrimal injuries.
- *Tissue loss:* Note if there is any tissue loss, as it may require mobilization of adjacent tissue or the use of skin flaps from neighboring areas or free skin grafts.
- *Infection:* If there is an infection, it may be necessary to postpone wound repair until the infection subsides.
- *Injury to the levator aponeurosis:* Injury to the levator muscle or aponeurosis can be diagnosed by assessing the patient's ability to look up and observing any absence of wrinkling in the upper lid skin. Radiologic evaluation is advised when necessary.

Goals of Eyelid Repair
- Restore the anatomical configuration
- Restore physiological function
- Improve cosmetic appearance

Timing of Surgery
- *Primary repair:* If patients present within 24 hours of the injury, immediate primary repair of the wound is performed to achieve the best cosmetic and functional outcomes.
- *Delayed primary repair:* If patients present >24 hours after the injury, or if there is significant lid edema or infection, a delayed primary repair is performed after 3–4 days. During this waiting period, measures such as cold saline compresses, anti-inflammatory drugs, and antibiotics are used to reduce tissue edema and control infection.
- *Secondary wound repair:* In cases where patients present long after the injury or in cases of chemical and thermal burns, healing by second intention is allowed to occur. A minimum waiting period of 5–6 months is necessary before planning a secondary wound repair.

Principles to Follow for Eyelid Repair
- Administration of local or general anesthesia
- Achieving sustained hemostasis with the infiltration of 2% xylocaine with adrenaline
- Thorough examination, with particular attention to special structures such as the canaliculi, canthal tendons, and levator function
- Cleansing the wound
- Removing foreign material from the wound
- Debridement of only clearly devitalized tissue
- Repairing special structures such as the canaliculi, canthal tendons, and levator aponeurosis
- Closure in two to three layers

■ PRIMARY WOUND MANAGEMENT

Primary wound management can be categorized as follows:
- *Repair of lid margin laceration:*
  - In cases with minimal tissue loss
  - In cases with moderate tissue loss
  - In cases with severe tissue loss
- Lid laceration with injury to the levator muscle or aponeurosis

- Injuries involving the medial canthus
- Injuries involving the lateral canthus
- Total avulsion of an eyelid
- Management of canalicular laceration
- Thermal and chemical injury
- Management of animal bites to ocular adnexa includes wound care and surgical repair of traumatized tissue, treatment of infection (most commonly *Pasteurella multocida*), appropriate tetanus and rabies prophylaxis, and notification of state public health officials.

REPAIR OF NONMARGINAL LID DEFECTS

Simple Lacerations

Smaller linear wounds can be sutured without undermining. However, round wounds should be converted into an elliptical shape. Tension or vertical pulling on the lid margins should be avoided. Nonabsorbable skin sutures should be removed after approximately 5 days. Vertical linear wounds can be converted into multiple Z-plasties to improve scar appearance.

Deep Lacerations

Deep nonmarginal lacerations require careful examination of each layer of the wound, including the orbital septum, levator aponeurosis, rectus muscles, and globe. Layer-by-layer closure is necessary.

Repair of Lid Margin Laceration with Minimal Loss of Tissue

If devitalized tissue is present, the lid margins should be freshened to create straight and smooth surgical edges while preserving as much tarsus as possible. The margin is repaired using the three-suture technique. The use of magnification aids in the repair process.

Lid margin sutures are passed first. A 6-0 silk suture is passed through the gray line 3 mm from the edge of the tear, to a depth of 3 mm. This is brought out of the wound and reinserted into the other side of the laceration 3 mm deep to the lid margin and emerging through the gray line 3 mm from the edge of the wound (**Fig. 9.15.1**). The same suture is then passed back into the gray line on the same side, 1 mm from the edge of the tear, to a depth of 1 mm (**Fig. 9.15.2**). The needle is brought out and reinserted into the opposite edge of the tear 1 mm deep to lid margins and emerging through the gray line 1 mm from the margin of the wound. Two more vertical mattress sutures are passed exactly in the same way through the posterior lash line and in the plane of the meibomian gland openings. These three sutures are triply tied and ends left long (**Fig. 9.15.3**).

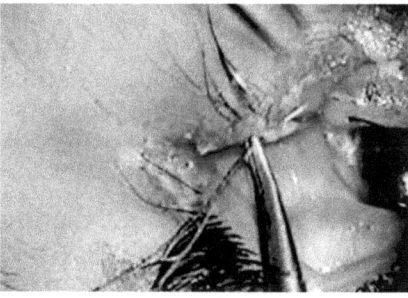

Fig. 9.15.1: A 6-0 silk suture is passed just behind the gray line through the firm tarsus 3 mm from the edge of the tear, to a depth of 3 mm and is being reinserted into the other side of the laceration 3 mm deep to the lid margin.

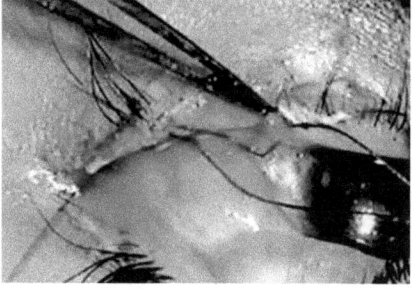

Fig. 9.15.2: The suture is then passed back into the gray line on the same side, 1 mm from the edge of the tear, to a depth of 1 mm.

5-0 polyglactin sutures are used to reapproximate the tarsus. There is no need to place sutures on the conjunctival surface since it will heal with the approximated tarsal edges. Skin sutures are removed in 4–5 days. Lid margin sutures are left in situ for 10–14 days.

With Moderate Loss of Tissue (One-fourth to One-half of Eyelid)

Closure can be achieved through various techniques, including lateral canthotomy and cantholysis, Tenzel flap, transconjunctival flap, or Mustarde's marginal pedicle rotation flap.

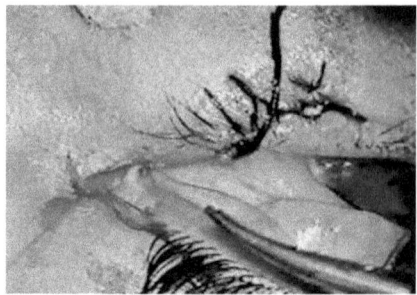

Fig. 9.15.3: Marginal sutures are passed and ends are left long.

With Severe Loss of Tissue (More than Half of Eyelid)

Repair involves using grafts from the opposite eyelid or surrounding tissue. Common techniques include the Cutler–Beard procedure, Hughes tarsoconjunctival advancement flap, Mustarde's cheek rotation flap, and free transconjunctival graft with mucocutaneous advancement.

Trauma to Levator Muscle or Aponeurosis

The levator palpebrae superioris (LPS) fibers, which run vertically, should be identified in comparison to the circumferentially oriented orbicularis muscle fibers. If the aponeurosis is disinserted from the tarsus, it can be reinserted by placing three sutures through the tarsus. Adjusting the level of aponeurosis can be done by having the patient look straight ahead during surgery. The orbital septum should not be sutured if it has been opened to prevent lagophthalmos. Eyelid crease recreation may be necessary for lacerations at the level of the lid fold.

Injuries Involving Medial Canthus

Reconstructing the medial canthal tendon (MCT) is important for lower lid avulsions at the medial canthus. The distal cut end should be sutured to its proximal part or the periosteum using sutures. Total avulsion may require the use of miniplates for anchorage of the MCT.

Associated nasolacrimal duct (NLD) obstruction injuries are often associated with naso-orbital fractures and can be managed with dacryocystorhinostomy (DCR) with or without repair of telecanthus or epicanthus. Difficulties may arise during surgery due to the identification of landmarks, difficult osteotomy, and increased bleeding.

Injuries Involving Lateral Canthus

Severed lateral canthal tendon (LCT) can be repaired by passing nonabsorbable prolene mattress sutures through both ends and anchoring them to the periorbita on the inner aspect of the lateral orbital tubercle (Whitnall's tubercle).

Total Avulsion of Eyelid

In cases of total avulsion, the avulsed segments should be found and stored in a sterile container with an antibiotic solution in the refrigerator until they can be surgically reimplanted.

Management of Canalicular Laceration

When the eyelid is injured at the medial canthus or has lacerations in that area, it can lead to discontinuity of the lacrimal passage (canaliculi). Several surgical techniques have been described in the past by different authors for repairing these lacerations. The main principle in repairing a lacerated canaliculus is to restore its drainage function. Advances in surgical techniques, such as the use of fine sutures, improved surgical methods, and the application of microscopes, have contributed to better outcomes.

Stenting is a technique used for repairing canaliculus injuries, which involves the insertion of a tube to maintain the drainage passage. Monocanalicular stenting, using silicone as the common material, is often preferred as it does not disturb the unaffected canaliculus. One option is the use of a Mini-Monoka stent, but due to cost and availability concerns, alternative techniques have been developed **(Fig. 9.15.4)**.

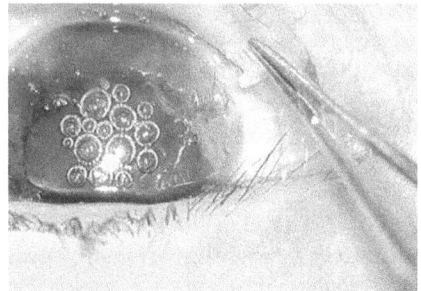

Fig. 9.15.4: Mini-Monoka being inserted through cut ends of the canaliculus.

The repair process begins by identifying the two cut ends of the canaliculi. The lateral end is located by passing a lacrimal probe through the punctum, while the medial end is identified by examining the wound under magnification, preferably with an operating microscope **(Fig. 9.15.5)**. If the cut end is not easily visible, sterile saline is pooled in the wound and air is injected from the upper canaliculus, observing for bubbles to identify the opening. The use of a pigtail probe for identifying the medial end should be avoided to prevent false passages and damage to the intact canaliculus. Once both cut ends are identified, a Mini-Monoka tubing or a 22-gauge (G) cannula sleeve is inserted up to the medial sac wall **(Fig. 9.15.6)**. Sutures are then taken around the canaliculus to secure it in place **(Fig. 9.15.7)**.

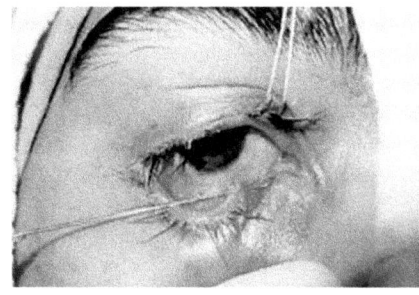

Fig. 9.15.5: Lacrimal probe is passed through the cut ends of the lower canaliculus.

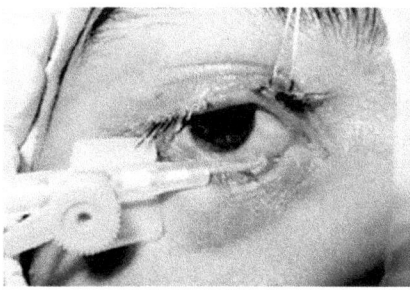

Fig. 9.15.6: 22-G cannula is passed through cut ends of canaliculus into medial sac wall.

The wound on the eyelid margin is closed using a marginal repair technique. It is crucial to repair the lacrimal drainage system if it has been disrupted. The silicone tubing or sleeve is left in place for a minimum of 3 months to facilitate healing. To prevent the extrusion of the tube, fixation sutures are passed through the tube and eyelid skin, providing traction to keep it in place. Alternatively, the silicone tubes can be passed into the nose using a Quickert–Dryden probing system, ensuring their retention for the required period.

In cases of *thermal and chemical injuries* to the eyelids, immediate and thorough irrigation with water or saline is essential.

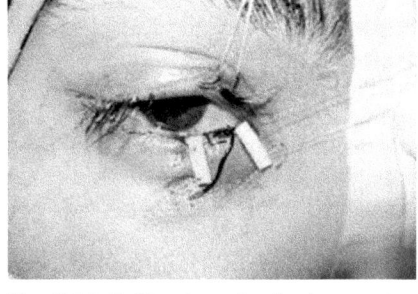

Fig. 9.15.7: Fixation of tube by passing double arm prolene through two polythene bolster and emerging toward the medial canthus and fixed to the skin of eyelid.

Neutralizing agents are not a priority, and irrigation should continue for at least 30 minutes. Debridement of necrotic tissue and foreign particles should be performed, and in burns affecting the medial canthal area, daily dilatation and the placement of a tube can help maintain patency.

As swelling subsides, lagophthalmos (incomplete eyelid closure) may occur, leading to corneal exposure. Tarsorrhaphy (surgical closure of the eyelids) can be performed to protect the eye. During the healing phase, cicatricial ectropion (outward turning of the eyelid) may develop due to the contraction of the scar tissue. Skin grafting is commonly used to correct these eyelid malpositions caused by wound contracture.

Secondary repair of eyelid injuries is typically performed 5–6 months after the initial injury, aiming to release contractures by removing scar tissue and replacing it with healthy skin.

In conclusion, proper primary repair of eyelid injuries yields the most satisfactory results, and meticulous repair is essential. However, in certain cases, a secondary repair can also provide significant functional and cosmetic improvements.

Orbital Trauma
This has been discussed in the section on orbital fractures.

■ SUGGESTED READING
1. Grover AK, Kaur S. Principles of oculoplastic surgery. In: Grover AK (Ed). Oculoplastic Surgery Practical Guidelines: CME series No. 5. New Delhi: All India Ophthalmological Society; 2001. pp. 11-4.
2. Herman DC, Bartley GB, Walker RC (1987). The Treatment of Animal Bite Injuries of the Eye and Ocular Adnexa. Ophthalmic Plast Reconstr Surg. 1987;3(4):237-41.
3. Shukla A, Singh M, Garg A. Epidemiological Profiling of Mechanical Ocular Trauma and Analysis Using Proposed New Classification for Ocular Adnexal Injuries. Beyoglu Eye J. 2021;6(2):102-7.

9.16 Newer Techniques in the Management of Orbital and Ocular Tumors

Santosh G Honavar, Rolika Bansal
Oculoplasty and Ocular Oncology, Centre for Sight, Hyderabad

■ INTRODUCTION
Orbital and ocular tumors include benign and malignant tumors ranging from involvement of the eyelids, ocular surface, uvea, retina, orbit, and adnexal structures. It is mandatory for the ocular oncologists to reach an accurate diagnosis by follow stepwise tailored management approach for the patients, i.e., clinical diagnosis, radiological investigations, histopathological confirmation, and adjuvant therapy as appropriate. Over the years, ocular oncology has evolved from radical measures for orbital and ocular tumors to a spectrum of conservative approaches, with excellent outcomes, pertaining to the revolutions in management techniques. In this chapter, we shall be discussing the newer techniques for treating the orbital and ocular tumors.

■ PERCUTANEOUS SCLEROTHERAPY
In cases with orbital lymphangioma and orbital dermoid cysts (especially dumbbell dermoids) where surgical intervention may not suffice due to diffuse presentation, posterior presentation or a possibility of functional deficit; sclerotherapy can be utilized. Sclerotherapy refers to treatment with sclerosing agents, i.e., Picibanil (freeze-dried

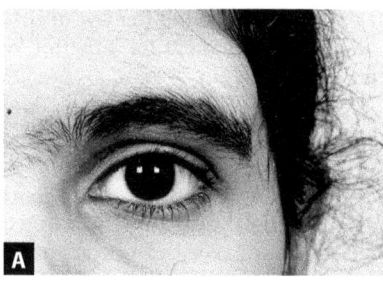 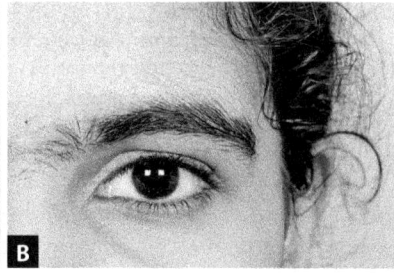

Figs. 9.16.1A and B: (A) Preoperative clinical image of an 18-year-old female presenting with an orbital dumbbell dermoid cyst at the superotemporal quadrant for 5 years, which was managed with foam sclerotherapy with sodium tetradecyl sulfate; (B) Excellent local tumor control was achieved at a final follow-up of 6 years with aesthetic outcomes.

biological product derived from *Streptococcus pyogenes*), sodium tetradecyl sulfate (STDS) (anionic surfactant), ethanol, ethanolamine oleate (combination of organic base and oleic acid), doxycycline (tetracycline), bleomycin A2 (antibiotic isolated from *Streptomyces verticillus*) and pingyangmycin (bleomycin A5).[1] The choice of sclerosing agent depends on the underlying pathology. Sclerosing agents act as tissue irritants leading to vascular thrombosis and endothelial damage causing endofibrosis and vascular obliteration. The therapeutic response usually occurs by 4–6 weeks.

Orbital dermoid cysts respond extremely well to foam sclerotherapy with STDS thus catering to the aesthetic requirements of the patients **(Figs. 9.16.1A and B)**. Often repeat injections of STDS may be required. Sclerotherapy in orbital lymphangioma (diffuse lesions or wrapped around neurovascular structures) can be done by injection Picibanil or injection bleomycin with or without cyst aspiration, along with CT guidance. Often minimal side effects such as inflammation and pain at site of injection or low-grade fever occur which resolve over few days without affecting the final outcome.[2] Sclerotherapy can be used either as monotherapy or as an adjunct to surgery, thus providing, excellent long-term response with low recurrence rates.

MULTILEVEL INCISIONAL BIOPSY

A systematic approach to the management of orbital tumors highly depends on accurate diagnosis. Therefore, it is warranted to perform a multilevel incisional biopsy with or without intraoperative frozen section; on lesions which are suspected to be malignant, are poorly localized, infiltrative, and associated with crucial structures which may cause functional deficit. The issues such as unrepresentative sample, nonuniform pathology, or tissue reaction get eliminated if the approach is schematic multilevel incisional biopsy, therefore eliminating misdiagnosis.

MINIMALLY INVASIVE SURGICAL APPROACH

After a detailed clinicoradiological analysis, the well-localized and circumscribed, benign or malignant orbital tumors can be approached by minimally invasive techniques for excision biopsy. These lesions are noninfiltrative without involvement of crucial structures and therefore carry minimal risk of functional deficit. Anterior orbitotomy by transconjunctival approach can be done by the following incisions:
- Medial perilimbal—Galbraith and Sullivan
- Lateral perilimbal
- Transcaruncular—Balch and Goldberg
- Lateral canthal
- Inferior forniceal with lateral canthotomy—McCord and Moses
- Inferior forniceal with transcaruncular approach

Transconjunctival approach **(Fig. 9.16.2)** provides a panoramic view of the orbit which can be utilized for tumors located in all quadrants except for superior lesions as that would lead to breach of the forniceal attachment of the levator, thus leading to complications like postoperative ptosis.

■ ORBITOTOMY WITHOUT BONE CUT

Lateral orbitotomy without bone cut is currently a preferred technique to minimize postoperative morbidity with better aesthetic outcomes, especially in lesions with a suspicion of lacrimal gland tumors, to avoid micrometastasis and temporal fossa infiltration postoperatively.

■ STEREOTACTIC EXTERNAL BEAM RADIOTHERAPY

Stereotactic external beam radiotherapy (EBRT) in ocular oncology refers to treatment of orbital tumors with an external radiation source which can be linear accelerator-derived, proton-beam, neutron, Gamma Knife, or intensity-modulated radiotherapy.[3] Radiation causes either direct damage to deoxyribonucleic acid (DNA) or interacts with the nearby molecules leading to free-radical formation.[4] EBRT can be preoperative to reduce the size of the tumor or postoperative as adjuvant therapy to the tumor bed and adjacent structures. The radiation depends on several factors, i.e., clinicoradiological diagnosis, histopathology, tumor site, the involvement of adjacent structures, and the radiation technique used.[5] This is an expensive form of treatment and even though the procedure has been widely accepted in developed countries, in the recent times, it has blended well in developing countries as well, with high acceptance by ocular oncologists as well the patients. This technique requires a well-crafted team including the surgeon, radiologist, histopathologist, radiation oncologist, as well as a radiation physicist.

Posterior benign tumors which are surgically inaccessible like cavernous hemangioma causing functional deficit **(Fig. 9.16.3)** can also be treated with creative techniques like Gamma Knife stereotactic EBRT. For example, in the **Figure 9.16.3**, the patient was treated with 4,000 cGy in 20 fractions, i.e., 200 cGy/fr. EBRT thus leads to reduction in tumor size and extent; and also causes lesser recurrence rates in malignant lesions with excellent outcomes.

A newer technique, i.e., after-loaded interstitial brachytherapy has also been utilized to provide radiation only to the bed of the tumor after excising the tumor. In this form of

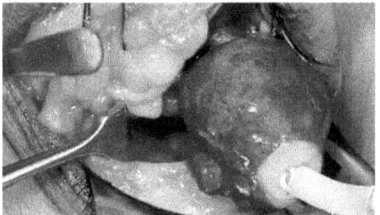

Fig. 9.16.2: Panoramic view achieved by the minimally invasive transconjunctival approach in a patient with cavernous hemangioma followed by excision biopsy with total tumor control, with lesser morbidity and excellent aesthetic outcomes.

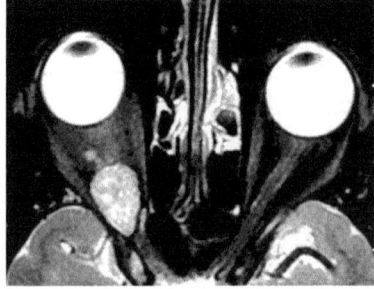

Fig. 9.16.3: Magnetic resonance imaging of the orbit showing a heterogeneous mass at the orbital apex, hyperintense on T2 with a flow void, in favor of the diagnosis of a posterior cavernous hemangioma. This lesion was pressing onto the optic nerve and was causing restriction of the visual field without affecting the best corrected visual acuity. Considering the inoperability, it was treated with stereotactic external beam radiotherapy (EBRT).

targeted therapy, silicone tubes are surgically attached to the target area and the patient is sent to the radiologist for brachytherapy sessions with iridium-192.

PLAQUE BRACHYTHERAPY

Plaque brachytherapy is an evolving yet effective globe and vision-sparing modality for the treatment of surface malignancies such as ocular surface squamous neoplasia, conjunctival melanoma, and intraocular tumors such as retinoblastoma, choroidal hemangioma, choroidal melanoma, and choroidal metastasis.[6,7] This is achieved by transscleral irradiation of the tumor base with a radioactive implant. The American Brachytherapy Society (ABS) along with the collaboration of the international multicenter Ophthalmic Oncology Task Force (OOTF) was assembled to reach a consensus regarding establishing practice guidelines and setting standards of care for intraocular tumors.[8-10] This technique provides the advantage of focal radiation thus eliminating the damage to the adjacent structures, minimal periorbital tissue damage, and absence of cosmetic disfigurement owing to lack of retarded bone growth as seen in EBRT. Thus, it reduces the risk of metastasis and with the recent advances it provides a shorter duration of treatment. A well-planned dosimetry for plaque brachytherapy results in achieving local tumor control and excellent prognosis **(Figs. 9.16.4A and B)**. The advent of indigenous plaque brachytherapy by the Bhabha Atomic Research Centre (BARC), in India, has revolutionized the outcomes in a cost-effective manner thus ensuring globe salvage; reducing morbidity and mortality; and avoiding cosmetic disfigurement.

MULTIMODAL MANAGEMENT

In several ocular tumors, multimodal management must be followed, i.e., a combination of debulking/en bloc excision/complete excision by surgical intervention, chemotherapy, and extended field stereotactic EBRT. This is useful for the malignant tumors with orbital retinoblastoma, rhabdomyosarcoma, adenoid cystic carcinoma, orbital squamous cell carcinoma, and orbital sebaceous gland carcinoma.[11] The sequence of intervention depends on the underlying etiology and the clinicoradiological assessment. This leads to good local tumor control, eye salvage, less morbidity with optimal functional preservation, higher survival, and minimized risk of systemic metastasis. Even in cases with recurrent lesions, the outcome with multimodal management has proven to be excellent.

CONCLUSION

A logical approach to the orbital tumors starting from accurate timely diagnosis with clinicoradiological diagnosis, meticulous planning, systemic evaluation, histopathological confirmation, and adjuvant therapy helps in optimizing the outcome.

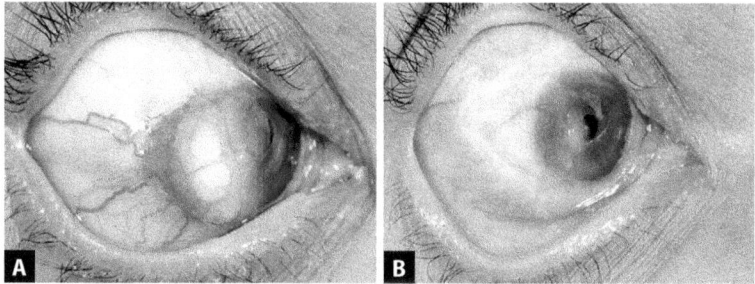

Figs. 9.16.4A and B: (A) A clinical picture of a patient with right eye ocular surface squamous neoplasia with corneoscleral invasion, who was treated with surgical excision with 4 mm clinically clear margins, lamellar sclerectomy, alcohol keratoepitheliectomy, followed by primary plaque brachytherapy and surface reconstruction with amniotic membrane graft and glue; (B) After 6 years, complete tumor control was achieved with no recurrence.

The newer advances have contributed significantly, in reducing the mortality and morbidity, and providing optimal functional outcome, with better aesthetic results and rehabilitation.

■ REFERENCES

1. Lam SC, Yuen HKL. Medical and sclerosing agents in the treatment of orbital lymphatic malformations: what's new? Curr Opin Ophthalmol. 2019;30(5):380-5.
2. Fasching G, Dollinger C, Spendel S, Tepeneu NF. Treatment of lymphangiomas by means of sclerotherapy with OK-432 (Picibanil®) is safe and effective—A retrospective case series. Ann Med Surg (Lond). 2022;81:104531.
3. Finger PT. Radiation therapy for orbital tumors: concepts, current use, and ophthalmic radiation side effects. Surv Ophthalmol. 2009;54(5):545-68.
4. Hall EJ. Radiobiology for the Radiologist. Philadelphia: Lippincott Williams & Wilkins; 2000. pp. 12-3, 439-42.
5. Marchand V, Dendale R. Normal tissue tolerance to external beam radiation therapy: eye structures. Cancer Radiother. 2010;14(4-5):277-83.
6. Walsh-Conway N, Conway RM. Plaque brachytherapy for the management of ocular surface malignancies with corneoscleral invasion. Clin Exp Ophthalmol. 2009;37(6):577-83.
7. Rao R, Honavar SG, Lahane S, Mulay K, Reddy VP. Histopathology-guided management of ocular surface squamous neoplasia with corneal stromal or scleral invasion using ruthenium-106 plaque brachytherapy. Br J Ophthalmol. 2023;107(5):621-6.
8. American Brachytherapy Society—Ophthalmic Oncology Task Force. The American Brachytherapy Society consensus guidelines for plaque brachytherapy of uveal melanoma and retinoblastoma. Brachytherapy. 2014;13(1):1-14.
9. Jampol LM, Moy CS, Murray TG, Reynolds SM, Albert DM, Schachat AP, et al. The COMS Randomized Trial of Iodine 125 Brachytherapy for Choroidal Melanoma: IV. Local Treatment Failure and Enucleation in the First 5 Years after Brachytherapy. COMS Report No. 19. Ophthalmology. 2020;127(4S):S148-57.
10. Simpson ER, Gallie B, Laperrierre N, Beiki-Ardakani A, Kivelä T, Raivio V, et al. The American Brachytherapy Society consensus guidelines for plaque brachytherapy of uveal melanoma and retinoblastoma. Brachytherapy. 2014;13(1):1-14.
11. Manjandavida FP, Honavar SG, Murthy R, Das S, Vemuganti GK, Mulay K, et al. Does Multimodal Treatment Improve Eye and Life Salvage in Adenoid Cystic Carcinoma of the Lacrimal Gland? Ophthalmic Plast Reconstr Surg. 2022;38(4):348-54.

9.17 Medical Management of Thyroid Eye Disease

Ashok Kumar Grover, Rwituja Thomas, Summy Bhatnagar
Vision Eye Centres, New Delhi
thomas.rwituja@gmail.com

■ ISSUES IN THYROID EYE DISEASE

Graves' orbitopathy or ophthalmopathy is an autoimmune condition. The disease process leads to proptosis due to activation of orbital fibroblasts. The proptosis is unilateral/bilateral. The disorder is also characterized by enlargement of extraocular muscles, fatty, and connective tissue volume. Due to this patient complains of:
- Irritation in the eye and a gritty sensation
- Photophobia
- Dry eye
- Discomfort
- Forward protrusion of the eye

When the disease process advances patient may complain of
- Retrobulbar pain (spontaneous/on movement)
- Double vision
- Blurred vision

Thyroid eye disease (TED) leads to eyelid retraction which is the most common presenting sign present in 90% of patients. Lid lag and lid edema is also present. Involvement of extraocular muscles leads to ocular misalignment and diplopia. Compressive optic neuropathy is an ocular emergency which occurs in <5% patients leading to fulminant visual loss.

Dry eye and exposure keratopathy resulting from proptosis and lagophthalmos, remain the most common and treatable conditions.

CLINICAL EVALUATION

This includes identification and quantifying the extent of ocular and orbital involvement:
- Lid lag
- Lateral flare
- Lid retraction (superior scleral show needs to be measured) or ptosis
- Lid edema (more frequently in the upper lid)
- Lagophthalmos **(Fig. 9.17.1)**
- Proptosis **(Fig. 9.17.2)** (Hertel's/Leudde's exophthalmometry)
- Motility restriction (quantification of restriction)—**Figure 9.17.3**
- Raised intraocular pressure (Goldmann applanation tonometry or Tonopen in opacified corneas)

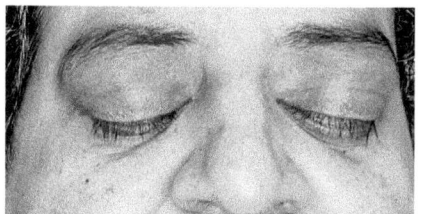

Fig. 9.17.1: Lagophthalmos.

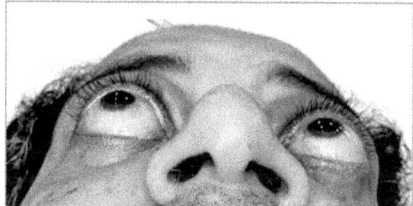

Fig. 9.17.2: Worm's-eye view to evaluate exophthalmos.

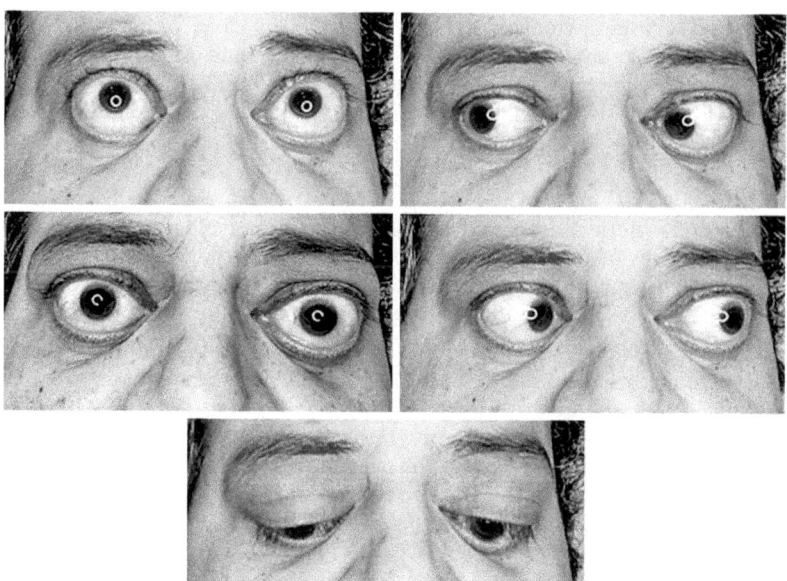

Fig. 9.17.3: Quantifying motility.

- Congestion
- Chemosis
- Exposure keratopathy/corneal ulceration
- Dysthyroid optic neuropathy with resultant visual field disturbances and diminution of vision

Scoring systems are used world-wide in order to decide on initiation of therapy.

Clinical Activity Score

Assign a value of 1 for each identified characteristic.

Symptoms
- Score 1 for the presence of pain or pressure in a periorbital or retroorbital distribution.
- Score 1 for experiencing pain during upward, downward, or lateral eye movement.

Signs
- Score 1 for swelling of lids.
- Score 1 for redness lids.
- Score 1 for conjunctival congestion.
- Score 1 for chemosis.
- Score 1 for inflammation observed in the caruncle or plica.

Changes
- Score 1 for an increase in measured proptosis by >2 mm over 1–3 months.
- Score 1 for a reduction in the limit of ocular motility by >8° over 1–3 months.
- Score 1 for a decrease in visual acuity by two Snellen chart lines over 1–3 months.

Clinical Activity Score >4
Has a positive predictive value of 80% and a negative predictive value of 64%.

■ INVESTIGATIONS

Thyroid eye disease diagnosis is mostly clinical based on the characteristic clinical picture and associated systemic thyroid disease.

The diagnosis may be supplemented by laboratory tests and orbital imaging.

Laboratory tests including thyroid hormone levels (FT3, FT4), thyroid-stimulating hormone (TSH), anti-thyroid antibodies (TRAb) and thyroid peroxidase antibody test (anti-TPO) are useful in making a diagnosis.

Imaging

Ultrasonography: Both A-scan and B-scan transocular echograms are capable of visualizing contents of the bony orbit and measuring the degree of increase in size of each rectus muscle. One benefit of this technique is its cost-effectiveness, absence of any ionizing rays, and short procedure duration.

Computed tomography (CT): A non-contrast CT image can help to differentiate thyroid eye disease from any localized lesions. It clearly delineates the spindle-shaped muscle bellies, which increased in size, along with the sparing of the tendons. Additionally, we can assess crowding of the muscles with respect to the optic nerve at the apex, which helps to decide which areas of the bony orbit need to be tackled. It also gives an idea of the fat volume, so that we can decide on fat decompression, as well as the bone, which helps to outline the amount of bone in each wall that may need to be drilled in order for bony decompression to be completed.

Magnetic resonance imaging (MRI): MRI can identify fusiform rectus enlargement and expansion of orbital fat. It is also useful in evaluating the water content in muscles and other soft tissues, which may correspond to active inflammation.

TABLE 9.17.1: Basic NOSPECS classification.

NOSPECS classification	
N	No symptoms or signs
O	Only signs
S	Soft tissue involvement
P	Proptosis
E	Extraocular muscle involvement
C	Corneal involvement
S	Sight loss due to optic nerve compression

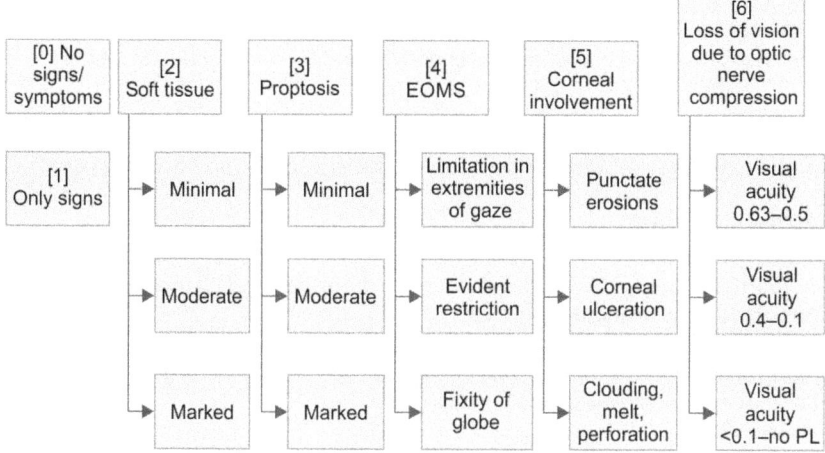

Fig. 9.17.4: Modified NOSPECS classification.

■ MANAGEMENT

Severity of Grave's orbitopathy classification is given in **Table 9.17.2**.

Both quitting smoking and maintaining a normal thyroid function contribute to preventing the worsening of the condition and reducing the duration of active disease. Additional lifestyle changes, such as reducing sodium intake to minimize water retention and tissue swelling, and sleeping with the head elevated to decrease swelling in the eye area, can also be beneficial. Oral nonsteroidal anti-inflammatory drugs (NSAIDs) can be used to manage pain around the eyes. Moreover, the use of selenium has demonstrated significant advantages in individuals with mild, noninflammatory orbitopathy.

The treatment of symptoms of thyroid eye disease is taking care of vision threatening conditions such as exposure keratopathy and compressive optic neuropathy. The protrusion of globe and lid retraction leads to dry eye and exposure keratopathy. Conservative therapy is the mainstay in mild symptoms. For corneal exposure, lubricants, taping and protective shields can be tried. Frequent lubrication with gel ointment at night is useful. If symptoms worsen tarsorrhaphy may be needed.

Eyelid retraction is one of the most common diagnostic signs of thyroid eye disease. Upper and lower eyelid retraction can both be present, which former being more common. Lid retraction may threaten vision in addition to esthetic alterations in the patients which affect the quality of life. Lid retraction is present in active disease as well as inactive disease. The treatment modalities can be divided into nonsurgical and surgical depending on the activity of the disease various modalities can be considered.

TABLE 9.17.2: Classification of Grave's orbitopathy as per European Group on Graves' Orbitopathy (EUGOGO).

Stage	Features
Mild GO	Minor lid retraction <2 mm
	Exophthalmos <3 mm above normal
	No or intermittent diplopia and corneal exposure responsive to lubricants
Moderate-to-severe GO	Lid retraction ≥2 mm
	Exophthalmos ≥3 mm above normal
	Inconstant or constant diplopia
Sight-threatening GO	Dysthyroid optic neuropathy and/or corneal breakdown

Source: Adapted from Bartalena L, Kahaly GJ, Baldeschi L, Dayan CM, Eckstein A, Marcocci C, et al. The 2021 European Group on Graves' Orbitopathy (EUGOGO) clinical practice guidelines for the medical management of Graves' orbitopathy. Eur J Endocrinol. 2021;185:G43-67.

The nonsurgical management is minimally invasive and provides rapid relief of the symptoms of the patients who wants to wait for the surgery or cannot undergo one.

Treatment Outline
- Smoking cessation
- Supportive measures such as lubricating eye drops, gels and lid taping, tarsorrhaphy
- Anti-thyroid medications
- Intravenous steroids (methylprednisolone)
- Neuromodulators, hyaluronic acid fillers
- Local triamcinolone acetonide injection
- Biological agents
- Radiotherapy

Systemic Steroids
According to EUGOGO guidelines, patients diagnosed with thyroid orbitopathy can receive a maximum cumulative dose of 8 g of intravenous steroids per treatment cycle. However, individuals with recent viral hepatitis, hepatic dysfunction, severe cardiovascular disease, or uncontrolled hypertension should not be administered intravenous glucocorticoids. It is important to ensure that diabetes is well controlled before initiating therapy.

There are two recommended regimens for steroid administration:
1. *Moderate dose:* This involves initiating treatment with a starting dose of 500 mg of intravenous methylprednisolone once weekly for duration of 6 weeks. Subsequently, the dosage is reduced to 250 mg once weekly for another 6 weeks. This regimen is suitable for patients with moderate cases of thyroid orbitopathy.
2. *High dose:* For severe cases, the treatment starts with a higher dose of 750 mg of intravenous methylprednisolone once weekly for 6 weeks. Following this, the dosage is reduced to 500 mg once weekly for an additional 6 weeks.

It is essential to follow these regimens as per medical guidance and individual patient needs.

Neuromodulators
Botulinum toxin injection in lid retraction patients who do not want to undergo surgery or in severe lid retraction can be very useful. Chemodenervation works on the

Müller's muscle more than the levator muscle causing lowering of the lids which help in relieving the symptoms in patients of exposure keratitis and conjunctivitis. It is more helpful in inactive disease showing more decrease in palpebral fissure height than patients with active disease. Transient ptosis is the most common complication which can be dealt with low volume and high concentration of injection techniques.

Hyaluronic Acid Fillers

Hyaluronic acid fillers are now the most commonly used noninvasive methods for both upper and lower eyelids retraction. The fillers help in lowering the upper lids when injected in subconjunctival space and lengthen the lower lid retractors in lower lids relieving the retraction. Fillers were proven to be more effective in patients who had active disease at the time of injection. Patients who underwent laparotomy surgery and had residual retraction can be given fillers postsurgery resulting in better lid position and contour.

Triamcinolone Acetonide Injections

Injectable glucocorticoids in the eyelids work via different mechanisms involving both Müller's muscle and the levator muscle. The net result is its anti-inflammatory and immunosuppressive effects. Triamcinolone acetonide is five times more potent than hydrocortisone. The steroid injection is more effective in active disease. The complications include intraocular pressure (IOP) elevation, superior sulcus deformity, high crease, transient ptosis and thinning of eyelids including both skin and tarsal plate. Intraorbital injections have also been tried with variable results. This would require further studies to quantify efficacy.

■ BIOLOGICALS

Rituximab: Rituximab is a monoclonal antibody that targets CD20, a marker found on B-cells. By depleting these CD20+ B-cells, it decreases the synthesis of pathogenic antibodies. The infusion dosage is two 1,000 mg/m^2 injections 2 weeks apart or 375 mg/m^2 injections weekly for 4 weeks. The decrease in B-cell numbers is noted within the first week itself, with reduction lasting up to 9 months. This however, does not affect the level of immunoglobulin M (IgM) antibodies in the body, thus preventing severe adverse effects. The level of anti-thyroid peroxidase (anti-TPO) antibodies was found to be reduced after the infusion. The level of the anti-thyrotropin receptor antibodies (TRAb) was also found to be altered, however, only for the fraction of stimulating TRAb that are pathogenic. Rituximab has resulted in improved CAS, but may result in occasional adverse effects such as transient fever and chills related to the infusion. Severe and rare adverse effects include worsening of TED and aggravation of inflammatory bowel disease.

Tocilizumab: Tocilizumab has been studied in cases with moderate to severe TED with cases resistant to systemic glucocorticoids. It targets the IL-6 receptor and thus inhibits the expression of thyroid stimulating hormone (TSH) receptors in fibroblasts located within the orbit. It has shown reduction in CAS and has shown a reduction of proptosis. Tocilizumab is administered intravenously at a dose of 4–8 mg/kg every 4 weeks. The efficacy and safety of tocilizumab have been demonstrated in numerous large-scale global studies for the treatment of rheumatoid arthritis, and it was first approved for TED in Japan in April 2008. Adverse effects include, neutropenia and hyperlipidemia. At present a multicentric study in ongoing in Italy, the results of which are expected soon.

Teprotumumab: This monoclonal antibody works by inhibiting the insulin growth factor-1 receptor (IGF-1R). It has been studied in two randomized controlled trials that are the OPTIC and its extension, the OPTIC-X. This was conducted in patients with active and moderate to severe TED. It showed a significant and rapid efficacy with a decrease in Clinical Activity Score (CAS), decrease in proptosis, improvement in diplopia, and improved quality of life. In the extension trial, patients who previously received the placebo were now treated with Teprotumumab, who also showed a very favorable response with 89% having some form of proptosis reduction. Some patients needed either retreatment or surgical management. It is now Food and Drug Administration (FDA) approved and has promising results in patients with chronic TED. Side effects include muscle spasms, hyperglycemia, hearing loss (variable degrees) and have been deemed severely teratogenic. Due its high cost and regulatory reasons, it is not yet available in countries other than the United States. Long-term studies are needed to study its usefulness in avoidance of surgery and longevity.

Other Biologicals

Several medications that have been tried and investigated for the treatment of thyroid orbitopathy include Cyclosporine, azathioprine, mycophenolate mofetil, and belimumab. Studies for secukinumab, hydroxychloroquine, sirolimus, tamsulosin, bimatoprost, and doxycycline in TED are ongoing.

Radiotherapy is also a viable second-line treatment option for moderate-to-severe and active thyroid orbitopathy, particularly in cases where there is restricted extraocular motility and severe proptosis. It is typically administered in conjunction with intravenous steroids.

■ SUGGESTED READING

1. Antonio AA, Santos RN, Abariga SA. Tocilizumab for giant cell arteritis. Cochrane Database Syst Rev. 2021;8(8):CD013484.
2. Bahn RS. Emerging pharmacotherapy for treatment of Graves' disease. Expert Rev Clin Pharmacol. 2012;5:605-7.
3. Bartalena L, Kahaly GJ, Baldeschi L, Dayan CM, Eckstein A, Marcocci C, et al. The 2021 European Group on Graves' orbitopathy (EUGOGO) clinical practice guidelines for the medical management of Graves' orbitopathy. Eur J Endocrinol. 2021;185:G43-67.
4. Chen H, Mester T, Raychaudhuri N, Kauh CY, Gupta S, Smith TJ, et al. Teprotumumab, an IGF-1R blocking monoclonal antibody inhibits TSH and IGF-1 action in fibrocytes. J Clin Endocrinol Metabol. 2014;99(9):E1635-40.
5. Costa PG, Saraiva FP, Pereira IC, Monteiro ML, Matayoshi S. Comparative study of Botox injection treatment for upper eyelid retraction with 6-month follow-up in patients with thyroid eye disease in the congestive or fibrotic stage. Eye (Lond). 2009;23:767-73.
6. Douglas RS, Francis-Sedlak M, Hold RJ, Dailey RA, Kossler AN. Real-World Adherence with Teprotumumab in TED. ASOPRS Fall Scientific Symposium; 2021.
7. Douglas RS, Gupta S. The pathophysiology of thyroid eye disease: Implications for immunotherapy. Curr Opin Ophthalmol. 2011;22(5):385-90.
8. Douglas RS, Kahaly GJ, Patel A, Sile S, Thompson EHZ, Perdok, R, et al. Teprotumumab for the treatment of active thyroid eye disease. N Engl J Med. 2020;382(4);341-52.
9. Dutton JJ. Anatomic considerations in thyroid eye disease. Ophthalmic Plast Reconstr Surg. 2018;34:S7-12.
10. Goldberg RA, Fiaschetti D. Filling the periorbital hollows with hyaluronic acid gel: Initial experience with 244 injections. Ophthalmic Plast Reconstr Surg. 2006;22:335-41.
11. Grisolia AB, Couso RC, Matayoshi S, Douglas RS, Briceño CA. Quality of life in Graves' ophthalmopathy. Best Pract Res Clin Endocrinol Metab. 2012;26:359-70.
12. Hegedüs L, Smith TJ, Douglas RS, Nielsen CH. Targeted biological therapies for Graves' disease and thyroid-associated ophthalmopathy. Focus on B-cell depletion with rituximab. Clin Endocrinol. 2011;74(1)1-8.
13. Kaneko A. Tocilizumab in rheumatoid arthritis: efficacy, safety and its place in therapy. Ther Adv Chronic Dis. 2013;4(1):14-21.
14. Kazim M, Gold KG. A review of surgical techniques to correct upper eyelid retraction associated with thyroid eye disease. Curr Opin Ophthalmol. 2011;22:391-3.
15. Lane LC, Cheetham TD, Perros P, Pearce SHS. New therapeutic horizons for graves' hyperthyroidism. Endocr Rev. 2020;41(6):873-84.
16. Li H, Yang L, Song Y, Zhao X, Sun C, Zhang L, et al. Comparative effectiveness of different treatment modalities for active, moderate-to-severe Graves' orbitopathy: a systematic review and network meta-analysis. Acta Ophthalmol. 2022;100(6):e1189-e1198.

17. Morgenstern KE, Evanchan J, Foster JA, Cahill KV, Burns JA, Holck DE, et al. Botulinum toxin type a for dysthyroid upper eyelid retraction. Ophthalmic Plast Reconstr Surg. 2004;20: 181-5.
18. Shen S, Chan A, Sfikakis PP, Hsiu Ling AL, Detorakis ET, Boboridis KG, et al. B-cell targeted therapy with rituximab for thyroid eye disease: closer to the clinic. Surv Ophthalmol. 2013;58(3):252-65.
19. Wiersinga WM. Quality of life in Graves' ophthalmopathy. Best Pract Res Clin Endocrinol Metab. 2012;26:359-70.
20. Young SM, Kim YD, Lang SS, Woo KI. Transconjunctival triamcinolone injection for upper lid retraction in thyroid eye disease – A new injection method. Ophthalmic Plast Reconstr Surg. 2018;34:587-93.

9.18 Image-guided Orbital Surgery

Kasturi Bhattacharjee, Vatsalya Venkatraman
Sri Sankardeva Nethralaya, Guwahati
kasturibhattcharjee44@hotmail.com, vatsalyavenkatraman24@gmail.com

■ INTRODUCTION

The role of image-guided surgery has been successfully established in several surgical domains of the head and neck region.

It elucidates a system comprising of hardware and software that utilize either infrared cameras or electromagnetic fields to enable the amalgamation of preoperative and/or intraoperative subject imaging with three-dimensional real-time localization of the surgical instruments on a computer screen in the operating room.

Its application in the fields of neurosurgery, skull base surgery, and sinus surgery are well known.

In the context of oculoplastic orbital surgeries, navigation serves to guide the operating surgeon in identifying bony landmarks, planning complex reconstructions with adequate symmetry, precisely localizing orbital tumors, and its bony and soft tissue relations to the surrounding structures.

■ PRINCIPLE OF IMAGE-GUIDED NAVIGATION SYSTEM

- In literature, the working of this image-guided navigation has been compared to the Global Positioning System (GPS) in order to simplify its understanding.
- The radiological scans of either computed tomography (CT) or magnetic resonance imaging (MRI) performed under the navigation protocol are loaded onto the console for isolation of the target area.
- The signal emitted from the hand-held pointer shows the surgeon's intraoperative position with respect to the fixed patient tracker.
- This aids the surgeon in easy maneuvering without any inadvertent injury to the surrounding tissues.
- The end point of the surgery is said to have reached when prefixed target and the mobile stylet placed at the tissue level overlap.
- Intraoperative navigation functions on the basic concept of stereotaxy which involves the use of external reference markers for location of internal surgical landmarks
- There are two such tracking modalities available:
  1. *Electromagnetic navigation:* The dynamic reference frame (DRF) is mounted onto the head of the patient, an electromagnetic field is created by the same around the surgical site and the movement of the navigation probe in relation to it provides the accurate location. While it is easy to set up, less expensive, and provides adequate surface registration, it is less accurate, has a narrower field, and it is associated with ferromagnetic interference of surgical instruments.

2. *Optical navigation:* Light sources such as infrared cameras emit beams which reflect the location of the probe using optical sensor thus making it more accurate. It has a larger field and offers both bony and soft tissue registration, but is more expensive, line of sight interference occurs and pinning of the DRF to the skull post is necessary.

■ INDICATIONS OF IMAGE GUIDANCE IN ORBITAL SURGERIES

- Orbital bony decompression in thyroid eye disease (TED)
- *Facial trauma:*
  - Internal orbital fracture
  - Midfacial fracture
- Orbital tumor resection
- Optic canal decompression
- Orbital foreign body extraction
- Endoscopic orbital and lacrimal surgeries

Orbital Bony Decompression in Thyroid Eye Disease

- Orbital decompression in TED is targeted at proptosis reduction or alleviating dysthyroid optic neuropathy.
- This can be attained by either thinning or removing the lateral wall, medial wall, orbital floor, and/or orbital fat.
- Navigation is useful in identifying bony landmarks for anatomical identification and channelized decompression.
- The inferomedial strut forms the lower boundary of the medial wall which is usually retained in order to sustain the integrity of the craniofacial skeleton while anterior and posterior ethmoidal arteries demarcate the upper border of the medial wall to avoid encroachment on the cribriform plate.
- The thickness of the greater wing of sphenoid can be quantified in order to estimate the extent of lateral wall decompression required.
- Orbital apex shows crowding in cases of compressive optic neuropathy in TED. This is an area having vital structures and navigation aids in safe steering through the apex.
- Preoperative marking and intraoperative correlation of the target areas aid to determine the end point of decompression.
- Postoperative and preoperative CT scans of the orbits can be compared to assess change in volume and globe position which measures the adequacy of decompression.

Facial Trauma

Internal Orbital Fracture

- Challenging orbital fractures include large orbital floor fractures with loss of posterior ledge and combined orbital floor and medial wall fractures.
- The goal of orbital wall fracture repair is to reinstate the normalcy of orbital structure and volume after meticulous repositioning of herniated contents back into the orbit and introducing an auto or allogenic barrier such as a plate to recreate the preexisting wall.
- Image guidance in the preoperative period can be utilized for virtual plate sizing and fitting or for designing a patient-specific implant (PSI). In case of unilateral fractures, the contralateral unaffected orbit is either manually or automatically segmented and mirrored onto the fractured orbit to yield a theoretical shape forming the necessary skeleton for a PSI.

- Intraoperatively, navigation aids the surgeon to delineate displaced orbital contents, adjacent important neurovascular bundles and the location of optic nerve to curtail unwarranted surgical manipulation, ensure appropriate enophthalmos correction, and relieve preoperative motility restriction.

Midfacial Fracture
- Complex orbitofacial fractures include zygomaticomaxillary complex, naso-orbito-ethmoid complex, Le Fort type fractures, and pan facial fractures.
- These fractures result in flattening or displacement of anterior malar prominence and there is incomplete visualization of the entire zygoma through transorbital approach which renders the challenge of precise reconstruction.
- Image guidance allows for preoperative three-dimensional CT-based reconstruction of the skull which helps plan for a functional and aesthetic midface restoration post trauma.
- Inadequate primary repair can increase the facial width from outward bending of the zygomatic arch and appearance of persistent enophthalmos due to inferiorly shifted malar eminence.
- Computer-assisted surgery also helps circumvent hurdles of delayed fracture repair such as malunion, nonunion, loss of surrounding soft tissue, callous formation, bony resorption, and fibrosis by accurately recognizing osteotomy sites and ensuring proper reduction despite the remodeling ensued.

Orbital Tumor Resection
- Navigation system can be used to fashion orbital bone flaps which are essential when large orbital tumors have to be excised. The margins of the tumor are defined using the feature of autosegmentation preoperatively. Tumor dimensions are noted both in the X and Y axes. Based on this, we can determine the size of the bone flap that needs to be raised. Intraoperatively, the site and size of the lesion can be seen on the console which guides the surgeon to the placement of the horizontal osteotomies. Postoperatively the appropriate repositioning of the flap can be gauged and any residual enophthalmos due to large bony defects left after tumor excision can be assessed for possible symmetrical secondary reconstruction.
- Dangerous zones can be identified preoperatively using the angiographic radiological scans and helps circumvent accidental trauma to the adjacent neurovascular bundles.
- When compared to soft tissue lesions, the spatial location of bony lesions is better with the navigation system whereby sites of thinning or secondary hyperostosis such as in the case of meningiomas can be accurately marked to avoid cerebrospinal fluid leakage or intracranial injury.
- To improve the visualization of soft tissue lesions, a CT and MRI fusion can be done on the console which is particularly useful in apical lesions to preserve visual function.

Optic Canal Decompression
- Stereotactic navigation technology provides enhanced precision and protection by elucidating intraoperative position and orientation of the optic canal anatomy for identification of impinging bone fragments, optic nerve edema, or optic nerve sheath hematoma during optic canal decompression for traumatic optic neuropathy.
- Along with the bony features, the vascular components can be highlighted with differential color coding in the navigation software on the CT angiogram, which acts as a guide intraoperatively to avoid damage to vital structures.
- A three-dimensional reconstruction can provide information regarding concurrent orbital wall fractures and a single stage surgery involving optic canal decompression and orbital wall reconstruction can be judiciously planned.

Orbital Foreign Body Extraction
- Improved image localization of intraorbital foreign body using the navigation system helps in incision site selection, especially in cases of delayed presentation.
- Using three-dimensional model of the patient, the nearest surface landmark to the foreign body can be measured to optimize the extraction procedure by chalking a surgical path and minimize collateral damage and foreign body displacement.
- Depth estimation of the foreign body in case of it being lodged in the orbital apex aids in safe removal safeguarding the optic nerve and apical vessels.

Endoscopic Orbital and Lacrimal Surgeries
- Navigation guidance accurately delineates the lacrimal sac and ensures correct resection of the medial wall of the sac avoiding long-term failure post endonasal dacryocystorhinostomy.
- Computer assistance intraoperatively tracks the surgeon's movements enabling him/her with real-time visualization of the patient's anatomy guaranteeing maximal tumor removal.
- Stereotaxy identifies bony anomalies along the lacrimal drainage system present congenitally or secondary to trauma and previous surgery.

LIMITATIONS
- Navigation console along with its software and other paraphernalia though easy to use, do incur a substantial capital, and necessitates an in-depth knowledge of the loading software and associated hardware.
- Preoperative planning and intraoperative utilization of the equipment requires time for set up and can therefore possibly prolong the surgeon's operative duration.
- CT and MRI scans compatible with the navigation system are usually of supreme quality and therefore poor-quality scans will be deficient for its evaluation using the software.
- There is a learning curve on the part of the operating surgeon to become proficient with the technology.

CONCLUSION
Image guidance has diverse applications in the field of orbital surgery and further advancements in the same shall continue to improve the operative precision and consequent patient outcomes.

SUGGESTED READING
1. Ali MJ, Singh S, Naik MN. Image-guided lacrimal drainage surgery in congenital arhinia-microphthalmia syndrome. Orbit. 2017;36(3):137-43.
2. Campbell AA, Mahoney NR. Use of computer-assisted surgery in the orbit. Orbit. 2022; 41(2):226-34.
3. Chang CH, Ku WN, Kung WH, Huang Y, Chiang CC, Lin HJ, et al. Navigation-assisted endoscopic surgery of lacrimal sac tumor. Taiwan J Ophthalmol. 2020;10(2):141-3.
4. Reichel O, Taxeidis M. Use of an image-guided navigation system for routine endonasal endoscopic dacryocystorhinostomy. J Laryngol Otol. 2019;133(8):685-90.
5. Udhay P, Bhattacharjee K, Ananthnarayanan P, Sundar G. Computer-assisted navigation in orbitofacial surgery. Indian J Ophthalmol. 2019;67(7):995-1003.
6. Zhao Y, Li Y, Li Z, Deng Y. Removal of Orbital Metallic Foreign Bodies with Image-Guided Surgical Navigation. Ophthalmic Plast Reconstr Surg. 2020;36(3):305-10.

9.19 Clinical Evaluation and Imaging of Lacrimal System

Prerna Sinha
Ophthalmic Plastic Surgery Services, LV Prasad Eye Institute, Hyderabad

Swati Singh
L V Prasad Eye Institute, Hyderabad
swatisingh@lvpei.org

INTRODUCTION

The lacrimal drainage system (LDS) is an integral part of the lacrimal functional unit, which involves tear production and drainage in the eye. The lacrimal gland produces tears, drained into the nasal cavity via the lacrimal punctum, canaliculi, sac, and nasolacrimal duct (NLD). Disorders affecting the LDS can result in epiphora associated with or without discharge. The spectrum of such disorders ranges from congenital aplasia and hypoplasia to congenital nasolacrimal duct obstruction (CNLDO) and acquired nasolacrimal duct obstruction (NLDO). To deal with such a varied presentation of various pathologies, one needs to be well versed with all the clinical and imaging modalities available for its evaluation. A detailed history, clinical examination, and investigations are necessary to make an accurate diagnosis. Recent advances have improved our understanding of the lacrimal system and added many diagnostic modalities to our armamentarium.[1] This chapter describes the tests that can be used in our clinical practice, techniques, and their interpretation, along with recent advances.

CLINICAL TESTS FOR LACRIMAL DRAINAGE SYSTEM

Clinical examination in the outpatient settings begins with external face assessment for clues such as gross nasal deformity, the laxity or other abnormalities of the eyelid, presence of scars and swellings around the lacrimal sac area, followed by detailed eyelids and lacrimal puncta examination on slit lamp and lacrimal syringing.[2] The preliminary slit lamp examination is followed by simple lacrimal irrigation. Further elaborate tests can be undertaken based on the clinical examination. **Table 9.19.1** summarizes the common indications of different tests employed in authors' practice.

Examination of Eyelids and Puncta

The position of eyelid and lashes is noted on diffuse slit lamp examination for entropion with trichiasis and punctal ectropion (either cicatricial or paralytic or mechanical), blepharitis, or meibomitis that can result in the reflex watering complaint **(Figs. 9.19.1A to C)**. The details of punctal anatomy, including its size, position, shape, and number, should be noted to rule out congenital abnormalities like aplasia or incomplete punctal canalization (IPC). The normal puncta position is at the lacrimal papilla's summit, facing the tear lake near the caruncle. The upper puncta lie 1–2 mm more medial to the lower puncta and they do not oppose each other when the eyelids are closed. An altered position can be noted in lax eyelids or facial palsy. The presence of edema and erythema in and around the puncta could indicate impending punctal stenosis secondary to topical antiglaucoma or chemotherapeutic medications, canalicular inflammatory disease, or if associated with discharge or concretions, as in canaliculitis.[2-4]

Examination of Conjunctiva and Caruncle

The presence of conjunctivochalasis can cause epiphora, where a fold of conjunctiva sits over the punctal opening and hinders tear drainage. It is commonly seen in the

TABLE 9.19.1: Common indications of different tests for LDS.

Indication	Tests done
Screening for sac infections before cataract surgery	ROPLAS/micro regurgitation
NLDO in pediatric age group and uncooperative patients	Fluorescein dye disappearance test
NLDO (PANDO/SALDO)	Lacrimal irrigation
Differentiating canalicular obstructions from NLDO	Lacrimal irrigation + probing
• Canalicular stenosis • Localizing site of NLDO	Dacryoendoscopy
Traumatic SALDO/post-traumatic NLDO	CT-DCG with 3D reconstruction
Lacrimal sac tumors	CT or MRI with contrast
Differentiate pre-sac and post-sac delay in patent LDS	Magnetic resonance dacryocystography (drop method)
Variety of punctal disorders	Optical coherence tomography

(CT-DCG: computed tomography dacryocystography; LDS: lacrimal drainage system; NLDO: nasolacrimal duct obstruction; PANDO: primary acquired nasolacrimal duct obstruction; ROPLAS: regurgitation on pressure over lacrimal sac; SALDO: secondary acquired lacrimal duct obstruction)

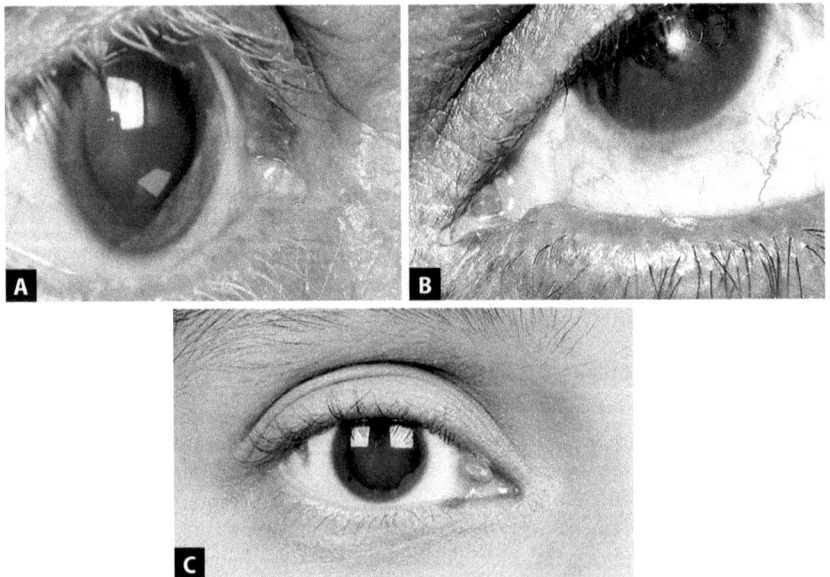

Figs. 9.19.1A to C: (A) Caruncular hypertrophy opposing the lower punctum; (B) Lower punctal ectropion; (C) Pigmented peripunctal nevus.

elderly population, and addressing the extra fold of conjunctiva usually takes care of most watering. The ocular surface should be closely examined for symblepharon that can distort the punctal morphology and anatomy. Any caruncular mass can also cause mechanical obstruction or ectropion of the punctal area **(Figs. 9.19.1A to C)**.[5] Also, micro regurgitation can be seen on the slit lamp after pressing over the medial canthal area in the eyes with complete NLDO.

Regurgitation on Pressure over Lacrimal Sac

It is a simple clinic-based test that can be positive in chronic dacryocystitis, mucocele, or NLDO. The sensitivity and specificity of regurgitation on pressure over lacrimal sac (ROPLAS) are 93.2% and 99.3% in diagnosing NLDO while screening cataract surgery patients. Pressure is applied over the lacrimal sac area by palpating the inferior orbital rim and tracing it superiorly and medially to reach the anterior lacrimal crest. Regurgitation can be either mucoid or purulent (NLDO) or blood tinged (dacryoliths or tumors) and can come from either one or both puncta or any fistulous opening in the area. However, there are certain occasions when ROPLAS might be damaging in the presence of NLDO when there is an encysted mucocele, fibrosed sac, incorrect technique, or sometimes due to the simple fact that the patient had emptied the sac before the examination. It can also be negative in an internal fistula or atonic sac where sac contents empty into the nose.[6,7]

Lacrimal Irrigation

Lacrimal irrigation, commonly referred to as syringing, is the most frequently performed procedure for LDS evaluation. The patient is positioned in a reclining or supine position, and a drop of 2% proparacaine is instilled. A 2 mL syringe is filled with normal saline or sterile water, and a smoothly curved cannula (~15°) or a straight cannula of 24 G or 25 G size is mounted onto the syringe. Straight cannulas are preferred over curved ones as they are less traumatic to the canaliculi. The patient is asked to look down or up (for upper and lower puncta, respectively), and the medial eyelid is gently pulled up (for the upper lid) or down (for the lower lid) to expose the punctum. The punctum is then dilated using a Nettleship punctum dilator if needed, and the cannula is inserted vertically in the punctum and then gently turned horizontally while maintaining traction laterally on the eyelid to straighten the canaliculus. The cannula is gently advanced into the horizontal canaliculus, slowly pushing a small amount of fluid to dilate the incoming lacrimal pathway to avoid inadvertent canalicular wall touch. The irrigation is then performed, and the passage or regurgitation pattern is noted. **Figure 9.19.2** displays the interpretation of lacrimal syringing. Lacrimal syringing shows good accuracy in

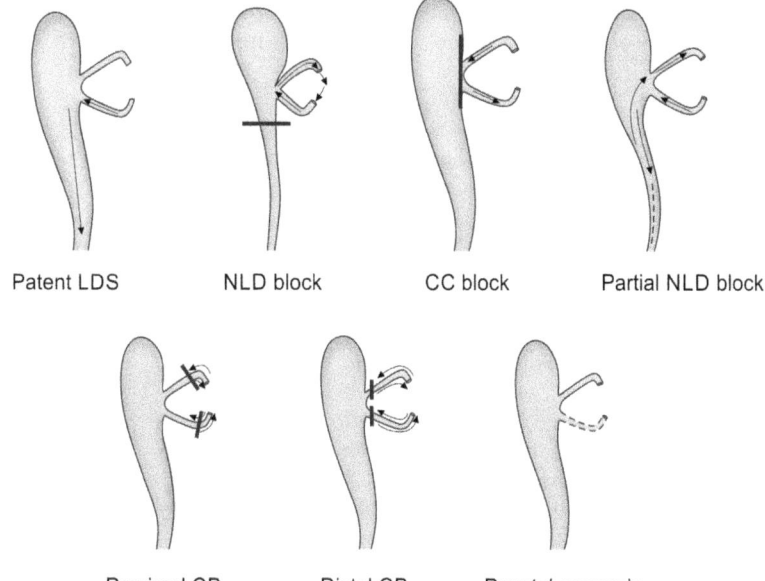

Fig. 9.19.2: Raised tear meniscus height along with retained dye in the right eye with functional nasolacrimal duct obstruction. (LDS: lacrimal drainage system; NLD: nasolacrimal duct)

diagnosing complete NLDO. However, in eyes with dacryostenosis, i.e., incomplete or partial NLDO, the diagnostic accuracy reduces. Even in the presence of patent irrigation, the possibility of functional delay or dacryostenosis might warrant further exploration of LDS using dacryoendoscopy (DEN) or dacryocystography (DCG), or dacryoscintigraphy (DSG).[7,8]

Differentiating Canalicular from Nasolacrimal Obstruction

After punctal dilatation, a Bowman's lacrimal probe is passed through the canaliculus while exerting lateral traction to keep it straight. The probe is gently advanced toward the sac, and the feel of stop is noted as "hard" or "soft". A hard stop indicates that the probe has passed beyond the common canaliculus and is against the bone, indicating that the regurgitation in syringing was due to distal NLD obstruction and not a common canalicular block. However, a soft stop usually indicates a proximal or common canalicular block. However, the findings of soft stop did not correlate well with DCG in eyes with common canalicular obstructions, but the correlation is good for proximal canalicular obstructions.[2,9,10]

Tear Film-based Tests

In eyes with patent LDS, one needs to perform tear film-based tests that can be secretory or excretory tests. Secretory tests such as Schirmer's test, tear film breakup time, and tear meniscus height are performed to rule out reflex watering in eyes with patent LDS. The excretory tests include the fluorescein dye disappearance test (FDDT) and the Jones test (I and II).

Fluorescein Dye Disappearance Test

It is a useful noninvasive test to assess NLDO, especially in children and uncooperative patients. 2% fluorescein dye is instilled in the nonanesthetized fornix, and after 5 minutes, the conjunctival cul-de-sac is examined under a cobalt blue filter for the presence of dye. The presence of remaining dye can be graded from 0 to 3, where "0" represents no dye, and "3" represents all the dye remaining **(Fig. 9.19.3)**. Similarly, a functional endoscopic dye test (FEDT) is performed to score the functional and anatomical patency of dacryocystorhinostomy (DCR) ostium.[11]

Jones Test

Jones, in 1961, described a simple test to assess the functional aspect of LDS. Jones dye test 1 is done to differentiate between hypersecretion of tears and partial obstruction of the NLD or a functional block. 2% fluorescein is instilled in the conjunctival sac and a cotton bud dipped in xylocaine is placed in the inferior meatus of the nose near the NLD opening. After 5 minutes, the cotton bud is checked for staining, or the patient is asked to blow out the nose on a piece of tissue. A stained bud or tissue indicates anatomical patency of the lacrimal drainage pathway. It is a physiological test, and a positive test strongly suggests a patent system but does not rule out physiologic dysfunction or mild anatomic obstruction. A negative test, on the other hand, indicates either a functional block or a partial NLD obstruction. To differentiate between these two, Jones dye test 2 is done. The conjunctival sac is flushed to remove all the fluorescein, and then syringing is done. In case of a lacrimal pump failure causing a functional block, no dye would have reached the lacrimal sac. Thus, in syringing, the fluid that will come out of the nose will be clear. A negative test thus suggests a functional block.

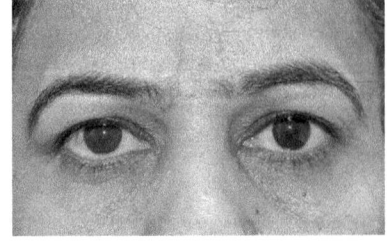

Fig. 9.19.3: Interpretation of different possibilities of lacrimal syringing.

In case of a partial NLD block, dye present in the sac from Jones test 1 will be washed out on syringing, and the fluid coming out of the nose will be stained. Hence, a positive Jones dye test II confirms a partial NLD block.[12]

Dacryoendoscopy

Dacryoendoscopy is the direct endoscopic visualization of LDS from canaliculi, common canaliculus, and lacrimal sac to NLD using a microendoscope. It can be performed as an outpatient procedure or operating room. Initially, the use of dacryoendoscope was limited to diagnostic purposes due to poor image quality and flexible fiberscope. The present-day dacryoendoscope, the rigid microendoscope, has larger diameters (0.9–1.1 mm), provides higher resolution images (15,000 pixels), and multiple ports for additional instrumentation, irrigation, laser port, and drill ports. On DEN, the normal canaliculi have a smooth pale pink appearing mucosa, and the lacrimal sac has a mucoid layer over its reddish mucosa and visible submucosal blood vessels **(Figs. 9.19.4A and B)**. DEN has enabled the exact localization and differentiation of mucosal edema, stenosis, strictures, and obstructions throughout the LDS. Therapeutic interventions that can be performed with DEN include guided expansion of the stenosis, laser dacryoplasty for strictures, microdrill removal of dacryoliths, and sheath-guided lacrimal intubation.[13]

■ IMAGING OF LACRIMAL DRAINAGE SYSTEM

The radiological evaluation of LDS is performed in situations like malignancies or traumatic NLDOs, or complex NLDO like after maxillectomy.

Dacryocystography and Dacryoscintigraphy

Digital subtraction dacryocystography (DS-DCG) has been traditionally used to localize the site of LDS obstruction, differentiate canalicular from proximal sac obstructions, and visualize the stenotic segments not negotiated by a cannula. However, lacrimal punctum and canaliculus are better visualized with optical coherence tomography (OCT) and DEN, respectively, and canalicular obstructions can be differentiated from proximal sac obstructions via lacrimal probing and syringing. 1 mL of radiopaque dye is injected into the canalicular system after cannulation and frames are obtained at 1 per second for 10 seconds. Anteroposterior, both oblique frontal and off-lateral projections are captured for better delineation of the system. DS-DCG gives an anatomical overview of LDS, whereas physiological assessment of contrast drainage is checked using DSG, where radionucleotides pass through LDS in real time. A pinhole-collimated gamma camera is used to image the lacrimal system after instilling 10 μL of technetium 99 pertechnetate in the conjunctival cul-de-sac. Patients are asked to blink normally,

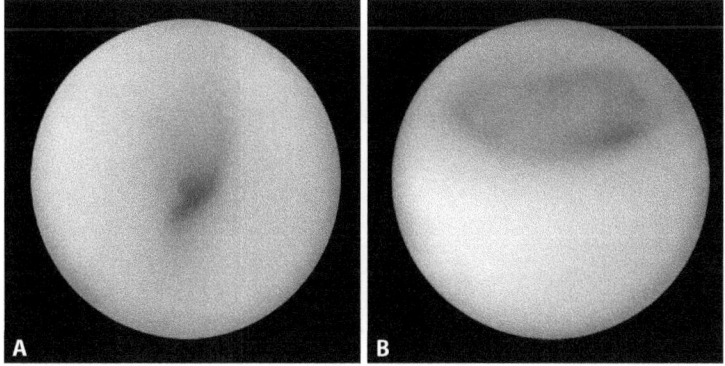

Figs. 9.19.4A and B: (A) Dacryoendoscopic appearance of normal canalicular mucosa; (B) Sac-nasolacrimal duct (NLD) junction.

and the duration of the first appearance of the dye in the nasal cavity is noted. Typically, the canaliculus and the sac are visualized by 30 seconds and NLD after 20–30 minutes. The current relative indications of DS-DCG or DSG are partial obstruction or functional NLDO, though the predictive value of DSG is still less in these eyes, and dacryoendoscopy is beginning to replace these modalities. Ultrasonography of the lacrimal system has been used in research but not much for clinical application.[14-16]

Computed Tomography and Magnetic Resonance Imaging

Computed tomography of the lacrimal system is extremely useful in cases with altered anatomy and lacrimal sac tumors **(Figs. 9.19.5A and B)**. The axial scans are used to study the lacrimal drainage pathways, and parasagittal cuts delineate the NLD anatomy the best in its entire length. The lacrimal sac fossa appears as a depression in the antero-inferior portion of the medial wall. When combined with DCG, a CT scan serves as an excellent tool for identifying the bony structures around the NLD. It is instrumental in cases of facial polytrauma (3D-CT DCG, **Fig. 9.19.6**), prior lacrimal or sinus surgeries and some congenital disorders like the lacrimal amniocele which can be seen as a dilated duct with bony changes. The disadvantage of CT is the poor visualization of the soft tissue around the NLD, which can be overcome by the use of magnetic resonance imaging (MRI). MRDCG is performed using 1, 1.5, or 3T MR scanners and T1-weighted fat-suppressed images are studied for LDS. The use of surface coils improves image quality. Gadolinium contrast media (1:100) is used either as a drop or cannulation method for MRDCG where drop method help in studying dye transition in real time **(Figs. 9.19.7A and B)**. The dye transit time is helpful in assessing the site of delay, whether pre-sac or post-sac, in a patient with a patent LDS. The average dye transit times are 15, 50, and 150 seconds for the lacrimal sac, NLD, and inferior meatus, respectively. The disadvantages of MRDCG include long acquisition time, expensive, and motion artifacts.[17-20]

Anterior Segment Optical Coherence Tomography

Optical coherence tomography techniques have been increasingly used in the study of the anatomy and pathology of proximal lacrimal disorders. It is a noninvasive and

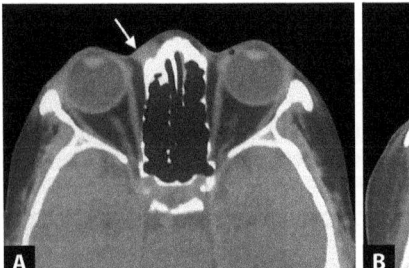
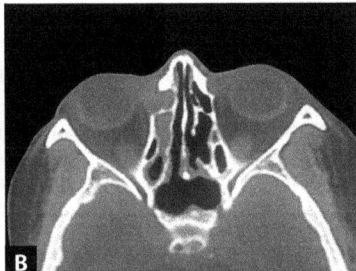

Figs. 9.19.5A and B: CT orbit shows well-defined lesion in the right lacrimal fossa mass that extends down the bony nasolacrimal duct (NLD) canal with opacification of ethmoid sinus.

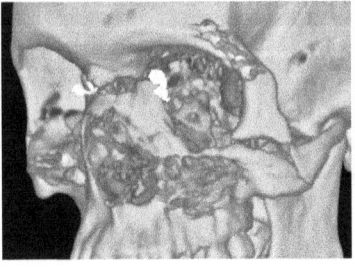

Fig. 9.19.6: 3D reconstructed computed tomography dacryocystography (CT-DCG) showing posteriorly displaced lacrimal sac along with naso-orbito-ethmoid and zygomatic bone fracture.

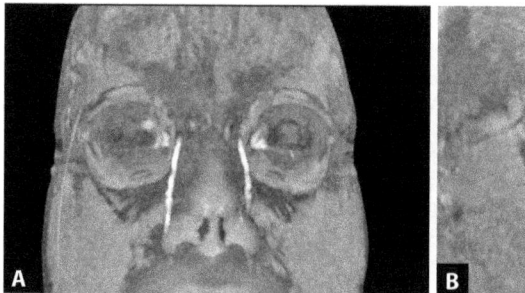
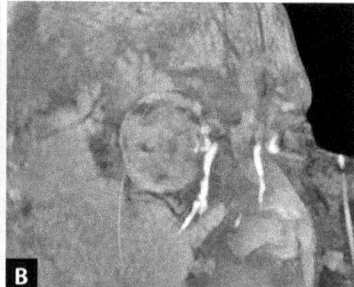

Figs. 9.19.7A and B: Magnetic resonance (MR) dacryocystography showing the patent lacrimal drainage system with narrow areas at sac-nasolacrimal duct (NLD) junction.

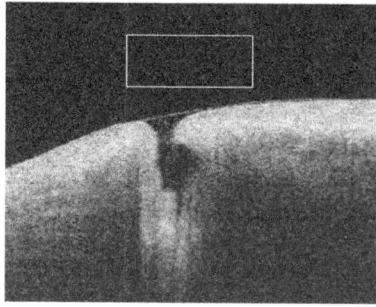

Fig. 9.19.8: Anterior segment optical coherence tomography (ASOCT) of the lacrimal punctum showing punctal opening continuing into the flask-shaped lacrimal canaliculus.

noncontact test with ease of acquisition and good penetration. The OCT is further enhanced by the use of contrast like rebamipide 2% suspension, which is instilled in the fornix [OCT dacryography (OCTD)]. During image acquisition, the patient is asked to look up, and images are acquired after 1 minute up to 10 minutes. Different punctal shapes, correlation of punctual outer and inner diameters, and angles of medial and lateral walls to the punctum have been described on OCT. The junction of the puncta and the vertical canaliculus is seen as an area of sudden lumen narrowing **(Fig. 9.19.8)**. The appearance of the vertical canaliculus has been described as flask shaped. A variety of punctual disorders can be confirmed on OCT, like the presence of a membrane in the case of IPC that can be noted as a hyper-reflective membrane over the puncta with table-top configuration and a patent underlying vertical canaliculus. A punctual keratinizing cyst can likewise be appreciated as a hyper-reflective globular lesion. The diagnosis of punctal stenosis can be made by measuring the outer and inner wall diameters of the puncta. OCTD can help in localizing the degree and site of obstruction in case of canalicular obstruction where the obstruction appears as a filling defect, and the normal flask-shaped segment of vertical canaliculus is lost.[21]

■ CONCLUSION

Diagnosing the functional and anatomical patency of LDS is essential for adopting an appropriate management strategy and for the proper counseling of the patient. The tests described earlier aid the ophthalmologist in arriving at a specific diagnosis while the possibilities of improving the accuracies of existing tests and adding newer tests continue to exist in the era of scientific and technological advancement.

■ CONFLICTS OF INTEREST

None of the authors have any conflicts of interest.

REFERENCES

1. Mahesh L, Ali MJ. Imaging modalities for lacrimal disorders. In: Ali MJ (Ed). Principles and Practice of Lacrimal Surgery, 1st edition. New Delhi: Springer; 2015.
2. Das S. Evaluation of epiphora. In: Ali MJ (Ed). Principles and Practice of Lacrimal Surgery, 2nd edition. Singapore: Springer; 2018. Pp. 147-61.
3. Soiberman U, Kakizaki H, Selva D, Leibovitch I. Punctal stenosis: definition, diagnosis, and treatment. Clin Ophthalmol. 2012;6:1011-8.
4. Ansari Z, Singh R, Alabiad C, Galor A. Prevalence, risk factors, and morbidity of eyelid laxity in a veteran population. Cornea. 2015;34(1):32-6.
5. Kamal S, Ali MJ. Primary Acquired Nasolacrimal Duct Obstruction (PANDO) and Secondary Acquired Lacrimal Duct Obstructions (SALDO). In: Ali MJ (Ed). Principles and Practice of Lacrimal Surgery, 2nd edition. Singapore: Springer; 2018.
6. Kim U, Vardhan A, Datta D, Mekhala A, Kishore N, Rathi G, et al. Regurgitation on pressure over the lacrimal sac versus lacrimal irrigation in determining lacrimal obstruction prior to intraocular surgeries. Indian J Ophthalmol. 2022;70(11):3833-6.
7. Thomas R, Thomas S, Braganza A, Muliyil J. Evaluation of the role of syringing prior to cataract surgery. Indian J Ophthalmol. 1997;45:211-4.
8. Shapira Y, Juniat V, Macri C, Selva D. Syringing has limited reliability in differentiating nasolacrimal duct stenosis from functional delay. Graefes Arch Clin Exp Ophthalmol. 2022;260(9):3037-42.
9. Liarakos VS, Boboridis KG, Mavrikakis E, Mavrikakis I. Management of canalicular obstructions. Curr Opin Ophthalmol. 2009;20(5):395-400.
10. Usmani E, Shapira Y, Macri C, Davis G. Soft stop on syringing and probing may have a high false-positive rate in diagnosing pre-sac obstruction. Int Ophthalmol. 2022;43(3):1127-33.
11. Kashkouli MB, Mirzajani H, Jamshidian-Tehrani M, Shahrzad S, Sanjari MS. Fluorescein Dye Disappearance Test: A Reliable Test in Assessment of Success After Dacryocystorhinostomy Procedure. Ophthalmic Plast Reconstr Surg. 2015;31(4):296-9.
12. Dutton JJ, White JJ. Imaging and clinical evaluation of the lacrimal drainage system. In: Cohen AJ, Mercandetti M, Brazzo BG (Eds). The Lacrimal System—Diagnosis, Management and Surgery. New York, NY, USA: Springer Verlag; 2006. pp. 74-95.
13. Singh S, Ali MJ. A Review of Diagnostic and Therapeutic Dacryoendoscopy. Ophthalmic Plast Reconstr Surg. 2019;35(6):519-24.
14. Singh S, Ali MJ, Paulsen F. Dacryocystography: From theory to current practice. Ann Anat. 2019;224:33-40.
15. Vonica OA, Obi E, Sipkova Z, Soare C, Pearson AR. The value of lacrimal scintillography in the assessment of patients with epiphora. Eye (Lond). 2017;31(7):1020-6.
16. Yan X, Xiang N, Hu W, Liu R, Luo B. Characteristics of lacrimal passage diseases by 80-MHz ultrasound biomicroscopy: an observational study. Graefes Arch Clin Exp Ophthalmol. 2020;258(2):403-10.
17. Singh S, Ali MJ. Imaging in Lacrimal Drainage Obstruction and Acute Dacryocystitis. In: Ben Simon G, Greenberg G, Landau Prat D (Eds). Atlas of Orbital Imaging. Edinburgh: Springer, Cham; 2022.
18. Ali MJ, Singh S, Naik MN, Kaliki S, Dave TV. Interactive navigation-guided ophthalmic plastic surgery: the utility of 3D CT-DCG-guided dacryolocalization in secondary acquired lacrimal duct obstructions. Clin Ophthalmol. 2016;11:127-33.
19. Manfrè L, de Maria M, Todaro E, Mangiameli A, Ponte F, Lagalla R. MR dacryocystography: comparison with dacryocystography and CT dacryocystography. AJNR Am J Neuroradiol. 2000;21(6):1145-50.
20. Singh S, Dhull A, Selva D, Ali MJ. Tear transit time evaluation using real-time technique for dynamic MR dacryocystography. Orbit. 2021;40(1):34-8.
21. Ali MJ, Singh S. Optical coherence tomography and the proximal lacrimal drainage system: a major review. Graefes Arch Clin Exp Ophthalmol. 2021;259(11):3197-208.

9.20 Congenital Nasolacrimal Duct Obstruction

Usha Kim
Aravind Eye Hospital and Postgraduate Institute of Ophthalmology, Madurai
usha@aravind.org

■ INTRODUCTION

It is a mechanical obstruction located distally in nasolacrimal duct (NLD) at level of valve of Hasner which covers it, seen in 50% of the newborn infants but most of the obstruction opens up spontaneously within 4-6 weeks after birth. Such obstruction becomes clinically evident in only 2-5% of full-term infants at 3-4 weeks of age. Approximately 90% of all symptomatic congenital NLD obstructions resolve by the first year of life.

■ EMBRYOLOGY

The development of the drainage system begins around 6 weeks of gestation. It starts by forming a rod of cells, between the medial canthus and the nasal cavity along the line of the cleft between the maxillary and lateral nasal processes. In the third month, canalization of this cord starts at the canthus and progresses toward both the eyelid margin and the inferior meatus. Communication between the drainage system and nose happens around 6 months into pregnancy. During the 7th month before separation of lids, lacrimal puncta open into the lid margin. The tear duct opening beneath the inferior turbinate in the nose becomes fully functional either at birth or shortly after birth. It is worth noting that blockage in this portion where tears enter into nose is an occurrence, which might not be recognized until several weeks, after birth when tears are normally produced.

■ CAUSES

In most of cases this happens because there is a layer of tissue located at the opening of the nasal passage called the valve of Hasner, present at nasal opening of the nasolacrimal duct. Sometimes commonly it can be caused by factors such, as a blockage in the tear duct that was present since birth (congenital atresia), a swollen sac in the tear duct (congenital lacrimal sac mucocele), congenital absence of valves, canaliculi and puncta or certain facial abnormalities like clefts.

■ CLASSIFICATION (BASED ON INTRAOPERATIVE FINDINGS)

- Simple CNLDO—membranous obstruction, canalicular valves
- Complex CNLDO—(variations of CNLDO as given by Jones and Wobig)
  - NLD in inferior meatus
  - Buried probe
  - Impacted anterior end of inferior turbinate
  - NLD ending in inferior end of inferior turbinate
  - NLD ending in maxillary wall
  - Absent NLD

■ DIFFERENTIAL DIAGNOSIS

The symptom that is most useful in distinguishing congenital nasolacrimal duct obstruction (CNLDO) from other causes of epiphora is the lack of photophobia. The history is important, because if the parents describe significant photophobia, one should look for other causes of epiphora. Congenital glaucoma is the most important entity that may be mistaken as CNLDO. Complete ophthalmological evaluation for corneal size and clarity, measurement of intraocular pressure and examination of the optic nerves has to be done to rule out congenital glaucoma. Other causes of epiphora include misdirected eyelashes, epiblepharon, and corneal abrasion **(Flowchart 9.20.1)**.

FREQUENCY

A total of 20% of newborns have CNLDO but only 1–6% of them have symptoms. Approximately 90–96% of diagnosed cases usually resolve by the age of 1 year.

SIGNS AND SYMPTOMS

- Epiphora and matted eyelashes, unilateral greater than bilateral—most common symptoms
- Mucous discharge from mucocele on regurgitation on pressure over lacrimal sac (ROPLAS)
- Periocular skin erythema and excoriation
- Acute/chronic dacryocystitis
  - Constant tearing with frequent mucopurulent discharge and matting of the lashes → suggests complete obstruction of NLD
  - Intermittent tearing with frequent mucopurulent discharge suggests intermittent obstruction of NLD → swollen inferior nasal turbinate as associated with upper respiratory tract infection **(Fig. 9.20.1)**.

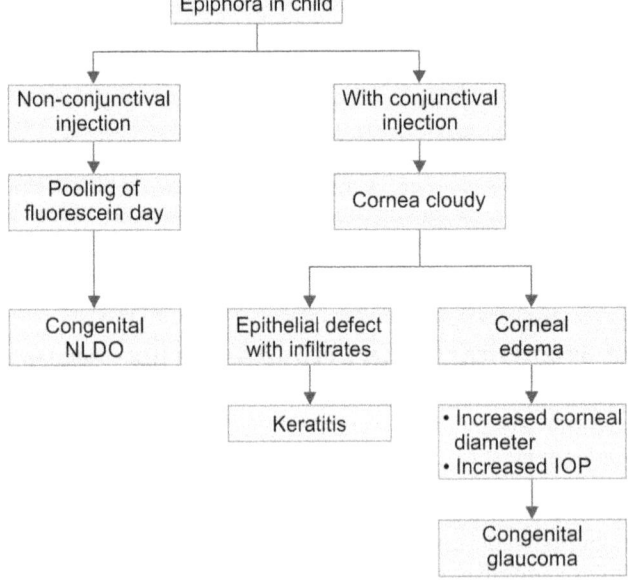

Flowchart 9.20.1: Differential diagnosis of epiphora.

(IOP: intraocular pressure; NLDO: nasolacrimal duct obstruction)

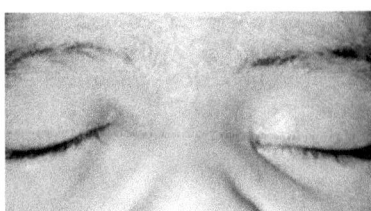

Fig. 9.20.1: Right congenital nasolacrimal duct obstruction.

FLUORESCEIN DYE DISAPPEARANCE TEST
- Outpatient Department (OPD) procedure in which 2% fluorescein dye is instilled in conjunctival cul-de-sac and checked for disappearance after 5 minutes (best appreciated when child is calm otherwise false result can be elicited)
- Graded from 0 to 3 based on amount of dye disappearance.

MANAGEMENT

Conservative
Conservative management includes observation, lacrimal sac massage, and topical antibiotics. Long-term use of topical antibiotics is needed to suppress chronic mucoid discharge. In most of the cases obstruction resolves and patency of NLD is obtained within 4–6 weeks.

Crigler's Massage
Slide the fingertip in posterior and inferior direction, placing moderate pressure over the lacrimal fossa just behind anterior lacrimal crest, and using the antibiotic ointment as a lubricant.
- 4 sittings per day
- 10–15 strokes per sitting
- Topical antibiotic drops only if purulent discharge is present on pressure over the sac.
- Mechanism of action—increases intraluminal pressure in sac and NLD causing break of membrane.

Surgical

Probing
The correct timing for initial probing has been controversial. Initial probing is done when the patient is approximately 1 year of age. It should not be delayed after 1 year as the success rate of probing decreases after the age of 1 year. This is based on a large study by Katowitz and Welsh, of 572 eyes, with initial probing success rate was 97% in patients younger than 13 months.

Procedure
Probing is usually done under short general anesthesia.
- Upper punctum is dilated. It is best to avoid the lower puncta as there is risk of traumatizing this channel **(Fig. 9.20.2A)**.
- Selection of probe is done according to age of the child
  - Size 00 probe—neonate
  - Size 0 probe—infant
  - Size 1 probe—older than 1 year
- Probe is lubricated with antibiotic ointment and passed into the canaliculus, while the lid is stretched to keep the canaliculus straight. It is passed as far as medial wall of lacrimal sac so as to touch the bone **(Fig. 9.20.2B)**.

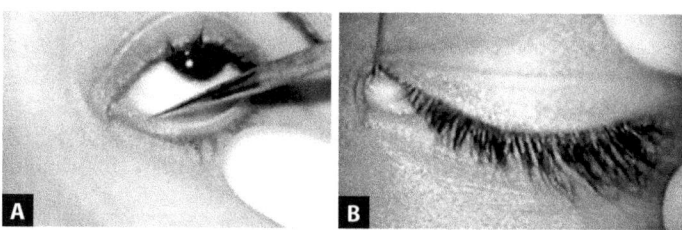

Figs. 9.20.2A and B: (A) Punctum dilatation; (B) Bowmen's probe in nasolacrimal duct.

- Then the probe is rotated inferiorly and is directed posteriorly and laterally down the NLD until it meets resistance at the lower end. A sense of membrane giving way is usually felt at the lower end as nose is entered. However, if it is a hard stop, which usually occurs in older children, there is high risk for failure of probing.
- To confirm the patency and correct passage of the probe, one of the following methods can be done:
  - Direct metal-to-metal contact with a larger second probe placed through the nares.
  - Direct visualization of the probe with an endoscope is particularly useful in complicated cases.
  - Inject fluorescein dye through the syringe of the cannula; retrieval of dye in the nose determines the patency of the system.
- Anterior rhinoscopy is done at the end of the procedure and if the inferior turbinate seems to be impacted on the NLD opening at the initial examination, it can be pushed medially by infracturing the turbinate toward the septum with a freer elevator.
- Patient is given topical antibiotic-steroid drops, Crigler's massage is continued, and is followed-up at 1 week.

COMPLICATIONS

- *False passage:* If there is formation of false passage, the procedure should be stopped and probing and irrigation should be rescheduled under a general anesthetic several weeks later to allow the postoperative inflammation to subside.
- *Failure of procedure:*
  - If initial probing has failed, procedure can be repeated after 6 weeks of primary procedure. It can be accompanied by turbinate infracture.
  - The secondary procedure may also involve a silastic intubation or balloon dacryoplasty.
  - If repeat probing or intubation fails, then external dacryocystorhinostomy (DCR) should be done with or without primary silicone intubation at 3–4 years of age.
  - Prognosis for probing decreases exponentially with the increasing number of probings and the age of the patient.

Difficult Probing

Causes
- False passage
- Tight bony obstruction

Management

"Graduated" or "stepwise" probing (increasing diameters probes are used progressively) or by "reaming" (probing is done in screwing fashion to enlarge the NLD).

Endoscopic Guidance for Probing

Recently many centers have initiated this procedure as it provided added benefit of identifying a complex CNLDO, causes minimal damage to nearby tissue and different modes of treatment trial can be done in same sitting.

Intubation

- *Indications:* Recurrent epiphora after failed probing, older children when initial probing reveals stenosis or scarring, upper drainage system abnormalities such as canalicular stenosis and punctal agenesis.
- Crawford stent is most commonly used. It is a silicon stent. Here a tube attached to a metal probe is inserted through the canaliculus into the nose and a silicon tubing

can be secured by a simple square knot or sutured to the lateral wall of the nose which allows stent retrieval through nose.
- Monocanalicular stents are used when patient has only one patent canaliculus. It is passed through punctum to nasal cavity. End of the stent is simply cut and allowed to retract loosely into nose. Proximal end has a smooth barb and is self-secured at the punctum.

Balloon Dacryoplasty
- A collapsed balloon catheter is passed in a manner similar to probing and inflated inside the duct at multiple levels. Reported success rate range from 80 to 100%.
- Useful adjunctive procedure in incomplete NLDO when probing has failed >13 months of age.
- Balloon is introduced till NLD – two cycles of balloon inflation and deflation to be done – balloon introduced through punctum till 15-mm mark reaches; inflated to eight atmospheres of pressure for 90 seconds, deflated for 10 seconds. In second cycle inflated to eight atmospheres of pressure for 60 seconds. Same procedure repeated at 10 mm marking.
- Generally limited to complicated cases or recurrence following standard probing techniques because of high success rates with simple probing and need of expensive equipment. Nowadays it is used as primary procedure as well. Alternate, cost-effective options with cardiac stents are in trial too.

Dacryocystorhinostomy
- When age of child reaches or crosses 4 years.
- Indications—reserved for children who have persistent epiphora following all of the abovementioned procedures, associated mucocele or dacryocystitis, congenital fistula, functional block, trauma, acquired obstruction
- Failure usually because of anatomic obstruction by granulation tissue.
- Success varies between 79% and 96%.

Endoscopic Dacryocystorhinostomy
- Done to avoid external scar
- Success rates—76–88%
- Advantage of treating concomitant sinonasal problems.

CONGENITAL LACRIMAL—CUTANEOUS FISTULA
- Arise from normal canalicular system or lacrimal sac, mostly at inferonasal to medial canthal area.
- Usually asymptomatic, requires no treatment if asymptomatic or associated with minimal tearing.
- One-third of the patients have underlying NLD obstruction or associated with mucoid discharge, which requires excision of fistulous tract along with silicon intubation of NLD.

CONGENITAL DACRYOCELE
Uncommon neonatal swelling of the lacrimal sac, typically tense, bluish, presents at birth, or beginning shortly after birth.
It occurs due to persistent non-canalization of lower end of NLD with functional obstruction at valve of Rosenmuller.
Associated with intranasal cyst resulting in respiratory distress

Management:
- Probing
- Cruciate incision for intranasal cyst

CONCLUSION

Crigler's massage should be performed in children <12 months of age unless early probing (in cases like. repeated sac infection) is needed. In children >12 months of age, probing needs to be done. Infracture of the inferior turbinate can be attempted, if the turbinate is impacted against the lateral nasal wall. In unresolved cases, repeat probing can be attempted. Silastic intubation to be considered if repeat probing fails. DCR is recommended where silastic intubation fails, in children with bony obstructions, craniofacial anomalies and is preferably done after 3–4 years of age.

9.21 | Chronic Dacryocystitis

Khushdeep Abhaypal, Manpreet Singh, Manpreet Kaur
Postgraduate Institute of Medical Education and Research, Chandigarh
drmanu83@gmail.com

Aditi Mehta
Grewal Eye Institute, Chandigarh
aditimehta7@gmail.com

INTRODUCTION

Dacryocystitis is a common ophthalmic condition (51.56% prevalence) confronted by ophthalmologists in their daily practice.[1] Most patients with dacryocystitis have epiphora with discharge as their chief complaint and a usual history ranging from months to years. The present chapter summarizes recent advances in understanding the pathophysiology of chronic dacryocystitis and discusses current management considerations.

Definition

Acute dacryocystitis is an acute infectious state of the lacrimal sac and perisac tissue, whereas chronic dacryocystitis results from prolonged inflammation of the lacrimal sac and surrounding tissues.[2,3] Chronic dacryocystitis is usually accompanied by nasolacrimal duct obstruction (NLDO) and needs a bypass surgical procedure like dacryocystorhinostomy (DCR). On the contrary, acute dacryocystitis may not always have coexisting NLDO.[4]

Applied Anatomy

- *Lacrimal sac:* It is housed in the bony lacrimal sac fossa with anterior and posterior lacrimal crests as boundaries formed by the frontal process of the maxillary and lacrimal bones, respectively.[5]
- *Cavernous body* (**Fig. 9.21.1**): It is a vascular plexus present inside the mucosal lining of the lacrimal sac and nasolacrimal duct (NLD). It plays a vital role in tear flow and systemic absorption. Malfunctions in the cavernous body may lead to disturbances in the tear outflow cycle, congestion, or total occlusion of the lacrimal passages.[6]
- *Bony lacrimal fossa changes:* In chronic dacryocystitis, extensive areas of periosteal, subperiosteal, and stromal fibrosis and irregular streaks of bone lying in maxillary and lacrimal bones can be noted.[7]

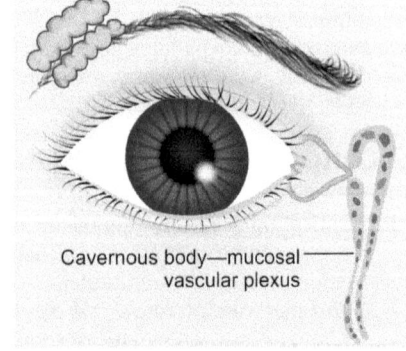

Fig. 9.21.1: Cavernous body.

SECTION 9: Oculoplasty

Defense Systems Against Dacryocystitis[6,8]

Various defense systems present in the lacrimal drainage system depicts in **Flowchart 9.21.1**.

Mucosa-associated lymphoid tissue present on the ocular surface and adnexa is shown in **Figure 9.21.2**.

Structure of the lacrimal duct-associated lymphoid tissue (LDALT) is presented in **Figure 9.21.3**.

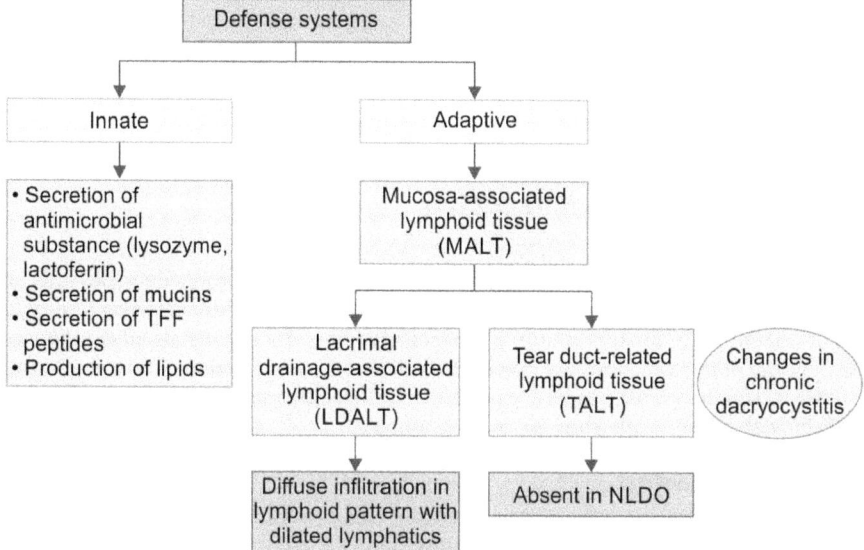

Flowchart 9.21.1: Various defense systems present in the lacrimal drainage system and how their derangements may lead to the genesis of chronic dacryocystitis.

(NLDO: nasolacrimal duct obstruction; TFF: trefoil factor family)

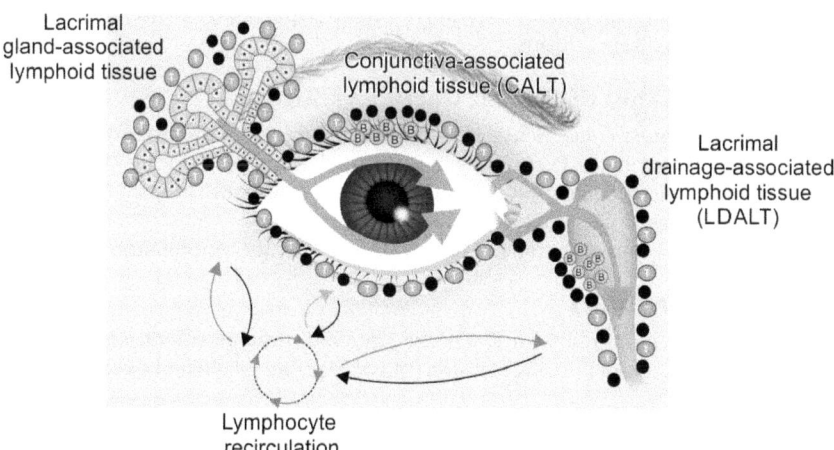

Fig. 9.21.2: Various mucosa-associated lymphoid tissue (MALT) present on the ocular surface and adnexa.

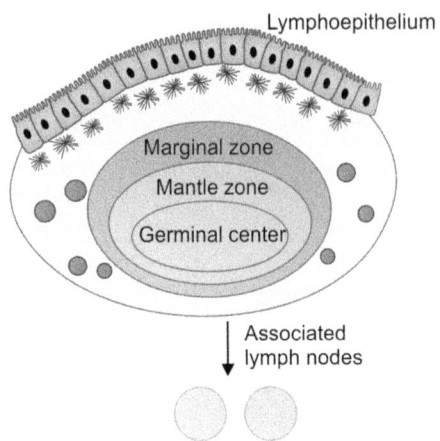

Fig. 9.21.3: Structure of the lacrimal duct-associated lymphoid tissue (LDALT).

■ ETIOPATHOGENESIS (FIG. 9.21.4)

Causative Organisms

The most common organisms isolated from the secretions of chronic dacryocystitis are gram-positive bacteria, with a predominance of *Staphylococcus* species accounting for 82% of infections.[9,10] Most common gram-negative bacteria is *Haemophilus influenza*. The majority of the infections are polymicrobial. Due to the high rate of microorganism-positive lacrimal sac cultures, every patient should be treated or operated on for their condition before performing any intraocular surgery.[11]

Predisposing Factors

- Age—more prevalent in the middle-aged and elderly population[1-3]
- Race and sex—more in females and whites (longer and narrower bony NLD)[5]
- Previous infections—history of recurrent viral or bacterial conjunctivitis[4]
- Other ophthalmic associations—antiglaucoma medications, allergic conjunctivitis, and severe dry eye[12]
- Nasal factors—concha bullosa, inferior turbinate hypertrophy, ostiomeatal complex disease, and maxillary sinusitis.[13]

Pathogenetic Stages of Chronic Dacryocystitis

- *Acute inflammatory stage:* Active inflammation and infiltration preceding infection lead to stenosis of the NLD, resulting in functional obstruction. In this stage, patients may benefit from topical antibiotics and anti-inflammatory eye drops.
- *Intermediate stage:* Intermittent symptomatic patients.
- *Fibrotic stage:* Fibrous obliteration of the NLD, persistently symptomatic patients.

■ CLINICAL FEATURES

Symptoms include epiphora with discharge (mucoid, mucopurulent, and purulent), irritation, and intermittent blurring of vision (raised tear film height and discharge stained tears).

Chronic dacryocystitis generally presents in three clinical types, i.e., catarrhal dacryocystitis, lacrimal mucocele, and chronic suppurative type (with or without lacrimal fistula). Chronic dacryocystitis can be due to either primary acquired nasolacrimal duct obstruction (PANDO) when the etiology is idiopathic or secondary acquired lacrimal duct obstruction (SALDO) secondary to various etiologies.

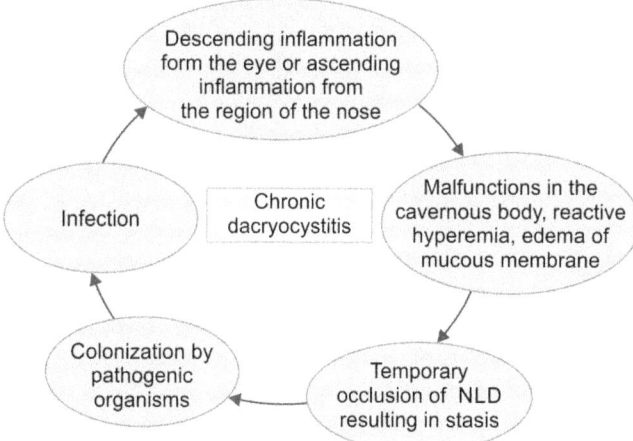

Fig. 9.21.4: Etiopathogenesis of chronic dacryocystitis. (NLD: nasolacrimal duct)

IMAGING (TABLE 9.21.1)
Radiology has made a 3D view of the lacrimal drainage system possible.[14-16] There is no single gold standard modality, and each of these comes with its own set of advantages and disadvantages.

INDICATIONS
- Midface trauma
- Medial canthal masses
- Previous sinonasal surgery
- Failed DCR—to look for the status of bony ostium and surrounding pathologies
- Possible anatomical variations—lacrimal sac diverticulum, etc.

MANAGEMENT (FLOWCHART 9.21.2)
Treatment for chronic dacryocystitis is usually elective, aiming at bypassing the blocked NLD and opening the lacrimal sac directly into the nasal cavity.[18,19] This surgical procedure is popularly known as DCR, which is performed via external or endonasal route as per the surgeon and patient's requirements.

Pearls for Good External Dacryocystorhinostomy
- *Anesthesia:* General or local anesthesia (infratrochlear, infraorbital, and dorsal nasal nerves).
- *Skin incision:* Keep it superficial, with no.15 surgical blade.
- *Blunt dissection:* Use blunt-tip tenotomy scissors, keep the blades horizontal and aim at bone; gently open the blades horizontally to get the desired exposure.
- *Muscle bleeders:* Change the position of Cats Paw Retractor for compressional hemostasis as vessels run within the muscle fibers.
- *Osteotomy:* Engage the bone punch gently to avoid nasal mucosal injury.
- *Dimensions of bony ostium:*
  - *Superior:* 3–4 mm superior to horizontally tented sac mucosa with Bowman's probe.
  - *Inferior:* Deroofing of the NLD.
  - *Anterior:* 3–4 mm anterior to anterior lacrimal crest.
  - *Posterior:* Complete removal of thin lacrimal bone.
- *Access to nasal cavity:* Always visualize nasal pack or tip of the instrument inserted from the nose.
- *Lacrimal stents:* In case of canalicular obstructions, revision DCR surgeries or SALDO.

TABLE 9.21.1: Various imaging modalities for lacrimal drainage system imaging.[17]

Imaging modality	Uses	Advantages	Disadvantages
Digital subtraction dacryocystography (DS-DCG)	• Study anatomical abnormalities • Evaluate results of dacryocystorhinostomy (DCR)	• Subtracts background images to give clear contrast-filled lacrimal images • Reduced radiation exposure • Understanding the flow dynamics	Invasive
Dacryoscintigraphy (DSG)	Assess flow dynamics	Describes physiological aspects	• Poor anatomical details • Poor resolution • Variable transit times
Ultrasonography (USG)[14]	• Detect lacrimal anomalies • Determine DCR ostium size	• Easy technique • Outpatient setting • No radiation exposure	• Lack of anatomical details • Inability to accurately localize abnormalities
Computed tomography dacryocystography (CT-DCG)	• Assessment of the anatomical variations • 3D lacrimal fossa evaluation • Evaluation of orbit and facial skeleton	• Delineating bony structures • Shorter acquisition time • Three-dimensional (3D) reconstruction	Contraindicated in pregnancy and in those with a history of Iodine allergy
Magnetic resonance imaging dacryocystography (MR-DCG)	Better soft tissue delineation	• High tissue contrast • Clear identification of fluid signals • No ionizing radiations	• Long acquisition times • Lack of bony details • Higher costs

External Dacryocystorhinostomy
- *Advantages:* Shorter procedure, the majority under local anesthetic (LA), no need for specialized instruments, and the shorter learning curve.
- *Disadvantages:* Skin scar, the possibility of compromised lacrimal pump function, functional epiphora, and slightly delayed recovery.

RECENT ADVANCES IN LACRIMAL SURGERY[20]
- To achieve better aesthetic outcomes—subciliary skin incision or transconjunctival route can be used.
- An ultrasonic bone scalpel can be used in either external or endoscopic DCR—useful in very thick bones. Ultrasonic waves act on the mineralized tissues, sparing the soft tissues.
- Nonendoscopic endonasal DCR—for viewing inside the nasal cavity, instead of using an endoscope, an endoilluminator and 23 G vitrectomy retinal light probe (inside canaliculus) is used as light sources. The other instruments remain the same.
- Primary endocanalicular laser DCR—a laser fiber optic is inserted via the punctum, canaliculus into the lacrimal sac. A nasal endoscope is used to visualize the laser

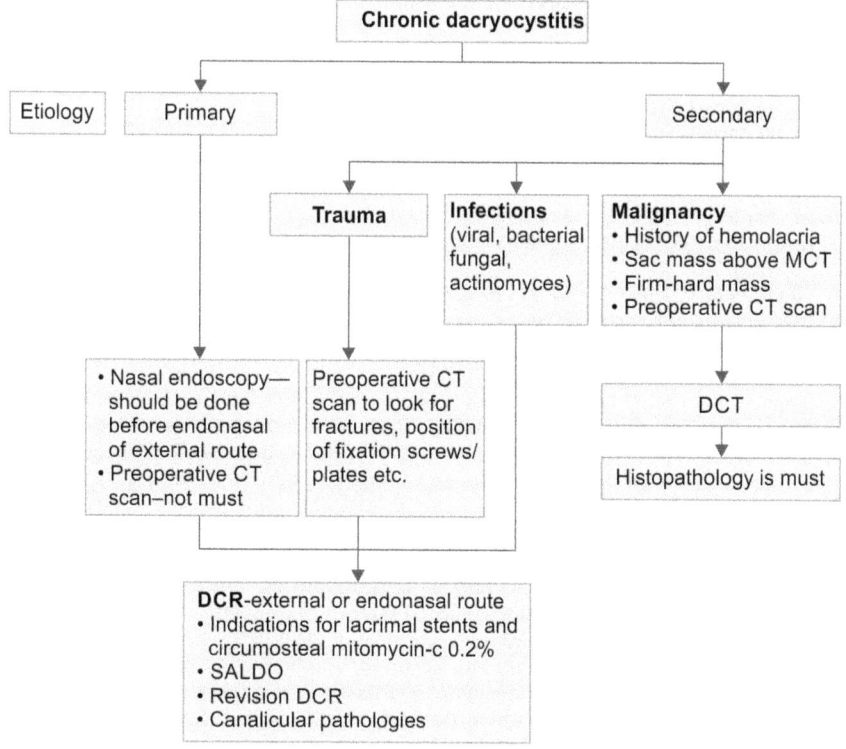

Flowchart 9.21.2: Management of chronic dacryocystitis.

(DCR: dacryocystorhinostomy; DCT: dacryocystectomy; MCT: medial canthal tendon; SALDO: secondary acquired lacrimal duct obstruction)

aiming beam from the nasal side. The holmium:yttrium-aluminum-garnet (Ho:YAG) laser is used to create the osteotomy.
- Balloon-assisted DCR—a 5 mm and 9 mm angled lacrimal balloon can be used via the nasal cavity to gradually enlarge the osteotomy.
- Conjunctivo-DCR—chronic dacryocystitis associated with complete canalicular obstructions, lacrimal pump failures, and severe lacrimal-facial trauma can be treated with this procedure. A bypass tube made up of Pyrex glass or acrylic (with modifications to prevent dislodgements) is placed for the drainage of tears from the conjunctival cul-de-sac directly into the nasal cavity.

REFERENCES

1. Das AV, Rath S, Naik MN, Ali MJ. The Incidence of Lacrimal Drainage Disorders Across a Tertiary Eye Care Network: Customization of an Indigenously Developed Electronic Medical Record System-eyeSmart. Ophthalmic Plast Reconstr Surg. 2019;35(4):354-6.
2. Ali MJ, Joshi SD, Naik MN, Honavar SG. Clinical profile and management outcome of acute dacryocystitis: two decades of experience in a tertiary eye care center. Semin Ophthalmol. 2015;30(2):118-23.
3. Badhu B, Dulal S, Kumar S, Thakur SK, Sood A, Das H. Epidemiology of chronic dacryocystitis and success rate of external dacryocystorhinostomy in Nepal. Orbit. 2005;24(2):79-82.
4. Vo KBH, Lucarelli MJ, van Landingham SW. Two cases of epidemic keratoconjunctivitis-associated dacryocystitis. Orbit. 2020;39(6):450-3.

5. Ali MJ, Schicht M, Paulsen F. Morphology and morphometry of lacrimal drainage system in relation to bony landmarks in Caucasian adults: a cadaveric study. Int Ophthalmol. 2018;38(6):2463-9.
6. Ayub M, Thale AB, Hedderich J, Tillmann BN, Paulsen FP. The cavernous body of the human efferent tear ducts contributes to regulation of tear outflow. Invest Ophthalmol Vis Sci. 2003;44(11):4900-7.
7. Ali MJ, Mishra DK, Bothra N. Lacrimal Fossa Bony Changes in Chronic Primary Acquired Nasolacrimal Duct Obstruction and Acute Dacryocystitis. Curr Eye Res. 2021;46(8):1132-6.
8. Ali MJ, Mulay K, Pujari A, Naik MN. Derangements of lacrimal drainage-associated lymphoid tissue (LDALT) in human chronic dacryocystitis. Ocul Immunol Inflamm. 2013;21(6):417-23.
9. Luo B, Li M, Xiang N, Hu W, Liu R, Yan X. The microbiologic spectrum of dacryocystitis. BMC Ophthalmol. 2021;21(1):29.
10. Eshraghi B, Abdi P, Akbari M, Fard MA. Microbiologic spectrum of acute and chronic dacryocystitis. Int J Ophthalmol. 2014;7(5):864-7.
11. Singh M, Kaur M, Abhaypal K, Gupta P. Commentary: Rule out lacrimal duct obstruction before every intraocular procedure. Indian J Ophthalmol. 2022;70(11):3836-7.
12. Ohtomo K, Ueta T, Toyama T, Nagahara M. Predisposing factors for primary acquired nasolacrimal duct obstruction. Graefes Arch Clin Exp Ophthalmol. 2013;251(7):1835-9.
13. Saratziotis A, Emanuelli E. Osteoma of the medial wall of the maxillary sinus: a primary cause of nasolacrimal duct obstruction and review of the literature. Case Rep Otolaryngol. 2014;2014:348459.
14. Karlin JN, Mustak H, Gupta A, Ramos R, Rootman DB. Cone Beam Computerized Tomography Dacryocystography (CBCT DCG) for the Evaluation of Lacrimal Drainage System Dysfunction. Ophthalmic Plast Reconstr Surg. 2020;36(6):549-52.
15. Timlin HM, Kang S, Jiang K, Ezra DG. Recurrent epiphora after dacryocystorhinostomy surgery: Structural abnormalities identified with dacryocystography and long-term outcomes of revision surgery: Success rates of further surgery following failed dacryocystorhinostomy surgery. BMC Ophthalmol. 2021;21(1):117.
16. Gore SK, Naveed H, Hamilton J, Rene C, Rose GE, Davagnanam I. Radiological Comparison of the Lacrimal Sac Fossa Anatomy Between Black Africans and Caucasians. Ophthalmic Plast Reconstr Surg. 2015;31(4):328-31.
17. Mahesh L, Ali MJ. Imaging modalities for lacrimal disorders. In: Ali MJ (Ed). Principles and Practice of Lacrimal Surgery, 2nd edition. Berlin, Germany: Springer; 2018. Pp. 93-102.
18. Sobel RK, Aakalu VK, Wladis EJ, Bilyk JR, Yen MT, Mawn LA. A Comparison of Endonasal Dacryocystorhinostomy and External Dacryocystorhinostomy: A Report by the American Academy of Ophthalmology. Ophthalmology. 2019;126(11):1580-5.
19. Ullrich K, Malhotra R, Patel BC. Dacryocystorhinostomy. Treasure Island (FL): StatPearls Publishing; 2023.
20. Ali MJ. Principles and Practice of Lacrimal Surgery, 1st edition. Berlin, Germany: Springer; 2015.

9.22 | Acute Dacryocystitis

Kamalpreet Likhari
RJN Eye Institute, Gwalior
kamalpreet.likhari@gmail.com

■ INTRODUCTION

Acute dacryocystitis (ADC) is an acute suppurative inflammatory condition of the lacrimal sac which usually follows stagnation of tears in the sac due to an obstruction within the nasolacrimal duct [*dacryocystitis* from Greek *dákryon* (tear), *cysta* (sac), and *itis* (inflammation)].

The mucous membrane-lined tract of the lacrimal excretory system extends onto two, the conjunctival and nasal mucosae, which are normally colonized with bacteria.

Under normal conditions, the mucosa of the lacrimal sac is highly resistant to infection. However, when the lacrimal drainage is obstructed, the resultant stasis of tears may trigger infection and acute or chronic inflammation. ADC is in general associated with infection and is a dramatic and clinically obvious condition characterized by the sudden emergence of severely painful erythematous swelling over the lacrimal sac, usually with a preceding history of epiphora and discharge. It can cause significant morbidity and, though rarely, mortality.

CLINICAL PROFILE

Although it may occur at any age, ADC is more commonly seen either below the age of 1 year or after 40 years. It is rare in neonates (<1%).

TERMINOLOGY

Acute dacryocystitis usually follows chronic, because of which the previous term for this was acute-on-chronic dacryocystitis. In 1986, Linberg and McCormick coined the term "primary acquired nasolacrimal duct obstruction (PANDO)" for nasolacrimal duct (NLD) obstruction caused by inflammation of unknown cause that eventually leads to occlusive fibrosis of the NLD; following this, Bartley proposed "secondary acquired lacrimal duct obstruction (SALDO)" for obstruction of NLD secondary to well-identified and known pathologies. SALDO may result from a wide variety of causes including infection, inflammation, neoplasm, and trauma, and ADC is the commonest type of SALDO. However, the most popular term remains ADC.

PREDISPOSING FACTORS

The predisposing conditions described for the development of acute/chronic dacryocystitis are:
- *Obstruction of the nasolacrimal duct:* This factor carries the highest risk and is almost a *sine qua non* for ADC to develop.
- *Age:* The incidence of ADC rises with increasing age with maximum prevalence in the fifth and sixth decades, but ADC affects slightly younger persons (the average age being about 5 years less than those with chronic dacryocystitis).
- *Gender:* Higher rates of both acute and chronic dacryocystitis have been reported among women (70–75% and 60–65%, respectively) than men.
- *Nasal pathologies:* An underlying nasal abnormality (the commonest being ipsilateral nasal septum deviation, rhinitis, and inferior turbinate hypertrophy) has been seen in over 25% of cases with dacryocystitis. Moreover, cultures obtained from nasal flora and lacrimal sac flora on the infected side are similar in about 50% of the patients.
- *Laterality:* The left side is slightly more commonly involved, probably because the nasolacrimal duct and lacrimal fossa form a greater angle on the right side than on the left side.
- *Race:* The anatomical characteristics of brachycephalic skulls like a longer nasolacrimal duct with a smaller inlet into it and narrower lacrimal fossa (as compared to dolichocephalic or mesocephalic skulls) predispose them to dacryocystitis. Also, the narrow osseous nasolacrimal canals seen in individuals with flat noses and narrow faces predispose them to this condition. As African skulls have a large nasolacrimal ostium and a shorter and straighter nasolacrimal canal, dacryocystitis is rarely seen in these races.
- *Dacryoliths:* Various studies have reported the presence of dacryoliths in 6–18% of patients with nasolacrimal duct obstruction undergoing external dacryocystorhinostomy. Dacryoliths are seen in patients with earlier presentation of clinical signs and symptoms (≤55 years).

CLINICAL FEATURES

Presentation
The presentation of ADC is usually dramatic, in the form of *severe hemifacial pain,* exquisite tenderness and erythematous edema overlying the lacrimal sac region. Ipsilateral conjunctival injection and chemosis may be seen. Although the symptoms can be mild in the initial stages or in subacute presentations, they are more commonly very severe with debilitating pain and extreme tenderness. The latter is characteristically localized in the medial canthal region (with maximal tenderness just below the medial canthal tendon or MCT). Pain may involve the ipsilateral half of the face including the side of the nose, cheek, teeth and extend to the side of head. The edema may spread to the contralateral eye. Severe reaction can be seen involving the entire facial tissues on the affected side by thermography. Epiphora is invariably present and purulent or mucoid discharge may be noted. A palpable mass may be noted inferior to the medial canthal tendon. As the disease progresses, the sac may rupture externally through the skin, but the resultant fistula commonly closes spontaneously within a few days, usually without a prominent scar. Fever, prostration, and a raised leukocyte count are usually seen. Preseptal cellulitis is commonly associated. Serious complications such as orbital cellulitis and sub-periosteal abscess formation can result leading to blindness (usually due to pressure atrophy of the optic nerve), cavernous sinus thrombosis, and even death.

Visual Acuity
A patient with ADC may complain of blurred vision due to altered refraction of incident light rays at the air-tear film interface caused by raised tear film height and debris. However, vision is not actually affected in ADC unless there is orbital cellulitis compromising optic nerve function, in which case contrast sensitivity and peripheral vision may be affected first.

Visible Sac Swelling
The inflamed sac in dacryocystitis can be seen as a visible swelling obvious even in the presence of lid edema. This is characteristically below the medial canthal tendon and is non-pulsatile.

Preseptal Cellulitis
In preseptal cellulitis the inflammation is anterior to the orbital septum; clinically this is seen as lid edema, erythema, and induration over the sac area which may be very severe but with normal ocular motility and pupillary reaction. There may be associated conjunctival congestion and chemosis, and tear film height is usually raised with purulent discharge from the puncta. Tear stasis with accumulation of debris and staphylococcal exotoxins results in inflammation. Periorbital edema is most pronounced in the morning due to inflammatory stasis of edema fluid and may decrease spontaneously as the day progresses.

Orbital Cellulitis
This is a rare, but serious, complication of both adult and pediatric ADC.

It presents with painful proptosis, restricted ocular motility, abnormal pupillary reaction and compromised visual function (as opposed to severe pain and edema with normal vision and extraocular motility seen in preseptal cellulitis). Vision and pupillary reaction are affected by raised intraorbital pressure causing ischemic damage of the pupillomotor fibers. Cellulitis probably occurs due to bacterial overgrowth causing the lacrimal sac to burst into the limited spaces of the surrounding soft tissues.

DIAGNOSIS

Acute dacryocystitis can almost always be easily diagnosed clinically with no ancillary tests required.

- *Laboratory analysis:* It has a supportive role in assessing the degree of leukocytosis and blood sugar levels. The causative organisms can be identified by cultures taken from blood and swabs from the conjunctival cul-de-sac and nose and thus guide the choice of appropriate antibiotic. However, samples from the conjunctiva and the debris overlying the punctum (even when it is obtained by pressure over the sac area) may be contaminated. The ideal method of sample collection is aspiration of the sac contents with a sterile 20G needle after disinfecting the surface skin. The needle should enter the skin below the medial canthal tendon and be oriented slightly below the horizontal. The sample should preferably be processed immediately and not later than 24 hours after collection. Till that time, it should be stored in an anaerobic transport medium at 4-8°C. the culture media preferred for direct inoculation are blood agar, chocolate agar, Sabouraud's agar, a medium for anaerobic microorganisms such as Schaedler's and thioglycolate broth.

    However, the value of blood culture is questionable. Possibly because many patients come after some form of prior antibiotic therapy, the culture positivity rate varies widely in various series (<10% to 100%).

    Blood cultures should be done in pediatric patients, immunosuppressed patients, and those with fever >38.5°C.

- *Syringing:* Syringing or probing should not be attempted during ADC in adults as it is extremely painful and may worsen the cellulitis and disseminate the infection.
- *Imaging:* The presence of orbital cellulitis, especially if it is not responding to treatment, is an indication for imaging. A computed tomography (CT) scan of the orbits should be asked for. Especially in children with orbital cellulitis, a scan should be obtained without delay. Its main importance is in patients suspected of harboring a mass or malignancy, and in posttraumatic ADC. Magnetic resonance imaging (MRI) is usually not as useful as CT but helps to differentiate solid from cystic masses and to identify sac diverticulitis.

BACTERIOLOGY

Gram-positive bacteria such as *Staphylococcus aureus* and *Streptococcus pneumoniae* are more commonly isolated in dacryocystitis cases than Gram-negative (the commonest being *Haemophilus influenzae, Serratia marcescens,* and *Pseudomonas aeruginosa*) in most studies. Methicillin-resistant *Staphylococcus aureus* (MRSA) is isolated more commonly in acute than chronic dacryocystitis; also, Gram-negative species are the commoner isolate in culture positive ADC. Gram-negative infection should primarily be suspected in patients who are diabetic, immunocompromised, or have atypical infections; for instance, persons residing in nursing homes. Among anaerobic microorganisms, *Bacteroides, Peptostreptococcus* species, *Propionibacterium* species, *Prevotella* species, and *Fusobacterium* species have been isolated.

Staphylococcus aureus, Haemophilus influenzae, beta-hemolytic streptococci, mycobacterial species, and pneumococci are the commonest pathogens isolated from pediatric dacryocystitis patients.

HISTOPATHOLOGY

Histopathological examination reveals inflammatory changes along the entire lacrimal pathway, extending to the nasolacrimal duct and nasal mucosa. Stasis and infection due to distal obstruction of the lacrimal outflow system can be identified. The sac itself may be affected by granuloma or abscess formation.

DIFFERENTIAL DIAGNOSIS

The clinical features of ADC are usually unmistakable; however, certain other conditions may confuse the clinician with a somewhat similar presentation, calling for further investigations. These include infective conditions (bacterial conjunctivitis, canaliculitis, and pediatric actinomycosis), inflammatory conditions such as chalazia, malignancies such as leukemias and basal cell carcinoma of the eyelids, and systemic conditions such as acute complications of sarcoidosis. Rarely, an occult tumor or cyst can cause medial canthal fullness.

TREATMENT

The treatment of ADC is in three phases:
- *Acute dacryocystitis with preseptal cellulitis:* It is treated with oral antibiotics, nonsteroidal anti-inflammatory drugs, topical antibiotics, and hot compresses. If the presentation is very severe or if impending orbital cellulitis is suspected, parenteral antibiotics and nonsteroidal anti-inflammatory drugs (NSAIDs) should be initiated. While systemic antibiotics are given for at least 5–7 days, oral NSAIDs may be continued for a longer duration, and topical antibiotics (though of limited value because of lacrimal stasis) applied four to six times daily till the obstruction is relieved. Wet or dry hot fomentation should always be instituted as it helps reduce the inflammation, and also provides symptomatic relief to the patient. Systemic comorbidities, especially diabetes mellitus and immune status, should be given due attention.
- *Acute dacryocystitis with a lacrimal abscess:* It needs an incision and drainage with empirical antibiotics, NSAIDs, and warm compresses. Surgical drainage of the abscess should be attempted only after the swelling becomes localized (with an obvious pus point) or fluctuant. Under local anesthesia, the skin over the softest part of the abscess is incised with an 11 number surgical blade. Pus is allowed to drain and its evacuation assisted by gentle pressure over the sides of the incision (a sample of pus can be collected on a sterile swab stick for culture and sensitivity at this stage). A small curved hemostat can be inserted in the cavity to break the loculi of the abscess by firmly spreading the tips of the hemostat. When no more pus can be expressed from the cavity, it is packed with a length of gauze soaked in 5% betadine solution. No sutures are required and the wound is allowed to heal by secondary intention. The pack can be removed after 24 hours, by which time the patient will have experienced considerable symptomatic relief. Concurrent oral or parenteral antibiotics and NSAIDs are a must, as are topical antibiotics.
- *Acute dacryocystitis with orbital cellulitis:* It necessitates hospitalization with intravenous (IV) antibiotics. Empirical antimicrobial therapy should be initiated immediately with broad spectrum antibiotics such as ampicillin-clavulanic acid or with drugs for penicillin-resistant *Staphylococcus* (such as nafcillin or cloxacillin). Samples for cultures should be obtained prior to antibiotic therapy. Topical antibiotics in the form of drops/ointment should also be given. Steroids may be added judiciously under cover of antibiotics to control the inflammation. While the patient is undergoing treatment, he should be watched daily for evidence of increasing inflammation refractory to the administered antibiotics. The pupillary reflex and the extraocular motility and if possible, the vision, should be checked and recorded. Signs of extension of the process to the central nervous system (CNS) should be looked out for.
- *Pediatric ADC:* ADC in neonates carries a high risk of serious complications such as sepsis, meningitis, and endocarditis, and may require IV antibiotic therapy and hospitalization or close observation. Urgent surgical intervention with nasolacrimal duct probing with or without nasal endoscopy for excision of intranasal cyst may be warranted, but should be performed after a minimum of 24 hours of IV antibiotic therapy. General anesthesia is usually not required. Blood cultures should be done before starting treatment.

- *Definitive treatment:* Definitive treatment is surgery (dacryocystorhinostomy). This may be external, endonasal, or endocanalicular laser-assisted dacryocystorhinostomy (DCR). Endocanalicular laser assisted and especially endonasal DCR may be done in the acute setting, but external DCR should only be done after the inflammation has resolved fully. Clinically this is seen as resolution of swelling and induration and an absence of tenderness over the sac area.

COMPLICATIONS

Lacrimal abscess with fistula, orbital cellulitis, subperiosteal abscess, optic atrophy, cavernous sinus thrombosis, meningitis, endocarditis, and death.

SUMMARY

Acute dacryocystitis is a condition which warrants immediate attention and treatment. Pediatric patients need special care because of the higher risk of serious complications. Diagnosis is mostly clinical and ancillary investigations are usually not required.

9.23 Canaliculitis

Ramesh Murthy
Axis Eye Clinic, Pune
drrameshmurthy@gmail.com

INTRODUCTION

Primary chronic canaliculitis is inflammation of lacrimal canaliculi. This can be caused by variety of bacteria, viruses, and mycotic organisms.

The most common causative organism is *Actinomyces israelii*, a filamentous gram-positive, non-acid-fast, cast forming, and nonspore forming anaerobic *Bacillus*. This *Bacillus* is difficult to isolate and to identify. This organism is found in soil more commonly in decayed organic matter like wet hay. It is also found in normal oral cavities, tonsillar crypts, dental plaques, and carious teeth.

- Other bacteria (*Fusobacterium* and *Nocardia* species)
- Fungal (*Candida, Fusarium*, and *Aspergillus* species)
- Viral (herpes simplex and varicella zoster)
- An important etiological factor is retained punctal plug
  Obstruction of the canaliculus can promote anaerobic bacterial growth secondary to stasis.

SYMPTOMS

- Watering
- Redness of eyes, especially at the medial canthus
- Mucopurulent discharge
- Irritation
- Medial eyelid and canthal pain

SIGNS

- Pouting and swollen punctum. A pouted punctum is a clinically diagnostic feature which occurs in <50% of patients.
- Discharge can be expressed out by exerting pressure over the canaliculus (confirmatory sign). Typically discharge contains concretions which consist of sulfur granules which may be expressed on canalicular compression with a glass rod or become evident following canaliculotomy.
- Pericanalicular inflammation is characterized by edema of the canaliculus.

- It can be characterized by swollen and congested plica, canalicular swelling, and overlying erythematous lid.
- In most cases, the lower canaliculus is affected, and the lacrimal sac and duct are not commonly involved.

INVESTIGATIONS
- Canalicular discharge and canaliculitis are subjected to Gram's stain and Giemsa stain.
- Culture and sensitivity testing is done (i.e., blood agar, Sabouraud agar, and anaerobic culture).
- Special staining (i.e., Calcofluor-white) can be performed.
- Imaging studies, though not routinely indicated can be done.
- Dacryocystography is a useful tool. This can be used to view the anatomy of the lacrimal drainage system.
- High-resolution ultrasonography using a 20 MHz transducer in chronic canaliculitis can show canalicular ectasia and sulfur granules usually measuring 1-2 mm in diameter.

MANAGEMENT
Medical Treatment
- Canaliculitis is difficult to treat medically. Initially treatment is started with broad-spectrum antibiotics, e.g., trimethoprim sulfate/polymyxin B, and moxifloxacin eye drops, and after culture reports specific treatment can be given.
- Oral doxycycline 100 mg twice a day can be used for 1-2 weeks.
- Fungal canaliculitis is treated with nystatin drops three times a day and nystatin solution irrigation several times per week.
- Herpes infection can be treated with trifluridine 1% drops five times per day.
- Actinomycetes are susceptible to penicillin and cephalosporin but have tendency to form stones; organism within the stones are safe from antibiotics and canaliculotomy is required to completely remove all stones.
- Canaliculitis can be completely cured only when all the stones and concretions are completely removed.

Surgical Care
- Canaliculitis not resolving on topical treatment required surgical intervention and removal of casts. A 2-snip punctoplasty and curettage is done to remove casts. Probing is performed to check for any diverticulum and remaining casts following which lacrimal irrigation should be done with antibiotic solution.
- Culture of the dacryoliths (after surgically obtained) and secretions will give confirmatory proof of *Actinomyces* which will help in proper treatment of the canaliculitis.
- After surgery patients may be treated with topical cefazolin for a month.
- Use of adjunctive hyperbaric oxygen has also been tried with success.

DIFFERENTIAL DIAGNOSIS
- Lacrimal diverticulum
- Lacrimal stone
- Herpes simplex infection can cause acute canaliculitis
- Giant fornix syndrome occurs in elderly, especially with levator disinsertion, where the upper fornix is colonized by *Staphylococcus aureus* and leads to purulent relapsing conjunctivitis.

PROGNOSIS
When the causative organism is confirmed and proper treatment is given, prognosis is excellent.

9.24 Tumors of Lacrimal Drainage System

Lakshmi Mahesh
Sakra World Hospital, Bengaluru
lakshmimahesh1@gmail.com

Smita Menon
Kamal Eye Clinic, Mumbai

Sonali Gaikwad
Sri Sankaradeva Nethralaya, Guwahati

Lacrimal sac masses are rare; hence, early recognition and management are of utmost importance as these tumors are locally invasive and potentially life-threatening.

EMBRYOLOGY

The lacrimal drainage system (LDS) is a complex anatomical structure that originates from the ectoderm and comprises the upper and lower punctum, the upper and lower canaliculi, the common canaliculus, the lacrimal sac, and the nasolacrimal duct. The epithelium lining the LDS undergoes a transition from the non-keratinizing, stratified squamous epithelium of the canaliculus to the stratified columnar epithelium with goblet cells that cover the lacrimal sac and nasolacrimal duct. The epithelium of the lacrimal sac and nasolacrimal duct exhibits apical specialization with microvilli and kinocilia. The LDS is surrounded by specialized lymphoid tissue, and there are also lymphocytes, macrophages, and immunoglobulin A (IgA) present in the epithelium. Intraepithelial melanocytes are present in the healthy LDS mucosa.

The primary function of the LDS is to drain tears from the ocular surface to the inferior meatus of the nasal cavity. Although the presence of apical microvilli suggests that the epithelium has an absorptive function, the exact mechanism of this process is not fully understood. Therefore, further research is required to elucidate the physiological significance of these microvilli.

AGE AND SEX PREDILECTION

The presence of benign tumors is commonly seen in the younger age group with malignant presentation seen commonly in the fifth decade of life. Male preponderance is noted.

PATHOGENESIS

The tumors are classified into three groups:
1. Primary epithelial
2. Primary nonepithelial
3. Inflammatory lesions

Epithelial Tumors

Epithelial tumors are the most common tumors of the lacrimal sac, constituting approximately 60–94% of all benign tumors.

Benign

Papillomas are the most common and comprise 36% of epithelial tumors. Other benign epithelial tumors include oncocytoma, adenomas and cylindromas however, these are extremely rare. These are believed to develop due to squamous metaplasia secondary to preexisting inflammation.

Malignant
Squamous cell carcinoma is the most frequently reported malignant tumor, followed by transitional cell carcinoma, oncocytic adenocarcinoma, mucoepidermoid carcinoma, and cystic adenoid carcinoma. Moreover, inverted papilloma is a tumor that has a tendency to recur locally and carries a high risk of malignant transformation transforming to squamous cell carcinoma. A common risk factor for both inverted papilloma and squamous cell carcinoma is human papillomavirus-6 (HPV-6) and HPV-18.

Nonepithelial Tumors

Rarer occurrence compared to epithelial tumors representing 25% of lacrimal sac tumors and is divided into three subtypes:
- *Lymphoproliferative tumors:* Commonly arising secondarily to systemic spread with leukemia or lymphomas, they account for 2–8% of lacrimal sac tumors.
- *Melanocytic tumors:* These tumors account for 4–5% of lacrimal sac tumors with benign lesions being rare in occurrence and malignant lesions accounting for 0.7% of ocular melanomas. Origin is said to be from the melanocytes in the epidermal lining of the lacrimal sac or secondary to seeding of conjunctival melanomas along the lacrimal drainage system.
- *Mesenchymal tumors:* This subtype forms 12–14% of the lacrimal sac tumors. The most common benign variant is the fibrous histiocytoma followed by fibroma, hemangiopericytoma, angiofibroma, lipoma, leiomyoma, and osteoma. Malignant variants include Kaposi sarcoma and rhabdomyosarcoma.

SIGNS AND SYMPTOMS

All patients present with one or more symptoms relating to a growing tumor mass at the site of the lacrimal sac. Others present with symptoms of chronic nasolacrimal duct obstruction like epiphora with blood-stained tears also known as hemolacria have also been reported. The triad of signs suspicious for malignancy include: (1) mass above the medial canthal tendon, (2) chronic dacryocystitis that irrigates freely, and (3) sanguinous reflux on irrigation.[1]

A firm, palpable, non-compressible mass may be present in the lacrimal sac area usually extending below the medial canthal tendon. When the mass is immobile, adherent to the deeper structures associated with pain and extending above the medial canthal tendon it is more likely to be malignant. Diagnosis of lacrimal sac tumors is usually incidental as discovered during dacrocystorhinostomy. Late-stage tumors may present with signs of orbital invasion, such as proptosis and nonaxial globe displacement, lymphadenopathy, overlying skin ulceration, and rarely, distant metastasis.[2-4]

DIAGNOSIS

Clinically, lacrimal sac tumors masquerade chronic dacryocystitis and often are misdiagnosed and managed conservatively until advanced stages of the disease. The median time for diagnosis is approximately 12 months and even longer for patients reporting epiphora as the only presenting symptom. Due to the delay in recognition and diagnosis, a large subset of patients present with locally advanced tumors and lymph node involvement at the time of diagnosis.

Involvement of the orbit, nose, and sinuses is common with late-stage diagnosis. Orbital invasion presents with proptosis, motility restriction with diplopia or optic neuropathy. Signs of sinonasal spread include ulceration of overlying skin, nose bleeds, anosmia, and nasal stuffiness. Lymphadenopathy and distant metastasis a common finding in late-stage presentation and should always be evaluated for.

Complete ocular examination of a patient presenting with epiphora suspicious of a lacrimal sac tumor includes inspection, palpation and digital expression of the lacrimal sac contents i.e. regurgitation on pressure over lacrimal sac (ROPLAS) test, sac syringing

SECTION 9: Oculoplasty

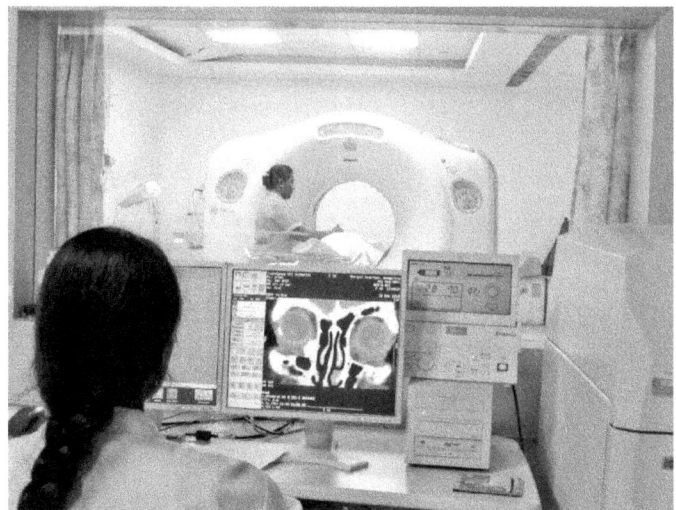

Fig. 9.24.1: Computed tomographic dacryocystography (CT-DCG) provides useful information in diagnosis of lacrimal tumors. Magnetic resonance dacryocystography (MR-DCG) allows better 3D visualization of the lacrimal drainage system (LDS) and dynamic functional evaluation.

which almost always reveals a patent LDS, probing of the lacrimal system and examination of the nasal cavity.

Differential Diagnosis
- Chronic dacryocystitis
- Nonspecific chronic inflammation "pseudotumor"
- Dacryolith

Imaging
In the evaluation of a suspected lacrimal sac mass, computed tomography (CT) imaging plays a key role in determining the presence of a mass, as well as its location and potential impact on adjacent structures. However, magnetic resonance imaging (MRI) offers superior tumor definition, allowing for a more nuanced understanding of the mass, including cystic or solid nature, and the degree of invasion into surrounding structures. Dacryocystography (DCG) can also provide useful information, although a negative result does not preclude the possibility of a tumor. A comprehensive approach utilizing multiple diagnostic modalities is often necessary to achieve an accurate diagnosis and guide appropriate treatment strategies.

A direct incisional biopsy with histopathologic assessment is recommended for a definitive diagnosis, tumor grading, staging, and for treatment. Metastatic workup can be commenced in coordination with an oncologist.

■ MANAGEMENT
Dacryocystectomy is the treatment of choice for benign epithelial or mesenchymal tumors confined to the lacrimal sac. In malignant lesions, en bloc tumor excision along with periosteum removal around the lacrimal sac and nasolacrimal duct is recommended. Tumor recurrence is attributed to the extension of premalignant lesions along the nasolacrimal duct. Postoperative radiotherapy or systemic chemotherapy can be delivered to prevent tumor dissemination and minimize recurrence.

In cases with radiological evidence of bony destruction beyond the lacrimal drainage system, resection of the orbital and nasal walls may be advocated. Radiotherapy is a

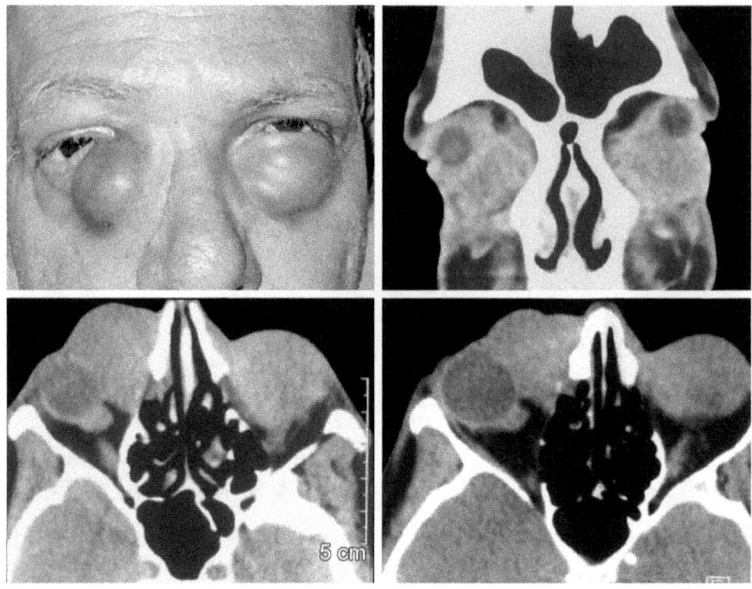

Fig. 9.24.2: A 56-year-old male patient with bilateral swellings at the medial canthal area. Biopsy confirmed non-Hodgkin's lymphoma of the orbit. The patient responded well to treatment.

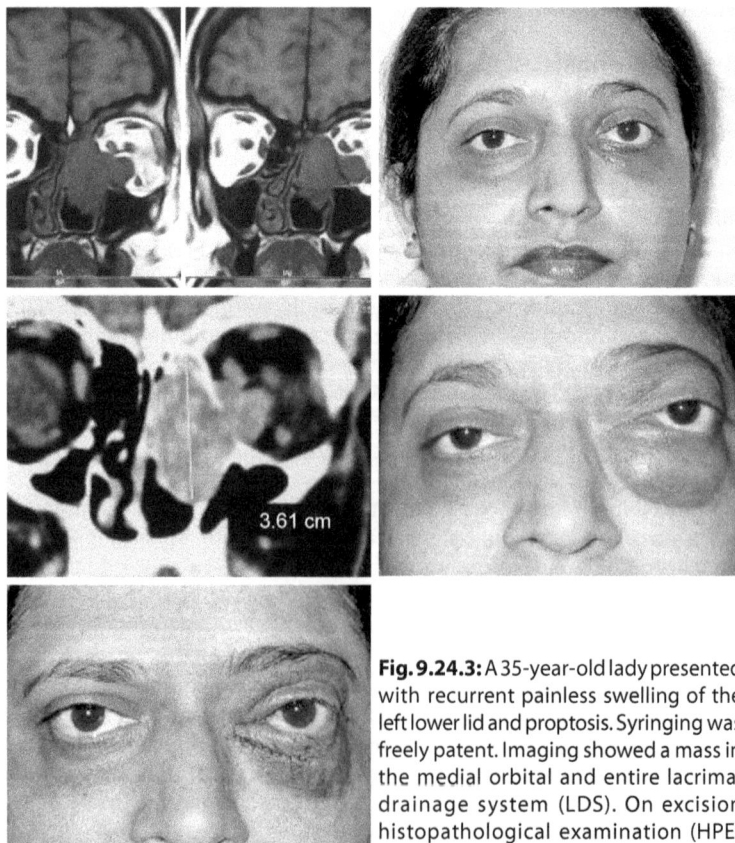

Fig. 9.24.3: A 35-year-old lady presented with recurrent painless swelling of the left lower lid and proptosis. Syringing was freely patent. Imaging showed a mass in the medial orbital and entire lacrimal drainage system (LDS). On excision histopathological examination (HPE) revealed solitary fibrous tumor.

SECTION 9: Oculoplasty

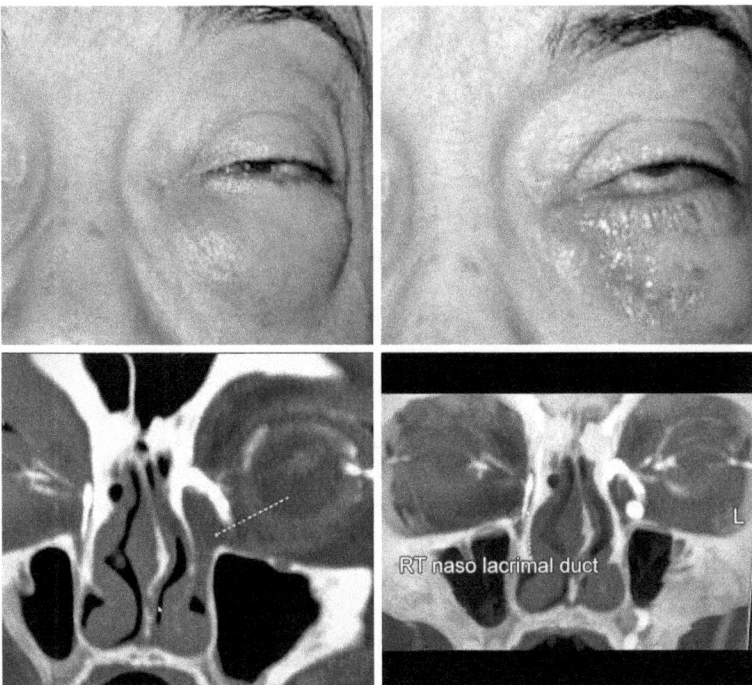

Fig. 9.24.4: A 60-year-old lady with left-sided painless progressive medial canthal swelling and proptosis. Histopathological examination (HPE) confirmed non-Hodgkin's lymphoma involving the lacrimal drainage system (LDS) extending into the orbit. The patient responded well to radiation treatment.

highly recommended treatment option in cases where there is clear evidence of bone or lymphatic invasion or when neoplastic cells are present in the resection margins. While radiotherapy alone is not typically considered the primary treatment, it can be an effective palliative option for patients with advanced cancer. The approach to the management of advanced stage disease requires a multidisciplinary team with short and long-term monitoring as recurrences and metastasis have been documented years after initial treatment.

PROGNOSIS

For malignant tumors confined to the lacrimal sac treated by dacryocystectomy and irradiation, the reported 5-year mortality rate is 44%, in contrast to those supplemented by lateral rhinotomy, with an associated mortality rate of only 13%.[5] Tumor type and growth pattern significantly impact prognosis and mortality. Papillary squamous carcinoma has a better prognosis (14% mortality), while transitional cell carcinoma has a poor prognosis (100% mortality).

REFERENCES

1. Flanagan JC, Stokes DP. Lacrimal sac tumors. Ophthalmology. 1978;85:1282-7.
2. Krishna Y, Coupland SE. Lacrimal sac tumors—a review. Asia Pac J Ophthalmol (Phila). 2017;6(2):173-8.
3. Kim HJ, Shields CL, Langer PD. Lacrimal sac tumors: diagnosis and treatment. In: Calvano CJ, Black EH, Nesi FA, Gladstone GJ, Servat JJ, (Eds). Smith and Nesi's Ophthalmic Plastic and Reconstructive Surgery. New York: Springer; 2012:609-14.

4. Schaefer DP. Acquired causes of lacrimal system obstructions. In: Calvano CJ, Black EH, Nesi FA, Gladstone GJ, Servat JJ, (Eds). Smith and Nesi's Ophthalmic Plastic and Reconstructive Surgery. New York: Springer; 2012:609-614.
5. Ni C, D'Amico DJ, Fan CQ, Kuo PK. Tumors of the lacrimal sac: a clinicopathological analysis of 82 cases. Int Ophthalmol Clin.1982;22:121-40.

9.25 Enucleation, Evisceration, and Exenteration

Kasturi Bhattacharjee, Deepika Kapoor
Sri Sankardeva Nethralaya, Guwahati
kasturibhattacharjee44@hotmail.com, deepika_kapoor14@yahoo.co.in

DEFINITIONS

- *Enucleation:* Enucleation is the removal of the globe and optic nerve from the orbit, along with the separation of all its connections.
- *Evisceration:* Evisceration involves removal of the contents of the eye, while leaving behind the scleral shell attached to the extraocular muscles.

ENUCLEATION

Indications

- *Malignant tumors in the eye:* In case a malignant tumor is suspected or conformed by imaging studies, *enucleation should be done and not evisceration*, e.g., retinoblastoma and melanoma.
- *Blind and painful eyes:* If possible, the cause must be identified as it may have an effect on the subsequent management.
- Severely injured blind eye
- Microphthalmia with cyst
- Phthisis bulbi
- Rarely few cases with autoenucleation have also been reported

EVISCERATION

Indications

- Anterior staphyloma
- Endophthalmitis
- Total sloughed out corneal ulcer in a blind eye

Contraindications

- Proven or suspected intraocular malignant tumors
- If precise histopathology of the specimen is needed
- Eyes with scleral contracture
- Severely mutilated eyes
- Evisceration in an injured eye carries a risk of sympathetic ophthalmia in the other eyes due to residual microscopic uveal tissue in the scleral canals.

PREOPERATIVE COUNSELING

- Patient requires psychological support, detailed and meticulous pre- and postoperative explanations as he/she has to undergo a permanent loss of the eye.
- Systemic evaluation by physician
- The concerns that can arise during immediate and late postoperative period due to anophthalmic socket should be explained to the patient, and he/she must also be

informed about the options of ocular prosthesis—stock shell and custom fit prosthesis. Patient should be explained regarding the time period after which the prosthesis (approximately 6 weeks)
- The indications for surgery should also be explained clearly and in detail.
- The exenteration candidate must be given detail information and counseled regarding the radicle nature of the surgery.

SURGICAL TECHNIQUE FOR ENUCLEATION

- *Principle:* The removal of the whole intact eye by excising the extraocular muscles and transecting the optic nerve **(Figs. 9.25.1A to E)**.
- *Method:*
  - It can be performed under local anesthetic with a retrobulbar block or peribulbar block. But for children, general anesthetic is necessary.
  - A speculum is inserted for adequate exposure.
  - Conjunctival peritomy is done for all 360° using forceps and corneoscleral scissors around the limbus separating the conjunctiva from the cornea.
  - The conjunctiva is separated from the globe in the four quadrants by blunt dissection.
  - Each of the four rectus muscles are then hooked using a squint hook.
  - Each muscle is then tagged with silk sutures (for traction) and Vicryl sutures for reattachment of the muscles for the socket reconstruction. The muscles should be separated about 1-2 mm from the globe.
  - Heavy scissors are then passed round the eye to bluntly dissect the soft tissue around the globe from the optic nerve either nasally or temporally. Once the optic nerve is free of all soft tissue attachments it is cut.
  - In cases of a suspected retinoblastoma, it is very important to obtain a long optic nerve stump (10-15 mm at least). This can be done by strong traction on the insertions of the recti muscles using artery forceps or sutures so that the eye is pulled forward and it stretches the optic nerve.
  - The eye is prolapsed forward from the orbit followed by dividing the remaining oblique muscles and attachments. The socket is packed with gauze and firm pressure should be applied for 4-8 minutes.

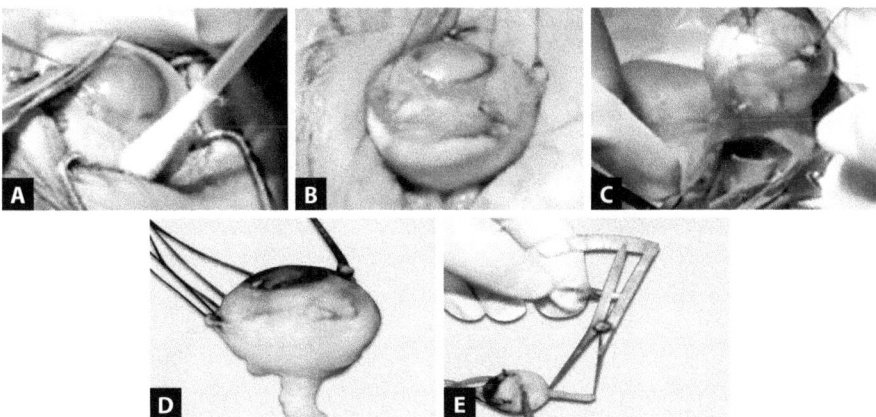

Figs. 9.25.1A to E: Steps of enucleation. (A) Conjunctival limbal peritomy; (B) Traction on the globe; (C) Soft tissue dissection prior to transecting the optic nerve; (D and E) Optic nerve stump measurement.

- The closure of the wound should be done in at least two layers, first the Tenon's capsule and then the conjunctiva. Continuous or interrupted absorbable sutures can be used for closing the wound.
- Antibiotic ointment, a firm pad, and bandage are then applied.

Myoconjunctival Technique for Enhanced Motility
- The initial steps are similar as for standard enucleation procedure
- Superior oblique tendon is sutured to superior rectus muscle
- Inferior oblique tendon sutured to lateral rectus muscle
- Optic nerve is cut using enucleation scissors
- Hemostasis is achieved
- Implant placed posterior to posterior Tenon's fascia
- Posterior Tenon's capsule closed
- Each rectus is sutured to opposite fornix by passing previously placed double armed Vicryl suture through Tenon's fascia and conjunctiva
- Recti should not cross midline
- Closure of anterior Tenon's fascia and conjunctiva is done
- This method provides good motility to prosthesis.

■ SURGICAL TECHNIQUE FOR EVISCERATION
- *Choice of anesthesia:* Local anesthesia (LA) with or without sedation, or general anesthesia (GA), especially in case of children **(Figs. 9.25.2A to D)**.
- *Peritomy:* The surgeon should be careful to preserve as much conjunctiva as possible.
- *Removal of corneal button:* A full-thickness stab incision at the limbus is made with an 11 number blade scalpel. This is followed by extending the limbal incision with corneoscleral scissors. Finally, the corneal button is excised.
- *Removal of intraocular contents:* Removed with the help of an "evisceration spoon", to separate the uveal tissue from the sclera. Special care is given to the complete removal of all uveal tissue.
- *Application of alcohol:* Inner surface of the sclera is then thoroughly cleaned with alcohol to denature any residual protein that may be a potential for sympathetic ophthalmia. Cautery should be avoided.
- *Sclerotomy:* Performing a sclerotomy, to allow for placement of larger implants, is now popular among many surgeons.

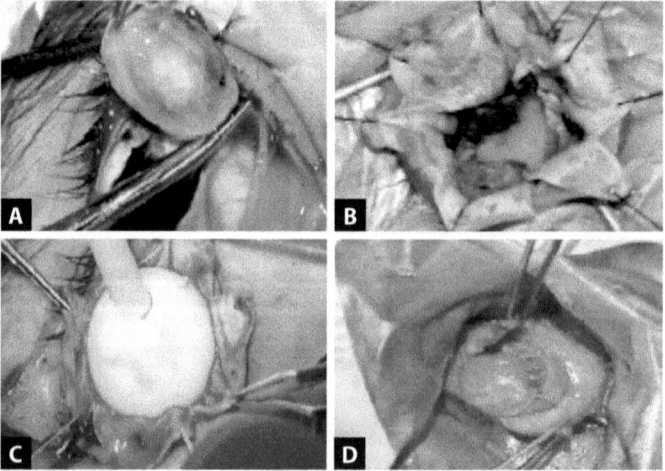

Figs. 9.25.2A to D: Steps of evisceration (sclerotomy quadrisection technique).

- *Implant placement:* The initial day practice was to place the largest implant possible. However, with the use of modern sclerotomy techniques, any size implant can now be used, depending on the prominence of the fellow eye. This results in a better cosmesis.
- *Closure:* The closure is done in multiple layers, including the sclera, Tenon's membrane, and lastly conjunctiva. This practice results in better retention of implant and the extrusion of implant is minimal as well.

SCLEROTOMY TECHNIQUES

- Classically with the evisceration technique, the largest implant that fits inside the scleral cavity without undue tension is 18 mm.
- Various sclerotomy techniques have been described, all aim to overcome this drawback:
  - *Multiple radial sclerotomy:* This has been described by Stephenson in 1987.
  - *Posterior sclerotomy:* This technique has been described by Kostick and Linberg in 1995.
  - *Disinserting optic nerve:* In 1997, Jordan and Anderson described disinserting the optic nerve and performing small radial sclerotomies.
  - *Scleral quadrisection:* By Yang et al., the technique left the optic nerve intact.
  - *Intraconal implant placement:* By Long et al., placing the implant behind the sclera in the muscle cone.
- In 2001, Massry and Hold described obliquely splitting the scleral cavity in two, and releasing the flaps from their optic nerve attachments.
- *Four petal technique:* In 2007, Sales-Sanz and Sanz-Lopez described this technique. Four complete sclerotomies from the limbus to the optic nerve have been performed. The optic nerve has been disinserted in this technique.
- For phthisis bulbi and microphthalmos, Georgescu et al. have described technique where a 5-mm wedge of sclera was excised nasally and temporally and a 360° equatorial scleral incision was made, dividing the scleral into anterior and posterior halves.
- Advantage of intraconal placement of implant is that it allows a large implant and gives an extra barrier of posterior sclera (**Fig. 9.25.3**).

COMPLICATIONS

Evisceration

- Postoperative infection, especially in cases of the procedure being performed in endophthalmitis or panophthalmitis
- Postoperative extrusion of the orbital implant
- Poor wound healing of the scleral edges
- Postoperative pain, more common in cases where the cornea is retained

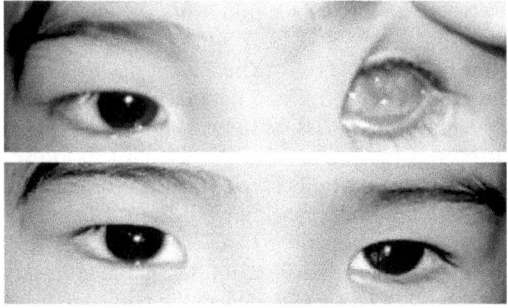

Fig. 9.25.3: Cosmesis after prosthesis fitting.

Enucleation

- Extrusion of orbital implant
- Volume deficiency of the anophthalmic socket
- Lower eyelid laxity leading to shelving of fornices resulting in poor prosthesis support
- Migration of orbital implant
- Upper eyelid ptosis
- Chronic conjunctivitis and mucoid discharge

Exenteration

- *Definition:* Orbital exenteration is surgical procedure that involves the removal of all the soft tissue contents of the orbit.
- *Types:*
  - *Total:* Removal of all of the soft tissues of orbit and periorbital adnexa.
  - *Subtotal:* Eyelid skin is preserved.
  - *Extended:* Resection of adjacent tissues (paranasal sinuses).
- *Indications:*
  - Malignant disorders:
    - Malignant eyelid tumors with orbital extension [basal cell carcinoma (BCC) and squamous cell carcinoma (SCC)]
    - Malignant eyelid tumors where simple surgical excision is not adequate [sebaceous gland carcinoma (SGC) with extensive conjunctival involvement]
    - Malignant conjunctival lesions (extensive conjunctival melanoma)
    - Malignant paranasal sinus tumors with orbital extension
    - Primary malignant orbital tumors (lacrimal gland carcinomas)
  - Nonmalignant disorders:
    - Benign orbital tumors (aggressive orbital meningioma)
    - Life-threatening infections (sino-orbital mucormycosis)
    - Severe nonsteroidal anti-inflammatory drug (NSAID) with intractable pain and blindness
    - Severe orbital deformity (neurofibromatosis)
    - End-stage socket contracture
- *Preoperative evaluation:*
  - Review of paraffin-fixed histopathological sections
  - Thorough ophthalmic examinations
  - General physical examination
  - Review of radiological imaging
  - Typing and cross-matching of blood
  - Complete blood count (CBC), platelet count, and coagulation profile
  - Discontinue antiplatelets 2 weeks prior to surgery
- *Anesthesia:* The procedure can be done under GA but under special circumstances it may be performed under LA with intravenous (IV) sedation.
- *Technique:* The steps for the surgical technique are as follows:
  - Total exenteration:
    - Along the line of the orbital rim, an incision is placed firmly down to the bone.
    - Firm pressure on wound edge and judicial use of diathermy along with use of diluted adrenaline into the tissues help to control bleeding at this point.
    - The periosteum is incised around the orbital rim to expose the bare bone, on which further dissection is carried on. Then the periosteum is separated from the underlying bone passing from the orbital rim toward the apex of the orbit.
    - It should be noted that the periosteum is adhered to the bone at the rim of the orbit, and it is hard to be separated from the bone, but is easier to be separated from the bone further back in the orbit right up to the apex of the orbit.

- The medial orbital wall which is the thinnest part requires careful handling. The dissection is completed as far back as possible to the apex of the orbit. The tissues at the orbital apex are then severed using curved scissors or a scalpel blade.
- Profuse bleeding is usually encountered at this stage, which can be controlled either with high-end cautery or by firm pressure applied for >4 minutes.
- The orbit may be left packed and a delayed skin graft performed, or it may be left to granulate and skin will gradually cover it from the edge.
- If the hemostasis is well controlled then on table split-thickness skin can be harvested and placed directly over the exposed socket. However, one can use a mesh graft with holes in it or a scattered application of small patches of skin as this allows drainage and is more likely to "take".
- The graft is applied over a damp pack which is pushed into the orbit. The edges of the graft may be stitched to the skin at the orbital rim.
- The graft will usually take even though it is applied directly to bone and if areas do fail they will re-epithelialize quite quickly.

- *Postoperative care:*
  - *Aquacel (cavity dressing):* Soft, sterile, hydrophilic, and nonwoven ribbon dressing made of hydrocolloid fibers.
  - *Allevyn cavity dressing:* Nonadhesive, hydrocellular cavity dressing. 5 cm in diameter, biconvex hydrophilic, polyurethane foam dressing covered in a nonadhesive polymeric wrapping.
  - *Medihoney:* Antibacterial wound gel containing 80% (80 mg/g) antibacterial honey, derived from group of plants leptospermum. It has high osmotic potential, having the characteristic property of wound cleaning, refreshes malodorous wounds, promoting autolytic debridement, and provides a shield that helps in easy wound dressing. Aids in healing of difficult sockets.
- *Subtotal exenteration:*
  - Eyelid skin is preserved
  - Skin incision placed 2 mm behind the lash line, skin and orbicularis flap is undermined till arcus marginalis
  - After completion of procedure skin is draped into the exenterated socket
  - Antibiotic ointment and dressing done
- *Extended exenteration:*
  - This is applicable in situation wherein there is extension of the diseases process to the adjacent adnexal tissues mainly the paranasal sinus and cranial cavity.
  - Multidisciplinary approach.

ORBITAL RECONSTRUCTION

1. *Laissez faire:* Healing by secondary intention. It has the following:
   Advantages:
   - Simple
   - Easy follow-up in cases where chances of recurrence exists
   - Reduced operating time
   Disadvantages:
   - Healing period is prolonged
   - Spontaneous fistula communicating with the ethmoid sinus may develop
   - Eyebrow may be drawn inferiorly by wound contracture
2. *Split-thickness skin grafts:*
   - *Local flaps:* Temporalis muscle transposition flap.
   - *Free flaps:* Radial forearm free flap.
3. *Osseointegration technique:* Using titanium implants, permits direct coupling of orbitofacial prosthesis to bony margin.

ORBITAL PROSTHESIS
- Customized orbital and orbitofacial prosthesis
- Standard black or customized patch
- *Spectacle prosthesis:*
  - Spectacles with opaque lens and side shield
  - Despite all the available options patients may not accept the prosthesis due to various reasons. Reasons for not accepting prosthesis include:
    - Lack of blinking and ocular movements resulting in unnatural appearance
    - Intolerance to local tissue adhesives
    - Difficulty in camouflaging the edges of the prosthesis
    - Rapid degradation of prosthesis
    - Cost for maintenance of prosthesis

9.26 | Anophthalmic Socket

Bipasha Mukerjee
Sankara Netralaya, Chennai
drbpm@snmail.org

Ruhi Jange

INTRODUCTION

Anophthalmic socket refers to an orbit without a clinically discernible eye. It can either be of congenital origin or acquired. Congenital anophthalmos is rare (0.3–0.6/10,000 births) and due to arrest of embryogenesis during formation of the optic vesicle.[1] Acquired anophthalmos can be due to trauma, but more commonly due to surgical removal (evisceration or enucleation).

PATHOGENESIS/PATHOPHYSIOLOGY

The absence of the eye or its contents leads to major changes in the physiology and dynamics of the orbit. Severe contraction of the socket may occur following trauma (accidental, or iatrogenic, due to surgical removal of the globe), non-replacement of orbital volume with an implant, recurrent inflammation due to an ill-fitting prosthesis, or radiotherapy. The pathophysiologic basis of the problems associated with anophthalmos is postulated to be a disturbance in the spatial architecture and interrelationships of the multiple tissue components of the orbit, and not orbital fat atrophy or a reduction of metabolic activity. No change in circulation dynamics or blood flow to orbital tissues was seen in anophthalmic sockets during experimental animal studies.[2]

CLINICAL EVALUATION

The general appearance and facial symmetry of the patient should be noted first **(Appendix 9.26.1)**. The prosthesis (if patient is using one) should be well centered, at the same level as the normal eye without any pseudoptosis or enophthalmos. The shell should have a "wet" look with normal blinking and absence of lagophthalmos. The ocular movements should be within the conversational range (10–15°).

Slit-lamp examination of the prosthesis should be done next to look for surface deposits, scratches, eyelid margins, and lash position. Any surface problem mandates a referral to the ocularist for polishing of the shell (entropion).

Socket should be examined after removal of the prosthesis. For this the lower lid is pulled downward and outward popping the inferior edge of the prosthesis forward slight pressure on the upper edge will pop the prosthesis out. The prosthesis edges should be rounded and smooth, the posterior surface should fit well with the anterior surface of the socket without redundant space in between. The conjunctival mucosa is examined for congestion, giant papillary conjunctivitis (GPC), excessive mucus or discharge. The implant, if present, should be well centered and the fornices should be adequate.

Do not forget to examine the normal eye and prescribe full-frame polycarbonate safety glasses.

INVESTIGATIONS

- B-scan ultrasonography:
    - To rule out any intraocular mass before evisceration
    - To measure the other normal eye axial length (A-scan)
    - To confirm the integrity of a microphthalmic globe
    - To evaluate an orbital cyst
- Computed tomography (CT) scan/magnetic resonance imaging (MRI):
    - In any suspected orbital mass, especially with history of retinoblastoma/irradiation
    - Volumetric measurements of the socket

MANAGEMENT

Nonsurgical Management

- *Optical illusion:* For the patient interested in a nonsurgical fixation, placing a +2 D sphere or higher over the affected side will magnify the eye socket making the enophthalmos less noticeable.
- Discharge is a common complaint of the anophthalmic patient, and the most common etiology is a lack of lubrication. If the discharge is white and ropy, the cause is GPC. The conjunctiva becomes edematous and excessive discharge can be seen. This condition is treated by prosthetic polishing and topical cromolyn sodium or topical steroids.
- The patient should be advised to review with the ocularist once a year for shell polishing and modifications as required. The average customized prosthesis should last for about 7 years and stock shells should ideally be changed every year.
- Artificial tears should be prescribed for lifelong use. Vitamin E oil with aloe vera has been used in dry sockets.

Surgical Management

- *Volume replacement:* Secondary implantation using alloplastic implants or autologous transplants can be done if there is no orbital implant.[3] However, extensive deep orbital soft tissue dissection for localizing and visualizing the extraocular muscles should be avoided. This can cause tissue alteration and persistent damage. It has been demonstrated that on frequent and extensive surgical dissection, there is a significant shrinkage of orbital fat tissue with a loss of orbital volume, defeating any volume augmentation initially intended. Hence, it is advisable to refrain from any unnecessary dissection of the orbital soft tissues, including the exposure of the extraocular muscles. An intraconal positioning of an alloplastic implant is recommended.

    A dermis-fat graft (DFG) comprises dermis of the skin with adjacent fat tissue. The preferable area for a DFG is the gluteal region. It is transplanted into the socket and attached to the soft tissues of the orbit (**Fig. 9.26.1**). It can be used

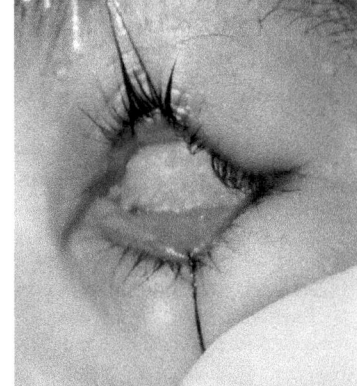

Fig. 9.26.1: Dermis fat graft in socket.

as a secondary orbital implant where it replaces the orbital volume and augments the conjunctival lining. The recipient conjunctiva can be attached to the very edge of the DFG. Hence, it can be advantageous to use DFG for the correction of combined conditions with post-enucleation socket syndrome (PESS) and socket contraction.[4]

- Surface reconstruction
- *Exposure and extrusion:* Break down of the overlying Tenon's capsule and conjunctiva can lead to exposure of the implant. Extrusion of the implant is seen in nonintegrated implants, when it extrudes out the socket. Early exposure or extrusion suggests improper surgical technique. Late exposure is commonly seen in porous implants due to constant rubbing of the prosthesis against the anterior rough surface of the implant.

    Small exposures are closed by either undermining the surrounding conjunctiva and Tenon's and directly suturing or placing a patch graft under the Tenon's capsule. Larger exposures and extrusion need implant exchange.

- *Migration:* It is usually seen with nonporous implants after enucleation. Typically the migration is inferotemporal. Sometimes, the prosthesis can be modified, but if the fit is unsatisfactory then an implant exchange is needed. DFG can be tried in recurrent implant migration.

- *Post-enucleation socket syndrome:* After an enucleation, there is a deficiency of the orbital volume and orbital soft tissue changes which lead to the clinical picture of PESS, consisting of:
    - Enophthalmos
    - Deep superior sulcus
    - Globe ptosis
    - Lax lower eyelid.

    The primary insertion of an orbital implant with an adequate volume (>20 mm) is the best way to prevent this undesirable condition. Deepening of the superior sulcus is the first sign of volume deficit. The management of this condition consists of replacing adequate volume; tightening the lower eyelid and avoiding large, heavy shells. Severe cases may need enophthalmic-wedge implants placed posterior to the equator of the implant to push the eye anteriorly.

- *Contracted socket:* It is defined as the shrinkage and/or shortening of the orbital soft tissue lining in an anophthalmic socket. It makes fitting a satisfactory cosmetic prosthesis impossible **(Box 9.26.1)**.
    - *Mild-socket contracture:* Retaining prosthesis is not a problem, but mild entropion of the eyelids may be seen:
        - Marginal rotation of the eyelid(s) with or without a scleral or cartilage graft is usually sufficient.
    - *Moderate-socket contracture:* Contracture of the inferior (most common), superior, or both fornices.

BOX 9.26.1: Classification of contracted socket.

- *Grade 1:* The socket is characterized by a shallow lower fornix which is converted into a downward sloping shelf that pushes the lower lid down and out, preventing retention of an artificial eye
- *Grade 2:* Loss of the upper and lower fornices
- *Grade 3:* Loss of the upper, lower, medial, and lateral fornices
- *Grade 4:* Loss of all fornices and reduction of the palpebral aperture in horizontal and vertical dimensions
- *Grade 5:* Recurrence of contraction of the socket after repeated trials of reconstruction

Malignant contracted socket: Most severe variety of contracted socket resulting from severe trauma or multiple surgeries.

- Mucous membrane graft followed by prosthesis or conformer application. Firm pressure patch (3-5 days) is applied to hold the lids closed and press the mucous membrane graft against the vascular bed. Prosthesis fitting is done by the ocularist after 3-4 weeks
- C-shaped conformer wrapped in mucous membrane graft (MMG)
- Volume replacement with implant/DFG/temporary muscle transfer
- *Severely-contracted socket:* Replacement of both volume followed by surface is needed in staged procedures:
    - Extensive craniofacial reconstruction may be needed in cases of congenital anophthalmos with temporary muscle transfer/microvascular flaps.
    - Fornix reconstruction is done by full thickness MMG if the socket is moist or split-thickness skin graft (STSG) in a dry socket.

(*Note for the skin graft:* Disadvantage—create poor socket hygiene. Advantage—heal successfully without excessive contracture)
- Volume replacement by implants which can be:
    - *Alloplastic:* Polymethylmethacrylate (PMMA), silicone, preformed wedge implant, room-temperature vulcanized silicone, hydroxyapatite, porous polyethylene, and hydrogel.
    - *Autogenous:* Bone graft (iliac crest, rib, split calvarium), cartilage, and DFG.

PREVENTION

- Treatment of congenital anophthalmos/microphthalmic sockets should be started as soon as possible after birth with:
  - Button conformers
  - Serially enlarging conformers/prosthesis/hydrogel self-expanding conformers/socket expanders.
- Removal of an eye should be avoided until growth of the bony socket is complete (8 years), unless absolutely indicated or the globe is rudimentary and is not providing any impetus for bony socket development.
- Evisceration is the preferred surgery over enucleation unless it is being removed for an intraocular tumor.
- During enucleation or evisceration conjunctiva should be preserved as much as possible; dissection should not extend to the fornices to minimize shortening; the extraocular muscles should be placed in their normal anatomic position; conformer should be placed in the socket after surgery and patient should be advised continuous wearing of a conformer or prosthesis, replacement of orbital volume by an implant should be done after enucleation or evisceration; to obtain the lightest prosthesis without creating anophthalmic enophthalmos largest possible implant (at least 20-22 mm) should be used.

COMPLICATIONS

- Recurrent socket contracture (most common complication in total socket reconstruction) may develop if the prosthesis is left out of the socket for a prolonged period of time. It requires reoperation with total socket reconstruction.
- *Malignant contracted socket:* Severe contracture with complete failure of all conventional techniques—best treated by nonsurgical means (glued or spectacle-mounted prosthesis).
- Post-enucleation socket syndrome
  - Ptosis
  - Enophthalmos
  - Entropion (due to foreshortening of the fornices)
  - Superior sulcus deformity
  - Socket contracture

- Graft failure (DFG/MMG/STSG)
- Oral cicatrix formation
- Mucous membrane granuloma formation
- Socket infection
- Ankyloblepharon
- Conjunctival inclusion cysts

REFERENCES

1. Stahnke T, Erbersdobler A, Knappe S, Guthoff RF, Kilangalanga NJ. Management of congenital clinical anophthalmos with orbital cyst: A Kinshasa case report. Case Rep Ophthalmol Med. 2018;2018:1-6.
2. Kronish JW, Gonnering RS, Dortzbach RK, Rankin JH, Reid DL, Phernetton TM. The pathophysiology of the anophthalmic socket part I. Analysis of orbital blood flow. Ophthal Plast Reconst Surg. 1990;6(2):77-87.
3. Custer PL, Kennedy RH, Woog JJ, Kaltreider SA, Meyer DR. Orbital implants in enucleation surgery: a report by the American Academy of Ophthalmology. Ophthalmology. 2003;110(10):2054-61.
4. Diab MM, Alahmadawy YA. Primary dermis fat grafting for socket reconstruction: Retrospective comparison of electrocoagulation versus scalpel dissection for epidermis removal. Clin Ophthalmol. 2020;14:2925-33.

Appendix 9.26.1: Socket examination.

OD/OS
Cosmesis: Good/fair/poor
- *Color match:* Good/fair/poor
- *Movements:* Good/fair/poor
- *Lagophthalmos:* .....mm
- *Pseudoptosis:* Present/absent
- *Enophthalmos:* Present/absent

Socket: Healthy/congested/congestion with papillae/granuloma
- *Volume:* Adequate/deficit
- *Implant:* Present/absent
- *Implant position:* Central/migrated
- *Implant exposure:* Present/absent
- *Superior fornix:* Well-formed/shallow/absent
- *Inferior fornix:* Well-formed/shallow/absent
- *Medial fornix:* Well-formed/shallow/absent
- *Lateral fornix:* Well-formed/shallow/absent

Shell
- *Discoloration:* Present/absent
- *Deposits:* Present/absent
- *Edges:* Sharp/blunt
- *Surface:* Smooth/rough/scratches

9.27 | Orbital Implants

Kasturi Bhattacharjee, Deepak Soni
Sri Sankaradeva Nethralaya, Guwahati
kasturibhattacharjee44@hotmail.com, deepaksoni20dec@gmail.com

INTRODUCTION

Orbital implants are defined as the medical prosthetics used to replace and augment the deficient orbital and allow reasonable movement of a prosthetic eye. Any patient who loses an eye following evisceration, enucleation, and exenteration experience a severe psychological setback. This suffering can be significantly reduced by using an appropriate implant and a mobile prosthesis that is properly placed. An orbital implant is usually inserted to replace the reduced orbital volume after evisceration or enucleation. In evisceration, the extraocular muscles are attached to the remaining sclera inside which the implant rests, whereas in enucleation either a direct or indirect (depending on the implant material) reattachment of the muscles with the implant is needed. Whereas, a custom-made prosthesis is typically implanted in exenterated patients. Since their introduction, orbital implants have significantly evolved in terms of material, design, shape, and size.

IDEAL ORBITAL IMPLANT

There are multiple widely-accepted prerequisites that should characterize an ideal implant; usually, it should be:
- Nondegradable,
- Biocompatible,
- Have noninflammatory potential to induce foreign body reaction,
- Easily sterilizable without undergoing degradation,
- Have reasonable mechanical resistance to allow safe intraoperative manipulation,
- Be capable of integrating with the remaining soft vascularized tissue,
- Cost effective, and
- Have an adequate motility to be transferred to the ocular prosthesis.

WRAPPING OF ORBITAL IMPLANTS

Before implantation, an orbital implant is enclosed in a sheet of a smooth material in order to reduce soft tissue abrasion, facilitate placement within the remaining soft tissues of the orbit, and aid in the precise attachment of the extraocular muscles to the implant surface. Various implants from different category have different chemical composition and hence may be responsible for varied complications. Roughness of the implant surface being abrasive to the soft tissues plays a key role in the initiation of conjunctival thinning and subsequent exposure and/or extrusion.

In case of ceramic and hydroxyapatite (HA) implants, where surface is rough and implant is stiff, efforts should be given to avoid a direct contact between implant and the conjunctiva. Usually, wrapping porous orbital implants—at least on their front side where the implant encounters the delicate conjunctival surface—is highly recommended. The type of wrapping and its material plays a significant role as it can induce a potential inflammatory reaction and, thus, seem unfavorable and increases the chances of implant exposure and extrusion.

Commonly used wrapping materials are:
- *Human donor sclera:* First choice for majority of surgeons, carries theoretical risk of virus transmission.
- *Especially processed human donor pericardium, fascia lata, and sclera:* Marketed as safe alternative implant, high cost remains an important consideration
- *Synthetic mesh of polyglactin [poly(lactic-co-glycolic acid)]:* Bioabsorbable synthetic material, preferred material for porous orbital implants, eliminates the risk of infectious disease transmission, does not require a second surgical site, and is readily available and simple to use.
- *Processed bovine pericardium (Peri-Guard® or Ocu-Guard™ Supple, Bio Vascular Inc., Saint Paul, MN, USA):* Food and Drug Administration (FDA) approved.
- *Autologous temporalis fascia, fascia lata, rectus abdominis sheath, and posterior auricular muscle complex graft:* Other alternatives, requires a second surgical site, prolonged operative time, and a potentially increased risk of morbidity.

CLASSIFICATION

Dermis Fat Graft

Dermis fat graft (DFG) is obtained from patient's own body tissue—gluteal region and non-hair-bearing anterior abdominal wall. It addresses both volume and surface deficiency. Use of DFG as autologous tissues to restore the orbit volume is recommended for its growth potential in both primary and secondary implantation with a preference in children, where anatomic structures will modify and enlarge over time.

Advantages

- DFG replaces both volume and surface deficiency, hence acts as best option for severely contracted sockets with severe forniceal shortening
- Preferred for children as it carries the potential to expand with the growth of the child
- No need to wrapping it before implantation
- Better substitute in situations where the patient is unable to tolerate a synthetic material in the socket

Disadvantages

- Donor site morbidity
- Recipient bed vascularity decides the graft uptake, which is most of the times is often unpredictable often unpredictable and could be compromised after surgery and radiotherapy.
- Risk of developing central ulceration, hence necrosis, and subsequent melting.
- Risk of fat atrophy which ultimately leads to suboptimal volume replacement.

Polymeric Implants

Polymeric agents are one of the most used orbital implants. They have advantage of low cost in comparison to other agents. Silicone because of its inertness, relative pliability, and excellent biocompatibility, is a highly suitable material for ocular implants. Another commonly used polymer for orbital implants is polymethylmethacrylate (PMMA) because of its outstanding biocompatibility, low cost, ease of surgical placement, and

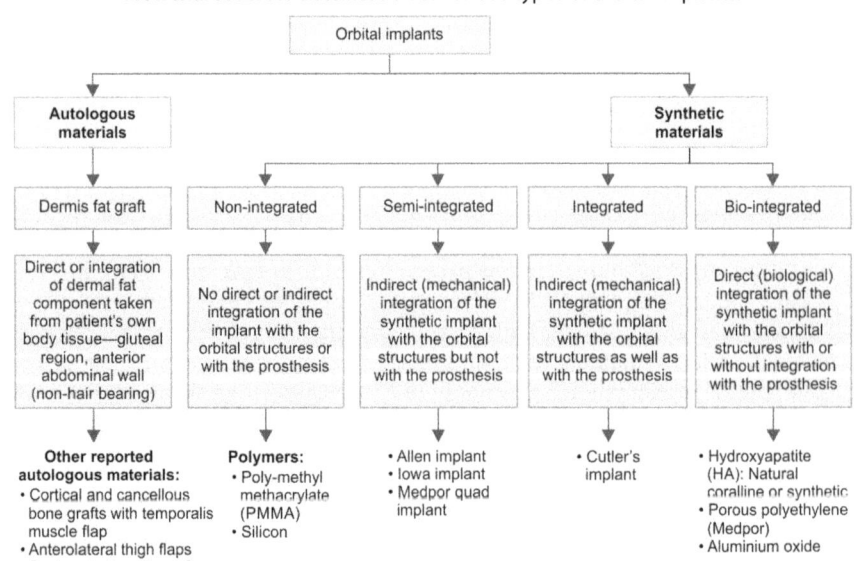

Flowchart 9.27.1: Classification of various types of orbital implants.

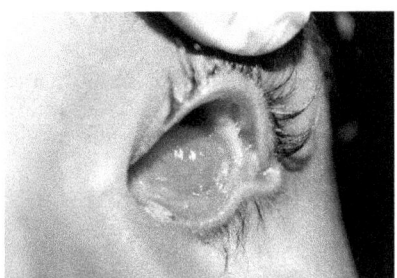

Fig. 9.27.1: Infection and subsequent inflammation of socket with symblepharon formation.

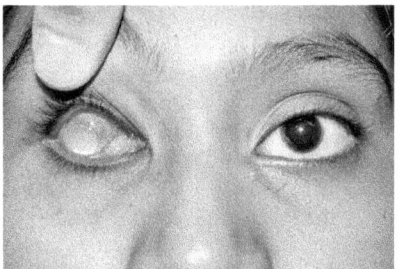

Fig. 9.27.2: Exposure of a nonporous polymethylmethacrylate (PMMA) orbital implant.

successful clinical outcomes. Nonporous PMMA and silicon spheres are suitable as both primary and secondary (or "definitive") orbital implants. Both silicon and PMMA implants are being used as a nonintegrated orbital implant.

Advantages
- Low cost
- Being inert carries lower chances of implant exposure
- Implants of choice for secondary exchange, if needed

Disadvantages
- As the anterior surface is completely covered by Tenon's and conjunctiva, there is no link with the ocular prosthesis, which results in poor prosthetic motility
- No fibrovascular growth and hence have higher rates of migration

Allen-type Family
It is another example of PMMA implants, which underwent significant modifications over the years. The pioneer design came with a peg intended to provide a mechanical integration between the implant and ocular prosthesis, however, results were unsatisfactory owing to short retention of the implant before extrusion.

Therefore, the Allen implant evolved quickly to the *"Iowa implant"* to integrate a "lock-and-key" coupling system that could support an ocular prosthesis with a simultaneous improvement in its motility. This new design had four anteriorly placed peripheral mounds to match four corresponding depressions on the prosthetic posterior surface. Results were comparatively superior in terms of low exposure and extrusion rates.

With this concern in consideration, a further adaptation of the Iowa implant was developed as *"Universal implant"* having smaller and more rounded protruding mounds. This has potentially reduced the complications while maintaining Iowa implant's motility advantages.

Another variation of the Allen-type devices is the *"Castroviejo implant"*. By serving as a smooth, convex pivotal surface for the prosthetic eye to move over, this implant gives the ocular prosthesis movement. The implant features four bridges surrounding a central depression; the four recti muscles are housed in tunnels directly beneath the bridges, and the ends of the opposing muscles are joined together to form an overlapping connection.

Ceramic Implants
Porous ceramic implants with highly interconnected pore network have gained increasing popularity in last few decades. HA ocular implant harvested from natural coralline. HA material is the most used ceramic ocular implant. The pore size of HA implant is

approximately 500 μm diameter which closely simulates structurally the Haversian system of human bone. These micropores act as a passive framework to offer fibrovascular in-growth therefore offering advantages of enhanced prosthesis motility and decreased complications. Natural coralline material is expensive and its harvesting disrupts the marine life ecosystem, hence synthetic HA implants were introduced, major commercial example being FCI implant.

The HA implant usually requires a wrapping material like donor sclera or fascia or synthetic mesh. Wrapping the implant adds approximately 1–2 mm to the overall dimensions. The scleral shell is trimmed to the required size and shape to cover the implant securely with a posterior the corneal window. Polypropylene sutures are used for securely closing the sclera; followed by creation of small windows cuts through the sclera and microholes are then drilled followed by suturing of the four horizontal recti muscles.

Bioceramic Orbital Implant

It is made of the porous, nonbrittle biomaterial alumina (Al_2O_3). The implant has uniform interconnected pores of approximately 500 μm in size. Unlike HA, it is manufactured with no disruption to marine ecosystems.

Polyethylene Implant

In contrast to other polymers, it can withstand high sterilization temperatures and contains interconnected pores which allow fibrovascular tissue in-growth. The most commonly used one is the "Medpor® implant", a low-cost substitute to ceramic porous implants. Unlike HA implants, polyethylene (PE) is much resilient, so muscles can be sutured directly over it without the need of wrapping.

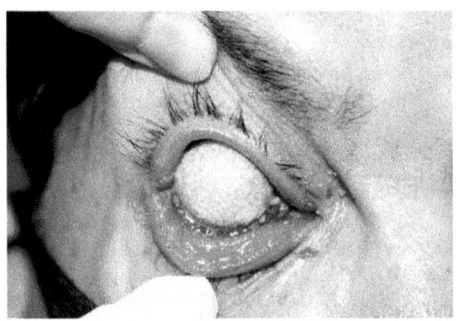

Fig. 9.27.3: Exposure of a porous Medpor® implant.

Advantages

- Fibrovascularization is allowed, hence theoretically, the implant is less likely to migrate or extrude
- Advantage of immune surveillance mediated via vascular supply which ultimately reduces the chances of postoperative infections with a better soft tissue healing.
- Overall, increased tolerance
- Superior prosthetic motility with comparatively few complications.

Disadvantages

- High cost
- Risk of conjunctival abrasion
- Requires a wrapping material
- Not recommended in pediatric patients

COMPLICATIONS

Complications of orbital implants are given in **Table 9.27.1**.

PEDIATRIC ORBITAL IMPLANTATION: CONSIDERATIONS

In pediatric evisceration or enucleation surgeries, the most significant factor to be considered is the need of stimulus for further adequate growth of the orbit. 80% of adult orbital volume is reached around 5–6 years of age, with adult volume achieved by 12–14 years. Typically, in a young child (<5-year-old), a wrapped nonporous sphere

TABLE 9.27.1: Complications of orbital implants.

Complications	Description
Conjunctival thinning	Conjunctival erosion caused by the movement of an underlying rough surface of orbital implant
Conjunctival granuloma	Overgrowth of tissue due to irritation or mechanical trauma; its appearance is usually a color ranging from red/pink to purple and can be painful
Inflammation/ infection	• Response of vascularized tissue to local irritation, serving to restrict, neutralize or wall off the stimulating agent or process • Due to bacterial penetration intraoperatively or postoperatively
Exposure/ extrusion	Breach in the anterior covering layer, mainly conjunctiva, leading to exposure of the implant and subsequent extrusion
Encapsulation	Typical foreign body reaction which involves the formation of a dense, avascular fibrous capsule surrounding the implant
Anophthalmic socket syndrome	Redistribution of orbital contents and subsequent rotatory displacement of the orbital tissues from superior to posterior and from posterior to inferior part leads to: • *Deep upper eyelid sulcus deformity:* Deeply sunken area between the upper eyelid and orbital rim due to loss of orbital volume and relaxation of soft tissues of the orbit • *Ptosis:* Drooping or falling of the upper eyelid • *Enophthalmos:* Inward axial displacement of the globe or implant due to inadequate volume replacement or redistribution of orbital contents • Lower eyelid elongation and laxity • *Ectropion:* Turning out of the eyelid (usually the lower eyelid) so that its inner surface is exposed

implant (acrylic or silicon) is preferred to be implanted within the muscle cone and to be attached with extraocular muscles. Later, when child achieves the adult orbital dimensions a volume augmentation can be performed using porous implant exchange with or without pegging subsequently.

SUGGESTED READING

1. Baino F, Perero S, Ferraris S, Miola M, Balagna C, Verné E, et al. Biomaterials for orbital implants and ocular prostheses: overview and future prospects. Acta Biomater. 2014;10(3): 1064-87.
2. Sami D, Young S, Petersen R. Perspective on orbital enucleation implants. Surv Ophthalmol. 2007;52(3):244-65.
3. Bhattacharjee K, Barman MJ, Ghosh S. Orbital implants. In: Chaugule SS, Honavar SG, Finger PT (Eds). Surgical Ophthalmic Oncology, 1st edition. Berlin, Germany: Springer; 2019. pp. 141-3.

9.28 Custom Fit Prosthesis

Usha Kim

Aravind Eye Hospital and Postgraduate Institute of Ophthalmology, Madurai

usha@aravind.org

INTRODUCTION

There are patients who have lost their eye/eyes and need special care at our hospital. We need to identify these patients and create awareness about the various modalities of treatment available for these patients at our prosthetics center in the orbit clinic. A basic idea about the types of ocular prosthesis available and their indications is essential to guide these patients. Ocular prosthesis fitting can help improve the quality of life of many in need. A custom-made ocular prosthesis provides better results functionally as well as aesthetically **(Figs. 9.28.1A and B)**.

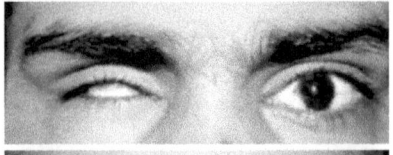
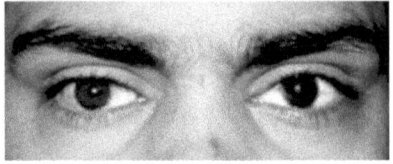

Figs. 9.28.1A and B: Improved cosmesis with custom fit prosthesis.

■ HISTORY

Making of artificial eye dates back to ancient times. In the 5th century, the first ocular prosthesis was made by Romans and Egyptians using clay attached to a cloth (Ectblepharons) later replaced by gold and colored enamel. Venetians used glass for making artificial in the 16th century. Later on acrylic prosthesis was made and now polymethylmethacrylate (PMMA) is used.

■ INDICATIONS OF OCULAR PROSTHESIS

- Anophthalmic socket **(Fig. 9.28.2)**
  - Enucleated socket
  - Eviscerated socket
- Phthisical eye (contracted eye) **(Fig. 9.28.3)**
- Exenterated socket **(Fig. 9.28.4)**
- Corneal scar
- Congenital anophthalmia/microphthalmia
 Deep fornices, healthy conjunctiva, and normal appearance of the lids are the short-term goals after both enucleation and evisceration.

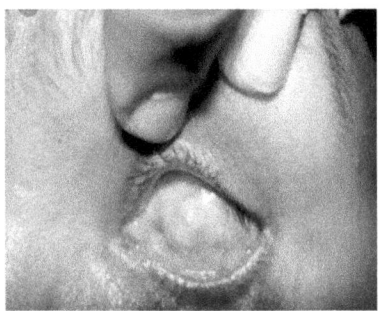

Fig. 9.28.2: Anophthalmic socket.

■ TYPES OF OCULAR PROSTHESIS

Types of ocular prosthesis include:
- Transparent/scleral cover shell/conformer
- Scleral lens
- *Custom fit prosthesis:* Making customized eye shells according to the socket dimension
- *Stock shell:* Readymade shells that are available in the market
- *Self-lubricating prosthesis:* It has a built in chamber containing ocular lubricant which is slowly released over ocular surface
 Comparison between custom-made prosthesis and stock shells is depicted in **Table 9.28.1**.

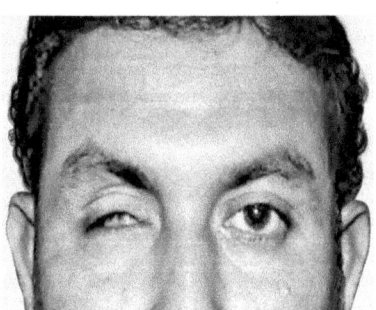

Fig. 9.28.3: Phthisis bulbi.

Conformer (Fig. 9.28.5)

- *Material:* Acrylic or silicone
- It is left for 4–6 weeks postoperatively, in the conjunctival fornices
- Helps to fit the prosthesis

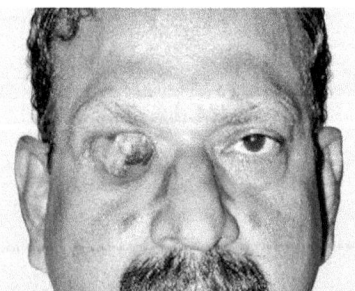

Fig. 9.28.4: Exenterated socket.

SECTION 9: Oculoplasty

TABLE 9.28.1: Comparison between custom-made prosthesis and stock shells.

Custom-made prosthesis	Stock eye
Prepared according to patient's measurement	Readily available in the market
Made of high-grade plastic	Made of low-grade plastic
Good symmetry with other eye	Poor symmetry with the other eye
Better eye movement with the prosthesis	Lesser eye movements
Modifications are possible to solve problems such as ptosis, proptosis, and socket expansion without surgery	No modifications are possible

- Helps to stabilize the implant during the healing process
- Reduces the risk of tissue contracture of an anophthalmic socket.

Stock Shell Prosthesis
- Stock shell prosthesis are ready to wear shells with prefixed (iris and scleral) colors.
- Fitting a stock shell does not give complete symmetry (**Figs. 9.28.6A and B**).

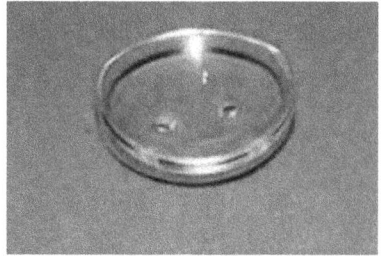

Fig. 9.28.5: Conformer.

Custom Fit Prosthesis
- Custom fit prosthesis is made for each patient according to their socket size and comfort (**Figs. 9.28.7A and B**).
- Material—PMMA
- They are hand painted
- Fits snugly
- It can be modified in order to expand the contracted socket. Also, ptosis shelf can be used to correct the ptosis.

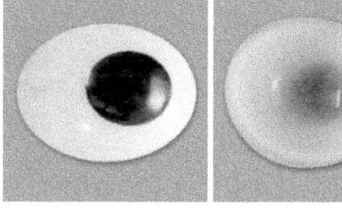

Figs. 9.28.6A and B: Stock shell.

Custom Fit Prosthesis Making
- Custom made prosthetic eye is preferred as it provides more stability and aids in movement.
- The ocularist decides the method of fitting.
- Most common technique is the impression fitting.
- It can be fitted after 6–8 weeks of surgical removal of eye.

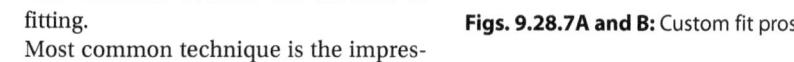

Figs. 9.28.7A and B: Custom fit prosthesis.

Impression Casting—Step 1 (Figs. 9.28.8A to D)
- Injecting alginate material directly into the patient's orbit using an impression tray.
- The substance hardens and removed from the orbit.
- Adjusted to from the front surface of the device using wax.

Wax Model Making—Step 2
Wax model is shown in **Figure 9.28.9**.

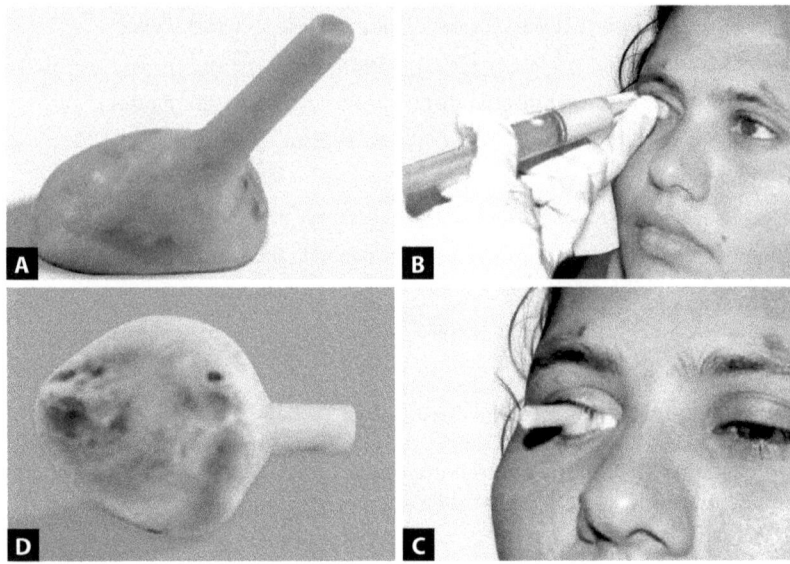

Figs. 9.28.8A to D: Steps of impression casting.

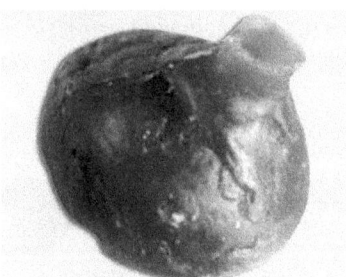

Fig. 9.28.9: Wax model.

Iris and Pupillary Marking—Step 3
Iris and pupillary marking is shown in **Figures 9.28.10A and B**.

Stone Mold Making—Step 4 (Figs. 9.28.11A to E)
- Wax model made is placed in a wet diastone powder in a metal flask to make a mold of appropriate size.
- Wax is removed after getting the impression once the diastone hardens.

Acrylic Preparation—Step 5
Acrylic preparation is shown in **Figures 9.28.12A to F**.

Acrylic Grinding—Step 6 (Figs. 9.28.13A and B)
Acrylic grinding is done using bur (metal bur-different sizes), stone bur, and sand paper to smoothen the edges and surface.

Painting on Iris Button—Step 7 (Figs. 9.28.14A and B)
Using:
- Selected iris button
- Pigments

SECTION 9: Oculoplasty

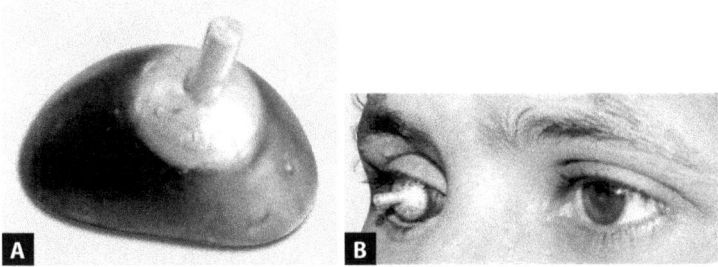

Figs. 9.28.10A and B: The iris and pupil positioned taking into account the appearance of fellow eye.

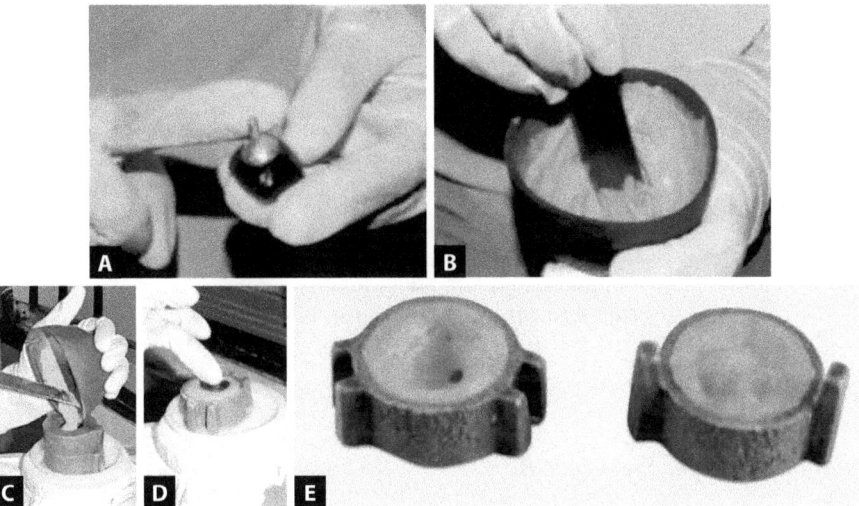

Figs. 9.28.11A to E: Impression over hard diastone powder.

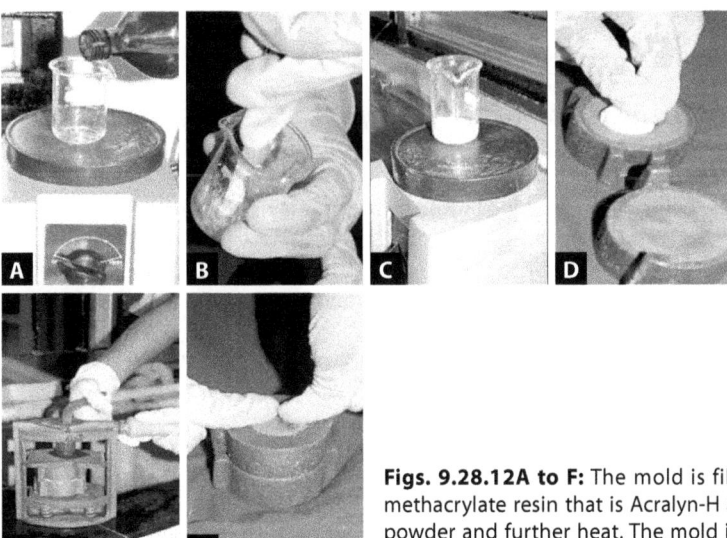

Figs. 9.28.12A to F: The mold is filled with methyl methacrylate resin that is Acralyn-H and white acrylic powder and further heat. The mold is heat treated to harden the liquid.

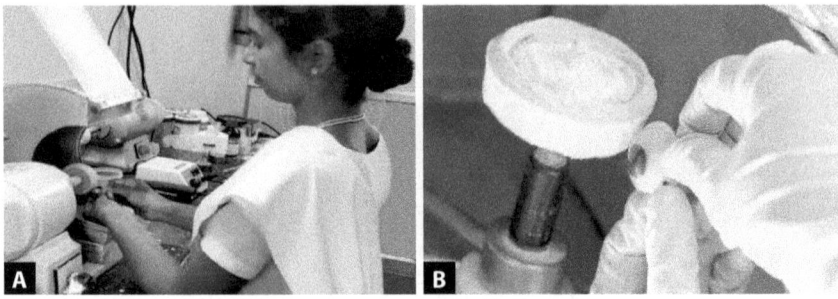

Figs. 9.28.13A and B: Acrylic grinding.

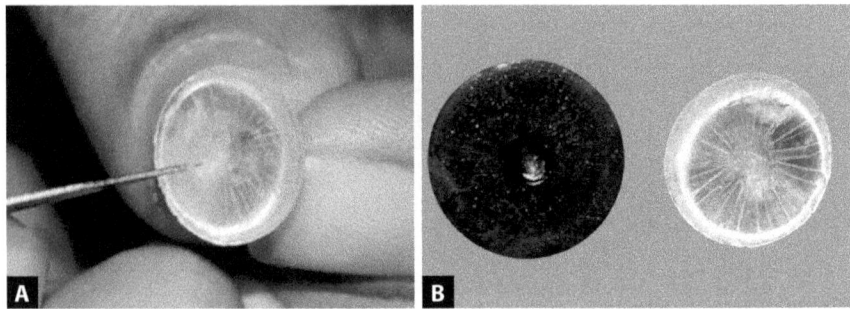

Figs. 9.28.14A and B: Painting on iris button.

- Blade
- Painting brush

Painting on Acrylic Eye—Step 8
Using:
- Already prepared acrylic eye
- Dry pigments
- Thread for veins
- Painting disk (pallet)
  After painting dried at room temp for 4 hours.

Clear Acrylic Coating and Final Polishing—Step 9
- Clear acrylic coating is done using clear acrylic powder and heat cure liquid (Acralyn-H).
- Final polishing done using polishing pumice powder and buffing wheel.

■ COMPLETED PROSTHESIS
The final prosthesis is then fit and evaluated with the following considerations:
- Size and lid contour
- Proper posterior fit over the anterior tissues in the ocular cavity for comfort and motility
- Color of the sclera (white)
- Position and plane of the iris
- Color of the iris and pupil size
- Movement of the artificial eye
- Patient's comfort and a pleasing cosmetic result.

Prostheses can be removed easily and replaced. It is ideal to wear the prosthesis full time but some patients prefer to remove it at night.

Hand hygiene and safe environment should be ensured while handling prosthesis. The prosthesis should be removed and cleaned as directed. Repeated handling can lead to socket irritation and discharge. A prosthesis should be replaced approximately every 8–10 years in adults and earlier in children.

The following signs should not be overlooked and must be corrected in order to maintain a healthy and cosmetically acceptable prosthesis.
- Conjunctival injection
- Copious yellow discharge
- Malpositioning of lids
- Socket contracture
- Poor cosmesis due to change in color of sclera and iris
- Discomfort on usage
- Discontinued/irregular usage for pain relief

Limitation of custom made prosthesis can be camouflaged using spectacles to disguise the asymmetry. This can be done by prescribing:
- Larger frames
- Tinted glasses
- Spherical, cylindrical lenses, and prisms

MAINTENANCE OF PROSTHESIS
- Hand hygiene while handling
- Continuous usage
- Weekly cleaning with clean water, air dried, and refitted
- Usage of lubricants to improve lid movements and closure
- Yearly polishing

SILICONE FACIAL PROSTHESIS
Facial prostheses are applied post exenteration and are made of materials like acrylic or silicone rubber. They can either be secured in place with adhesives or can be spectacle mounted. Wax is used to make a symmetrical mold similar to contralateral orbital area.
- A white acrylic shell is chosen to match the other eye and the prosthesis is carved in modeling wax. It is tried on the patient's face to check the orientation in comparison with the other eye.
- The anteroposterior position is adjusted and verified on the patient on observing from front and from above the head.
- Once the orientation is confirmed, the adnexal structures (like lids) are sculpted in wax and prosthesis is placed in the exenterated socket.
- Then wax model is duplicated in a sectional cast and acrylic extension is used to stabilize the eye shell and dewaxed. Room temperature vulcanizing (RTV) medical-graded silicone material (factor II) is mixed according to manufacturer's instructions.
- Pigment stains are mixed into the base color for better staining to gain the accurate skin shade of the patient, then the mold is packed and kept at room temperature for setting.
- Then it is removed and hand painting of iris and sclera is done.
- Ready-made eye lashes are glued to the prosthesis.

PRESSURE CONFORMERS
In certain cases with repeatedly shallow fornix and scar contracture secondary to multiple socket surgeries a pressure conformer can be fit.

Periosteal Stock Shell Fixation
In severely contracted sockets, the stock shell can be directly sutured to the periosteum.

Three-dimensional Printed CFP

After taking an impression mold of an anophthalmic socket as in conventional method—3D scanning and modeling followed by 3D printing with polymeric resin is done. Using dye sublimation transfer system, iris and vessels as other eye are printed on the prosthesis. It offers the advantages of less making time and patient's socket data storage for future use.

9.29 | Orbital Imaging

Akshay Gopinathan Nair
Dr Agarwal's Group of Eye Hospital, Mumbai
R Jhunjhunwala Sankara Eye Hospital, Panvel

■ INTRODUCTION

Imaging of the orbit gives us clues about the structural characteristics of the orbit which are not visible to the naked eye. And therefore, it is a useful adjunct in the diagnosis of tumors, infections, fractures, inflammation, and other abnormalities of the orbit. This article will discuss about the basic indications of each of the different imaging modality is used to image the orbit. Additionally, this will also discuss the anatomical landmarks that one should look for while interpreting these imaging studies.

■ COMPUTED TOMOGRAPHY SCAN

Computed tomography (CT) scans of the orbit involves visualizing the bone and the soft tissue structures of the orbit. Most commonly, this modality is performed as a noncontrast scan. The standard CT scan protocols for the orbits are usually performed with 2 mm cuts. Coronal, axial, and sagittal reconstructed slices are usually procured. CT scan is extremely useful and ideal for orbital imaging because the intraconal fat appears hypointense and therefore provides a natural contrast to visualize the surrounding structures, namely the extraocular muscles and the optic nerve. Additionally, high density bone appearance enables visualization of metallic foreign bodies, calcification, bony lysis, and displaced fractured bones.

The typical indications for a CT scan of the orbit are:
- *Congenital or pediatric orbital anomalies:* Congenital abnormalities of the orbit usually involve bony structural malformations such as craniosynostosis and are better visualized on the CT scan. Additionally, 3D reconstructed images always give a better view for the spatial configuration of the orbits and the surrounding cranial fossa. Neurofibromatosis is another congenital condition that can be assessed and diagnosed on a CT scan. Characteristic lesions such as the absence of the greater ring of the sphenoid; the presence of plexiform neurofibromas over the eyelid, eyebrow, and face; as well as optic nerve gliomas are seen clearly on CT scans.
- *Orbital trauma:* CT scans help in diagnosing orbital wall fractures and associated extraocular muscle entrapments. Additionally, intraoperative imaging or postoperative imaging is useful to assess the placements of plates or implant in the orbit. While evaluating trauma, one must remember that salvaging the globe takes precedence over management of orbital fractures, and other deformities. **Figure 9.29.1** shows a CT scan showing a fractured floor of the orbit.

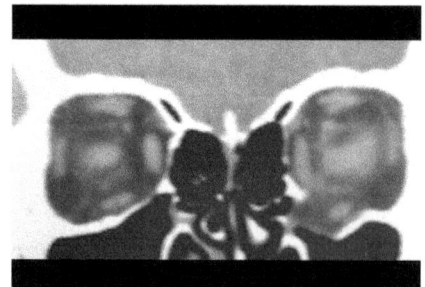

Fig. 9.29.1: CT scan of orbital floor fracture.

- *Suspected intraocular or intraorbital foreign bodies:* In cases of suspected orbital foreign bodies, especially when a metallic foreign body is suspected—a CT scan should be performed. Magnetic resonance imaging (MRI) in the setting of an intraocular foreign body is contraindicated. **Figure 9.29.2** shows a hyperdense speck—representing a metallic intraocular foreign body.
- *Orbital infections:* In orbital cellulitis, infection or abscessed that are seen in the orbit are usually spill over inflammation from surrounding structures such as the sinuses, the eyelids, or the lacrimal apparatus. The most common epicenter of such infections remains the paranasal sinuses; namely the ethmoidal and the maxillary sinuses. It is important to identify this such that concurrent specific treatment, if any, for the orbital cellulitis can be planned. Other orbital infections such as fungal infections like mucormycosis require MRI for disease assessment and treatment planning. **Figure 9.29.3** shows pansinusitis with associated orbital cellulitis.
- *Orbital tumors:* Orbital tumors are a wide spectrum of lesions. In many cases, a CT scan may be adequate to understand the size, shape, location, and relations of the tumor with respect to the surrounding structures. However, there may be cases where even the CT scan may be requested first and MRI is often needed subsequently for further analysis and better soft tissue delineation. Understanding if the tumor is intraconal or extraconal is important. **Figure 9.29.4** shows the intermuscular septum which divides the orbital space into intraconal versus extraconal space. **Figure 9.29.5** shows an intraconal mass close to the optic nerve; however, the optic nerve cannot be clearly delineated from the mass. But in **Figure 9.29.6** which is an MRI of another orbital intraconal mass, the nerve can be seen distinctly from the tumor mass.
- *Orbital inflammation:* Orbital inflammation such as idiopathic orbital inflammatory disease (IOID) can be assessed on CT scans. Additionally, thyroid eye disease is

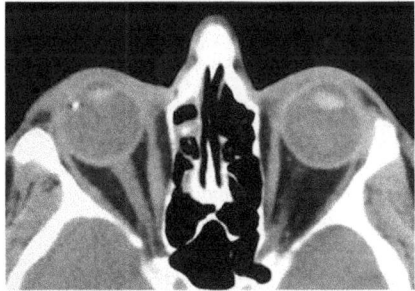

Fig. 9.29.2: Metallic intraocular foreign body.

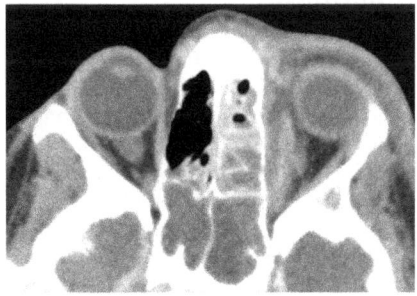

Fig. 9.29.3: Pansinusitis with associated orbital cellulitis.

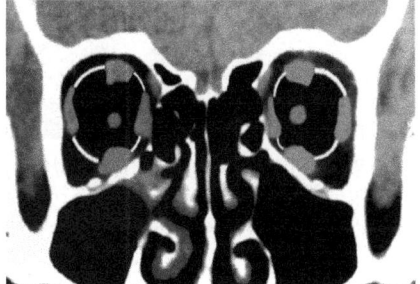

Fig. 9.29.4: Intermuscular septum which divides the orbital space into intraconal versus extraconal space.

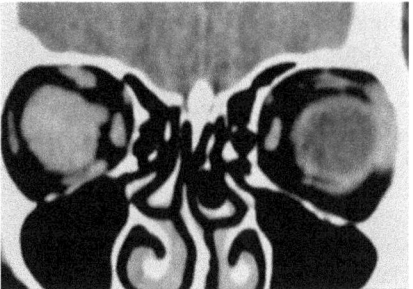

Fig. 9.29.5: Intraconal mass close to the optic nerve; however, the optic nerve cannot be clearly delineated from the mass.

another condition where a CT scan is very useful in diagnosis as well as surgical planning. The classical enlargement of the extraocular muscles that is tendon-sparing and typically involves the belly of the muscle can be seen on the axial slices in a CT scan. Additionally, while planning a surgical decompression of the orbit in burnt out thyroid eye disease or dysthyroid optic neuropathy, a CT scan is useful to understand the amount of space is available in the sinuses surrounding the orbit. **Figure 9.29.7** shows classical extraocular muscle enlargement seen in thyroid eye disease, below the axial slices show the typical tendon sparing enlargement of the muscle belly. **Figure 9.29.8** is an MRI of active thyroid eye disease—note how the inferior rectus (arrow) is hyperintense indicative of activity and edema as compared to the other muscles which are enlarged but not hyperintense indicating no activity in those muscles.

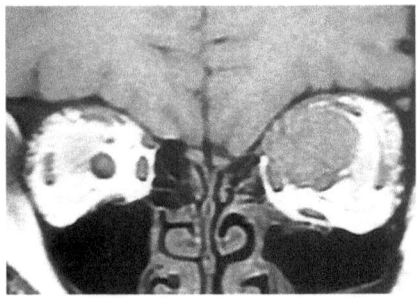

Fig. 9.29.6: Intraconal mass close to the optic nerve; the optic nerve can be clearly delineated from the mass.

MAGNETIC RESONANCE IMAGING

Magnetic resonance imaging is a relatively newer technique of imaging that does not involve patient exposure to ionizing radiation. In MRI, T1- and T2-weighted images are obtained by altering the parameters to create a contrast difference between the tissues. For example, it is good to remember that vitreous appears black in T1 images **(Fig. 9.29.9)** and white in T2 images **(Fig. 9.29.10)**. In principle, T1-weighted images are used to show normal anatomy whereas pathology is better visible and assessed on T2-weighted images. MRI has multiple advantages over CT scan in that it is not altered by artefacts such a small dental fillings or jewelry like nose rings. The lack of ionizing radiation remains the biggest advantage of MRI. However, MRI is more sensitive to motion artefacts, such as eyeball and eyelid movements as compared to CT scans. CT scans however show bony delineation better. **Figure 9.29.11** shows bone window of a bone cyst and **Figure 9.29.12** shows bony erosion arising from a lacrimal gland tumor.

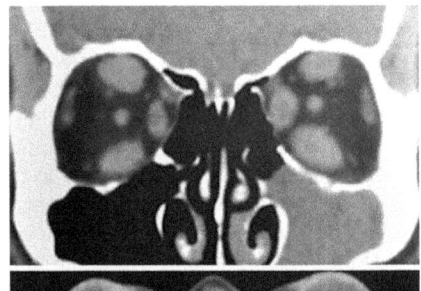

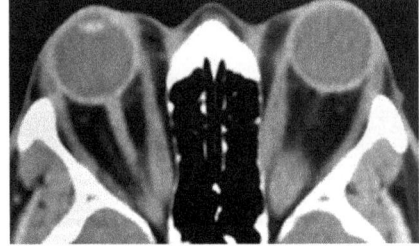

Fig. 9.29.7: Extraocular muscle enlargement seen in thyroid eye disease.

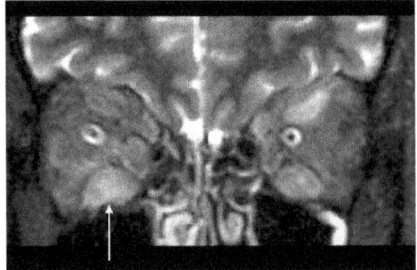

Fig. 9.29.8: MRI of active thyroid eye disease—the inferior rectus (arrow) is hyperintense indicative of activity.

Indications for MRI for orbital pathologies are:
- *Intraocular tumors:* Intraocular tumor such as retinoblastoma is melanomas and other lesions or better. CT scan is not the modality of choice for diagnosis and

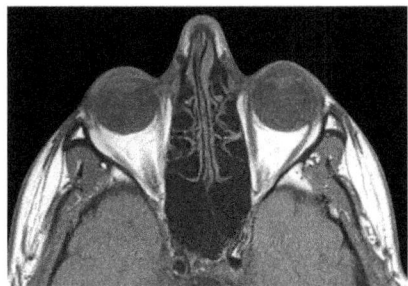

Fig. 9.29.9: T1 image—vitreous is white.

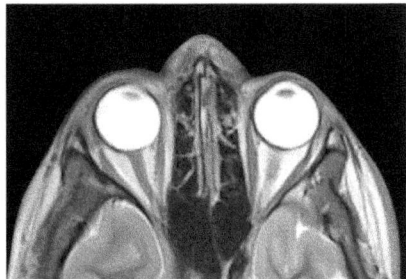

Fig. 9.29.10: T2 image—vitreous is black.

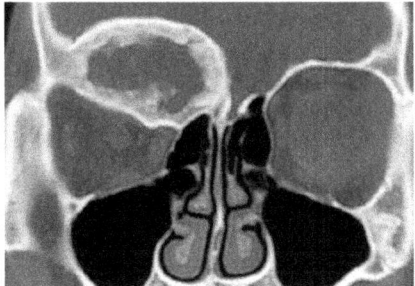

Fig. 9.29.11: Bone window of a bone cyst.

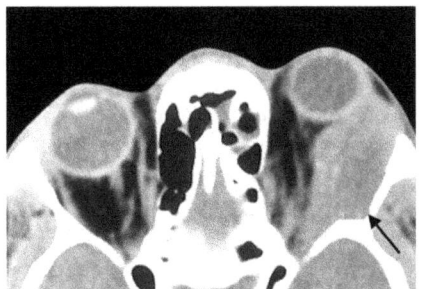

Fig. 9.29.12: Bony erosion arising from a lacrimal gland tumor.

follow-up of children with retinoblastoma due to radiation exposure. And because of its superior soft tissue contrast, MRI is more sensitive and specific than CT in detection of tumor extent and metastatic risk factors. In choroidal melanomas, MRI is useful for identifying tumor size, extraocular extension, and ciliary body infiltration. In addition, MRI is better than CT in the identification of retinal detachment and extrascleral spread.

- *Intraconal and orbital apical mass lesions:* In the orbit, MRI allows better visualization of structures at the orbital apex and also helps in differentiating mass lesions and tumors from the optic nerve which a CT scan cannot. Cavernous hemangiomas are common intraconal masses and radiologically they are seen as homogenous masses with smooth margins and uniform enhancement. They can be easily separated from the optic nerve and extraocular muscles.
- *Optic nerve diseases:* Optic nerve lesions such as optic neuritis or lesions abutting the orbital apex and orbital masses that have extended intracranially are indications for MRI. For example, in cases of mucoceles or dermoids that have eroded the roof of the orbit and have gone intracranially, a MRI can help delineate the intact dura which is useful in surgical planning.

    Sudden-onset visual disturbances indicative of optic nerve pathology is one of the most common indications for MRI. Optic neuritis is typically seen as unilateral optic nerve swelling in its retrobulbar/intraorbital segment, with high T2-weighted image signal, and contrast enhancement. In chronic cases, the optic nerve might become atrophied rather than swollen. Contrast enhancement is best detected with fat-suppressed T1-weighted images and contrast enhancement associated with optic neuritis may be seen in >90% of patients within 20 days of visual loss.
- *Optic nerve tumors:* While CT scans may also help in demonstrating the fusiform enlargement typically associated with optic nerve tumors, MRI gives a clear picture. Meningiomas can originate either from the optic nerve sheath or the periosteum of

SECTION 9: Oculoplasty

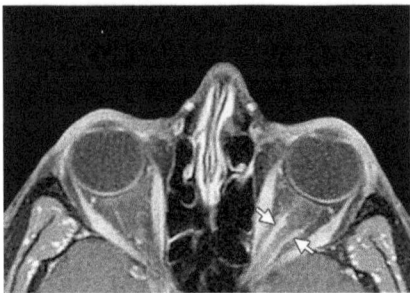

Fig. 9.29.13: Tram track appearance in optic nerve sheath meningioma.

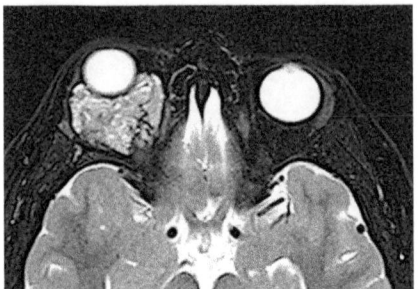

Fig. 9.29.14: Orbital venolymphatic malformation.

the orbital wall (primary meningioma). Tram-track enhancement along the optic nerve sheath is an imaging characteristic for meningiomas **(Fig. 9.29.13)**.
- Nonmetallic foreign bodies
- *Trauma/traumatic optic neuropathy:* Blunt trauma not involving penetrating foreign bodies, optic nerve avulsion, optic nerve hemorrhage, and intrasheath hemorrhage are well diagnosed in MRI.
- *Mucormycosis:* Recently the use of contrast assisted MRI imaging in the management of fungal diseases such as mucormycosis has also come to the fore.
- *Orbital inflammatory disease:* Thyroid eye disease, IOID, myositis can be differentiated based on the involvement of the tendons of the extraocular muscles. Additionally, MRI can help understand the level of disease activity in thyroid eye disease.
- *Vascular malformations:* For orbital venolymphatic malformations such as lymphangiomas, MRI is superior to CT in the evaluation and assessment of their extension and depicting various components. MRI signal is variable, depending on the fluid contents and the age of internal blood. Intralesional phleboliths are occasionally seen and appear as small dense foci within the solid venous part of the lesion; which are actually seen better on CT scans **(Fig. 9.29.14)**.

Preferred imaging modalities for specific clinical conditions are as follows:
- *Caroticocavernous fistula:* CT angiography
- *Idiopathic intracranial hypertension:* MR venography (to look for cerebral venous sinus thrombosis/aplasia/hypoplasia)
- *Hemifacial spasm:* MRI + MR angiography (to look for mass lesions/vascular loops abutting the facial nerve, especially at cerebellopontine (CP) angle)
- *Third nerve palsy:* MRI + MR angiography (to diagnose aneurysms that may cause isolated III N palsy)
- *Rhino-orbital-cerebral mucormycosis:* MRI

SUMMARY

If the clinical picture suggests a specific lesion or localization and initial imaging is "normal" or is not representative of the clinical picture, one must consider repeating the imaging with thinner slices and higher magnification. One must discuss with the radiologist to see if any other imaging modality can be performed. At the end, we must be mindful of the possibility that the lack of an imaging abnormality does not exclude pathology. This is because imaging is not the end of the diagnostic process. There are many imaging modalities that are available but this should not shift the focus away from the traditional techniques of diagnosis that involve detailed history taking and clinical examination. Careful evaluation and interpretation of the imaging studies should be done in detail before jumping to a diagnosis—there are new prizes awarded for the fastest diagnosis made by looking at scans.

9.30 Surgical Approaches to the Orbit

Obaidur Rehman
Sri Sankaradeva Nethralaya, Guwahati, Assam, India
obaid.rehmann@gmail.com

■ INTRODUCTION

The orbit is a small, confined space yet houses several important structures (apart from the eyeball) and is affected by a variety of pathologies, ranging from benign growths to malignant masses. A thorough understanding of the orbital anatomy can help the surgeon delineate the most appropriate surgical approach for management of an orbital pathology. The orbit houses five distinct surgical spaces: 1. *Sub-Tenon's space:* Lying between the globe and the Tenon's fascia. 2. *Intraconal/central space:* Lying within the recti muscle cone. 3. *Extraconal/peripheral space:* Lying outside the muscle cone. 4. *Subperiosteal space:* A potential space between periorbita and bony walls of the orbit. 5. *Subarachnoid space:* Lying between the optic nerve and its surrounding sheath.

One or multiple surgical spaces may be involved by a single disease process. Depending on the location of the lesion, the type of procedure required (complete excision or incision biopsy) and the extent of the lesion, a suitable surgical approach can be decided. Radiological imaging findings, patient counseling, and type of anesthesia to be used (local/sedation/general anesthesia) should be kept in mind before proceeding to surgery.

"Orbitotomy" implies entry into the orbit through a surgical procedure to gain access to orbital contents. Depending on approach utilized, orbitotomies can be classified as follows:
- Anterior orbitotomy
- Lateral orbitotomy
- Medial orbitotomy
- Transcranial orbitotomy
- Endoscopic orbitotomy
- Combined orbitotomies

■ ANTERIOR ORBITOTOMY

Surgically approaching the orbit from the anterior aspect is preferred for lesions lying anteriorly in the orbit (mostly anterior to the equator). Different surgical incisions for this approach can be:
- *Through the skin*: Transcutaneous
- *Through the conjunctiva*: Transconjunctival
- *Cutting through the eyelid vertically*: Lid split

Depending on the site of lesion, anterior orbitotomy may involve the upper eyelid or the lower eyelid and may be superior, medial, inferior, or medial. Combination of lower eyelid transconjunctival incision with lateral cantholysis can be utilized to approach the inferolateral orbit. Similarly, combining a lower eyelid transconjunctival incision with a transcaruncular approach can help the surgeon reach into the medial orbit.

■ LATERAL ORBITOTOMY

Lateral approach to the orbit can be employed to gain access to the intraconal space, the lateral extraconal space or the optic nerve. It can also be combined with other approaches depending on the surgical goal. The classic lateral orbitotomy approaches that have been described include:
- Berke-Reese incision
- Bicoronal flap
- Upper lid crease extended laterally
- Stallard-Wright incision

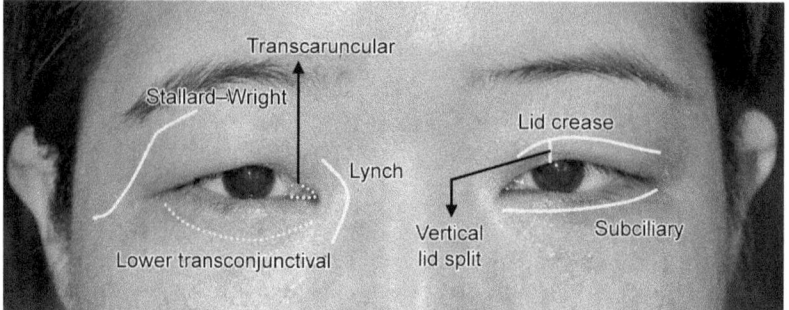

Fig. 9.30.1: Various orbitotomy incisions.

Smaller triangular incisions, based on the lateral canthus have also been used for lateral orbitotomy. The gentle S-shaped Stallard–Wright incision is most preferred for lateral orbitotomies. It starts from the lateral part of the brow and curves laterally to end at the anterior zygomatic arch. Part of the lateral orbital rim can be removed or burred for access to the deeper parts of the orbit or to remove larger lesions. The removed bone fragment can be preserved and reposited back at the end of the surgery.

MEDIAL ORBITOTOMY

This approach can be used to access the sub-Tenon's space and medial wall of orbit.
- *Transcaruncular:* Incision between the caruncle and plica semilunaris
- *Transconjunctival:* Medial peritomy of the conjunctiva medially
- *Transcutaneous:* Lynch incision is a curved incision midway between the medial canthus and root of the nose.

TRANSCRANIAL ORBITOTOMY

This approach is used when a surgeon intends to reach the deep orbit or the orbital apex.
- *Transcranial frontal orbitotomy:* A hemicoronal or bicoronal flap is created to reach the frontal bone, which is then removed as a hinged flap.
- *Pterional approach:* Bone flap based on the pterion is created.
- *Eyebrow incision:* Removal of frontal bone to access superior orbit and apex.

Endoscopic Orbitotomy

Transethmoidal endonasal endoscopic route can be utilized to reach the medial wall of the orbit, orbital apex, and the optic canal. Optic nerve sheath fenestration or optic canal decompression can be performed using this technique. This approach to the orbit is best utilized by ear, nose, and throat (ENT) surgeons.

WHAT IS NEW?

- *Transorbital neuroendoscopic surgery (TONES):* It is a set of minimally invasive procedures, that can be performed via a variety of approaches, namely upper eyelid crease, lower eyelid, caruncular, retrocanthal, and preseptal. Using endoscopes in TONES, a surgeon can gain access to the orbit or the base of skull without undue manipulation or large incisions.
- *Image-guided orbital surgeries:* Intraoperative imaging using CT or MRI can prove to be a useful aid to surgeons, when dealing with critical structures in the small confines of the orbit. Real-time tracking and visualization can enhance the precision of surgery and prevent inadvertent collateral damage. The various machines utilized in this approach include InstaTrak (Visualization Technology Inc., Woburn, MA, USA), LandmarX (Xomed-Medtronic, Jacksonville, FL, USA), Cygnus PFS System (Compass

International, Rochester, MN, USA), and Stealth Station (Medtronics, Memphis, TN, USA).
- *Cavitron ultrasonic surgical aspirator (CUSA):* A novel device that uses ultrasound energy to fragment tissues of interest while irrigating and aspirating the surgical field at the same time. It has been used for a long time by neurosurgeons, but recently found its way into orbital surgeries also. CUSA can create precise bony orbitotomies using the bone-cutting handpiece and also aid in removal of orbital masses with the soft tissue handpiece. The ability to not harm blood vessels and nerves is an added advantage of the CUSA system.

ACKNOWLEDGMENT
Vatsalya Venkatraman, MD.

SUGGESTED READING
1. Abussuud Z, Ahmed S, Paluzzi A. Surgical Approaches to the Orbit: A Neurosurgical Perspective. J Neurol Surg B Skull Base. 2020;81(4):385-408.
2. Campbell AA, Grob SR, Yoon MK. Novel Surgical Approaches to the Orbit. Middle East Afr J Ophthalmol. 2015;22(4):435-41.
3. Leatherbarrow B. Oculoplastic Surgery, 2nd edition. London: CRC Press; 2010.

9.31 Pathologies and Surgeries Related to Punctum and Canaliculus

Nandini Bothra, Mohammad Javed Ali
Govindram Seksaria Institute of Dacryology, LV Prasad Eye Institute, Telangana
drjaved007@gmail.com

INTRODUCTION
Punctum, canaliculus, and common canaliculus form the proximal lacrimal drainage system. There are multiple anomalies associated with these structures and can be congenital or acquired.

CONGENITAL ANOMALIES OF THE PROXIMAL LACRIMAL DRAINAGE APPARATUS

Punctal and Canalicular Agenesis (Fig. 9.31.1)
There is failure of out-budding from the upper end of the solid lacrimal cord in an embryo of 18-24 mm, which leads to canalicular and punctal agenesis. Clinically, there is absence of punctal papilla, flattening the canalicular region, presence or absence of hair follicles in the pars lacrimal area of the eyelid, and sometimes in the canalicular area. There can be other ocular associations such as lacrimal fistula, blepharitis, distichiasis, eyelid tags and strabismus or systemic associations like ectodermal dysplasia and Hay-Wells and Levy-Hollister syndromes.

Treatment for punctal agenesis depends on the severity of symptoms (epiphora). Mild cases can be observed, whereas symptomatic

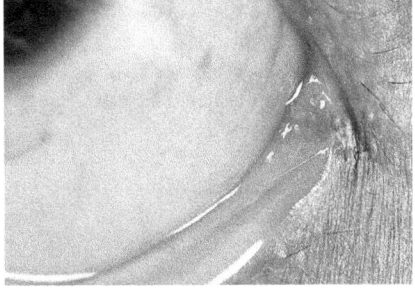

Fig. 9.31.1: Clinical photograph of the right eye showing lower punctal and canalicular agenesis with absence of punctal papilla, concavity in the area of the canaliculus, and hair in the pars lacrimalis portion of the eyelid.

cases will need either conjunctivodacryocystorhinostomy (CDCR) or lacrimal gland measures like botulinum toxin or needling of the lacrimal gland or lacrimal gland debulking.

Incomplete Punctal Canalization (Fig. 9.31.2)

Failed dehiscence of epithelium over the normal underlying canaliculi or failure of canalization of the proximal-most part of the lacrimal apparatus leads to formation of membranes in the punctal area. This is referred to as punctal dysgenesis with membranes. Three varieties of membranes have been described, i.e., external, internal, and balloon variant. Treatment is a simple membranotomy using Nettleship's punctum dilator.

Sometimes, it has been associated with canalicular stenosis and congenital nasolacrimal duct obstructions but is rare. No known systemic associations exist.

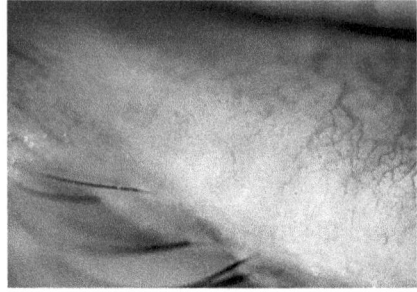

Fig. 9.31.2: Clinical photograph of the left eye lower eyelid showing a translucent membrane in the punctal papillary region with blood vessels traversing over the membrane—no indentation of the blood vessels is seen signifying the external membrane variant.

Supernumerary Puncta and Canaliculi (Fig. 9.31.3)

These result due to multiple epithelial buds developing from the upper end of the solid lacrimal cord in an 18–24 mm embryo. These cases are mostly asymptomatic and the findings are generally incidental. Known ocular associations are lacrimal fistula and lacrimal sac diverticula and systemic associations are Down's syndrome and preauricular sinus.

Canalicular Wall Dysgenesis

Dysregulation of the mesenchymal condensation around the canalicular primordium and

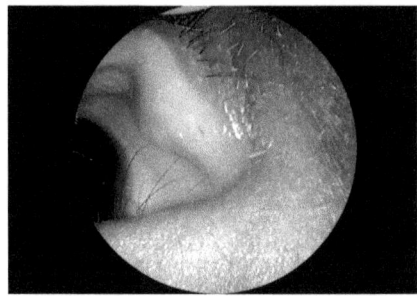

Fig. 9.31.3: Clinical photograph of the right eye upper eyelid showing the presence of two punctal openings.

its contiguity with the subadjacent mesenchyme of the surface ectoderm during embryonic development leads to canalicular wall dysgenesis. There are eight subtypes of canalicular wall dysgenesis described in literature depending on the wall (anterior, posterior, superior, and inferior) of the canaliculi affected.

Symptomatology varies from being asymptomatic to having minimal epiphora. No treatment is generally required, however, when associated with congenital nasolacrimal duct obstructions, care is to be taken during intervention as the walls are exceptionally thin and chances of cheese wiring of the punctal opening is a possibility.

ACQUIRED ANOMALIES OF THE PROXIMAL LACRIMAL DRAINAGE APPARATUS

Idiopathic Canalicular Inflammatory Disorder

Idiopathic canalicular inflammatory disorder (ICID) is an idiopathic and noninfective disorder affecting the puncta and canaliculi with no ocular or systemic association. These patients have a female preponderance and present in the fifth to sixth decades of life. The presentation is with epiphora, generally asymmetric with one eye being affected earlier than the other. There is absence of any discharge, congestion, or any other sign of acute infection. There is no history of any other ocular or systemic disease or association with any topical or systemic drug use. The collagen vascular profile and microbiological workup is negative in these cases.

On examination, five distinct stages have been defined:
1. *Stage of progressive punctal edema:* Puncta and vertical canalicular mucosa shows pearly white edema causing mechanical punctal occlusion which can be corroborated on Fourier-domain ocular coherence tomography (OCT) of the puncta.
2. *Stage of progressive centripetal vascularization:* There is a host of dilated and tortuous vessels seen in the peripunctal area encroaching the punctum.
3. *Stage of pouting vascularized mucosa:* The vertical canalicular and punctal mucosa starts pouting in the punctal papillary area with no signs of underlying punctal orifice.
4. *Stage of dense membrane formation*: The punctal papilla shows a translucent to dense white membrane formation over the punctal orifice. Peripunctal vasculature may or may not be present.
5. *Stage of progressive scarring:* The punctal papillary area shows complete scarring with atrophic conjunctiva and absence of peripunctal vasculature. This scarring of proximal lacrimal drainage passage can also be corroborated on Fourier-domain OCT of the puncta.

Treatment of this condition depends on the staging of the disease. In the early stages, tapering dose of topical steroids and topical cyclosporine eye drops is started till resolution of the edema. If membranes are present, membranotomy with or without stenting is then done under continuous influence of topical cyclosporine. Stent extubation is done after 1 month and topical cyclosporine is continued for 3-6 months after clinical resolution. Better success rates are obtained in early stages (1-3) of the disease. Once the disease reaches stage 5, there is complete scarring, and is not amenable to further treatment. In this stage, CDCR or lacrimal gland measures are the only modality of treatment for continued epiphora.

Punctal Stenosis

Punctal stenosis refers to a condition where narrowing of the punctal orifice is present. Normal punctal size varies from 0.2 to 0.5 mm. Some studies have classified punctal stenosis to occur when the size is <0.3 mm or when there is inability to cannulate the punctum with a 26 G cannula without dilatation. The incidence of the condition varies from 8 to 55% in various studies. Physiologically, the puncta undergoes stenosis in the sixth decade of life and exaggerates in the seventh decade of life, reversing thereafter. Thus, one should be conscious of this fact prior to making a diagnosis of punctal stenosis. Etiology of punctal stenosis varies from chronic blepharitis (most common cause), lid conditions such as ectropion and entropion, antiglaucoma drugs and chemotherapeutic drugs such as 5-fluorouracil, docetaxel and paclitaxel, infections such as herpes simplex and trachoma, and ocular surface diseases such as ocular cicatricial pemphigoid and Stevens-Johnson syndrome.

Symptomatology is mainly epiphora of various grades depending on the degree of stenosis. When associated with inflammatory disorders, other symptoms such as redness, burning, and discharge can accompany. Punctal orifice in order to understand punctal stenosis has been graded as follows:
- *Grade 0*: No punctum identified, punctal atresia or effacement
- *Grade 1*: Punctal papilla covered with a membrane or fibrosis
- *Grade 2*: Less than normal size but recognizable
- *Grade 3*: Normal (easily recognized)
- *Grade 4*: <2 mm
- *Grade 5*: >2 mm, larger than usual punctum

Diagnosis is mainly clinical. Various treatment modalities have been described in literature. Dilatation of the puncta using Nettleship's punctal dilator followed by punctal plug placement or stent placement for 6-8 weeks ensures long duration of punctal dilatation and thus, may prevent restenosis. Balloon punctoplasty using a 1.5 mm cardiac balloon has also been described without stent placement to have good effect. Other more invasive techniques employed are 1-snip or 3-snip punctoplasty, wedge or punch punctoplasty with or without stents. These techniques disturb the architecture of the punctum and hence the peripunctal anatomy including the Horner-Duverney's muscle, hence compromising on the functioning of the lacrimal pump. Thus, care has to be taken before practicing more invasive techniques and disturbing the architecture of the puncta.

Canaliculitis (Figs. 9.31.4A to D)

Canaliculitis is a common disorder, constituting about 0.8–2% of the lacrimal disorders. There is a noted female preponderance and commonly affects the lower canaliculus. The common presenting symptoms are epiphora, pain, swelling, and redness in the medial aspect the eyelid and discharge. Punctal pouting is the pathognomonic sign of canaliculitis, however, this may be absent in chronic cases. Other signs seen are swelling of the canalicular area with congestion of the conjunctiva and eyelid medially and presence of discharge.

The treatment includes medical and surgical modalities. Punctal dilatation or punctal snip with complete canalicular curettage followed by specific topical antibiotics gives the best results. As far as possible, it is important to maintain the integrity of the puncta and canaliculi (avoid snip) so as to minimize the postinfective epiphora. The common microorganisms involved in the causation include actinomycetes, *Staphylococcus*, and *Streptococcus* species.

Canalicular Obstructions

Canalicular obstructions are mainly acquired obstructions of the canaliculus. According to studies, 16–25% of the patients with epiphora may present with canalicular obstructions. Etiology varies from ocular surface infections such as ocular cicatricial pemphigoid and

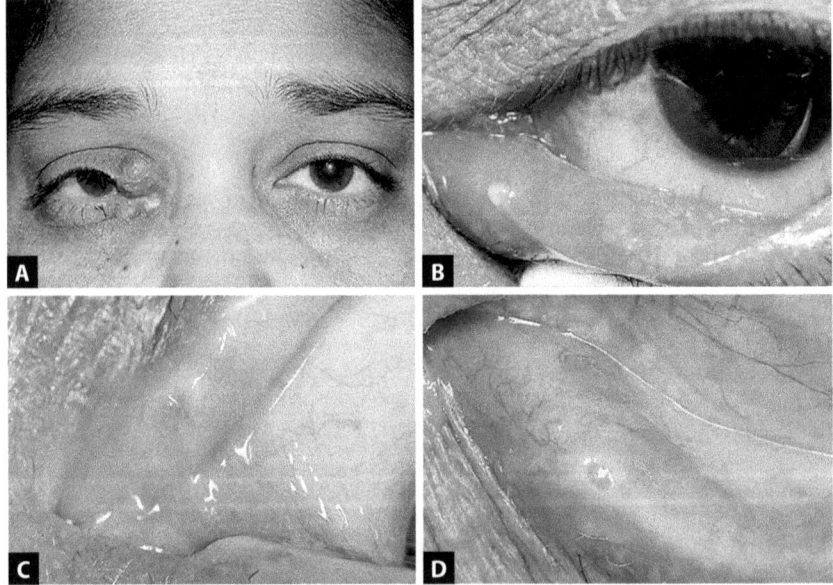

Figs. 9.31.4A to D: (A) Clinical photograph of the right eye upper eyelid redness and swelling medially with discharge in the palpebral fissure area; (B) Clinical color photograph of the everted left lower eyelid showing punctal pouting with discharge and conjunctival congestion with swelling of the medial part of the eyelid; (C and D) Signifies chronic canaliculitis cases with minimal external signs and no punctal pouting.

Stevens–Johnson syndrome, chronic blepharitis, dermatologic diseases like lichen planus, chemical and thermal burns, trauma, local radiation therapy, topical antiglaucoma medications, chemotherapeutic drugs like 5-fluorouracil, docetaxel and paclitaxel, imatinib, etc.

Canalicular obstructions have been classified as proximal canalicular obstructions (<4 mm), mid-canalicular obstructions (>4 mm and <8 mm), and distal canalicular obstruction (>8 mm). Treatment will depend on symptomatology and the anatomic location of the obstruction.

Proximal obstructions are difficult to treat as the condition of the remaining canaliculus is uncertain. Techniques such as retrograde intubation with dacryocystorhinostomy and canalicular trephination with intubation have been attempted with moderate success. In cases where there is failure to attain patency, CDCR or lacrimal gland measures can be attempted in cases with excessive epiphora. Mid-canalicular obstructions can be overcome with canalicular trephination with or without stenting. In case of failure, dacryocystorhinostomy with trephination and stenting or CDCR can be attempted. Distal canalicular obstructions give the best result with canalicular trephination with stents or dacryocystorhinostomy with stent.

■ FINANCIAL DISCLOSURE
Mohammad Javed Ali receives royalties from Springer for his treatise "Principles and Practice of Lacrimal Surgery", "Atlas of Lacrimal Drainage Disorders", and "Video Atlas of Lacrimal Drainage Surgery".

■ CONFLICT OF INTEREST
None.

■ FUNDING SOURCES
Hyderabad Eye Research Foundation.

9.32 | Peripheral Nerve Sheath Tumors

Maya Hada, Nikita Jain
Oculoplasty and ocular oncology services, SMS Medical College, Jaipur
mayahada@gmail.com

■ INTRODUCTION
Orbital peripheral nerve sheath tumors (PNSTs) are a diverse group of mostly benign neoplasms, arising from the neural ectoderm. In the orbit, these tumors involve the branches of III, IV, V, VI, or VII cranial nerves.[1,2] These were first described by Akenside in 1768. "neurofibromatosis" term was coined by von Recklinghausen in 19th century.

Peripheral nerve sheath tumors comprise approximately 2-4% of orbital tumors. The most common PNST of the orbit is neurofibroma, which is further classified as plexiform, diffuse, and localized or isolated. The second most common PNSTs are schwannomas. In addition, other rare PNSTs of the orbit are neuroma, granular cell tumor (GCT), nerve sheath myxoma (NSM), and malignant peripheral nerve sheath tumor (MPNST). Benign PNSTs are characteristically slow growing and noninvasive in nature.

■ NEUROFIBROMA
Neurofibromas are the most common benign PNSTs, which can present in the orbit in following three forms:[3]
1. Plexiform neurofibroma
2. Diffuse neurofibroma
3. Solitary neurofibroma

Plexiform Neurofibromas

Plexiform neurofibromas are the most common subtype of neurofibromas, which are composite network, or "plexus", of infiltrative, poorly circumscribed, and thickened nerve bundles. Plexiform neurofibromas of the orbit usually appear in first decade of life. These tumors have a characteristic "bag of worms" consistency and lead to a typical "S-shaped upper eyelid" deformity **(Figs. 9.32.1A to D)**. These infiltrative, multinodular masses grow along the course of peripheral nerves.[4]

Plexiform neurofibromas have been stated as pathognomonic for neurofibromatosis type 1 (NF1) **(Box 9.32.1)**. It is inherited in an autosomal dominant fashion, but 50% of cases may be sporadic. Biallelic loss of the tumor suppressor gene *NF1* located on chromosome 17q11.2 in Schwann cells is seen as the molecular mechanism.[5]

Neurofibromatosis type 2 (NF2) is characterized by multiple nonmalignant nervous system tumors, including schwannomas, meningiomas, ependymomas, and gliomas, with the cardinal feature being bilateral vestibular schwannomas **(Table 9.32.1)**

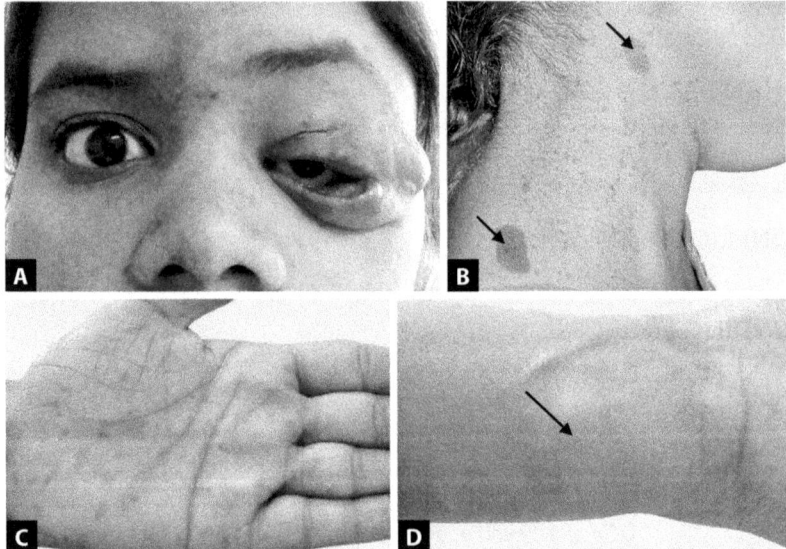

Figs. 9.32.1A to D: Neurofibromatosis. (A) Clinical photograph of a 16-year-old female showing infiltrative, nodular mass involving left upper and lower eyelid with a "bag of worms" consistency; (B) Multiple large (>15 mm) café-au-lait spots (black arrows); (C) Multiple small hyperpigmented lesions suggesting freckles; (D) Subcutaneous nodule (black arrow).

BOX 9.32.1: Diagnostic criteria for neurofibromatosis type 1 (NF1).[6]
- The diagnosis of NF1 is made with the presence of two of the following:
  - Six or more café-au-lait macules >5 mm in diameter in prepubertal individuals, and >15 mm in diameter in postpubertal individuals
  - Two or more neurofibromas of any type, or one plexiform neurofibroma
  - Freckling in the axillary or inguinal regions
  - Optic nerve glioma **(Figs. 9.32.2A to D)**
  - Two or more Lisch nodules (iris hamartomas)
  - A distinctive bony lesion such as sphenoid dysplasia or thinning of the long bone cortex with or without pseudoarthrosis
  - A heterozygous pathogenic *NF1* variant with a variant allele fraction of 50% in apparently normal tissue such as white blood cells
- A child of a parent who meets the diagnostic criteria specified in A merits a diagnosis of NF1 if one or more of the criteria in A are present

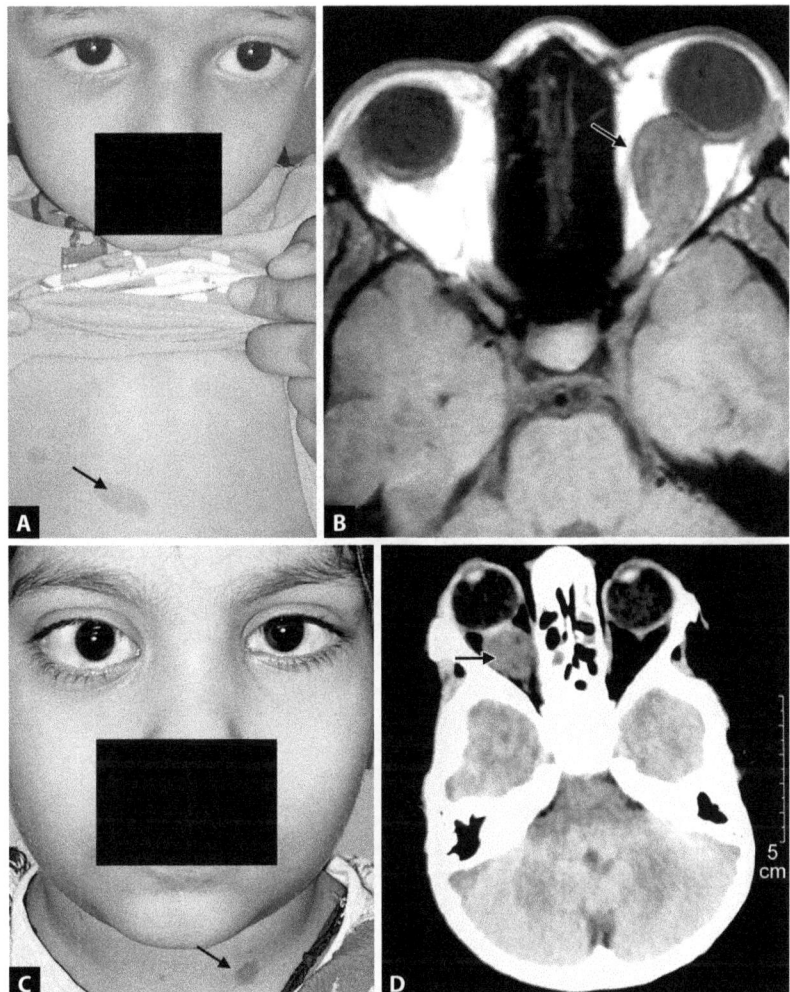

Figs. 9.32.2A to D: Neurofibromatosis type 1 (NF1). (A) A 3-year-old male presented with vision loss in left eye, on examination multiple café-au-lait spots (arrow) were present. (B) Axial section of T1-weighted MRI showing fusiform enlargement of the optic nerve suggesting optic nerve glioma; (C) A 5-year-old female presented with right eye axial proptosis, café-au-lait spots (arrow) seen on examination; (D) Axial section of computed tomogram scan showing fusiform enlargement of optic nerve suggestive of optic nerve glioma.

TABLE 9.32.1: Manchester criteria for clinical diagnosis of neurofibromatosis type 2 (NF2).

	Additional findings needed for diagnosis
Bilateral vestibular schwannomas	None
First-degree family relative with NF2	Unilateral vestibular schwannoma or two NF2-associated lesions (meningioma, glioma, neurofibroma, schwannoma, or cataract)
Unilateral vestibular schwannoma	Two NF2-associated lesions associated with the disorder (meningioma, glioma, neurofibroma, schwannoma, or cataract)
Multiple meningiomas	Unilateral vestibular schwannoma or two other NF2-associated lesions (glioma, neurofibromas, schwannoma, or cataract)

SECTION 9: Oculoplasty

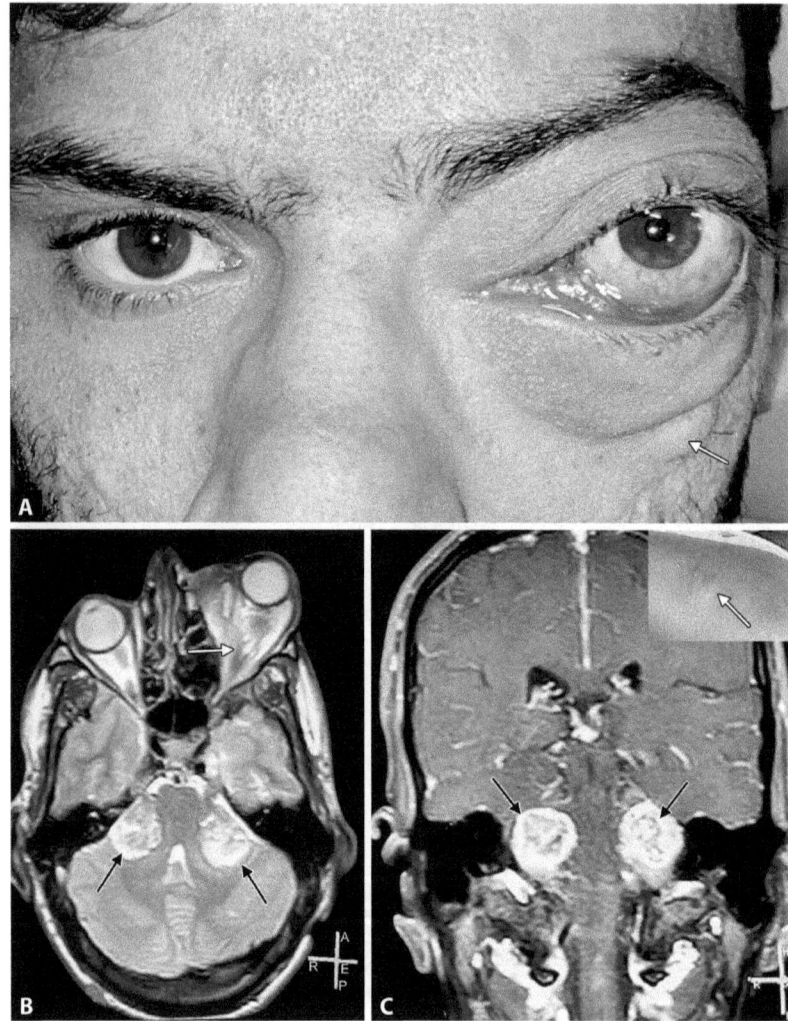

Figs. 9.32.3A to C: Neurofibromatosis type 1 (NF2). (A) A 20-year-old male presented with left eye abaxial proptosis, bilateral hearing loss, and multiple cutaneous nodules (white arrow); (B) Axial MRI T2-weighted (T2W) image showing left optic nerve sheath meningioma (white arrow) with bilateral vestibular schwannoma (black arrow); (C) Coronal MRI T2W showing enhancement of bilateral acoustic schwannoma post gadolinium contrast (black arrows). Multiple cutaneous neurofibromas (white arrow, inset) were also noted.

(Figs. 9.32.3A to C). It has autosomal dominant inheritance and is caused by mutation in the *NF2* gene, which is a tumor suppressor gene located on chromosome 22q12. This gene encodes a protein known as merlin or schwannomin.

Imaging

On CT, plexiform neurofibromas appear as diffuse, infiltrative soft tissue masses which may be associated with bony orbital expansion. Characteristically, there may be absence of one or both sphenoid wings[7] **(Figs. 9.32.4A to D)**. On T2-weighted MRI, plexiform neurofibromas appear hyperintense and show heterogeneous enhancement on contrast administration material.[8]

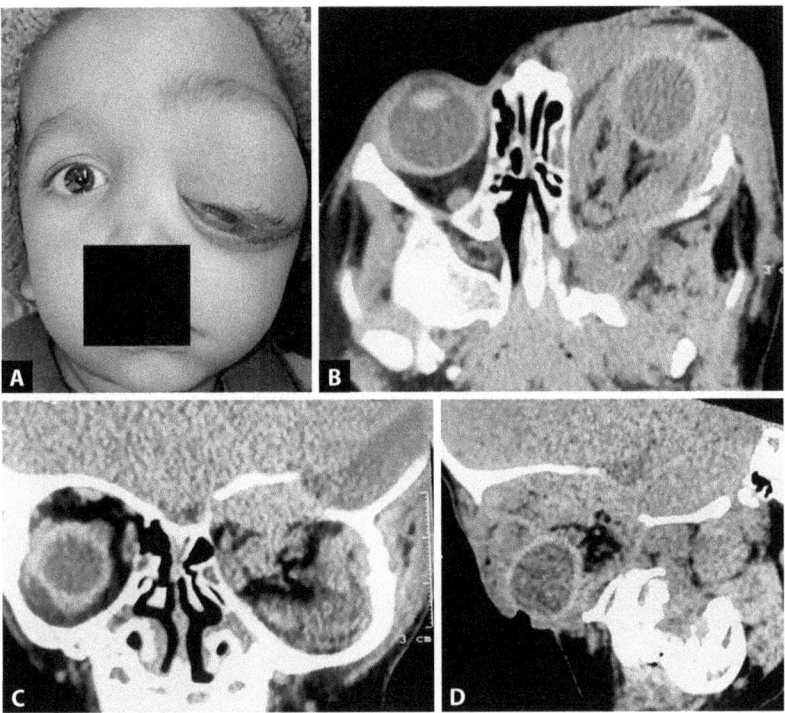

Figs. 9.32.4A to D: Plexiform neurofibroma with sphenoid wing dysplasia. (A) A 3-year-old male presented with left-sided enlarged orbital dimensions with elongated eyebrow, large eyelids, and inferiorly displaced large eyeball. Computed tomogram scan showing absence of a part of greater wing of sphenoid associated with ill-defined diffuse soft tissue density in the left orbit in axial (B), coronal (C), and sagittal (D) sections.

Pathology

On histopathology, these are comprised of nonencapsulated, randomly oriented thin spindle cells with characteristic "crab grass" pattern of growth. Variable amount of myxoid material with collagen is present in the surrounding ("shredded carrots") matrix.[9] In addition, there is a mixture of neural and non-neural elements such as axons, perineural cells, mast cells, and fibroblasts.[10]

Management

The treatment for plexiform neurofibroma depends on many factors including the age of the patient, rate of progression, and extent of involvement by the tumor and presence of a functional deficit (vision loss, strabismus, proptosis, ptosis, amblyopia, or glaucoma) **(Box 9.32.2)**. Nonprogressive plexiform neurofibromas without any associated functional deficit can be best managed with observation and serial clinicoradiological evaluation. 3D MRI can be used to measure the volume of plexiform neurofibromas of the orbit, as higher volume correlates with presence of anisometropia, ptosis, and amblyopia in these cases. Debulking surgery is done for progressive tumors that compromise critical structures, lead to functional issues or cause disfigurement. A multidisciplinary approach is required for the surgical management of orbitotemporal plexiform neurofibroma which includes tumor resection or debulking, sphenoid wing defect correction with grafting, ptosis correction **(Figs. 9.32.5A and B)**, and rarely enucleation in the setting of a painful and deformed eyeball.

BOX 9.32.2: Orbital periorbital plexiform neurofibroma (OPPN) working group consensus statement for ophthalmic monitoring and management.[11]

- Comprehensive ophthalmic evaluation is recommended every 6 months until the age of 8 in children with OPPN
- Patients with OPPN confined to the upper eyelid may not need to undergo neuroimaging
- Early intervention is recommended for associated ophthalmic issues such as ptosis, amblyopia, and lacrimal involvement with the exception of strabismus surgery, as strabismus caused by orbital tumor involvement while the tumor is in its rapid growth phase carries a high risk for recurrence after strabismus surgery
- Debulking surgery is indicated in presence of following conditions:
  – Visual decline
  – Progressive tumor growth involving a vital structure
  – Progressive disfigurement or functional decline
- Clinical trials using biologic agents (i.e., MEK inhibitors) are underway but no definitive recommendations can be made at this time

The recent development includes the targeted medical therapies as MEKi, the mitogen-activated protein kinase inhibitor (selumetinib or trametinib), targeting a downstream effector of rat sarcoma virus (RAS).

Isolated or Localized Neurofibromas

Isolated or localized neurofibromas are well-defined, nonencapsulated, and slowly progressive lesions that usually present in the third to fifth decades. Isolated neurofibromas are the least vascular of the three types.[12]

Isolated neurofibromas are mostly located in the superior orbit that corresponds to the presence of higher number of sensory nerves. Typically, these tumors do not affect visual acuity unless the optic nerve is compressed. Pain, if present, may signal nerve root compression, globe indentation, or rarely malignant transformation. Clinical and imaging features of isolated neurofibromas are usually indistinguishable from schwannomas.[13]

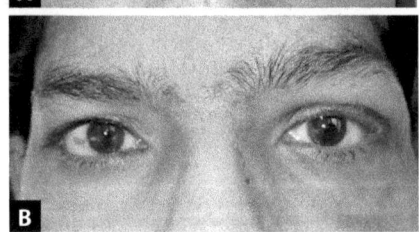

Figs. 9.32.5A and B: (A) Clinical photograph of a 32-year-old female presented with "S"-shaped swelling of the left eyelid associated with ptosis and thickened eyelid margin suggestive of plexiform neurofibroma; (B) Postoperative photograph after debulking and levator resection surgery of the eyelid.

Imaging

On CT, isolated neurofibromas appear to be homogenous, smoothly marginated, round, ovoid, or lobulated masses. They are usually located in the extraconal compartment as they originate from the sensory branches of the trigeminal nerve. On T1-weighted MRI, these are isointense to the extraocular muscles and hyperintense to orbital fat. On T2-weighted imaging (T2WI), these are hyperintense to orbital fat and can display a "target sign" due to a peripheral ring of hyperintensity.[14]

Management

In toto, excision is recommended without breaking the capsule for benign isolated neurofibromas.

Pathology
On histopathology, these appear as well-circumscribed lesions with a pseudocapsule consisting of a cellular perineural sheath.

Diffuse Neurofibromas
Diffuse neurofibromas are slow growing, infiltrative masses which present at young age. These are characterized by plaque-like thickening of the dermal and subcutaneous tissues due to tumor infiltration into the subcutaneous fat.[15]

Imaging
These are ill-defined and irregular masses with variable enhancement on CT scan.

Pathology
On histopathology, diffuse neurofibromas shows higher vascularity and also infiltrate into the adjacent subcutaneous tissues, fat, and structures of the ocular adnexa.

■ SCHWANNOMA
Schwannomas are benign, slow growing PNSTs originating from proliferation of Schwann cells, which produce the myelin sheath around peripheral axons. These tumors arise most frequently from the supraorbital and supratrochlear nerves. The orbital schwannomas commonly present in the second to fourth decade of life and evolve over a period of several months to years. Unlike neurofibroma, multiple schwannoma or schwannomatosis is associated with various genetic syndromes with different alterations including NF2 and Carney complex.[16]

Clinical Features
Orbital schwannomas present with gradual onset proptosis and lid fullness. Other manifestations include diplopia, ocular movement limitation, especially in elevation, and diminution of vision on optic nerve compression. As these tumors are mostly located in the superior quadrant, inferior globe dystopia with proptosis is seen **(Figs. 9.32.6A to D)**. Paresthesias, or deep, dull pain may also be perceived in the distribution of the affected nerve. There have been reports describing rapid growth of orbital solitary schwannomas during pregnancy. It has been attributed to the presence of progesterone receptors on immunohistochemistry (IHC) on these tumors. Sometimes intratumoral hemorrhage may also lead to rapid expansion.[17]

Imaging
Schwannomas appear homogenously dense, isodense to extraocular muscles, smooth round or elongated masses, which demonstrate enhancement with contrast on CT. Schwannomas are often extraconal and may extend through the superior orbital fissure, which helps in differentiating these tumors from cavernous hemangioma and meningioma. Schwannomas typically produce a hypointense signal on T1-weighted MRI and a hyperintense signal on T2-weighted MRI. MRI can reveal both homogenous and heterogeneous enhancement and correlate with histology and morphology of tumor. Antoni A regions have intermediate intensities with T1 and T2, but Antoni B regions are hypointense on T1 and hyperintense on T2.[18,19]

Pathology
Schwannomas are well-circumscribed, encapsulated, and vascular tumors. Histologically, they are composed of biphasic morphologic areas: Antoni A and Antoni B. While Antoni A areas are more cellular comprising of spindle-shaped cells with nuclear palisading, Antoni B areas display loose, stellate, and vacuolated cells suspended in a mucinous matrix

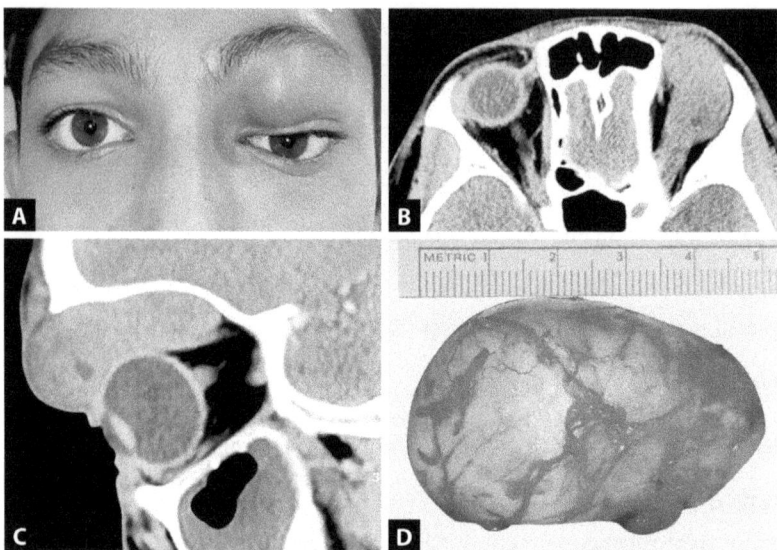

Figs. 9.32.6A to D: Schwannoma. (A) Clinical photograph of a 19-year-old male with superior orbital mass and inferior globe dystopia on the left side; (B) Axial section of computed tomogram scan showing well defined, homogenous, elongated mass in superior orbit; (C) Sagittal section of computed tomogram scan showing the oblong mass having smooth borders with no globe indentation or bony erosions in the extraconal superior orbit; (D) Well-encapsulated elongated mass with remnants of nerve attached to the capsule.

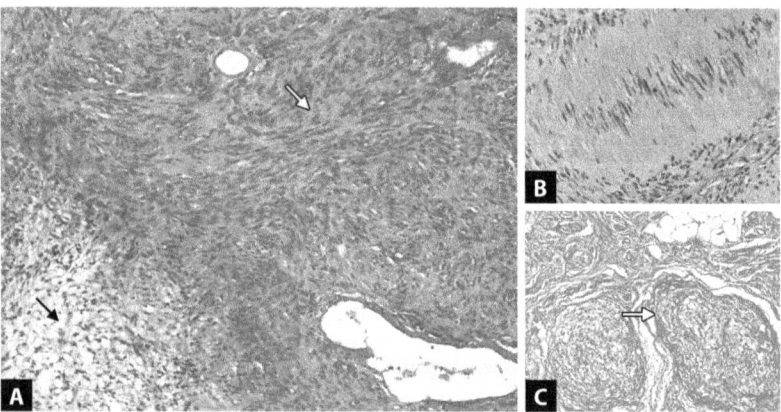

Figs. 9.32.7A to C: (A) Photomicrograph showing schwannoma displaying spindle-shaped cells with nuclear palisading forming solid cellular Antoni A areas (white arrow) and loose, vacuolated cells suspended in a mucinous matrix forming Antoni B areas (black arrows); (B) Photomicrograph showing clusters of elongated spindle cell nuclei arranged in palisades suggesting Verocay bodies; (C) Photomicrograph showing loose spindle cells interspersed with wavy collagen and section of myelinated axon (white arrow) suggesting neurofibroma.
(*Courtesy:* Professor Seema Kashyap, AIIMS)

in a sheet formed arrangement. Antoni A patterns also have Verocay bodies, which are nuclear areas surrounded by clusters of elongated spindle cell nuclei arranged in palisades (Figs. 9.32.7A to C). These tumors stain positively for S-100 protein on IHC.[20]

Schwannomas are known to have four types of histological variants: cellular, melanotic, plexiform, and neuroblastoma.[21]

- The cellular schwannoma has minimal to absent Antoni B tissue pattern with cells that are packed tightly in fascicles. They have poorly formed Verocay bodies. Cells may also show atypia and increased mitoses which might raise suspicion for malignancy.[22]
- Plexiform schwannomas are predominantly comprised of Antoni type A patterns.
- Cystic schwannoma displays degenerative microcystic and myxoid areas that have coalesced to form a large cyst.[23]
- Other rare subtypes are melanotic and neuroblastoma.

Management

The primary treatment of orbital schwannoma is excision while maintaining the capsular integrity. Incomplete excision may lead to recurrence. The most common approach is anterior orbitotomy through an eyelid crease incision because majority of these tumors are located in the superior orbit. Extension of schwannoma into the superior orbital fissure may complicate the surgical approach and limit full extraction from the orbital approach. In such scenario, pterional-extradural approach in collaboration with neurosurgeon provides adequate exposure to the superior posterior orbit, superior orbital fissure, and optic canal, which increases the chances of complete excision. During the excision of the tumor, effort should be made to avoid sacrificing the nerve by microsurgical techniques or careful capsular dissection.[24]

In patients with documented serial imaging suggests slow growing schwannoma affecting the orbital apex or where resection is not feasible, orbital decompression can be done.

The role of radiotherapy in orbital schwannomas is evolving. High incidences of optic neuropathy have been earlier reported with radiation doses above 8-12 Gray. Multisession Gamma Knife surgery is an appropriate modality to treat small, unresectable, inaccessible, or postsurgical benign schwannomas.[25]

MALIGNANT PERIPHERAL NERVE SHEATH TUMOR

Malignant PNSTs are biologically aggressive soft tissue sarcomas of neural origin that constitutes 5-10% of all soft tissue sarcomas. These have also been referred to as neurogenic sarcoma, neurofibrosarcoma, malignant schwannoma, or malignant neurilemmoma. Malignant PNSTs may originate from preexisting neurofibromas or schwannomas. Association with NF1 is seen in up to 50% of cases.[26] Others may arise sporadically or postradiation therapy.

Clinical Features

The clinical history is usually that of rapid tumor growth causing pain, redness, hyperesthesia in the distribution of the nerves involved, and rapidly progressing proptosis. Rapid recurrence of previously diagnosed benign PNSTs following partial excision should raise a clinical suspicion of MPNST. These tumors are usually cystic on palpation. Early metastasis with spread along peripheral nerves to the cranium may lead to the presentation of neurological changes in addition to orbital complaints.[27]

Imaging

Imaging characteristics that differentiate MPNSTs from benign PNST include large diameter of the mass, peripheral enhancement, perilesional edema, and intratumoral cysts or lobulations. Bone destruction, if present, also favors malignancy. On MRI, orbital MPNSTs appear isointense to muscles on T1-weighted images and demonstrate heterogeneous enhancement.[28]

Pathology

Malignant PNSTs are generally cellular and consist of dense fascicles of monomorphic spindle cells alternating with less cellular areas (referred as marbling at low magnification).

Epithelioid cytomorphology is seen less commonly. The spindle cells demonstrate abundant eosinophilic cytoplasm and large pleomorphic or wavy nuclei with prominent nucleoli. Malignant PNSTs as compared to the benign neurofibromas, demonstrate high mitotic activity, cellularity, pleomorphism, and less extracellular matrix material. The tumor cells stain focally positive for S-100 and SOX10 on IHC and negatively for keratin. Cytogenetically, NF1 mutations can be seen in setting of NF1, associated with other mutations as the precursor lesion transform, in multiple tumor suppressor genes (*TP53* and *CDKN2A*) and receptor tyrosine kinase amplification (e.g., *EGFR*).[29]

Management
Radical excision or orbital exenteration is required once the histopathological diagnosis is confirmed with preoperative biopsy. It has a high rate of recurrence if there is incomplete excision. Recurrent tumors may spread intracranially or metastasize to regional lymph nodes and the lungs. Radiation therapy is recommended after surgery, especially when complete resection is difficult or when the resection margin is uncertain.

GRANULAR CELL TUMOR
Granular cells tumors are the benign tumors, believed to arise from Schwann cells due to their frequent association with peripheral nerves and electron microscopic findings of a basal lamina around cells and cytoplasmic inclusions resembling degenerated myelin. They often occur in the extraocular muscles because of their dense neural supply.[30]

Clinical Features
Granular cell tumors typically present as slow-growing, solitary, and painless lesions associated with proptosis. These are frequently associated with extraocular muscles; most commonly the inferior and medial rectus muscles are involved leading to diplopia at presentation. They usually present in the third to sixth decade of life and have female preponderance.[31]

Imaging
These are well-demarcated solitary masses characteristically hypointense on T2WI MRI with higher signal along the periphery, with avid peripheral enhancement. These may have globular or fusiform appearance and are often inseparable from the extraocular muscles. Low central apparent diffusion coefficient (ADC) values may be seen due to the tumor's higher cellularity.[32]

Pathology
Granular cell tumors are nonencapsulated and have invasive borders. Histologically these are comprised of polygonal and spindle cells arranged in nests and clusters with abundant eosinophilic, granular periodic acid-Schiff (PAS)-positive, and diastase resistant cytoplasm. The tumor cells stain positively for S-10059, CD68, and leu-7 on IHC.

Management
Complete surgical removal is the treatment of choice.

FINANCIAL DISCLOSURE
None.

REFERENCES
1. Sweeney AR, Gupta D, Keene CD, Cimino PJ, Chambers CB, Chang SH, et al. Orbital peripheral nerve sheath tumors. Surv Ophthalmol. 2017;62:43-57.
2. Lyons CJ, McNab AA, Garner A, Wright JE. Orbital malignant peripheral nerve sheath tumours. Br J Ophthalmol. 1989;73:731-8.

3. Lee LR, Gigantelli JW, Kincaid MC. Localized neurofibroma of the orbit: a radiographic and histopathologic study. Ophthal Plast Reconstr Surg. 2000;16(3):241-6.
4. Karcioglu Z. Clinicopathologic correlates in orbital disease. In: Duane TD, Tasman W, Jaeger EA (Eds). Duane's Foundations of Clinical Ophthalmology on CD-ROM. Philadelphia: Lippincott Williams & Wilkins; 2006.
5. Gutmann DH, Ferner RE, Listernick RH, Korf BR, Wolters PL, Johnson KJ. Neurofibromatosis type 1. Nat Rev Dis Primers. 2017;3:17004.
6. Legius E, Messiaen L, Wolkenstein P, Pancza P, Avery RA, Berman Y, et al. Revised diagnostic criteria for neurofibromatosis type 1 and Legius syndrome: an international consensus recommendation. Genet Med. 2021;23(8):1506-13.
7. Rennert RC, Scott Pannell J, Levy ML, Khalessi AA. Sphenoid wing dysplasia and plexiform neurofibroma in neurofibromatosis type 1. ANZ J Surg. 2018;88(7-8):E615-6.
8. Santaolalla F, Sanchez JM, Ereño C, Lecumberri G, Valdes C. Severe exophthalmos in trigeminal plexiform neurofibroma involving the orbit and the infratemporal fossa. J Clin Neurosci. 2009;16(7):970-2.
9. Kindblom LG, Meis-Kindblom JM, Havel G, Busch C. Benign epithelioid schwannoma. Am J Surg Pathol. 1998;22(6):762-70.
10. Fine SW, McClain SA, Li M. Immunohistochemical staining for calretinin is useful for differentiating schwannomas from neurofibromas. Am J Clin Pathol. 2004;122(4):552-9.
11. Avery RA, Katowitz JA, Fisher MJ, Heidary G, Dombi E, Packer RJ, et al. Orbital/Periorbital Plexiform Neurofibromas in Children with Neurofibromatosis Type 1: Multidisciplinary Recommendations for Care. Ophthalmology. 2017;124(1):123-32.
12. Cannon T, Carter K, Folberg R. Neurogenic Tumors of the Orbit. In: Duane TD, Tasman W, Jaeger EA (Eds). Duane's Clinical Ophthalmology on CD-ROM, Philadelphia: Lippincott Williams & Wilkins; 2006.
13. Cheng SF. Malignant peripheral nerve sheath tumor of the orbit: malignant transformation from neurofibroma without neurofibromatosis. Ophthal Plast Reconstr Surg. 2008;24(5):413-5.
14. Kottler UB, Conway RM, Schlötzer-Schrehardt U, Holbach LM. Isolated neurofibroma of the orbit with extensive myxoid changes: a clinicopathologic study including MRI and electron microscopic findings. Orbit. 2004;23(1):59-64.
15. Van Zuuren EJ, Posma AN. Diffuse neurofibroma on the lower back. J Am Acad Dermatol. 2003;48(6):938-40.
16. Cantore G, Ciappetta P, Raco A, Lunardi P. Orbital Schwannomas: Report of Nine Cases and Review of the Literature. Neurosurgery. 1986;19(4):583-8.
17. Singh M, Singh U, Zadeng Z, Pathak A, Sukhija J. Clinico-Radiological Spectrum and Management of Orbital Schwannomas: A Tertiary Care Institute Study. Orbit. 2013.
18. Kashyap S, Pushker N, Meel R, Sen S, Bajaj MS, Khuriajam N, et al. Orbital schwannoma with cystic degeneration. Clin Experiment Ophthalmol. 2009;37(3):293-8.
19. Khan SN, Sepahdari AR. Orbital masses: CT and MRI of common vascular lesions, benign tumors, and malignancies. Saudi J Ophthalmol. 2012;26(4):373-83.
20. Pekmezci M, Reuss DE, Hirbe AC, Dahiya S, Gutmann DH, von Deimling A. Morphologic and immunohistochemical features of malignant peripheral nerve sheath tumors and cellular schwannomas. Mod Pathol. 2015;28(2):187-200.
21. Huang H-Y, Park N, Erlandson RA, Antonescu CR. Immunohistochemical and ultrastructural comparative study of external lamina structure in 31 cases of cellular, classical, and melanotic schwannomas. Appl Immunohistochem Mol Morphol. 2004;12(1):50-8.
22. Kurtkaya-Yapicier O, Scheithauer B, Woodruff JM. The pathobiologic spectrum of Schwannomas. Histol Histopathol. 2003;18(3):925-34.
23. Morgenstern KE, Vadysirisack DD, Zhang Z, Cahill KV, Foster JA, Burns JA, et al. Expression of sodium iodide symporter in the lacrimal drainage system: implication for the mechanism underlying nasolacrimal duct obstruction in I(131)-treated patients. Ophthal Plast Reconstr Surg. 2005;21(5):337-44.
24. Goldberg RA, Rootman DB, Nassiri N, Samimi DB, Shadpour JM. Orbital Tumors Excision without Bony Marginotomy under Local and General Anesthesia. J Ophthalmol. 2014;2014:424852.
25. Kim BS, Im Y-S, Woo KI, Kim Y-D, Lee J-I. Multisession Gamma Knife Radiosurgery for Orbital Apex Tumors. World Neurosurg. 2015;84(4):1005-13.

26. D'Agostino AN, Soule EH, Miller RH. Sarcomas of the peripheral nerves and somatic soft tissue associated with multiple neurofibromatosis (von Recklinghausen's disease). Cancer. 1963;16:1015-27.
27. Wanebo JE, Malik JM, VandenBerg SR, Wanebo HJ, Driesen N, Persing JA. Malignant peripheral nerve sheath tumors: a clinicopathologic study of 28 cases. *Cancer.* 1993;71:1247-53.
28. Farid M, Demicco EG, Garcia R, Ahn L, Merola PR, Cioffi A, et al. Malignant peripheral nerve sheath tumors. Oncologist. 2014;19(2):193-201.
29. Daimaru Y, Hashimoto H, Enjoji M. Malignant peripheral nerve-sheath tumors (malignant schwannomas): an immunohistochemical study of 29 cases. Am J Surg Pathol. 1985;9:434-44.
30. Elkousy H, Harrelson J, Dodd L, Martinez S, Scully S. Granular cell tumors of the extremities. Clin Orthop Relat Res. 2000;(380):191-8.
31. Rekhi B, Jambhekar NA. Morphologic spectrum, immunohistochemical analysis, and clinical features of a series of granular cell tumors of soft tissues: a study from a tertiary referral center. Ann Diagn Pathol. 2010;14:162-7.
32. Blacksin MF, White LM, Hameed M, et al. Granular cell tumor of the extremity: magnetic resonance imaging characteristics with pathologic correlation. Skeletal Radiol. 2005;34:625-31.

SECTION 10

Pediatric Ophthalmology and Strabismus

Editor: Lav Kochgaway

- 10.1 **Pediatric Refraction** 892
  Kavitha Kalaivani, Nikunj Kalodiya
- 10.2 **Amblyopia Treatment** 895
  Lav Kochgaway
- 10.3 **Sensory Functions: Evaluation and Clinical Usefulness of the Assessment in Diagnosis and Treatment of Strabismus** 898
  Rohit Saxena
- 10.4 **Evaluation of Accommodative Convergence to Accommodation Ratio** 905
  Pradeep Sharma
- 10.5 **Diagnosis and Management of Esotropic Deviations** 906
  HM Ravindranath
- 10.6 **Infantile Esotropia** 909
  Sumita Agarkar, Gayathri J Panicker, Roshni Desai
- 10.7 **Exodeviations** 912
  Saurabh Mittal
- 10.8 **A-V Pattern Deviations** 915
  KS Santhan Gopal, V Jyothi
- 10.9 **Paralytic Strabismus** 916
  Meenakshi Swaminathan, Srikanth Ramasubramanian, Arun Samprathi
- 10.10 **Dissociated Vertical Deviations** 918
  Ramesh Kekunnaya
- 10.11 **Restrictive Strabismus** 921
  Kalpana Narendran
- 10.12 **Strabismus Surgery: Planning, Executing, and Complications** 922
  TS Surendran
- 10.13 **Clinical Management of Nystagmus** 924
  Mihir Kothari
- 10.14 **Pediatric Cataract Management** 933
  Lav Kochgaway
- 10.15 **Pediatric Eye in Various Systemic Syndromes** 935
  Jitendra Jethani
- 10.16 **Pediatric Epiphora** 944
  Rajesh Chaudhuri
- 10.17 **Myopia Progression in Children** 945
  Jitendra Jethani

10.1 Pediatric Refraction

Kavitha Kalaivani, Nikunj Kalodiya
Sankara Nethralaya, Chennai
kavithakalaivani@yahoo.com

■ INTRODUCTION

Refractive error is the most common cause of visual impairment in children. So, early diagnosis and treatment can reduce visual impairment and other ocular morbidities.

■ PREREQUISITES

- Visual assessment and refraction in the pediatric patient is always a challenge due to limited cooperation, low reliability in subjective response.
- We need to develop a rapport with children.
- We should use attention-getting targets.
- We should examine the child in presence of parents or attender.

■ BRÜCHNER TEST

- It is a quick method to estimate refractive error by examining the red-reflex.
- Procedure
  - Shine a light of scope directly into pupils from a distance so that the circle of light lights-up both pupils at the same time.
- Interpretation
  - Observe the red-reflex from each eye. If the whole pupil is lightened-up a child is emmetropic. Inferior crescents indicate myopia. Superior crescents indicate hyperopia.

■ CYCLOPLEGIC REFRACTION

- Retinoscopy is superior to autorefraction in pediatric refraction.
- When the child is too young for subjective refraction, glass prescription should be given on basis of retinoscopy reading alone.
- Cycloplegic (wet) refraction is very useful in children due to the presence of strong accommodation. Cycloplegic refraction should be carried out in every patient with or without strabismus. The total refractive status of the eye with the accommodation at rest can be assessed by wet refraction. A dry retinoscopy can be done prior to cycloplegia to get a rough estimate of the refractive error and to assess the accommodative effort.

Drugs Used for Cycloplegia and Mydriasis (Table 10.1.1)

TABLE 10.1.1: Drugs for cycloplegia and mydriasis.

Drug	Cycloplegia		Mydriasis	
	Maximum	Recovery	Maximum	Recovery
Cyclopentolate	30–80 minutes	6–24 hours	30–60 minutes	6–24 hours
Tropicamide	30–40 minutes	2–6 hours	30–50 minutes	2–6 hours
Homatropine	30–60 minutes	1–3 days	50–90 minutes	1–3 days
Atropine	1–3 hours	3–14 days	3–6 hours	7–14 days
Phenylephrine	No cycloplegia		20 minutes	2–3 hours

Side Effects of Drugs (Table 10.1.2)

TABLE 10.1.2: Ocular and systemic side effects of drugs.

Drug	Ocular side effects	Systemic side effects
Cyclopentolate (C)	• Transient stinging • Allergic reaction • Irritation • Diffuse redness	• Hallucination • Drowsiness • Ataxia • Disorientation
Tropicamide (T)	• Transient stinging • Raised intraocular pressure (IOP) • Hypersensitivity reaction	• Confusion • Skin rash • Dryness of mouth
Atropine	• Allergy • Risk of angle closure • Raised IOP	• Cutaneous flush/fever • Tachycardia • Urinary retention • Decreased secretion
Homatropine (HA)	Same as atropine	
Phenylephrine	• Transient pain • Lacrimation • Rebound meiosis	• Increased blood pressure • Tachycardia • Ventricular arrhythmia • Occipital headache

PREFER CYCLOPLEGICS IN CHILDREN

- Based on child-age requirement, presence or absence of squint and side-effect profile of the drug, we should choose the appropriate drug or combinations of drugs in appropriate dosage and for the appropriate duration.
- Ideal cycloplegic drug should have rapid onset, sufficient duration of action, rapid recovery, absence of side effect and should cause full paralysis of accommodation.
- *Up to 1 year:* Retinopathy of prematurity (ROP) drops (equal volumes of tropicamide plus + lubricant).
- *1–16 years:* CTC provided no contraindication for it (convulsions, cerebral palsy, mental retardation, Down's syndrome, Trisomy 13 and 18).
- *HA + T:* If contraindication for CTC.
- *T-plus (tropicamide 0.8% + phenylephrine 5%):* In aphakic and pseudophakic patient.

Open-field autorefractor with the distant nonaccommodative target will also be useful in pediatric refraction. It can also be used to measure accommodation by presenting target at various distances.

After finalizing refractive status, we need to treat it if needed.

WHAT TO PRESCRIBE?

The refractive status of a child is constantly changing with age. We should consider all factors such as age-related emmetropization, magnitude and type of refractive error, visual needs of the child, strong accommodation, strabismus, and amblyopia before prescribing glasses.

HYPEROPIA WITH ORTHOTROPIA

- Hyperopia is more amblyogenic than myopia. It can cause ametropic amblyopia, accommodative esotropia.
- Mild hyperopia can be observed as most young children are hyperopia with large accommodative reserve.
- Moderate-to-high hyperopia should be treated with glasses. Infant more than +6D, 1–2 year-old child with more than +5D, and 2–3-year-old child with more than +4.50D hyperopia should be treated with age appropriate under-correction.

- Postmydriatic test can be done in children who are capable of giving subjective response for optimal hyperopic correction.
- Hyperopes can be prescribed cycloplegic to relax accommodation and get used to high-plus power.

Hyperopia with Esotropia with Normal Accommodative Convergence to Accommodation Ratio

Full correction without under-correction should be prescribed in such children.

Hyperopia with Esotropia with High Accommodative Convergence to Accommodation Ratio

Full correction with near-add should be prescribed in such children in the form of executive bifocal. Executive bifocal has to be designed in such a way that the line of segment sits at or just below the center of the pupil.

MYOPIA

- Low-to-moderate myopia (less than 4D) may not need to be prescribed in infants as they are not expected to view distant objects and objects in fine detail.
- Children having myopia more than 4D should be prescribed glasses with full correction without over or under correcting it.
- Children with intermittent divergent strabismus can be under corrected for myopia with close follow-up.

ASTIGMATISM

- The prevalence rate of astigmatism is higher in infants than adults because of the steep cornea. Astigmatism reduces up to a certain age as the child grows up. Symmetrical mild-to-moderate meridional astigmatism up to 1.5D can be observed.
- Oblique astigmatism is more amblyogenic, so it should be corrected.
- Children >3 years of age should be corrected for astigmatism of 1.0D also.

APHAKIC PATIENT

- Aphakic infants should be prescribed single vision glass for near. Bifocal glass can be prescribed as they grow older.
- Contact lens can be considered as an option in infants with unilateral aphakia.

PSEUDOPHAKIC PATIENT

Pseudophakic children should be given full correction in form of bifocal or progressive glass as there is no residual accommodation after cataract surgery.

ANISOMETROPIA

- Anisometropia is very powerful amblyogenic factor. One diopter of spherical and 1.5D of cylindrical anisometropia can cause amblyopia.
- Hyperopic anisometropia should be treated with age appropriate under-correction with full correction of astigmatism in an orthotropic child.
- Hyperopic anisometropia should be treated with full correction of hyperopia and astigmatism in an esotropic child.
- Contact lens can be considered if anisometropia is significant to cause aniseikonia. Children can tolerate aniseikonia more than adults so glass should be prescribed in children who are intolerant to contact lens.

Full-frame glasses should be prescribed. A tinted or photochromatic glass should be prescribed in children with albinism, aniridia, and cone dystrophy.

10.2 Amblyopia Treatment

Lav Kochgaway
Netralayam, Kolkata
lav.kochgaway@netralayam.com

INTRODUCTION

Amblyopia, often called "lazy-eye", is defined as unilateral or bilateral decrease of visual acuity caused by pattern vision deprivation or abnormal binocular interaction which is reversible if appropriately treated in time. Prevalence estimates range from 1 to 5% depending on the population studied and the definition used. Amblyopia is usually found in the setting of causative factors such as strabismus, refractive error, sensory obstacles such as congenital cataract, opacities in the media, and associated with nystagmus.

MANAGEMENT

The approach to therapy includes:
- Removal of the amblyopiogenic
- Appropriate refractive correction
- Treatment of amblyopia by appropriate method
  - Occlusion
  - Penalization
    - Optical
    - Pharmacological (atropine)

The following options mentioned below have not been proven to be sufficiently effective and are not routinely used:
- Pleoptics
- CAM vision stimulator
- Red-filter treatment
- *Medical:* Levodopa
- Active-vision therapy

Removal of Amblyopiogenic Factor

Early recognition and treatment of amblyopiogenic risk factors in period of plasticity may increase the chance of development of binocular vision. The therapy needs to be individualized according to the age, baseline vision, and cause of amblyopia for a particular child. The basic strategy is to allow the formation of sharp and clear image by removing amblyogenic factor and then to increase the visual stimulation of the worse eye. This can act as prevention for amblyopia if done early. Pediatric cataracts especially in unilateral ones are highly amblyopiogenic. A mean visual acuity of 20/60 can be achieved by operating on a unilateral congenital cataract within 2 months as against hand movements to 20/160 by waiting further. In some cases where amblyopiogenic risk factors are present (e.g., unilateral keratopathy), a small monocular cataract, or ocular conditions that can cause anisometropia such as unilateral ptosis and hemangioma, it may be useful to institute preventive therapy using spectacles to correct refractive error and/or occlusion therapy.

Appropriate Refractive Correction

A proper cycloplegic refraction and optimal correction is the most important intervention in amblyopia. It is the only treatment required for an ametropic amblyopia. In the case of refractive amblyopia, a progressive improvement in acuity for up to 16–22 weeks has been shown in some patients after refractive correction, prior to implementation of other measures. **Table 10.2.1** shows the guideline given by American Academy of Ophthalmology (AAO) for prescription of glasses in infants and young children.

TABLE 10.2.1: Guidelines for refractive correction in infants and young children (AAO preferred practice methods 2012).

Condition	Refractive errors (diopters)		
	Age <1 year	Age 1–2 years	Age 2–3 years
Isoametropia (Similar refractive error in both eyes)			
Myopia	–5.00 or more	–4.00 or more	–3.00 or more
Hyperopia (no manifest deviation)	+6.00 or more	+5.00 or more	+4.50 or more
Hyperopia with esotropia	+2.50 or more	+2.00 or more	+1.50 or more
Astigmatism	3.00 or more	2.50 or more	2.00 or more
Anisometropia			
Myopia	–4.00 or more	–3.00 or more	–3.00 or more
Hyperopia	+2.50 or more	+2.00 or more	+1.50 or more
Astigmatism	2.50 or more	2.00 or more	2.00 or more

(AAO: American Academy of Ophthalmology)

Treatment of Amblyopia

Occlusion

Occlusion of the good eye remains the mainstay of treatment, the basis of which is that it removes the inhibitory influences of the better eye and ameliorates the abnormal binocular interaction. The patient is forced to use the worse eye, which causes constant positive reinforcement of the vision in the worse eye.

Duration of Occlusion

Full-time (all waking hours) occlusion is considered as gold standard for the treatment of amblyopia by a group of pediatric ophthalmologists.

The regimen commonly followed for full-time occlusion therapy goes with the age of patient, as follows:
- 1:1 for a child up to 2 years of age
- 2:1 up to 3 years of age
- 3:1 up to 4 years of age
- 4:1 up to 5 years of age
- 5:1 up to 6 years of age
- 6:1 for 6 years and above.

The US Pediatric Eye Disease Investigator Group (PEDIG) tested two patching regimens. For the treatment of moderate (20/40 to 20/80) amblyopia in 3–7-year-old children: 2 hours versus 6 hours/day (plus 1 hour/day of near visual activities during patching) was compared. Visual acuity in the amblyopic eye improved a similar amount in both groups. In a further study of severe (20/100 to 20/400) amblyopia, no significant difference was found in the visual outcome in the amblyopic eye following full time compared to 6 hours patching per day (each combined with at least 1 hour of near visual activity during patching). Both studies reported similar improvement in visual acuity following 4 months of treatment. Part-time occlusion can be used in milder cases of anisometropic amblyopia, cases not compliant with full time use and as maintenance therapy after resolution of amblyopia.

Total occlusion is a complete obstruction of visual input from the better eye by applying an opaque patch and is the most effective method of the therapy. Adhesive patches stuck directly onto the periorbital skin of the eye are the most commonly used.

They are cheap, easy to apply and remove, and prevent peeping over the patches. Patches can also be stuck onto spectacle lenses, but this gives the child an opportunity to peep around them. Occlusive contact lens is an alternative with better cosmetic appeal but is expensive, can be difficult to maintain and carries risk of corneal problems.

The risks or side effects of occlusion are the following:
- Skin irritation
- Increased risk for accidents when the child is wearing the patch.
- Precipitation of or an increase in the magnitude of strabismus.

Occlusion Amblyopia

Occlusion amblyopia is a rare but important complication of occlusion therapy. Therefore, frequent follow-ups are required. The parent should be informed of potential risks before occlusion is initiated and the child should be actively monitored for side effects of occlusion. Partial occlusion with the help of translucent patch or nail varnish can be given for maintenance. This is better accepted cosmetically and ensures better compliance.

Penalization

This technique may be particularly helpful for children with mild-to-moderate amblyopia. Penalization is achieved by defocusing the eye with better vision by using cycloplegia or by altering the spectacle lens to cause decreased vision in the non-amblyopic eye. The major advantage of atropine penalization is that it is cosmetically more acceptable and as the drug can be instilled by the parent, compliance can be ensured. But it should be used with caution as systemic side effects, such as flushing, hyperactivity, and tachycardia, may occur.

The PEDIG study compared occlusion versus atropinization and concluded that atropine is as effective as patching in the treatment of moderate (20/40 to 20/100) amblyopia in children-aged from 3–7 years. It also compared the daily atropine regimen versus weekend regimen in moderate amblyopia and found both the groups comparable in terms of gain in visual acuity. However, for penalization to be successful cycloplegia must be sufficient enough to decrease the vision of the sound eye to less than that of the amblyopic eye, which may not be feasible in cases of severe amblyopia. In cases of strabismic amblyopia a switch of fixation to the amblyopic eye is important to ensure stimulation of that eye.

Near Activity During Patching

Pediatric Eye Disease Investigator Group study showed that near activity during patching had no added advantage over a child doing only distance activity during patching.

Patching in Older Children

Pediatric Eye Disease Investigator Group study also evaluated effect of patching on older children. They found out that children between 7 and 12 years may benefit with patching even if it was done earlier. But children between 13 and 17 years benefitted only if they were never treated earlier. So children above 13 years should be offered patching therapy if they have never been treated earlier.

Active Vision Therapy

A wide range of active treatments for amblyopia has become available, using a variety of methods. For example, active treatment may involve the patient doing near work; completing word puzzles, dot-to-dot drawings or coloring-in parts of patterns.

In recent years, computer-based software and games are available where monocular and binocular, including dichoptic; perceptual training treatments have been developed to improve binocular dysfunction.

FOLLOW-UP

Follow-up is to be planned according to the age of the child with younger children evaluated early to monitor compliance and observe for side effects especially occlusion amblyopia. In general, the child should be reviewed after 1 month of starting treatment to see the response to the therapy; and then every 2 months to assess the progression. Therapy is continued till maximum vision is achieved.

Once the vision in the amblyopic eye becomes stable for two consecutive visits one should consider for weaning off the therapy and giving the maintenance therapy (in anisometropic amblyopia) especially during the period of plasticity. In case of strabismic amblyopia, 1:1 ratio of occlusion is continued until surgery aligns the eyes.

Around 25% of successfully treated amblyopic children experience a recurrence within the 1st year of treatment, the risk of which is greater when patching is stopped abruptly. Many children will have a residual visual deficit despite compliance with treatment. Failure of visual acuity to improve within 6 months of the commencement of amblyopia treatment should prompt re-refraction and re-examination of the fundus, looking in particular for sub-clinical pathology.

10.3 Sensory Functions: Evaluation and Clinical Usefulness of the Assessment in Diagnosis and Treatment of Strabismus

Rohit Saxena
Dr RP Centre for Ophthalmic Sciences, AIIMS, New Delhi
rohitsaxena80@yahoo.com

INTRODUCTION

Binocular vision is one of the greatest assets that evolution has given mankind as it gives us the third dimension to our world around us. Binocularity has many advantages, it gives us a wider field of view than a monocular field, binocular summation in which the ability to detect faint objects is enhanced and most important stereopsis in which horizontal disparity between the two eyes because of their different positions on the head give precise depth perception.

To visualize an object as singular perception the two eyes require sensory fusion and motor fusion. A proper sensory evaluation would help us to decide about management in certain cases especially in cases of intermittent divergent. A documented deterioration in stereopsis may be an indication of worsening of binocular sensory status and thus an indication for surgery. On the contrary a good fusion or stereopsis sometimes may be present in cases like MED (monocular elevation defect) or DRS (duane's retraction syndrome) which do not warrant any kind of intervention except for observation.

Preoperative sensory evaluations allow us to judge the patient's potential for fusion and thus predict the postoperative results. A patient having superior binocular status preoperatively is more likely to maintain long-term alignment of eyes than patient without any binocularity.

Sensory fusion is by the virtue of retinal correspondence such as that when an object stimulates corresponding points on two different retinae it is seen as one. The process of seeing an object binocularly requires simultaneous perception of that object by two different retinae, fusion of the image formed by the two retinae and perception of the depth of that object.

ABNORMAL SENSORY ADAPTATION

Suppression
The disruption of fusion between two eyes results in the suppression of image from the deviating eye or from the eye with poorer vision. Suppression to begin with is facultative, i.e. present only under binocular condition, but if allowed to persist eventually becomes obligatory and is present even when the fixing-eye is closed. Suppression is usually associated with esotropia and affects the postoperative outcome in terms of residual deviation or recurrence therefore antisuppression exercises should be given to the patient before surgery.

Abnormal Retinal Correspondence
In presence of retinal rivalry when suppression does not occur, a non-foveal point takes over the functions of fovea. This usually takes place in presence of constant small-angle squint where two foveae cease to be corresponding point and fovea of normal eye shares a common visual direction with the non-foveal point of squinting eye. It is important to look for abnormal retinal correspondence (ARC) preoperatively as these patients are more likely to show postoperative drift and thus recurrence of squint.

Diplopia
While suppression and abnormal retinal correspondence are adaptation of immature visual system, any disruption of fusion in matured visual system causes diplopia.

Assessment of Sensory System
The foremost objective behind evaluating sensory system is to look for presence or absence of suppression, ARC, and diplopia which not only aid in surgical decision but are important factors determining the postoperative results.
1. Test for suppression
   a. Synoptophore simultaneous prescription (SMP) slides
   b. After image test
   c. Bagolini's striated glasses
   d. Worth's four-dot test (WFDT)
   e. 4-prism base-out test
   f. Red filter test
   g. Optical test chart
2. Test for abnormal retinal correspondence
   a. Synoptophore
   b. Bagolini's striated glasses
   c. WFDT
   d. After-image test
   e. Polaroid dissociation
3. Stereopsis evaluation
   a. Distance stereopsis test
      i. Frisby–Davis distance
      ii. Distance Randot
      iii. Mentor B-VAT
   b. Near stereopsis
      i. TNO
      ii. Randot
      iii. Titmus
      iv. Frisby-Davis near test.

Synoptophore

Based on haploscopic principle the synoptophore is an instrument in which all three components of deviation can be neutralized (**Fig. 10.3.1**). It consists of different series of slides which can be used for simultaneous perception, fusion and stereopsis depending upon the type of target projected.

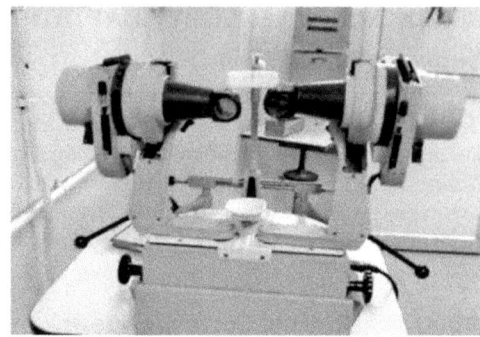

Fig. 10.3.1: Synoptophore.

Simultaneous macular perception slides (**Fig. 10.3.2**): These slides consist of two dissimilar objects, substending an angle of 5° at macula. One solid and one hollow object, like lion and cage is projected in either eye. If both the images superimpose and patient perceives lion in cage indicates simultaneous perception absence of either target suggests suppression of that eye. Any deviation if present should be corrected so that both the images fall on fovea. If patient can perceive both the images in presence of manifest squint it is suggestive of ARC. Subjective angle is measured when patient is asked to superimpose the images by moving the bar. Objective angle is measured when examiner finds no movement of eyes on switching the flashes.

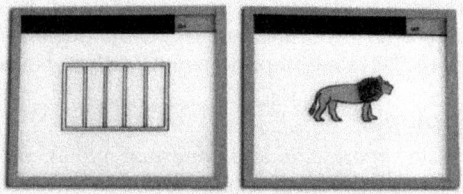

Fig. 10.3.2: Simultaneous macular perception slides.

- If subjective angle is equal to objective angle → normal retinal correspondence (NRC).
- If subjective angle is less than objective angle → ARC.
- If angle of anomaly is equal to objective angle → harmonious ARC (full sensory adaptation).
- If angle of anomaly is less than objective angle → unharmonious ARC.

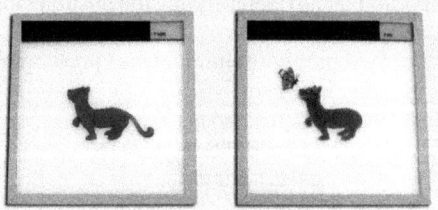

Fig. 10.3.3: Fusion sides.

Fusion: The targets used are same in all respect except for some part either missing in one slide or addition in the other one. The patient should be able to fuse the two targets sees both the target as one complete figure. For example as seen in **Figure 10.3.3**, where one slide shows a cat with tail but without fly and the other slide consists of cat and fly but the tail is absent. A patient with normal fusion would see the picture as a complete cat with tail and fly as well.

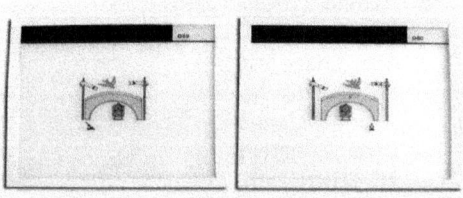

Fig. 10.3.4: Depth perception (stereopsis) slides.

Stereopsis: These slides consist of two similar slides with horizontal disparity which gives depth perception when seen as one (**Fig. 10.3.4**).

After image slides (**Fig. 10.3.5**) this is the most dissociating test in which battery-powered camera flash is used to produce a vertical after image in right eye and a horizontal after image in the left eye. Each eye is stimulated separately and patient is asked to draw the relative position of the lines.

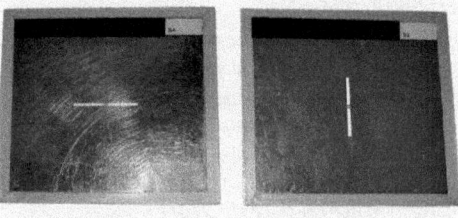

Fig. 10.3.5: After image slides.

- A cross response at center indicates NRC.
- An asymmetrical cross response is suggestive of ARC.
- Absence of vertical line and horizontal line indicates suppression of right and left eye, respectively.

Bagolini's Glasses

These are plastic discs with regular micro-Maddox cylinder which convert a point source of light seen as a streak. Striations in right eye are at 135° while in left it is 45°. This is the least dissociating test. A point source of light is shown for either distance or near and results can be interpreted as follows:
- Crossing of the lines at right angles to each other without deviation is NRC.
- Crossing of lines in presence of manifest deviation indicates harmonious ARC.
- Foveal suppression scotoma (fixation point scotoma) is seen as defect in center.
- Single line represents suppression.

Worth's Four-Dot Test

It is based on red-green color dissociation. It consists of box with four internally self-illuminating panes of colored glasses, arranged in diamond shape (two green, one red, and one white). Patient wears red in front of right eye and green in front of left eye. Patient is then asked to view the box. The result can be interpreted as follows:
- The patient sees all the four dots.
  - Normal binocular response with no manifest deviation → NRC.
  - With manifest squint → harmonious ARC.
- The patient sees five dots.
  - Red-dots appear to the right → uncrossed diplopia with esotropia.
  - Red-dots appear to the left of the green dots → crossed diplopia with exotropia.
- The patient sees three green-dots → suppression of right eye.
- The patient sees two red-dots → suppression of left eye.

The similar test is done for near with the help of red and green goggles and Worth's four-dot torch.

Four Prism Base-out Test

This test is of great aid in detecting the small scotoma in case of monofixation syndrome. A 4-diopter prism is placed base-out in front of one eye as the patient fixes at a distance target. The base-out prism causes sudden displacement of an image onto the parafoveal temporal retina this will elicit a nasal refixation movement and simultaneous temporal movement of the other eye. Next a slower vergence movement directed nasally in both eye will occur to maintain bifoveal fixation. But no refixation movement will occur in the eye with prism if the image has been shifted to scotomatous area. In cases of inattentiveness or defective fusion the normal movement is delayed for few seconds.

Red Filter Test

A red filter is placed over one eye and patient is asked to look at a point source of light.
- Presence of diplopia suggests NRC,
  - If crossed diplopia → exotropia.
  - If uncrossed diplopia → esotropia.
- If patient sees one pinkish light then it indicates harmonious ARC.

Optical Polarized Test Chart

The chart has three lines of text, with the middle line printed or marked in letters characters which have no polarizing effect. The line above this middle line is marked in letters or characters which have the effect of polarizing light reflected from them, in a plane of polarization in one direction, while the line below the middle line is similarly marked with letters or characters having the effect of polarizing reflected light but with the plane of polarization at a right angle to the direction of polarization caused by the upper line. The patient views the test chart through polarizing spectacles, the spectacle in front of one eye having a plane of polarization corresponding to that of the upper line of text on the chart, and the spectacle in front of the other eye having a plane of polarization corresponding to that of the lower line of the text.
- All three lines perceived → NRC.
- A difference in contrast between the different lines on the chart, or if he is unable to read either the top or bottom line, suggest suppression depending upon the polarization of the line.

Extent of Scotoma

Prism: Prisms of increasing strength are placed in front one eye till patient reports diplopia. One can chart the horizontal extent of scotoma by placing base-in or base-out prism and vertical extent can be determined by placing base-up or base-down prisms. The power of the prism indicates the diameter of scotoma.

Worth's four-dot test: The size of scotoma can be quantified using WFDT. The size is calculated from the distance at which the flash light is held from the patient. **Table 10.3.1** gives the size of scotoma.

Other methods are:
- Synoptophore
- Lees or Hess screen
- Polaroid scotometer

TABLE 10.3.1: Size of scotoma.

Distance at which flashlight is held (in feet)	Scotoma size
1	6.4
3	2.3
6	1.1
8	0.9
10	0.7
15	0.5
20	0.3

Depth of Scotoma

The illuminance of the image perceived by deviating eye is reduced by placing the red filters of increasing density in front of the normal fixating eye, while the patient fixes at small light source. The increasing density-filters are placed till patient complains of diplopia. Strength of filter gives the strength of the scotoma.

Stereoacuity

Stereopsis is the appreciation of depth due to horizontal disparity between stimulated retinal points located in the Panum's area of fusion. Stereopsis that can be resolved by minimal horizontal separation is known as stereoacuity. The mean stereoacuity with normal binocularity is 20 seconds of arc with standard deviation of ±10 seconds arc. Most of the clinical tests that have been used to measure stereopsis have 40 seconds arc as cut-off between normal and abnormal stereopsis. Stereoacuity is maximal about 0.25° in center in the foveola, and diminishes exponentially with increasing eccentricity. Stereopsis is nil beyond 15° eccentricity.

Distance Stereopsis Tests

Distance stereotesting is proved to be highly sensitive to small refractive error changes, heterophorias and strabismus. Distance stereopsis evaluation aids in assessment of control of deviation and deterioration of fusion in cases of intermittent exotropia.

Distance Randot test: This test is designed to evaluate three levels of disparity (800, 200, and 60 arcsec) using vectographic random dot stimuli and are mounted on books to be viewed through polarizing glasses. The test consists of six books (two books for each level of disparity; each book containing two vectographs). For each disparity level, there are three vectographs that contain a stereotarget and one vectograph is blank. The stereotargets are simple geometric shapes. The subjects have to view the books at a distance of 3 m. Testing is started with the coarse disparity (800 seconds of arc) and proceeded to progressively smaller disparity. To enhance testing in small children, matching cards can be provided. If the subject identifies or matches two out of three of the stereotargets, the level is passed.

Frisby–Davis 2 Test

The Frisby-Davis 2 (FD2) test is based upon the near Frisby Stereotest but with various modifications for distance presentations. The FD2 test comprises a box containing four back illuminated and differently shaped plastic objects mounted on rods. These are either four animal or four geometric shapes set in a transparent frame pointing toward the observer. The shapes are translucent but sufficiently dark to obscure the rods, giving the appearance that the shapes are free floating. One shape is set by the examiner to be nearer to the observer at each presentation and the test requirement is to identify this target. The amount of disparity presented can be altered by the depth differences provided in the test which ranges from 1 to 13.4 cm, and by the distance of the observer from the targets. These two features provide the disparities ranging from 200-4 seconds of arc. The test has targets in form of animals which make it friendly for young children.

Near Stereopsis Tests

Frisby–Davis Test

The Frisby-Davis test is based on real depth test. The targets are printed on the two sides of transparent plexiglass plates of different thicknesses. There are three plates, 1 mm, 3 mm, and 6 mm thick, respectively. Each plate has printed on it four random-texture patterns and "hidden" in one of these is a circular-shape. The patient has to decide in which pattern the hidden shape lays a task that can be done successfully only if stereopsis is present. In this case it is the difference between the two levels, related to the distance from the observer, and the PD, which gives the measure of the stereo acuity. As there are four patterns on each plate, they can be presented in any one of four positions and with either side facing the patient, so that the small area may appear in front of or behind the level of the surrounding pattern. This reduces the possibility false-positive response from the patient. The test can be held at any of six distances, from 30 to 80 cm, the distance being controlled by the use of a tape attached to the test and held by the patient against the check. The six positions, combined with the three thicknesses of plates, provide 18 values of stereo acuity, ranging from 880 seconds of arc to 20 seconds. The test has various advantages over other tests of stereoscopic depth perception.
- No special glasses are required.
- There are no monocular clues as the test has target presented in actual depth although the motion parallax is a limiting factor.

- Large stereo acuity range.
- Suitable for a wide age range, even young preschoolers.
- Good visual acuity is not essential.

Lang Stereotest

The Lang Stereotest is also a real-depth test based on panographic principle where fine cylinder gratings are used on which random dots are imprinted. This was created to simplify stereopsis screening in children. There are three stereoscopic shapes, cat, star, and car which measure stereopsis of 1,200, 600, 550 seconds of arc, respectively. In the new Lang II test, the random dots are smaller and less dense. This disparity is finer, namely 200 seconds of arc for the moon and the star, 400 for the car, and 600 for the elephant. The test is administered at 40 cm exactly at right angle to remove monocular clues. The major advantage of the test is that it does not require any special glasses, but difficulty in recognition of form and monocular parallax clues are major disadvantages.

Titmus Stereotest

The test consists of vectographic stereograms which has contour pattern that use crossed polarized filters locates at axis 45° and 135° in front of either eye. The test consists of three parts. The fly test consists of a picture of a large housefly. It is used for small children. The child is asked to pick a wing of the fly. In presence of gross stereopsis, he will attempt to hold at a level above the plane of the book. It is a test for gross stereopsis about 3,000 seconds of arc.

The animal test is performed if gross stereopsis is present. It has three rows each having a picture of five animals. In each row one animal is imaged disparately and as a misleading clue one animal is also printed heavily. The disparate images account for thresholds of 10, 200, and 400 seconds of arc, respectively. A patient with stereopsis feels the particular disparate image to be standing out while the one with no stereopsis feels the heavily marked animal to be standing out.

The circle test consists of nine squares each having four circles. In each square one circle is disparately imaged. The patient is asked to point out the circle which stands out. The square in which he finds no circle standing out is the limit of his stereoacuity. It tests a range of stereoacuity from 800 to 40 seconds of arc. It is the most widely used test as it is easy to administer but sometimes false presence of stereopsis can be elicited as some patients may point out to the specific disparate images as they look different from the rest and not due to stereopsis.

Randot Stereotest

Randot stereotest is similar to Titmus fly test except that the stimulus for pattern used is a random dot stereogram rather than the contour stimulus. This theoretically removes the lateral displacement cue found in the Titmus fly test. The test has three parts. The right hand side has eight stereograms, all of 660 seconds of arc. The left side has circles and animal patterns interposed in random dot pattern. The various modifications of Randot test includes: Randot preschool test and Randot stereosmile test. The test is performed at 40 cm as with all other near stereopis test.

TNO test uses red-green anaglyph for viewing random dot stereograms. It consists of a booklet with seven plates. The plates contain red and green dots on gray background thus red lens filters green light and sees red dots and vice versa. Each plate has stereoscopic as well as monocular targets that serve as control. The first three plates determine gross stereopsis (1,980 seconds of arc) while the last four determine the stereoacuity.

10.4 Evaluation of Accommodative Convergence to Accommodation Ratio

Pradeep Sharma
Centre for Sight, New Delhi
drpsharma57@yahoo.com

■ INTRODUCTION
Before we consider accommodative convergence to accommodation (AC/A) ratio we need to be familiar with the different types of convergence.

■ DIFFERENT TYPES OF CONVERGENCE
1. Voluntary convergence
2. Reflex convergence
   a. *Tonic convergence:* It is brought about by the tonus of the extraocular muscles and remains stable throughout life. However, in a nonaccommodative convergence excess esotropia, it is postulated that tonic convergence is increased.
   b. *Accommodative convergence:* It is the convergence brought about by an act of accommodation.
   c. *Fusional convergence:* When accommodative convergence does not meet the full requirement of convergence, fusional convergences are brought into play. The stimulus for it is the disparate retinal imagery.
   d. *Proximal convergence:* It is induced by the awareness of nearness of an object and does play a significant role in the near convergence response. AC/A ratio is defined as the change in convergence induced by a unit stimulus to accommodation.

■ METHODS OF DETERMINATION OF ACCOMMODATIVE CONVERGENCE TO ACCOMMODATION RATIO

Heterophoria Method
In this method, through the alternate prism bar cover test with the patient wearing his/her full refractive correction, deviations are measured both for distance (6 m) and near (33 cm) and the AC/A ratio calculated as follows:

$$AC/A = IPD + \frac{\Delta n - \Delta d}{D}$$

Where
IPD is interpupillary distance (cm).
Δn is the deviation at near (33 cm).
Δd is the deviation at distance (6 m).
D is the fixation distance at near in diopters.
Sign convention: Esodeviations are considered positive (+) Exodeviations are considered negative (–)
Normal range: 4–7Δ/1 diopter
Example: IPD = 5.5 cm, Δn = 30 PD base out, Δd = 25 PD base out
$\quad$ AC/A = 5.5 + [(+30) – (+25)]/3
$\quad\quad\quad$ = 5.5 + (30–25)/3
$\quad\quad\quad$ = 5.5 + 1.6
$\quad\quad\quad$ = 7.1Δ/D

Gradient Method
In this method, through the alternate prism bar cover test with the patient wearing his full refractive correction, deviation is measured multiple times at one particular distance

after the interposition of additional lenses (minus lenses when measuring for distance and plus lenses when measuring for near) and the AC/A ratio is calculated as follows:

$$AC/A = \frac{\Delta 1 - \Delta 0}{D}$$

Where $\Delta 0$ is the deviation with the patient wearing only his refractive correction if any $\Delta 1$ is the deviation with the patient wearing additional lenses over and above his refractive correction.

D is the power of the additional lens in diopters.
Normal range: $3\text{-}5^{\Delta}/1$ D
Example: $\Delta 0 = 15$ PD base in, $\Delta 1 = 7$ PD base in, $D = -2.00$ Dsph
$$AC/A = (-7) - (-15)/2$$
$$= (-7 + 15)/2$$
$$= +8/2 = 4\Delta/D$$

Other Methods

Other methods are the fixation disparity method and the haploscopic method.

■ EXAMPLE

A 3-year-old patient presents with alternating inward squinting of eyes for past 6 months. His vision is 6/12 OU. On cycloplegic refraction his retinoscopy is +6.00 Dsph OU at 50 cm and was prescribed +4.00 D OU. His distance deviation with and without glasses is 30 PD and 70 PD, respectively. His near deviation with glasses is 45 PD. His IPD is 5 cm.

With the help of heterophoria method his AC/A ratio is

$$AC/A = \frac{5.00 + (45-30)}{3} = 10$$

Hence, this patient is a case of refractive accommodative esotropia with high AC/A ratio. The practical utility of knowing the AC/A ratio is when it is found to be high as in esotropias the patient needs to be prescribed appropriate bifocals.

There is another situation of intermittent exotropia with high AC/A ratio, which can manifest as esodeviation for near after squint surgery and for which again a bifocal will need to be prescribed.

This can be evaluated preoperatively by doing 3D test to distinguish the simulated divergence excess (SDE) exotropia, but this 3D test should be done after the patch test. If this is not done some cases of SDE exotropia with high AC/A ratio will be falsely labeled as true divergence excess exotropia.

Care should be taken while measuring deviations in primary position in patients with A/V pattern; if incidentally down gaze deviations are measured artifactual error will come in the calculation of AC/A ratio.

10.5 Diagnosis and Management of Esotropic Deviations

HM Ravindranath
Drishti Speciality Eye Clinic, Davangere
echenmar2110@yahoo.com

■ TYPES OF ESOTROPIAS

- Comitant esodeviations
- Incomitant esodeviations

Comitant Esodeviations

Accommodative
- Refractive accommodative (Normal AC/A)
- Nonrefractive accommodative (High AC/A)
- Partially accommodative

Nonaccommodative
- Infantile esotropia
- Acquired esotropia

Incomitant Esodeviations
- Paralytic squints
- Restrictive squints

EVALUATION OF A CASE OF ESOTROPIA

Evaluation of a case of esotropia should include proper history, complete ophthalmic examination, and investigations whenever necessary.

History
- Family history of strabismus
- Age of onset
- *Medical history:* Birth weight, developmental, neurological
- *Which eye:* Same eye or alternates
- *Mode of onset:* Sudden or gradual
- Constant or intermittent
- Diplopia
- *Medical illness:* Viral fever
- *Prior treatment:* Glasses, occlusion, surgery.

Inspection of the Patient
- Observe for the head posture, usually present in A and V pattern esotropia, restrictive and paralytic squints and nystagmus blockade syndrome
- Facial asymmetry
- Constancy of deviation
- Nystagmus

Cover Test and Cover-Uncover Test
- Diagnosis of pseudosquint can be made.
- Primary and secondary deviations can be observed.
- Fixation preference is documented.

Vision Assessment
- Assessment of vision in children is crucial to diagnose and treat amblyopia early.
- Objective methods for patients too young, tumbling E or letter chart are used for little older children.

Refraction
- Hypermetropia can coexist or induce esotropia (accommodative esotropia). It is important to do cycloplegic refraction in all children with esotropia especially to unmask hypermetropia
- Cyclopent 1% is most commonly used cycloplegic agent. It can be combined with tropicacyl 1% to obtain good mydriatic effect. In our country atropine is still used

in many centers. Bizarre behavior is observed in some children after cyclopent instillations, it is dose dependent and self-limiting. Digital occlusion over punctal area can be done soon after administration of cyclopent.

Evaluation of Ocular Motility
- To look for oblique muscle overaction, usually seen in infantile esotropia.
- Limitation or restriction of movement as in cases of Duane's retraction syndrome and lateral rectus palsy.
- Dissociated vertical deviation (DVD) can coexist with infantile esotropia.
- Bilateral abduction limitation and crossed fixation in infantile esotropia.
- Nystagmus.

Measurement of the Amount of Deviation
- Amount of deviation is measured by prism bar cover test. If the patient is uncooperative or having very poor vision or having gross limitation of movement, corneal light reflex assessment gives the approximate assessment of amount of deviation.
- The amount of deviation is measured both for near and distance fixation. In nonaccommodative squints like infantile esotropia and acquired basic esotropia the deviation is almost same for near and distance fixation. In accommodative and convergence excess type esotropia, the deviation is more for near than distance fixation suggesting high AC/A ratio.
- Measure the amount of deviation in upgaze, primary and downgaze to diagnose A and V pattern, in lateral rectus palsy the amount of deviation is more when patient looks toward affected eye.
- Measure the angle of deviation with glasses and without glasses.
  - If the squint is controlled fully it is refractive accommodative esotropia.
  - If the squint is partially controlled it is partially accommodative esotropia.
  - If the squint is more for near but unchanged with glasses it is nonaccommodative convergence excess.
  - If the squint is controlled by glasses after addition of plus three diopters lenses it is nonrefractive accommodative esotropia.

Assessment of Binocular Status
Binocular status for distance and near is assessed by worth four dot test and Bagolini's striated glasses and stereopsis is assessed by Titmus fly test. Complete ocular examination including anterior segment, lenticular status, media and fundus evaluation by direct and indirect ophthalmoscope is done. Corneal opacity or congenital cataract can cause sensory esotropia in children usually associated with nystagmus. Disc and macular pathology also cause sensory esotropia in early childhood. Retinoblastoma though rare, needs to be ruled out in all children with strabismus.

Investigation
In cases of acute esotropia of both comitant and incomitant form (6th nerve palsy) neuroimaging often gives clue toward etiology.

TREATMENT
Glasses
Refractive errors are promptly corrected in esotropia especially hypermetropia. Hypermetropia is fully corrected in cases of refractive accommodative esotropia.

When high AC/A ratio is noted, addition of +3 lenses can be tried and if squint is controlled fully bifocals can be prescribed.

It is better to avoid small fancy frames for children; as children try to peep over the frames. Large oval or round size optics is preferred. Proper optical centration should be checked while testing the glasses. Head band prevents the decentration of the frame. While prescribing bifocals, high executive bifocals are prescribed with near segment at the lower pupillary border.

Cycloplegic refractions are repeated annually for any change in hypermetropia.

Treatment of Amblyopia

Occlusion therapy is the most effective treatment for amblyopia. It is better to advice complete full time occlusion as it removes the possible abnormal binocular interaction which is one of the mechanisms of development of amblyopia. Other eye is occluded periodically to prevent occlusion amblyopia. It is better to treat amblyopia before the patient is taken up for surgery. Periodic follow-up is necessary to monitor the response.

Surgical Treatment

Timing of Surgery

In infantile esotropia there is a growing trend toward early intervention. Some surgeons suggest surgery <1-year of age. Surgery can be done at very young age if the ocular motility, oblique overactions, and amount of deviation are noted and documented properly.

Procedure

Bimedial recession is most effective surgery in young children. Inferior oblique myectomy or recessions are combined whenever necessary. Recession and resection procedure is usually reserved for older children or adults. Late-onset DVD or oblique overactions are common after squint surgery. Parents should be well-informed about the possible second or even third surgery.

10.6 | Infantile Esotropia

Sumita Agarkar, Gayathri J Panicker, Roshni Desai
Sankara Nethralaya, Chennai
drsar@snmail.org

■ DEFINITION

Infantile esotropia is defined as a large constant inward deviation of the eyes presenting within first 6 months of life in a neurologically normal child. It is rarely present at birth. In addition to misalignment, it is often associated with abnormal motion processing and binocularity.

■ EPIDEMIOLOGY

It is believed that it affects 1% of normal full-term neonates but prevalence increases in children with prematurity, low birth weight, and those with stormy perinatal period.

■ GENETICS

Genetic basis is multifactorial as no specific gene has been identified.

However monofixation syndrome is seen much more frequently in first degree relatives of children with infantile esotropia and could be a partial expression of a genotype that codes for infantile esotropia.

■ CLINICAL FEATURES

Diagnosis is mostly clinical though it must be differentiated from other esotropia seen in infancy. Patients usually present by 2–4 months of age. Examining photographs of the child in the first few months of life can assist in documenting the onset, detecting the stability of the condition, and confirming the diagnosis.

Esotropia
Esotropia may be intermittent initially, cyclic and then becomes constant later. Once stabilized, the angle of deviation is usually constant and larger than 30 PD. Cross fixation is often noted. Cross fixation is also partly responsible for apparent abduction limitation.

Abduction Limitation
Limitation is usually seen due to the tight medial rectus and cross fixation. In infants, normal abduction can be demonstrated by rapidly spinning the head of the baby (Doll's maneuver) or by monocular occlusion.

Latent Nystagmus
The incidence is reported to be 50–100%. Nystagmus is predominantly horizontal jerk nystagmus elicited by occluding either eye. The slow phase is toward the side of the occluded eye.

Dissociated Vertical Deviation
Dissociated vertical deviation (DVD) occurs in approximately 75% of patients and is usually bilateral but asymmetrical. Rarely detected in infants despite careful examination and usually appears after the first birthday.

Inferior Oblique Overaction and V-Pattern
Inferior oblique overaction and V-pattern is a common association. Prevalence has been reported to be as high as 70% in patients.

Pursuit Asymmetry on Optokinetic Nystagmus
The pursuit from temporal-to-nasal is normal, while the nasal-to-temporal pursuit movement is cogwheel. Persistence of this asymmetry beyond 6 months age is often noted in association with infantile esotropia.

Refractive Error
Majority of children have low-to-moderate age-appropriate hyperopia. A small percentage of children can have high hyperopia or high myopia.

Amblyopia
Amblyopia occurs in approximately 40–50% of children with infantile esotropia. Constant deviation of one eye or a strong fixation preference usually indicates amblyopia. Fixation preference can be checked in office by vertical prism test (10-prism diopter base down test).

Differential Diagnosis
- Prominent epicanthal folds and wide-nasal bridge can give an appearance of esotropia. Cover test is usually diagnostic.
- *Accommodative esotropia:* Rarely children can present with accommodative esotropia earlier than 1 year of age. These children have high hyperopia and glasses may correct the esotropia.
- *Congenital sixth nerve palsy:* It is very rare and is accompanied by large esotropia and abduction limitation.

SECTION 10: Pediatric Ophthalmology and Strabismus

- *Nystagmus blockage syndrome:* This syndrome is associated with variable angle esotropia and nystagmus. During inattentive phase children may be orthophoric with nystagmus.
- *Type I Duane's syndrome:* Duane syndrome can present with esotropia and abduction limitation. It is associated with characteristic features such as palpebral fissure changes and upshoot or downshoot.
- *Ciancia syndrome:* This syndrome occurring in infants has large angle esotropia associated with face turn and abduction deficit and nystagmus. Medial recti are often tight on forced duction.
- Sensory esotropia is common in infants with poor vision due to variety of causes. Hence it is imperative that all children with esotropia should have a comprehensive ophthalmic evaluation including fundus examination.
- Congenital fibrosis of extraocular muscles.
- Mobius syndrome.
- Infantile myasthenia gravis.
- Associated with neurologic diseases, e.g., cerebral palsy, periventricular encephalomalacia.

MANAGEMENT

Refractive Correction
Trial of glasses should be considered if hyperopia is >3 diopters.

Amblyopia Management
Amblyopia should be suspected in cases where there is strong fixation preference for one eye. These children should receive occlusion therapy or atropine penalization as deemed appropriate.

Alternate Patching
Some investigators have proposed a period of alternate patching prior to surgery but subsequent work by Ing et al. showed that it did not influence postoperative alignment.

Botulinum Toxin
Botulinum toxin injection in medial rectus muscle has been tried in infantile esotropia. Injection may or may not be electromyography (EMG)-guided and up to 2.5–5 units can be injected. Multiple injections may be required with decremental response to subsequent injections. Advantages include relative safety, simple procedure with less anesthetic exposure and help to reduce the angle of deviation and therefore necessitating lesser surgical dosage.

Extraocular Muscle Surgery
Surgical correction is still the gold standard and should be done as early as possible ideally before 2 years of age to achieve better functional outcomes in terms of binocularity. There is evidence to suggest that functional outcomes were related to the duration of misalignment. Presence of stereopsis can prevent DVD. Recent evidence is in favor of very early surgery, i.e., within 6 months of onset of infantile esotropia as the benefits of restoring binocularity and reduced incidence of DVD and inferior oblique overaction outweighs the challenge of estimation of angle of deviation. (*Source:* Bhate M, Flaherty M, Martin FJ. Timing of surgery in essential infantile esotropia: What more do we know since the turn of the century? Indian J Ophthalmol. 2022;70(2):386-95.)

Bilateral medial rectus recession is the procedure of choice for most surgeons. Unilateral recession-resection procedure has also been described. During surgery, it is recommended to use limbus as landmark as medial rectus insertion can be anterior.

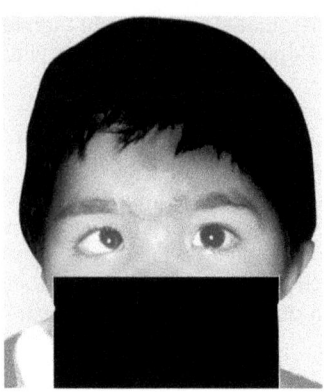
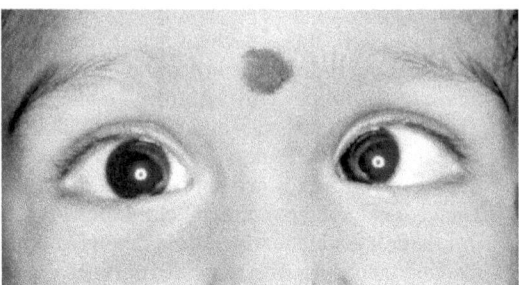

Fig. 10.6.1: Infantile esotropia with inferior oblique overaction.

Fig. 10.6.2: Infantile esotropia without inferior oblique overaction.

For deviation larger than 50 prism diopter three muscles surgery may be required. Surgical plan should include inferior oblique weakening if there is inferior oblique over action or V-pattern. If not addressed initially it may lead to consecutive exotropia. DVD may not be present at the initial surgery as it often develops after the first year of life and the parents should be counseled for possible later surgeries.

The surgical goal is to achieve a deviation within 10 PD of orthotropia. This usually results in some binocularity with gross stereopsis.

Surgical success with bilateral medial rectus recessions in infantile esotropia is limited by the high variability in surgical dose-response.

Undercorrection and overcorrection are the most commonly noted complications. Many of these are transient. The number of children requiring a second operation varies between 15 and 30%.

■ FOLLOW-UP

Patients should be followed closely for amblyopia, even if they achieve good motor alignment. Close follow-up is required especially in cross fixating children as amblyopia in one eye usually develops after surgical alignment. Occlusion therapy or penalization may need to be continued for a while even after surgical alignment.

Amblyopia, residual esotropia or consecutive persistent exotropia may occur. These unfavorable outcomes should be addressed early to get the best possible visual and fusion potential.

10.7 | Exodeviations

Saurabh Mittal
Thind Eye Hospital, Jalandhar
dr_saurabhmittal@hotmail.com

■ INTRODUCTION

Exotropia, also known as divergent squint, is characterized by outward deviation of visual axis.

It was of three main types:
1. *Primary:* Intermittent or constant
2. *Secondary:* Due to visual loss
3. *Consecutive:* Seen after overcorrection of esotropia

■ INTERMITTENT EXOTROPIA

The deviation usually begins as an exophoria; patient is able to fuse his eyes straight when open, but they drift outward on dissociation. Patient can maintain bifoveal fixation during this phase.

This usually starts around 2–3 years of age, more commonly in female, seen first for distance, noted more when the child is inattentive, after sleep, day dreaming, during illness or if he loses focus. Most frequent initial complaint is closure of one eye in bright daylight.

During the natural course of disease patient develops bitemporal suppression, reduced-tonic convergence, increased-divergence of bony orbit, reduced-accommodative power, intermittent periods of diplopia, and finally constant exotropia.

The course of intermittent deviation is variable; some can maintain the frequency and size of deviation, and keep them unnoticed for many years. A few can deteriorate quickly resulting in constant or decompensated exotropia. Measurement of stereoacuity for distance is a good measure for assessing worsening of deviation.

Burian's classified exodeviation into four groups:
1. *Basic pattern:* Distance and near deviation measurements are equal (D=N).
2. *Convergence insufficiency type:* Near deviation exceeds distance deviation by more than 10 PD (N>>D).
3. *Divergence excess type:* Distance deviation exceeds near deviation by 10 PD or more (D>>N).
4. *Simulated divergence excess:* Distance deviation initially exceeds near deviation but after prolonged occlusion of one eye the near and distance deviations are equalized.

Management

Assessment of Deviation

- Extraocular movements should be assessed to look for any associated pattern deviation or DVD.
- Measurement of deviation should be done for both distance and near.
- Near point of convergence should be recorded.
- Monocular occlusion for 45 minutes should be done and deviation is measured with +3.0D lenses.

Treatment

- Correct any refractive error (even small degrees of myopia/astigmatism).
- Deterioration of distance stereopsis is indication for surgery.
- Patients can assess worsening of condition if they note increase in frequency, size of angle or if the deviation becomes noticeable among family or friends.

Surgery

- Recess-resect procedure of lateral and medial recti of one or both eyes is indicated in the basic type.
- Bilateral lateral rectus recession is preferred for true divergence excess.
- Associated vertical deviations should be addressed at the time of surgery.

■ CONSTANT EXOTROPIA

Primary Infantile or Early-Onset Exotropia

It may be present before 1 year of age. Angle of deviation is usually large and stable. It can be either constant unilateral or alternating bilateral exotropia types **(Figs. 10.7.1 and 10.7.2)**. In constant unilateral exotropia patient may have amblyopia, binocular single vision is absent. Patient may have associated DVD.

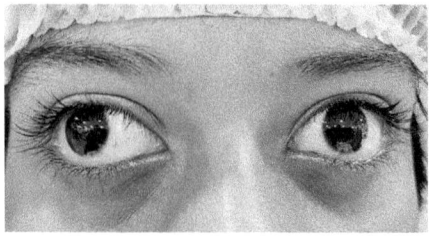
Fig. 10.7.1: Unilateral exotropia.

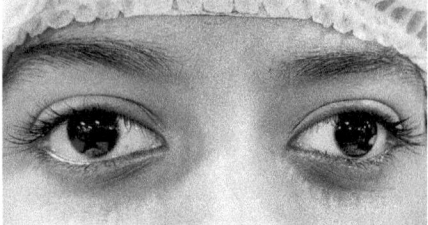
Fig. 10.7.2: Bilateral exotropia.

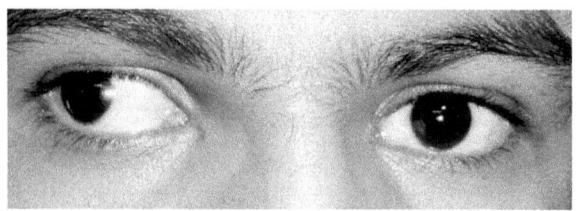
Fig. 10.7.3: Decompensated exotropia.

Secondary Infantile or Early-Onset Exotropia
These are usually associated with cerebral palsy, craniofacial disorders, ocular conditions such as high myopia, retinoblastoma, congenital cataract, etc. Patients usually have poor vision in affected eye.

Decompensated Exotropia
This is most commonly seen in teenagers and adults **(Fig. 10.7.3)**. This usually presents as a sequel to primary intermittent exotropia. Patient presents for the cosmetically unacceptable deviation. Complaints of asthenopia or diplopia are usually absent.

Management
- Treatment of constant exotropia is primarily surgical.
- Prior to surgery correction of any refractive error, amblyopia, or ocular comorbidity is must.
- Surgery is aimed at slight overcorrection (at least 10 prism diopter) in case of severe visual loss.
- Surgical procedure choices:
  - *Recession or resection:* Preferred choice in unilateral constant exotropia.
  - *Bilateral lateral rectus-recession:* For alternating exotropia some surgeons prefer this over recession or resection procedure.
  - Associated DVD and oblique overactions should also be managed.
- Postoperative convergence exercise may be instituted to prevent recurrence of exotropia.

■ CONSECUTIVE EXOTROPIA
This can be seen as a result of unfortunate surgical overcorrection of esotropia or mismanaged hypermetropia.

Management
- Hypermetropic correction should be reduced with age depending upon the requirement of patient to maintain 6/6 vision. This should be done as with advancing age,

hypermetropia along with decreasing accommodation amplitude, convergence insufficiency, and active divergence will induce exodeviation.
- Convergence exercise should be started early.
- Resurgery may be needed for surgical-related consecutive exotropia.
  - Evaluate for the previous surgical procedure (surgical records, old photos, surgery marks, knowing surgeons choice will help).
  - Magnetic resonance imaging (MRI) can be performed to look for slipped-medial rectus.
  - Prefer medial rectus advancement with or without resection.
  - If deviation is large lateral rectus-recession can be planned.
  - Conjunctival resection can be performed if there is excess of conjunctiva over the medial rectus.
- Surgical target is aimed at orthophoria or slight esotropia.

10.8 | A-V Pattern Deviations

KS Santhan Gopal, V Jyothi
Kamala Nethralaya, Bengaluru
santhangopal@gmail.com

INTRODUCTION

A and V patterns are horizontal deviations that change in magnitude with upgaze and downgaze. Recognition of these patterns is of importance in effectively managing ocular deviations.

An A-pattern is present when there is increasing convergence in upgaze and increasing divergence in downgaze. Converse is true for V-pattern. One in five of all strabismus has an associated A or V pattern.

Various etiological factors play a role in causing A and V patterns. These factors are extraocular muscle dysfunction (horizontal, vertical, and oblique muscles have been implicated facial characteristics and abnormal muscle insertions). The extraocular muscles dysfunction can be innervational, anatomical or both. Current school of thought is that oblique muscle dysfunction plays a major role in the etiology of A and V pattern. A pattern is generally associated with overaction of superior oblique and/or underaction of inferior oblique. V-pattern is found to be generally associated with overaction of inferior oblique or weakness of superior oblique.

Diagnosis of A and V pattern is made by measuring the deviation by prism and cover tests in position of 25° elevation and 35° depression. The patient fixates on an accommodative target wearing full-refractive correction. A pattern is considered clinically significant if it measures 10 prisms or more difference in up gaze and down gaze. V pattern is considered clinically significant if it measures 15 prism diopters or more in gaze up and gaze down. Anomalous head position and facial asymmetry may be associated. Oblique muscles overactions and underactions are carefully observed during versions.

Only clinically significant A-V patterns need to be treated surgically. Primary and reading positions are functionally most important. The goal of treatment is to restore blood stage vaccines (BSV) if possible and to correct head posture if any. If there is no oblique overaction unilateral or bilateral surgical procedure for horizontal strabismus is performed. The vertical incomitance is corrected by vertical transposition of the horizontal recti by one or half tendon width. The medial rectus is always shifted to apex of the pattern, i.e. where convergence is greater. The lateral rectus is always transposed to the end of the pattern, i.e. where divergence is greater. If there is oblique dysfunction with V-pattern inferior oblique weakening or tucking of superior oblique is performed. Similarly in A-pattern with superior oblique overaction bilateral superior oblique tenotomies are employed. Slanting recession of horizontal recti has also been tried.

SAMPLE TREATMENT PLANS

V-Esotropia

Without Inferior Oblique Overaction

Bilateral medial recti recession with downward transposition of medial recti; in recess or resect procedure medial rectus is transposed downward and lateral rectus is transposed upward.

With Inferior Oblique Overaction

Inferior oblique weakening procedure is combined with horizontal muscle surgery.

A-Exotropia

With Superior Oblique Overaction

Bilateral tenectomy of superior oblique combined with horizontal muscle surgery is performed to correct residual deviation.

V-Exotropia With Inferior Oblique Overaction

Bilateral inferior oblique recession and lateral rectus-recession and medial rectus resection in one or both the eyes.

V-Exotropia Without Inferior Oblique Overaction

Lateral rectus recession and upshift and medial rectus resection with down shift.

10.9 Paralytic Strabismus

Meenakshi Swaminathan
Visiting Professor, Sri Ramachandra Institute of Higher Education and Research, Chennai
meenakshiswaminathan@gmail.com

Srikanth Ramasubramanian
Leela Eye Clinic, Chennai
dr_sri1981@yahoo.com

Arun Samprathi
Samprathi Eye Hospital and Squint Centre, Bengaluru
arunsamprathi@yahoo.com

INTRODUCTION

Paralytic squint is strabismus occurring secondary to damage to the cranial nerves (3rd, 4th, and 6th) supplying the extraocular muscles. It may be congenital or acquired. Diplopia is usual in the acquired forms and is maximal in the direction of gaze of the paralytic muscle. It results in incomitant squint. It may be caused by isolated nerve palsy or multiple nerve involvement.

SEQUELAE OF MUSCLE PALSY

- *Motor Sequelae*
    - Agonist underaction (paralyzed), e.g., right lateral rectus (LR) paresis
    - Ipsilateral antagonist overacts (Sherrington law), e.g., right medial rectus (MR)
    - Contralateral synergist overacts (Hering's law), e.g., left MR
    - Underaction of the contralateral antagonist—inhibitional palsy, e.g., left LR.
- *Sensory Sequelae*
    - Onset in an adult (visually mature patient)
        - Diplopia will be the presenting symptom

- Onset in a child
  - Results in diplopia followed later by suppression and amblyopia.

HISTORY (SYMPTOMS)
- Double vision—onset, duration, direction of greatest separation
- Abnormal head posture
- Associated pain and vomiting
- History of injury
- Alteration in eyelid position
- Blurred vision
- Strabismus

SYSTEMIC HISTORY
- Diabetes
- Hypertension
- Thyroid disorder
- Associated neurological symptoms if any, like weakness of limbs, altered consciousness, etc.

CLINICAL EXAMINATION
- Record visual acuity
- Refraction
- Note the head posture (face turn or head tilts)
- Look for ptosis
- Cover tests in all the nine cardinal positions of gaze
- Ocular motility examination including ductions and versions
- Clinical saccadic testing differentiates paretic from restrictive strabismus—ask the patient to change fixation between two targets 20–300 apart—eye with weak muscle will show floating saccade
- Pupillary examination
- Fundus evaluation to rule out disc edema.

SPECIAL TESTS
- Diplopia chart
- Park's three step test if cyclovertical muscles are involved.
- Forced duction test to differentiate restrictive from paralytic strabismus
- Forced generation test to determine the residual power of the muscle
- Hess chart
- Evaluation of torsion (subjective by Double Maddox Rod, objective by fundus examination).

SYSTEMIC EXAMINATION
- Full neurological examination to localize the site of lesion
- In patients with suspected 4th nerve palsy, perusal of old photographs, family album
- Ear, nose, throat (ENT) examination.

INVESTIGATIONS
- Fasting and postprandial blood sugars
- Blood pressure
- Computed tomography/magnetic resonance imaging (CT/MRI) scan if indicated (neuroimaging in young patients, posthead trauma, no clear vasculopathic history, pupil involvement, uncertain congenital onset)
- Thyroid profile if indicated.

MANAGEMENT
- In a visually immature child, occlusion of one of the eyes to prevent suppression and loss of binocular vision and also prevent amblyopia.
- Active duction and version exercises.
- Patching of affected eye in adults to relieve diplopia.
- Prisms may be useful to relieve diplopia.
- Botulinum toxin injection into the antagonist muscle in selected cases.

GUIDELINES FOR SURGICAL INTERVENTION
- Delayed for at least 6 months to allow for spontaneous recovery.
- Choice of procedure depends on the muscle involved.
- Weakening the antagonist or the yoke muscle of the paretic muscle gives the best improvement.
- This may be combined with a resection of the affected muscle if the paralysis is partial.
- Strengthening of totally paralyzed muscle is usually ineffective.
- Muscle transposition may be considered. Superior rectus transposition with or without medial rectus recession has gained acceptance in the management of lateral rectus palsy. Transposing the split lateral rectus to the medial rectus has shown favorable results in complete third nerve palsy.
- Fixation of the globe to the nasal periosteum with non-absorbable sutures is another alternative in complete third nerve palsy.
- In patients with aberrant regeneration, (widening of palpebral fissure on attempted adduction) surgery may be considered in the unaffected eye.
- Faden sutures or adjustable-Faden sutures are an option in the management as it corrects the incomitance without affecting the primary gaze measurement.
- Adjustable suture surgery may be needed where results are less predictable due to contractures in long-standing cases or if the patient is diplopic.
- Patients with ptosis associated with complete third nerve palsy may need a conservative ptosis surgery due to poor Bell's phenomenon.

CONCLUSION
Acquired paralytic strabismus should be carefully evaluated to rule out associated neurological disorders which could sometimes be life threatening.

10.10 | Dissociated Vertical Deviations

Ramesh Kekunnaya
LV Prasad Eye Institute, Hyderabad
drrk123@gmail.com

INTRODUCTION
Dissociated vertical deviation (DVD) is characterized by elevation, abduction and excyclotorsion of the nonfixing eye without corresponding hypotropia in the other eye. It is a dissociated strabismus complex consisting of DVD, dissociated horizontal deviation (DHD) or dissociated torsional deviation (DTD).

SYNONYMS
Alternating hypertropia, alternating sursumduction, and dissociated vertical divergence.

CLINICAL CHARACTERISTICS
- On cover test, there is upward and outward movement of the occluded eye (Fig. 10.10.1)

- Amount of deviation when eye is covered is variable, tending to increase on prolonged occlusion, often differing between the two eyes.
- It violates the Hering's law.
- Usually asymptomatic because of poor fusion and suppression.
- Latent nystagmus present in 50% of cases.
- Mostly associated with esotropia (46-92%) or exotropia.
- Mostly bilateral but asymmetrical due to overaction of either the inferior oblique or the superior oblique.
- A or V pattern may be present.
- Sometimes excycloduction of each eye under cover may be the only manifestation, when it is termed as dissociated torsional deviation.
- Unilateral DVD usually seen with profound amblyopia in the involved eye.
- Bielschowsky phenomenon present. When the fixing eye is presented with light of decreasing density, the eye with DVD falls. It is present in at least 50% of patients with DVD, a strong evidence suggesting that it is a sensory anomaly.

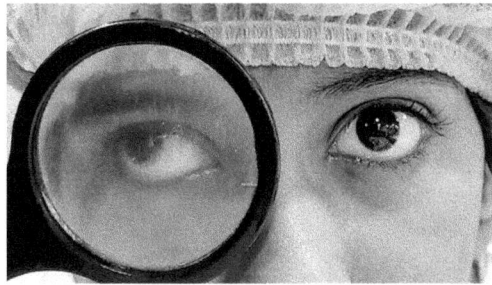

Fig. 10.10.1: Cover test.

ETIOLOGY

The etiology of DVD is still obscure. Several mechanisms have been postulated.
- Bielschowsky explained this on the basis of a vertical vergence signal that elevates the occluded eye and depresses the fixing eye by cancelling the simultaneous supraversion impulse and increasing the innervational flow to the elevators of the occluded eye further (as according to Hering's law).
- Another hypothesis explains this on the basis of an abnormal excitation of vertical divergence centers, the cause of which still remains unknown.
- Spielman assumed it to be caused by an imbalance of binocular stimulation. This may explain its frequent occurrence with infantile esotropia and sensory heterotopias.

MEASUREMENT

An accurate quantitative assessment can be obtained provided each eye has sufficient visual acuity to fix at a target. The patient is asked to fix at a target at 6 m distance, the occluder is quickly shifted to the fixing eye, so that the dissociated-eye takes up fixation and the amount of excursion noted. An increasing amount of base down prisms is held under the occluder, until the downward fixation movement is neutralized on alternate cover test (simultaneous prism cover test). The same steps are repeated with the fellow eye fixing. It is graded as +1 to +4, depending upon the amount of excursion varying from 5 prism diopters to 25 prism diopters **(Table 10.10.1)**.

MANAGEMENT

Usually asymptomatic, therefore, may be left alone.

Indications for Surgery

Cosmetic disfigurement in primary position manifests hyperdeviation DVD-associated with horizontal deviation.
   DVD with coexisting inferior oblique overaction.

TABLE 10.10.1: Differential diagnosis.

	Dissociated vertical deviation	Inferior oblique over action
Elevation	In abduction and adduction	Maximal in adduction, never in abduction
Superior oblique action	May overact	Usually under action
V-pattern	Absent	Often present
Pseudoparesis of contralateral superior rectus	Absent	Present
Incycloduction on refixation	Present	Absent
Saccadic velocity of refixation movement	10–200°/sec	200–400°/sec
Latent nystagmus	Often present	Absent
Bielschowsky phenomenon	Often present	Absent

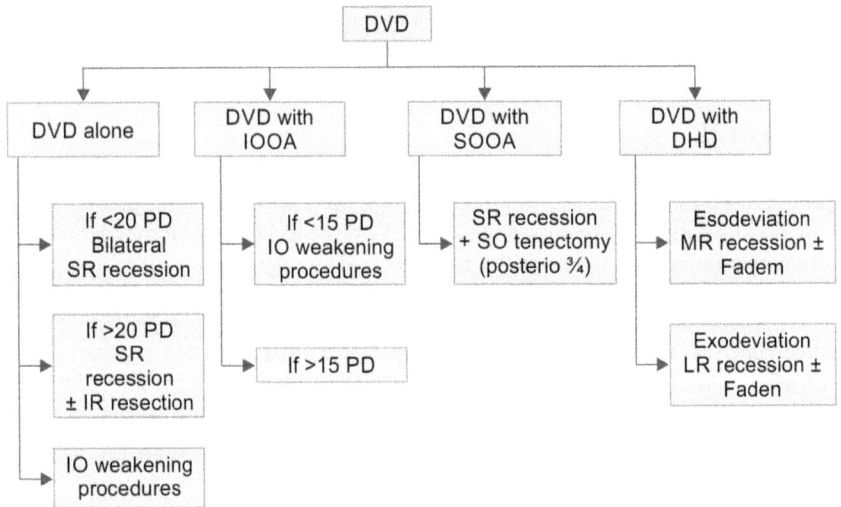

Flowchart 10.10.1: Treatment options for dissociated vertical deviations.

(DHD: dissociated horizontal disorder; DVD: dissociated vertical deviations; IOOA: inferior oblique overaction; LR: lateral rectus; MR: medial rectus; SOOA: superior oblique overaction; SR: superior Jrectus)

Goal of Surgery
Minimize dissociation and improve control, favoring depression.

■ TREATMENT
Various treatment options are available as summarized in the **Flowchart 10.10.1**.

Although in most of the patients with a conspicuous DVD, surgery is the recommended treatment, the possible effectiveness of conservative approach should not be ignored.

10.11 | Restrictive Strabismus

Kalpana Narendran
Aravind Eye Hospital, Coimbatore
kalpana@cbe.aravind.org

■ INTRODUCTION

Restrictive strabismus is a form of incomitant strabismus characterized by limitation of movement. Restriction may be muscular contracture, persistent abnormal position of globe in the orbit, postsurgical scar or adhesion due to multiple operations. Common characteristics include marked limitation of movement, incomitant strabismus, and a positive forced duction test (FDT). Few of them are of particular importance.

■ DUANE'S SYNDROME

Commonly seen, the incidence of this is 1-4%. Condition is generally unilateral with female preponderance and left eye involvement. Few characteristic features are limitation of abduction, globe retraction and narrowing of palpebral fissure on adduction, widening of palpebral fissure on adduction and upshoot or downshoot on adduction. Fibrotic lateral rectus and cocontraction of medial and lateral recti have been implicated in the pathogenesis. Esotropia is the commonest presentation. Patient may adopt a face turn. Other ocular findings include nystagmus, dermoid, anisocoria, ptosis, congenital cataract, heterochromia, and optic nerve hypoplasia. DRS may be part of many systemic anomalies such as Wildervanck syndrome, Okihiro syndrome, Goldenhar syndrome, and Holt–Oram syndrome. Differential diagnosis includes 6th nerve palsy, Moebius syndrome, infantile esotropia, and congenital oculomotor apraxia. The indications for surgical intervention include abnormal head-posture, deviation in primary gaze, marked globe retraction, and upshoots and downshoots.

Various surgical techniques include recession of the medial and lateral recti, Y-splitting of the lateral rectus to improve upshots. Vertical recti transposition to lateral rectus can be done to improve abduction.

■ BROWN SYNDROME (SUPERIOR OBLIQUE SHEATH SYNDROME)

Characteristic feature is limitation of elevation in adduction and V-pattern. It is caused by tight superior oblique tendon which prevents the eye from moving-up in adducted position. The child may be orthophoric in primary position. Elevation is normal in primary position and abduction but absent in adduction. FDT is positive. Acquired forms have been seen following trauma, blowout fractures, and superior oblique (SO) tucking. In some congenital cases spontaneous recovery has been noted around 10-12 years. Treatment options include SO tenectomy or SO lengthening by silicon expanders but the results are not satisfactory.

■ CONGENITAL FIBROSIS OF EXTRAOCULAR MUSCLES

Autosomal dominant condition characterized by fibrosis of muscles of the eye and the orbit. Clinical features include ptosis with chin-up posture, absence of elevation with downward fixation, and perverted convergence on attempted upgaze. Family history is usually positive.

Treatment options include inferior rectus (IR) recession with frontalis sling for ptosis correction.

■ DYSTHYROID OPHTHALMOPATHY

Restrictive limitation of ocular movements is seen in dysthyroid eye disease. Other features include proptosis, chemosis, dilated-conjunctival vessels, and vertical strabismus.

Limited ocular movements are due to muscle fibrosis. IR and MR are commonly involved. CT scan shows fusiform enlargement of extraocular muscles (EOM). Management includes systemic therapy including steroids, immunosuppressive agents or radiotherapy. Surgical treatment includes orbital decompression, recessions of the recti (as affected), and lid surgery for lid retraction.

ORBITAL BLOWOUT FRACTURE

Blunt trauma over the eye or the maxilla can lead to fracture orbital floor or medial wall with entrapment of the IR, IO, and the surrounding tissue. The patient presents with limitation of elevation and depression with hypoesthesia over the infraorbital nerve distribution. No surgery is indicated in the first 2 weeks. In case of severe enophthalmos with orbital tissue prolapse the fractured floor is sealed with supramid sheet and the IR is freed from incarceration. The ocular motility may be improved by recessing the IR till FDT becomes negative and resecting the SR.

STRABISMUS FIXUS

A rare condition in which the eyes are fixed in extreme adduction or abduction FDT confirms the immobility. Supramaximal recessions of the horizontal recti have been found to be of cosmetic benefit.

Other restrictive conditions include adherence syndromes following trauma or retinal detachment surgery and orbital myositis.

10.12 Strabismus Surgery: Planning, Executing, and Complications

TS Surendran
Sankara Nethralaya, Chennai
t_surendran@yahoo.co.uk

INTRODUCTION

Well-planned surgery in strabismus requires a thorough planning and a comprehensive knowledge about the anatomy of the extraocular muscles. A detailed orthoptic evaluation and a good cycloplegic refraction as an obligatory preoperative requirement cannot be over emphasized. The parents have to be informed about all the risks and possibility of under and overcorrections. A preoperative consultation with pediatrician for anesthesia will go a long way.

The parents sign an informed consent.

INDICATIONS FOR SQUINT SURGERY

- Cosmetic purposes.
- To restore binocular functions.
- Correct diplopia in cases of incomitant squints.
- Lastly to correct head postures, face turn and chin elevation and depression.

WEAKENING PROCEDURES ON THE MUSCLES

- Recession
- Marginal myotomy and myectomy
- Fadenization
- Tenotomy and tenectomy
- Denervation and extirpation
- Recession and anteriorization
- Shifting the muscles up or down by 1/2 breadth

MUSCLE STRENGTHENING PROCEDURES
- Resection
- Advancement of the muscle
- Harada-Ito procedure
- Tucking of the muscle tendon

Adjustable sutures are used usually after recession on a muscle to give a more predictable result. The purpose of the adjustable suture is to achieve a desired surgical alignment reducing over or under corrections. A good binocular function is necessary to do this adjustable suture. The adjustment is done in the immediate preoperative period using the exteriorized sutures and knots. If the operation is carried under general anesthesia a short-acting reversal agent is given and the adjustment is made.

Under topical anesthesia the adjustment can be made by asking the patient to focus on the light or the operating microscope light. The adjusting procedure requires a very cooperative patient.

STAY SUTURES
Temporary stay sutures attached to limbus and the globe secured to periocular skin and the eye is fixed in desired position for restrictive strabismus.

TRANSPOSITION PROCEDURES
Muscle transpositions are indicated in paralytic strabismus such as transposing the lateral halves of superior and inferior recti to the upper and lower border of the lateral rectus in 6th nerve palsy.

HORIZONTAL COMITANT STRABISMUS
One millimeter of recession or resection of MR corrects up to 3-4 prisms of deviation. One millimeter of recession or resection of lateral rectus corrects up to 2-3 prisms of deviation. Symmetrical surgery such as bilateral or bimedial rectus recession or resection is done for comitant horizontal deviations (esotropias or exotropias). The lateral rectus can be recessed up to a maximum of 10 mm and medial rectus can be recessed up to a maximum of 7 mm.

TYPE OF ANESTHESIA
The squint cases can be easily operated on under local or general anesthesia. Topical anesthesia is being tried in selected cases only with an anesthetist standby.

CONJUNCTIVAL INCISION
The conjunctival fornix incision is made in either superior or inferior quadrants 2 mm from the limbus and 8 mm in length.

For oblique muscles, the incisions are made obliquely in the intermuscular area, between inferior and lateral recti for the inferior oblique muscle and between the lateral and superior recti for the superior oblique. Tackling the superior oblique on the nasal side is generally avoided, due to the severe degree of scarring induced in this area.

COMPLICATIONS
The complications in a well-planned and executed strabismus surgery are rare. But it is important to remember the following can occur, rarely in experienced hands as well.
- Under or over corrections
- Refractive changes induced, though small are well-known
- Postoperative diplopia
- Scleral perforation/s
- Orbital cellulites
- Granuloma
- Inclusion cyst and conjunctival scarring

- Adherence syndrome
- Corneal dellen
- Anterior segment ischemia
- Enophthalmos or exophthalmos
- Lost or slipped muscle
- Oculocardiac reflex
- Malignant hyperthermia
- Wrong muscle tackled.

SUGGESTED READING

1. Noorden GK, Campos EC. Binocular Vision and Ocular Motility, 6th edition. St. Louis: Mosby; 2002.

10.13 Clinical Management of Nystagmus

Mihir Kothari
Jyotirmay Eye Clinic and Ocular Motility Laboratory, Thane
drmihirkothari@gmail.com

INTRODUCTION

If the patient has: (1) rhythmical, (2) involuntary, (3) repetitive, (4) to-and-fro movement or oscillations of the eyes,[1] it is "Nystagmus"!

CRITICAL EXAMINATIONS IN NYSTAGMUS

The critical examination in nystagmus has been described in **Table 10.13.1**.

TABLE 10.13.1: Critical examination in nystagmus.

Examination	Technique	Interpretation	Diagnostic utility/ relevance
Vision under partial fogging	+4D lens in front of the eye to be occluded after the full optical correction	Prevents latent nystagmus to become manifest	Necessary to assess monocular vision in FMNS/LN
Binocular vision vs. monocular vision	Assess best corrected vision of both eyes open and with each eye covered	If binocular vision is better than best monocular vision there is a latent component	Patient can be benefitted by improving the fusion
Near vision vs. distance vision and convergence dampening	Use logMAR vision assessment for both near and distance testing	In 10% patients there is a true convergence dampening that leads to better vision for near	These patients are highly benefitted by base in prisms or MR recessions (artificial divergence surgery)
Vision in preferred head position	Monocular occlusion and subject reads the optotypes	• Reads with head posture • Reads with eye in adduction	• Look for null zone • Look for FMNS
Gaze-dependent acuity	Best corrected binocular visual acuity is measured with straight ahead posture and then progressively with face turned/tilted/chin-up and down 10, 20, and 30° eccentric	Significant change in vision is noted in INS with change of gaze	Very good clinical parameter to assess visual functions in nystagmus

Contd...

Contd...

Examination	Technique	Interpretation	Diagnostic utility/relevance
OKN	Smart phone app (viz. eye hand book) OKN drum	Abnormal vertical OKN (absent in up and/or down gaze) indicates neurological anomaly	The patient will need MRI brain
Abnormal head posture (Static/dynamic)	Ask the child to read at distance or resolve a target. Use a goniometer (e.g., simple protractor with scale or an android app) to measure	Face turn or chin up or down or mixed or pure head tilt	• Indicates eccentric null, (associated with) better vision • Absence of AHP is more likely with sensory defects
Cover test	Apply a cover in front of one eye and alternate		Will reveal any squint or latent nystagmus
Head nodding	Ask the patient to read or resolve	• Associated with spasmus nutans where holding the head increases nystagmus. • No increase in nystagmus on holding head if INS with or without sensory defects	Only in spasmus nutans, it is compensatory and 180° out of phase with nystagmus that leads to improved vision
Pupil	Direct reaction to light, RAPD and near distance dissociation	Sluggish reaction/RAPD indicates Anterior visual pathway disease	Warrants further investigation–ERG/MRI
Optic disc evaluation	Pallor/Hypoplasia		Warrants further investigation–ERG/MRI
Prism test 1	Keep prisms with apex toward the head posture in front of both/dominant eye	Improvement in head posture	Helps to measure the effect of surgery on face turn and attendant squint/induction of squint
Prism test 2	Keep prism bar apex in to induce convergence	Dampening of nystagmus and improvement in distance visual acuity	Helps to measure the maximum improvement in visual acuity with artificial divergence surgery. Also helps to calculate the amount of bimedial recession

(AHP: anomalous head posture; ERG: electroretinography; FMNS: fusion maldevelopment nystagmus syndrome; INS: infantile nystagmus; LN: latent nystagmus (old terminology for FMNS); MRI: magnetic resonance imaging; OKN: optokinetic nystagmus; RAPD: relative afferent pupillary defect)

GRAPHIC RECORDING OF THE NYSTAGMUS (FIG. 10.13.1)

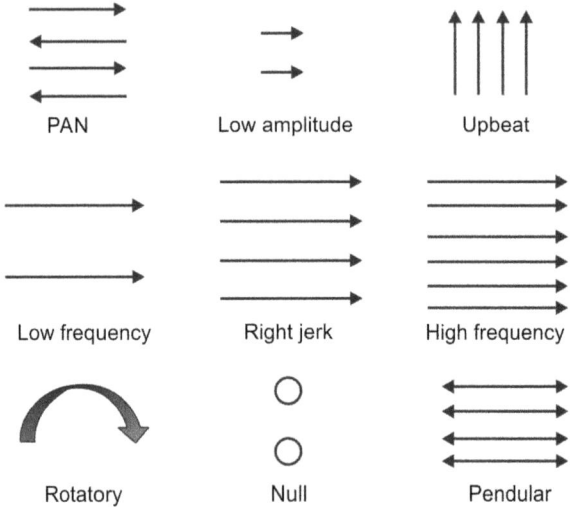

Fig. 10.13.1: Graphic recording of nystagmus. (PAN: periodic alternating nystagmus)

COMMON INVESTIGATIONS

Common investigations that are needed in patients with nystagmus have been described in **Table 10.13.2**.

TABLE 10.13.2: Common investigations needed in patients.

Name of the investigation	Indications	What can it reveal?
Video nystagmography/ eye movement recording	Preferably in every patient of nystagmus to objectively assess → Nystagmus with strabismus (to differentiate INS from FMNS)	• Type of nystagmus (classify accurately) • Potential for vision improvement with treatment (NAFX/ANAF) • Objective documentation of response to treatment • Null point evaluation • Identifies vertical components in seemingly horizontal nystagmus • To understand the natural history of the disease and progression/regression in individual patient
OCT	Retinal dystrophy/ maldevelopment	• Foveal hypoplasia • Schisis cavity • Accumulation of deposits • Retinal/choroidal thinning
ERG	Sensory nystagmus	• Achromatopsia • CSNB • LCA • Other atypical retinal dystrophies
MRI brain	Neurological disorder	• Space occupying lesions • Demyelinations • Perinatal damage • Congenital malformations/infections

Contd...

Contd...

Name of the investigation	Indications	What can it reveal?
Red-free fundus photography (autofluorescence)	Macular dystrophy	Accumulation of lipofuscin in various macular dystrophies

(ANAF: automated nystagmus acuity function; CSNB: congenital stationary night blindness; ERG: Electroretinography; FMNS: fusion maldevelopment nystagmus syndrome; INS: infantile nystagmus; LCA: Leber congenital amaurosis; MRI: magnetic resonance imaging; NAFX: expanded nystagmus acuity function; OCT: optical coherence tomography)

INVESTIGATIONS IN NYSTAGMUS: NEUROLOGICAL OR RETINAL—WHAT IS THE CAUSE?

Detailed and routine electroretinography or magnetic resonance imaging (ERG/MRI) and optical coherence tomography (OCT) in patients with nystagmus may reveal that as many as 90% patients with nystagmus have associated neurological or retinal disease. However, the sensory defect is not the cause of nystagmus in them rather an association.

When to suspect a "neurological" cause in nystagmus and get an MRI brain has been described in **Table 10.13.3**.

TABLE 10.13.3: Signs and symptoms of "neurological" cause in nystagmus.

	Symptoms or signs that warrant investigations	Disease suspected
See-saw nystagmus	All patients need MRI	Chiasmal pathology
Pendular nystagmus	Optic atrophy, relative afferent pupillary defect and/or visual field loss	Chiasmal glioma
Pendular nystagmus	Wasting despite a normal appetite, excessive food intake, diabetes insipidus, euphoric affect, headache or lethargy	Hypothalamic tumors
Spasmus nutans: "Minimal" head nodding, the small-amplitude and the high-frequency of the oscillations, and the asymmetry of the nystagmus are typical for spasmus nutans. A head turn and tilt is common in congenital nystagmus, but it also occurs in about two-third of patients with spasmus nutans	Age of onset <4 months or >2 years, significant vertical component, any systemic/ocular signs of neurological deficit. Café-au-lait spots/stigmata of neurofibromatosis	Gliomas/subacute necrotizing encephalopathy
Vertical nystagmus	Vertical pendular, Down beat, Upbeat	• Brainstem and cerebellar disease • Craniocervical junction/cerebellar disease • Anticonvulsants • Cerebellar/pontomedullary abnormalities

Contd...

Contd...

	Symptoms or signs that warrant investigations	Disease suspected
Asymmetric horizontal nystagmus		Nonlocalizing may need ERG also
Abnormal (absent in upgaze and/or downgaze) vertical OKN6		Nonlocalizing

(ERG: electroretinography; MRI: magnetic resonance imaging; OKN: optokinetic nystagmus)

The features that indicate abnormal retina in a "normal appearing fundi"—warrant an ERG **(Table 10.13.4)**.

TABLE 10.13.4: Features indicating abnormal retina.

Disease	Features	ERG
Leber's congenital amaurosis (LCA)	Paradoxical pupil reaction (pupil constrict when room lights are switched off), oculodigital sign +, enophthalmos	ERG – extinguished (rule out mental retardation, SNHL, cardiomyopathy, medullary cystic renal disease, cerebellar vermis hypoplasia)
Achromatopsia	Pronounced paradoxical pupil reaction, light sensitivity, dyschromatopsia	Photopic ERG-attenuated. Scotopic ERG normal
Congenital stationary night blindness	Paradoxical pupil reaction, nyctalopia	Negative-wave ERG (attenuated "a" wave)
Joubert syndrome	Developmentally-delayed infants, breathing problems	Attenuated or nonrecordable ERG, MRI brain–cerebellar vermis hypoplasia
Peroxisomal disorders	High, bulging forehead, hepatomegaly, renal cysts, a sensorineural hearing loss, hypotonia, retinal dystrophy	ERG extinguished

(ERG: electroretinography; MRI: magnetic resonance imaging; SNHL: sensorineural hearing loss)

■ OPTICAL MANAGEMENT OF NYSTAGMUS

The optical management of nystagmus has been described in **Table 10.13.5**.

TABLE 10.13.5: Optical management.

Type of defect	Correction measure	Remark
Refractive error	Full correction	
Contact lenses	Soft (bandage or powered)/ Semisoft clear or tinted contact lenses can be prescribed	There may/may not be significant improvement in visual acuity, foveation and light sensitivity
Convergence dampening	Base out prism	Typically 7 PD base out with -1 DS in non-presbyopic
Accommodation failure	Bifocals	Patients with aniridia, albinism, cerebral vision impairment, foveal hypoplasia, etc., may have significant defects in accommodation

Contd...

Contd...

Type of defect	Correction measure	Remark
Head postures	Prisms with apex in the direction of the head (will move the eye to center)	Good for small (<20 PD) postures. More useful for the vertical torticollis
Nystagmus/Refractive error and light sensitivity	Contact lenses (CL)	CL material does not matter, correct the refractive error and use painted CL for aniridia or albinism
Low vision	Optical and nonoptical aids	
Light sensitivity	Photogray/tinted lenses	In spectacles or CL
Oscillopsia	Apex toward head posture (e.g., apex up for down beat nystagmus)	With image stabilization (high – contact lens with high + spectacles)

PHARMACOLOGICAL TREATMENT OF NYSTAGMUS (TABLE 10.13.6)

TABLE 10.13.6: Pharmacological treatment of nystagmus.

	Downbeat nystagmus (DBN)	Upbeat nystagmus (UBN)	Acquired pendular nystagmus (APN)	Periodic alternating nystagmus (PAN)	Infantile (congenital) nystagmus
Direction of nystagmus (quick phase)	Downward, may be diagonal with lateral gaze	Upward	Mainly horizontal, may have vertical and/or torsional components	Horizontal	Mainly horizontal; may have torsional and small vertical components
Waveform (slow phase)	Jerk, constant, increasing, or decreasing slow phase velocity	Jerk, constant, increasing, or decreasing slow phase velocity	Pendular, sinusoidal slow phase	Jerk, mostly constant slow phase velocity	Accelerating slow phases; foveation periods when the eye is transiently still
Special features	Increased intensity during lateral and downward gaze; sometimes influenced by convergence	Increased intensity during upward gaze; may convert to DBN on convergence	Associated with other oscillations (e.g., palate) and with hypertrophic degeneration of the inferior olive	Changes direction every 90–120 seconds	Null zone, in which nystagmus is minimal; often suppressed with convergence
Sites of lesion	Cerebellum (bilateral floccular hypofunction); rarely lower brainstem lesions	Medial medulla, pontomesencephalic junction, rarely cerebellum	Pontomedullary, probably affecting components of neural integrator for gaze holding	Cerebellum (nodulus, uvula)	Uncertain; some cases are associated with afferent visual system anomalies

Contd...

Contd...

	Downbeat nystagmus (DBN)	Upbeat nystagmus (UBN)	Acquired pendular nystagmus (APN)	Periodic alternating nystagmus (PAN)	Infantile (congenital) nystagmus
Etiology	Cerebellar tumors, degenerations, Chiari malformations, and stroke; idiopathic; often associated with bilateral vestibulopathy and neuropathy	Brainstem or cerebellar stroke and tumors; Wernicke's encephalopathy	Multiple sclerosis, oculopalatal tremor due to brainstem or cerebellar stroke involving Guillain–Mollaret triangle	Cerebellar degeneration, craniocervical anomalies, multiple sclerosis, cerebellar tumors and stroke	Uncertain; may be associated with afferent visual system anomalies; hereditary in some patients (e.g., FRMD7 mutations)
Treatment (dose, frequency)	• 4 aminopyridine (5–10 mg, tid) • 3, 4-diaminopyridine (10–20 mg, tid) • Baclofen (5–10 mg, tid) • Clonazepam (0.5–1 mg, bid)	Often transient, treatment often not necessary • Memantine (10 mg, qid) • 4 aminopyridine (5–10 mg, tid) • Baclofen (5–10 mg, tid)	• Gabapentin (300 mg qid) • Memantine (10 mg, qid)	• Baclofen (5–10 mg, tid) • Memantine (5–10 mg qid)	• Gabapentin (300 mg qid) • Memantine (10 mg qid)
Side effects	• Dizziness, paresthesias, incoordination • Dizziness, paresthesias, incoordination • Drowsiness, dizziness, lethargy • Drowsiness, dizziness, incoordination	• Lethargy, dizziness, headache • Dizziness, paresthesias, incoordination • Drowsiness, dizziness, lethargy	• Dizziness, incoordination, drowsiness • Lethargy, dizziness, headache	• Drowsiness, dizziness, lethargy • Lethargy, dizziness, headache	• Dizziness, incoordination, drowsiness • Lethargy, dizziness, headache
See-saw nystagmus	Clonazepam (0.5–1 mg, bid)/Memantine (10 mg, qid)—drowsiness, dizziness, incoordination/lethargy, dizziness, headache					
Torsional	Gabapentin (300 mg, qid)—dizziness, incoordination, drowsiness					

■ SURGICAL PROCEDURE

- To try to improve visual acuity (usually by 1–3 logMAR lines), contrast vision, reaction time (improves by 0.3 seconds) and gaze-dependent acuity by improving the foveation.

SECTION 10: Pediatric Ophthalmology and Strabismus

- To transfer the nystagmus null zone from an extreme position to a frontal one, in order to improve abnormal head position and spectacle centration.
- To correct strabismus when it is present to restore binocular fusion and stereopsis.

▪ MY PROTOCOL (TABLE 10.13.7)

TABLE 10.13.7: Protocol of nystagmus.

Abnormality	Procedures	Principle	Benefits of surgery	Indication
Nystagmus ONLY	Tenotomy and reattachment (large 4-muscle recessions or muscle extirpations are not preferred)	4-horizontal recti are detached and resutured at the same insertion	• 25% reduced intensity of nystagmus • Broadening of null zone • 1–3 lines (logMAR) improvement in vision in 50% patients • 40% increase in NAFX in 90% patients	• Nystagmus with no null, primary position null or alternating null (periodic or aperiodic). • Nystagmus with or without sensory/neurological defects
Convergence dampening (near vision better than distance vision)	Artificial divergence surgery	Bilateral medial rectus recession only suitable in patients with confirmed presence of fusion and stereoacuity after measuring the fusional convergence amplitudes	• 70–90% dampening of nystagmus • Magnificent improvement in vision	Patients with INS and convergence dampening with near vision > distance vision
Combined with abnormal head posture (move the eyes in the direction of head turn/tilt/chin)	Augmented Anderson procedure	9 mm MR recession and 12 or 13 mm LR recession	• 20° correction of face turn • 2.5° reduction in amplitude of nystagmus • 1.5 Hz reduction in frequency of nystagmus	Patients with INS and moderate face turn (<25°)
	Augmented Kestenbaum–Anderson procedure	Classic 5, 6, 7, 8 recess resect augmented with degree appropriate to the face turn to move the null to the center (20% augmented for 20° face turn, 30% for 30°, so forth and so on)	• 20–60° correction of face turn • 25% reduction in amplitude and frequency of nystagmus • 1–3 lines (LogMAR) improvement in vision	Patients with INS with moderate to severe face turn

Contd...

Contd...

Abnormality	Procedures	Principle	Benefits of surgery	Indication
	Oblique/torsional Kestenbaum–Anderson procedure	Inferior oblique advance or recess and superior oblique anterior fibers tenotomy or advancement (Harada–Ito)	Correction of head tilt – approximately 5°/mm of surgery	Head tilts
	Elevator weakening or depressor weakening	IO myectomy with SR recession 5 mm for chin down or SO tenectomy with IR recession 4 mm for chin up	1. Correction of the head posture	Chin up or down
Combined squint and nystagmus	FMNS with squint (diagnosis in VNG/EMR)	Correct the squint only	• Correction of squint and recovery of fusion and stereopsis • Conversion of manifest nystagmus to a latent nystagmus • Improvement in vision	VNG/EMR needed for any patient with squint and nystagmus to identify this type
	INS with squint	Correct the squint and add T and R	Benefits of both—squint surgery and nystagmus surgery	
Combined squint, abnormal head posture and nystagmus	FMNS/INS with squint and abnormal head posture	Squint surgery on nondominant eye and head; posture surgery on dominant eye	Benefits of squint surgery, nystagmus surgery, and correction of abnormal head postures ++	Use prisms to correct the head posture in front of dominant eye and then correct the squint with prisms in front of nondominant eye and then calculate the amount of surgery

(EMR: electronic medical records; FMNS: fusion maldevelopment nystagmus syndrome; INS: infantile nystagmus; IO: inferior oblique; LR: lateral rectus; MR: medial rectus; NAFX: expanded nystagmus acuity function; SO: superior oblique; SR: superior rectus; VNG: videonystagmography)

REFERENCE

1. Sarvananthan N, Surendran M, Roberts EO, Jain S, Thomas S, Shah N, et al. The prevalence of nystagmus: the Leicestershire nystagmus survey. Invest Ophthalmol Vis Sci. 2009;50(11):5201-6.

10.14 Pediatric Cataract Management

Lav Kochgaway
Netralayam, Kolkata
lav.kochgaway@netralayam.com

■ INTRODUCTION

Pediatric cataract management is one of the most complex situations in eye diseases. To complicate the matter, most of these patients are from poor socioeconomic background who have less understanding of the disease and its management. There are many differences in management protocol of pediatric cataract, as compared to adult cataract. Decisions related to timing of surgery, intraocular lens (IOL) implantation, target postoperative refraction, refraction, and amblyopia management after surgery are all complex issues that need to be clear to us before we attempt pediatric cataract surgery. During surgery, pediatric eye is different from adult eyes as it has lower scleral rigidity, capsule is more elastic and it is a growing eye which makes surgical decisions different from those in adult eyes.

■ SURGICAL DECISION MAKING

Decisions in pediatric cataract surgery are influenced by multiple factors, few of which are outlined below:
- *Location of the cataract:* The cataract has to be significant enough to subject the child to dangers of stimulus deprivation amblyopia, then only we should decide about surgery. Some variety of cataracts such as blue-dot cataract, small pin-head sized cataract in visual axis and cataract-off visual axis need not be operated as they do not obstruct passage of light to the retina.
- *Status of fellow eye:* Especially in unilateral cataract is important, in terms of its refractive status. We should be aware of it when deciding about the postoperative refraction of the eye to be operated. It is also important when take decision about IOL implantation in infants. If parents are motivated enough to use contact lens, then we can leave them aphakic, otherwise we have to take decision in favor of IOL implantation to avoid gross anisometropia.
- *Age of the patient:* Surgical decisions related to IOL implantation and postoperative target refraction are taken based on the age of the child. For bilateral cataract, the consensus is that IOL should be implanted in children aged 2 years and above, though many surgeons are implanting IOL at younger age as well. In younger patients, the target postoperative target refraction can be slightly higher hyperopia considering the rapid myopic shift that is expected in them. As the child grows older the rate of myopic shift is expected to be slower, so we can target for a lower hyperopia.
- *Presence of strabismus and nystagmus:* Presence of squint and nystagmus is a poor prognostic indicator. It indicates that dense stimulus deprivation amblyopia has already set in. In presence of these two features, the eye with a maintained fixation has better visual prognosis postoperatively compared to the other eye with unmaintained fixation.
- *Systemic syndromes:* Identification of associated systemic syndromes is very important to assess the fitness of the child to undergo surgery under general anesthesia. Special attention should be given to cardiac status of the child, as many of them may have cardiac malformations as well. In such cases fitness for surgery under general anesthesias should be taken from the pediatrician or pediatric cardiologist. Preoperative checkup by anesthetist is also important for them to plan the precautions well in advance.
- *Ocular comorbidities:* Like features of torch infection, coloboma, anterior segment dysgenesis, microphthalmos, etc., should be identified before surgery so that prognosis is explained to the parents and surgical planning is done accordingly.

INVESTIGATIONS

Children with pediatric cataract should undergo the following investigations to determine the cause of cataract and to ensure fitness for surgery under general anesthesia:
- Complete blood count
- Chest X-ray
- Toxoplasmosis, Rubella, Cytomegalovirus and Herpes (TORCH) Titer
- Urine for reducing sugars, amino acids, calcium, and phosphorus
- Red cell galactokinase
- Echocardiography (if cardiac anomaly is suspected).

INTRAOCULAR LENS POWER CALCULATION

Considerations

There are various formulas that have been advised for IOL power calculation in children. It still remains a dilemma as there is rapid change in axial length and keratometry in the first 2 years of life. Eyeball growth is achieved up to 90% by 2 years of age and keratometry changes stabilize by 18 months. There is broad consensus on use of SRK T formula for routine purposes and Hoffer Q for eyes with smaller axial length. Postoperatively we have to aim for hyperopia in children, as their refraction undergoes myopic shift as they grow. Myopic shift is faster in operated eye of patients with unilateral cataract. In bilateral cataract there are various suggestions which recommend *higher hyperopia in younger children*. But when there is doubt about compliance with spectacles after surgery—we should aim for a lower hyperopia as uncorrected high hyperopia itself would be amblyogenic and would defeat the purpose of the surgery.

Intraocular Lens Surprise

In spite of all care taken for accurate biometry, we do face situations in which the final refraction is significantly different from what we had aimed for.

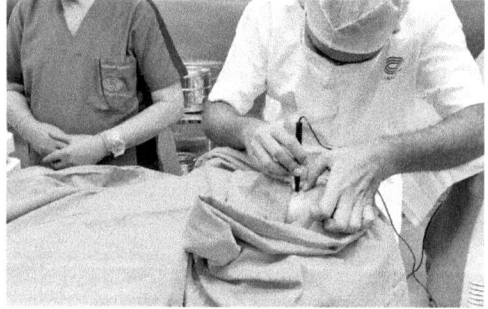

Fig. 10.14.1: Biometry in OT.

MANAGEMENT PROTOCOL

Lensectomy

In infants, when IOL is not being planned, lensectomy is the procedure of choice in which only the rim of anterior capsule is left behind for future secondary IOL implantation. Pars plana or limbal route can be taken.

Lens Aspiration, Intraocular Lens Implantation with Primary Posterior Capsulorrhexis and Anterior Vitrectomy

This is the procedure of choice for majority of children beyond infancy. There is broad consensus in favor of IOL implantation in children beyond 2 years of age, but can even be done in between 1 and 2 years in safe hands.

Lens Aspiration with Intraocular Lens Implantation

In children older than 7 years of age, nowadays surgeons are doing posterior capsulorrhexis and anterior vitrectomy in older children as well.

COMPLICATIONS

- Anterior segment inflammation in early postoperative period
- Visual axis opacification
- IOL decentration due to uneven contraction of bag
- Pupillary capture of optic—if IOL is placed in sulcus.
- Glaucoma
- Retinal detachment

VISUAL REHABILITATION AND FOLLOW-UP

This is the most important aspect of pediatric cataract management. Postsurgery the child has to be given refractive correction in the form of spectacles or contact lens. Contact lens is used mainly after unilateral cataract surgery in which IOL has not been implanted. If parents are motivated enough it can be prescribed for bilateral aphasia as well. Amblyopia therapy forms an integral part of pediatric cataract management. Initially these children have to be followed up every 3 months to check for refraction, visual axis clarity, IOL, fundus, and compliance with amblyopia treatment protocol. Once the final outcome in terms of vision has been achieved they should be followed up every 6 months for life.

10.15 Pediatric Eye in Various Systemic Syndromes

Jitendra Jethani
Baroda Children Eye Care and Squint Clinic, Vadodara
xethani@rediffmail.com

INTRODUCTION

A syndrome is a pattern of anomalies thought to be pathologically-related. The term implies a single cause. A malformation is a morphological defect of an organ or part of an organ resulting from an intrinsic abnormal developmental process. Eyes are the mirror to the brain and body. A variety of systemic diseases may affect eye and its functioning. The most common is the diabetes mellitus in adults. However, the pattern of these diseases is different in children than in adults. The examination of eyes would point toward various systemic diseases and syndrome in children. The careful examination of eyes in children is very important along with the history and development of various signs in pediatric eye. These conditions may not only give a clue and have vision saving effect but sometimes may even end-up being life-saving.

The common systemic disease presenting with various ocular manifestations in eye can be broadly divided into:
- Chromosomal abnormalities
- Craniofacial malformations
- Connective tissue, skin, and bone disorders
- Neurocutaneous syndromes
- Metabolic diseases
- Genetic syndrome
- Syndromes associated with lens
- Retinitis pigmentosa and allied syndromes
- Syndrome associated with lids.

CHROMOSOMAL ABNORMALITIES

Humans have 23 pairs of chromosomes, out of which two are sex chromosomes namely X and Y and they determine the gender. Deoxyribonucleic acid (DNA) has the information which is transcribed to ribonucleic acid (RNA) which is finally translated into a protein generating sequence and finally a protein. Each nucleated cell of an organism would contain the similar DNA. During the cell duplication, nuclear DNA is duplicated and each daughter cell receives the same information as the parent unless a mutation or chromosomal anomaly occurs.

There are two major types of anomalies namely:
- *Numerical:* When chromosomes do not segregate properly, cells may have missing like monosomy or extra chromosomes like trisomy. Such anomalies where the number of chromosomes is atypical are called aneuploidy.
- *Structural:* There are five types of structural chromosomal anomalies namely, deletions, duplications, inversion, and translocations and occasionally ring chromosome. This could occur in various chromosomes and we have included only the common syndromes here.

Trisomy

Trisomy 13 (Patau's Syndrome)
The major diagnostic criteria include microphthalmia, cleft lip or palate, ectodermal scalp defect (cutis aplasia), and polydactyly. Other eye anomalies include holoprosencephaly, cyclopia, persistent fetal vasculature, retinal dysplasia. Systemic abnormalities will include polycystic kidneys, undescended testis, and biseptate uterus in females.

Trisomy 18 (Edward's Syndrome)
Common eye problems include epicanthus, hypertelorism, cataract, corneal opacities, and microphthalmia. Other systemic features include microcephaly, fawn-like ears, midfacial hypoplasia with flat occiput, poor muscle development, rocker-bottom feet, webbing of toes, and ventricular septal defect.

Trisomy 21 (Down's Syndrome)
It is one of the most common trisomies. Eye findings include epicanthus, upward slanting of the palpebral fissures (mongoloid slant), myopia, strabismus, nystagmus, keratoconus, and cataracts. Brushfield's spots may be seen on iris. Congenital nasolacrimal duct obstruction is common and is resistant to treatment with probing.

Systemic features include hypotonia, brachycephaly, a large protruding tongue, small nose with a small bridge and a short-thick neck. Clinodactyly of the fifth digit; short and stubby feet with a wide-gap between the first and the second toes; cardiac malformations; delayed milestones; Simian crease seen in trisomy 13 and fetal alcohol syndrome also; Turner's syndrome.

Monosomy

Monosomy 21
It may cause epicanthus, downward slanting of palpebral fissures, Peter's anomaly of the anterior segment, and cataract.

Deletions
Cri-du-chat syndrome or deletion 5p syndrome children have a typical cat-like cry mainly due the structural abnormality of larynx. Eye features include blepharoptosis, myopia, and reduced-tear production. The child may have associated cataract, strabismus, glaucoma, tortuous retinal vessels, foveal hypoplasia, and optic atrophy. Other features may include wide and flat nasal bridge, sex determining chromosomal syndromes.

Turner's Syndrome (Monosomy, 45 XO)
Eye findings include blepharoptosis, strabismus, cataract, blue sclera, and color blindness.
Systemic findings include cardiac abnormalities, coarctation of aorta, autoimmune diseases especially thyroid and diabetes. The appearance is of a female with short and

webbed-neck, low-set ears, low-hairline at the back of the neck, short stature, cubitus valgus, and swollen hands and feet. It is one the most common causes of primary amenorrhea.

Klinefelter's Syndrome (Duplications, 47 XXY)
Two or more X chromosomes in a male.

Eye findings include myopia, upward slant of palpebral fissure, Brushfield's spots on iris, and coloboma microphthalmia.

Systemic findings include weaker muscles, tall stature, poor coordination, less body hair, smaller genitals, and breast growth. Intelligence is usually normal; however, reading difficulties and problems with speech are more common.

■ CRANIOFACIAL MALFORMATIONS
Craniostenosis
The most important ocular finding is to look for the optic nerve status in such patients. The eye findings would be proptosis, refractive errors, V-pattern strabismus, keratoconus and nasolacrimal duct problems and occasionally corneal-exposure problems. A fundus examination is a must in these cases.

The various syndromes are Crouzon's and Apert's which are common apart from the Carpenter's syndrome and Pfeiffer and Saethre-Chotzen syndrome. Midface abnormalities, syndactyly of hands and feet (Apert's), short-broad thumb (Pfeiffer's) obesity, hypogonadism, intellectual disability (Carpenter's) progressive hydrocephalus with no hand and feet anomalies (Crouzon's).

Fibroblast growth factor receptor 1 (FGFR 1) mutation is commonly seen in Pfeiffer type 2 and 3 and FGFR mutations are seen commonly in Crouzon's and Apert's syndrome.

Plagiocephaly
It is defined as the asymmetry of the skull mainly due to the abnormal fusion of the anterior or posterior coronal suture or due to a deformation defect from compression on the head (deformational plagiocephaly).

The plagiocephaly is divided into the frontal (coronal suture) or posterior (lamboid suture) type.

The frontal type would commonly have vertical strabismus with hypertropia on the affected side mainly due to the mechanical underaction of superior oblique. The head tilt would be toward the unaffected side.

Mandibulofacial Dystosis (Treacher Collins Syndrome)
Eye findings (mostly bilateral) include coloboma or notching of outer part of lower lid, antimongoloid slant.

Systemic findings include large mouth, abnormal dentition, and abnormal palate; malformation of external or middle ear, parrot beak nose, atypical hairline, and blind fistulas between angle of mouth and ear.

Oculo-auriculo-vertebral Syndrome (Goldenhar Syndrome)
Eye findings include epibulbar and conjunctival lipodermoids with vertebral anomalies, ptosis and narrow palpebral fissure in children with facial microsomia; upper lid colobomas, anophthalmia with severe central nervous system (CNS) anomalies; visual loss due to refractive error, amblyopia and strabismus. Also may have associated Duane's retraction syndrome, uveal coloboma and corneal anesthesia and resulting corneal ulcer and optic nerve hypoplasia.

Systemic findings include the most common ear malformations from anotia to preauricular tags, supernumerary tags, unilateral facial involvement, mandibular ramus and condyles are frequently severely involved. Other associations include spina bifida, preauricular pits, trigeminal and facial nerve involvement, Klippel–Feil anomaly and scoliosis (fusional anomalies).

Oculo-mandibulo-dyscephaly (Hallermann–Streiff Syndrome)
Eye findings include congenital cataracts which spontaneously resorb. This may be associated with microphthalmia, nystagmus, and strabismus. Glaucoma may be primary or secondary. Less common are uveitis, blue sclera, and downslanted palpebral fissures.

Systemic findings include dyscephaly, small stature, dental anomalies, and hypotrichosis. The face is small with a thin, pointed, pinched nose. A double-chin with a central cleft and high-arched palate is also noted.

Mobius Sequence
There is a combination of bilateral sixth nerve with facial nerve involvement with or without systemic abnormalities. The restriction of horizontal movement may be variable with only abduction limitation, both adduction and abduction limitation, associated with retraction (Duane's retraction syndrome), asymmetric or unilateral ocular motility restrictions and both horizontal and vertical motility restriction.

Systemic anomalies include limb deformities especially feet. The child may have micrognathia, tongue malformations; deficiency of sternal head of pectoralis major muscle (Poland syndrome) may be associated.

Cervico-oculo-acoustic Syndrome (Wildervanck Syndrome)
The triad includes hearing loss secondary to inner ear anomaly, Klippel–Feil anomaly (fusion of one or more cervical vertebrae resulting in short webbed-neck) and Duane's retraction syndrome may be associated with epibulbar dermoids, subluxation of lens and pseudopapilledema.

Waardenburg Syndrome
Telecanthus with displacement of puncta and synophrys is the common finding. Partial or complete heterochromia of one or both irides is seen in both types. The fundi may also be albinotic. It may be associated with cataracts, microphthalmia, and ptosis.

Systemic association includes white-forelock which disappears with age and premature graying of hair, nasal root is broad with hypoplastic alar cartilage and sensorineural deafness.

CHARGE Association
CHARGE association would include coloboma involving iris, choroid or optic nerve, heart defects, choanal atresia, retarded growth, development or central nervous anomalies, genital hypoplasia, and ear malformations or deafness; may be associated with microphthalmia, high myopia, strabismus, cleft palate, facial palsy, autism, and swallowing difficulties.

Amniotic Band Syndrome
Eye-findings include lid coloboma, corneal opacities, contiguous facial clefts, hypertelorism, palpebral fissure changes, microphthalmia, and strabismus.

Systemic findings include facial clefts, skull defects, asymmetric encephaloceles, constrictive anomalies of limbs, umbilical cord abnormalities, and visceral malformations.

■ CONNECTIVE TISSUE, SKIN, AND BONE DISORDERS

Pseudoxanthoma Elasticum
It first affects the retina through a dimpling of the Bruch's membrane (a thin membrane separating the blood vessel-rich layer from the pigmented layer of the retina),

that is only visible during ophthalmologic examinations. This is called peau d'orange. The mineralization of the elastic fibers in the Bruch membrane creates cracks (angioid streaks) that radiate out from the optic nerve. Pseudoxanthoma elasticum (PXE) affects the skin first, often in childhood but frequently later. Small, yellowish papular lesions form and cutaneous laxity mainly affects the neck, axillae (armpits), groin, and flexural creases (the inside parts of the elbows and knees). Skin may become lax and redundant.

Pseudoxanthoma elasticum may affect the gastrointestinal and cardiovascular systems. In the digestive tract, the principal symptom is gastrointestinal bleeding, usually from the stomach.

Ehlers–Danlos Syndrome

Ehlers-Danlos type VI has the eye findings commonly associated with it which includes rupture of globe or retinal detachment following trivial trauma. Other findings include myopia, microcornea, and keratoconus.

Systemic findings include hyperflexible joints, fragile skin, atrophic "cigarette-paper scar" skin, hiatal hernia, valvular heart disease, and sleep apnea.

Marfan's Syndrome

The most common eye-finding is ectopia lentis and the cause for it is weak zonules. The lens may shift upward and outward. Other signs and symptoms affecting the eye include increased length along an axis of the globe, myopia, corneal flatness, and strabismus. Systemic findings include most readily visible signs of the skeletal system. Many individuals with Marfan syndrome grow to above-average height, and some have disproportionately long, slender limbs with thin, weak wrists and long fingers and toes; undue fatigue, shortness of breath, heart palpitations, racing heartbeats, or chest pain radiating to the back, shoulder, or arm. Cold arms, hands, and feet can also be linked to Marfan syndrome because of inadequate circulation. The signs of regurgitation from prolapse of the mitral or aortic valves result from cystic medial degeneration of the valves, which is commonly associated with Marfan syndrome.

Weill–Marchesani Syndrome

Ocular findings include microspherophakia and ectopia lentis.

Systemic findings include short-stature, brachycephaly, short stubby spade-like hands and feet.

Stickler Syndrome

Eye findings include congenital and occasionally stable high myopia, presenile cataract, and vitreoretinal degeneration. Retinal detachment is common. Radial patches of lattice degeneration are seen.

Screening for hearing loss is mandatory in children with stickler syndrome. Other findings include cleft palate, progressive arthropathy, and mitral valve prolapse.

Homocystinuria

Subluxation of lens with broken zonules may be seen.

Skin Disorders

Albinism

It is an absence of or reduction in the amount of melanin pigment in the skin, eye lashes, iris, hair or fundus; broadly two types but lot of variants. The tyrosinase negative variant is more severe one and the defect involves the enzyme tyrosinase which is responsible for conversion of tyrosine to dihydroxyphenylalanine (DOPA).

The hairbulb incubation test can be done to classify the type. Other important findings include:
- Refractive errors
- Nystagmus
- Strabismus
- Foveal hypoplasia
- Absence of pigment in *retinal pigment epithelium* (RPE), iris, uveal tissues
- Abnormal decussation of nerve fibers

Two important syndromes should be looked for in these patients.

Chédiak–Higashi Syndrome
- Tyrosinase positive
- Susceptible to gram-positive infections
- Neuropathy

Hermansky–Pudlak Syndrome
- Defective platelet aggregation
- Restrictive lung disease
- Bowel disorders

Cockayne Syndrome
Eye findings include pigmentary retinopathy with optic atrophy, strabismus, and nystagmus though the visual acuity may be preserved. The dilator muscle of iris is the cause for poor response to dilating drops in these patients.

Systemic features include growth retardation, progeroid facies, disproportionately long limbs, and photodermatitis.

Xeroderma Pigmentosum
Eye findings are restricted mainly to the anterior chamber only; photophobia secondary to conjunctivitis, keratitis, and dryness of ocular surface. Lid lesions with ectropion of entropion may occur. Squamous cell carcinoma is common.

Systemic lesion over skin starts with freckling, dryness, and scaling and then to hypopigmentation and telangiectasia along with actinic keratosis. Malignant skin neoplasms are common.

Juvenile Xanthogranuloma
Mostly affects infants in first few years of their life. Eye lesions mainly involve the iris and ciliary body; may involve lid, orbit, and extraocular muscles. The child may develop spontaneous hyphema mostly unilateral.

Skin lesions may also be seen which regress spontaneously by 3-6 years of age.

Neurocutaneous Syndromes (Covered in Phakomatosis Section)
- Neurofibromatosis type I
- Neurofibromatosis type II
- Tuberous sclerosis
- Von Hippel-Lindau disease
- Ataxia-telangiectasia
- Sturge-Weber syndrome

METABOLIC DISEASES

Wilson's Disease
The disease is secondary to the disorder of copper transport.

Eye findings include the Kayser–Fleisher ring due to the copper deposition in Descemet's membrane; associated with sunflower cataract (infrequently); may be associated with jerky oscillations of eyes, gaze paresis and involuntary movements, impairment of accommodation and convergence, apraxia of lid opening and night blindness.

Systemic features include mainly episodes of jaundice, vomiting, progressive hepatic insufficiency, splenomegaly, gastroesophageal varices, and ascites.

The most common neurological manifestations are dysarthria and incoordination of voluntary movements. Renal tubular damage is common and cardiac involvement may lead to arrhythmias and heart failure.

Mucopolysaccharidoses

The group of syndromes is caused by deficiency of specific lysosomal enzymes involved in the degradation of dermatan sulfate, heparin sulfate, and keratin sulfate.

Eye findings include progressive clouding of cornea except in type II, III, and IV (mild haze); associated with pigmentary retinal degeneration, papilledema and optic atrophy and in some cases glaucoma.

Systemic findings include bone anomalies, joint contractures, skeletal deformities, and dwarfing. Typical dysmorphic facies, visceromegaly, cardiac problems, hearing impairment, and intellectual disabilities are associated.

The Gangliosidoses

It results from defect in degradation of gangliosides which causes accumulation of these lipids. They are found in high concentration in the gray cells of brain and in extraneural tissue.

Eye findings include cherry-red spot in most of the cases associated with visual loss and optic atrophy. The frequency may vary depending upon the type of gangliosidosis. There may be associated impairment of convergence, horizontal and vertical defects in chronic cases.

Systemic findings include neurological abnormalities with progressive deterioration. May have seizure, dystonia.

Albinism (mentioned above).

Galactosemia

The enzymes involved to convert galactose to glucose are galactokinase, galactose-1-phosphate-uridyltransferase (GALT) and uridine diphosphate galactose-4-epimerase (GALE).

Galactokinase deficiency may lead to cataract and pseudotumor cerebri.

GALT deficiency may lead to cataract in eyes and hepatomegaly and ovarian failure. If left untreated may lead to intellectual disability and speech anomaly.

GALE deficiency is confined to erythrocytes and does not cause cataract.

■ MISCELLANEOUS COMMON GENETIC SYNDROMES

Alport's Syndrome

It is characterized by defect in the type IV collagen which makes up the basement membrane in many body systems. Eye findings include anterior lenticonus which is most common and may be associated occasionally with posterior lenticonus, perimacular yellow flecks, cornela arcus, posterior polymorphous dystrophy, and recurrent nontraumatic corneal erosions.

Systemic findings include deafness, sensorineural, especially affecting high frequencies, hypertension, glomerulonephropathy, hematuria, gross and microscopic proteinuria, thinning of the glomerular basement membrane (early in the disease), thickening of the glomerular basement membrane (later in the disease), thrombocytopenia, and hypoparathyroidism.

Aicardi's Syndrome

Eye findings include microphthalmia, optic nerve coloboma, bilateral chorioretinopathy, chorioretinal lacunae, retinal detachment, cataract, nystagmus optic atrophy, sparse lateral eyebrows. Good visual prognosis if the lesions do not involve macula.

Systemic findings include microcephaly, upturned nasal tip, spinal bifida, butterfly vertebrae, proximally placed limbs, precocious puberty, intellectual disability, infantile spasms, seizures, hypotonia, Dandy–Walker malformation, Arnold–Chiari malformation, intracranial cysts, delayed-myelination, agenesis of corpus callosum, enlarged lateral and third ventricles, hypoplastic cerebellar vermis, dysplasia of the cerebellar hemispheres.

Alstrom Syndrome

The child normally presents with profound loss of vision and nystagmus. Eye findings include cone-rod dystrophy, pigmentary retinopathy, subcapsular cataracts, waxy-optic disc pallor, hyperopia, central vision loss precedes peripheral visual loss, visual field constriction, abnormal cone and rod functions at birth seen on electroretinogram (ERG). Systemic findings include short stature, hearing loss, gingivitis, cardiomyopathy, gynecomastia, hepatitis, nephropathy, kyphosis, scoliosis, developmental delay, alopecia, diabetes insipidus, and growth hormone deficiency.

Prader–Willi Syndrome

Eye findings include almond-shaped eyes, strabismus, upslanting palpebral fissures, refractive errors, and bilateral cataracts.

Systemic findings include obesity, short stature, small hands and feet, hypotonia in infancy, hypogonadism with intellectual disability, thin upper lip, hypopigmentation and high-pain threshold, and childhood polyphagia.

Rubinstein–Taybi Syndrome

Eye findings include highly arched-eyebrows with long eyelashes, ptosis, epicanthal folds, strabismus, nasolacrimal duct obstruction, cataracts, glaucoma, coloboma, downward slanting palpebral fissures.

Systemic findings include short stature, microcephaly, grimacing or unusual smile with almost closing of the eyes, beaked-nose, deviated nasal septum, broad nasal bridge, small opening of the mouth, narrow palate, delayed skeletal maturation joint hypermobility, atrial septal defects, ventricular septal defects, broad thumbs with radial angulation, fifth finger clinodactyly, persistent fetal fingertip pads.

Walker–Warburg Syndrome

The various findings include hydrocephalus, argyria, and retinal dysplasia with or without encephalocele (HARD +/-E). Total agenesis of optic nerve and pathway has been described. Posterior lenticonus and ectopia lentis have been associated.

Systemic associations include lissencephaly, congenital muscular dystrophy, and encephalocele

Noonan Syndrome

Individuals who have Noonan syndrome have normal chromosome studies. Four genes—*PTPN11*, *SOS1*, *RADF1* and *KRAS*—are the only genes that are known to be associated with Noonan syndrome.

The child may have wide spaced eyes, light colored eyes, short neck, and low set ears. It involves short stature, heart defects present at birth, bleeding problems, developmental delays, and malformations of the bones of the rib cage. The intelligence is normal and the complication includes leukemia.

RETINITIS PIGMENTOSA AND ALLIED SYNDROMES

Usher Syndrome
Retinitis pigmentosa associated with deafness. Usher syndrome type I (congenital profound deafness, absent vestibular function, and prepubertal onset of retinitis pigmentosa). Usher syndrome type II (congenital moderate-severe deafness, normal vestibular dysfunction, and onset of retinitis pigmentosa in late-second to early-third decade). Usher syndrome type III (postlingual progressive deafness, variable vestibular dysfunction, and progressive retinitis pigmentosa with variable age of onset).

Bardet–Biedl Syndrome
Eye findings include rod-cone dystrophy, retinitis pigmentosa, retinal degeneration, strabismus, and cataracts.

Systemic findings include high-arched palate, dental crowding, hepatic fibrosis, hypogonadism, renal anomalies, polydactyly, usually postaxial, learning disabilities, developmental delay, intellectual disability, ataxia, and poor coordination.

Lawrence–Moon Syndrome
Eye findings include pigmentary retinopathy, nystagmus, and choroidal atrophy. Systemic findings include short stature, obesity, polydactyly, micropenis, hypoplastic scrotum, ataxia, intellectual disability, and spastic paraplegia.

Refsum Disease
It is an inborn error of lipid metabolism characterized by a tetrad of clinical abnormalities: (1) retinitis pigmentosa, (2) peripheral neuropathy, (3) cerebellar ataxia, and (4) elevated protein levels in the cerebrospinal fluid (CSF) without an increase in the number of cells.

Other findings include cardiomyopathy, shortening of the metacarpals, ichthyosis, peripheral sensorimotor neuropathy, hyporeflexia, limb atrophy, limb weakness, sensory impairment, and nerve hypertrophy.

Abetalipoproteinemia
People affected by this disorder are not able to make certain lipoproteins, which are molecules that consist of proteins combined with cholesterol and particular fats called triglycerides.

Apart from retinitis pigmentosa, the other findings may be fatty, pale-foul smelling stools, developmental delay, muscle weakness, slurred speech, scoliosis, progressive decreased vision, balance and coordination problems, and acanthocytosis and hypocholesterolemia.

Kearns–Sayre Syndrome
It has a mitochondrial inheritance.

Eye findings include progressive external ophthalmoplegia, pigmentary retinopathy, and ptosis.

Systemic findings include short stature, microcephaly, sensorineural hearing loss, complete heart block, cardiomyopathy, muscle weakness, ragged-red fibers seen on muscle biopsy, cerebellar ataxia, basal ganglia calcifications, diabetes mellitus, hypoparathyroidism, Addison disease, and diffuse signal abnormality of central white matter.

Cockayne syndrome (mentioned earlier).

Alstrom syndrome (mentioned earlier).

10.16 Pediatric Epiphora

Rajesh Chaudhuri
Netralayam, Kolkata
rajeshmchaudhuri@hotmail.com

INTRODUCTION

Epiphora is originally a Greek word meaning a sudden outflow.

It indicates an overflow of tears on the cheek, due to either excess tear production or impaired drainage by the tear ducts.

The most common cause of childhood epiphora is a membranous obstruction at the valve of Hasner at the distal end of the nasolacrimal duct (NLD). This has an incidence of 5–20% of the newborns depending on the study we look into.

Of course, we must remember that watery-eye in an infant or a child may indicate other serious ocular pathologies like congenital glaucoma and entropion which must be ruled out by thorough clinical examinations.

EMBRYOLOGY

Nasolacrimal duct develops from a solid cord of neuroectodermal cells buried in the cleft between the lateral nasal and maxillary processes. Canalization of the cord starts about 3 months of gestation and completes just before birth. The canalization starts at the middle of the cord and proceeds to the top and bottom. Therefore, the most common developmental anomalies are in the intrameatal NLD and the punctal area.

CLINICAL EVALUATION

- Thorough history, both ocular and general
- Clinical examination, both ocular and general
- Fluorescein dye disappearance test
- Regurgitation on pressure over the lacrimal sac (ROPLAS) test
- To rule out any congenital midline facial anomalies

MANAGEMENT PLAN FOR DISTAL NASOLACRIMAL DUCT BLOCK

- No universally structured protocol available
- Literature based on lower level evidence such as case reports and expert opinion
- Lack of higher level evidence such as randomized controlled trials and meta-analysis

The Prevailing Consensus Regarding Treatment of Congenital Nasolacrimal Duct Block

Plan for the First 12 Months

- Lacrimal sac massage (Kushner's modification of Crigler's technique) and topical antibiotic drops
- Probing within 1 year of age if the patient gets recurrent, severe infections

No Improvement in Condition after Proper Sac Massage and the Child is about 12 Months of Age

- The first probing may be attempted around 12–13 months of age.
- Primary probing procedure is successful in 70–97% of cases.
- Decreasing success with bilateral cases and increasing age of the child.

If the First Probing is Not Successful
- Repeat probing with or without inferior nasal turbinate infracture may be attempted 3–6 months after the initial failed probing.
- Success rate between 40 and 60%.

Other Options
- Silicone intubation
- Balloon dacryoplasty

These two procedures may be tried as a primary procedure or after previous failed probing. Literature does not really show any major difference in outcome compared to repeat probing.

FINALLY
Dacryocystorhinostomy is indicated in cases of failed repeat probing or intubation or complex (bony) lower lacrimal system obstruction. The procedure is usually performed around 4–5 years of age and has an excellent success rate in trained hands.

10.17 Myopia Progression in Children

Jitendra Jethani
Baroda Children Eye Care and Squint Clinic, Vadodara
xethani@rediffmail.com

INTRODUCTION
Myopia or short-sightedness is a condition where the rays coming from infinity are focused and anterior to retina and need an appropriate diverging or a concave lens to focus on retina for a sharp and focused image.

PROGRESSION OF MYOPIA
Myopia increases typically in school-going age children mainly due to axial elongation of eyeball as the age grows. Around 15–40% of children between 5 and 15 years of age have myopic progression. A child progressing >0.5 diopter myopia in a year is said to be a progressor.

AXIAL MYOPIA
When the myopia is secondary to axial elongation it is said to be axial myopia. The other types are curvature and index myopia.

PREMYOPIA (MYOPIA SUSPECT)
Though there is no consensus on premyopia, it is a condition where there is evidence that a particular child who may be hyperope or emmetrope has a history or axial elongation or reduction in hyperopia with age more than expected. There may be a history of myopia in siblings and parents.

PREVALENCE OF MYOPIA (IN INDIA)
- The prevalence of myopia in 5–15 years old urban children increased from 4.44% in 1999 to 21.15% in 2019.
- The prevalence of myopia will increase to 31.89% in 2030, 40.01% in 2040, and 48.14% in 2050.
- There will be an overall increase in myopia prevalence across all age groups of 10.53% in the next three decades (2020–2050).

TABLE 10.17.1: Factors affecting progression of myopia.

Natural factors	Environmental factors	
Genetic factors	Low outdoor timings	Increased near work
Family history	Using LED lamps	Reduced reading distance
Increasing age	Dim light exposure	More screen time
Prematurity (only in early years)	Urban environment	More reading time

■ MANAGEMENT

TABLE 10.17.2: History taking for a child with myopia/premyopia.

Birth history	Family history	Developmental history	Visual environment
Term/Preterm	Parental/Sibling myopia	Cerebral palsy	Number of hours of near work
Low birth weight	Progressive myopia	Delayed milestones	Type of near work and type of screen used
	Complications of myopia such as squint, amblyopia and peripheral retinal degenerations	Rule out syndromes such as Down's, Marfan's, etc.	Light condition at school and home

TABLE 10.17.3: Test done for a child with myopia.

Mandatory	Preferred	Helpful	Investigative
Visual acuity	Axial length	Aberrometry	Open-field autorefraction
Intraocular pressure	Keratometry	Corneal topography	Peripheral refraction
Slit lamp examination	• Binocular vision assessment including	Macular OCT	Tear-film assessment
Fundus evaluation	• Near point of accommodation, near point of convergence and accommodative lag	Pupillometry	Vitamin D levels
Cycloplegic refraction			

Risk Factors
- Younger age and higher baseline myopia
- Past myopia progression rate of >0.50 D/year
- Parental and sibling myopia (single parent two times risk)
- Environmental risk factors
  - Decreased outdoor activities
  - Increased near work and digital screen time
  - Vitamin D levels (indirect evidence of low outdoor activities)

First Time Evaluation
- Wait for progression if no family history of myopia.
- Compare their refractive error to the age-normal values.
- Measure accommodative lag, axial length and compare with normal values.

- Based on risk factor identification advice reduced near work and increased outdoor activities.
- Follow up after 3 months.

Environmental Modifications
- Reduce near work in dim light.
- Increased outdoor activities.
- Improved diet and physical activities.
- Improve sleep habits.
- Rule of 20-20-20 as mentioned in computer vision syndrome.

Pharmacological Intervention
Low concentration atropine (LCA) (0.01%)
- Most recommended and easy alternative at present. It is a nonselective irreversible antimuscarinic agent which reduces myopia progression by slowing axial length elongation.
- Easy availability, affordable, and minimal side effects. Few side effects are blurred vision and sensitivity to light, allergic conjunctivitis, etc.
- Some children may exhibit rebound phenomenon (there is rebound increase in the progression of myopia) after stopping the drug may be noted so needs tapering the dose and/or frequency of the drug when planning to discontinue its usage.
- Non-responders to atropine (0.01%) are children who progress despite putting the drops regularly.
- Young age of onset, high myopia children are more frequently non-responders to LCA.

Which children are suitable for LCA (0.01%)?
- Based on the risk factors if the child is a progressor or there is a history of axial progression noticed, LCA drops can be started once a day at bed time.
- The child is then called for follow-up after 2 weeks to assess near point of accommodation and near point of convergence and accommodative facility. Accommodative lag and pupil size also evaluated. Cover test to look for esophoria.
- If child complains of near vision problems or allergy then LCA drops are stopped and optical intervention can be tried.
- If child has no complains, the follow-up visit is at 3 months and then 6 months.
- Cycloplegic refraction is done along with axial length measurements and tests recommended in every 6 months.
- If there is no progression LCA drops are to be continued till 2 years. After two years, the drops are tapered off gradually to prevent any rebound phenomenon over a period of 3-6 months. The child is followed up and if there is a progression again LCA drops can be started till 15 years of age.
- If there is a progression despite putting the drops, then one of the following can be done.
  - The frequency of drops can be increased to two times a day. Again follow-up after 1 month to look for any complains of blurring of vision, photophobia, accommodative facility, and pupil size.
  - The concentration of atropine can be increased to LCA (0.05%) once a day. Follow-up should be done to look for any complains of blurring of vision, photophobia, accommodative facility, and pupil size. Progressive add on lens can be prescribed in selected children if complains of blurring of vision for near.
  - Peripheral refraction with retinoscope or open field autorefractometer can be done and optical interventions can be added along with LCA drops.
- Contraindications for starting atropine therapy
  - *Down's syndrome:* Cycloplegic effects and potential systemic toxicity
  - Congenital heart disease

- Cerebral palsy
- History of asthma or other lung diseases
- Already on other medications that may have anticholinergic or antimuscarinic effects, e.g., some antidepressants and antihistamines.

Optical Measures

Spectacles

- Miyosmart (Hoya) (defocus-incorporated multiple segment spectacles)
- *Stellest (Essilor) (highly aspheric lenslets spectacles):* Special spectacles are designed with the aim to reduce or eliminate peripheral hyperopic defocus. Children with high peripheral hyperopic defocus may have axial growth due to this. These spectacles have peripheral add on hyperopic power which causes a myopic defocus and thereby reduce the stimulus for growth.
- *Progressive add on lenses:* These may work by reducing accommodation lag during extended near work by inducing relative myopic shifts in peripheral refractive error. May be useful when the child is on LCA and has complains for near vision blur due to effect of LCA drops on accommodation, children with esophorias and accommodative lag **(Table 10.17.4)**.

TABLE 10.17.4: Advantages and disadvantages of progressive spectacles for myopia progression.

Advantages	Disadvantages
Simple and easy to fit	Efficacy with peripheral hyperopic defocus patient
Well tolerated	Expensive compared to monovision

Contact Lenses

- *Orthokeratology:* The rigid lenses are reverse geometry lenses which act by reshaping and flattening the central part of the cornea. This causes a relative myopic shift in peripheral retina.

TABLE 10.17.5: Advantages and disadvantages of contact lens use for progressive myopia.

Advantages	Disadvantages
The need to wear glasses is eliminated	Risk of microbial keratitis
	Needs trained practitioner
	May have rebound effect

- *Soft multifocal contact lenses*
  Not readily available in India there are multiple companies which claim benefit. The disadvantages are similar to abovementioned for orthokeratology. This would be under off label usage. The children may experience blurring of vision initially.

  MiSight® 1 day (CooperVision) and NaturalVue® (Visioneering Technologies) are daily disposable lenses specially designed and approved for use in myopia in some countries.

  SEED 1 dayPure EDOF soft contact lens is a center-distance contact lens with peripheral add working on extended depth of focus principle to control myopia and is available in India.

  Proclear® toric multifocal (CooperVision) lenses have been used in myopia with astigmatism.

SELECTION OF TREATMENT STRATEGIES

A lot of treatment strategies are now available for control of myopia progression. Here are few points to know which one would be useful. This would be based on following considerations:

- *Rate of progression:* Estimation of the rate at which myopia progresses for a given individual may help identify an appropriate strategy. One can combine the two modalities such as LCA eye drops with progressive add-ons or with Stellest lenses along with low concentration atropine eye drops.
- Baseline refractive error and age (younger age generally leads to faster myopia progression). One needs to be more aggressive when the child has progression at a younger age. One should keep an eye open for progression in children who have been diagnosed with myopia at a younger age.
- Binocular vision status (greater myopia control effects with progressive spectacles were reported in children with larger lags of accommodation and near esophoria). All patients should undergo a check of accommodative lag and peripheral refraction to have an appropriate strategy.
- Environmental and lifestyle modifications must be advised with any form of optical or pharmacological intervention and have been discussed above.
- Children who possess multiple risk factors may require more strategic management and frequent review, compared to those with little or no associated risk factors.
- Maintain follow-up at the scheduled time and record the parameters accordingly. Keep an eye on the ocular health of the child and examine whenever necessary.

*"If you can't explain it simply,
you don't understand it well enough".*

—**Albert Einstein**

Index

Page numbers followed by *f* refer to figure, *fc* refer to flowchart, and *t* refer to table.

A

Ab externo suture fixation
    technique 166, 167*f*
    modifications of 167
    small-incision 167
Ab interno
    canaloplasty 300, 300*f*
    technique 168
Abatacept 439, 440
Abduction, bilateral 908
Aberrations 348
    free intraocular lenses 185
    order of 349
    spherical 155, 185, 370
Aberrometry 307
    intraoperative 190
Abetalipoproteinemia 494, 943
Abicipar 571
Ablation zone, decentration of 383
Abscess
    choroidal 629
    corneal 541*f*
    formation 837
    intraorbital 778, 781
    lacrimal 838, 839
Acanthamoeba 28, 72, 447
    keratitis 28, 37, 55
Acetazolamide 245
    oral 266
Acetylcholine 730
    deficiency of 709
Achromatopsia 594, 620, 928
Acid 78
    burn 79*f*
    fast bacilli 448*f*
Acinetobacter baumannii 544
Acquired immunodeficiency syndrome 77, 735
Acquired lacrimal duct obstruction, secondary 816, 830, 833, 835
Acquired nasolacrimal duct obstruction, primary 816
Acrochordon 745
Acrylic eye, painting on 866
Acrylic grinding 864, 866*f*
Acrylic plate 289

Actinomyces 22, 23, 840
Actinomycetales 22
Actinomycetes 878
Actinomycosis 424
Activated partial thromboplastin time 432
Active fluidics system 109, 372
Active vision therapy 895, 897
Acute angle-closure
    crisis 228
    glaucoma 228
Acyclovir 32, 33, 54
Adalimumab 438, 439, 440
Add-on sulcoflex lens 397*f*
Adenocarcinoma, ciliary 450
Adenoid cystic carcinoma 454, 455, 455*f*, 763
    pathology of 455
Adenosine deaminase 593
Adenoviruses 9
Adherence syndrome 924
Adhesion, prevent 80
Adjacent conjunctiva, biopsy of 45
Adnexa 746*fc*, 829*f*
Adnexal trauma 795
    classification of 795, 795*fc*
Advanced glaucoma 273
    intervention study 145
Advanced macular traction maculopathy 589*f*
Adventitious sheath 478
A-exotropia 916
Afferent pupillary defect 482
    relative 467, 680
Aflibercept 480, 483, 486, 517, 569, 587
Age-related cataract, risk factors for 83
Age-related eye disease
    modification in 633
    study 633, 634
Age-related macular degeneration 83, 368, 484, 495, 503, 511, 532, 542*f*, 563, 568, 580, 594, 612, 631, 633*f*, 634*fc*, 646, 666
    advance 632, 632*f*
    early 631, 632*f*

intermediate 631, 632*f*
nonexudative
    neovascular 485
    non-neovascular 646*f*
Ahmed glaucoma valve 290, 292, 294
Aicardi's syndrome 942
Air bubble
    dimpling 57
    entrapment of 57
Albendazole, oral 37, 785
Albinism 939
Albright's syndrome 762
Albuminuric retinitis 621
Alcaftadine 13
Alcian blue stained slide 448*f*
Alcohol
    application of 848
    consumption 83
    keratoepitheliectomy 803*f*
Alefacept 439, 440
Alemtuzumab 439, 440
Alizarin stain 449*f*
Alkali
    burn 78*f*
    injuries 78
Alkedol 98
Alkyl nitrate abuse 620
Allen-type devices 859
Allergic conjunctivitis, seasonal 12
Allergic disease 22
Allergic disorder 12
Allergy 56
Allevyn cavity dressing 851
Allogenic corneal implants 377
Alloplastic implant 853
Alopecia 438, 942
Alpha-hemolytic streptococci 23
Alport's syndrome 941, 942
Alveolar soft part sarcoma 761
Alzheimer's disease 702
Amadeus microkeratome 318*f*
Amblyopia 95, 267, 708, 737, 765, 768, 883, 895, 910
    chance of 710
    management 911
    treatment of 895, 896, 909

Amblyopic 95
    eyes 653
Amblyopiogenic factor,
    removal of 895
Ambrósio relational
    thickness 307
Amebic deoxyribonucleic
    acid 29
Amethocaine 54
Ametropia, modified
    formulas for 218
Amikacin 24, 25
Amino acids 934
Aminoglycosides 29, 55
Amniotic band syndrome 938
Amniotic membrane 54
    transplantation 80
Amoaku classification 530
Amphotericin B 27
    topical 27
Ampicillin-clavulanic acid 838
Amplitude scan 603
Amyloidosis 415, 769
Anakinra 439, 440
Analgesics 230
Ancillary tests 421, 424, 680
Anderson's criteria 275
Anderson's Whitnall
    advancement
    surgery 713
Ando iridectomy 551
Anemia 437, 596
Anesthesia 104, 136, 144, 279,
        292, 725, 831, 850
    choice of 848
    facial 105, 106
    general 105, 107, 584
    intracameral 104, 106
    intraconal 106
    local 93, 584
    retrobulbar 104, 106
    segmental 71
    topical 104, 105, 260
    type of 923
Aneurysms 426, 502
Angiofibromas 750
Angiogenesis 568
Angiogram, phases of
    normal 500
Angiography 476, 477f
    oral 503
Angioid streaks 657
Angiolymphoid hyperplasia 747
Angiomas 751
Angiotensin-converting
    enzyme 44, 418, 678,
    771, 792
Angle kappa 369
Angle-closure glaucoma 268
    primary 262
    secondary 257

Anhidrosis, facial 685
Aniridia 182
Aniridic eyes,
    phacoemulsification
    in 182
Aniridic prosthetic devices 184
Anisocoria 680, 684, 685, 685t
    pathological 684
Anisometropia 267, 894, 896
Ankyloblepharon 856
Ankylosing spondylitis 413,
        424, 439
Anophthalmic socket 852,
        862, 862f
    syndrome 861
Anophthalmos, congenital 855
Anorexia 437
Anterior chamber 119, 122,
        126, 147, 152, 158, 165,
        174, 200, 244, 249f, 260,
        289, 345f-347f, 395,
        413, 469f, 680
    angle, distortion of 246
    depth 150, 217, 254, 339, 343
        assessment 340
    flare 228, 414t
    intraocular lens 131, 158, 159f
        current status of 162
        Strampelli tripod 159f
    moderate to severe 539
    normal 287
    paracentesis 414
    postoperative shallow 255
    reformation 287
    shallowing of 126
    stable 111
Anterior segment 416
    disease, active 339
    ischemia 924
    manifestations 431
    optical coherence
        tomography 66, 85,
        135, 312, 340, 347f, 360,
        371, 373, 401, 607, 820,
        821f
    procedure 519f
Anterior stromal
    infiltrates 34
    puncture 17
Anterior synechiae, peripheral
        161, 232, 249, 257
Antiamebic agents 29
Antibacterial regimen 39
Antibiotic 5, 17, 629
    broad-spectrum 782, 840
    chronic use of 238
    intracameral 101
    intravenous 24, 543
    intravitreal 65, 540f, 546, 546f
    lid scrubs 720

ointment 825
    postoperative 64
    prophylaxis 80, 99
    steroid eye drops 282
    therapy
        modified 25t
        oral 721
Antibodies 44, 71
Anticardiolipin
    immunoglobulin G 432
Anticonvulsants 927
Anti-deoxyribonucleic acid 71
Antiemetics 230
Antifibrotic
    agents 238
    therapy 235
Antifungal
    agents 575, 576t
    drugs 540f
Antigens
    bacterial 39
    viral 430
Antiglaucoma drugs 877
Antiglaucoma medications 54
    topical 35, 879
Antiglaucoma surgery 551, 560
Anti-inflammatory
    therapy 5, 406
Anti-interleukin 440
    therapies 438, 441
Antimetabolite 234, 280
    application of 280, 281f, 284
    toxicity 253
    treatment 284
    use of 236, 255
Antimicrobial treatment 247
Antineutrophil cytoplasmic
        antibody 44, 427, 678
Antinuclear antibodies 44, 71,
        678, 771
Antioxidant 632
    lutein 633
Antiphospholipid
    antibodies 428
Anti-thyrotropin receptor
    antibodies 809
Antitubercular therapy 418,
        423, 425, 428
Anti-tumor necrosis
    factor-alpha 441
    agents 440
Antivascular endothelial
    growth factor 433, 464,
    468, 515, 535, 568-570,
    580, 626
    agents 556, 569, 613, 615
    drugs 517, 564
    injection 499
    intravitreal injections of 556
    preoperative 497

Index

therapy 258, 485f, 504f, 531, 565
treatment of 587
Antiviral agents 32
topical 32t
Apert's syndrome 759
Aphakia 161, 291, 292, 549
Aphakic bullous keratopathy 18, 50
Aphakic eye 222, 248
Aponeurosis 798
Appetite, loss of 675
Applanation tonometry 228
Apraclonidine 21
Aquacel 851
Aqueous humor 264, 270
sub-tenon drainage of 301
Aqueous misdirection
glaucoma 246f
syndrome 231
Aravind aqueous drainage implant 251
Arboviruses 429
Arciform translation 317
Arcuate scotoma, superior 277f, 278f
Argon laser
cilioplasty 2
trabeculoplasty 145
Argyria 942
Arlt's triangle 413
Arnold-Chiari malformation 942
Arteriovenous malformation 747, 766, 767
Arteritic anterior ischemic optic neuropathy 673-675
Arthritis 412
juvenile idiopathic 412, 426, 440
Artificial eye 862
Artificial intelligence 556
Artificial tear 406, 720
lubricating drops 49
A-scan 603
Asepsis, maintenance of 96
Aspergillosis 424, 784
Aspergillus 575, 629, 630
cell wall component of 575
endophthalmitis 628
flavus 784
fumigatus 628, 784
niger 784
Aspiration flow rate 108-110, 137
Astigmatism 59, 339, 494, 894, 896
corneal 58
correction 352
irregular corneal 265

management of 189
surgically induced 151
toric intraocular lenses for 186
Ataxia-telangiectasia 940
Atopy 387
Atresia, congenital 823
Atrophic hole 459f
Atrophy
foveal 506f, 507
geographical 633f
macular 586f
Atropine 892
low concentration 947
Aurolab aqueous drainage implant 290, 290f
Autograft, conjunctival 237
Autoimmune
diseases 436, 718, 770
disorders 526, 718
inflammations 786
Autologous blood injection 237, 260
Autologous bone marrow, use of 495
Autologous neurosensory retinal free flap 492
Autorefractometry 395
A-V pattern deviations 915
Avascular retina, peripheral 504f, 553, 582f
Avastin 569
Axial length 370
measurement 218
Axial myopia 945
Azathioprine 45, 72, 436, 437, 792
Azelastine 13
Azithromycin 9, 39, 721
oral 25, 39, 418
Azotobacter 22

B

Bacillocid rasant 97
Bacillus
cereus 629
subtilis 64
Bacteria 20, 100, 447, 834, 839
gram-negative 23
gram-positive 830
Bacterial keratitis 26, 43
management of 22
Bacteriology 837
Bacteroides 22, 837
Baerveldt implant 290, 290f
Baggy lower eyelids 728
Bagolini's striated glasses 899, 901
Baiocchi-Calossi-Versad front and back index 311

Balanced salt solution 112, 113, 147, 152, 280, 382
Balloon
dacryoplasty 827
punctoplasty 878
Bandage contact lens 17, 19, 35, 45, 47, 50, 80
Band-shaped keratopathy 53, 53f, 394, 413, 415, 416, 419
management of 551
Bardet-Biedl syndrome 494, 943
Barraquer microkeratome 317
Barrett true-K formula 335, 336
Bartonella henselae
immunofluorescence assay 418
Bartonella neuroretinitis 423
Basal cell carcinoma 443, 443f, 734, 735
Basal lamina around cells 888
Basement membrane damage 79
Basiliximab 439, 440
Bassen-Kornzweig syndrome 494
B-cells 440
inhibitors 439
Beard flap 742f, 743f
Bebie curve 275
Behçet's disease 423, 424, 426-428, 436, 437, 439, 440, 478
Belin-ambrósio enhanced ectasia display total deviation value 311
Bell's phenomenon 711
Bellinvia's incision 724
Benedikt's syndrome 681
Bent 25-gauge needle 300f
Bent ab interno needle goniectomy 299
Benzalkonium chloride 21, 54, 57, 98
Berke-Reese incision 775, 873
Berlin's edema 661
Best-corrected visual acuity 131, 462, 540f, 541f, 543f, 624f, 699f, 802f
Beta-blockers 54, 230, 251
topical 245, 266
Beta-glucans 38
Betamethasone 70
Betaxolol 266
Bevacizumab 439, 480, 483, 486, 566, 569, 587
Bhabha Atomic Research Centre 803
Biarcuate scotoma 278f
Bicoronal flap 873

Biguanides 29
Bimatoprost 245
Binkhorst's formula 217, 218
Binkhorst's lenses 160*f*
Binocular indirect
    ophthalmomicroscope
    519*f*, 520*f*
Binocular vision 898
Bioabsorbable synthetic
    material 857
Bioceramic orbital implant 860
Biodegradable agents,
    temporary 732
Biomechanical assessment
    313, 315, 316*f*
Biomechanical index 307
Biometry 87
    preoperative 396
Biomicroscopy 528
Biopsy 45, 418, 844*f*
    conjunctival 45
    intralesional steroids 763
    preoperative 888
Biplanar corneal
    incision 116, 214*f*
Bipolar cells 495
Birdshot
    chorioretinopathy 426, 440
    choroidopathy 420
    retinochoroidopathy 427
    retinopathy 439
Birt-Hogg-Dubé syndrome 750
Black spots 359
Bladder 438
Blau syndrome 412
Bleb
    failure 236, 285, 287
    fibrosis 234
        early 234
    leaks
        early-onset 237
        late-onset 237
    needling of 235
    resuturing of 237
Blebitis 236, 238, 571
Bleeding 92
Bleomycin 736, 801
Blepharitis 4, 8, 238, 718, 719*f*,
    723, 875
    anterior 5, 719
    posterior 719
    treatment for 720, 736
Blepharoconjunctivitis 722, 736
Blepharophimosis syndrome
    713, 713*f*, 715, 715*f*
Blepharoptosis 708
Blepharospasm, benign
    essential 731
Blind eyes 846
Blindness worldwide,
    causes of 83*f*

Blood 296
    ocular-barrier 623
    pressure 84, 624*f*, 625*f*, 917
        control 623
        monitor 423
        retinal barrier 524
    sugar 423, 678
        fasting 917
        profile 596
    transfusions 66
    vessels, endothelial
        cell of 761
Bloodstream 571
Blue field entoptoscopy 89, 653
Blue light-filtering intraocular
    lenses 188
Blue nevi 748
Blunt
    dissection 831
    keratome 19
    phaco tip 124
    trauma 50, 661, 922
Blurred vision 49, 244, 415,
    656, 804, 830, 917
Body's immune system 56
Bone
    cyst, bone window of 871*f*
    decompression 790
    disorders 935, 938
    graft 855
        autogenous 756
    marrow 80
        suppression 437, 438
    spicule retinal
        pigmentation 494*f*
Bony lacrimal fossa changes 828
Bony ostium, dimensions of 831
Borreliosis 424
Bortezomib 4
Botox injection 7
Botulinum toxin 730, 911
    injection 808, 911
Bovine pericardium,
    processed 857
Bowel disorders 940
Bowman's lacrimal probe 818
Bowman's layer 60
    transplantation 60
Bowman's membrane 18, 53,
    60, 393
    lack of 53
    transplant 52
Bowmen's probe 825*f*
Brachytherapy 558, 559*f*
Bradycardia 765
Brain
    computed tomography scan
        of 682, 690
    magnetic resonance
        imaging of 674
    tumor 528*f*
Brainstem disease 927

Branch retinal vascular
    occlusion 478
    risk factor for 478
Branch retinal vein occlusion
    478, 480*f*, 531, 665
    signs of 478
Brightness scan 603
Brimonidine 230, 245, 266
Brinzolamide 266
Broad adherent epiretinal
    membrane 600
Brolucizumab 487, 569
Bromfenac 104
Bronchoalveolar lavage 418
Brow ache 239
Brown syndrome 921
Brucella 446
Brucellosis 11
Bruch's membrane 619, 657
Brüchner test 892
B-scan 417, 603
    ultrasonography 244
    role of 562
Buckle placement 198
Bulbar conjunctiva, superior 57
Bull's eye 507
    appearance 134
    pattern 506*f*
Bullous keratopathy 18
    current management of 204
    therapy for 19
Bullous pemphigoid 74
Bunny's line 731, 731*f*, 732*f*
Burst mode 124
Buttonholes 400

C

Café-au-lait spots 770, 880*f*
Calcineurin inhibitors 436
    topical 13
Calcium 794, 934
    deposits 54, 449*f*
Calcofluor white stain 37*f*
Caldwell's view 753
Canakinumab 439
Canalicular inflammatory
    disorder, idiopathic 876
Canalicular laceration,
    management of 798
Canalicular mucosa,
    normal 819*f*
Canalicular obstructions
    831, 878
Canalicular trephination 879
Canaliculi 876
Canaliculitis 839, 840, 878
    primary chronic 839
Canaliculus
    current status of 799*f*
    injuries 799
    lower 799*f*

Candida 630
  albicans 628, 723
  endogenous
    endophthalmitis 573*f*
  glabrata 630
  krusei 630
  septicemia 628*f*
  tropicalis 628
Cannula, smoothly curved 817
Canthal tendon 717
  severed lateral 798
Cantholysis 741*f*
  lateral 873
Canthopexy 716
  lateral 717
Canthotomy 741*f*
  closure of 741*f*
  orbitotomy, lateral 777
Canthus subcutaneous
    tissue 776
Cap lenticular adhesion 360
Capillary closure 528
Capillary nonperfusion 421, 622
Capillary plexus, superficial 477*f*
Capsular bag 129
  dialysis 114
  distension syndrome
    114, 398
Capsular delamination 269
Capsular hooks 128
Capsular tension
  ring 114, 128, 129, 131, 184
  segment 114, 128
Capsule rupture, signs of pre-
    existing posterior 138
Capsulopalpebral ligament 707
Capsulorhexis 113, 121, 127,
    136, 214, 371
  extension of 114
  incomplete 131
  primary posterior 934
Capsulotomy
  anterior 119, 209, 213
  posterior 212
  primary posterior 210*f*
Carbon dioxide
    accumulation 56
Carbonic anhydrase inhibitor,
    oral 27
Cardiomyopathy 942
Cardiovascular disease 627
Carlevale lens 171, 171*f*
Caroticocavernous fistula 872
Carotid
  artery disease 257
  cavernous fistulas 690
Carpenter's plane 317
Carriazo pendular
    microkeratome 318,
    319*f*

Carriazo-Barraquer
    microkeratome 318
Cartilaginous tumors 454, 762
Caruncle, examination of 815
Caruncular edema 789
Caruncular hypertrophy
    opposing lower
    punctum 816*f*
Castroviejo electrokeratome 317
Castroviejo implant 859
Cat paw retractor 831
Cat scratch disease 415, 418
Cataract 13, 78, 81, 83, 88, 90,
    91, 95, 131, 132, 145,
    175, 196, 292, 267, 339,
    346, 416, 419, 528, 570,
    617, 654
  age-related 84, 86
  bilateral 208
  evaluation 143
  extraction 146, 247
  family history of 83
  formation 288, 483
  location of 933
  maturity, level of 270
  mild 85
  moderate 85
  procedure 246
  progression of 196
  risk factors for 83, 84*f*
  severe 85
  simultaneous 197
  surgery 88, 99, 104, 131,
    140, 143, 145, 146, 175,
    182, 196, 197, 203, 204,
    212, 312, 413, 462*f*, 521,
    551, 591, 592, 652
    base of 91
    indications for 208
    indications of 95
    informed consent for 91
    perform 131
    risks of 91
    techniques of anesthesia
      for 104
    type of 522
  surgical management of 127
  traumatic 149, 200
  type of 143
  unilateral
    complete 208
    partial 208
  wound neovascularization
    247
Cataractous lens absorbs 617
Catheter angiography 682
Cavernous body 828, 828*f*
Cavernous hemangioma 453,
    454*f*, 747, 760, 769
  pathology of 454
  posterior 802*f*

Cavernous sinus 781
  lesions 681, 682, 684
  thrombosis 778, 781, 836
Cavernous venous
    malformation 767
Cavitron ultrasonic surgical
    aspirator 875
Cefazolin 25, 64
Ceftazidime 25, 178
Ceftriaxone 9, 25
Cefuroxime 101
  intracameral 101
Cell
  carcinoma, transitional 845
  count 427
  melanoma, mixed 451
  membrane damage 526
  tumors, round 448
Cell-to-cell movement 30
Cellular schwannoma 887
Cellulitis 836
Centraflow technology 342*f*
Central foveal
  cavitation 509*f*
  thickness 474, 615
Central iridocorneal touch 253
Central macular
    thickness 506*f*, 618
Central nervous system 412,
    419, 838
  severe 937
Central retinal
  apposition 562
  artery 528
    occlusion 431
  thickness 588*f*, 615
  values 483
  vein occlusion 431, 481,
    481*f*, 482*t*, 531
    risk factors of 481
    signs of 482
    treatment of 484
Central serous
    chorioretinopathy
    408, 502*f*, 579, 615, 648,
    649*f*
  extramacular variant of 651*f*
  pregnancy-induced 651
  types of 648, 651
Central serous retinopathy 515
Centripetal vascularization,
    stage of progressive 877
Centurion syndrome 715
Centurion vision system 110
Ceramic implants 859
Cerebellar disease 927
Cerebellar hemispheres,
    dysplasia of 942
Cerebral venous sinus
    thrombosis 675

Index

Cerebrospinal fluid 616, 755
  analysis 427
Certolizumab 439, 440
Cervical dystonia 731
Cervical lymph nodes 708
  anterior 734
Cervico-oculo-acoustic
  syndrome 938
Cetuximab 736
Chalazia 3
  chance of 4
  recurrent 39
Chalazion 3, 441, 442f, 721
Chandler's classification 778
Chédiak-Higashi syndrome 940
Chemical
  disinfection 97
  injury 50, 78, 240, 242, 799
Chemosis 10, 22, 780f-782f,
  787f, 789
Chemotherapeutic
  drugs 877, 879
Chemotherapy
  concurrent 526
  topical 76
Chest
  computed tomography
    scan of 414,, 427
  high-resolution computed
    tomography scan of 422
  X-ray 414, 422, 934
Chiasmal compressive
  lesions 690
Chiasmal glioma 927
Chikungunya 420, 429
Chin augmentation 733
Chirped pulse amplification 321
Chlamydia 447
  trachomatis 74
  infection 9
Chlorambucil 436
Chloramphenicol 37
Chlorhexidine 29, 37
Chlorobutanol 21
Chondroitin sulfate 152
Chop pattern 214
Choriocapillaris 434f, 476, 610
  atrophy 646
  ischemia 648
Chorioretinal atrophy 585,
  586, 586f
Chorioretinal scars 242
Chorioretinitis 420
Chorioretinopathy
  chronic central serous 650f
  idiopathic central serous
    645, 645f
Choristomas 453
Choroid
  inflammatory diseases of 647f

malignant melanoma of
  451, 451f
patch technique 566
Choroidal atrophy 588
Choroidal detachment 287,
  549, 604, 604f, 661, 662
  pre- and postoperative 549
Choroidal effusion 232, 236, 254
Choroidal flush 500
Choroidal lymphoma,
  primary 450
Choroidal melanoma 451, 531,
  536, 557, 559f, 604f, 669f
  brown mushroom-
    shaped 557f
  management of 558
Choroidal neovascular
  membrane 408, 421,
  424, 464, 484, 485, 485f,
  542f, 586f, 587, 588f,
  590, 590f 631, 647, 665
  causes of 655
  risk of 651
  signs of 632
Choroidal neovascularization
  419, 421, 485, 569, 570,
  613
  causes of 655
  idiopathic 659
  treatment of 271
Choroidal nevus 558, 655
Choroidal rupture 656
Choroidal schwannoma 450
Choroidal vascular beds 623
Choroidal vessels 622
Choroideremia 595
Choroiditis 420, 659
Choroidopathy,
  hypertensive 622, 623
Chromatopsia 618
Chromosomal aberrations 451
Chronic dacryocystitis 828,
  829fc, 830, 831, 842, 843
  etiopathogenesis of 831f
  management of 833fc
  pathogenetic stages of 830
Churg-Strauss syndrome 426
Ciancia syndrome 911
Cicatricial conjunctivitis 2, 74
Cicatricial pemphigoid 74
  drug-induced 21
Cicatrix formation, oral 856
Cicatrization, conjunctival 74
Cilia, loss of 737
Ciliary artery, posterior 561
Ciliary body 247
  leiomyoma 450
  melanoma 450
  schwannoma 450
  tumors 605

Ciliary nonpigment epithelium
  adenoma of 450
  Fuchs' adenoma of 450
Ciliary pigment epithelium,
  adenoma of 450
Ciliary processes
  diffuse ablation of 303
  swelling of 231
Ciliary sulcus fixation 167, 196
  knotless ab externo
    technique for 168
  two-point 168
Ciliochoroidal detachment
  253, 255, 606
Cilio-vitreo-lenticular
  block 231
  glaucoma 231
Ciprofloxacin 24
  oral 178
Cirrhosis 437
Cisplatin 736
Claude's syndrome 681
Claustrophobia 773
Clear corneal incisions 212
Clear lens extraction 368
Climatic droplet
  keratopathy 393
Clotrimazole 29
Cluster endophthalmitis 543,
  545, 546
  suspicion of 546
Coats' disease 503, 531, 579, 581
Coaxial corneal light reflex 359
Coccidioides immitis 572
Cochlear implants 773
Cockayne syndrome 940, 943
Cogan's lid twitch sign 709
Cogan's syndrome 42
Cola bottle sign 787f
Colchicine 436
Colenbrander's formula 218
Colistin
  methanesulfate 544
  sulfonylmethate 544
Collagen cross-linking 386,
  387, 390, 394
  complication of 386, 387
  indications of 386
  progression after 389
Coloboma 581
Color fundus photography 421
Color vision 678, 770
Comitant esodeviations
  906, 907
Commotio retinae 661, 753
Compartment syndrome 727
Complete blood count 71,
  674, 934
Compression sutures 260
Compressive lesions 695

Index

Computed tomography 820
 dacryocystography 816
 scan 418, 433, 445, 689, 754, 772, 868, 917
Conbercept 571
Concha bullosa 830
Cone dystrophy 507
 progressive 494
Cone outer segment
 tips 489, 489*f*
Conformer 862, 863*f*
Congenital glaucoma 823
 treatment of 266
Congenital nasolacrimal duct
 block, treatment of 944
 obstruction 8, 815, 823, 876
Congenital nevi 748
Congestion 413
 chronic cicatricial 573
 conjunctival 785, 786*f*
 pattern of 413
Congo red stained slide 449*f*
Conjunctiva 282, 288, 413, 559, 707, 708, 713, 744, 753, 848, 859, 873
 avascular 260
 examination of 815
 fold of 815
 palpebral 708
Conjunctival closure 282, 282*f*, 284, 295, 295*f*
Conjunctival defect 255
Conjunctival dissection 285
Conjunctival flap 280
Conjunctival graft 738
Conjunctival incision 283, 728, 923
Conjunctival injection
 bilateral 8
 unilateral 8
Conjunctival leaks 286
Conjunctival lesions,
 malignant 850
Conjunctival mobility 292
Conjunctival mobilization 237
Conjunctival redness 22, 789
Conjunctival resection 45
Conjunctival retraction 284
Conjunctival sac 818
Conjunctival scarring 79, 923
Conjunctival shrinkage 21
Conjunctival thinning 861
Conjunctivitis 8, 10, 238, 431, 433, 809
 adenoviral 10*f*
 allergic 12
 bacterial 7, 12
 chronic 21, 74
 follicular 11
 infective 74

neonatal inclusion 11
 viral 69
Conjunctivochalasis 815
Connective tissue 935, 938
Contact lens 46, 52, 55, 255, 406, 520, 894, 928, 948*t*
 complications 8
 materials 56
 method 219
 over refraction 334
 rehabilitation 398
 users 55
 wear 55
Continuous curvilinear
 capsulorhexis 113, 122, 127, 136, 149, 151, 195, 209
 size of 121
Contoura vision 352
 technology 392
Contracted socket 854
 malignant 854, 855
Contrast magnetic resonance
 imaging 692
Convergence, types of 905
Cornea 1, 10, 15, 42, 56, 57, 66, 250, 254, 294, 332, 332*f*, 333*f*, 413, 703
 cross-section of 379*f*
 peripheral donor 67
 punctate staining of 22
Corneal aberrations 528
Corneal abrasion 55, 729
Corneal allogenic intrastromal
 ring segments 52
Corneal arcuate incisions 213
Corneal basement
 membrane 79
Corneal biomechanical
 assessment 307
 index 315
Corneal button, removal of 848
Corneal changes 55, 71
Corneal collagen
 cross-linking 47, 52, 132, 383
 technique of 52
Corneal cross-linking
 progression after 387
 types of 386
Corneal decompensation 159, 236, 291, 346
Corneal deformation, stages
 of 314*f*
Corneal dellen 69, 924
Corneal dermoids 265
Corneal diameter 265
Corneal diseases 368
Corneal dissecting blebs 261
Corneal dystrophies 393
 anterior 393

Corneal ectatic disorders 339
Corneal edema,
 chronic stromal 264
Corneal endothelial
 cell damage 150
 count 396
 defect 55, 402
 desiccation 57
 erosions 393
 healing 79
 pathology 161
 punctate 57
 status 292
Corneal graft 65, 292
 infection 63
 rejection 18
 treatment of 68
Corneal guttata 153
Corneal haze 265, 383, 387, 389
Corneal incision
 advantages of 118*t*
 disadvantages of 118*t*
 placement 213*f*
 sutureless clear 118
Corneal infiltration 383
Corneal injury, traumatic 22
Corneal inlays 376, 407
Corneal involvement 544*f*
Corneal irritation,
 consequence of 264
Corneal lenticule extraction 322
Corneal melt 387, 390
 disorders, peripheral 46
Corneal mucus plaques 34
Corneal neovascularization 31
Corneal opacification 528, 553
Corneal opacities 414
 extensive central 149
 subepithelial 11
Corneal pachymetry 87
 evaluation 313
Corneal patch graft 295*f*
Corneal pathologies 214, 312
Corneal perforation 20, 387, 390
Corneal power 217, 218
 measurement, true 334
Corneal procedures 376
Corneal protection,
 temporary 7
Corneal scars 267, 393
Corneal sensations 31, 770
Corneal stromal
 dystrophies 48*t*
 healing 79
Corneal surface,
 applanation of 327*f*
Corneal surgery 309
Corneal thickness spatial
 profile 311
Corneal topography 46, 307, 343, 353*f*, 361*f*

Index

Corneal toxicity 54
Corneal ulcer 20, 22
    development of 14
    management of 22
Corneal vascularization 5
Corneal warpage 56
Corneal wound
    construction 213
Corneoscleral invasion 803f
Coronal brow lift 730
Coronavirus disease 2019
    (COVID-19) 40, 420,
    430, 432
    ocular manifestations of
        430
    ophthalmic
        manifestations of 433
    orbital manifestation of 432
    pandemic 628
    uveitis in 432
    vaccination 40
Corpus callosum,
    agenesis of 942
Corrected near visual acuity 379
Corticosteroids 32, 75, 271,
    272, 418, 425, 428, 433,
    523, 777, 793
    oral 792
Corynebacterium 22, 25, 64
Cosmetic eyelids surgeries 723
Cotrimoxazole 418
Cotton-wool spots 528, 530f,
    533f, 534f, 622, 625f
Cover test 711, 907, 919f
Cover-uncover test 907
Coxsackievirus B infection 424
Cranial nerve palsy 679, 690
Craniocervical junction 927
Craniofacial dysostosis 759
Craniofacial malformations
    935, 937
Craniostenosis 937
C-reactive protein 427, 674,
    675, 678
Cribriform 455
Crigler's massage 825, 828
Crocodile tears 731
Crohn's disease 439
Crouzon's syndrome 759
Cruise control 141, 141f
Cryotherapy 2, 460, 736
Cryptococcus neoformans 628
Crystalens 186
    intraocular lens 186
Crystalline keratopathy,
    infectious 64
Crystalline lens 254
    dislocation of 661
Cube scan, three-
    dimensional 640
Cul-de-sac, conjunctival 819

Custom fit prosthesis 861, 862,
    862f, 863, 863f
Cyanoacrylate tissue 255
Cyclitic membrane 419
Cyclocryotherapy 233
Cyclodestruction
    procedures 267
Cyclodialysis 242, 253
    cleft 256
Cyclooxygenase 181
    regulation of 522
Cyclopentolate 17, 892
Cyclophosphamide 45, 423,
    436, 437, 438
Cyclophotocoagulation 233
    endoscopic 303
Cycloplegia 892
    drugs for 892t
Cycloplegic 17, 543
    discontinuation of 232
    mydriatic agent 27
    refraction 306, 892, 946
    stabilize choroidal
        vasculature 562
Cyclosporine 306, 423, 436,
    437, 792
    ophthalmic emulsion,
        topical 41
    oral 68
    role of 68
Cyst 759, 771, 785
    conjunctival inclusion 856
    dormant 28
    intracranial 942
    multilobulated 785
    single 785
Cystic bleb, thin 237f
Cystic eye, congenital 759
Cystitis, hemorrhagic 438
Cystoid macular edema 93,
    103, 160, 162, 173, 177,
    180, 417, 419, 421, 424,
    428, 499, 502, 522f, 643f
    classic petaloid appearance
        of 502f
    postoperative 521
Cytomegalovirus 414, 420,
    427, 429, 437
    retinitis 423, 430, 579

D

Daclizumab 439, 440
Dacrocystorhinostomy 842
Dacryoadenitis 790
Dacryocele, congenital 827
Dacryocystectomy 833, 843
Dacryocystitis 828-830, 835, 836
    acute 834, 835, , 838
    chronic 828, 829fc, 830, 831,
        842, 843

Dacryocystography 819, 821f
Dacryocystorhinostomy 798,
    827, 833, 879
    endoscopic 827
    pearls for good external 831
Dacryoendoscopy 819
Dacryoliths 835
    microdrill removal of 819
Dacryops 763
Dacryoscintigraphy 819
Dalen-Fuch's nodule 434
Dandy-Walker
    malformation 942
Deep anterior lamellar
    keratoplasty 49, 60, 61
Deep retinal vascular
    plexuses 610
Deep upper eyelid sulcus
    deformity 861
Demodex 5, 723
    blepharitis 720
    folliculorum 723
    infestation 5
Demyelinations 926
Dendritic ulcer, peripheral 40
Dengue 420
    fever 579
    virus 429
Dense membrane formation,
    stage of 877
Deoxyribonucleic acid 9, 382,
    446, 636, 935
Depth perception slides 900f
Dermal fillers 730, 732
Dermatitis herpetiformis 74
Dermis fat graft 853, 853f, 858
Dermoid 769
    cyst 758
Dermolipoma 759, 762
Descemet's folds 197
Descemet's membrane 42, 48,
    52, 60, 193, 941
    detachment 19, 119, 193
    management of 193
    endothelial keratoplasty 19,
        60, 62, 205
Descemet's stripping
    automated endothelial
    keratoplasty 19, 60,
    61, 204
Descemet's wrinkling 49
Desmarres lid retractor 795
Dexamethasone 68, 70, 178, 484
    implant, sustained-
        release 484
Dextrose, intravenous 628f
Diabetes
    insipidus 942
    mellitus 16, 257, 387, 432,
        464f, 543, 571, 601, 620,
        677, 917

Index

Diabetic macular edema 522f,
591, 592, 595, 597f,
598fc, 599, 642
  initial assessment of 596
Diabetic retinopathy 256, 368,
463, 502, 506f, 531,
569, 591, 595, 612, 624,
665, 666
  study, early treatment
for 462, 591
  progression of 591
Diabetic traction retinal
detachment 496
Dialysis 498
Diamidine 29
Diamond burr polishing 18
Diarrhea 14
Diclofenac 104
  intravitreal 524
Dietary deficiency 14
Diffuse lamellar keratitis 330,
360, 375, 405
Digital calipers 340, 344
Digital ocular compression
235, 285
Digital subtraction
angiography 690
Dipivefrin 21
Diplopia 86, 755, 786, 842, 899
  acquired 729
Direct argon laser
photocoagulation 233
Direct brow lift 729
Direct light reflex,
perform 684
Direct macular
evaluation 88, 652
Disciform
  endotheliitis 32
  keratitis 34
Disease-modifying anti-
rheumatic drugs 438
Disk
  edema 621, 622, 624f, 701
    bilateral 624f
    segmental 673
    unilateral 673
  glaucomatous 278f
  hemorrhage 277f
  neovascularization
of 421, 463
Disodium cromoglycate 13
Dissociated horizontal
deviation 918
  disorder 920
Dissociated torsional
deviation 918
Dissociated vertical deviation
908, 910, 918, 920
  etiology of 919

Distal nasolacrimal duct block,
management plan
for 944
Distance randot test 903
Distance stereopsis test 899, 903
Distichiasis 2, 875
  congenital 716
Distinct clinical syndrome 9
Diurnal variation 87
Docetaxel 877
Docking 213, 365
  problems 330
Dog tapeworm 785
Dolichocephalic skulls 835
Doll's maneuver 910
Donor
  cornea 60, 61
  corneal patch graft 237
  graft preparation 63
  preparation 61, 62
  recipient interfaces,
types of 60
  tissue 61, 66, 738
Dorzolamide 245, 266
  topical 40
Double layer sign 513
Double vision 755, 804, 917
Down's syndrome 936, 947
Doxorubicin 736
Doxycycline 5, 428, 801
  oral 25, 423, 721
Drainage devices 145
Drugs
  against cytokine
tumor necrosis factor
alpha 438
  toxicity 17
Drusen bodies, types of 631
Drusenoid deposits 646
Dry age-related macular
degeneration 631, 667f
  stages of 631
Dry eye 55, 73, 175, 336, 360,
390, 406, 732, 804
  development of 712
  evaluation 306
  signs of 528
  syndrome 7
  treatment of 75
Dual Scheimpflug imaging 310
Dual-linear foot pedal 124, 125f
Duane's syndrome 911, 921
Duke elder classification 135
Dye disappearance,
amount of 825
Dye-enhanced capsulotomy 120
Dynamic corneal response 313
Dyschromatopsia 676
Dysfunctional lens
syndrome 368
Dysplasia, fibrous 762

Dysplastic nevi 748
Dysthyroid
  ophthalmopathy 921
  optic neuropathy 786
Dystrophia myotonica 687
Dystrophies 16, 265
  endothelial 18
  macular 49f

E

Eales disease 435, 478
Ecchymosis 726, 753, 779f
  superficial 726
Eccrine spiradenoma 749
Echinococcus granulosus 785
Echocardiography 934
Echothiophate 54
Eclampsia 580
Ecoshield 98
Ectasia 361, 375, 383, 406
  corneal 61
  graft 59
  risk score system 307, 308
Ectropion 714-716, 716f,
757, 861
  management of 714
Edema 783f, 791
  corneal 35, 228, 244, 381,
413, 539, 629
  graft 58
  simulating congenital
glaucoma 265
Edward's syndrome 936
Efalizumab 439, 440
Ehlers-Danlos syndrome 939
Eight-ball hyphema 241
Electroepilation 2
Electronic medical records 932
Electroretinogram 422
Electroretinography 495,
925, 928
Elevated episcleral venous
pressure 241
ELITA femtosecond laser 331f
Ellipsoid zone 619
Elschnig's pearls 216
Elschnig's spots 625f
Embryology 823, 841, 944
Emmetropia 218
Encapsulated cell
technology 487
Encephalitozoon 36
Encephalocele 759, 942
Endocyclophotocoagulation
302, 303f
Endophthalmitis 59, 65, 236,
245, 408, 539, 541f, 542,
543, 543f, 544f, 570,
575, 603, 608, 846
  bacterial 571
  chronic 543

endogenous 575, 627, 628
infectious 539
metastatic 627
pathophysiology of
 postoperative 100
postoperative 99, 538, 539,
 540f, 547
prevention 100
severe 541f
treatment of 546
vitrectomy study 100, 178
Endoscopy-assisted scleral-
 fixated intraocular
 lenses 169
Endothelial blebs 56
Endothelial cell 524
count 339
 progressive loss of 165
Endothelial damage 387, 389
Endothelial disorders 153
Endothelial dysfunction
causes of 50
descemet's membrane
 for 205
Endothelial protection 122, 152
Endotheliitis 34
diffuse 32
viral 50
Endothelium 152, 343, 623
Endotracheal tube 561
Enophthalmos 753, 755, 854,
 855, 861, 924
apparent 685
Enterobacteriaceae 22, 23
Enterococcus 25, 545
Enterocytozoon 36
Entopic visualization 90, 654
Entropion 11, 714, 717, 855, 877
management of 714
medial 715
Enucleation 76, 846, 850
steps of 847f
surgical technique for 847
Enzyme-linked
 immunosorbent assay
 416, 418, 422
Ependymomas 880
Ephelis 747
Epiblepharon 2, 715, 716f
Epidermidis 239
Epidermis 746f
Epigastric burning 438
Epi-laser in-situ
 keratomileusis 382
Epinastine 13
Epinephrine 21, 144
Epinucleus 110t
removal 108
Epiphora 815, 824, 830, 835,
 836, 875, 877, 944
causes of 823

differential diagnosis of 824fc
excessive 879
pediatric 944
recurrent 826
Epiretinal membrane 408, 421,
 430, 488f, 645, 646f,
 665, 665f
primary 665f
Episclera 79
Episcleritis 69, 70
Episode, acute on chronic 262
Epithelial abnormalities 312
Epithelial abrasion 31, 56
Epithelial debridement 17
 alcohol-assisted 382
Epithelial defect 40, 64, 360, 402
Epithelial down growth 241, 250f
Epithelial healing 80
Epithelial ingrowth 359f,
 375, 404
Epithelial microvilli, loss of 54
Epithelial thickness 373
Epithelial tumors 841
benign 745, 763
Epithelial wrinkling 57
Epithelioid 435
cell 451
 melanoma 451
Epitheliopathy, surface 5
Epithelium 841
ciliary 78
edematous 19, 20
failed dehiscence of 876
Epstein-Barr virus 42
infection 11, 450
Erosion 296
recurrent 48
Erysipelas 721
Erythema 791
multiforme 74
Erythrocyte sedimentation rate
 414, 427, 438, 674, 675
Erythropoietin, role of 257
Escherichia coli 387, 628
Esotropia 894, 896, 907, 910
accommodative 910
acquired 907
infantile 907, 909, 912f
types of 906
V-pattern 683
Esotropic deviations, diagnosis
 of 906
Etanercept 438, 439, 440
Ethmoid sinus 780f
 opacification of 820f
Ethylenediaminetetraacetic
 acid 53
Euryblepharon 715, 715f
Evisceration 846
steps of 848f
surgical technique for 848

Ewing's tumor 763
Excimer laser
 phototherapeutic
 keratectomy 49
Exenteration 777, 850
extended 778, 851
Exfoliation 268f
syndrome 231
Exodeviations 912
Exophthalmos 805f, 924
Exotropia 913
bilateral 914f
consecutive 914
decompensated 914, 914f
early-onset 913, 914
intermittent 913
unilateral 914f
Expanded nystagmus acuity
 function 932
Exposure keratopathy 6, 7,
 35, 723
management of 7
External beam radiation
 therapy 535
External eye
examination 86
infection 239
Extracapsular cataract 140
extraction 18, 146, 175, 176,
 200, 522f
surgery 175f
Extraconal space,
 superior 774f
Extramacular tractional retinal
 detachment 496f
Extraocular movements,
 likelihood of
 improvement of 784
Extraocular muscle 853,
 885, 922
congenital fibrosis of 911, 921
enlargement 870f
normal 787f
surgery 911
Extraocular needle-guided
 haptic insertion
 technique 471
Exudative retinal detachment
 420, 578, 579f
Eye 88, 90, 633, 652, 654
absence of 852
anatomy 301
anterior segment of 85
characteristics of 268
contralateral 781
diabetic 591
disease, adenoviral 10
drop 245
 prednisolone
 phosphate 177
 tropicamide 177

Index

glaucomatous 699f
hygiene, poor 545
hyperopic 231
increasing redness of 92
infection 545
injury, perforating 664
inner corner of 724
movement recording 926
painful 846
pathology in 603
pediatric 161, 935
plan fellow 398
postvitrectomy 199
prosthetic 856
protrusion of 804
removal of 855
rubbing of 12
soft 144
Eyeball 753
  cut section of 452f
  deformed 883
  normal 666
  protrusion of 753, 755
  sinking 753
Eyebrow
  elongated 883f
  incision 874
Eyecryl phakic intraocular lens 342
Eyelash 2, 4, 503, 703
Eyelid 7, 703, 740f, 749, 777, 799
  abscess 778
  anatomy of 707
  applied anatomy of 744
  bruising 755
  cleansing agents 720
  crease 776f
  defects 738
    full-thickness 739, 741f, 742f
  disturbances 6
  edema 785
  examination of 734, 815
  hygiene measures 720
  infections 718
  inflammation 41
  injury 795
    secondary repair of 800
  large 883f
  laser therapy of 884f
  lesions 744
    benign 744, 745
  lower 739, 755
  manifestations 431
  margin 4
    direct closure of 741f
  marginal rotation of 854
  movable 707
  movements 870

pars lacrimalis portion of 875f
pathology of 441
position of 815, 917
reconstruction 738
  goals of 738
repair
  goals of 796
  principles for 796
retraction 807
  ipsilateral 769
skin of 723, 799f
split technique 775
tags 875
total avulsion of 798
tumors 734, 736, 746f
  benign 744, 750
  laser therapy of 750
  malignant 850
  vascular 744
Eylea 569

F

Face examination 734
Facial
  anatomy 739
  bony defects 754f
Familial exudative vitreoretinopathy 473, 503, 504f, 581, 582f, 582t
Faricimab 487
Fasanella-Servat surgery 711
Fascia lata 237, 294, 857
Fascicular sixth nerve palsy 682
Fat excision, endpoint of 728
Fatigue 437
Feeder vessels, large 76f
Fellow eye 228, 865f
  asymptomatic 638fc
  status of 933
Femtosecond laser 212, 213, 214, 321, 324, 332
  action, mechanism of 326f
  assisted
    capsulotomy 120
    cataract surgery 129, 138, 212, 213f, 215, 371
    flap 327f, 329t
    in situ keratomileusis 319, 352, 358, 362
  flap making procedure, steps of 326
  photo disruption 322f
Femtosecond machines 323t
Fibrin 296, 608
  formation 32
Fibroadenoma 438
Fibroblast 435
  growth factor 656

Fibroma, ossifying 762
Fibrosis, subconjunctival 261
Fibrous connective tissue tumors 762
Fibrovascular membrane 241, 256, 497
Fibrovascular proliferation 464f, 554f
  components of 570
Fibrovascularization 860
Filtration failure,
  risk factors for 279
Fine keratin nodules 76
Finger
  classification 529
  staging system 529t
Fish tail sign 134, 138
Fissures, asymmetric palpebral 769
Fistula, lacrimal 875
Fixation losses,
  percentage of 274
Flap
  dislocation 404
  striae 403
  suturing 285
  tears 402
Flash visual evoked potential 694
Flat anterior chamber 236
Fleck dystrophy 47
Fleischer ring 51
Floppy
  eyelid syndrome 716, 716f
  iris syndrome 112
Fluconazole 37
  intravenous 629
Fluid
  accumulation, progressive 650
  air exchange 550
  attenuated inversion recovery 674, 679
  specimens 574
Fluorescein
  angiogram 480f, 586, 649f
  angiography 181f, 254, 476f, 477f, 479, 485, 485f, 498f, 499, 504f, 511, 530, 533f, 610t, 666f
  dye leakage 527f
  imaging, application of 665
  dye 818
    disappearance test 818, 825
  meniscus height after instillation of 175
  patterns of abnormal 501
Fluorometholone 70, 272
Flurbiprofen 103, 104

Index

Focal laser 581
  photocoagulation 648, 650*f*
Foldable intraocular
    lens 184, 185
  design of 185
Foot switch 364
Forced duction test 921
Formaldehyde 98
  fumigation 97
Formalin
  fumigation, methods of 97
  spray 97
  vaporizer 97
Forme fruste
    keratoconus 307, 406
Fornix-based conjunctival flap,
    creation of 280*f*
Four petal technique 849
Four-point suture fixation 167
Four-prism base-out
    test 899, 901
Foveal avascular zone 598
  abnormal 477*f*
Foveal reflex 181*f*
Foveal roof 490*f*
Foveal tractional retinal
    detachment 644*f*
Foville's syndrome 682
Fracture, midfacial 813
Fragmatome 661
Freckles 747
Fresh vitreous hemorrhage 468
Frisby-Davis
  distance 899
  test 899, 903
Frontalis sling
  pentagon technique 712*f*
  surgery 712
Frontoethmoidal mucoceles 760
Frosted branch angiitis 426
Fuchs' endothelial dystrophy
    49-51, 204, 311
Fuchs' marginal keratitis 40
Fuchs' spot 586*f*, 587
Fugo plasma blade 120
Fumagillin 37
Fundus 250, 382, 496*f*, 498*f*, 587
  autofluorescence 421, 462*f*,
    488, 495, 632, 664
    imaging 508*f*
  evaluation 339, 946
  examination 244, 557, 753
  fluorescein angiography
    180, 417, 421, 424, 427,
    432, 473, 499, 510*f*,
    512*f*, 513*f*, 523, 523*f*,
    528*f*, 530*f*, 564, 567*f*,
    580, 586*f*, 590, 598, 620,
    659, 664
  peripheral 630*f*

Fungal endophthalmitis 542,
    543, 543*f*, 571, 573*f*,
    575, 577
  endogenous 571
  exogenous 571
  Ishibashi's classification
    of 572*t*
  management of 577*fc*
Fungal infection, mode of 572*fc*
Fungal keratitis 26, 28, 43
  forms of 26
  incidence of 26
Fungi 20, 447
Fusiform rectus
    enlargement 806
Fusion 900
  maldevelopment nystagmus
    syndrome 925, 932
  Panum's area of 902
Fusobacterium 837, 839
Fyodorov's formula 218

G

Gadolinium, intravenous 772
Galactokinase 941
Galactose-1-phosphate-
    uridyltransferase 941
Galactosemia 941
Gallium scan 418
Ganciclovir 32
Ganglion cell 495
  complex thickness 277*f*, 701
  layers 640
Gangliosidoses 941
Gas
  bubbles, intracameral 401
  cataract 551
  fluid exchanges 520
Gastrointestinal intolerance 437
Gatifloxacin 178, 239
Gaze, direction of 617
Gene therapy 487, 593
  agents, systemic delivery
    of 593
  development of 593
Genetic 635
  syndrome 885, 935
Genitourinary tract 412
Gevokizumab 439
Ghost cell
  arteritis 43, 257, 426
  glaucoma 241, 468
Giant
  fornix syndrome 840
  hairy pigmented nevi 748
  papillary conjunctivitis 12
Giemsa stain 36, 574
Gingivitis 437, 942
Glare 86
Glasses 406, 908
  power of 86

Glaucoma 13, 27, 79, 83, 145,
    162, 227, 228, 236, 242,
    245, 267, 269, 271, 273,
    276, 291, 276, 312, 339,
    346, 419, 483, 551, 601,
    613, 883, 935
  advanced 273
  alpha-2 agonist for 251
  anemia-associated 241, 243
  ciliary block 231
  ciliolenticular block 231
  congenital 823
  congestive 256
  corticosteroid-induced 270
  detection of 270
  drainage devices 267, 289,
    292, 291, 292*fc*
    selection of 292
    surgery 258
  end-stage 53
  evaluation 143
  exfoliative 267
  following cataract surgery
    246, 252*t*
  hemifield test 275
  hemorrhagic 256
  juvenile 238
  late-onset 264
  lens-induced 229
  malignant 229, 231, 244,
    249, 287
  mechanism of 244
  medical therapy 271
  medications 55
  pigmentary 269
  postoperative 246
  preexisting 145
  primary congenital 264
  procedure 145
  progression 271
  pseudoexfoliation 269
  recurrent 267
  secondary 159, 265, 558
  steroid-induced 272
  surgery 143, 145
  treatment for 272
  type of 143
  typical field defects in 276
  uncontrolled 18, 368
Glaucomatous damage 275, 279
Glaukomflecken 262
Glioma 690*t*, 880, 927
Globe perforation 157
Glomus tumor 747
Glucocorticoids 809
Glucose-6-phosphate
    dehydrogenase
    deficiency 75
Glutaraldehyde 98
Glycosaminoglycan 48, 79, 733

Index

Goldenhar's syndrome 762, 921, 937
Golimumab 439, 440
Gömöri-Methenamine silver 574
Gonadal atrophy, irreversible 438
Gonioscopy 228, 234, 239, 250, 256, 257, 288, 343, 413, 467
Goniotomy 266, 298
Gonococcal conjunctivitis 9
  systemic antibiotic for 9
Graft
  failure 65, 856
  rejection 65, 68f
    clinical diagnosis of 66
    differential diagnosis of 68
    risk factors for 65
    sudden episode of 59
    symptoms of 66
    treatment of 67fc
Gram's iodine 446
Gram's stain 36, 446
Granular cell tumor 888
Granular dystrophy 49f
Granular periodic acid-Schiff 888
Granulocytic sarcoma 763
Granuloma 420, 837, 923
  conjunctival 861
  eosinophilic 763
Granulomatous reaction 435f
Grave's orbitopathy
  classification 808f
  severity of 807
Graves' disease 769
Graves' hyperthyroidism 786
Graves' orbitopathy 788, 789, 808t
Grid macular laser photocoagulation 535
Grocott methenamine silver stain 446, 449f, 574
Growth hormone deficiency 942
Gynecomastia 942
Gyrate atrophy 595

H

Haab's striae 264
Haemophilus influenza 64, 830, 837
Haigis formula 87, 222
Hair follicle 5, 746f
  tumors, benign 749
Hallermann-Streiff syndrome 938
Hamartomas 453
Handshake technique 171f
Hansatome microkeratome 318, 319f

Hansen's disease 413
Haptic rubbing 247
Harada-Ito procedure 923
Hard cataract 112, 122
  phacoemulsification 122
Hard nucleus 109t, 153
  moderately 470
Hay-Wells syndromes 875
Head
  and neck cancers 525
  contrast-enhanced magnetic resonance imaging of 679
  posture
    abnormal 917
    anomalous 683, 925
Headache 239, 651, 675, 680
Healing, conjunctival 79
Hearing loss 810, 942
Heart disease, congenital 947
Helium-neon laser 653
Hemangioendothelioma
  epithelioid 765
  malignant 761
Hemangioma 558, 580, 737, 765, 769
  capillary 453, 737, 737f, 747, 750, 760, 765
  choroidal 527f, 655
  epithelioid 747, 765
  infantile 765, 766f
  type of congenital 765
Hemangiopericytoma 448, 453, 747, 760, 766
Hematoma 755
Hematoxylin and eosin stained slide 448f
Hemicentral vein occlusion 481
Hemifacial pain, severe 836
Hemifacial spasm 731, 872
Hemoglobin, glycosylated 596
Hemolacria 842
Hemorrhage 92, 174, 247, 532, 533f, 563, 622, 629, 661, 662, 795
  absence of 621
  choroidal 259, 590
  coin-shaped 657
  duration of 564
  focal 586f
  gray vitreous 663
  intralesional 766
  large
    submacular 564
    subretinal 510f
  macular 408, 530f, 534f
  multiple 479f
  postoperative 570
  recurrent 250
  subconjunctival 330, 570, 753
  thickness of 564

Hemorrhagic choroidal detachment 604f
Hemosiderosis bulbi 468
Hepatitis 942
  B surface antigen 44
  C 43
Hepatotoxicity 437
  reversible 437
Hermansky-Pudlak syndrome 940
Herpes simplex 420, 722, 839
  infection 840
  keratitis 43, 64
  virus 11, 30f, 31f, 41, 64, 414, 429, 437
    endotheliitis 31
    epithelial keratitis 30
    infection prophylaxis 32
    iridocyclitis 32
    keratopathy 30
    manifestations 33
    trabeculitis 32
    types of 30
Herpes zoster 34t, 71, 722
  manifestations of 33
  ophthalmicus 33f, 55, 413, 718
  viral infection 424
  virus 11, 42
  keratitis 33
Herpetic eye disease 387
Hertel's exophthalmometry 805
Hess screen 902
Heterophoria method 905
Hidradenitis 438
High efficiency particulate air 96
High vacuum flow restricted tubing 141, 142f
Higher order aberration 156, 189, 349, 350, 352
Highly aspheric lenslets spectacles 948
Histiocytic lesions 763
Histiocytoma, fibrous 762, 842
Hodgkin's disease 42
Hodgkin's lymphoma 525
Hoffer mean-value method 219
Hoffer Q formula 221, 218
Hoffman elbowed Baerveldt implant 290, 290f
Hoffman pockets 169f
Hoffman technique 169
Holladay formula 221, 369
Holladay system 221
Holt-Oram syndrome 921
Homatropine 892
Homocysteine levels 428
Homocystinuria 939
Hordeolum, external 3
Horgan classification 531

Index

Hormone
  adrenocorticotrophic 271
    therapy 5
Horner's syndrome 682,
    684-686, 710
Horner-Trantas dots 12
Hoya optimized aspheric
    intraocular lens with
    aspheric balanced
    curve design 156, 186
Hughes flap 743*f*
Human donor sclera 857
Human embryonic stem cell 495
Human eye, monochromatic
    aberrations of 349*t*
Human herpes virus 429, 766
Human immunodeficiency
    virus 43, 77, 418, 420,
    427, 627, 734
Human leukocyte antigen 412,
    426, 436
  concentration of 66
Human papillomavirus 842
  infection 75
Humphrey visual field 673, 700
Hurricane keratopathy 55
Hyaloid
  attachment, posterior 489*f*
  membrane, taut
    posterior 644*f*
Hyaluronic acid 732, 733
  derivatives 733
  fillers 809
Hydrocephalus 675, 942
Hydrochloroquine
  maculopathy 507
Hydrodelineation 136, 371
Hydrodissection 126, 128, 130,
    136, 139, 200, 209, 371
Hydrogel 855
  hydrophilic acrylate 185
Hydrophobic acrylate 185
Hydroxyapatite 855
  implants 857
Hydroxychloroquine
    retinopathy 666
Hydroxypropyl
    methylcellulose 152
Hydrus microstent 300, 301*f*
Hyper-autofluorescence,
    abnormal regions
    of 666
Hyperbaric oxygen 535
Hypercapnia 56
Hypercortisolism,
    endogenous 651
Hyperemia 10, 624*f*
Hyperemic disk edema 673
Hyperfluorescence 500, 501
Hyperglycemia 810
Hyperhidrosis 731

Hyperlipidemia 677
Hypermetropia 339, 907
Hypermetropic correction 914
Hyperopia 401, 893, 894, 896
Hyperopic anisometropia 894
Hyperosmotic agents 17
Hyperplasia, epithelial 19
Hyperpulse 124
Hypersensitivity response,
    type of 65
Hypertension 257, 271, 432,
    438, 526, 561, 677, 917
  accelerated 622
  acute 622
  chronic 622, 626
  malignant 580, 625*f*
  pregnancy-induced 623
  retinochoroidopathy 625*f*
  severe 622
Hypertensive retinopathy 531,
    621, 623, 624*f*, 626,
    626*t*
  pathophysiology of 622*t*
Hyperthermia, malignant 924
Hypertrichoism 438
Hypertrophy, inferior
    turbinate 830
Hyperviscosity syndromes 625
Hyphema 32, 162, 173, 241,
    242, 247*f*, 285, 295, 753
  postoperative 298
  recurrent attacks of 605*f*
Hypoesthesia
  corneal 56
  infraorbital 753, 755
Hypofluorescence 50, 501, 616
Hypophosphatasia 53
Hypophthalmos 755
Hypoplasia, foveal 940
Hypoplastic cerebellar
    vermis 942
Hypopyon 32, 248*f*, 573, 606, 608
  resolution of 541
Hypotonia 942
Hypotony 253, 255, 288, 296,
    430, 551, 577
  causes of 237
  chronic 288, 606
  effects of 253
  maculopathy 236, 252, 254
Hypoxanthine-guanine phos-
    phoribosyltransferase,
    symptoms of 593
Hypoxia 56
Hysteresis 313

I

Iatrogenic retinal damage 560
Ichthyosis 715, 716*f*
Idiopathic anterior uveitis,
    recurrent bilateral 432

Idoxuridine 21, 54
Iliac crest 855
Illuminated near card
    assessment 89, 653
Image-guided
  navigation system,
    principle of 811
  orbital surgery 811, 874
Imidazole 29
Imipenem 545
Immobile lens syndrome 57
Immune
  recovery vitritis 415
  ring 31
Immunoglobulin
  A 841
  G 416
  G4-related disease 793
  intravenous 427, 433,
    439, 440
Immunohistochemistry
    447, 765
Immunosuppressive therapy,
    indications of
    primary 436
Impetigo 721
Implantable collamer lens
    338, 342, 342*f*, 345*f*
  implantation 347*f*
  length determination 344
Implantable phakic contact
    lens 337, 338, 342
Implanted contact lenses 312
In vitro kills retinoblastoma 636
Incision 4, 127, 136, 366*f*,
    371, 756
  biopsy 873
  closure 209
  construction 208
  external 118
Incisional biopsy,
    multilevel 801
Incisional tear 360
Inclusion cyst 923
Incomitant esodeviation
    906, 907
Incomitant hypertropia 683
Incomplete eyelid closure 800
Incomplete punctal
    canalization 876
Indocyanine angiography 664
Indocyanine green 120, 465
  angiography 421, 427, 485,
    512, 512*f*, 513*f*, 529,
    564, 648, 649*f*, 657,
    668*f*, 669*f*
  imaging, application
    of 666
Indomethacin 104

Index

Infections 412, 729, 796, 861, 877
  acute 247
  bacterial 26, 42
  bleb-related 288
  causes of 547
  cluster 545
  congenital 926
  corneal 56
  graft 64*f*
  prevent 80
  secondary 438
  source of 30, 545, 545*t*
Infectious disease 575
Infectious epithelial keratitis, recurrent 33
Infectious keratitis 361, 387, 405
  causes of 28
Inferior bleb 238
Inferior oblique overaction 910, 912*f*, 916, 920
Inferior retinal nerve fiber layer defect 277*f*
Inferior retinal tracts 650*f*
Inferior subconjunctival antibiotic-steroid injection 282
Inferotemporal branch retinal vein occlusion 479*f*
Inflammation 79, 241, 243, 247, 254, 288, 861
  acute suppurative 4
  conjunctival 5, 788
  degree of 254
  severe 253
  suppression of 428
Inflammatory bowel diseases 426
Infliximab 438, 439, 440
  intravitreal 524
Infusion 284
  bottle placement 199
Injury 917
  mechanical 240
Inner limiting membrane 590
Inner retinal
  development 474
  layers 474
Integrins 656
Intense vitritis 573
Interferometry, principle of 639
Interferons 439, 441, 596
  alpha 440
Intermediate uveitis 415, 415*t*, 416, 416*t*, 419, 426, 439, 440
  etiology of 415
Intermuscular septum 869*f*
Internal hordeolum 3
Internal limiting membrane 199, 466*f*, 491*f*, 492*f*, 616*f*
Internal orbital fracture 812

Interno needle goniectomy 299
Interstitial keratitis 35, 41, 41*f*
  active 41
  inactive 42
Intracapsular cataract extraction 176, 247, 522*f*
Intraconal implant placement 849
Intraconal mass 869*f*, 870*f*
Intracranial hypertension, idiopathic 675, 872
Intracranial tract 772
Intraocular contact lens 391
Intraocular foreign body 560, 604, 606, 608, 869
Intraocular inflammation 245
Intraocular lens 47, 91, 119, 131, 136, 140, 147, 153, 156, 156*t*, 158, 162, 165, 170, 174, 183, 186, 195, 197, 205, 212, 215, 219, 220*t*, 248*f*, 270, 332, 368, 397, 413, 471*f*, 541*f*, 520, 661, 933
  accommodating 186, 217, 224
  aspheric 185
  biocompatible 246
  calculation methods 334
  choice of 185, 592
  diffractive 187
  dislocation 172
  emmetropic 218*t*
  evaluation of 395
  exchange 396
  fourth-generation 160
  glued intrascleral haptic fixation of 171
  glued sutureless scleral fixation of 471
  haptic of 605*f*
  implantation 114, 128, 138, 195, 198, 209, 210, 371, 934
    secondary 210
    type of 18
  malposition 398
  management of posteriorly dislocated 469
  power 222, 223
    calculation 87, 207, 220, 332, 334, 340, 369, 934
    formulas 217, 335
  scleral fixation of 168
  selection 144
  sutured scleral fixation of 166, 470
  sutureless scleral fixation of 471
  third-generation 159
  toric phakic 344
  transscleral suture fixation of 470

Intraocular lymphoma 418, 426, 427, 452, 453, 453*t*, 580
Intraocular mass lesion 472
Intraocular pressure 41, 87, 110, 128, 158, 166, 177, 178, 194, 206, 228, 231, 234, 243, 244, 256, 259, 262, 267, 270, 339, 340, 363, 399, 413, 467, 483, 539, 629, 753, 770, 795, 809, 824
  assessment of 254
  control of 143, 279
  elevation 246*f*
    mechanism of 246
    transient 246
  high 241, 287
  low 286
  measurement 242
  raised 287, 415
    postoperative 114
  risk factors for 243
  spikes, postoperative 203
Intraocular silicone oil 53
Intraocular tamponade 198
Intraocular tumors 450, 503, 604, 763, 870
  malignant 450
  most common 452
Intra-operative posterior capsular rupture 161
Intraretinal fluid 650*f*, 656*f*
  accumulation 645
Intraretinal microvascular abnormalities 600
Intrastromal corneal ring 322
Intrastromal presbyopia correction 322
Intravenous pulse therapy 72
Intravitreal antibiotics, newer 544
Intravitreal antivascular endothelial growth factor 476*f*, 524, 533*f*, 565
  monotherapy 565
Intravitreal avastin 543, 544*f*
Intravitreal corticosteroid injections 271
Intravitreal dexamethasone implant 523
Intravitreal injections 272, 540*f*, 580
Intravitreal triamcinolone 244
  acetonide, use of 271
Intrinsic tumor vessels 76
IOLMaster 700 Barrett suite calculation 336*f*
Ionizing radiation 526

Index

Iowa implant 859
Iridectomy 250, 285
  complications 286
  peripheral 282, 282f, 284, 285
Iridocorneal angle 339
Iridocorneal apposition,
    peripheral 259
Iridocorneal endothelial
    syndrome 50, 291
Iridocorneolenticular
    adhesions 553
Iridocyclitis 33
Iridodialysis 146, 242
Iridoschisis 242
Iridotomy, peripheral 145, 346
Iris 247, 413, 605, 864, 865f
  anomalous 339
  atrophy 174, 242
  button, painting on 864, 866f
  claw lens 162, 163, 173
    design of 163
    fixation sites of 164
    retrofixation of 129
  corneal touch, peripheral 253
  diaphragm, single-piece 183f
  fixation 470
  heterochromia 685
  hooks 128
  leiomyoma 450
  melanocytic tumors 450
  melanoma 450
  mid-peripheral 269
  neovascularization of 256f, 257, 591
  pigment epithelial
    adenocarcinoma 450
  pigmentation 617
  retractors 144
  sphincter tears 242
  sphincterotomies 144
  sutures 147
  tissue 296
  vasculature, abnormal 174
  whirling 262
Iritis 242
Iron ring 51
Irreversible trabecular
    meshwork damage 250
Irrigation
  aspiration 128
  lacrimal 817
Irritation 31, 36
Irvine–Gass syndrome 522, 592
Ischemia 257, 537, 600, 601
  acute choroidal 622
  choroidal 622
  macular 600
Ischemic optic neuropathy 695, 696, 696f, 701

Isoametropia 896
Itching 22
Itraconazole 29, 37

J

Jarisch–Herxheimer
    reaction 429
Jaw claudication 675
Jones test 818
Joubert syndrome 928
Juvenile xanthogranuloma 763, 940

K

Kahook dual blade
    glide 299, 300f
Kaplan–Meier graph 526f
Kaposi sarcoma 42, 765, 766
Kaposiform hemangioendo-
    theliomas 765
Kasabach–Merritt
    phenomenon 765
Kawasaki disease 431
Kaye's dots 67
Kayser–Fleisher ring 941
Kearns–Sayre syndrome 494, 943
Keith–Wagener–Barker
    systems 621
Kelly's punch 282f
Kelman needle 133
Keratectomy
  photorefractive 312, 333, 335f, 336, 339, 374, 381, 384, 389, 392, 397
  superficial 48
  phototherapeutic 17, 48, 393, 394
Keratic precipitates 228, 413
Keratin, central plug of 747
Keratitis 55, 89, 387, 571
  bacterial 26, 43
  epithelial 9
  fungal 26, 28, 43
  geographical 30f
  infectious 361, 387, 405
  marginal 5, 39, 40, 44
  medicamentosa 54, 54f
  punctate 34, 36
  severe 25
  sicca 21
  superficial 55
  toxic 55
  viral necrotizing 31
Keratoacanthoma 747
Keratoconjunctivitis 8, 37
  adenoviral 9
  atopic 12
  chronic atopic 74
  epidemic 10

Keratoconus 47, 51, 52, 131, 132, 200, 339, 356, 381, 386, 393, 394, 494
  mild-to-moderate 132, 357
  progression of 52
  severe 132
Keratoglobus 46
Keratomalacia 14, 15
Keratometric index error 333
Keratometry 340, 396
Keratopathy 21, 718f
  band-shaped 53, 53f, 394, 413, 415, 416, 419
  epithelial 30
  punctate 19
  toxic 21
Keratoplasty 35, 49, 52
  conductive 380
  endothelial 60, 66, 204
  postpenetrating 538
Keratoprosthesis 75, 544
Keratorefractive surgery 310
Keratouveitis 34
Ketoconazole 29
  oral 27
Ketorolac
  intraoperative injection 103
  tromethamine 13, 104
Ketotifen 13
Keyhole iridectomy 144
Khaw small descemet
    membrane punch 284
Khodadoust line 67, 68f
Kidney function test 596
Kimura's spatula 36
Kissing choroidal 255, 662
Klebsiella 628, 630
Klinefelter's syndrome 937
Koch method 219
Kranenburg syndrome 615
Krill's disease 420
Krimsky tests 680
  modified 680
Krukenberg spindle 269
Kyphosis 942

L

Lacerations
  deep 797
  simple 797
Lacquer crack 586, 586f
Lacrimal apparatus 703
Lacrimal canaliculus,
    flask-shaped 821f
Lacrimal drainage pathway 818
Lacrimal drainage system 799, 815-817, 829f, 832t, 841, 843, 843f-845f
  imaging of 819
  tests for 816t
  tumors of 841

Lacrimal duct-associated
     lymphoid tissue 829
     structure of 830f
Lacrimal fossa 835
     mass, right 820f
Lacrimal gland 455, 763
     carcinomas 850
     enlarged 791f
     mass 772f
     pleomorphic adenoma
          of 455f
     tumor 454, 763, 769, 871f
     removal of 775
Lacrimal probe 799f
Lacrimal punctum 821f
Lacrimal sac 828, 843, 845
     fossa 820
     mucocele, congenital 823
     tumor 842
Lacrimal stents 831
Lacrimal surgery, recent
          advances in 832
Lacrimal syringing 815,
          817, 818f
Lacrimal system 815
Lacrimation 41
Lactic-co-glycolic acid 857
Lagophthalmos 6, 7, 727,
          734, 805f
Laissez faire 851
Lamellar corneal
          transplantation 63
Lamellar keratoplasty 48, 49,
          51, 59, 60
     anterior 60, 322
     posterior 322
Lamellar macular hole 488,
          644, 645f
Lamina cribrosa 481
Laminar flow 500
Laser 535, 592
     application 365
     arm and vacuum system 364
     blended vision 379
          principle of 379f
     indirect ophthalmoscope 460
     interferometry 89, 653
     photocoagulation 468, 479,
          483, 515
     pocket, creation of 327f
     therapy 233, 237, 750
     trabeculoplasty 269
          selective 145, 270
     treatment 263, 555
     type of 323
     vision correction 333, 368
          effects of 333, 333f
Laser-assisted in situ
          keratomileusis 321,
          333, 335f, 336, 387, 391,
          399, 571
     flap 324

procedures 376
     thin flap 374
Laser-assisted subepithelial
     keratectomy 382
     keratomileusis 381
Lash
     appendages 719f
     loss 722f
     position of 815
Latanoprost 54, 245
Lattice dystrophy 49f
Lawrence-Moon syndrome 943
Lax lower eyelid 854
Leber's congenital amaurosis
          494, 593, 928
Leber's hereditary optic
          neuropathy 594, 676,
          699, 702
Lees screen 902
Leflunomide 436
Leiomyoma 448
     choroidal 450
Leiomyosarcoma 448
Leishmaniasis 42
Lens 413, 703, 753
     aspiration 934
     capsule, anterior 268f
     corneal touch 288
     epithelial cell 174
     epithelium 78
     first-generation 158
     fragment during
          phacoemulsification,
          posterior dislocation
          of 206
     fragmentation 213, 214, 583
          patterns 214f
     management 550
     opacities 262
          classification system 85,
               85f, 133, 312
          mild-to-moderate 88, 652
     particle glaucoma 247
     position of 241, 243
          effective 195, 196, 214
     power calculation errors 396
     removal 198
     scleral fixation of 168f
     second-generation 159
     status 292
     subluxation,
          spontaneous 270
     substance removal 209
     syndromes with 935
     use of posterior 491
     vault 341
     vitreous admixture 583
Lensectomy 556, 934
Lens-iris diaphragm 259
     retropulsion syndrome 133

Lenticule
     cut 366f
     diameter 364
     dissection of 365
     extraction of 365
          small-incision 322
     minimum thickness of 364
     parameters 364
     retained 360
     thickness
          minimum 364
          total 364
Lenticulocorneal touch 253
Lentigo simplex 747
Lentiviral vectors,
          tropism of 593
Leprosy 424
Leptochoroid 665
Leptospirosis 415, 417
Leser-Trélat sign 747
Lesions
     benign 744, 762, 777
     clinical characteristics of 420
     malignant 744, 765, 777
     site of 873
     structural 758
     treatable 600
     vascular 760
Leudde's exophthalmometry
          805
Leukemia 438, 454, 763
     chronic lymphocytic 439
Leukocoria 579
Leukocytoclastic angiitis,
          cutaneous 426
Levator
     aponeurosis 710, 796, 797
     function, assessment of 711
     muscle 798
     palpebra superioris 708,
          714, 798
          function 712
     resection 712, 884f
Levobunolol 230, 266
Levy-Hollister syndromes 875
Lid
     contour 866
     defects, repair of
          nonmarginal 797
     edema 789
     examination of 710
     injury, evaluation of 796
     lag 805
     level assessment 711f
     malpositioning of 867
     position, assessment of 710
     redness 789
     retraction 808
     scars 2
     scrubs 5

swelling of 806
syndrome with 935
tumors, benign 745*t*
Lid margin 503, 708, 717, 797, 797*f*, 823
  anomalies 714
    surgical correction of 75
  disease 5
  laceration, repair of 796, 797
  posterior 737
  sutures 797
  ulceration of 722*f*
Lidocaine 105
Light adjustable lens 189
Light-emission diode illumination system 473
Lignocaine 105
Limbal bleed 401
Limbal deficiency 5
Limbal infiltrates 5
Limbal inflammation 41
Limbal ischemia 78*f*
Limbal peritomy, conjunctival 847*f*
Limbal phaco incision 116
Limbal relaxing incisions 213, 322
Limbal scarring 149
Limbal stem cell transplantation 80
Limbal vasculature 66
Limbal vasculitis 31
Limbic keratoconjunctivitis, superior 57, 69
Lin's formula 218, 220*t*, 222
Lincoff's rules 459, 460*f*
Linear endotheliitis 32
Linear immunoglobulin disease 74
Linear translation 317
Linear wounds, smaller 797
Linezolid 39
Lip
  augmentation 733
  mucosa 738
Lipid
  keratopathy 35
  laden dermal histiocytes 441*f*
Lipogranulomatous inflammation 442*f*
Liquid biopsy 635
Lissamine green staining 76
Listeria monocytogenes 628, 629
Liver
  abscess 628
  enzymes, elevation of 437
  function test 596
  ultrasonogram 575
Lock-and-key coupling system 859

Loteprednol 13, 272
Lotmar visometer 89, 653
Low endothelial cell count, preexisting 18
Lower lid 707
  avulsions 798
  blepharoplasty 723, 728
  cicatricial ectropion of 717*f*
  ectropion 717*f*
  elongation 861
  entropion 717*f*, 757
    bilateral 718*f*
  laxity 718*f*
  malpositions 729
  margin, repair of 741*f*
  mechanical ectropion of 717*f*
  retractor 708, 741*f*, 793*f*
  swinging 777
  transconjunctival incisio 873
Lower punctal ectropion 816*f*
Lower-order aberrations 349
Lubricants 5, 16, 17
Lucentis 569
Luminescence 499
Lung
  disease, restrictive 940
  interstitial fibrosis of 438
Lyme's disease 415, 418, 427, 428, 677
  serology 427
Lymph node examination biopsy 418
Lymphangiomas 453, 747, 761, 766, 767*f*, 769, 777
Lymphedema 727
  prolonged postoperative 757
Lymphocytes 440
Lymphocytic infiltration, diffuse 434, 434*f*
Lymphocytopenia 437
Lymphoid cells, atypical large 452*f*
Lymphoid lesions 769
Lymphoid tissue
  lymphoma, part of mucosa-associated 450
  mucosa-associated 829*f*
Lymphoid tumors 454, 455, 763
Lymphoma 455, 737, 769, 771
Lysozyme 418, 794

M

Macroform erosions 16
Macrophages swollen 247
Macrostriae 403
Macuclear eye drops 635
Macugen 569
Macula 496, 599
  central 648
  scans of 640
  sensory detachment of 649*f*

  serous detachment of 615
  status of 143
Macular buckling 589, 590
Macular degeneration 495
Macular dysfunction 652
Macular edema 198, 479, 481, 482, 507*f*, 528, 532, 533, 533*f*, 534*f*, 592, 600, 602, 701
  chronic 440
  ischemic 601
  progression of 533
  resolution of 533*f*
  tomography of 645
  treating 483
Macular function tests 87, 88, 652
Macular hole 199, 242, 488, 490, 490*f*, 491*f*, 492, 642, 665*f*
  base of 490*f*
  full-thickness 408, 590, 644, 645*f*, 665*f*
  management of 642
  staging of 489*t*
  surgery 490-492
  surgical repair of 490
Macular infarction 408
Macular neovascularization, extrafoveal 567*f*
Macular neuroretinopathy, acute 431
Macular pigment optical density 633
Macular telangiectasia 505, 505*t*, 506*f*, 619
  classification of 505
  idiopathic 505
  signs of 508
  staging of 505
Macular traction
  maculopathy 585, 589*f*
  stages of 588
  retinal detachment 592
Maculopathy 591, 615*f*
  complication of 590
  dome-shaped 590
  hypotonic 256
  ischemic 597*f*
  preexisting 620
Maddox rod test 90, 654, 680
Magnetic resonance
  angiography 692, 773
  spectroscopy 689
  venography 693
Magnetic resonance imaging 433, 674
  scan 418, 427, 445, 682, 689, 690, 691, 694, 772, 820, 870, 915, 917, 925, 928
  sequences 691

Malignancy, secondary 437
Maloney topography
  method 219
Malyugin ring 144
Mandibulofacial dystosis 937
Mantoux test 414, 422, 427
Manual continuous curvilinear
  capsulorhexis 120
Manual small incision cataract
  surgery 146, 148-151
  preventing endothelial
    damage during 153
Marcus Gunn jaw-winking
  phenomenon 713
Marfan's syndrome 939
Marionette lines 731, 733
Masquerade syndrome 412,
  424, 452
Massive suprachoroidal
  hemorrhage 561
  spontaneous 561
Masson trichrome stained
  slide 449f
Mast cell degranulation 12
Measles 14, 429
Mechanical epithelial
  debridement 382
Medial canthal
  defects 739
  masses 831
  region 836
  swelling, painless
    progressive 845f
  tendon 798, 833, 842
    injuries 758, 758f
Medial orbitotomy 774, 775,
  873, 874
Medial rectus muscle 775, 932
Medial sac wall 799f
Medication, preoperative
  changes in 144
Medihoney 851
Medulloepithelioma 450, 451
Megalocornea 164f
Meibomian gland 720, 721
  disease 359
  dysfunction 5, 306, 719
  orifices 720
Meibomian
  orifice abnormalities 431
  seborrhea 5
Meibomitis 39
  primary 5
  secondary 5
Meige syndrome 731
Melaleuca alternifolia 720
Melanocytes 747
Melanocytic eyelid tumors,
  benign 747
Melanocytic nevi 744, 748

Melanocytic tumors,
  primary 454
Melanocytoma, choroidal 450
Melanoma 448, 580, 737
  cutaneous 763
  extensive conjunctival 850
  large 558
  malignant 451, 451f, 737
  small 558
Membrane surgery,
  extensive 462f
Meningioma 690t, 762, 769, 880
  multiple 881
  primary 872
Meningitides 25
Meningocele 759
Mesenchymal condensation,
  dysregulation of 876
Mesocephalic skulls 835
Metabolic diseases 508,
  935, 940
Metallic foreign body 609, 773,
  868, 869f
Metamorphopsia 488, 490,
  506, 656, 659
Metastasis
  choroidal 558, 580
  secondary 769
Metastatic colorectal cancer 439
Metastatic disease 769
Methamphetamine,
  inhalation of 427
Methotrexate 45, 72, 436,
  437, 736
Methyl methacrylate resin 865f
Methylcellulose, mixture of 345f
Methylprednisolone,
  intravenous 68, 422, 788
Meticulous anterior
  chamber 247
Microaneurysms 532, 533f
Microbial keratitis 56
  differential diagnosis of 23
Microbial spectrum 627
Microbiologic procedure 239
Microcephaly 942
Microcirculation, coronary 621
Microcoaxial phaco 141
Microcystic macular edema 701
Microcysts, epithelial 56
Microform erosions 16
Microhyfrecation 2
Microincisional cataract
  surgery 140, 141, 142f
  platform 140
Microincisional vitrectomy
  surgery 169, 660
Microkeratome 317, 401
  devices 319
  disposable 320
  flap 329t, 399
  mechanical 317

Microphacoemulsification,
  bimanual 138
Microphthalmos 759
Micropulse laser 303, 304
  machine 303f
  therapy 536
Micropulse transscleral
  cyclophotocoagulation
  303
Microspora 36
Microsporidia 29, 36, 387
Microsporidial keratitis 36, 37
Microsporidial
  keratoconjunctivitis
  36, 36f, 37
Microsporidial stromal
  keratitis 37, 37f
Microsporidiosis 37
Microstriae 404
Mid-canalicular
  obstructions 879
Midface trauma 831
Migraine, chronic 731
Mild-socket contracture 854
Milk-alkali syndrome 53
Millard–Gubler syndrome 682
Miniature visual acuity
  chart 653
Minimal incision cataract
  surgery 371
Minimal inhibitory
  concentration 100
Minimally classic choroidal
  neovascularization 513f
Minimally invasive glaucoma
  surgery 146, 297
  complication of 304
Minimally invasive surgical
  approach 801
Minimizing phaco times,
  technology upgrades
  for 124
Mini-monoka tubing 799
Minocycline 5
Mitomycin 254
  C 76, 234, 382, 393
  role of 382, 385
MK-2000 318
  microkeratome 318f
Mobile conjunctiva 252
Mobius sequence 938
Mobius syndrome 911
Moderate-socket
  contracture 854
Modern anterior chamber
  intraocular lenses 160
Mohs micrographic surgery
  735, 736
Moiré fringes 653
Molding procedures 380
Molecular techniques 575

Molecular weight 490
Molluscum contagiosum 442, 442f, 722
Molteno double plate implant 289f
Molteno implant 289, 289f
Monocanalicular stents 827
Mononucleosis 42
 infectious 11
Monosomy 936
Mooren's ulcer 43, 43f, 46
Moorfields safer surgery system 283, 283f
Moraxella 22, 23, 64
 lacunata 719
Morgagnian cataract 149
Moria one-use plus microkeratome 319f
Motility restriction 842
Motion
 artifact 612
 correction technology 504
Motor sequelae 916
Moxifloxacin 37
 eye 101, 239, 388f, 840
 hydrochloride 177
Mucocele 760, 769
 lacrimal 830
Mucoepidermoid carcinoma 455
Mucopolysaccharidoses 941
Mucormycosis 783f, 872
Mucosal grafts 738
Mucous membrane 834
 grafting 3
 granuloma formation 856
Müller's cells 593
Müller's muscle 708, 710, 713, 809
Multifocal central serous chorioretinopathy 651, 651f
Multifocal choroiditis 420, 424, 440, 659
Multifocal contact lenses, soft 948
Multifocal electroretinogram 90, 654
Multifocal hemorrhagic retinal vasculitis, acute 426
Multifocal intraocular lens 187, 369
 mix and match 191
 pearls for mixing 192
Multifocal placoid pigment epitheliopathy, acute posterior 420
Multimodal management 803
Multiple antivascular endothelial growth factor injections 588f

Multiple cotton-wool spots 528f
Multiple cutaneous neurofibromas 882f
Multiple drug therapy 29
Mumps 42
Munson's sign 51
Muscle
 bleeders 831
 layer 623
 of Riolan 714
 palsy, sequelae of 916
 protractive 707
 spasms 810
 strengthening procedures 923
 tendon, tucking of 923
 weakening procedures on 922
Musculoaponeurotic system, superficial 714
Mustarde's marginal pedicle rotation flap 798
Myasthenia gravis 686, 687, 709
 infantile 911
Mycobacteria 447
 atypical 23
 species 837
Mycobacterium 23
 fortuitum-chelonae 25
 leprae 447
 tuberculosis 72, 628
Mycophenolate mofetil 436, 788, 792
Mycosis fungicides 42
Mycotic ulcer treatment 27
Mydriasis 242, 892
 drugs for 892t
Myectomy 922
Myocardial infarction 601
Myocilin 272
Myoconjunctival technique 848
Myocysticercosis 769
Myogenic ptosis 709
Myogenic tumors 762
Myoneural junction 709
Myopathy, forms of 710
Myopia 271, 339, 637, 657, 894, 896, 946f, 946t
 early life 83
 high 200, 253, 494
 phaco in high 133
 prevalence of 945
 progression of 945, 948t
 suspect 945
 with early-stage keratoconus 368
Myopic choroidal neovascular membrane 657

Myopic maculopathy 590fc
 management of 585
Myopic retinoschisis 587
Myopic traction maculopathy 587
Myositis 790
Myotomy, marginal 922
Myotonic dystrophy 686
Myxoid tumors 454
Myxomatous tumors 762

N

Nasal bone 754
Nasal cavity 815, 831
Nasal deformity 815
Nasal detachment, superior 459
Nasal mucosae 834
Nasal pathologies 835
Nasal tip, upturned 942
Nasolacrimal canal 835
Nasolacrimal duct 815, 817, 820f, 823, 825f, 831, 843, 944
 obstruction 238, 815, 816, 818, 824, 828, 829, 835
 functional 817f
 right congenital 824f
Naso-orbito-ethmoid bone fracture 753, 758, 820f
Nasopharyngeal bacterial colonization 8
Natamycin 27, 28
Natural coralline 859
Natural crystalline lens, dislocation of 229
Nausea 228, 437, 438
Navigation system 774
Near stereopsis 899
 tests 903
Near vision 506
 chart 654
Neck stiffness 675
Necrosed tissues 782f
Necrosis 413
Necrotic herpetic retinopathies 426
Necrotizing encephalopathy, subacute 927
Necrotizing fasciitis 721, 781
Necrotizing scleritis 70, 72
 surgically-induced 71
Negative aberration Alcon IQ, Tecnis 185
Neisseria gonorrhoeae 9, 23, 25
Neodymium-doped yttrium-aluminum-garnet 263, 555
 laser 17, 212
 capsulotomy later 137
 iridotomy 251
 posterior capsulotomy 249

Index

Neodymium-doped yttrium orthovanadate 750
Neomycin 29
Neoplasia 769
  malignant 737
Neoplastic lesions 761, 765
Neovascular age-related macular degeneration 485, 485f, 647f
  management of 484, 487
Neovascular glaucoma 229, 241, 256, 291, 570
Neovascularization, course of 256
Nepafenac 103, 104
Nephropathy 942
Nerve
  fibers, abnormal decussation of 940
  sheath myxoma 879
Nerve palsy
  fourth 683
  nuclear
    sixth 682
    third 681
  sixth 682
  third 680, 710, 872
Netaherpetic keratitis 31f
Nettleship's punctal dilator 877
Neurilemmoma 761
Neuroblastoma 886, 887
Neurocutaneous syndromes 935, 940
Neurodegenerative nature 509
Neurofibroma 454, 737, 737f, 761, 777, 879, 884, 885
  choroidal 450
  diffuse 879, 885
  isolated 884
  preexisting 887
Neurofibromatosis 850, 880, 880f, 881f, 940
  clinical diagnosis of 881t
Neurogenic ptosis 709, 710
Neurogenic tumors 749
Neurological disorder 926
Neuromodulators 808
Neuronal ceroid lipofuscinoses 494
Neuro-ophthalmic manifestations 431
Neuro-ophthalmology 671
  electrophysiology in 693
Neuropathy 940
  glaucomatous 699f
Neuroretinal rim 278f
Neuroretinitis 420, 426, 625, 673, 674
  diffuse unilateral subacute 420, 424, 426

Neurosensory
  detachment 514, 649f
  retina persists 492
Neurotrophic keratitis 19, 20f, 31f, 381
  stages of 19
Neurotrophic keratopathy 31, 33, 35
  complication of 31
Neurovascular dysfunction 766
Neutrophils 434
Nevus 580, 737
  cells, number of 747
  flammeus 747, 750
New cut technologies 320
New generation formulas 221
Newer agents 481
Newer technologies 85
Newer vitrectomy systems 560
Niacin 596
Night blindness 494
  congenital stationary 928
Night glare and haloes 383
Nocardia 22, 23, 25, 446, 447
  keratitis 24
Nodular episcleritis 69
Nodular scleritis 70, 72
Nodules 413
Nonarteritic anterior ischemic optic neuropathy 673, 674
Noncentral macular subfields 599
Noncontact systems 518
Noncontact wide-angle viewing system 519f, 521
Non-distensible malformations 767
Nonepithelial tumors 455, 842
Non-fellow eyes, asymptomatic 639fc
Nongonococcal 8
Nongranulomatous anterior uveitis 413
Nonhealing foot ulcer 602
Non-Hodgkin's lymphoma 439, 448, 449f, 844f, 845f, 456
Noninfectious conditions 43
Noninfectious scleritis, types of 70
Noninflammatory orbitopathy 807
Noninterventional management 46
Nonischemic central retinal vein occlusion 481
Nonmalignant disorders 850
Nonpigment epithelium 450

Nonporous poly-methylmethacrylate orbital implant 859f
Nonproliferative diabetic retinopathy, moderate-to-severe 591
Nonrestrictive implants 289
Nonretinal ocular diseases 595
Nonspecific orbital inflammatory disease 792
Nonsteroidal anti-inflammatory drug 13, 71, 177, 180, 272, 523, 807, 850
  application of 102
  role of 102
  topical 104
Nonsurgical management 853
Nontuberculous mycobacterial keratitis 24
Nonvalved implants 289, 294
Noonan syndrome 942
Nosema and microsporidium 36
NOSPECS classification, modified 807f
Nothnagel's syndrome 681
Nucleal rotation 139
Nuclear
  cataract 268
  emulsification 113
  fragment removal 108
  opalescence 85
  piece 584
  ribonucleoprotein 44
Nucleotomy techniques 137
Nucleus
  chopping of 201
  course of 200
  dropped 469, 469f
  management 152
  phacoemulsification of 126
  rotation of 200
  soft 110t
Nutritional supplements 5
Nyctalopia 14
Nystagmus 908, 924, 924t, 926f, 927t, 929, 933, 940
  asymmetric horizontal 928
  blockage syndrome 911
  clinical management of 924
  graphic recording of 926
  infantile 925, 932
  latent 910, 925
  optical management of 928
  periodic alternating 926f
  pharmacological treatment of 929, 929t
  protocol of 931t
  vertical 927

Index

O

O'brien techniques 106
Occlusion
　amblyopia 897
　arterial 624
Occupational exposure 83
Ocriplasmin 465
Ocular association 257
Ocular changes 144
Ocular cicatricial pemphigoid 74, 878
Ocular comorbidities 522, 933
Ocular examination 413, 527, 596, 770
Ocular features 10
Ocular fundus 621
Ocular herpes simplex 30
Ocular histoplasmosis syndrome 655
Ocular hypertension 162, 601
Ocular hypotony 252, 419
　postoperative 252
Ocular inflammatory diseases 368
Ocular ischemic syndrome 531, 625
Ocular management 11
Ocular manifestations 180
Ocular motility 753, 770, 771, 791f
　disorders 690, 728
　evaluation of 908
　examination 680
　normal 836
　restricted 779f
Ocular movement 711, 790
　limitation 885
Ocular neovascularization 256
Ocular pain, severe 18
Ocular pathology 441, 445, 446t
Ocular preparations, topical 271
Ocular prosthesis
　indications of 862
　types of 862
Ocular sarcoidosis 426, 478
Ocular signs 621, 779
Ocular structures 703
　radiation tolerance of 702
Ocular surface 829f
　disease index 363
　disturbances 259
　evaluation of 395
　infections 878
　reconstruction 75
　squamous neoplasia 75, 76f
Ocular surgery 413
Ocular tissues 21, 430
Ocular trauma
　nonpenetrating 424
　types of 240

Ocular tumors 800, 803
　management of 800
Oculo-auriculo-vertebral syndrome 937
Oculocardiac reflex 924
Oculocerebral lymphoma 427
Oculodermal melanocytosis 748
Oculo-mandibulo-dyscephaly 938
Oculoplasty 705
Oil droplet sign 51
Okihiro syndrome 921
Old phaco tubings 124
Oleic acid 801
Olopatadine 13
Olson formula 222
Omega 3 fatty acid 633
Onchocerciasis 42
Oncolytic adenovirus, modified 636
Oncolytic virus VCN-01 treatment 636
Onion ring appearance 134
Opaque bubble layer 324, 330, 358, 401
Open globe injury 661, 664
Open haptic loops 159
Open-angle glaucoma 268, 269, 482
　preexisting 250
　primary 50, 270, 494
Operate pediatric cataract 208
Operating room
　etiquette 99
　sterilization of 96
　ventilation in 96
　waste disposal 99
Operation theater 214
　cleaning schedule 98
Operculum, complete detachment of 490f
Ophthalmia neonatorum 8f, 9
Ophthalmic evaluation, routine 262
Ophthalmic instruments, retinal phototoxicity from 620
Ophthalmic oncology task force 803
Ophthalmic radiation therapy 537
Ophthalmic vein, superior 781, 781f
Ophthalmic viscoelastic device 112, 129, 395
　complication of 114
Ophthalmic viscosurgical device 18, 120, 152, 203
　types of 115t

Ophthalmoplegia, chronic progressive external 686, 687
Ophthalmoscopy 770
　indirect 467, 637
Opportunistic infections 437
Optic atrophy 242, 430
　dominant 699
Optic canal decompression 688, 813
Optic disk 616
　congenitally anomalous 675
　damage 262
　　glaucomatous 262
　drusen 494, 667f
　edema, bilateral 674
　photography 262
　pit 581
Optic nerve 87, 454, 666, 704, 802f, 814, 836, 849
　avulsion 688, 689
　damage, degree of 143
　diseases 871
　disorders 689, 693, 695t
　glioma 454, 454f, 690, 761, 881f
　pathology of 454
　head
　　drusen 701
　　granuloma 421
　　involvement 436
　　pit 615
　injury 606
　lesions 503
　meningioma 690
　pits 615
　sheath 616
　　meningioma 525, 872f
　straightening of 787f
　stump measurement 847f
　transecting 847f
　tumors 689, 690, 761, 871
Optic neuritis 421, 431, 433, 678, 679, 689, 694, 695, 696f, 700
　acute phase of 698
Optic neuropathy 689, 842
　anterior 688
　compressive 697, 697f
　posterior 688
　radiation-induced 704
　toxic-nutritional 702
　traumatic 661, 663, 687, 689, 690, 698, 702, 872
Optic pit 615f, 616, 616f
Optical aberrations 348
Optical coherence
　pachymetry 329

Optical coherence tomography
 88, 180, 181*f*, 193, 213,
 213*f*, 214*f*, 269, 323, 334,
 417, 421, 425, 427, 488,
 489, 495, 497*f*, 513, 514*f*,
 516*f*, 523, 530, 564, 567*f*,
 580, 587, 590, 590*f*, 592,
 598, 610*f*, 619, 625*f*, 630*f*,
 633, 639, 642, 643*f*, 647,
 649*f*, 652, 657, 663, 676,
 700
  angiography 422, 479, 485,
 504, 509*f*, 531, 564, 599,
 609, 610, 612, 657, 666
  algorithms 611
  platforms 611
  work 610
  devices, physics of 640*f*
  intraoperative 135, 492*f*
  limitations of 702
  optic nerve head 277*f*
   analysis 277*f*, 278*f*
  role of 700
  scanning 640
Optical effects 197
Optical fiber free intravitreal
  surgery system 518
Optical illusion 853
Optical management 928*t*
Optical measures 948
Optical microangiography 611
Optical navigation 812
Optical phenomenon 200
Optical polarized test chart 902
Optical quality analysis
  system 391
Optical rehabilitation 27
Optical test chart 899
Optimal chemoprophylaxis 100
Optimal phaco machine
  settings 199
Optineurin 272
Optokinetic nystagmus 925, 928
  pursuit asymmetry on 910
Optos pseudocolor fundus
  imaging 488*f*
Ora serrata 638
Oral acyclovir 722
  indications of 32
Oral supplementation of
  carotenoids, treatment
  efficacy of 633
Orbicularis muscle 740*f*
  fibers 798
Orbicularis oculi 707, 744
Orbit 873
  computed tomography scan
  of 682, 690
  contrast-enhanced
  magnetic resonance
  imaging of 679

infectious disorders of 778
infective disorders of 778
inflammatory disorders
  of 778, 786
magnetic resonance
  imaging of 674
neoplastic lesions of 758
vascular lesions of 765
Orbital apical mass lesions 871
Orbital approach,
  advantage of 755
Orbital arteriography 773
Orbital biopsy 773
Orbital blowout fracture 922
Orbital bony
  decompression 812
Orbital cellulitis 770, 778, 836-
  839, 869*f*, 923
Orbital cephaloceles 759
Orbital compartment
  syndrome 766
Orbital complaints 887
Orbital congestion,
  secondary 767
Orbital contents,
  incarceration of 754*f*
Orbital cysticercosis 785
Orbital decompression 7
Orbital deformity, severe 850
Orbital dermoid cysts 800, 801
Orbital diseases, infiltrative 773
Orbital dumbbell dermoid
  cyst 801*f*
Orbital emphysema 755
Orbital examination 770
Orbital extension 777
Orbital fat 707
Orbital floor fracture 754*f*, 868*f*
Orbital foreign body
  extraction 814
Orbital fracture 752-754
  diagnosis of 752
  isolated 753
  management of 752
Orbital hematoma 727, 729
Orbital hydatid cyst 785
Orbital imaging 771, 868
Orbital implantation cysts 759
Orbital implants 856, 859
  complication of 861*t*
  types of 858*fc*
  wrapping of 857
Orbital infections 869
  bacterial 778
  fungal 783
Orbital inflammation 869
  specific 793
Orbital inflammatory
  disease 872
  idiopathic 790
  disorder, idiopathic 769

Orbital large floor fracture,
  right-sided 754*f*
Orbital lesions 681, 682, 760
Orbital lymphangioma 800
Orbital lymphoid tumors 456
Orbital lymphoma 455*f*, 456, 763
  B cell type 455*f*
  T cell type 456*f*
Orbital manifestations 432
Orbital mass, superolateral 764*f*
Orbital meningioma 454, 454*f*
  aggressive 850
  pathology of 454
Orbital myositis 432
Orbital pain 784
Orbital peripheral nerve
  sheath tumors 879
Orbital prosthesis 852
Orbital pseudotumor 579
Orbital reconstruction 851
Orbital schwannomas 887
Orbital septum 707, 797
Orbital surgery 773, 774, 812
  endoscopic-guided 774
Orbital tissues,
  displacement of 755
Orbital trauma 800, 868
Orbital tumor 453, 800, 811, 869
  benign 850
  management of 800
  primary 453
  resection 813
  secondary 763
Orbital varix 761
Orbital venography 773
Orbital venolymphatic
  malformation 872*f*
Orbitotomy 777, 823
  anterior 774, 873
  endoscopic 873, 874
  incisions 874*f*
  lateral 775, 802, 873
  without bone cut 802
Orbscan 344
Organ transplants 734
Orifices, loss of 720
Orthokeratology 948
Orthotropia 893
Oscillopsia 929
Osmotic 232
  effects 57
Osseointegration technique 851
Osseous tumor 454, 762
Osteoma 580, 762
Osteosarcoma 762
Ostiomeatal complex disease
  830
Outer lamellar macular
  hole 589*f*
Outer nerve fiber layer,
  dissociation of 492

Index

Outer retina 476
  disruption of 644
Outer retinal
  atrophy at macula 198
  hyper-reflective 508
    lesions 507
  layers 474
  necrosis, progressive 430
  tubulations 665
Oval intracellular bodies 37
Overfiltering bleb 261f
  assessment of 254
Overfunctioning blebs 259
Overhanging bleb 288, 296
Ovine hyaluronidase 468
Ozurdex 429

P

Pacemakers 773
Pachymetric progression
    index 311
Pachymetry 343
  assessment 314f
  evaluation 313
  thinnest 357
Paclitaxel 877
Paget's disease 53
Pain 31, 36, 41, 383, 651, 791
  excessive 92
  severe 244
  sudden onset of 228
Painless swelling, recurrent 844f
Pale discs 676
Palpebral fissure 809
Pan uveitis 435
Panophthalmitis 627
Pan-retinal laser
    photocoagulation 535
Pansinusitis 869f
Panuveitis 174, 424, 655
  causes of 424t
  idiopathic 440
  noninfective 425
Papanicolaou's stain 574
Papillary dilation 160
Papillary distortion 160
Papillary endothelial
    hyperplasia 747
Papillary hypertrophy 10
Papillary reaction 22
Papillary squamous
    carcinoma 845
Papilledema 674, 675, 701
Papilliform 76
Papillitis 673, 674
Papilloma 737, 841, 842
Papillomacular bundle 702
Papillopathy 602
Papillophlebitis 602

Par planitis 436
Parabulbar anesthesia 104,
    106, 559
Paracain eye drops 555
Paracentesis 282, 284
Paracentral acute middle
    maculopathy 431
Parachiasmal lesions 701
Parafoveal telangiectasia 659
Paranasal sinus tumors 763
  malignant 850
Parapontine reticular
    formation 682
Parasitic cysts 604
Parasitic diseases 785
Parasitic infections 42
Parathyroid hormone 53
Paresthesia 437
Parinaud's near vision chart 654
Parinaud's syndrome 722
Pars plana
  inferotemporal 563f
  insertion 294
  lensectomy 469, 471
  snowbanks 416
  vitrectomy 198, 258, 292,
    429, 461f, 462, 462f,
    464f, 468, 471, 524,
    541f, 588, 608, 661
  primary 460, 461
Pars planitis 415, 416t, 426, 436
  evidence of 416
  no evidence of 416
Pasteurella multocida 797
Patau's syndrome 936
Patching 17, 897
  near activity during 897
Patient information sheet 91
Pattern standard deviation 275
Pattern visual evoked
    potential 694
Pediatric apparent diffusion
    coefficient 838
Pediatric cataract 208
  management 933
  surgery 207, 210
Pediatric orbital
  anomalies 868
  implantation 860
Pediatric retina 477
  imaging 472
Pegaptanib 569
Pelli-Robson chart 154
Pellucid marginal
    corneal degeneration
    46, 47, 386
Pemphigus vulgaris 74
Pendular movement 317
Pendular nystagmus 927

Penetrating keratoplasty 35,
    48, 49, 58, 63, 64f, 164f,
    168, 291, 544
  procedures 165
Penicillin-resistant
    Staphylococcus 838
Pentacam equivalent
    K-reading report 334f
Pentacam map, normal 308f
Pentasodium
    colistimethanesulfate
    544
Pentoxifylline, oral 535
Peptococcus 22
Peptostreptococcus 22
Percutaneous sclerotherapy 800
Perennial allergic
    conjunctivitis 12
Perfluorocarbon liquid 470
  silicone oil exchange 520
  use of 550
Peribulbar anesthesia 104,
    105, 157
Pericanalicular
    inflammation 839
Pericardium 294
Pericentral retinitis
    pigmentosa 494
Perifoveal telangiectasia 531
Perifoveal vitreous
    detachment 489
Perineuritis 792f
Periocular anesthesia 157,
    158fc
Periocular steroids 523
Periocular tissues 782f
Periodic acid-Schiff
    stain 446, 574
  slide 448f
Periodic intravitreal
    lucentis 534f
Perioperative massive
    suprachoroidal
    hemorrhage 561
  risk factors for 561
Periorbital ache 618
Periorbital changes 771
Periorbital edema 780f, 791f
  right 779f
Periorbital swelling 22
Periosteal stock shell
    fixation 867
Periosteum 776f, 867
Peripapillary atrophy 658f
Peripapillary retinal nerve
    fiber layer thickness
    700
Peripheral nerve 454
  sheath tumor 761, 879
    malignant 887

Peripheral retina 553
  breaks 498
  persistent vascularity of 504f
Peritomy 848
  conjunctival 62, 293f, 470
Perivascular sheathing 528
Permanganate method 97
Peroxisomal disorders 928
Persistent epithelial
    defect 387, 389
Persistent inflammation 250
Personalized surgeon factor 222
Petaloid pattern, typical 523f
Peter Choyce lens 159
Phaco 146
  burst 108f
  incision 116, 117
    architecture of 116
    types of 116
  parameters, low 133
  pulse 107f
  time, pearls for
      minimizing 124
Phacoanaphylactic lens 435
Phacoaspiration 210f
Phacodonesis 153
Phacodynamics 107
Phacoemulsification 122, 123,
    128, 132, 140, 155, 178,
    197, 200, 201, 205, 371
  machine, parameters of 137
  postoperative treatment of
      uncomplicated 177
  steps of 113
  surgery 112
Phacosection 150
Phagocytosis, metabolic
    residue of 508
Phakic intraocular lens 52,
    161, 337, 339, 341, 342,
    348, 374
  classification of 337
  contraindications of 339
  implantation 344, 374
  indications of 339
  power calculation,
      parameters
      required for 340
  removal of 346
  surgery 311, 342
  types of 338f
Phakomatosis section 940
Pharmacologic testing 686
Pharmacological
    immunosuppression 77
Pharyngitis 8
Pharyngoconjunctival fever 10
Phenolic compounds 97
Phenylephrine 103, 892
  test 711

Pheral iridotomy 415
Phlyctenular inflammation 5
Phosphorus 934
  levels 414
Photic retinopathy 617
  index 618
Photo stress test 89, 652
Photochemical injury 619
Photodisruption 212
Photodynamic therapy 486,
    509, 516, 516f, 581, 613
  treatment of 587
Photographic
    documentation 771
Photophobia 31, 41, 54, 618, 804
Photopic negative response 699
Photoreceptor layer 474
  development 475
Photorefractive keratectomy,
    topo-guided 382
Phototoxicity, macular 408
Phthiriasis 722
Phthisis bulbi 53, 430, 846, 862f
Phylum straminipila 38
Picibanil 800
Piezoelectric bone surgery 774
Piggyback intraocular lens
    188, 223, 225t, 397
  calculation 397
  power 217, 224
Pigment
  absence of 940
  deposition 248, 262
  epithelial
    atrophy 506f
    derived factor 656
    detachment 485, 514f,
        625f, 648, 657
    epithelium 450, 594
    intraocular tumors 450
    peripunctal nevus 816f
Pigtail probe, use of 799
Pilocarpine 21, 54, 230, 685
Pilomatrixoma 749
Pingyangmycin 801
Pinhole acuity 88, 652
Pinhole-collimated gamma
    camera 819
Piperacillin 544
Pityrosporum orbiculare 723
Pizza pie retinopathy 430
Placido
  lesions 76
  topography, incorporation
      of 310
Plagiocephaly 937
Plaque brachytherapy 525,
    526, 803
Plasma
  cells 434, 435
  membrane changes 618

Platelet aggregation,
    defective 940
Pleistophora 36
Pleomorphic
    adenocarcinoma 763
Pleomorphic adenoma 454,
    455, 748, 763
  pathology of 455
Pleoptics 895
Plexiform
  layers 640
  neurofibroma 749, 879, 880,
      883f, 884f
Plus disease 553
  severe 553
Pneumatic displacement 565
Pneumatic retinopexy 459, 462
  vs. vitrectomy 462
Pneumocystis carinii 446
Pneumonia 14
Pneumonitis, acute 437
Pneumotonometer 244
Polaroid dissociation 899
Polaroid scotometer 902
Polyarteritis nodosa 43, 72, 426
Polyarticular juvenile
    idiopathic arthritis 439
Polychondritis, relapsing
    43, 426
Polyetheretherketone 756, 757f
Polyethylene 860
  implant 860
Polyglactin, synthetic
    mesh of 857
Polyhexamethylene
    biguanide 29, 37
Polyimide 185
Polymegathism, endothelial 56
Polymerase chain reaction 37,
    422, 427, 453f, 575
Polymeric implants 858
Polymerized
    glycosaminoglycans,
    accumulation of 272
Polymethylmethacrylate 56,
    174, 184, 185, 209, 376,
    855
Polymorphonuclear
    neutrophils 79
Polymorphous corneal
    dystrophy, posterior 50
Polymyxin B 840
Polyopia 86
Polypoidal choroidal
    vasculopathy 510, 516,
    563, 668f
  subclassification of 515
Polypoidal lesion 745
Polypropylene 185
Polytetrafluoroethylene 757f

Polytrauma, facial 820
Polyvinylidene fluoride 185
Polyvinylpyrrolidone 100
Pontomedullary abnormalities 927
Pork tapeworm 785
Porous ceramic implants 859
Porous Medpor® implant 860*f*
Porous polyethylene 756, 855
Porphyria cutanea tarda 74
Port-wine stain 747, 750, 767
Posner–Schlossman syndrome 229
Post-adenoviral subepithelial infiltrates 11
Post-cataract surgery 177, 538
  cystoid macular edema 180, 181*f*
  endophthalmitis 541*f*
Post-Descemet's membrane endothelial keratoplasty 62*f*
Post-enucleation socket syndrome 854
Posterior aqueous diversion syndrome 231
Posterior capsular
  dehiscence 137
  opacification 121, 198, 304, 408
  rupture 122, 131
  tear 195
Posterior capsule
  fibrosis, management of 199
  opacification 207, 209, 215, 369
  rupture 583
Posterior chamber defect, preexisting 200
Posterior chamber intraocular lens 161, 165, 206
  implantation 128
Posterior continuous curvilinear capsulorhexis 137, 209
Posterior polar
  cataract 134, 138, 200
  cortical disc defect 135
Posterior vitreous
  cavity 583
  detachment 407, 470, 488, 603, 607, 644, 662
  acute 638, 638*fc*
Post-fever retinitis 423
Postintravitreal bevacizumab 498*f*
Postintravitreal injection 538
Post-laser-assisted in situ keratomileusis 387, 390
  adjustment, topography-based 334

Post-pars plana vitrectomy 589*f*
Postprandial blood sugars 917
Postrefractive surgery 332, 335
  complications 394
  ectasia 386
Post-trabeculectomy 538
Post-traumatic macular holes 490
Postvitrectomy 538
Potential acuity meter 89, 652, 653
Pouting vascularized mucosa, stage of 877
Povidone iodine 100
Power calculation 218*t*, 340
Prader–Willi syndrome 942
Preauricular glands 708
Precise incision construction 199
Precocious puberty 942
Pre-Descemet's endothelial keratoplasty 60, 63
Prednisolone 70, 422
Preeclampsia 623
Preinjection fluorescence 501
Premalignant lesions 744
Prematurity, aggressive retinopathy of 477*f*, 553, 554*f*, 555
Premyopia 945, 946*t*
Preplus disease 553
Preretinal hemorrhage 498*f*
Preretinal neovascularization 475
PresbyLASIK, peripheral 378
Presbyond laser blended vision 379
Presbyopia 341, 376
  correction of 376
Presbyopic allogenic refractive lenticule implantation procedure 377
Presbyopic laser-assisted in situ keratomileusis 378
Presbyopic phakic intraocular lenses 341
Preseptal cellulitis 721, 778, 836, 838
PreserFlo microshunt 302*f*
Pressure conformers 867
Pressure over lacrimal sac test 842
  regurgitation on 816, 817
Pressure patch 255
Presumed ocular histoplasmosis syndrome 420
Presumed sterile 23
Pretrichial brow lift 730
Prevotella species 837

Primary angle-closure glaucoma, chronic 262
Prism test, vertical 910
Progressive scarring, stage of 877
Projection artifact 611
Proliferative diabetic retinopathy 463, 496, 498*f*, 592
Proliferative vitreoretinopathy 459, 462*f*, 468, 548, 551, 609
  postoperative 549
  prevention of 551
  primary 549
  severe 560
Promote epithelial healing 80
Promote stromal healing 80
Propamidine 29, 54
Prophylaxis 637
  preoperative 100
Propionibacterium acnes 100, 206, 542, 719
Proptosis 753, 755, 767*f*, 769, 783*f*, 784, 786, 790, 793*f*, 842, 844*f*, 845*f*, 883
  bilateral 787*f*
  evaluation of 771
  measurement of 771
  right 779*f*
  surgical management of 769
  types of 770, 771
  variability of 771
Prostaglandin analogs 596
Prostheses, facial 867
Prosthesis 852, 866
  custom-made 863, 863*f*
  maintenance of 867
Prosthetic devices 183
Protein
  C 481
  S deficiency 481
Proteus 71
Proton magnetic resonance spectroscopy 693
Protracted epithelial ulceration 27
Proximal lacrimal
  disorders 820
  drainage apparatus
    acquired anomalies of 876
    congenital anomalies of 875
Proximally placed limbs 942
Pseudocyst, foveal 644
Pseudodendrites 34
Pseudodendritic keratitis 21
Pseudodendritic lesions, fungal 26

Pseudoexfoliation 143
  material 268
  syndrome 153, 267, 268
Pseudoholes 488
Pseudomembrane 10f
Pseudomonas 23, 71, 545
  aeruginosa 22, 56, 387, 544, 837
  infection 545
  species 25
Pseudopapilledema 674, 675
Pseudophakia 249f, 291, 292, 605f
  pigment dispersion with 248
Pseudophakic bullous keratopathy 18, 50, 62f, 159, 162
Pseudophakic cystoid macular edema 521, 522f
Pseudophakic patient 894
Pseudophakic pigmentary glaucoma 248
Pseudophakos 254
Pseudoproptosis 769
  causes of 769
Pseudoptosis 755
Pseudotrachoma 55
Pseudotumor 448, 448t
  cerebri 675
Pseudoxanthoma elasticum 938, 939
Psoriasis 439
Psoriatic arthritis 439
Pterional approach 874
Pterygium 77
Pterygopalatine fossa 784f
Pthirus pubis 5, 722
Pthisis bulbi 303
Ptosis 679, 686, 708, 713, 727, 779f, 780f, 784, 784f, 855, 861, 883
  amount of 710
  aponeurotic 709, 710, 710f
  apparent 709
  bilateral 681
  causes of 709
  congenital 712
  contralateral 769
  evaluation of 710
  globe 854
  mechanical 710
  mild 710
  moderate 710, 712
  right 782f, 794f
    complete 791f
  severe 710
  S-shaped 761
  surgery, complication of 713
Pulsatile tinnitus 675

Pulse 107, 124
  high-intensity focused ultrasound 487
  per second 109
  sequences 691
  steroid 68
Puncta 876
  examination of 815
Punctal agenesis, treatment for 875
Punctal and canalicular agenesis 875
Punctal edema, stage of progressive 877
Punctal occlusion 406
Punctal papilla, absence of 875f
Punctal papillary region 876f
Punctal stenosis 877
Punctate epithelial granularity 10
  keratopathy 30
  staining, superior 57
Punctate inner choroidopathy 420
Punctate keratitis, superficial 56
Punctate keratopathy, superficial 12
Punctum dilatation 825f
Pupil 244, 339, 865f
  abnormal 684
  diameter 617
  dilators and hooks 144
  distortion of 162
  fixation 382
  poorly dilating 153
  small 112, 114, 174, 685
  unequal 684
  white 579
Pupillary assessment 90, 654
Pupillary block 249, 287
  glaucoma 232, 249, 249f
Pupillary dilatation, degree of 143
Pupillary dilation 268, 620
Pupillary margin 257
Pupillary reaction 770, 836
Pupillary reflexes 753
Pure clear corneal incision 116
Purse-string sutures 284
Putterman surgery 713
Pyoderma gangrenosum 439
Pyogenic granuloma 442, 443f, 750, 765, 766f
Pythium 38, 39
  cell wall 39
  hyphae 39
  insidiosum 38
  keratitis 38

Q

Quantiferon test 414
Quantiferon-TB gold tests 422
Quantifying motility 805f
Quantitative optical coherence tomography angiography 613
Quinolone antibiotic 25

R

Rabies prophylaxis 797
Radial keratotomy 332, 369
  effects of 332, 332f
Radial sclerotomy, multiple 849
Radial thermal keratoplasty 380
Radiation
  retinopathy 524, 525, 528f, 625
  side effects of mild 525
  treatment, effects of 525
  type of 525
Radiation maculopathy 524
  cumulative incidence of 526f
  treatment of 531
Radiation optic neuropathy 525, 528
  treatment of 531
Radiation therapy 525, 793
  local 879
Radical vitrectomy 542f
Radiofrequency 120, 209
  ablation 120
  cautery device 725
Radiologic examination 753
Radiotherapy 76, 702, 810
  consequence of 524
  intensity-modulated 703
  role of 887
Radius measurement error 333
Rainbow glare 330
Randot stereotest 904
Ranibizumab 480, 483, 486, 516, 517f, 534f, 569, 587, 615
  efficacy of 480
  injection 533f
  intravitreal 615
Ranizurel 569
Rapid plasma reagin test 414
Rapidly progressive diffuse suppurative infiltrate 23
Rash 437
Raymond's syndrome 682
Razumab 569
Recent dental procedures 412
Receptor antagonists, specific 439

Recession 922
Recirculation phase 500
Rectus muscles 797
　isolation of 293f
　lateral 932
Recurrent corneal erosion 393
　classification 16
　syndrome 16
Red cell galactokinase 934
Red filter test 899, 902
Red reflex, reduced 629
Redness 244
　lids 806
Reducing sugars, urine for 934
Rees incision, classic 724
Refillable reservoir devices 487
Refraction 86, 262, 339, 340, 382, 395, 907
　pediatric 892
Refractive correction 911
　advanced 322
Refractive error 892, 910, 929, 940
　high 341, 617
　visual field test 276
Refractive implantable lens 337, 342, 343
Refractive intraocular lens 187
Refractive lens exchange 368, 369, 372, 376
　preoperative for 369
Refractive lenticule extraction 362
Refractive multifocal intraocular lens, rezoom 192f
Refractive surgery 217, 219t, 305, 309, 321, 350, 350t, 383, 407
　modern 321
　newer procedures in 391
　preoperative work-up for 306
　retreatment options following 372
　techniques 332
Refractive surprise after cataract surgery 394
Refractory glaucoma
　treatment of 303
　types of 303
Refractory infantile glaucoma 291
Refsum disease 494, 943
Regression 553
　formulas 217
Renal disease 596
Renal failure, chronic 625f
Renal function 592

Renal rejection,
　prophylaxis of 439
Renal toxicity 438
Residual mass 527f
Resight system 518f
Respiratory distress syndrome 782, 827
Resultant fistula 836
Retina 457, 558, 573, 619, 645, 704
　abnormal 928t
　avascular 477f
　causes 648
　causing schisis 616
　inflammatory diseases of 647, 647f
　normal 640
　photothermal damage to 618
　portion of 468, 626
　society classification 548
　thin 588
　ultrasound energy on 584
Retinal abscesses, multiple 628f
Retinal artery
　macroaneurysm 467, 564
　occlusions, risk for 623
Retinal breaks 242, 577, 637
Retinal changes, monitor 641
Retinal conditions 568
Retinal correspondence, test for abnormal 899
Retinal cotton wool spots 629
Retinal detachment 158, 198, 206, 242, 339, 408, 461f, 462f, 464f, 468, 520, 541f, 548, 562, 577, 590, 604, 604f, 605, 606, 629, 630, 637, 753, 935
　advanced tractional 496f
　configuration of 472
　long duration of 548, 549
　postperforating injury 548
　previous 561
　revision surgeries for recurrent 551
　risk factors for 368
　subtotal 459f, 460f
　surgery 12, 291
　tear with 662
　total aphakic 461f
　tractional 498f, 528
Retinal dialysis 661, 662
Retinal diseases 196, 594
Retinal disorders 339
　management of 647
Retinal drug toxicities 666
Retinal dysplasia 942
Retinal dystrophy 926
Retinal edema 622

Retinal ganglion cells 593
Retinal gene therapy
　delivery 594f
Retinal hard exudates 528
Retinal hemorrhages 528
Retinal hole, full-thickness 488
Retinal imaging 664
　techniques 664
Retinal inner layer,
　disorganization of 665
Retinal ischemia 257
Retinal layers 641f
Retinal microaneurysms 528
Retinal microvascular
　lesions 627
　signs 624
Retinal morphology,
　quantitative
　measurements of 642
Retinal necrosis 630
　acute 423, 429
Retinal neovascularization 419, 479, 528
Retinal nerve fiber
　analysis 251
　layer 640, 700
　　defects 278f
　　hemorrhages 624f
　　superior wedge-shaped 277f
　　thickness 278f
Retinal ocular diseases 595
Retinal pathology 642
　co-existent 492
Retinal photography,
　role of 627
Retinal pigment
　epitheliopathy, diffuse 650f
　epithelitis 420, 620
　epithelium 434, 474f, 495, 508, 514f, 528, 566, 593, 612, 617, 622, 625f, 632, 634, 640, 646, 666, 940
　　detachment 517f
Retinal pigment epithelial 558
　adenocarcinoma 451
　detachment 510
Retinal surgery 556
　retrofixation after 164f
Retinal tamponade 491
Retinal tears 661
　large 549
Retinal telangiectasia 505
　idiopathic juxtafoveolar 505
Retinal telangiectatic
　vessels 528
Retinal thickening 599, 665f
Retinal thickness, spongy 643f
Retinal tomography 647

Index

Retinal vascular
 changes 624
 disease 424, 481, 620
 occlusion 568, 569, 645
Retinal vasculitis 420, 425, 426, 428, 437
 idiopathic 426
 infective 428
Retinal vein occlusion 256, 483, 646f
Retinal-choroidal
 architecture 625f
Retinectomies 550
Retinitis 420
 arboviral 430
 herpetic 423
 pigmentosa 198, 493, 667f, 935, 943
  transplantation for 495
  triad of 494
  variants of 494
 punctata albescens 494
 viral 429
Retinoblastoma 448, 449f, 452-452, 580, 635, 636, 769
 classification of 452
 eye ball appear, cut section of 451
 prenatal diagnosis of 636
Retinochoroiditis 420
Retinopathy 620, 621
 anemia-associated 531
 cancer associated 427
 hypertensive 531, 621, 623, 624f, 626, 626t
 mixed 602
Retinopathy of prematurity 473, 475, 504f, 552, 554f, 555, 570, 665
 classification of 552
 early treatment for 555, 556
 screening 554
 staging 552
 treatment 555
Retinopexy 550
Retinoschisis 588
 advanced stage of 589f
 X-linked 594, 595
Retinoscopic reflex, poor 208
Retinoscopy 51, 892
Retinotomy
 drainage 550
 relaxing 550
Retractors 708, 775f
Retrobulbar pain 804
Retrofixation 164f
Retroiris claw lens 164f
Retroiris-fixated lens 164
Retro-orbicularis oculi fat 725
Rhabdomyoma 454

Rhabdomyosarcoma 448, 454, 762, 769
Rhegmatogenous retinal
 detachment 419, 496, 459, 662
 management of 462
 subtotal 460f
 surgical management of 459
Rheumatoid arthritis 43, 413, 424, 426, 439, 579
 juvenile 174
Rheumatoid factor 44, 71, 427, 678
Rhino-orbital-cerebral
 mucormycosis 783, 872
Rhizopus oryzae 783
Rhomboid flap 739
Rib 855
Ribavirin 433
Riboflavin 26, 47, 52
 variation in 384, 385
Ribonucleic acid 935
Ribosomal ribonucleic acid 37
Rickettsial diseases 427
Right eye 470, 817f, 875f
 conjunctival congestion 792f
 ocular surface squamous
  neoplasia 803f
 upper eyelid 876f, 878f
Rigid gas permeable 52
Ringer lactate 79
Rituximab 45, 439, 440, 793, 809
River blindness 42
Rizzuti phenomenon 51
Rod-cone dystrophies 666
Room-temperature vulcanized
 silicone 855
Root mean square 311
Rosacea 39
Rosai-Dorfman disease 793
Rose Bengal
 photodynamic therapy 26
 stain 31, 76
Rotation flap 739
Roth's spots 629, 630f
RPE65 gene 495
Rubella 429, 655
Rubeotic glaucoma 256
Rubinstein-Taybi syndrome 942
Ruptured lens capsule 435f
Ruptured normal vessel 467

S

Sac-nasolacrimal
 duct 819f, 821f
Sacroiliac joint, X-ray of 427
Saline lavage 9
Sampaolesi line 269
Sample treatment plans 916

Sarcoidosis 43, 53, 412, 415, 417, 418, 420, 422, 424, 426, 436, 440, 677, 771, 793, 794
Scalp tenderness 675
Scalpel-shaped incision 724
Scanning electron
 microscope 120
Scanning laser
 ophthalmoscopy 504
 based angiography 504
Scans, types of 605
Scar related issues 727
Scatter laser photocoagulation 429, 479
Scharioth technique 169, 170f
Scheie systems 621
Scheimpflug device 309
Scheimpflug image 85, 310f, 332
 device
  disadvantages of 312
  limitations of 312
  single 310
Scheimpflug principle 309
 application of 309
Scheimpflug topographers 311
Scheimpflug-based systems,
 variations in 310
Schirmer's test 175, 306, 818
Schlemm's canal 300
Schnyder's crystalline
 dystrophy 47
Schroeder classification 135
Schwannoma 448, 454, 750, 761, 880, 885, 886f, 887
 displaying spindle-
  shaped 86f
 extension of 887
 multiple 885
Schwannomatosis 885
Sclera 71, 294, 295f, 413, 703, 857
 based procedures 376
 thin 149
Scleral buckle 459, 460f, 462, 549, 580
Scleral disease 149
Scleral expansion 376
Scleral fixation 470
 sutureless 169
Scleral flap 283, 285
 closure of 282, 282f
 creation 281
 of triangular 281f
 partial thickness 281
 related complications 285
 sutures 284
Scleral incision 376
 advantages of 118t
 disadvantages of 118t

Scleral indentation 467
Scleral lamella pocket 171*f*
Scleral lens therapy 75
Scleral melt 606
Scleral patch 294
Scleral perforation 923
Scleral pockets, partial
    thickness 471
Scleral quadrisection 849
Scleral tear 295
Scleral thinning 291, 292
Scleral tunnel 295*f*
    incision 116, 118
    superior 470
Scleral-fixated intraocular
    lens 165, 166
    techniques of 166, 167*fc*
Sclerectomy, lamellar 803*f*
Scleritis 25, 69, 70, 413, 579, 606
    complication of 71
    diffuse 72
        anterior 70
    infectious 71
    posterior 71, 424
    treatment of infective 72
Sclerocornea 265
Scleroderma 769
Sclerokeratitis 34
    fungal 573
Scleromalacia perforans 70
Sclerosing agents 800
Sclerosis, multiple 415, 417,
    418, 426, 439, 700, 701
Sclerostomy 281, 282*f*, 284, 285
Sclerotomy 472, 563*f*, 848
    incision 608*f*
    placement 559
    posterior 849
    quadrisection technique 848*f*
    site of 559
    techniques 849
Scoliosis 942
Score trial 479
Scotoma 415, 656
    central 488
    depth of 902
    extent of 902
    size of 902*t*
Scotomata, paracentral 618
Sculpting 108
Sealing phaco incision 117
Sebaceous cell carcinoma 777
Sebaceous gland
    acute infection of 721
    adenoma 749
    carcinoma 444, 444*f*,
        736, 736*f*
    hyperplasia 749
    tumors, benign 749
Seborrheic alone 5

Seborrheic blepharitis 5
Seborrheic dermatitis 719
Seborrheic keratosis 744, 747
Sectoral retinitis
    pigmentosa 494
Secukinumab 439
See-saw nystagmus 927
Segmentation artifact 612
Seidel's sign 237*f*
Seidel's test 239, 259
Seizures 942
Self-lubricating prosthesis 862
Semipermanent biodegradable
    compounds 733
Sensorineural hearing loss 928
Sensory
    adaptation, abnormal 899
    functions 898
    nystagmus 926
    retinal thickening 514
    sequelae 916
    system, assessment of 899
Serous
    choroidal effusion 255
    macular detachment 590*f*
    retinal detachment 616,
        644*f*, 645, 665
Serpiginous choroiditis 420, 440
    reactivation of 432
Serpiginous choroidopathy 659
Serpiginous ulceration 34
Serratia 22, 23, 629
    marcescens 56, 64, 837
Serum
    angiotensin-converting
        enzyme 53, 427
    levels 414
    calcium 414
    immunoglobulin G4 771
    lipid levels 596
    lysozyme levels 414
Severe acute respiratory
    syndrome
        coronavirus 2 430
Shaken baby syndrome 475
Shallow anterior chamber 161,
    228, 263, 286, 287
Shallow inferior
    detachment 459
Shallow staphyloma 657
Shallow subretinal fluid,
    chronic 650
Shamma's fudged formula 218
Shamma's method 219
Shamma's refraction
    method 219
Shapirno and Leen, modified
    technique of 168, 168*f*
Sheath-guided lacrimal
    intubation 819
Sheathotomy, arteriovenous 481

Short stature 942
Short tau inversion recovery 692
Short tube 295
Siedel's test 254
Siepser slipknot technique 148*f*
Silent sinus syndrome 760
Silicon 185
    facial prosthesis 867
    intraocular lenses 100
    material 867
    oil 244, 577
        injection 461*f*, 462*f*
        removal of 551
    tires 12
    tubing 826
Simmons shell 287
Simple limbal epithelial
    transplantation 80
Simulated divergence
    excess 913
Simultaneous macular
    perception slides 900,
        900*f*
Singh classification 135
Singh's modified iris-claw
    lens 163
Singh-worst design 163*f*
Single visual field data 274
Sino-orbital mucormycosis 850
Sinus
    cavities 784
    superior discharging 779*f*
Sinusitis 8
    maxillary 830
Sirolimus 436, 635
Sixth nerve palsy,
    congenital 910
Sjögren's syndrome 426, 793
Skin 707, 714, 738, 873, 935, 938
    abscess 721
    closure 741*f*
    disorders 939
    epithelium 744
    excoriation of 779*f*
    Fitzpatrick type of 734
    graft 855
        full-thickness 740*f*
        split-thickness 851
    incision 725, 831
    infection, superficial 721
    marking 724
    necrosis of 782*f*
    tag 745
    ulceration 842
Slack zonules 231
Slit-lamp 815
    biomicroscopy 239, 262, 416
    evaluation 259, 339
    examination 44, 86, 250,
        382, 413, 540, 606, 753,
        852, 946

Small hard drusen 631
Small incision lenticule
  extraction 350, 357,
  362, 363, 367, 372, 377,
  391, 392
  complication of 357, 358*fc*
  secondary 374
Small pupil, pseudoexfoliation
  with 201
SMILE to flap 374
SMILE Xtra 385
Smoking 596
Smooth muscle tumor 450
Snellen's vision 652
Snuff out 287
Socket contraction 854
Socket contracture 855, 867
  end-stage 850
Socket infection 856
Socket irritation and
  discharge 867
Sodium
  chloride 17, 50
  injection 730
  fluorescein 473, 499
  hyaluronate 113
SofPort advance optics 155, 186
Soft shell technique 113
Soft tissue 753
  dissection 847*f*
  lesions, visualization of 813
  sarcomas 887
Solar lentigo 747
Solar maculopathy, chronic 619*f*
Solitary fibrous tumor 448, 844*f*
Solitary neurofibroma 749, 879
Solitary trichoepithelioma 749
Spasms, infantile 942
Spastic lid disorders 730
Spatial presaturation inversion
  recovery 692
Specific disease,
  treatment of 428
Speckle variance 611
Spectacle 398, 948
  prosthesis 852
Spectral-domain optical
  coherence tomography
  472, 474*f*, 479, 489*f*-491*f*,
  506*f*, 522*f*, 598, 619*f*
  postoperative 491*f*
Specular microscopy 50, 66,
  87, 340, 343
Sphenoid wing dysplasia 883*f*
Spheroidal degeneration 393
Sphincter sclerosis 174
Spinal bifida 942
Spindle cell 451
  hemangioma 765
  melanoma 451

Split calvarium 855
Split nevus 748
Split spectrum 611
  amplitude decorrelation
  angiography 504, 611
Spondyloarthritis 426
Sports-related injuries 752
Squamous cell carcinoma 442,
  444, 444*f*, 448, 450*f*,
  735, 744, 842
Squamous metaplasia 841
Squamous papilloma 442,
  443*f*, 745
Squint 710
  divergent 912
  paralytic 907, 916
  restrictive 907
  surgery 922
SRK formula 221
Stain, type of 447
Stallard-Wright
  incision 775, 873
Standard fluorescein
  angiography 503
Staphylococcal
  blepharitis 74
  bullous impetigo 721
  keratitis 388*f*
  lid disease 722*f*
Staphylococcus 25, 40, 239,
  288, 878
  aureus 4, 22, 39, 56, 64, 100,
    101, 239, 387, 539, 628,
    719, 837, 840
  antigens 40
  methicillin-resistant 628
  epidermidis 23, 64, 100, 539
  epidermis 628
  species 830
Staphyloma
  anterior 846
  posterior 586*f*, 587
  progressive 589
Stargardt disease 594, 666
  early 620
Static rhytides 732
Static wrinkles 732
Stay sutures 923
Steep-walled blebs 261
Stem cell 635
  damage 79
  therapy, role of 495
  transplantation 493
Stereoacuity 902
Stereopsis 900
  evaluation 899
Stereoscopic diagonal
  inverter 518
Stereotactic external beam
  radiotherapy 802

Stereotactic navigation
  guidance 774
Sterile air 460*f*
Sterile keratitis,
  development of 387
Steroid 32, 80, 232, 271, 306
  administration,
  regimens for 808
  antibiotic combination 245
  delivery, route of 271
  drops 230
  induced glaucoma 229, 249,
    270, 271
  injection 4
  intravitreal 423, 479, 523
  oral 422
  preoperative 549
  response 243
  subconjunctival 68
  types of 271
  use of 412
Stevens-Johnson
  syndrome 74, 718
Stickler syndrome 939
Stock shell 862, 863*f*, 863*t*
  prosthesis 863
Stomatitis 437
Stone mold making 864
Stored tissue 66
Strabismus 267, 833, 875, 891,
  917, 933, 940
  fixus 922
  horizontal comitant 923
  paralytic 916
  restrictive 921
  surgery 922
  treatment of 898
  types of 731
Streptococcal
  infections 721
  species 239
Streptococci viridans 100
Streptococcus 25, 288, 721, 782
  pneumoniae 56, 64, 628, 837
  pyogenes 801
  species 100
  viridans 64
Streptomyces verticillus 801
Striated muscle 744
Stringy discharge 22
Stroke, ischemic 431
Stroma 79
  progressive destruction of 45
  vascularization of 41
Stromal degeneration 387, 389
Stromal dystrophies 47
Stromal edema 56, 267
Stromal healing 80
Stromal interstitial keratitis 31
Stromal invasion stage 28

Index

Stromal keratitis 37, 69
  pressure-induced 405
Stromal keratopathy 31
Stromal lesions 28
Stromal necrosis 31
Stromal rejection 67
Stromal scarring 19, 31, 61
Stromal striae 56
Stromal tumors 735
Stromal ulceration 31
Stryker saw 776, 776*f*
Sturge-Weber syndrome 253, 291, 737, 767, 940
Stye 3, 4
Subarachnoid portion 681, 682
Subarachnoid space 684
Sub-basal corneal nerves, transection of 363
Sub-cap lenticule extraction 374
Subcapsular cataract, posterior 494
Subconjunctival 5-fu 285
Subconjunctival injection 24, 234
Subcutaneous emphysema 753
Subcutaneous tissue 707, 744
Subdural hemorrhage 467
Subepithelial infiltrates 9, 67
Subepithelial reticular dot infiltrates 38*f*
Subfoveal melanomas 532
Subglottic lesions 765
Subhyaloid hemorrhage 661, 663
Subluxated capsular bag, severely 131
Subluxated cataract 112
  management of 127
Submacular bleed 662
Submacular hemorrhage 563, 566*f*
  displacement of 566*f*, 567*f*
  small 564
Submandibular nodes 734
Suborbicularis oculi fat 707
Subperiosteal abscess 778, 780, 780*f*, 839
Subretinal abscess 630
Subretinal fibrinous material 511
Subretinal fibrosis 420
Subretinal fluid 517*f*, 588*f*, 590*f*, 625*f*, 647, 650, 650*f*
  drainage 461
  macula 648
  persists 648
Subretinal gliosis 462*f*
Subretinal hemorrhage 590, 661
Subretinal hyperreflective membrane 656*f*, 665
Subretinal injection 593

Subretinal lipid exudation 514
Subretinal material 648
Subretinal membranes 548
  removal of 550
Subretinal neovascularization 505, 506*f*
Subretinal pneumatic displacement 566
Subretinal transplantation, tolerability of 495
Sub-Tenon
  anesthesia 104, 106
  space 873
Suction loss 358, 400
Sulcus
  deformity, superior 809, 855
  to sulcus scan 605
Sulfa allergy 75
Sulfamethoxazole 25, 418
Summit-Krumeich-Barraquer-microkeratome 317, 318*f*
Superior oblique sheath syndrome 921
Superior rectus 932
  levator palpebrae superioris 794*f*
  traction suture 280, 280*f*
  weakness 709
Superonasal quadrant 280, 772*f*
Superotemporal branch retinal vein occlusion 480*f*
Superotemporal neuroretinal rim 277*f*
Superotemporal pars plana 562*f*
Superotemporal quadrant 277*f*, 557*f*
Superotemporal vessels 462*f*
Suprachoroidal drainage 297
Suprachoroidal drug delivery 487
Suprachoroidal fluid 255
Suprachoroidal hemorrhage 232, 244, 255, 286, 287, 295, 296, 561, 562*f*, 563*f*, 590
  pathogenesis of perioperative 561
Supracor 378
Supratrochlear nerves 885
Surface ablation 373, 374, 381
  techniques 382
  complication of 383
Surgery 20, 76, 536
  complication of 93
  after 92
  during 92
  cornea-based 407
  goal of 920
  indications of 86, 588, 755, 919

  site of 283
  steps of 757*f*
  timing of 755, 796, 909
  type of 238
Surgical care 840
Surgical complications 522
Surgical endothelial trauma 18
Surgical excision 76
Surgical options 549
Surgical precautions 133
Surgical procedure 7, 80, 204, 756
Surgical steps 208
Surgical technique 136, 214, 292, 365, 584, 724, 728, 755
Surgical treatment 19, 27, 263, 524, 711
Susac's syndrome 426
Suture
  adjustment 58
  discomfort 284
  gonioscopy-assisted transluminal trabeculotomy 299*f*
  granuloma 713*f*
  lysis 235
  material 166
  removal and replacement 58
  tarsal plate 741*f*
  tight 59
  with infiltrate 59
Suture-related problems 172
Swan's syndrome 247
Sweat glands, benign tumors of 748
Sweating 228
Swelling 93
Swiss-cheese
  appearance 53
  pattern 455
Swollen cataractous lens 241
Symblepharon 11, 528
  formation 21, 757, 859*f*
  ring 287
Sympathetic ophthalmia 421, 424, 434, 436, 440, 579
  pathology of 434
Sympathetic palsy 685
Symptoms gastrointestinal tract 412
Synchrony intraocular lens 186
Syndromic retinitis pigmentosa 494
Synechiae
  anterior 242, 262
  formation 236
  posterior 32, 143, 174, 250
Synechiolysis 144

Index

Synkinetic movements, abnormal 711
Synkinetic ptosis 710
Synoptophore 899, 900, 900f, 902
 simultaneous prescription slides 899
Syphilis 418, 420, 423, 424, 427, 428
 acquired 42
 congenital 42
 serology 427
Syringomas 748
Syrup glycerol 230
Systemic acetazolamide 230
Systemic antibiotic 9
 role of 607
 therapy 9
Systemic diseases 418, 770
Systemic disorders 494
Systemic examination 596, 770, 917
Systemic hypertension 596
Systemic immunomodulating agents 72
Systemic infliximab 45
Systemic leukemia 763
Systemic lupus erythematosus 43, 424, 426, 427, 677, 771
Systemic metastasis 803
Systemic sclerosis, progressive 43
Systemic steroids 616, 808
Systemic syndromes 933, 935
Systemic therapy 414, 630
Systemic thyroid disease 806
Systemic vascular diseases 257
Systemic vasculitides, primary 426

T

Tacrolimus 68, 436
 oral 75
Taenia solium 785
Takayasu arteritis 426
Tamoxifen 596, 620
Tamponading agents, short-term 550
Tangential traction 491
Tarsal fraction 718
Tarsal plate 707
Tarsoconjunctival flap 738
Tarsoconjunctival junction 711
Tarsorrhaphy 21, 35
 lateral 7
Tarsus 744
Taurine 633
Taxanes 596

Tazobactam 544
T-cells inhibitors 439
Tear
 breakup time 5, 363
 meniscus, raised 817f
 supplements 7
 trough deformity
  posthyaluronic acid filler 733f
  prehyaluronic acid filler 733f
Tear film 711
 based tests 818
 break-up time 175
Tearing 244
Technical aspects 325
Tecnis multifocal intraocular lens 192f
Teflon block 61
Telangiectasia 502, 751
 hereditary hemorrhagic 767
Temporal artery biopsy 674
Temporal brow lift 729
Temporal detachment, superior 459
Temporal fossa infiltration 802
Temporal retinal traction 582f
Temporal triangular flap 470
Temporalis muscle 776, 776f
Tendency-oriented perimetry 274
Tendons, sparing of 787f, 806
Tenectomy 922
Tenon's capsule 285, 854
Tenon's cyst 288
Tenon's fascia 237, 848
Tenon's space 775
Tenotomy 922
Tension glaucoma, normal 315
Tentacular projections 38f
Tenzel flap 742f, 798
Teprotumumab 809
Teratomas 759
Terson's syndrome 467
Tetracaine 54
Tetracycline 5, 801
Theoretical formulas 217
Therapeutic bandage contact lens 7
Therapeutic penetrating keratoplasty 39
Thermal injuries 78, 799
Thermal keratoplasty 380
Thermal laser, treatment of 587
Thiazolidinediones 596
Thiomersal hypersensitivity 57
Thrombocytopenia 437
Thromboembolic events 571
Thrombotic glaucoma 256

Thyroid
 disorder 596, 769, 770, 917
 eye disease 771, 786, 804, 805, 812, 870, 870f
  medical management of 804
  treatment for 788
 orbitopathy 731
 profile 917
 stimulating hormone 809
Timolol 21, 230, 266
 maleate 245
 gel 765
Tinnitus 651
Tissue
 addition 376
 adhesives 45
 altered, percentage of 308
 direct smear of 574
 loss 796
 minimal loss of 797
 moderate loss of 798
 plasminogen activator 565, 663
 severe loss of 798
Titanium implants 851
Titmus 899
 stereotest 904
Tobramycin 388f
Tocilizumab 25, 439, 809
 safety of 809
Tomographic notch sign 513
Tonic convergence 905
Tonometry 314f, 382
 evaluation 313
Tonopen 244
Topical antibiotic 75, 100
 therapy 720
Topical carbonic anhydrase 245
 inhibitors 251
Topical corticosteroid 35, 234, 523
 therapy 720
Topical steroid 11, 33, 41, 45, 388f, 414
 drops 68
 mild 41
 ointment 68
Topographer 311
Topography 340
 abnormal preoperative 406
 treatment pattern 254f
Topography-guided ablation 355
 in keratoconus 356
Torch light examination 413
TORCH titer 934
Toric intraocular lens 189, 372
 position of 395
Torpedo patch 260

Torsional oscillations 125*f*
Torsional phacoemulsification 111
Torsional ultrasound 124
Tortuous retinal veins 254
Toxic anterior segment syndrome 18, 114, 151, 179, 539
Toxic epidermal necrolysis 74
Toxic keratitis, central 406
Toxicity 21, 56
  recognition of 21
  solution 57
  surface 21
Toxin inhibits 730
Toxocara canis 427
Toxocara uveitis 606
Toxocariasis 415, 418, 420, 423, 655
Toxoplasma antibodies 422
Toxoplasmic retinochoroiditis 426
Toxoplasmosis 415, 418, 420, 422, 423, 424, 428, 478, 579, 655
  serology 427
Trabectome 299
  machine 299*f*
Trabecular damage 249
Trabecular meshwork 79, 299
Trabeculectomy 145, 146, 236, 252, 258, 259, 266, 279, 291, 304
  bleb, preexisting 149
  steps of 279
  surgery modification 233
  topical corticosteroids 234
Trabeculitis 33
Trabeculodysgenesis, isolated 264
Trabeculoplasty 270
Trabeculotomy 266
Trachipleistophora 36
Trachoma 11, 718
Traction suture 280, 283
Tram track appearance 872*f*
Transconjunctival 25-gauge vitrectomy 559
Transconjunctival approach 728, 756, 802
Transconjunctival flap 798
Transconjunctival müllerectomy 711
Transcranial frontal orbitotomy 874
Transcranial orbitotomy 777, 873, 874
Transcutaneous incision 774, 775
Transepithelial photorefractive keratectomy 358, 382
Transfrontal craniotomy 759

Transient hypopyon 27
Transient light sensitivity 330 syndrome 324
Transient visual
  loss 675
  obscurations 675
Transillumination defect 160, 242
Transluminal trabeculotomy, Gonioscopy-assisted 298
Transorbital neuroendoscopic surgery 874
Transpalpebral browpexy 729
Transposition flap 739
Transposition procedures 923
Transpupillary thermotherapy 509, 581
Transscleral delivery 487
Transverse forehead lines post-Botox 731*f*
Trauma 16, 605, 658, 680, 872
  facial 812
  nonpenetrating 241
  posterior segment sequelae of 661
Traumatic glaucoma 240, 241, 291
  mechanism of 241
Travoprost 245
Treacher Collins syndrome 937
Trefoil factor family 829
Trephination, borders of 61
Treponema pallidum hemagglutination 418 test 414, 418, 422, 427
Treponema pallidum infection 42
Triamcinolone
  acetate 359*f*, 429
  acetonide 483, 535
    injections 809
  acetonide therapy 535
  crystals 244
  intravitreal 244
  periocular injection of 536
Triangular flap 470
Trichiasis 2, 75
Trichilemmoma 749
Trichloroacetic acid 237
Trichoepithelioma, desmoplastic 749
Trichofolliculoma 749, 751
Trifluorothymidine 21, 54
Trifocal intraocular lens 188
Trimethoprim 25, 418
  sulfate 840
  use of oral 25
Trimethoprim-sulfamethoxazole 24
Triplanar incision 116, 117*f*
Trisomy 936

Tropicamide 892
Truly knotless technique 168
Trypan blue 490
Tube
  insertion 294
  ligation 294*f*
  retraction of 296
  truncation 295
Tubercles, choroidal 435
Tubercular granuloma 579
Tuberculosis 42, 412, 415, 417, 418, 424-428, 722
  syphilis 43
Tuberculous panuveitis 425
Tuberculous uveitis 435
Tuberous sclerosis 940
Tubular structure 289
Tumor 771
  adnexal 735
  benign 744, 841
    mixed 455
  choroidal 580
  epidermal 735
  fibro-osseous 454, 762
  hypothalamic 927
  intracranial 675
  lipocytic 454
  lipomatous 762
  location, function of 526*f*
  lymphoproliferative 842
  malignant 803, 846
    mixed 455
  melanocytic 842
  mesenchymal 842
  metastatic 451, 735, 763
  necrosis factor 439
    alpha 419
  painless progression of 737
  posterior benign 802
  progressive 883
  proximity of 525
  secondary 735
Tunica vasculosa lentis 570
Turner's syndrome 936
Tyrosinase positive 940

U

Ulcer 735
  corneal 20, 22
  dendritic 30
  dendrogeographic 30
  geographical 30
  marginal 31
  metaherpetic 31
  regular debridement of 27
Ulcerative colitis 439
Ulcerative keratitis, peripheral 43, 43*f*
Ulcerative keratopathy, severe 21

Index

Ultra soft shell technique 113
Ultrasonography 158, 422, 427, 468, 472, 603, 772
  B-scan, application of 666
Ultrasound 424
  biomicroscopy 256, 417, 422, 425, 427, 605, 605*f*
Ultraviolet radiation 98
Ultra-wide field
  angiography 503, 598
  fluorescein angiogram 504*f*
  imaging 664
  retinal imaging 473
Uniplanar incision 116, 117
Universal implant 859
Upper eyelid 739, 740*f*
  blepharoplasty 726
  crease incision 776
  retracted 791*f*
  sebaceous carcinoma, right 743*f*
  S-shaped deformity of 791*f*
  sulcus, deformity of 755
Upper lid 7
  blepharoplasty 723
    surgical steps of 725*f*
  chalazion of 442*f*
  crease extended laterally 873
  ptosis, mild 685
  retractors 708
Uridine diphosphate galactose-4-epimerase 941
Usher syndrome 594, 943
Usual presentation 511
Utrata forceps 120
Uvea 703
Uveal effusion syndrome 579
Uveal melanocytic proliferation, bilateral diffuse 451
Uveal melanoma 451
  molecular classification of 451
Uveal prolapse 27
Uveal tract, malignant melanoma of 451
Uveitic
  conditions 579
  glaucoma 229, 291
  mass lesions 421
  pathology 434, 579
Uveitis 159, 161, 162, 173, 248*f*, 269, 411, 412, 414, 426, 435, 439*t*, 440, 441, 503, 570
  anterior 412, 413, 415, 436, 528
  bilateral recurrent anterior 175*f*

chronic 53, 339, 346
co-existing 548
glaucoma hyphema syndrome 159, 247, 251, 605
granulomatous 414
  anterior 412, 414
infectious 412
  intermediate 418
infective 423
intermediate 415, 415*t*, 416, 416*t*, 419, 426, 439, 440
lens-induced 435
nomenclature, standardization of 413, 415
noninfectious 439
noninfective posterior 422
posterior 420, 612
recurrent 205
syndrome 420
treatment
  for noninfectious intermediate 418
  of anterior 414
viral 414

V

Vacryocystorhinostomy, external 832
Valve 290
  implants 289
Van der Heijde's formula 218
Van Lint technique 106
Vancomycin 25, 629
  intravitreal 178
Varicella 722
Varicella-zoster 420, 839
  keratitis 43
  virus 414, 429
Vascular endothelial
  cells 495
  damage 78
  growth factor 256, 292, 480, 483, 542*f*, 553, 590, 594, 598, 656
  inhibitors 439
  role of 257
Vascular filling defect 501
Vascular loop formation 582*f*
Vascular malformations 872
Vascular occlusions 503, 612
Vascular tortuosity 504*f*
Vascular tumors, benign 750
Vasculitic entities 579
Vasculitis
  essential cryoglobulinemic 426
  peripheral 417
  primary 426
  secondary 426

Vasculogenic tumors 453
Vasoproliferative tumor 494
Vasospastic manifestations 623
Vein, obstruction of 478
Venereal disease research laboratory 418
  test 422
Venous hemangioma 747
Venous malformation 453
Venous obstruction 622
Venous occlusions 624
Venous phase 500
Venturi chamber 290
Vernal gerontoxon 12
Vernal keratoconjunctivitis 12, 271, 387
Versatility combines safety 162
Verteporfin photodynamic therapy 486
Vertical traction 491
V-esotropia 916
Vestibular schwannoma
  bilateral 880, 881
  unilateral 881
Vibrational circular dichroism 277*f*
  ratio 278*f*
Vicryl suture 848
Vidarabine 21
Videonystagmography 926, 932
Vinciguerra screening report 313, 315, 316*f*
Viral disease 42
  active 32
Viral keratitis 26, 28
  scars of 413
Virchow's triad 482
Virgin cornea 355
Virus 20
  direct invasion of 430
VISA inflammatory index 789*t*
Viscoadaptive viscoelastics 113
Viscoanesthesia 114
Viscodispersive viscoelastics 113
Viscoelastic 112, 144
  closure 197
  removal at end of procedure, techniques of 114
  substances 114
    influence of 246
  types of 113, , 247
Visible sac swelling 836
Vision 142, 412, 579, 784, 789
  assessment of 753, 907
  fool proof prognosis for 652
  functional 153
  impairing diabetic macular edema, lower rates of 464

Index

impairment, mild-to-moderate 42
improving 600
inflammation, strabismus, and appearance (VISA) 789
intraocular lens, extended range of 188
likelihood of improvement of 92
loss of 92, 529t, 537, 563, 625f, 757, 883
low 929
occasional blurring of 31
poor 14
potential 653
related problems 362
sudden blurring of 624f
sudden loss of 241
threatening, care of 807
Visual acuity 86, 134, 259, 262, 339, 461f, 480, 483, 536, 539, 596, 615, 675, 678, 770, 777, 836, 884, 946
poor 525
presenting 606
recovery of 651
reduced 54
postoperative 387, 390
unaided 190
Visual axis opacification 935
Visual disturbances 438
sudden-onset 871
Visual evoked potential 678, 693, 695t, 787
interpretation of 694
Visual field 272, 273, 276, 277f, 278f, 495, 678
assessment 87
consequence of 494
defect 273, 579
examination 228
index 275
loss 262, 273
glaucomatous 271
progression 276
testing 422
Visual function, deterioration of 47
Visual impairment 528
Visual loss 259, 675, 676, 762
mild 482
permanent 303
proportional 663
Visual outcome 585
risk factors for 591
Visual recovery, prognostic factors of 492
Visual rehabilitation 46, 211f, 935

Visual scotoma 506
Visually significant cataract 204
VisuMax
500 platform 365f
laser system 364
machine, components of 363
platform 353, 358
Vital stains 490
Vitamin
A 14, 620
A deficiency 14, 15
causes of 14
treatment regimen 15t
B$_2$ 52
C
deficiency 620
supplementation 20
deficiency, severe 14
E 853
Vitelliform maculopathies 666
Vitrectomized eyes 601
Vitrectomy 198, 255, 285, 462, 496, 543, 546, 556, 565, 566, 581, 616f, 661
anterior 131, 209, 934
bimanual 497
complication of 492
conventional 560
core 470
endoscopic 544, 577
indications of 584
samples 574
timing of 584
undergone 271
Vitrectorhexis 120
Vitreolysis, enzymatic 465
Vitreomacular adhesion 465, 465f, 665
Vitreomacular interface 665
Vitreomacular traction 465, 466f, 488, 600, 619, 665
syndrome 464
trypan blue staining of 466f
Vitreoretinal assessment 197
Vitreoretinal disease 196, 603
treatment of 197
Vitreoretinal disorder management 647
tackle cataract with 197
Vitreoretinal facilities 609
Vitreoretinal lymphoma 450, 451
Vitreoretinal precursors of retinal detachment 637
Vitreoretinal procedures, principles of 550
Vitreoretinal surface abnormalities 600
Vitreoretinal surgery 197, 549

Vitreoschisis 496, 497f
cavity 497f
anterior leaf of 497f
identification of 491
Vitreous 248, 249f, 291, 296, 498, 558, 573, 871f
abscess 629
anterior 413, 583
base, supporting 549
biopsy 427
cells 417, 494
chamber 669
filling anterior chamber 248
incarceration, peripheral 608
inflammation 231
needle biopsies 574
opacities 242
prolapse 583
reaction 629
retained lens fragments in 583
snowballs 416
surgery 620
white 871f
Vitreous hemorrhage 173, 244, 467, 525, 528, 549, 557, 570, 603, 661, 663
causes of 467
clearance of 468
grading of 468
nonclearing 592
Voclosporin 436
Vogt's striae 51
Vogt-Koyanagi-Harada disease 421, 424, 436, 439, 440
pathology of 434
Vogt-Koyanagi-Harada syndrome 424, 579
Vogue 100
Vomiting 228, 437, 438
von Hippel-Lindau disease 940
Voretigene neparvovec 593
Voriconazole 27, 37, 629
Vortex vein obstruction 561
Vryghem macular function test 90, 654
V-Y plasty 739

W

Waardenburg syndrome 938
Walker-Warburg syndrome 942
Wart, viral 442
Water's view 753
Waterjet system 320
Watery discharge 31
Watzke-Allen test 488
Wavefront-guided ablation 351
Wavefront-optimized ablation 350
Wax model 864f

Index

Weber's syndrome 681
Wegener's granulomatosis 43, 72, 426, 437, 579, 771, 793
Weight loss 675
Weill-Marchesani syndrome 939
West Nile
  disease 420
  virus 429
Whipple's disease 427
White acrylic powder 865f
White dot syndrome 420, 655
  multiple evanescent 420
Whitnall's ligament 712
Whitnall's tubercle 798
Whorl-shaped punctate keratopathy 21
Wide-angle
  endoilluminators 521
  systems 520
    types of 518
  viewing systems 518
Wildervanck syndrome 921, 938
Wilms' tumor 763
Wilson's disease 940
Worm, bag of 880, 880f
Worm's eye 783f
  view 805f
Worst iris-claw lens 163
  design 163f

Worth's four-dot
  test 899, 901, 902
  torch 901
Wound
  burn 119
  closure 197
    meticulous 254
  construction 118
  dehiscence 59, 250
  infection 59
  leak 255, 284
    assessment of 254
    management, primary 796
  margin of 797
  modulation 235
  repair, secondary 796
  site thermal injury 111, 122
  stability 142
Wyburn-Mason syndrome 767

X

Xanthelasma 441, 441f
  palpebrarum 751
Xanthogranulomatous inflammation 793
Xen gel stent 301, 302f
Xeroderma pigmentosum 77, 940
Xerophthalmia 14
Xerotic keratitis 14

Y

Yamane technique 172, 172f
Yellow filter test 89, 653
Yttrium aluminum garnet laser capsulotomy 193
Y-V plasty 739

Z

Zeis gland 721
  infection of 721
Zeiss keratometers 333
Zero aberration 185
Zero power phaco chop 123, 125
Ziehl-Neelsen stain 446, 448f
Zinc 633
Zonular apparatus, weak 174
Zonular breaks 242
Zonular dialysis, surgical principles for 127
Zonular fibers, weakness of 270
Zonular weakness 268
Zonules, integrity of 143
Zoster ophthalmicus 722
Z-plasty 739
Zygoma 754, 813
Zygomatic arch 776, 813
Zygomatic bone fracture 820f
Zygomatic complex fractures 757
Zygomaticomaxillary complex fractures 753

EU GSPR Authorised Reprsentative
Logos Europe, 9 rue Nicolas Poussin
1700, La Rochelle, France
Phone: +33 (0) 6 67 93 73 78
E-mail: contact@logoseurope.eu

www.ingramcontent.com/pod-product-compliance
Ingram Content Group UK Ltd.
Pitfield, Milton Keynes, MK11 3LW, UK
UKHW060949220426
5322IPUK00030B/173